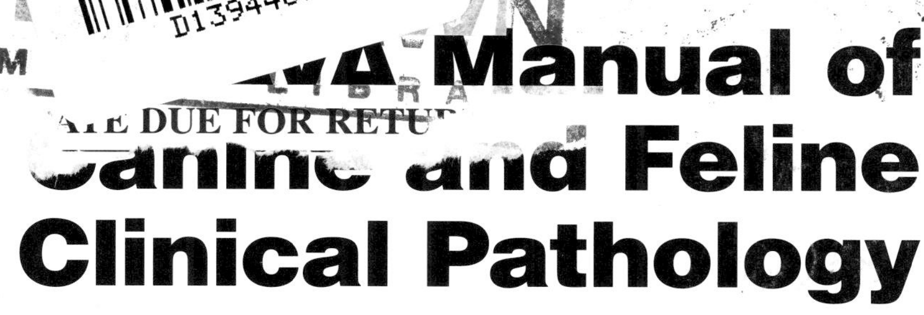

BSAVA Manual of Canine and Feline Clinical Pathology

Second edition

Editors:

Elizabeth Villiers

BVSc DipRCPath CertVR CertSAM MRCVS

Department of Veterinary Medicine, University of Cambridge
Madingley Road, Cambridge CB3 0ES

and

Laura Blackwood

BVMS PhD MVM CertVR MRCVS

Small Animal Hospital, Department of Veterinary Clinical Science
University of Liverpool, Crown Street, Liverpool L7 7EX

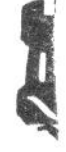

Published by:

British Small Animal Veterinary Association
Woodrow House, 1 Telford Way,
Waterwells Business Park, Quedgeley,
Gloucester GL2 2AB

A Company Limited by Guarantee in England.
Registered Company No. 2837793.
Registered as a Charity.

First edition published 1998
Second edition published 2005
Reprinted with corrections 2010

The drawings in Figures 4.1, 4.4, 5.1, 5.2, 15.2, 20.65 and 21.2 were drawn by S.J. Elmhurst BA Hons and are printed with her permission.

The drawings in Figure 22.3 were designed and created by Vicki Martin Design and are printed with their permission.

A catalogue record for this book is available from the British Library.

ISBN 0 905214 79 X

The publishers and contributors cannot take responsibility for information provided on dosages and methods of application of drugs mentioned in this publication. Details of this kind must be verified by individual users from the appropriate literature.

Typeset by Fusion Design, Wareham, Dorset, UK
Printed by: Replika Press Pvt. Ltd, India

Other titles in the BSAVA Manuals series:

Manual of Canine & Feline Abdominal Imaging
Manual of Canine & Feline Abdominal Surgery
Manual of Canine & Feline Advanced Veterinary Nursing
Manual of Canine & Feline Anaesthesia and Analgesia
Manual of Canine & Feline Behavioural Medicine
Manual of Canine & Feline Cardiorespiratory Medicine
Manual of Canine & Feline Dentistry
Manual of Canine & Feline Emergency and Critical Care
Manual of Canine & Feline Endocrinology
Manual of Canine & Feline Endoscopy and Endosurgery
Manual of Canine & Feline Gastroenterology
Manual of Canine & Feline Haematology and Transfusion Medicine
Manual of Canine & Feline Head, Neck and Thoracic Surgery
Manual of Canine & Feline Infectious Diseases
Manual of Canine & Feline Musculoskeletal Disorders
Manual of Canine & Feline Musculoskeletal Imaging
Manual of Canine & Feline Nephrology and Urology
Manual of Canine & Feline Neurology
Manual of Canine & Feline Oncology
Manual of Canine & Feline Rehabilitation, Supportive and Palliative Care: Case Studies in Patient Management
Manual of Canine & Feline Thoracic Imaging
Manual of Canine & Feline Wound Management and Reconstruction
Manual of Exotic Pets
Manual of Farm Pets
Manual of Ornamental Fish
Manual of Practical Animal Care
Manual of Practical Veterinary Nursing
Manual of Psittacine Birds
Manual of Rabbit Medicine and Surgery
Manual of Raptors, Pigeons and Passerine Birds
Manual of Reptiles
Manual of Rodents and Ferrets
Manual of Small Animal Dermatology
Manual of Small Animal Fracture Repair and Management
Manual of Small Animal Ophthalmology
Manual of Small Animal Reproduction and Neonatology
Manual of Wildlife Casualties

For information on these and all BSAVA publications please visit our website: www.bsava.com

Contents

Contributors

Joy Archer VMD/MS PhD MRCPath DipECVCP MRCVS
Department of Veterinary Medicine, University of Cambridge, Madingley Road, Cambridge, CB3 0ES

Laura Blackwood BVMS PhD MVM CertVR MRCVS
RCVS Recognised Specialist in Veterinary Oncology
Small Animal Hospital, Department of Veterinary Clinical Science, University of Liverpool, Crown Street, Liverpool L7 7EX

Sue Dawson BSc BVSc PhD
University of Liverpool, Veterinary Teaching Hospital, Leahurst, Chester High Street, Neston, CH64 7TE

Emma Dewhurst MA VetMB DipRCPath MRCVS
Petsavers Resident in Clinical Pathology, Department of Clinical Veterinary Science, University of Bristol, Langford House, Langford, Bristol, BS40 5DU

Joan Duncan BVMS PhD DipRCPath CertVR MRCVS
IDEXX Laboratories, Grange House, Sandbeck Way, Wetherby, West Yorkshire, LS22 4DN

John K. Dunn MA BVM&S MVSc DSAM DipECVIM-ca MRCPath MRCVS
Axiom Veterinary Laboratories, 5 George Street, Teignmouth, Devon, TQ14 8AH

Gary England BVetMed PhD DVetMed DVRep DipACT FRCVS
Guide Dogs for the Blind Association, Tollgate House, Banbury Road, Bishops Tachbrook, Warwickshire, CV33 8QJ

Derek Flaherty BVMS DVA DipECVA MRCA MRCVS ILTM
RCVS Recognised Specialist in Veterinary Anaesthesia. European Veterinary Specialist in Anaesthesia
Faculty of Veterinary Medicine, University of Glasgow, Bearsden Road, Glasgow, G61 1QH

Kathleen Freeman DVM MS PhD DipECVCP MRCVS
RCVS Specialist in Veterinary Pathology (Clinical Pathology); European Veterinary Specialist in Clinical Pathology
Rynachulaig Farm, Killin, Perthshire, FK21 8TY

Karen Gerber BVSc BVSc (Hons) DAVCP (Clinical Pathology) MRCVS
Axiom Veterinary Laboratories, 5 George Street, Teignmouth, Devon, TQ14 8AH

Alexander J. German BVSc (Hons) PhD CertSAM DipECVIM-CA MRCVS
Department of Veterinary Clinical Sciences, University of Liverpool, Small Animal Hospital, Crown Street, Liverpool, L7 7EX

Peter A. Graham BVMS CertVR PhD MRCVS
North Western Laboratories, Lancefield House, 23 Mains Lane, Little Singleton, Poulten-le-Fylde, FY6 7LJ

Edward J. Hall MA PhD VetMB MRCVS
Department of Clinical Veterinary Science, University of Bristol, Langford House, Langford, Bristol, BS40 5DU

Michael Herrtage MA BVSc DVR DVD DSAM DipECVIM-CA DipECVDI MRCVS
Department of Veterinary Medicine, University of Cambridge, Madingley Road, Cambridge, CB3 0ES

John F. Innes BVSc PhD CertVR DSAS (Orth) MRCVS
Small Animal Hospital, Department of Clinical Veterinary Science, University of Liverpool, Crown Street, Liverpool, L7 7EX

Tim Jagger BVM&S MSc DipRCPath MRCVS
Leeds Veterinary Laboratory, Millcroft, Gateway Drive, Yeadson, Leeds, LS19 7XY

Clare Knottenbelt BVSc MSc DSAM MRCVS
Division of Companion Animals, Institute of Comparative Medicine, University of Glasgow, Faculty of Veterinary Medicine, Bearsden Road, Glasgow, G61 1QH

Yvonne McGrotty BVMS CertSAM MRCVS
Internal Medicine and Critical Care, VRCC, 1 West Mayne, Bramston Way, Southfield, Laindon, Essex, SS15 6TP

Richard Mellanby BSc BVMS DSAM ECVIM-CA MRCVS
Department of Pathology, Immunology Division, University of Cambridge, Tennis Court Road, Cambridge, CB2 1QP

Carmel T. Mooney MVB MPhil PhD DECVIM-ca MRCVS
RCVS Specialist in Small Animal Medicine (Endocrinology)
Department of Small Animal Clinical Studies, Faculty of Veterinary Medicine,
University College Dublin Veterinary College, Belfield, Dublin 4, Republic of Ireland

Kate Murphy BVSc (Hons) DSAM DipECVIM-CA MRCVS
Small Animal Hospital, School of Clinical Veterinary Science, University of Bristol, Langford, Bristol, BS40 5DU

Tim Nuttall BSc BVSc PhD CertVD CBiol MIBiol MRCVS
University of Liverpool, Small Animal Hospital, Crown Steet, Liverpool, L7 7EX

Natasha Olby MA VetMB PhD DipACVIM MRCVS
University College of Veterinary Medicine, North Carolina State University, 4700 Hillsborough Street, Raleigh, NC 27606, USA

Kostas Papasouliotis DVM PhD DipRCPath DipECVCP MRCVS
Langford Veterinary Diagnostic Laboratories, School of Clinical Veterinary Science, University of Bristol, Langford, Bristol, BS40 5DU

Alan Radford BSc BVSc PhD
University of Liverpool, Veterinary Teaching Hospital, Leahurst, Chester High Street, Neston, CH64 7TE

Ian Ramsey BVSc PhD DSAM MRCVS
Department of Veterinary Clinical Studies, University of Glasgow, Bearsdon, Glasgow, G61 1QH

Marco Russo DVM PhD
Department of Clinical Science, Section of Clinical Obstetrics, Faculty of Veterinary Medicine,
University of Naples, Italy

Barbara Skelly MA VetMB PhD CertSAM DipACVIM MRCVS
Department of Veterinary Medicine, University of Cambridge, Madingley Road, Cambridge, CB3 0ES

Richard A. Squires BVSc PhD DVR DipECVIM-ca MRCVS
Institute of Veterinary Animal and Biomedical Sciences, Massey University, Palmerston North, New Zealand

Tracy Stokol BVSc PhD DipACVP (Clinical Pathology)
Department of Population Medicine and Diagnostic Sciences, College of Veterinary Medicine, Cornell University, Ithaca, NY 14853, USA

Kathleen Tennant BVetMed CertSAM CertVC DRCPath MRCVS
Department of Pathology, Royal Veterinary College, Hawkshead Lane, North Mymms, Hatfield, AL9 7TA

Elizabeth Villiers BVSc DipRCPath CertVR CertSAM MRCVS
Department of Veterinary Medicine, University of Cambridge, Madingley Road, Cambridge, CB3 0ES

Penny Watson MA VetMB CertVR DSAM DipECVIM-ca MRCVS
Department of Veterinary Medicine, University of Cambridge, Madingley Road, Cambridge, CB3 0ES

Foreword

Clinical Pathology forms the cornerstone of veterinary internal medicine. The careful selection, processing and analysis of clinical specimens, and the accurate interpretation and application of results are essential to enable a diagnosis to be made and for appropriate treatment to be prescribed.

The second edition of the *BSAVA Manual of Clinical Pathology* provides a complete revision and update of the previous volume which, in its turn, replaced the Manual of Laboratory Techniques produced by BSAVA in the 1970s and 1980s. Each of these texts in their day provided practitioners with current, practical and relevant material. Likewise, this completely new volume will deliver the same high quality of information to today's practitioners.

The authors of the chapters are internationally recognized experts. The text is supported with clear illustrations and algorithms to guide the reader. The early chapters cover general areas of clinical pathology, such as the interpretation of laboratory data, haematology and urine analysis. Subsequent chapters deal with clinical pathology using either a problem-based approach or by organ system. The emphasis, as is the case for all BSAVA Manuals, is to provide readily accessible, authoritative and up-to-date material for the busy clinician.

The editors, authors and, of course, the staff of the Publications Department at BSAVA are to be congratulated for having produced an exceptionally user-friendly manual that should find itself well-thumbed and in use every day in the small animal practice.

Ian Mason **BVetMed PhD CertSAD DipECVD MRCVS**
BSAVA President 2004–2005

Preface

This second edition of the *BSAVA Manual of Canine and Feline Clinical Pathology* builds on the strengths of the first edition, and incorporates new information unavailable at the time of the original publication in 1998. The primary aim of the manual is to provide accessible information for busy clinicians in general practice: which tests should be done, how they are carried out, and how to interpret results. Clinical case examples have been added in many chapters to illustrate how test selection and interpretation are used in real cases, and to give readers the opportunity to apply for themselves the information presented in the chapters.

The first chapters summarize very important information for anyone using or establishing laboratory tests, and are concise and relevant. Chapters on haematology and haemostasis are followed by the biochemical chapters. These chapters are based on clinical approach, and include individual chapters for important body systems or organs which have particular clinicopathological profiles (renal, hepatic, gastrointestinal, pancreatic and skin), in addition to separate chapters covering proteins and electrolytes. Blood gas analysis and urinalysis are discussed in dedicated chapters. The subsequent chapters deal with clinical and reproductive endocrinology.

Cytology is a vital and growing part of clinical pathology, and a large chapter reviews cytological sampling and interpretation. There is a separate chapter covering body cavity effusions, and another on CSF analysis. These, and the chapters on joint and muscle, and skin, include both biochemical and cytological information.

The final chapters summarize the role of clinical pathology in the diagnosis of infectious diseases (bacterial, fungal, viral and protozoal).

Lastly, we have included quick reference appendices summarizing the samples required for common tests, differential diagnoses of many of the abnormalities discussed in detail elsewhere in the book, and conversion factors for international readers.

We would like to thank the chapter authors for their hard work, and for meeting virtually all our unreasonable demands. As a team of one clinical pathologist and one clinician, we hoped to create a truly useful manual which contains the applicable information that clinicians, budding clinical pathologists and students need.

Butty and Laura
(Elizabeth Villiers and Laura Blackwood)

February 2005

1

Making the most of in-clinic and external laboratory testing

Joan Duncan

Introduction

In recent years, increased use and understanding of clinical pathology has led to more accurate disease detection and the use of rational therapeutic approaches. It is now possible to perform a wide range of analyses in the practice laboratory and veterinary surgeons are often faced with the choice of external or internal laboratory services. This chapter outlines the benefits and disadvantages of commercial and practice laboratories, and details the factors that should be considered when establishing a practice laboratory. Detailed information regarding specific analysis and interpretation of test results can be found in later chapters.

In-clinic testing or external laboratory?

Many clinicians, practice managers and veterinary partners struggle with the choice of in-clinic laboratory testing *versus* submission of samples to an external laboratory (commercial, university or government facility). There is no single formula that can be applied to determine whether a practice should invest in a clinic laboratory. However, it is likely that the combination of internal and external laboratory analyses provides the essential mix of speed, accuracy, quality and professional support necessary for a timely and accurate diagnosis. Highlighted here are some of the benefits and disadvantages to be considered.

Quality

The production of accurate results with a meaningful, valid interpretation of the laboratory findings is essential for the commercial survival of diagnostic laboratories. Therefore, considerable time and financial commitments are made to ensure that such quality is maintained. In the UK, diagnostic laboratories may apply for quality accreditation, e.g. ISO 17025 (General requirements for the competence of testing and calibration laboratories). The laboratory must demonstrate:

- Validity and acceptable performance of equipment and assays
- Optimal procedures to identify, correct and reduce technical or interpretation error
- Adequate staff training and continuing education time to maintain necessary skills
- Procedures to ensure that the promised quality of service is maintained
- Adequate documentation to prove that all of the above are carried out.

Such accreditation does not apply to practice laboratories but the accuracy of results and interpretations is central to the diagnosis of disease. For in-clinic testing it is the practice's responsibility to ensure production of reliable results and implementation of procedures to identify and correct error, and to ensure that the interpretations provided by the veterinary surgeons are valid and helpful to the management of the case.

Availability of results

There is a clear medical benefit for the patient if accurate test results are delivered quickly to the clinician. Even if a practice does not have facilities for extensive laboratory testing, there are basic tests that are easily and reliably performed in the practice, and which provide valuable information. These include:

- Packed cell volume (PCV)
- Blood film examination
- Total protein
- Blood glucose
- Urea (and creatinine if possible)
- Urinalysis. The results of urinalysis (pH, cells, crystals, casts) change with time, and analysis in the practice is valuable
- Electrolytes
- Blood gas analysis.

In other circumstances, where immediate analysis may not be essential on medical grounds, the rapid availability of in-clinic results may still be considered of value to the practice, for example, in terms of client appreciation and communication. However, the pressure of providing an instant diagnosis may lead to erroneous interpretation of results and the benefit of a rapid diagnosis should be balanced against the need for adequate time to consider fully the details of the case.

Although the delay in the availability of results is considered a major disadvantage when using external laboratories, most have taken significant efforts to improve turnaround time for routine assays by using courier services, phone or FAX reports and e-mail reports. If such a laboratory service is readily available, then it may not be necessary for a practice to invest the time and effort in providing extensive patient-side testing.

Range of tests

The tests listed above are priceless with regard to the information they provide in emergency situations. Beyond these tests, there is a range of others that may be performed in the practice, including haematology, biochemistry, endocrinology and serological testing. With such a wide range of tests available it is tempting to include facilities for all of these in the practice laboratory. However, if it is not essential or valuable that the test is done at the patient side, then perhaps a more circumspect approach is prudent. Many of these investigations require technical skill and a focus on laboratory procedures that may not be possible for nursing and veterinary staff who also have responsibilities elsewhere in the practice.

Motivation and staffing

The focused attention and motivation of nursing and veterinary staff is central to the success of the veterinary laboratory. Errors and mechanical breakdown will occur, and staff should be prepared to spend time correcting such problems. Irrespective of the volume of laboratory testing performed in the clinic, it is essential to maintain a close link with veterinary pathologists and clinical pathologists who can provide additional expertise and information regarding test interpretation, further investigations and recent scientific advances.

Cost and marketing of laboratory testing

In general terms, commercial laboratories are able to provide a wide range of tests at highly competitive prices when compared to the cost of in-clinic analysis. The price advantage of commercial laboratory profiles becomes of great importance where extensive investigations are envisaged.

Irrespective of where the analysis is performed, consideration should be given to charges for blood sampling and interpretation of results. In-clinic testing is often charged at a higher rate, justified on the basis of more rapid availability of results. However, large 'mark-ups' for in-clinic or commercial laboratory testing may limit the uptake of testing.

Pre-anaesthetic laboratory screening is commonly performed in veterinary practices, although patient selection, and the range of tests to be included in the profile, are controversial issues. Proponents believe that, in addition to the identification of subclinical disease, pre-anaesthetic laboratory testing improves practice profitability. However, it is essential to realize that such testing may reveal clinically insignificant, abnormal test results (see Chapter 2) which may in turn trigger unnecessary, extensive laboratory investigations.

Establishing a relationship with a commercial laboratory

When selecting a commercial laboratory it is important to consider both scientific and personal factors. For example, two laboratories may provide a similar service, but the practice may already have a trusting relationship with a pathologist in one facility. In general terms, the following are realistic expectations of the service that should be received when using a commercial diagnostic laboratory:

- Accurate, repeatable results. Commercial laboratories should be expected to demonstrate to clients that the performance of laboratory tests (measured by accuracy and repeatability) is acceptable
- Valid and meaningful interpretation of results. Clinicians should be confident that the interpretations provided and suggestions for follow-up testing are helpful with regard to the investigation of the disease, and are consistent with the clinical presentation and subsequent outcome
- Advice readily available from technical, professional and support staff
- Expertise of pathologists. Pathologists should have a commitment to continuing professional development, through attendance or presentation at scientific meetings, personal study and publication. Pathologists may have a particular field of interest which is valuable to the practice, and, in most cases, are happy to talk to local veterinary groups
- Sampling advice and protocols
- Regular updates regarding new tests
- Quality assurance systems should be in place to ensure that the laboratory upholds its commitment to quality in the above areas.

The evaluation of different laboratories is difficult. It is best to select one option and work with that laboratory for some months to ensure that the clinic has gained an insight into its full potential before trying another option. Attempting to compare two laboratories in parallel makes it difficult to establish a relationship with either. Irrespective of the final choice made, the following tips should help the clinic to maximize the services of most commercial laboratories:

- Plan test and sample selection with care; otherwise, the first, and often most important, diagnostic opportunity may be lost
- Call for advice before sampling. This advice is usually provided by support or technical staff and it is often not necessary to speak to a pathologist
- Provide the information requested by the laboratory. This includes details of: patient and practice; species; test required; clinical history; and specific lesions
- Where possible, comply with laboratory advice regarding sample collection and always comply with appropraite national postal regulations. Details of these are available from the diagnostic laboratory
- Keep a referral log of the samples despatched. It is useful to include the expected turnaround time of each sample and details of any conversations with the laboratory, so that other staff members do not have to duplicate patient follow-ups
- Discuss the cases with the clinical pathologists; further interpretation or advice may be available after a full case discussion
- Ask for a review of the report or a second opinion if necessary. Human error is always possible
- Provide immediate feedback to staff and management regarding any problems encountered.

Running a practice laboratory

It is first necessary to decide on the tests that will be offered in the practice laboratory. It is essential that these assays will provide accurate results when performed in the practice, by the staff available. Tests that are based upon simple principles, which use relatively robust equipment, and are highly repeatable, are easily transferred to the practice laboratory. However, clinicians must always have realistic expectations of the accuracy and repeatability of more complex in-clinic testing. There are many occasions where it is prudent to confirm abnormalities identified in the clinic, by follow-up testing at a commercial laboratory, and it is helpful to formulate a plan for such follow-up testing.

Irrespective of the range of tests that will be performed in the practice laboratory, it is necessary to consider the additional responsibilities of complying with Health and Safety regulations, equipment maintenance, laboratory documentation and staff training.

The practice laboratory: general

Laboratory work should only be carried out in rooms or areas dedicated to that use. Ideally, a practice laboratory should provide the following:

- Dedicated laboratory space (not a thoroughfare or extension or a room used for other purposes)
- Non-slip, impervious flooring which can withstand cleaning with strong disinfectants
- Dust-free environment, with good ventilation
- Quiet
- Sufficient work space to allow easy manipulation of samples and equipment
- Refrigerator. This should be kept tidy with adequate space between contents to allow optimal performance. Flammable material and food should not be stored in the laboratory refrigerator. The temperature should be recorded regularly. Where sampling protocols indicate that a sample should be frozen, the recommended temperature is usually –20°C. The freezer units within refrigerators and some domestic freezers do not reach this temperature
- Sink
- Storage space for consumables and chemicals. The latter should not be stored on high shelves
- A wash basin, preferably with elbow or foot operation, situated close to the exit. Bactericidal hand wash and paper towels should be provided. A mirror above the basin is helpful to check for splashes on the face and use of the eyewash
- Eyewash, first aid kit, first aid notice advising staff where to get first aid help and an accident book
- Appropriate fire extinguishers
- Colour-coded waste bins (household waste in black bags, clinical waste in yellow bags or rigid containers)
- Spillage kit. This should include paper towels, cloths, disinfectant, gloves and forceps for picking up glass and a disposal container for the materials used
- Flammable solvents cupboard (if flammable substances are used)
- Protective clothing. A clean, long-sleeved laboratory coat should be worn. A disposable apron and gloves are recommended when working with blood, and safety goggles should be available for use while handling hazardous chemicals
- Library space for textbooks, standard operating procedures (SOPs), equipment logs and sample logs.

Health and safety

Health and safety at work is the responsibility of both the employer and employee. Employers have a responsibility to protect their staff from hazards, but employees have a responsibility to take reasonable care of themselves and others. Employers, or the Practice Safety Officer, should ensure that staff understand and comply with the detailed contents of the practice Health and Safety Policy Document. All veterinary practices must comply with the regulations listed below.

Health and Safety at Work Act 1974 and Management of Health and Safety at Work Regulations 1999

It is important that anybody working in the practice laboratory is either suitably trained or is working under the supervision of a trained person. Training includes not only technical proficiency, but training in safe systems of work, including operation of all laboratory equipment. It is the employer's duty:

- To provide equipment which is free of risk
- To provide an environment which is free of risk
- To ensure that materials are used, moved and stored safely
- To ensure safe systems of work are implemented
- To provide the information and training necessary for health and safety
- To provide protective clothing
- To provide adequate first aid facilities
- To ensure that the appropriate safety signs are present and maintained
- To monitor safety.

In order to comply with the above, it is necessary for the employer to assess the risks to employees' health and safety, to record that risk assessment (if there are five or more employees) and to take the actions identified as necessary. There are specific regulations covering provision of protective clothing, manual handling, visual display units, provision of the equipment and the display of safety signs. The reader is referred to the Health and Safety Executive for detailed current information.

The Advisory Committee on Dangerous Pathogens produces guidelines that relate to the handling of specific pathogens **(Advisory Committee on Dangerous Pathogens 1995 and 2000)**. These guidelines should be available to staff performing microbiological testing. Pathogens are categorized into four pathogen groups, based upon their ability to produce disease in humans. Some organisms of veterinary importance are included in Hazard Group

3 and must be handled in a safety cabinet. These include *Brucella*, *Chlamydophila* (formerly *Chlamydia*) *psittaci*, *Mycobacterium*, *Echinoccocus* and *Toxoplasma gondii*. In veterinary diagnostic laboratories, most risk comes from faeces or urine although it is important to remember that the risk of handling individual samples is often not known, and that all samples should be handled as if they have a potential risk. Avian tissues, ovine abortion material and feline faeces are considered to present a significant risk of infection (*C. psittaci*, *T. gondii*) and should not be handled by pregnant women. In addition, primate samples may pose a risk to laboratory staff and it is essential to confirm that the diagnostic laboratory is happy to receive such samples before dispatch.

Control of Substances Hazardous to Health (COSHH) 2002, Control of Pollution Act and Environment Protection Act

Employers should assess all products used in the veterinary practice, with regard to the COSHH regulations **(Control of Substances Hazardous to Health 2002)**. The aim is to identify risks associated with the use of individual products and to take steps to reduce that risk. If there are five employees or more, the assessment should be made in writing or stored on a computer. For each individual chemical or group of chemicals, the assessment should contain information regarding the storage, spillage and disposal procedures, and any specific first aid requirements in the event of an accident (Figure 1.1). They should be read

RISK ASSESSMENT FORM

Ref No ....

Initial assessor ....

Signed ....
Date ....

HAZARD ....
RISK ....

1. *Who is at risk?* ....
2. *How serious is the risk?* Insignificant [ ] Minor [ ] Potentially major [ ]

   Details ....
3. *What is the probability of it occurring?* Very unlikely [ ] Unlikely [ ] Likely [ ] Very likely [ ]

   Comments ....
4. *Is there a risk to health?* Yes [ ] No [ ]

   Details ....
5. *Is there a risk to the environment?* Yes [ ] No [ ]

   Details ....
6. *Who is responsible for this area, procedure or task?* ....
7. *What control measures are in place?* ....
8. *What protective equipment is provided?* ....
9. *Are special procedures needed for the following, and if so are they in place?*:

First aid	Yes [ ]	No [ ]	Details ....
Fire	Yes [ ]	No [ ]	Details ....
Spillage	Yes [ ]	No [ ]	Details ....
Storage	Yes [ ]	No [ ]	Details ....
10. *Are current controls or measures satisfactory?* Yes [ ] No [ ]
11. *If not, what additional controls or measures are needed?* ....

Target date for implementation ....
Who monitors this risk? ....

Action to be taken by ....
Date for next review ....

Supervisor ....
Date ....

Signed ....

1.1 An example of a risk assessment form (BSAVA, 2000).

by employees and be readily available at all times. Assessments should be reviewed at regular intervals, but also where there is reason to question the validity of the assessment or when working practices change.

The categories of information included in a COSHH assessment include:

- Identification and name of activity
- Identification and list of hazardous substances
- Identification of route by which they are hazardous
- Protection required
- Means of disposal
- Assessment of risk.

Collection and Disposal of Waste Regulations 1992

Clinical waste and chemical waste from the laboratory must be disposed of correctly. Clinical waste is defined as any waste which consists of, or is contaminated by, animal tissue, blood or other body fluids. It should be placed in yellow bags or containers, ready for collection by a licensed waste disposal company. Rigid yellow containers are used for the disposal of 'sharps' and glass slides. Used plastic materials, such as pipette tips, should be discarded into a suitable disinfectant for a minimum of 12 hours before transfer to a bag for incineration. Bacteriological media and samples should be autoclaved, using a 'dirty' autoclave, before disposal.

Reporting of Injuries, Diseases and Dangerous Occurrence Regulations 1995 (RIDDOR)

Under these regulations, it is essential to report to the Health and Safety Executive any death, major injury, work-related disease or injury that causes an absence of greater than 3 days (including non-working days). In addition, the details and nature of any accident should be logged in an accident book and the book regularly reviewed by the Safety Officer or employer to determine if changes in working practices are required. The accident book should be kept for 3 years and should include:

- Date and time of accident
- Name and address of personnel involved
- Place and nature of incident
- Description of the incident.

First Aid Regulations 1981

The minimum first aid provision on any work site is a suitably stocked first aid box and an appointed person to take care of first aid issues. If it is considered that there is a significant risk of accidents then one or more staff should be trained in first aid techniques.

Local laboratory rules

All staff members should be familiar with the general safety rules (fire, accident, cleanliness) detailed in the practice Health and Safety Policy. It is essential to establish and enforce a set of local laboratory rules which decrease the risk of accidents and error in the laboratory. Copies of the local safety rules must be available to all members of staff and visitors entering the designated laboratory area. Local rules will commonly include:

- Protective clothing should be worn
- No food or drink should be consumed in the laboratory or stored in the laboratory refrigerator
- Cosmetics should not be applied in the laboratory
- Hands must be washed frequently, and before leaving the laboratory
- Any cuts or grazes must be covered with a waterproof dressing
- Smoking is not permitted
- Nothing should be placed in the mouth, e.g. pipettes, pens, pencils
- Open-toed sandals should not be worn
- Visitors should be accompanied at all times
- The laboratory should be kept tidy (including floors and walkways) and work tops should be disinfected after each work session
- Instructions on equipment must be followed. Do not attempt to over-ride safety systems on equipment, e.g. centrifuges
- Standard operating procedures for specimen handling and laboratory methods must be read and complied with
- COSHH assessments for chemicals used, and tasks performed within the laboratory must be read
- All chemicals should be clearly labelled with appropriate hazard warning signs
- All spillages must be cleaned up immediately. Refer to the COSHH assessments for specific information
- Waste must be disposed of in the correct container.

Equipment

The following pieces of equipment form the core of the laboratory. When used appropriately, they can provide a large amount of diagnostic information, or are used for optimal preparation of samples for further analysis.

Centrifuge

A microhaematocrit centrifuge, for measurement of PCV, and a variable speed centrifuge, for centrifugation of other sample types, are required. A centrifuge is essential for effective separation of plasma and serum for biochemical testing and also allows preparation of sedimented samples of cells from urine and body cavity fluids. However, the centrifugal force required to separate blood is greater than that required to sediment the cells in urine and body cavity fluids, and it is essential to follow manufacturer's guidelines for each sample type.

The noise and vibration of a centrifuge can create workplace stress so it is also useful to trial equipment before purchase. Newer centrifuges have a locking device to prevent opening during operation. Older centrifuges must have a warning label indicating that they should not be opened while the rotor is still spinning. The safety plate of a microhaematocrit centrifuge should always be screwed in place before operation. The contents of the centrifuge should be balanced adequately before operation to prevent excess vibration.

The equipment should be kept clean and regularly checked for signs of wear. If a breakage or spill occurs the machine should be stopped and any aerosols allowed to settle for 30 minutes before opening; it should then be decontaminated with a disinfectant recommended by the manufacturer.

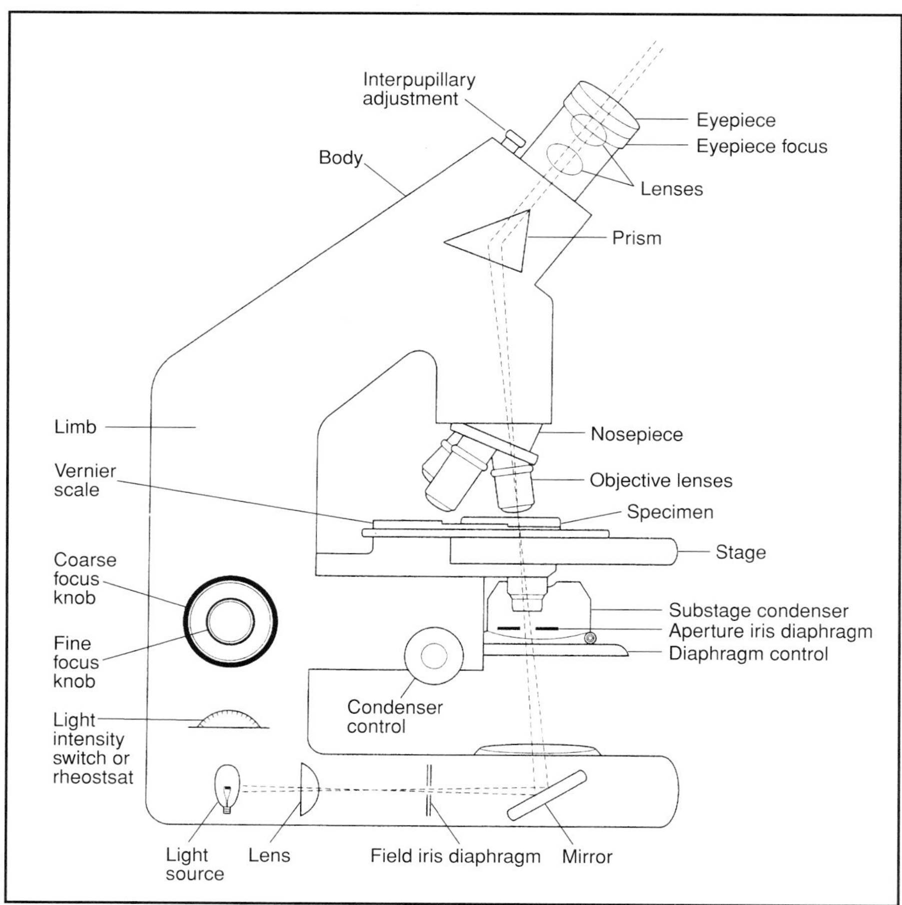

1.2 The optical features of a microscope. (Reproduced from *Veterinary Nursing, 3rd edn*, 2003, edited by DR Lane and B Cooper, with permission from Elsevier.)

Refractometer

A refractomer (total solids meter) is used to measure the specific gravity (SG) of urine and the total protein (TP) concentration of plasma and body fluids. Although refractometers measure the refractive index of a solution, they are calibrated to measure SG and TP. They are easy to use, provide very valuable information and require just a single drop of urine/fluid, or the plasma from a microhaematocrit centrifuge tube. The calibration should be checked regularly using distilled water (SG = 1.000). The prism should be wiped with soft tissue after each use and should be handled with care to avoid scratching the surface.

Microscope

Monocular or binocular microscopes are available but the latter are preferred for prolonged use. In addition, there should be comfortable viewing positions for spectacled and non-spectacled operators. Facilities for photomicrography are available and may be helpful for training purposes.

The objectives required are determined, in part, by the expected use. The most commonly used combination is two scanning objectives (4X, 10X), a high dry objective (40X) and oil immersion (100X). However, a 20X objective and a 50X (oil immersion), although expensive, are valuable if a large volume of haematology or cytology is expected. When using the 40X objective, a coverslip or thin layer of oil is required for optimal image quality. However, this lens must be kept free from oil. For optimal use the microscope should be set up according to the principles of Koehler (Figures 1.2 and 1.3). The following tips should help keep the microscope in good condition and solve some of the common microscopy problems:

1. Place a slide on the microscope stage.
2. Rotate the 10X objective into position.
3. Position the eyepieces so that there is a single image.
4. Bring the cellular material on the slide into focus.
5. Locate the field iris diaphragm control. Close the field iris, bring the blades of the iris (which appear as a black image at the edges) as far as possible into the field of view. When fully closed a small area of light is still visible.
6. Locate the condenser focus control. Alter the height of the condenser to bring the edge of the field iris blades into sharp focus.
7. Use the condenser centring screws to move the area of interest to the centre of the field of vision.
8. Open the field iris until the light fills the field of vision.
9. Take out one of the eyepieces and view the disc of light directly down the tube.
10. Alter the aperture iris diaphragm so that the disc of light fills approximately 80% of the maximum diameter. Replace the eyepiece.

1.3 Setting up a microscope for optimal image quality. The controls mentioned are common to all good quality microscopes, although their appearance and location vary slightly.

- The microscope should be covered to protect it from dust
- It should not be subject to intense vibration
- The light rheostat should be turned down to the lowest level before switching off; ensure it is at the lowest level before switching on
- Any oil should be cleaned from the lenses immediately, and from the immersion lens at the end of each session. Lint-free tissues can be used to remove excess oil and then the lens cleaned with lens cleaning fluid. Lens fluid should be used sparingly, because, over time, any solvents used may loosen the adhesive which holds the lens in place
- The microscope should be serviced regularly by a trained engineer
- Replacement bulbs must not be handled with bare fingers (whether hot or cold)
- Before viewing a slide, it should be checked that the cellular material is on the uppermost side. If not, then one will be able to focus at low power, but not at high power or using oil immersion
- The condenser position should be checked (Figure 1.2, 1.3) if the image appears refractile or there is a lighting problem
- There may be considerable heat output from some microscopes and they should be handled carefully after prolonged use.

Portable blood glucose meter

Portable blood glucose meters (PBGMs) are available for the measurement of blood glucose in whole blood. In two studies, the performance of individual meters in relation to a laboratory reference measurement was found to be variable (Cohn *et al.*, 2000; Wess and Reusch, 2000) and it is difficult to give definitive guidelines, since individual studies have used different experimental design and statistical methods. Information regarding the possible bias of an individual PBGM may be obtained from the manufacturer or the veterinary literature. It is recognized in human and veterinary medicine that the use of insufficient blood, and failure to use control material, are major potential sources of error.

Stains

Rapid haematology stains, e.g. RapiDiff II, give staining characteristics similar to the Romanowsky stains commonly used in large laboratories. The colour of the cells may be adjusted by altering the length of contact time with each stain. With use, the stain becomes exhausted and the staining times should be increased. Thick preparations, such as lymph node aspirates, also require increased contact with the individual stains. Other stains commonly used in the practice laboratory include new methylene blue, which is used for identification of reticulocytes (see Chapter 4), and Sedistain urine stain, for identification of cells and casts in urine sediment.

Microscope slides

Good quality microscope slides are essential. Poor quality slides may be greasy, thus preventing cellular adhesion and optimal staining. In addition, a bevelled edge makes blood film preparation easier, and a frosted end allows easy identification of the patient, date and type of sample.

Selecting a biochemistry or haematology analyser

When selecting an individual piece of equipment it is essential to consider all of the factors in Figures 1.4 and 1.5; above all, the equipment should be validated for the species for which it will be used, and should produce consistent, accurate and helpful results.

General
Validated for species?
Robust?
Footprint and workspace available?
Range of assays available (check the usefulness of unfamiliar assays)
Operation
Technical skill required for operation and training for new operators?
Batch or single samples only?
Large 'hands-on' time?
Profiles determined by manufacturer or can individual tests be selected?
Volume of sample required?
Sample requirements, i.e. plasma *versus* serum (serum takes longer to prepare)?
Interferences, i.e. lipaemia and haemolysis? Methods which are significantly affected by lipaemia require more attention to the sample collection protocol and may require additional preparation steps
Reagents – number of tests per reagent bottle?
Shelf-life for wet reagents once reconstituted?
Plumbing requirements?
Electrical requirements?
Transfer of data to patient records?
Health and Safety
Check COSHH assessment for reagents
Disposal of waste?
Safety of equipment operation?
Technical support and repair
Technical support available?
Speed of advice?
Value of advice offered and success of recommended interventions?
Is troubleshooting possible at the practice or will equipment have to be returned to manufacturer?
Replacement equipment available if equipment has to be returned to manufacturer?
Warranty?
Service agreement available?
Cost of repairs (discuss with other users)?
Spare parts available?

1.4 Factors to consider when investing in a laboratory analyser.

Capital cost
Capital; lost interest
Running cost
Calibration; consumables per maintenance cycle; consumables per patient sample; waste reagent
Labour cost
Analysis; maintenance; reviewing quality procedures; troubleshooting
Quality cost
Quality control material; audit of performance (equipment and operators)
Training cost
Initial staff training; subsequent staff training; continuing professional development for veterinary staff providing interpretations
Building cost
Space for equipment and consumables

1.5 Costs to consider when selecting an analyser.

At least two or three options, where available, should be considered, and the potential advantages and disadvantages researched thoroughly before arranging an equipment trial. Unfortunately, there are currently only a small number of independent validation studies for some of the more commonly used veterinary analysers but information may be obtained from sales representatives, personal contact with other users and postings on internet fora. A trial period is recommended to select equipment tailored to the individual practice, and to determine the usefulness of technical support and training. It should be noted, however, that some equipment (especially haematology analysers) requires a critical level of laboratory skills and the full benefit of this equipment may not be realized during a trial period.

When considering the cost of in-clinic equipment prior to purchase, it is essential to evaluate the full potential cost (Figure 1.5), which should be compared to the expected number of tests per week or month, and expected revenue.

All equipment should be installed according to the manufacturer's guidelines. Installation is likely to be performed by the sales representative or technical staff and may require special attention to water supplies, electrical supply and computer linkages. Equipment should be maintained according to manufacturer's instructions and serviced by a competent engineer.

Systems of work

A standard operating procedure (SOP) details information regarding a specific task or set of tasks. There should be an SOP to cover all tasks that are commonly undertaken, such as use and maintenance of the centrifuge, and performing a urinary sediment examination. Staff should follow the SOP at all times, allowing a safe and standardized approach to laboratory testing and operation of equipment. It is necessary for supervisors to check that staff comply with the SOP and that the documents are regularly reviewed for possible improvements. Changes in instrumentation or method may require a change in the SOP. The time taken to prepare this documentation is considerable, but the long-term value with regard to safety, training and quality cannot be overstated. The following information is commonly included in technical SOPs:

- Purpose of SOP – the scope of the SOP and if necessary, why the task is performed
- Principle of test
- Health and Safety – summary of, or referral to, COSHH assessments for individual reagents. Awareness of the risks of operating equipment
- Equipment required – major equipment required and any specific operating instructions
- Reagents – list of reagents, calibration and control material required
- Samples – list of the preferred sample type and alternatives which might be used. Any sampling considerations should be highlighted, e.g. animal must be fasted, sample must be collected 2 hours after feeding
- Method – detailed steps of the method of performing the task and the disposal of any waste
- Results – how results should be reported, e.g. total protein reported in g/l
- Interpretation – guidelines for interpretation and reference intervals
- References
- Appendix – any worksheets required, e.g. blood film examination results sheet.

Staff training

The range of tests offered by a practice laboratory determines the level of expertise required by staff, and the training requirements. It is important that anybody working in the practice laboratory is either suitably trained or is working under the supervision of a competent person. Training should include:

- General safety procedures (fire, first aid, manual handling of loads) and local laboratory rules
- The use of COSHH assessments
- Disposal of waste and treatment of spillages
- Underpinning scientific knowledge related to the analyses performed
- Training for each SOP, task or group of tasks (technical proficiency).

It is important to maintain training records for each member of staff. These should include details of training in each item listed above, CPD records and, ideally, a current CV.

Early in the training period it is likely that all work will be checked, followed by a period of 'self-referral'. Even highly experienced staff seek other opinions, especially in haematology and cytology, and it should be easy for practice staff to have access to a second opinion, whether on-site, or from a commercial laboratory. Once a member of staff has been fully trained and deemed competent to perform an analysis it is still necessary to monitor his or her performance, as it is easy for staff to work independently and gradually modify the procedure over time. Observation and audit are the main methods of ensuring that staff produce consistent work of an acceptable quality.

Training resources

A range of textbooks and haematology atlases are available, which detail methods for the practice laboratory. An excellent array of images can also be found on the websites of many veterinary schools and institutes. However, the availability of practical courses or workshops that provide hands-on experience of practical tasks is limited.

Quality management

Quality assurance, or total quality management, refers to a set of procedures, systems of work and documentation that is in place to limit the risk of laboratory error and to maintain the quality of a service or product. Details of quality management are provided in Chapter 2, but the following components are important in large diagnostic laboratories and are relevant to the practice laboratory.

Quality processes

The formulation of clear and relevant SOPs, compliance with those SOPs, adequate staff training and proper selection and care of laboratory equipment should produce accurate, reliable results most of the time. However, the use of quality control materials and quality assessments detect the potential for error (before it becomes important to the patient) and ensure that any errors which do occur are thoroughly evaluated.

Quality control

Quality control (QC) involves the use of solutions with a known analytical composition and of statistical methods to document that equipment, reagents and operators are performing within expected limits. The use of this material is outlined in Chapter 2. In addition, external QC schemes can be used to check the performance of the practice laboratory against others using similar equipment. Although external QC schemes are used by most commercial laboratories, to the author's knowledge, there is only one such scheme in the UK for practice equipment.

Quality assessment

The practice should have a review policy for all QC procedures, including SOPs and QC results. It is important to solicit and record feedback from all the clinicians using the practice laboratory. Do they have confidence in the results? Does the service answer their laboratory needs? Ideally, feedback from clinicians and quality processes should be used to plan improvements in the service. Changes in systems should then be monitored to ensure that they do actually deliver the expected improvement. Some of the most common problems encountered are highlighted in Figure 1.6 and it may be useful to consider these while planning quality systems for a laboratory.

Laboratory documentation checklist

The following logs are helpful to ensure that all aspects of the quality management process are recorded:

Problem and cause	Action
Inaccurate results: limitations of equipment or method	Select equipment that is validated Understand its uses and limitations Plan follow-up testing at a diagnostic laboratory
Laboratory error due to failure of proper use or maintenance of equipment	Produce SOPs for equipment use and maintenance Ensure compliance with SOPs Run QC material
Laboratory error due to lack of standardized methods, training and verification of unexpected results	Write SOPs for technical tasks Plan staff training Verify unexpected results/seek advice from a veterinary clinical pathologist
Results attributed to wrong patient	Label sample clearly, immediately after sample collection Keep laboratory tidy Reduce risk of transcription error where possible Plan follow-up testing where test results are not consistent with the clinical presentation
Incorrect interpretation due to inadequate training, insufficient clinical or therapeutic information, or assumptions regarding sample timing	Ensure sampling protocols are followed Interpret results in the light of prior drug therapy Ensure sufficient underpinning knowledge and ongoing CPD Invest in good textbooks and educational resources
Failure to order appropriate follow-on tests	It is easy to limit test selection to those tests available in the practice laboratory and to repeat those tests when others may be more appropriate. Seek advice from a veterinary clinical pathologist
Extensive laboratory investigations in healthy patients	Not all abnormal test results indicate disease. Mild abnormalities may be noted in healthy patients. See Chapter 2

1.6 Common pitfalls and limitations of in-clinic laboratory testing.

- SOPs
- Training records
- Equipment calibration, maintenance and service records
- QC results for both internal and external schemes. The actions taken when problems are encountered should also be recorded
- Reagent preparation sheets, detailing preparation, expiry, QC checks, storage requirements and lot numbers
- Microscope log (details of service and electrical checks)
- Fridge/freezer log (record of temperatures and action taken if a problem is detected)
- Laboratory diary (to include reminders for maintenance)
- Audit reports
- 'Problem log' with details of action taken to correct problem.

References and further reading

Advisory Committee on Dangerous Pathogens (1995) *Categorisation of Biological Agents according to Hazard and Category of Containment, 4th edn.* Health and Safety Executive, Caerphilly

Advisory Committee on Dangerous Pathogens (2000) *Second supplement to: Categorisation of Biological Agents according to Hazard and Category of Containment, 4th edn.* Health and Safety Executive, Caerphilly

BSAVA (2000) *BSAVA Practice Standards Scheme: Everything You Need to Know, 2nd edn* (CD-ROM). BSAVA, Gloucester

Cohn LA, McCaw DL, Tate DJ and Johnson JC (2000) Assessment of five portal blood glucose meters, a point-of-care analyser and colour strips for measuring blood glucose concentrations in dogs. *Journal of the American Veterinary Medical Association* **216,** 198–202

George JW (2001) The usefulness and limitations of hand-held refractometers in veterinary laboratory medicine: an historical and technical review. *Veterinary Clinical Pathology* **30,** 201–210

Health and Safety Executive Website: www.hse.gov.uk

Jagger T (1999) Home or Away? The veterinary laboratory. *In Practice* **21,** 152–154

Wess G and Reusch C (2000) Evaluation of five portable blood glucose meters for use in dogs. *Journal of the American Veterinary Medical Association* **216,** 203–209

2

Interpretation of laboratory data

Joy Archer

Introduction

Laboratory test results form part of the database from which a clinical diagnosis may be made. History, clinical examination and ancillary tests (laboratory tests, radiographs, etc.) are interpreted in conjunction with each other to obtain the best possible diagnosis. Laboratory data should not be interpreted in isolation but with an understanding of the laboratory methods used, and the potential errors caused by inappropriate sample collection and handling. Appropriate quality control systems should be implemented in every laboratory to minimize error. Test results are interpreted by comparison with reference values for a group of healthy animals and with knowledge of how disease processes can change these results. The principles of the methodology of data analysis, and identification of abnormal results, should also be appreciated in relation to clinical decision making.

Errors may be introduced into diagnostic tests at three main stages:

- Pre-analytical: involving sample collection and handling
- Analytical: involving sample testing and result reporting
- Post-analytical: involving analysis and interpretation of test results.

Pre-analytical errors

Poor quality or inappropriate samples can lead to the generation of poor quality results and serious errors. Errors may be introduced during:

- Sample collection
- Sample handling
- Sample submission to the laboratory.

Sample collection

Every effort should be made to obtain the best possible sample for testing. Sampling is influenced by the testing required. For example, urine for microbiology testing should be collected aseptically by cystocentesis, while for routine urinalysis an uncontaminated voided sample collected into a clean container is often appropriate. Urine from the cage floor is unsuitable for either analysis and could introduce artefacts.

Blood

With blood collection for haematology, biochemistry and special tests, venipuncture should be performed as atraumatically and as rapidly as possible, and the sample submitted in the correct container for the test. If blood is collected from indwelling catheters, the correct protocol for flushing and sampling should be carefully followed. Traumatic or delayed collection can cause platelet activation and formation of microthrombi in the collected sample which may not be visible to the naked eye, but will interfere with haematological analysis. Trauma can also damage erythrocyte membranes and cause haemolysis.

Unless a vacutainer system for blood collection is used, the needle should be removed from the syringe before the blood is transferred *gently* to the tube to avoid damage to the cells and to minimize haemolysis. With vacutainer tubes, once the needle has pierced the cap, blood should be allowed to transfer from the syringe to the tube without added pressure on the plunger.

If a single sample is to be divided between several collecting tubes it is good practice to collect into an empty (serum) tube first before collection into tubes containing anticoagulant agents, to prevent possible contamination, especially with ethylenediamine tetraacetic acid (EDTA) as this affects many analytes. EDTA contamination causes increases in potassium, and decreases in calcium, magnesium, creatine kinase (CK) and alkaline phosphatase (ALP). Tubes should be filled to the correct volume and gently inverted to mix the blood with the pre-measured contents (e.g EDTA, sodium citrate, lithium heparin). It is important to collect an adequate volume of blood for the tests required, remembering that approximately 50–60% of the volume is plasma/serum.

Haematology: For routine haematology, the anticoagulant of choice is EDTA (potassium or sodium salt). It causes the fewest artefactual changes in the morphology of blood cells in most mammalian species, though it is unsuitable for many avian and reptilian blood cells. If the concentration of EDTA is excessive in relation to blood volume, cells will shrink and a falsely low packed cell volume (PCV) will be obtained. EDTA tubes less than half full (>3.0 mg EDTA/ml blood) reduce the PCV by 5%, while machine-measured haematocrit is unaffected because the red cells re-expand when they are mixed with diluent in the analyser (Cornbleet, 1983). If liquid EDTA is used this can add to the error by diluting the sample, thus further lowering cell counts. Conversely, insufficient EDTA in relation to blood will lead to clot formation. Small clots in the sample, which might be missed by visually inspecting the sample, can cause errors in machine-measured parameters, in particular the platelet count and white cell count.

Biochemistry: Biochemical tests can be performed on either serum or plasma. Many laboratories prefer serum since this reduces the probability of microfibrin clot formation in the sample and interference with instrument automatic sampling. Heparin salts (sodium, ammonium or lithium) bind and inhibit thrombin, preventing clot formation; therefore the blood can be processed rapidly to yield plasma, which is used for many hormone tests as well as routine biochemistry. Plasma from stored blood or unseparated samples can often contain small clots which interfere at the analysis stage.

If serum is needed, a plain tube or one containing a separator gel can be used and samples should be held at room temperature until full clot formation has occurred, usually 15 minutes for small animals, before centrifugation. If a full clot does not develop or there is inadequate centrifugation, fibrin clots may develop in the sample and cause problems during analysis. Clots, whether large or small, can cause errors in haematology, biochemistry and blood gas analyses, and also with coagulation screening and should, therefore, be avoided. With separator gel tubes no further manipulation is required after centrifugation as the gel is inert and separates the cells and their continued metabolism from the serum/plasma. Most analytes are not affected by this substance, but gel tubes are inappropriate for therapeutic monitoring of many drugs. For other tubes the serum/plasma should be carefully removed from the sedimented cells and placed in the correct tube (plastic/glass) as soon as possible.

All tubes should be labelled with the animal's name, hospital number date and collection time (if important for the test) as soon as possible after they are filled to prevent errors in sample identification.

If samples for glucose are to be stored or sent to a laboratory, the blood should be collected into fluoride/oxalate which inhibits enolase and, when centrifuged, prevents the oxidation of glucose. Sodium citrate binds calcium and citrate plasma is used for coagulation testing. Details of sample volumes required and choice of tubes for a range of tests can be found in Appendix 2.

Sample timing

Physiological changes can affect samples, therefore the time of sample collection can be important, depending on which test is to be performed.

- Exercise or excitement/fear can cause changes in haematology and may lead to increased neutrophil and decreased lymphocyte counts. These changes are most often seen in young stressed cats.
- Hyperglycaemia is also commonly seen in cats as a result of stress.
- Dehydration may lead to increased PCV.
- Food consumption can affect biochemistry tests, in particular cholesterol, triglyceride and glucose. Unless postprandial samples are required (e.g. for bile acid measurement) an overnight (12 hour) fast is best for general biochemical tests. In some animals a longer fast, up to 24 hours, may be needed to eliminate such effects.
- There are normal diurnal variations in some hormone levels, therefore a set time may be indicated for collection of samples for measurement of these hormones, especially if they are to be sequential.

If samples are to be collected for monitoring drug therapy, collection times can be important and should be timed to correspond with peak and trough drug levels; the times should be carefully recorded. Special tests, such as glucose tolerance tests and hormone stimulation tests, should have protocols defining test substance dosage and times of administration and sample collection. Times should be carefully recorded on the sample containers.

Sample handling

Once a sample has been collected into the correct tube it should be processed promptly. For haematology it is always best to make one or more blood films close to the time of collection and air dry them. Although EDTA preserves cell morphology, changes begin to appear within hours, especially in white cells. Samples should be held in the refrigerator before shipping and/or analysing. Blood films and cytology smears should not be refrigerated or kept close to formalin. Samples for plasma and serum should be handled carefully to avoid haemolysis and should be transferred to suitable storage tubes and stored at the correct temperature for the test (either refrigerated or frozen).

Certain samples require special and timely handling. If reliable results are to be obtained from samples that should arrive at the special testing laboratory frozen, these samples must be maintained in this condition from the time of collection and preparation until analysis. Similarly, if there is delay between collection and analysis of whole blood samples for blood gas analysis, gas can diffuse and pH changes occur. Samples for ionized calcium and magnesium measurement must also be handled according to strict temperature and time protocols for reliable results. Samples for glucose determination need to be placed in fluoride/oxalate, or be separated promptly and frozen if analysis is to be delayed. Glucose decreases at a rate of 3% per hour if unseparated samples are held at room temperature.

Sample submission

Submission of inappropriate samples can be the source of numerous laboratory errors and, in extreme cases, will lead to the rejection of the samples by the laboratory. The correct volume of sample should be submitted in the appropriate container, clearly labelled with sample and patient identification and date of collection. Along with the samples there should be a clearly legible submission form. This should indicate the tests requested, patient identification (name, number, species, age, breed and sex) and a brief history and clinical findings, including information on any drug therapy or blood replacement products given. Samples should be sent to the testing laboratory using courier services or reliable mail services; they should arrive with the shortest possible time delay to avoid ageing artefacts in the samples. Many laboratories have set criteria for sample rejection in order to minimize sources of laboratory analytical and reporting error. Amongst these are:

- Inadequate sample identification
- Sample in poor condition due to improper collection, tubes, sample volumes, handling and transportation
- Severe haemolysis
- Severe lipaemia
- Marked icterus
- Microbiology samples in incorrect transport medium
- Sample too old.

At the pre-analytical stage, the greatest numbers of errors for haematology tests are introduced by sample ageing, and the primary sources of error for biochemical tests are sample haemolysis, lipaemia and icterus.

Analytical error

Analytical error can be introduced at the analysis stage as a consequence of pre-analytical sample factors (e.g. haemolysis, lipaemia), or can result from problems with equipment or reagents, or test methodology. Most laboratories have standard operating procedures (SOPs) for every stage of the analytical process. In addition, laboratories document any unexpected changes and deviations at each stage of the process, which can be reviewed on a regular basis or when a problem is detected.

Equipment and reagents

Detailed records of equipment maintenance according to the manufacturer's instructions should be kept and any failures of performance addressed. Reagents and materials for calibration and control should be inventoried with dates of receipt and lot and batch numbers; they should be stored under the conditions recommended by the manufacturers and discarded when outdated. When a new batch or lot of reagents/calibrators/controls is started, its performance should be compared with the old batch and sample tests run in parallel to ensure that there are no significant changes in test performance.

Calibration

Daily or more frequent checks on instrument and reagent performance are required to ensure correct analysis of samples. Because most instruments and reagents are designed for use with human samples, most of the calibrators for both equipment and reagents are designed to check performance while testing human samples. Most calibration materials are made to resemble human blood, serum or plasma. Few still contain these products, unless in denatured form. They are produced by the manufacturers to conform to National Standards guidelines and are usually pre-assayed for performance using the equipment and/or test procedure for which they are provided. Manufacturers provide information on the expected performance of such materials. If the results obtained in a laboratory are outside these limits, patient samples should not be run on the instruments in question until the cause has been found and corrected and the instrument or test has been recalibrated.

Controls

Aqueous and protein matrix 'serum'-based control materials are commercially available. These contain multiple analytes and have been pre-tested and validated by the manufacturer. They are available for all common haematological and biochemical tests and can be obtained for test values at low, medium and high levels of the expected test results range. A range of expected values is provided with the control material and the results obtained in the laboratory should be within this range.

Two control materials for each analyte should be run at least once every 24 hours. Usually one control has values representative of a reference 'healthy' value and the other has abnormal high or low values. These materials are designed to produce values in ranges suitable for human samples, which are not always similar to the ranges seen in dogs and cats. Therefore control sample pools prepared from animal serum/plasma may also be used with each batch of patient samples. Usually, if the control samples give results within the expected range then it is assumed that the patient test results are also valid and can be accepted.

Accuracy and precision in laboratory tests

For interpretation of laboratory tests to be useful, it is important to know and set the accuracy, precision and allowable error in those tests and then to monitor test performance with quality control procedures.

Accuracy

In a group of replicate values obtained on a sample, the closer the mean of these comes to the true or known value, the more accurate is the measurement or method. This is a measure of the systematic error (bias) (Figure 2.1).

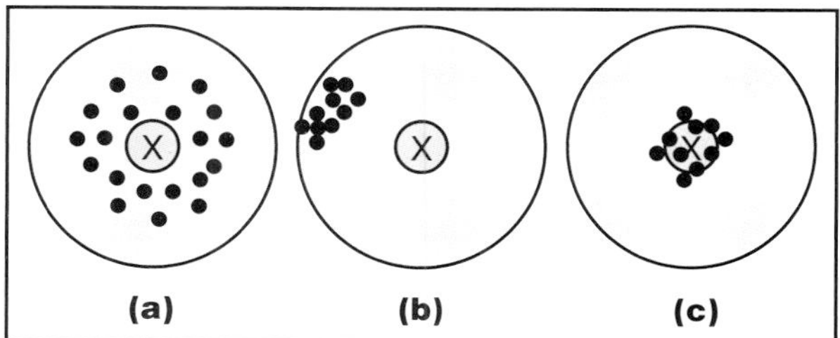

2.1 In the three circles, X is the true value and the dots represent results obtained from sequential analysis of the sample. (a) An accurate but imprecise method: the dots are evenly distributed around the true value and the mean of all the values is equal to the true value. (b) A precise but inaccurate method: the dots are closely clustered together, showing that there is good repeatability, but the results are consistently biased. (c) A method which is both accurate and precise: all the dots are close to the true value and are tightly clustered together.

Precision

In a group of replicate values obtained on a sample, the closer these are to each other the more precise is the measurement or method. This is a measure of reproducibility or random error.

Accuracy and precision are important in the interpretation of test results. Assessing accuracy (systematic analytical error) and precision (random analytical error) allows the determination of the total analytical error of a method (see Figure 2.1).

Allowable error

This is defined as the maximum amount of error allowable in a test result for it to have any clinical diagnostic usefulness or value. Once the level of allowable analytical error has been determined, quality goals can be set and an internal quality control system can be used to monitor achievement of these.

Quality control systems

Quality control (QC) systems usually monitor test performance quality at three levels:

- Daily (short-term) monitoring for systematic and random errors in each run to ensure that patient sample test results are acceptable
- Weekly to monthly (medium-term) monitoring for the development of systematic errors (bias) and to ensure that the analytical methods remain free of random error
- Monthly to yearly (long-term) monitoring that analytical methods remain as accurate and precise as possible. This usually uses an internal QC and an external proficiency testing control system. The most widely used external QC systems are based on human samples. These include UK National External Quality Assessment Service (NEQAS) for haematology and biochemistry and Randox Quality Assessment Service (RQAS) for biochemistry. A veterinary microbiology QC service is provided by the Veterinary Laboratory Agency (VLA).

Internal quality control

Each test method has a characteristic inherent variability which can be expressed as the standard deviation (SD) or as the coefficient of variation (CV) (calculated from SD/mean x 100%). The higher the SD and CV, the greater the inherent variability within the test. Typically the SD and CV are small for analytes such as electrolytes, moderate for enzymes and much larger for most hormones. Instrument-measured haematology parameters have smaller CVs than those derived from manual procedures.

The SD can be established for a given test or instrument by recording values obtained on control materials over 20–30 runs. Most analysers can store this information and calculate the SD and CV values. These are then used to set control limits. Commonly the mean ± 2SD is set as the limit for rejection of patient test data, and this is referred to as the 1_{2S} rule under the Westgard QC system (see below). Using the 2SD limit, 95% of control values are expected to fall within the limits but 5% of values will fall outside the limits and so be falsely rejected. Thus, this limit has a good detection rate for error but will falsely detect error in 5% of 'good' control runs. For many tests the limit is increased to 3SD (1_{3S}) before rejection is indicated. Using the 1_{3S} limit there will be a lower rate of false rejection (around 1%), but also a lower rate of error detection. The choice of rule used is based on the accuracy and precision of the specific test and the number of controls used (i.e. low, medium and high, or close to 'normal' and high or low). For example the 1_{2S} rule is suitable for electrolytes, as these methods have small SDs and CVs, while the 2_{2S} (see below) or 1_{3S} rule or multiple rules would be more appropriate for enzymes and hormone tests, which have larger SDs and CVs.

Control data can be monitored using Levey–Jennings control charts (Figure 2.2). These can be produced by manually plotting data, but most modern instrument computers generate and store these charts and perform statistical analysis of the data in them automatically. Most charts are constructed to cover a period of 1 month or 30 days of data collection and analysis.

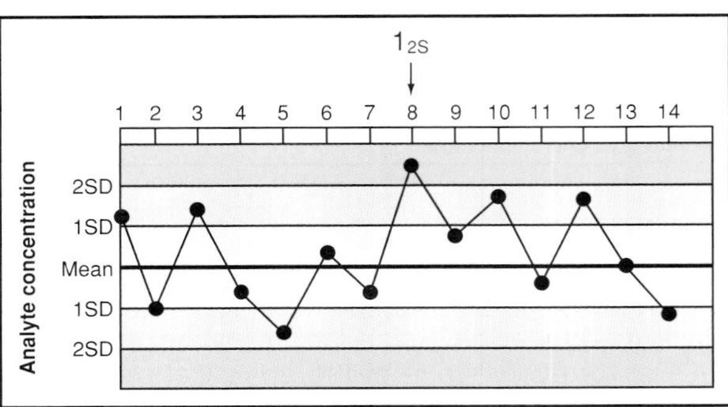

2.2 A Levey–Jennings plot system with an allowable error of ± 2SD from the mean (1_{2S}). The first seven values appear 'in control' and are close to the mean, evenly distributed either side of it. The eighth value is outside the control limits (as indicated by the arrow), but subsequent values are within control limits.

For the detection of both random and systematic error, more effective multiple rule quality control charts, involving cumulative mean values and a wider range of control limits, can be used. The Westgard control rules are the most widely used multiple rule charts and are summarized below ($\bar{x}$ = mean value.)

- The 1_{2S} rule (one control value exceeding $\bar{x}$ ± 2SD) is an early warning for further testing using other control rules.
- The 1_{3S} rule (one control value exceeding $\bar{x}$ ± 3SD) is sensitive to random error (i.e. imprecision).
- The 2_{2S} rule (two consecutive values exceeding $\bar{x}$ + 2SD or 2 consecutive values less than $\bar{x}$ – 2SD) is sensitive to systematic error (i.e. bias).
- The R_{4S} rule rejects a run if one observation exceeds $\bar{x}$ + 2SD and one observation is less than $\bar{x}$ – 2SD within one run. (Two controls, the high level and the normal or low level control, are used in each run.) This rule is sensitive to random error (i.e. imprecision).
- The 4_{1S} rule rejects a run if 4 consecutive control observations all exceed $\bar{x}$ + 1SD or are all less than $\bar{x}$ –1 SD and is sensitive to systematic error (i.e. bias).

- The 10X rule rejects a run if 10 consecutive control observations fall on one side of the mean, and is sensitive to systematic error (bias).

These rules help to classify the type of error (random error or systematic error). The analysis process can then be inspected for causes of that error, the problem corrected and the control sample re-run. Figure 2.3 shows a Levey–Jennings chart with several rules being violated.

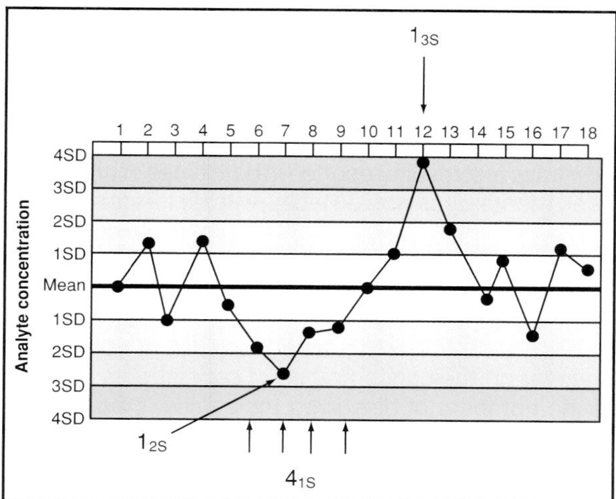

2.3 A Levey–Jennings plot using the Westgard Multirules system. The first five readings are 'in control'. Readings 6–9 all exceed 1SD on the same side of the mean, violating the 4_{1S} rule. This is an indicator of systematic error (bias). In addition, reading 7 violates the 1_{2S} rule. Following recalibration of the analyser, readings 10 and 11 are in control, but reading 12 exceeds 3 SDs, violating the 1_{3S} rule, reflecting random error. Trouble shooting revealed an error in test procedure. Subsequent readings are 'in control'.

Some large laboratories have recently adopted a more sophisticated control system also developed by Westgard, called the 6 Sigma Rules System (Westgard, 2001), which was originally used for industrial manufacturing processes. Most laboratory testing does not as yet extend much beyond the control rules described above.

External quality control

Most large veterinary laboratories also participate in external QC programmes. In these a central agency provides each laboratory in the programme with 'unknown', often pretested, materials for both haematology and biochemical testing. The results obtained by the laboratory are returned to the agency, which, in turn, issues statistical evaluations of all the results, providing an external unbiased measure of the accuracy of the laboratory's test procedures.

Use of patient data in quality decisions

In human testing laboratories patient data are commonly used as a method of monitoring test performance, as large numbers of their samples are from normal healthy individuals. Unfortunately, in veterinary laboratories it is not as easy to use this method as the majority of samples are from sick animals. However, deviations from usual test result patterns can probably still be used to monitor performance.

The delta check

Using computer-based systems it is possible to check results for the current sample in relation to previous samples from the same patient. A delta check can test for results that vary by a set amount or set percentage and is valuable for monitoring analytes that change little from day to day for an individual patient, for example creatinine or PCV. It is unlikely that a consecutive series of tests would show marked changes unless there had been a major change in the clinical condition.

Effects of pre-analytical error in compounding analytical error

Changes in the sample that occurred at the pre-analytical stage and affected the condition of the sample upon arrival at the laboratory, can compound analytical error. Both sample ageing and haemolysis can affect haematology results. Common conditions that affect analytical performance of biochemical assays are haemolysis, lipaemia and icterus (Figure 2.4). Most laboratories report the presence of haemolysis, lipaemia and icterus with the results, and usually state whether it is mild, moderate or severe, or denote this in terms of 1+ to 4+. Frequently they will also report the

Analyte	Effect of haemolysis	Effect of lipaemia	Effect of icterus
RBC count	Decreased		
Haemoglobin concentration	Increased	Increased	
Haematocrit	Decreased		
MCHC	Increased	Increased	
Potassium	Increased		
Glucose	Decreased	Increased	
Creatinine	Decreased	Increased	
Calcium	Increased	Increased	
Inorganic phosphate	Increased	Increased	
Total protein (refractometer)		Increased	
Albumin		Decreased	
ALT	Increased	Increased	
AST	Increased	Increased	
ALP	Increased	Increased	
GGT	Decreased	Variable	
Creatine kinase	Increased		
Amylase	Decreased	Decreased	
Lipase	Decreased	Decreased	
Bile acids	Decreased	Increased	
Bilirubin		Increased	Increased

2.4 Examples of common interferences. The effects vary depending on the analyser and test method being used.

expected type and severity of interference and to which analytes. In cases of extreme contamination the tests may not be performed.

Many laboratories have developed **interferogrammes** for use with their instruments and for all biochemical tests. To construct an interferogramme a serum/plasma sample is split into aliquots in which varying amounts of haemolysis/lipaemia/icterus are created. To create haemolysis a blood clot is macerated and the haemolysed fluid harvested by centrifugation and its haemoglobin content determined. This is then added to clear serum/plasma at varying concentrations, which can be measured using a haematology analyser and subjectively visually graded as 1+ through to 4+, just as clinical samples are graded. A panel of biochemical tests is run on the samples and the effect of the varying levels of haemolysis on the results is plotted graphically. In a similar way the effects of lipaemia are assessed by adding varying quantities of a fat emulsion, and the effects of icterus are assessed by adding varying quantities of purified bilirubin.

Tests for some analytes are affected more profoundly than others; the effect varies depending on the method and analyser being used, and some tests are not affected until haemolysis and lipaemia are very severe.

Interfering substances may interfere directly in a chemical reaction or, more commonly, with colorimetric methods and enzyme assay kinetic detection methods. For example, haemoglobin may absorb at the same wavelength as the colour product of a reaction, or lipid may interfere with a turbidimetric assay by increasing the turbidity. Hormone assays, including those which rely on immunological methods, may also be affected.

Lipaemia and haemolysis also lead to errors in haematological parameters (Figure 2.4). Lipaemia may interfere with the spectrophotometric assay for haemoglobin (Hb), resulting in falsely high Hb and mean corpuscular haemoglobin concentration (MCHC). Large lipid droplets may be falsely counted as leucocytes or platelets by some analysers (e.g. the Cell-Dyn). Haemolysis falsely raises MCHC and lowers PCV and the red cell count. Blood replacement products prepared from bovine haemoglobin interfere with tests in a similar way to haemolysis (directly in a reaction or with colorimetric methods). The effects are dose-dependent and persist for 48 hours or more after administration.

External quality assurance schemes

Many large laboratories also belong to quality assurance (QA) schemes, which provide assurance that the laboratory tests are performed and managed according to set standards. In the UK the major system is United Kingdom Accreditation Service (UKAS) which follows international guidelines set down by the International Organization for Standardization (ISO) for laboratory performance.

Post-analytical errors

Errors can occur due to reporting of incorrect values or ascribing the results to the wrong patient. Occasionally the incorrect reference values for the species may be provided, e.g. dog values for a cat sample. The majority of errors at this stage are, however, related to interpretation. Error may occur because the person interpreting the results is a third party and is incompletely informed (for example, of a history of drug therapy), or because the clinician in charge of the case is unaware of certain changes that can occur in laboratory tests in certain conditions.

Units of measurement

In many countries, laboratory test results are reported in SI units (Système International d'Unites), while in the USA they are still widely reported in conventional units (non-SI units) based on mass gravimetric measurements. Most recent textbooks and veterinary journals now have test results reported in both types of unit. Many books contain conversion tables with factors for converting values in either direction for the most commonly encountered analytes. A few non-SI units have been retained, either because of the complexity of converting them into SI units or because of their widespread use.

Litre (l) is the designated measure of volume. SI units report the concentration of constituents in terms of the numbers of dissolved molecules, measured in moles (with decimal units mol, mmol, μmol, pmol). A *mole* of a chemical contains the number of grams equivalent to its molecular weight. Conventional units report concentrations of constituents in terms of dissolved mass in grams (g, mg, μg, pg).

SI units are not used for total protein, for example, because this is a complex of molecules of different molecular weights. Therefore it is usually reported as g/l. Albumin is also reported in g/l (although it could be reported in μmol/l), largely because the relationship between total protein and albumin is close and they are considered together when test results are evaluated.

The SI unit of enzyme activity is the *katal*, which is defined as the amount of enzyme that will catalyse the transformation of 1 mole of substrate per second in an assay system. This is the accepted reporting unit by the IUPAC (International Union of Biochemistry), but not for clinical tests, and the international unit (IU) continues to be used. There is a constant relationship between katal and IU when measured under identical conditions: 1 katal = 60 million IU.

Some conversion factors are shown in Figure 2.5. A more complete conversion table can be found in Appendix 3.

Gravimetric unit conversion	SI unit
g/100 ml x 10	g/l
g/100 ml x $\frac{10}{\text{mol wt}}$	mol/l
pg/ml x $\frac{10^3}{\text{mol wt}}$	pmol/l
mEq/l x $\frac{1}{\text{valency}}$	mmol/l

2.5 Conversion factors from gravimetric units to SI units. See also Appendix 3.

Interpretation of test results

For the interpretation of test results other pieces of information are required. These include a history, clinical examination, list of differentials, reference values generated by the testing laboratory and other guidelines, such as clinical cut-off limits. Some of these may be provided by the testing laboratory or they can be generated by the clinician. Outlines of some of these are given below. Detailed methods can be found in referenced special texts and are beyond the scope of this chapter.

Reference values/reference intervals

These are usually referred to as normal values, expected values or, more commonly, as 'reference ranges'. They are usually derived from a reference population of normal 'healthy' animals, but for in-house and patient-side analysers they may be supplied by the manufacturer. They are used by the clinician in the evaluation of the test results and in the formulation of a diagnosis for the patient. Therefore it is important that the clinician understands their origin and derivation, and he or she should request this information from the testing laboratories, or manufacturers of laboratory equipment and test kits. Ideally, reference values should be constructed using the guidelines of the National Committee for Clinical Laboratory Standards (NCCLS, 1995). However, this is difficult in veterinary medicine because of the large number of species and breeds encompassed. The major difficulty is identifying an adequate population for use as the reference population. Some compromises have, therefore, been made in methodology and in acceptable minimum numbers of animals. Another consideration is the not inconsiderable cost of establishing reference values for the large number of tests performed by the average veterinary clinical pathology laboratory.

A **reference range** is defined as the entire range of values (actual minimum to maximum measured values) obtained for a test on a population of healthy, non-diseased animals. In practice, a **reference interval** is used, which is the interval between an upper and lower limit and commonly includes the central 95% of the apparently healthy 'normal' reference population determined by statistical methods. The reference population from which samples are to be obtained should be predefined and tight clinical parameters for 'healthy' established. Ideally this population should be representative of the animals from whom samples are sent to the individual laboratory. In practice this is difficult to obtain. Bias may occur if a restricted group of animals is used, for example values from a colony of young Beagle dogs or from cattery cats. The reference population should represent a general mix of breeds, sexes and ages living in different environmental conditions. The reference values generated by the laboratory or instrument from which the results were obtained should always be used.

Reference values are affected by pre-analytical and analytical variables, so these stages should be subject to rigorous quality control before establishment of reference values.

Determination of reference interval: Once the population of healthy normal animals has been selected, the reference values obtained from these are subjected to statistical analysis to determine the reference intervals for each test. The values can be analysed by parametric methods if they form a Gaussian or 'normal' symmetrical bell-shaped curve distribution when a histogram is plotted (Figure 2.6a). With a Gaussian distribution, a reference interval is established based on the mean and 2SDs from the mean (Figure 2.7).

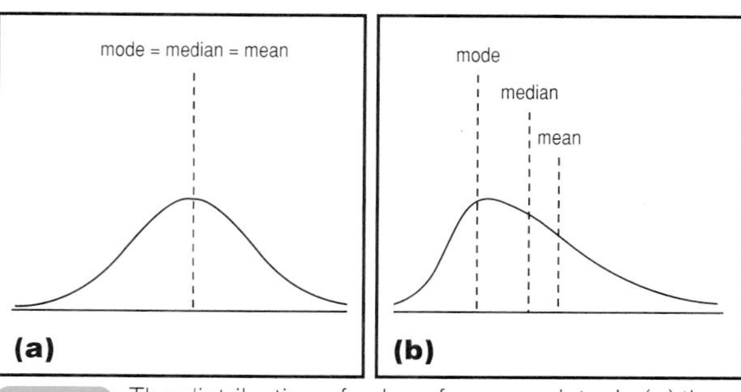

2.6 The distribution of values for an analyte. In (a) there is a Gaussian symmetrical distribution and the median, mean and mode are in the same central position. These data could be analysed by parametric methods, calculating the mean and 2SD to produce reference values. (b) The data points are not in a symmetrical distribution and the mode, median and mean are different. These data would be analysed by non-parametric methods (usually using percentiles) to produce reference values.

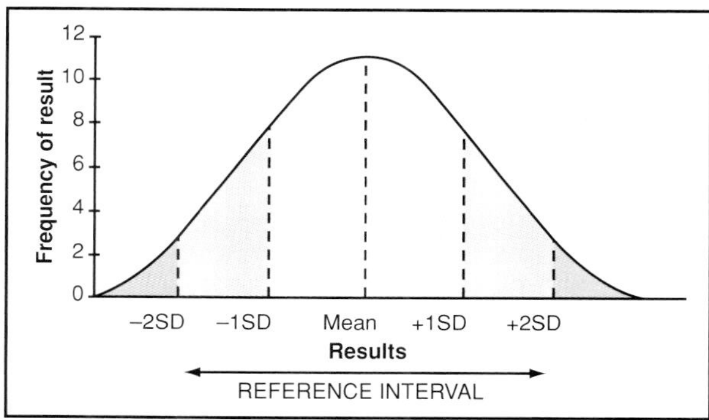

2.7 The usual reference intervals, using the central values with exclusion of the lowest and highest 2.5% of the reference values.

If the distribution is a skewed asymmetrical distribution (Figure 2.6b), the values are transformed using logarithmic or root transformation to produce a more Gaussian distribution and then the interval is defined. Alternatively, non-parametric statistical methods can be used (Solberg, 1987). This commonly involves ranking values and using percentile limits. The value at the 97.5th percentile is the upper reference limit and the value at the 2.5th percentile is the lower reference limit. The values obtained from the reference population are put into ascending order. If n is the number of samples, the position of the sample result lying on the 2.5th percentile is calculated $(n + 1) \times 0.025$, and that on the 97.5th percentile is calculated $(n + 1) \times 0.975$. For example, if there are 78 dogs in the reference population the 2.5th percentile is calculated as $(78 + 1) \times 0.025 = 1.975$ = approximately 2. The samples are ranked in ascending order from 1 to 78. The value of the second result in the ascending series is the lower limit of the reference interval. The 97.5^{th} percentile is (78 + 1) x 0.975 = 77. The value of the 77th sample is the upper limit of the reference interval (Figure 2.7).

When preparing the histograms of values, one or more 'outliers' may be recorded. Unless these values are known to be the result of pre-analytical or analytical error they should be retained. Non-parametrically derived reference limits would be only slightly changed by the exclusion of a single outlier if they were based on a minimum of 120 samples (which is unlikely in veterinary medicine). With smaller populations special statistical tests for outliers can be applied (Dixon, 1953). Ideally, when the outlier is removed it is appropriate to retest the remaining values for any additional outliers. It has been suggested that 200 subjects are required for the construction of reference intervals with an acceptable confidence interval (margin of error). This has been adjusted downward to 60 or above for parametric and 120 or above for non-parametric derived intervals. However, in veterinary medicine a more achievable number is a minimum of 40 subjects.

It should be borne in mind that a reference interval represents expected results in 95% of healthy animals, and using these methods 5% of the truly normal or healthy animals would be classified as abnormal (2.5% below the limit for measured values and 2.5% above the limit for measured values). Therefore, in every 20 healthy animals there will be one animal with test results outside the reference normal values. However, as this is a normal healthy animal the test result would be expected to be close to the set limits. For most tests and analytes this is acceptable, as truly diseased animals will be expected to have values far higher or lower than these intervals. When evaluating a panel of test results from a single animal there is a probability of $1 - 0.95^n$ (where n is the number of tests in the panel) that not all values will be within the set reference interval. Thus, for 20 results there is a 64% chance that one result will be 'abnormal', $[100 \times (1 - 0.95^{20})]$. This becomes important when evaluating results from potentially clinically healthy animals for pre-anaesthetic screens or geriatric profiling, for example.

Limitations of reference intervals

Most laboratories provide reference intervals for the tests performed, based on a wide-ranging general healthy population. A narrow selection of healthy subjects split into subgroups (for example, age and breed groups) would be ideal but this is not practical. It is important to be aware of deviations from the provided ranges, particularly in young animals, for analytes such as haematocrit (HCT), mean cell volume (MCV), total protein, globulins, calcium, phosphorus and alkaline phosphatase. Likewise certain hormone levels, electrolyte and protein values will be at variance with the quoted values in pregnant animals, depending on the stage of gestation, and lactating animals. Specific breed-related anomalies should also be considered, e.g. increased HCT in Greyhounds, increased MCV in some Miniature Poodles, large platelets and thrombocytopenia in Cavalier King Charles Spaniels. Certain narrower breed- and age-related reference intervals can be sourced from the veterinary literature but, without knowledge of the selection of subjects, tests and instrumentation used, it is difficult to transfer these for use with other laboratories' test results or other populations (see below).

Alternative methods of determining reference intervals

Computer-based analysis of normal subpopulation: Because of the difficulties encountered establishing reference intervals, alternatives to the methods described have been sought. The introduction and increasing use of computer databases and laboratory information management systems (LIMs), has allowed stored patient data to be used to construct reference intervals. If a large proportion of the patient samples are from healthy individuals, computerized methods based on a combination of laboratory and diagnostic data can be used to select data from healthy patients to produce reference ranges (Kouri *et al.*, 1994). This system could be adapted using the Systemized Nomenclature of Medicine (SNOMED) coding system for characterization of diseases to exclude all 'clinical patients' and select apparently healthy animals. Statistical methods could be applied to these values. This method would better represent the population of animals tested at the individual laboratory or hospital and would make acquisition of adequate numbers of values (results) easier. However, it would be critical to ensure that the animals selected were in fact clinically normal at the time of testing. Also, this type of data accumulation has inherent increased levels of error related to pre-analytical and analytical factors. Further analysis and documentation of this method is needed before widespread use is encouraged.

Transference: This is another more widely used and accepted method. When new instrumentation or methods are introduced into a laboratory, reference intervals can be obtained from:

- An existing reference interval generated in the same laboratory on an old instrument or using an old method
- Values from another laboratory using the same instrument and or method
- The literature.

These intervals are transferred using a process of validation. In order to do this certain conditions must be met in regard to instrumentation, method and animal population. If these overlap then a minimum of 20 'healthy' animals should be tested and a mini reference interval created. If no more than two of the results are outside the transferred intervals then it can be adopted. Recommendations are to use a sample of 40–60 individuals in human medicine, which would be equivalent to producing a new reference interval in veterinary medicine. The transference of established reference intervals can be statistically validated using Monte Carlo significance testing (Holes *et al.*, 1994).

Intra-individual reference interval: A method favoured in human medicine and research is the intra-individual reference interval, using the subject to create his or her own reference 'healthy' interval. Not unexpectedly the range of results obtained in an individual over time is consistently less than the population-based reference interval (Figure 2.8). The variability of results over time means that a healthy individual may obtain results outside the population reference interval when healthy and inside the population interval when ill.

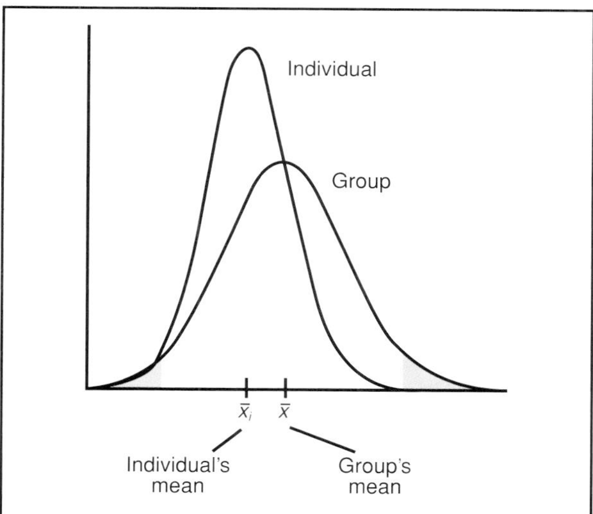

2.8 Illustration of the problems with population-based reference intervals when applied to the individual. It can be seen that in individuals 'healthy values' fluctuate much less than the values for a population. The shaded areas represent results falling outside 2SD of the mean, which equates to the lower and upper 2.5% of the reference values.

Clinical decision limits

The relevance of results in clinical decision making is based on clinical information and the clinical relevance of a laboratory test, not just on a test result outside the reference interval. Test results may be used to:

- Establish, exclude or confirm the presence of a particular disease
- Monitor disease progression
- Monitor therapy or progression or regression of a disease
- Provide prognostic information
- Screen populations of healthy animals.

The importance of certain test characteristics depends on the use to which the test is to be put. If a test is to be used to screen for a disease of low prevalence in a healthy population then it must be very sensitive (identify a high proportion of affected animals), whilst specificity is less important (animals which test positive can be subjected to further, more specific tests). Screening tests also need to be safe and inexpensive. For tests that are used to confirm a diagnosis, specificity is more important (the test should not incorrectly identify non-diseased animals), especially if the consequences of a positive result are serious (e.g chemotherapy, surgery or even euthanasia).

Decision analysis in this context involves the concepts of the sensitivity, specificity and predictive value of the test results (see also Chapter 26):

- The diagnostic **sensitivity** of a test is the probability of obtaining a positive test result in an animal that has the disease
- The diagnostic **specificity** of a test is the probability of obtaining a negative test result in an animal that does not have the disease
- A **true positive** result (TP) correctly identifies a diseased animal as having the disease
- A **true negative** result (TN) correctly identifies an unaffected animal as free from the disease
- A **false positive** result (FP) occurs when an unaffected animal is incorrectly identified as having the disease
- A **false negative** result (FN) occurs when a diseased animal is incorrectly identified by the test as free from disease.
- **Positive predictive value** is the probability that an animal with a positive test result has the disease (expressed as a percentage)
  $$= \frac{TP}{TP + FP} \times 100\ (\%)$$
- **Negative predictive value** is the probability that an animal with a negative test result does not have the disease (expressed as a percentage)
  $$= \frac{TN}{TN + FN} \times 100\ (\%)$$
- **Prevalence** is an estimate of the frequency of a disease in a population at a point in time
  $$= \frac{TP + FN}{TP + FP + TN + FN} \times 100\ (\%)$$

Prevalence is important in determining the predictive value of a test. For a test with a diagnostic sensitivity of 95% and a diagnostic specificity of 95%, the predictive value of a positive test result within a population, with a disease prevalence of 50%, is 95%. However, if the prevalence is only 5% then the predictive value of a positive test falls to only 50%, causing the predictive value for the test to be no better than chance or flipping a coin.

A test that has reasonably high sensitivity and specificity and is a good diagnostic test in a population with a high probability of having the disease will, therefore, be very poor in a population where disease prevalence is very low, i.e. as a screening test in a healthy population. Illustrative examples of this can be found in Chapter 26.

Generally the aim is to maximize both sensitivity and specificity, but no test is 100% sensitive and 100% specific. As one is maximized, the other is decreased. In the diagnostic situation a test with 100% sensitivity may generate unacceptable numbers of false positive test results. Likewise, when a test is 100% specific it may generate unacceptable numbers of false negative results. In the clinical diagnosis of disease, other medical decision limits can be used, and where results have a numerical value (i.e. not just positive or negative) cut-off values can be selected to maximize the discriminatory power of the test (Figure 2.9).

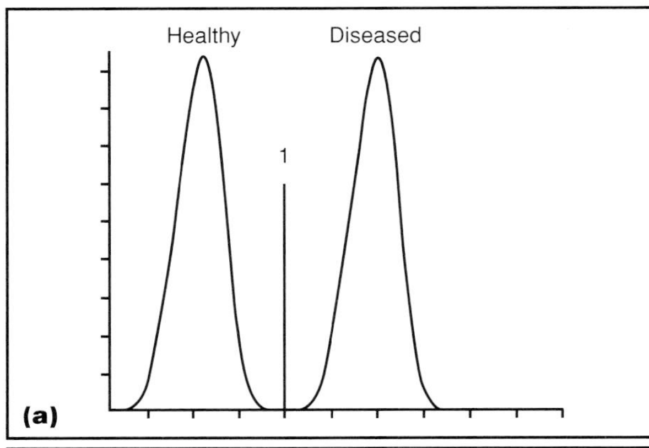

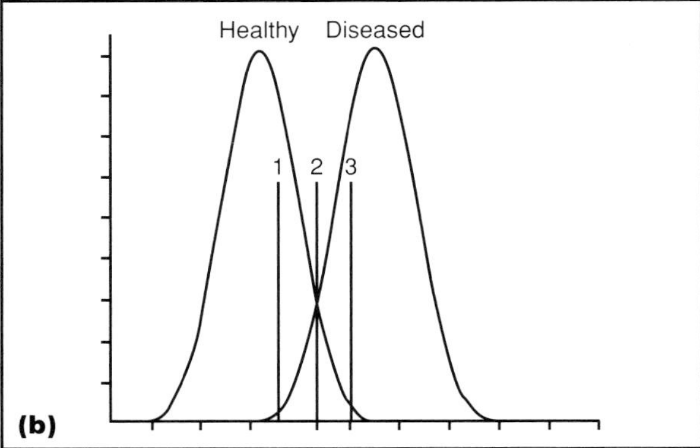

2.9 Demonstration of the problem of trying to establish cut-off points for any test between healthy individuals and diseased individuals. In (a) the test results from healthy animals do not overlap the test results from diseased animals and so there is a clear cut-off indicated by line 1.This test has 100% sensitivity and specificity. In (b) the test results from healthy animals overlap those from diseased animals. If the cut-off is set at line 1 the test is sensitive but not specific, because a high proportion of healthy animals will have results above the cut-off. Conversely, if the cut-off is set at line 3 the test becomes more specific (very few non-diseased animals have results above the cut-off), but is much less sensitive (a significant proportion of diseased animals have results below the cut-off). If line 2 is selected as the cut-off, the test has moderate sensitivity and specificity.

Cut-off values: There is rarely a perfect separation of test results for healthy and diseased animals, and some degree of overlap of the two populations occurs, so there is usually a need for 'trade-offs' in the clinical decision process. This involves setting cut-off values which minimize the number of false negatives or false positives for a particular test. Cut-off values are determined using the concepts of sensitivity, specificity and predictive value, based on distribution of test results from healthy animals, animals with the disease of interest, and, in certain situations, a third group with a different disease which gives a test result different to a healthy animal.

For example, if one uses the urine cortisol:creatinine ratio for the diagnosis of hyperadrenocorticism and sets a *low* cut-off value, the test will have close to 100% diagnostic sensitivity (there will be very few false negative results) but a low specificity with many false positive results. This can be interpreted clinically to mean that if the test result is negative then it is highly likely to be a true negative and the animal does not have the disease. However, there are many false positive results and these animals would have to have another diagnostic test, such as an ACTH stimulation test, to confirm the presence of disease. If a *high* cut-off value is set, the specificity will be increased to close to 100% with very few false positive results but sensitivity will decrease and more false negatives will be generated.

In cases where tests are affected by more than one disease, setting cut-off limits becomes difficult. For example, many enzymes produced by the pancreas are handled by the kidney for inactivation and excretion. In this instance, to obtain high specificity for diagnosis of pancreatitis in an animal with renal compromise, a very high cut-off limit for the pancreatic enzyme tests would have to be set, and false negatives would be likely. In general, cut-off limits are set at levels that produce the highest diagnostic efficiency for a particular disease.

Receiver-operating characteristic curve analysis: This can be used to show graphically the ability of a test to discriminate between disease and non-disease, or to compare the efficiency of two tests in the diagnosis of a disease. To form a receiver-operating characteristic (ROC) curve, sensitivity (true positive rate) is plotted against 1–specificity (false positive rate). Different cut-off values can then be applied to generate the best values for decisions about diagnosis (Dawson-Saunders and Trapp, 2000). A perfect diagnostic test would have 100% sensitivity and 100% specificity and be close to the top left corner of the graph. A diagonal (lower left corner to upper right corner) would indicate a useless test. The point on the curve which is closest to the upper left corner is the cut-off value or decision limit that provides the greatest diagnostic accuracy (efficiency of the test) (Figure 2.10). The area under the curve describes the accuracy of the test; therefore, the greater this area, the more accurate is the test in diagnosing the disease in question.

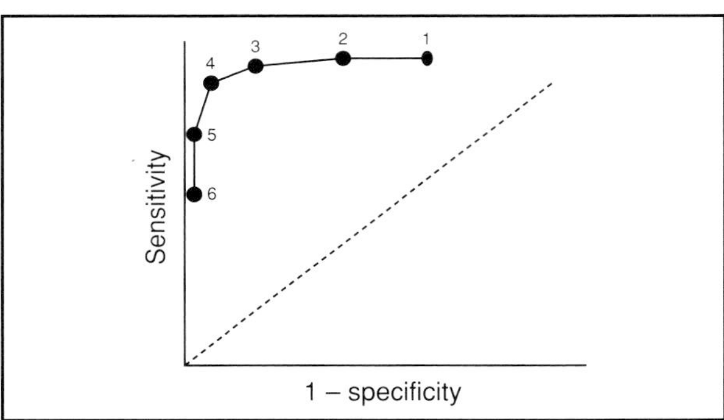

2.10 The receiver-operating characteristic (ROC) curve is a graphic way of plotting diagnostic sensitivity and specificity for a test at varying selected cut-off values, in this example numbered 1–6. Cut-off level 1 is the lowest cut-off plotted and gives a high sensitivity but low specificity. Cut-off level 6 is the highest cut-off plotted. The specificity is much higher (close to Y axis) but the sensitivity is lower. Cut-off level 4 has the best compromise of sensitivity and specificity, lying closest to the top left corner of the graph. A good test has values close to the upper left corner of the graph. Test results around the diagonal dotted line would indicate a useless test.

Likelihood ratios: These, with pre-test probability of the disease, can provide post-test information about the disease (Cockroft and Holmes, 2003):

- The likelihood ratio (LR) for a positive test result measures how many times more likely it is to obtain a positive test result from an animal that has the disease than from an animal who does not have the disease
- The LR for a negative test result measures how many times more likely it is to obtain a negative result from an animal who does not have the disease than from an animal who has the disease.

An evidence-based medicine approach to the interpretation of the results of diagnostic tests utilizing practice records and meta analysis (comparison of studies, methods and results by sophisticated statistics) can be found in Cockroft and Holmes (2003).

Biological variation

It is presumed that in health there is a homeostatic environment for most analytes, with analyte levels fluctuating around a fixed homeostatic set point and that in disease this fluctuation will be greater. This leads to biological variation within an animal and between animals at any particular time point. In humans it has been shown that within- or between-individual variation is largely of the same magnitude in healthy people and in people with chronic stable disease conditions. It is also assumed that this is largely independent of analytical method used to measure any analyte, and is not affected by the number of individuals in a population or regional, country or race differences. Making these assumptions, if there is a difference between two consecutive measurements in an individual this may be due to:

- Pre-analytical variation
- Analytical variation
- Biological variation
- The patient becoming diseased
- The patient recovering from the disease.

The coefficients of variation (CVs) for commonly used analytes in dogs are shown in Figure 2.11. The low CVs for electrolyte and protein levels reflect the narrow regulation of these parameters in the body and the high precision of analytical tests for these parameters. Conversely, urea and creatinine have much higher CVs. Urea is affected by diet and creatinine is affected by muscle mass and exercise and their levels are not so closely controlled in the body. Hormones have greater variability due to circadian rhythms and the test methods are not as accurate and precise as in other biochemical tests.

Knowledge of the variation in CVs for different analytes is important when monitoring specific parameters. For example, in a dog with hypoadrenocorticism an increase in potassium of > 3.3% (approximately 0.25–0.30 mmol/l) would reflect a 'real' increase and not be attributable to intrapatient biological variation or assay variation. However, a similar small increase in urea may simply reflect biological or assay variation, which could account for variations of up to 19% within one animal.

Analyte	Coefficient of variation (%)		
	Between dogs	***Within a dog***	***Analytical variation***
Red blood cell count	4.4	5.4	2.8
Haematocrit	5.2	6.4	1.1
White blood cell count	12.3	12.1	3.7
Sodium	3.5	3.2	0.1
Potassium	3.6	3.3	0.1
Urea	35.1	16.1	3.8
Creatinine	12.9	14.6	2.9
Total protein	3.1	2.6	1.1
Albumin	3.0	2.4	1.6
ALT	23.7	9.7	3.2
ALP	34.2	8.6	1.7
Total T4	17.2	17.0	4.0
Free T4	24.3	20.2	6.7
Thyroid stimulating hormone	43.6	13.6	8.8

2.11 Biological variation in dogs for selected diagnostic tests. Analytical variation is the variation in results produced by an analyser when a single sample is run repeatedly.

Biological variability, analytical variation and test error

There are statistical methods for incorporating biological variation into test analysis, using the method of nested analysis of variance which will provide a CV of intra-animal and between-animal variability. This biological variability, expressed as the coefficient of variation, can be factored into the maximal allowable imprecision of a test. Analytical variation alone usually contributes around 10% of test result variation, and can also be factored into the maximum allowable bias of an assay and hence into the maximum total allowable error of a test before the result is rejected in a QC programme (Fraser *et al.*, 1997). These methods are not widely used in veterinary medicine but they help to explain the critical difference between an animal's results and those of the population of healthy animals when the animal is assumed healthy or should not have an expected change in a particular test result.

Rational laboratory data interpretation

This is an art, based on experience and knowledge of physiology and pathology of disease processes, as well as an understanding of error factors that can occur at any stage of test result production. Laboratory test results are only a small part of the database on which a clinical diagnosis is made and so should be interpreted in conjunction with as much other information about the patient as possible. When an abnormal test result is obtained it is good practice to consider it in relation to:

- The history and clinical examination, and differential diagnoses previously formulated
- The magnitude of the abnormality: is it close to the provided reference values, in a grey zone or is it markedly lower or higher than this?
- Could the result be related to pre-analytical error, such as inadequate fasting, immediate postprandial sampling, effects of exercise?
- Is the sample of poor quality, e.g. errors due to ageing, haemolysis, lipaema or icterus, microclot formation? (Many of these factors will be reported upon by a good laboratory)
- Could an abnormal result be due to a particular breed-specific effect? For example, hyperkalaemia may occur in samples from Akitas due to *in vitro* haemolysis and the high potassium content of their red cells
- Is it an isolated abnormal result and related to probability (as discussed above, in a panel of 20 tests there is a 64% chance of one result being abnormal)? In that case it may be wise to repeat the test with a fresh sample before any further decision is made
- Is the result in an 'inconclusive range' when clinical cut-off limits are provided by the reporting laboratory? For example, an inconclusive post-ACTH stimulation test cortisol level in an animal with suspected hyperadrenocorticism. In this case an alternative test could be chosen, e.g. a low-dose dexamethasone suppression test
- Is the unexpected result due to the effects of intercurrent illness? Examples would be a T4 level within the reference interval for a cat with a high index of suspicion for hyperthyroidism but which also has intercurrent disease, or a low T4 level in a dog with normal thyroid function affected by other disease
- Is the unexpected result due to current drug therapy? Glucocorticoid therapy, in particular, can interfere physiologically with many tests. In dogs, glucocorticoids can induce the steroid isoenzyme thus increasing the total alkaline phosphatase levels and also affect plasma glucose levels and urine specific gravity. Glucocorticoids increase lipase levels and, depending on duration of therapy, they can also affect many tests that measure liver parameters. They can also profoundly affect the complete blood count (CBC), again depending on duration and dose level, and several specific tests, such as T4 levels. Many anticonvulsants can affect liver enzyme levels through induction. Bromide compounds can directly affect analytical tests for chloride and cholesterol through interference.

Because of the rapidity of sample analysis by automated methods and the economic advantage of requesting many tests at one time it is common practice to obtain a database including CBC, biochemistry profile or organ-specific profile and urinalysis. This is frequently described as a minimum database. For initial evaluation this can be helpful and all the components of the laboratory data should be analysed and interpreted in relation to each other. This can assist formulation or re-ranking of differential diagnoses. It can also prompt further more specific tests targeted to a particular organ or disease process. For monitoring of progress a more limited selection of specific tests is usually adequate. The results of these can be evaluated in conjunction with prior test results for the same analytes.

References and further reading

Bellamy JEC and Olexson DW (2000) *Quality Assurance Handbook for Veterinary Laboratories.* Iowa State University Press, Ames

Cockcroft PD and Holmes MA (2003) Appraising the evidence. In: *Handbook of Evidence-Based Veterinary Medicine,* pp.84–106. Blackwell Publishing, Oxford

Cornbleet J (1983) Spurious results from automated hematology cell counters. *Laboratory Medicine* **14,** 509–514

Dawson-Saunders B and Trapp RG (2000) Evaluating diagnostic procedures. In: *Basic and Clinical Biostatistics, 2nd edn,* pp. 232–247. Appleton and Lange, Norwalk

Dixon WJ (1953) Processing data for outliers. *Biometrics* **9,** 74–89

Fraser CG, Hyltoft-Petersen P, Luibeer JC and Ricos C (1997) Proposal for setting generally applicable quality goals based solely on biology. *Annals of Clinical Biochemistry* **34,** 8–12

Holes EW, Kahn SE, Molnar PA and Bermes WE (1994) Verification of reference ranges by using a Monte Carlo sampling technique. *Clinical Chemistry* **40,** 2216–2222

Kouri T, Kairisto V and Virtanen A (1994) Reference intervals developed from data from hospitalized patients: computerized methods based upon combination of laboratory and diagnostic data. *Clinical Chemistry* **40,** 2209–2215

National Committee for Clinical Laboratory Standards (1995) How to define and determine reference intervals in the clinical laboratory. Approved guidelines NCCLS document C28-A. NCCLS, Villanova

Smith RD and Snelling BD (2000) Decision analysis: dealing with uncertainty in diagnostic testing. *Preventative Veterinary Medicine* **45,** 139–162

Solberg HE (1987) Establishment and use of reference intervals. In: *Fundamentals of Clinical Chemistry, 3rd edn,* ed. NW Tietz, pp.197–212. WB Saunders, Philadelphia

Westgard JO (2001) Six Sigma Quality Design and Control. Westgard QC, Madison

3

Introduction to haematology

Elizabeth Villiers

Introduction

The complete blood count (CBC) is an integral part of the diagnostic investigation of any systemic disease process. It consists of two components:

- **Quantitative examination** of the cells, including: packed cell volume (PCV), total red blood cell count (RBC), haemoglobin (Hb) concentration; total white blood cell count (WBC), differential WBC count, and platelet count. In addition, the red cell mean corpuscular volume (MCV), mean corpuscular haemoglobin (MCH) and mean corpuscular haemoglobin concentration (MCHC) are evaluated and total plasma protein is measured
- **Qualitative examination** of blood smears for changes in cellular morphology.

It cannot be over-emphasized that **both** these elements should always be performed.

Blood sampling

Jugular, rather than peripheral, vein venipuncture is recommended in order to minimize the potential for cell damage during blood sampling; 21 gauge needles are usually used in dogs, whilst 23 gauge needles are generally preferred in cats. However, smaller needles are more likely to cause cell damage and subsequent haemolysis. The phlebotomist should try to ensure a slick venipuncture technique, with minimal movement of the needle in and out of the vein, and should avoid excessive suction on the syringe during sampling. After the sample has been obtained, the needle is removed from the syringe and the sample is gently expressed into the appropriate anticoagulant tube. Ethylenediamine tetra-acetic acid (EDTA) is generally the anticoagulant of choice for haematology because cells are well preserved and smears stain well. However, in cats EDTA may, on occasion, induce platelet clumping, resulting in falsely low automated platelet counts. Sodium citrate can be used as an alternative in this situation and this anticoagulant is also used in coagulation tests. Heparin is unsuitable for haematology since it results in poor leucocyte staining on blood films.

The EDTA tube should be filled precisely to the level indicated. Underfilling, resulting in EDTA excess, may artefactually reduce red cell size and alter cell morphology. If liquid anticoagulant is being used, underfilling may also result in significant sample dilution. Overfilling may lead to clot formation.

The sample should be mixed carefully by gently inverting it several times to ensure adequate distribution of the anticoagulant. The tube should not be shaken since this may cause haemolysis.

Blood smears should be made soon after obtaining the blood sample or cellular degeneration will impede interpretation. Cell morphology begins to deteriorate within 12 hours, so if blood is being mailed to an external laboratory, a blood smear should be made at the time of sampling (see below) and mailed along with the EDTA sample. The EDTA sample should be kept in the fridge until it is put in the post.

Haemolysis

Damage to the cells during or after sampling may lead to haemolysis (Figure 3.1). This results in a falsely low RBC and PCV, and a falsely high MCHC. Plasma protein measured using a refractometer is also falsely elevated. Causes of haemolysis include:

- Narrow gauge needle
- Excessive suction on the syringe
- Excessive agitation of the blood in the tube
- Prolonged storage
- Storage at high temperatures.

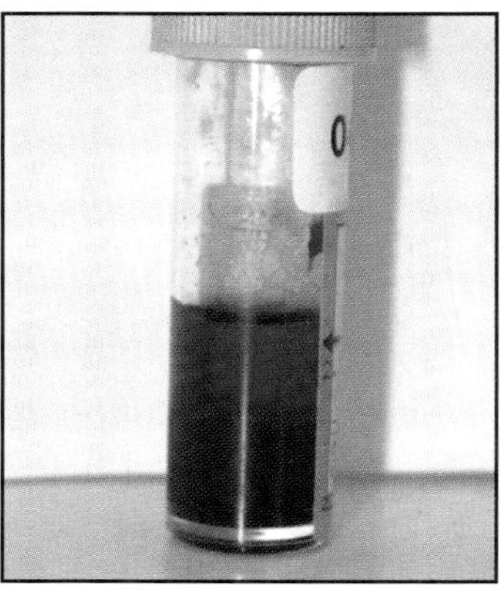

3.1 Haemolysed blood: the plasma is red.

Basic quantification techniques

Packed cell volume

The PCV accurately reflects the red cell count as long as the mean volume of the red cells (MCV) is within reference limits. PCV is readily measured using a microhaematocrit centrifuge. Blood in an EDTA tube should be well mixed and a microcapillary tube filled to about 65–75% by placing the haematocrit tube into the EDTA tube and tilting the latter. The base of the microhaematocrit tube is plugged with clay and it is then centrifuged for 5 minutes at high speed (12,500–15,000 rpm). The red cells are packed at the bottom of the tube above the clay plug. The white cells form the buffy coat, which sits on top of the red cells and is seen as a grey/cream layer. The platelets lie at the top of the buffy coat and may be discernible as a thin, cream-coloured layer adjacent to the slightly greyer buffy coat. The plasma is found above the platelet layer (Figure 3.2).

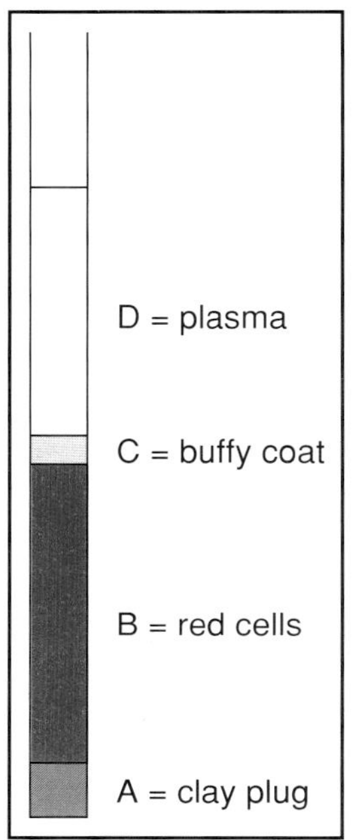

3.2 Diagrammatic representation of a microhaematocrit tube following centrifugation. The PCV is calculated by dividing the length of the packed red cells (*B*) by the total length of the packed red cells, buffy coat and plasma (*B* + *C* + *D*). A sliding measuring device (haematocrit reader) can be used.

In addition to the PCV, examination of the microhaematocrit tube provides other useful information. Gross examination of the plasma detects **icterus**, **haemolysis** or **lipaemia**. A very broad estimate of the white cell count can be made by calculating the percentage of the tube occupied by the buffy coat:

$$\% \text{ tube occupied by buffy coat} = \frac{C}{B + C + D}$$

where B = width of red cells, C = width of buffy coat and D = width of plasma.

The first 1% equates to approximately 10 x 10^9/l; and each percent thereafter equates to approximately 20 x 10^9/l.

Plasma protein

This can be measured using a refractometer (Figure 3.3). The microhaematocrit tube is scored and broken above the buffy coat. A drop of the plasma is expressed on to the prism and the protein value read from the scale. Most refractometers have an internal scale for plasma protein and urine specific gravity. If the scale is graduated only for refractive index a conversion chart is necessary. Plasma protein may also be measured using a biochemical analyser. Note that haemolysis, lipaemia and marked icterus falsely elevate plasma protein.

Interpretation of PCV and plasma protein

Plasma protein and PCV should be interpreted together. In an anaemia caused by reduced production of red cells, the number of red cells falls whilst the volume of plasma present is unchanged and so the PCV is low. In contrast, acute haemorrhage results in loss of both red cells and plasma and so initially the PCV does not fall. Following the shift of interstitial fluid into the circulation, plasma volume expands and the PCV falls, reaching its nadir by 24 hours after the haemorrhage.

- **Low PCV and low plasma protein**: recent or ongoing external haemorrhage. Plasma protein is being lost from the body along with red cells. Internal haemorrhage may initially cause only a mild reduction in plasma proteins, and then proteins are rapidly reabsorbed.
- **Low plasma protein with normal PCV** usually indicates hypoproteinaemia (usually hypoalbuminaemia) due to causes other than haemorrhage. These include failure of production (e.g. chronic liver disease) or protein loss (e.g. glomerulonephropathy).
- **High PCV with high plasma protein** is seen with dehydration. Water lost from the body results in increased concentration of both red cells and protein. However, these parameters provide only a crude estimate of an animal's hydration status.

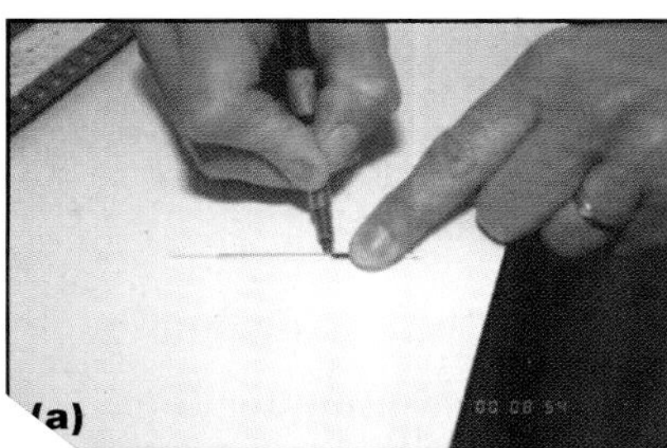

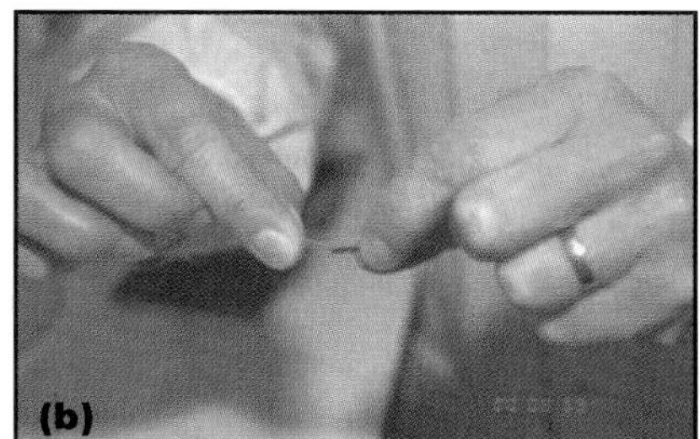

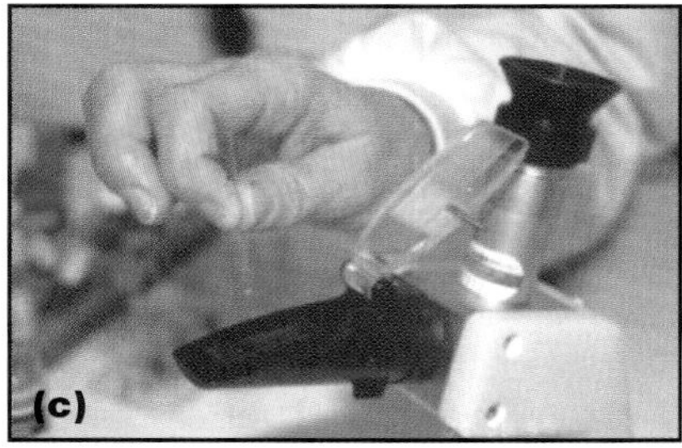

Measuring plasma protein using a refractometer. (a) The microhaematocrit tube is scored just above the buffy coat, using a diamond writer or razor blade. (b) The tube is broken at the scored line. (c) The plasma is expelled on to the refractometer prism by swiftly flicking the tube downwards towards the prism, taking care not to [illegible] with the tube. The prism cover is then replaced and the plasma protein read from the internal scale.

3

Introduction to haematology

Elizabeth Villiers

Introduction

The complete blood count (CBC) is an integral part of the diagnostic investigation of any systemic disease process. It consists of two components:

- **Quantitative examination** of the cells, including: packed cell volume (PCV), total red blood cell count (RBC), haemoglobin (Hb) concentration; total white blood cell count (WBC), differential WBC count, and platelet count. In addition, the red cell mean corpuscular volume (MCV), mean corpuscular haemoglobin (MCH) and mean corpuscular haemoglobin concentration (MCHC) are evaluated and total plasma protein is measured
- **Qualitative examination** of blood smears for changes in cellular morphology.

It cannot be over-emphasized that **both** these elements should always be performed.

Blood sampling

Jugular, rather than peripheral, vein venipuncture is recommended in order to minimize the potential for cell damage during blood sampling; 21 gauge needles are usually used in dogs, whilst 23 gauge needles are generally preferred in cats. However, smaller needles are more likely to cause cell damage and subsequent haemolysis. The phlebotomist should try to ensure a slick venipuncture technique, with minimal movement of the needle in and out of the vein, and should avoid excessive suction on the syringe during sampling. After the sample has been obtained, the needle is removed from the syringe and the sample is gently expressed into the appropriate anticoagulant tube. Ethylenediamine tetra-acetic acid (EDTA) is generally the anticoagulant of choice for haematology because cells are well preserved and smears stain well. However, in cats EDTA may, on occasion, induce platelet clumping, resulting in falsely low automated platelet counts. Sodium citrate can be used as an alternative in this situation and this anticoagulant is also used in coagulation tests. Heparin is unsuitable for haematology since it results in poor leucocyte staining on blood films.

The EDTA tube should be filled precisely to the level indicated. Underfilling, resulting in EDTA excess, may artefactually reduce red cell size and alter cell morphology. If liquid anticoagulant is being used, underfilling may also result in significant sample dilution. Overfilling may lead to clot formation.

The sample should be mixed carefully by gently inverting it several times to ensure adequate distribution of the anticoagulant. The tube should not be shaken since this may cause haemolysis.

Blood smears should be made soon after obtaining the blood sample or cellular degeneration will impede interpretation. Cell morphology begins to deteriorate within 12 hours, so if blood is being mailed to an external laboratory, a blood smear should be made at the time of sampling (see below) and mailed along with the EDTA sample. The EDTA sample should be kept in the fridge until it is put in the post.

Haemolysis

Damage to the cells during or after sampling may lead to haemolysis (Figure 3.1). This results in a falsely low RBC and PCV, and a falsely high MCHC. Plasma protein measured using a refractometer is also falsely elevated. Causes of haemolysis include:

- Narrow gauge needle
- Excessive suction on the syringe
- Excessive agitation of the blood in the tube
- Prolonged storage
- Storage at high temperatures.

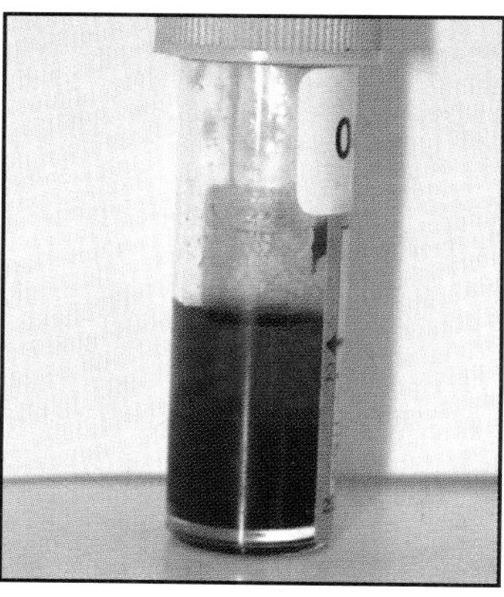

3.1 Haemolysed blood: the plasma is red.

Basic quantification techniques

Packed cell volume

The PCV accurately reflects the red cell count as long as the mean volume of the red cells (MCV) is within reference limits. PCV is readily measured using a microhaematocrit centrifuge. Blood in an EDTA tube should be well mixed and a microcapillary tube filled to about 65–75% by placing the haematocrit tube into the EDTA tube and tilting the latter. The base of the microhaematocrit tube is plugged with clay and it is then centrifuged for 5 minutes at high speed (12,500–15,000 rpm). The red cells are packed at the bottom of the tube above the clay plug. The white cells form the buffy coat, which sits on top of the red cells and is seen as a grey/cream layer. The platelets lie at the top of the buffy coat and may be discernible as a thin, cream-coloured layer adjacent to the slightly greyer buffy coat. The plasma is found above the platelet layer (Figure 3.2).

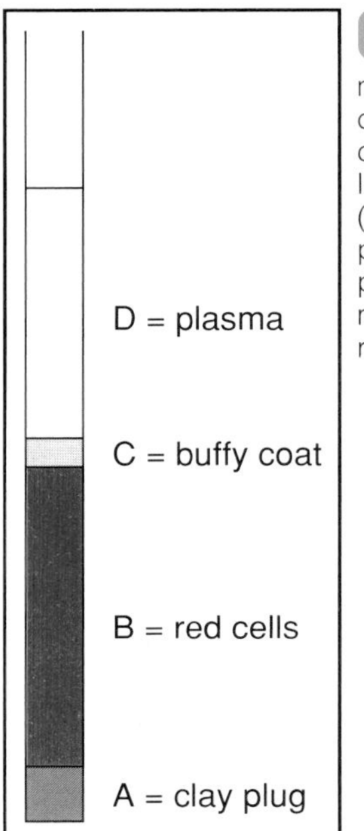

3.2 Diagrammatic representation of a microhaematocrit tube following centrifugation. The PCV is calculated by dividing the length of the packed red cells (*B*) by the total length of the packed red cells, buffy coat and plasma (*B* + *C* + *D*). A sliding measuring device (haematocrit reader) can be used.

In addition to the PCV, examination of the microhaematocrit tube provides other useful information. Gross examination of the plasma detects **icterus**, **haemolysis** or **lipaemia**. A very broad estimate of the white cell count can be made by calculating the percentage of the tube occupied by the buffy coat:

$$\%\text{ tube occupied by buffy coat} = \frac{C}{B + C + D}$$

where B = width of red cells, C = width of buffy coat and D = width of plasma.

The first 1% equates to approximately 10 x 10^9/l; and each percent thereafter equates to approximately 20 x 10^9/l.

Plasma protein

This can be measured using a refractometer (Figure 3.3). The microhaematocrit tube is scored and broken above the buffy coat. A drop of the plasma is expressed on to the prism and the protein value read from the scale. Most refractometers have an internal scale for plasma protein and urine specific gravity. If the scale is graduated only for refractive index a conversion chart is necessary. Plasma protein may also be measured using a biochemical analyser. Note that haemolysis, lipaemia and marked icterus falsely elevate plasma protein.

Interpretation of PCV and plasma protein

Plasma protein and PCV should be interpreted together. In an anaemia caused by reduced production of red cells, the number of red cells falls whilst the volume of plasma present is unchanged and so the PCV is low. In contrast, acute haemorrhage results in loss of both red cells and plasma and so initially the PCV does not fall. Following the shift of interstitial fluid into the circulation, plasma volume expands and the PCV falls, reaching its nadir by 24 hours after the haemorrhage.

- **Low PCV and low plasma protein**: recent or ongoing external haemorrhage. Plasma protein is being lost from the body along with red cells. Internal haemorrhage may initially cause only a mild reduction in plasma proteins, and then proteins are rapidly reabsorbed.
- **Low plasma protein with normal PCV** usually indicates hypoproteinaemia (usually hypoalbuminaemia) due to causes other than haemorrhage. These include failure of production (e.g. chronic liver disease) or protein loss (e.g. glomerulonephropathy).
- **High PCV with high plasma protein** is seen with dehydration. Water lost from the body results in increased concentration of both red cells and protein. However, these parameters provide only a crude estimate of an animal's hydration status.

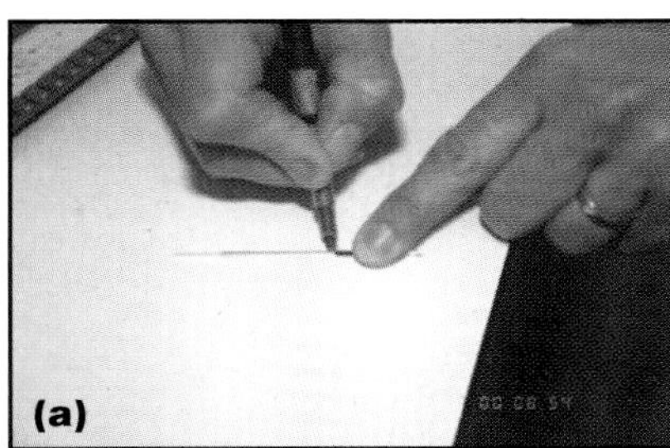

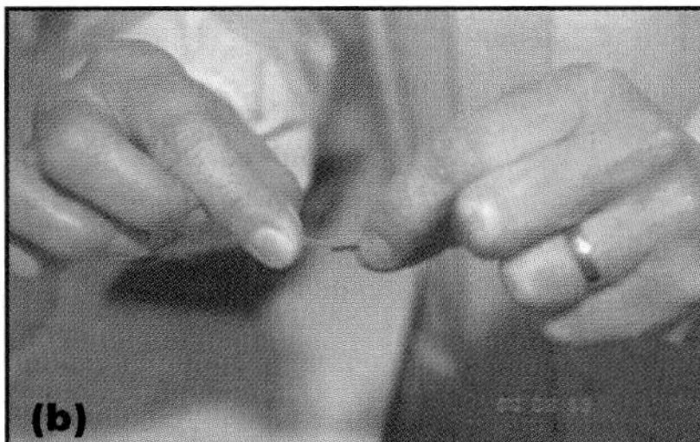

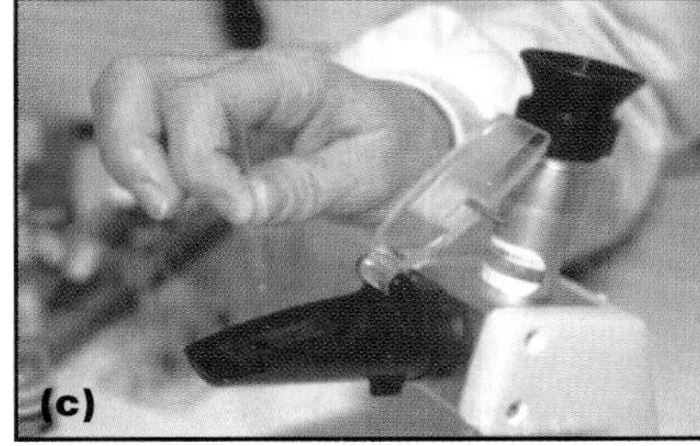

3.3 Measuring plasma protein using a refractometer. (a) The microhaematocrit tube is scored just above the buffy coat, using a diamond writer or razor blade. (b) The tube is broken at the scored line. (c) The plasma is expelled from the tube on to the refractometer prism by swiftly flicking the tube downwards towards the prism, taking care not to touch the prism with the tube. The prism cover is then replaced and the plasma protein read from the internal scale.

- **High plasma protein with normal or low PCV** is usually due to hyperglobulinaemia. Marked hyperglobulinaemia is seen with myeloma and some B cell lymphomas, as well as some infectious diseases, such as ehrlichiosis. Evaluation of albumin and globulin, and protein electrophoresis are indicated to investigate persistently low or high plasma protein values (see Chapter 7).

Automated cell counts

Prior to using any analyser the blood should be thoroughly mixed and checked for clots. This is best achieved by using a small wooden stick (an 'orange stick'). This is wiped around the inside of the tube and then removed and examined. Any clots in the sample should be scooped up by the stick (Figure 3.4). Samples containing clots should be discarded since they will have falsely low platelet and leucocyte counts and red cell counts may be increased or decreased.

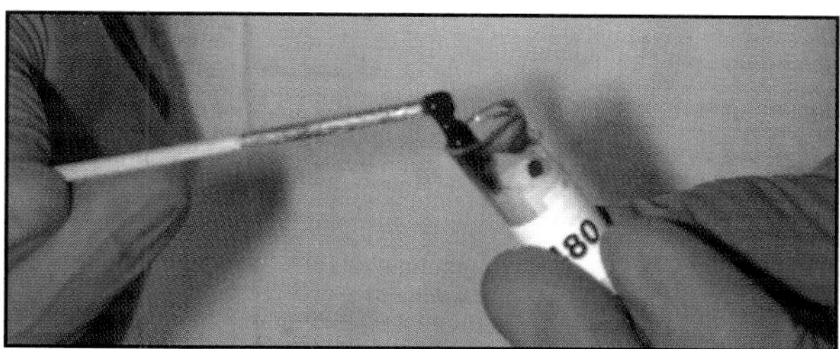

3.4 A blood clot in an EDTA sample is detected by wiping a wooden stick around the inner surface of the tube. Clotted samples should be discarded.

Manual haemocytometer techniques are rarely used nowadays and have been superseded by a choice of several in-house haematology analysers or large flow cytometry analysers in commercial laboratories. Impedance cell counters and quantitative buffy coat (QBC) analysers are the main types of haematology analysers available for practice use; a flow cytometer has also recently become available.

Impedance cell counters

In these analysers a chamber containing an electrically conductive fluid is divided into two areas connected by a small aperture. An electric current is passed into this fluid and flows through the aperture. A stream of cells is directed towards the aperture; as cells pass through they interfere with the flow of current, creating a pulse (Figure 3.5). The pulse height is proportional to cell size; pulse frequency is proportional to cell number. The RBC, MCV and platelet count are determined in diluted blood, platelets being distinguished from red cells by their smaller size. Haemoglobin (Hb) is measured spectrophotometrically after red cell lysis. Thus, for red cells the analyser measures RBC, MCV and Hb. It then calculates the haematocrit (HCT), mean corpuscular haemoglobin (MCH), and mean corpuscular haemoglobin concentration (MCHC) using the formulae shown in Figure 3.6.

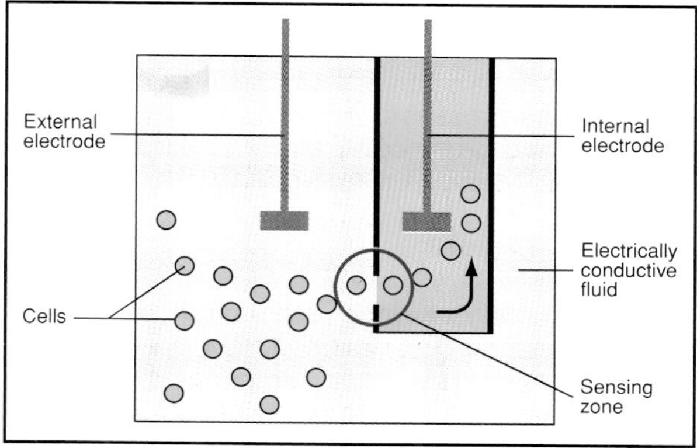

3.5 Diagrammatic representation of an impedance counting chamber. Cells within an electrically conducting fluid are passed through an aperture; in so doing they impede the flow of electricity through the aperture, creating a pulse.

$$\text{HCT (l/l)} = \frac{\text{MCV (fl)} \times \text{RBC } (\times 10^{12}/\text{l})}{1000}$$

$$\text{MCHC (g/dl)} = \frac{\text{Hb (g/dl)}}{\text{HCT (l/l)}}$$

$$\text{MCH (pg)} = \frac{\text{Hb (g/dl)} \times 10}{\text{RBC } (\times 10^{12}/\text{l})}$$

3.6 Calculation of red cell parameters.

Since the distinction between platelets and red cells is made on the basis of cell size, errors may occur when large platelets (macroplatelets or 'shift' platelets) are miscounted as small red cells or *vice versa*. This is more common in cats, since they have smaller red cells and often have variably sized platelets. If very large numbers of macroplatelets are present this may falsely increase the RBC and HCT and lower the MCV and platelet count (Figure 3.7). Conversely, if microcytic red cells are present, they may be miscounted as platelets, resulting in a falsely high platelet count.

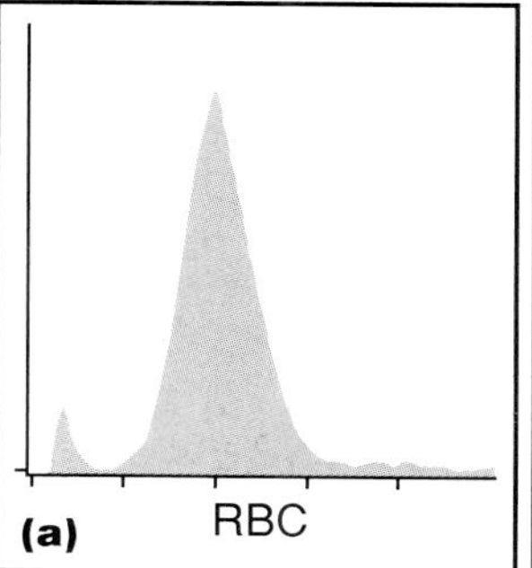

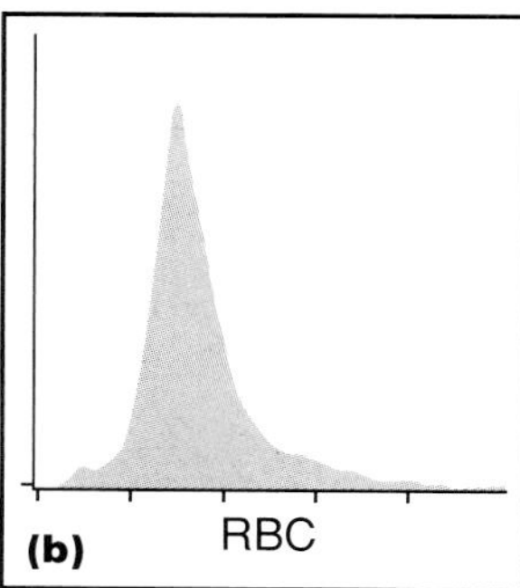

3.7 Histogram plots produced by the Cell-Dyn 3500 showing separation of platelets and red cells based on size. Plot (a) from a dog, shows good separation with a well defined peak of platelets to the left and red cells to the right. However on plot (b), from a cat, the two peaks are not well defined. The analyser gave a platelet count of 1481 x 10^9/l. Inspection of the blood film suggested the count was much lower than this, with approximately 34 platelets per high power field, equivalent to a count of 510 x 10^9/l. The MCV was low and some of the microcytic red cells were being counted as platelets.

Leucocytes are counted after lysing red blood cells. In some analysers cell-specific lysing solutions are used to produce a differential white cell count. In others the lysing agent results in shrinkage of the lymphocyte, monocyte and granulocyte nuclei at different rates, facilitating a three-part differential count.

Flow cytometers

Large commercial laboratory analysers, such as the Bayer H1 (formerly known as Technicon H1) and the Cell-Dyn 3500 analyser, are essentially flow cytometers. An in-house analyser (Lasercyte, Idexx) has also recently become available. A stream of cells is directed through a laser beam and, as cells pass through the beam, they scatter light at different angles. The amount of low angle or forward scatter correlates with cell size and the amount of high angle or side scatter correlates with cell granularity or density. The H1 uses this technology to count red cells and platelets as well as white cells. Since red cells are packed with haemoglobin they are much denser than platelets and so there is better separation of these two cell types than when using impedance analysers. For counting leucocytes the H1 combines flow cytometry and cytochemistry: leucocytes are distinguished on the basis of their size, granularity, peroxidase activity and also their susceptibility to lysing reagents. The plots produced by these analysers are very useful for identifying abnormal cells populations, left shifts and regenerative anaemias (Figure 3.8). The Cell-Dyn differs in that it uses impedance technology to count red cells and platelets and flow cytometry to count white cells.

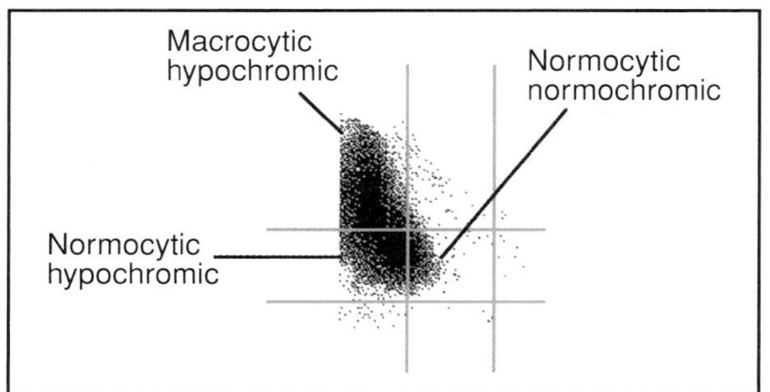

3.8 Scatter plot of red cells using the Bayer H1 haematology analyser. The grid shows red cell size on the *y* axis and haemoglobin content on the *x* axis. Normocytic normochromic red cells fall into the central box. In a regenerative anaemia, the macrocytic hypochromic cells fall into the upper left box and so the plot is shifted up and to the left. (Courtesy of Heather Holloway, Idexx Laboratories, Wetherby, UK.)

Quantitative buffy coat analysers

QBC machines rely on separation of red cells, granulocytes, monocytes/lymphocytes and platelets into various layers in a microhaematocrit tube containing the vital stain, acridine orange, which is taken up by DNA, RNA and lipoprotein in the cells. The tube contains a cylindrical float that forces the cells to spread out in a thin layer between the float and the tube. After centrifugation ultraviolet light is directed at the stained cells which then emit fluorescent light. Nucleated cells, which contain DNA, emit green fluorescence, whilst cells containing lipoprotein or RNA emit red light.

Reticulocytes can be distinguished from mature red cells because they have more RNA. Eosinophils can be distinguished from neutrophils because they have more lipoprotein. Platelets are rich in lipoprotein and so emit red light. The amount of red or green light emitted is proportional to the number of cells present in the space between the float and the tube, which, in turn, is dependent on cell size. Hence a cell layer consisting of smaller cells (e.g. lymphocytes) will emit relatively more light that a layer of larger cells (e.g. neutrophils), as shown in Figure 3.9. The QBC analyser thus calcu-

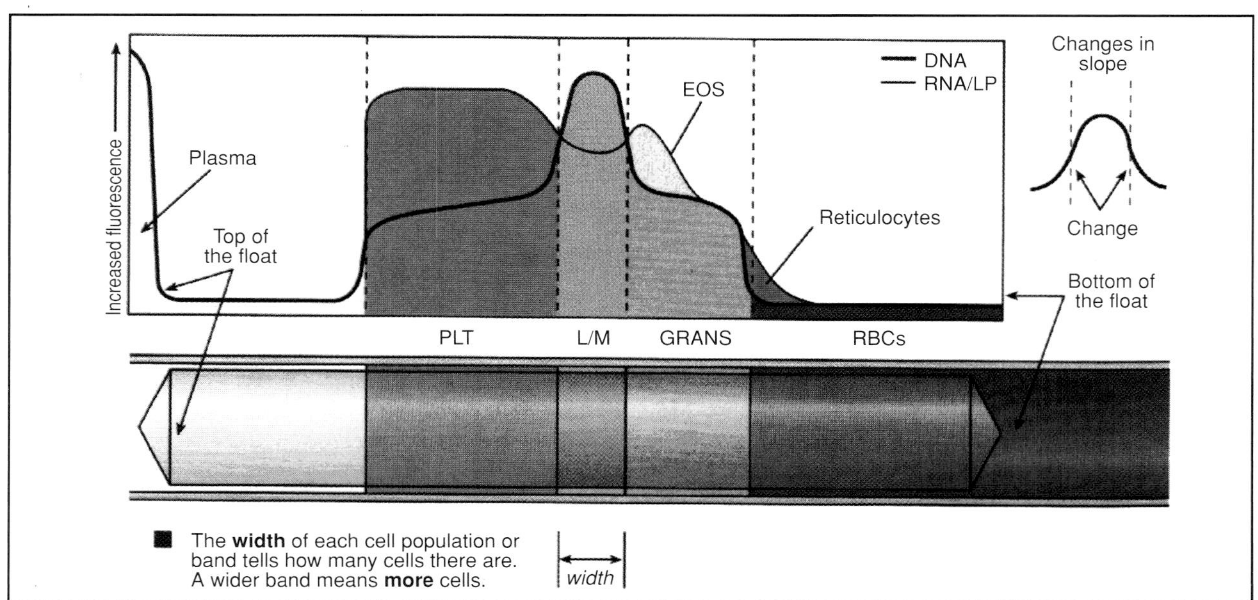

3.9 Diagrammatic representation of the buffy coat, expanded by a cylindrical float, and a histogram showing the amount of fluorescence emitted by DNA (in nucleated cells) and RNA/lipoprotein (in reticulocytes, platelets (PLT) and eosinophils (EOS)) in the various layers of the buffy coat. (Courtesy of Idexx laboratories, Wetherby, UK.) GRANS = granulocytes; L/M = lymphocytes and monocytes.

lates the PCV, WBC, neutrophil, eosinophil, mononuclear cell (lymphocytes and monocytes) and platelet counts from the width of the various bands of fluorescence. The MCHC can be calculated because it is inversely correlated with the distance the float has sunk into the packed red cell layer. Hb is calculated from the PCV and MCHC: Hb (g/dl) = MCHC x PCV% /100. All calculated cell counts are based on the assumption that cell volumes are normal, so, in disease states where cell volumes are altered (e.g. in leukaemia), inaccuracies may occur.

Red blood cell parameters

HCT, RBC and Hb all give an indication of the red cell mass. As discussed above, HCT is a calculated value produced by the analyser and is usually expressed as l/l. It is equivalent to the PCV, which is usually expressed as a percentage, i.e. a HCT of 0.25 l/l is the same as a PCV of 25%. All three parameters rise in dehydrated animals and fall in anaemic animals. In microcytic anaemia the reduction in HCT is more marked than that in RBC because the former is reduced further by the small cell size. Haemolysis falsely lowers the RBC and HCT but Hb will not be affected since the already 'free' haemoglobin from the previously lysed cells will be measured along with Hb released from cells lysed in the analyser. Since mean cell haemoglobin concentration (MCHC) is calculated by dividing Hb by PCV, this parameter is falsely elevated in haemolysis. Hb is falsely elevated in lipaemic samples.

Red cell indices

Mean corpuscular volume

MCV indicates the average size of the red cells. Increased MCV is seen in regenerative anaemia, along with decreased MCH and MCHC. Macrocytic anaemia may also be seen with a non-regenerative anaemia caused by myelodysplasia in cats, often in association with FeLV infection. Sample ageing (e.g. samples 2 or more days old) results in red cell swelling and increased MCV. Non-regenerative anaemia is usually normocytic. Low MCV is seen in iron deficiency. These are discussed in detail in Chapter 4.

Red cell distribution width

The red cell distribution width (RDW) describes the variability in red cell size. It is a more sensitive indicator of altered red cell size than the MCV, since, in the latter, a relatively large number of cells must have altered size before the *mean* value is altered. The RDW describes the entire population of red cells instead of one average value (Figure 3.10).

Mean corpuscular haemoglobin

MCH is expressed in picograms (pg) and indicates the mean quantity (weight) of haemoglobin per average red cell. It does not take into account the volume of the red cell since it is calculated by dividing the Hb by the RBC.

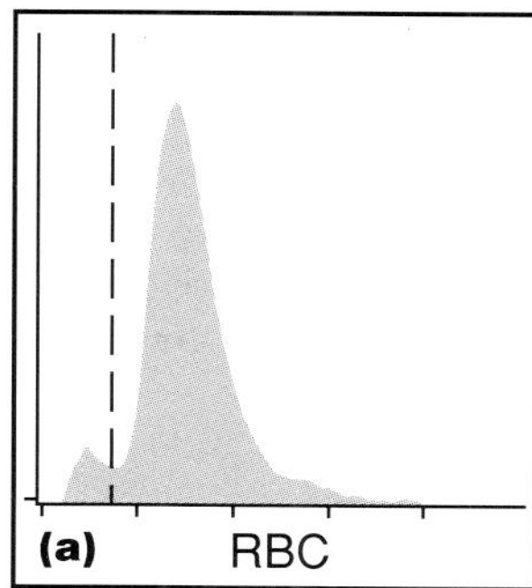

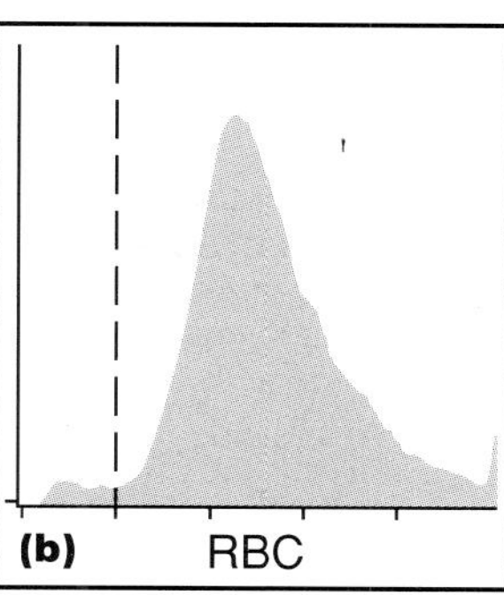

3.10 Using the Cell-Dyn the RDW is calculated from the frequency distribution plot of red cell size (size on *x* axis, frequency on *y* axis). RDW is the coefficient of variation of red cell size and is expressed as a percentage. (a) Healthy dog (RDW=15%). (b) A dog with a markedly regenerative anaemia (RDW=25%): the red cell curve is much wider and extends further to the right, reflecting the numerous larger red cells present.

Mean corpuscular haemoglobin concentration

MCHC indicates the mean concentration of haemoglobin per red cell. It is calculated by dividing the Hb by the HCT and, since the latter is affected by red cell size, MCHC is a more useful indicator of the amount of haemoglobin present in red cells. If a normal animal has an MCV towards the bottom of the normal range the MCH may be low, even though the cells contain a normal amount of haemoglobin relative to their size (smaller cells should have less total haemoglobin than big cells). The MCHC, which corrects for this variation in cell size, would be normal.

- Normal MCHC defines the red cells as normochromic and is seen in non-regenerative anaemia as well as in normal animals
- Decreased MCHC is synonymous with hypochromasia and is seen in regenerative anaemia and iron deficiency
- Raised MCHC is almost always due to haemolysis, and may be seen artefactually in lipaemic samples.

White cell counts

All haematology analysers can determine the total white cell count and this is usually expressed as cells x 10^9/l. Most modern impedance analysers give a three-part leucocyte differential count (granulocytes, monocytes and lymphocytes) and some give a five-part differential count. QBC machines count neutrophils, eosinophils and mononuclear cells, but cannot distinguish lymphocytes and monocytes (these are lumped together as mononuclear cells). High tech flow cytometry analysers give a full white cell differential count, i.e. the number and percentage of neutrophils, lymphocytes, eosinophils, monocytes and basophils are determined. The H1 analyser can also identify band neutrophils.

Whilst the total WBC is generally accurate, differential counts are not always accurate. Some analysers have problems identifying monocytes, eosinophils or basophils. Blast cells (e.g. in leukaemia) may be missed.

Except in the H1 analyser, band neutrophils are not distinguished from mature neutrophils. These factors highlight the importance of blood film examination.

Nucleated red cells (nRBCs) and even large platelets may be miscounted as leucocytes. Some analysers may identify nRBCs and correct the white cell count accordingly, others may have flags for these, which prompt the clinician to examine a blood film and then correct the reported WBC using the formula:

$$\text{Corrected WBC} = \frac{100}{100 + \text{Number of nRBCs per 100 WBCs}} \times \text{Automated white cell count}$$

Platelet counts

All analysers can perform a platelet count, although the accuracy of these counts is very variable depending on the analyser used. As discussed above, analyser error is more likely in cats because their small red cells can be falsely counted as platelets or large platelets can be miscounted as small red cells. Significant laboratory error can also occur if platelets form clumps *in vitro*: platelets in clumps are not counted by the analyser and so lead to a falsely low count. This is a common laboratory error and is more likely to occur if the blood sampling procedure does not go smoothly; in cats it can occur even following atraumatic venipuncture, possibly due to the effects of EDTA. Clumping may be reduced by sampling into sodium citrate tubes. Whenever a low platelet count is recorded by an analyser, a blood film should be examined: if platelet clumps are found at the tail of the smear (Figure 3.11) this is the likely cause of the apparent thrombocytopenia and a fresh blood sample is required to obtain an accurate platelet count.

Macroplatelets or shift platelets are often present if there is an accelerated rate of thrombopoiesis and may be miscounted as small red cells (see above).

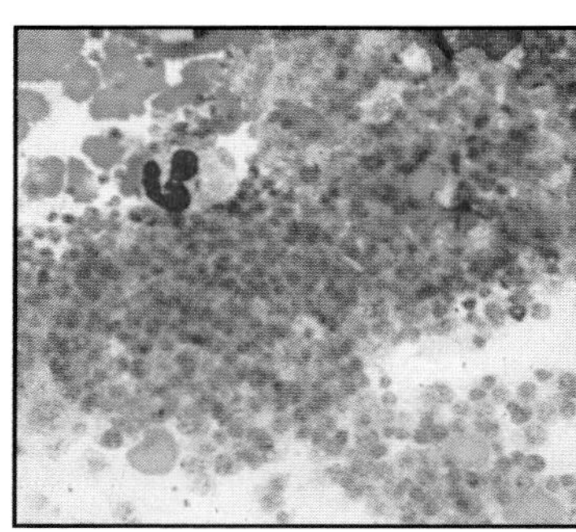

3.11 A platelet clump seen at the tail of a blood smear from a dog. Platelets are round with slightly grainy cytoplasm but no nucleus. (May–Grünwald–Giemsa stain; original magnification X1000.)

Blood films

A blood smear should always be evaluated in conjunction with automated cell counts. This is required:

- To check the leucocyte differential count
- To assess cell morphology, e.g. polychromasia, anisocytosis, fragmented red cells, spherocytes, Heinz bodies, red cell parasites
- To assess white cell abnormalities, e.g. toxic neutrophils, left shifts, blast cells
- To assess platelet abnormalities, e.g. macroplatelets and platelet clumps.

Blood film examination is essential in commercial laboratories, even where high tech, quality controlled, 'gold standard' analysers are being used. In the practice laboratory, where in-house analysers may provide less accurate leucocyte differential and platelet counts, blood film examination is perhaps even more important; failure to perform blood film examination may result in frequent serious errors in clinical decision making.

Preparation of blood films

Blood sample smears should be prepared soon after taking the blood sample. Polished glass slides with frosted ends are preferred since pencil can be used for easy labelling. Slides should be handled by their edges/ends since grease from fingers can result in poor smearing. If in doubt the slide can be wiped clean using a tissue before use. The technique for smear preparation is shown in Figure 3.12.

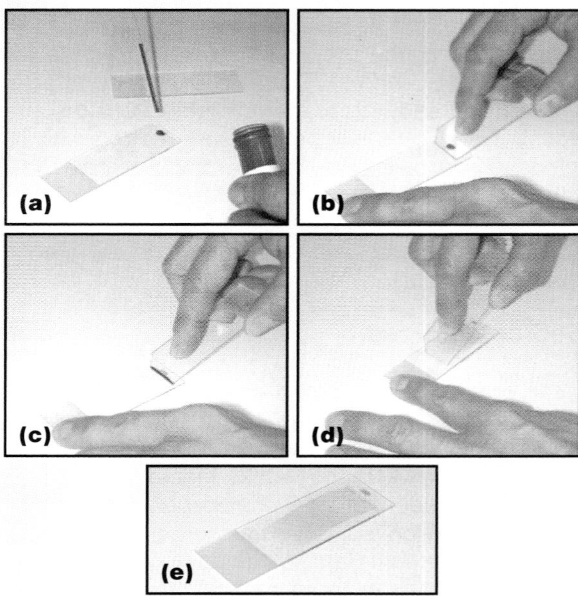

- A spreader slide is required to make the smear: this is narrower than the smear slide to avoid spreading the cells over the edge of the slide. Spreader slides can be made by breaking off a corner of a normal slide having first scored it with a blade or diamond writer. The spreader slide should be washed in water and dried regularly and should be replaced periodically as the edge can become roughened
- The blood sample is mixed carefully and then a sample harvested using a microhaematocrit tube. A drop of blood is placed on to the end of a slide (a)
- The spreader slide is held between the thumb and second finger, placing the index finger on top of the spreader. This helps to apply even pressure on the spreader when smearing (b)
- The spreader is placed at an angle of about 30 degrees in front of the blood spot and slid backwards until it comes into contact with the blood, which then rapidly spreads out along the edge of the spreader slide (c). The moment this occurs, the spreader is advanced forwards smoothly and quickly. As the smear is made a 'feathered edge' forms; do not lift the spreader slide until the feathered edge is completely formed (d)
- Ideally the smear should extend to approximately two thirds of the length of the slide and should a have fairly square feathered edge (e)
- The smear should be allowed to fully air dry prior to staining.

3.12 Preparation of blood films.

Causes of poor quality smears are discussed and illustrated in Figures 3.13 and 3.14.

Problem	Cause	Solution
Smear too long (feathered edge has disappeared off the end)	Spreader speed too slow Low viscosity blood, i.e. anaemia Excess blood applied to slide	More rapid spreader speed Apply smaller blood spot
Smear too short/thick	Spreader speed too fast High viscosity blood, i.e. high PCV	Slower spreader speed
Feathered edge consists of long streaked tails (Figure 3.14a)	Uneven contact of spreader with slide Spreader has roughened edge	Apply even pressure using index finger on top of spreader Replace spreader
Smear has holes or gaps	Grease on slide Lipaemia	Clean slides before use
Smear thick at feathered edge end of film	Blood in front of spreader	Ensure firm contact of spreader and slide when pulling spreader backwards towards blood spot

3.13 Causes and solutions of poor quality blood films.

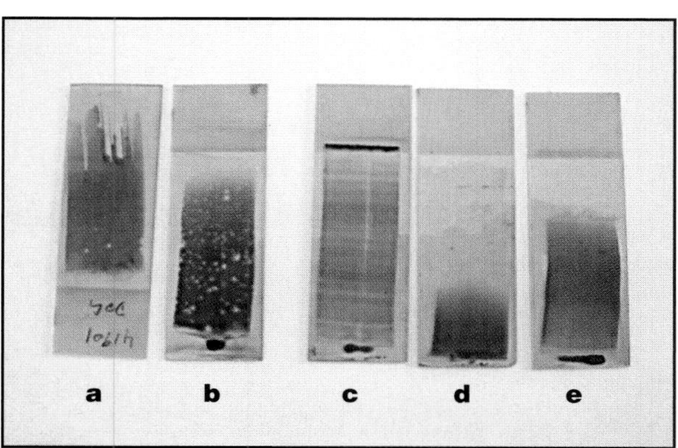

3.14 Examples of blood smears. (a) Smear has a ragged feathered edge due to uneven contact of the spreader with the slide, possibly because the spreader is dirty or roughened. (b) Smear has holes in, which may be due to grease on the slide or lipaemia. (c) Smear is too long because too much blood has been applied to the slide. Blood in front of the spreader has resulted in the dense line at the tail. (d) Smear is too short, which may be because insufficient blood was applied to the slide or the spreader speed was too fast. (e) A good smear with an even 'square' end.

Stains

Several types of rapid 'dunking' kits (e.g. Diff-Quick) are available. Hema-Gurr (BDH) is recommended by the author. These stains are more than adequate for in-house use. These kits have a three-stage staining procedure which incorporates a fixative pot (usually five dips), an orange/pink dye in the second pot (usually three dips) and a blue dye in the third pot (usually six dips). The intensity of the blue and orange staining can be altered by varying the number of dips in each pot and it is worth experimenting to determine optimum staining. Smears are dipped in buffered water to rinse and then air dried. It is helpful to add a coverslip and a mounting medium glue can be used. One or two drops of the mounting medium are placed on a coverslip and the smear slide is slowly lowered onto the coverslip. N.B. Make sure the glue has set prior to examination, and avoid getting it on the microscope lenses.

Film examination

A set procedure should be followed for blood film examination to ensure that all cell lines are examined properly. Initially the smear is checked for large platelet clumps (Figure 3.11) by examining the feathered edge at low power (X20 or X40). The smear is then examined at higher power in the thin area in from the feathered edge where the cells are evenly distributed in a monolayer (Figure 3.15). In this 'examination area' the red cells should not usually be touching one another. Do not examine cells at the feathered edge (distorted) or in thick areas of the smear where the cells are in clumps (cells do not lie flat in these areas). The red cells, white cells and platelets are examined in turn.

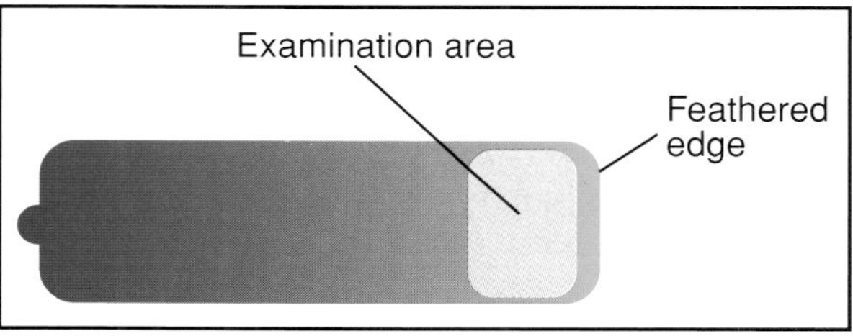

3.15 Diagrammatic representation of a blood film showing the area of the blood film in which cell examination should be performed.

Examination of red cells

Evaluation of the red cells should include an assessment of colour, size and shape, and examination for inclusions. Red cells from dogs and cats are anucleate and stain pink. Canine red cells have a pale area in the centre of the cells (central pallor) which is not obvious in feline red cells. Canine red cells are larger (diameter 7 μm) than feline red cells (diameter 5.5 μm) (Figure 3.16).

Anisocytosis refers to a variation in cell size. Some variation in cell size is normal in feline blood. Immature red cells (reticulocytes) are larger (macrocytic) than mature cells and also stain a blue–grey colour, which is described as polychromasia. Only small numbers (<1%) of immature red cells are seen in normal animals.

Poikilocytosis refers to altered red cell shape, e.g due to the formation of acanthocytes or schistocytes. Red cell abnormalities are discussed in Chapter 4.

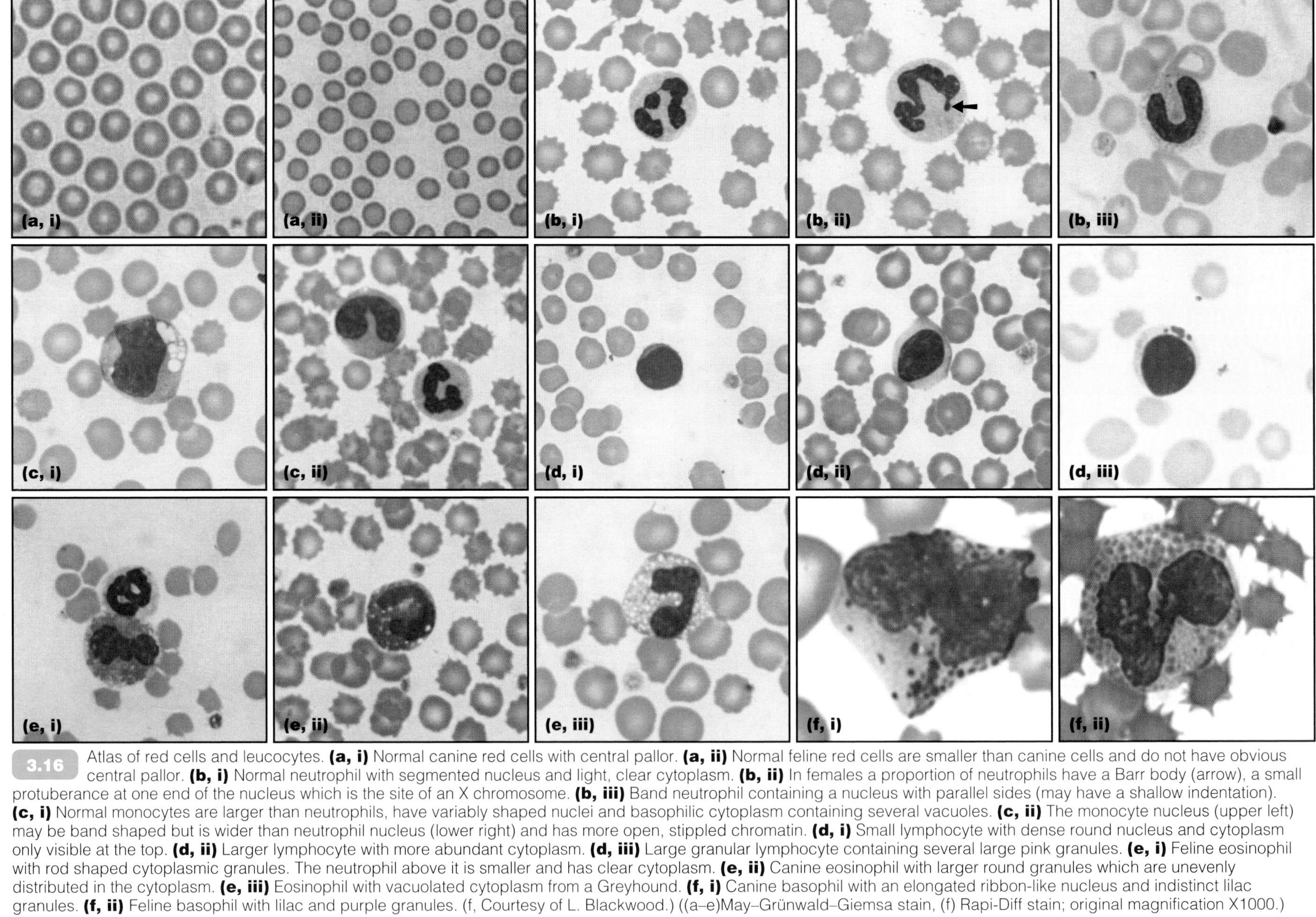

3.16 Atlas of red cells and leucocytes. **(a, i)** Normal canine red cells with central pallor. **(a, ii)** Normal feline red cells are smaller than canine cells and do not have obvious central pallor. **(b, i)** Normal neutrophil with segmented nucleus and light, clear cytoplasm. **(b, ii)** In females a proportion of neutrophils have a Barr body (arrow), a small protuberance at one end of the nucleus which is the site of an X chromosome. **(b, iii)** Band neutrophil containing a nucleus with parallel sides (may have a shallow indentation). **(c, i)** Normal monocytes are larger than neutrophils, have variably shaped nuclei and basophilic cytoplasm containing several vacuoles. **(c, ii)** The monocyte nucleus (upper left) may be band shaped but is wider than neutrophil nucleus (lower right) and has more open, stippled chromatin. **(d, i)** Small lymphocyte with dense round nucleus and cytoplasm only visible at the top. **(d, ii)** Larger lymphocyte with more abundant cytoplasm. **(d, iii)** Large granular lymphocyte containing several large pink granules. **(e, i)** Feline eosinophil with rod shaped cytoplasmic granules. The neutrophil above it is smaller and has clear cytoplasm. **(e, ii)** Canine eosinophil with larger round granules which are unevenly distributed in the cytoplasm. **(e, iii)** Eosinophil with vacuolated cytoplasm from a Greyhound. **(f, i)** Canine basophil with an elongated ribbon-like nucleus and indistinct lilac granules. **(f, ii)** Feline basophil with lilac and purple granules. (f, Courtesy of L. Blackwood.) ((a–e)May–Grünwald–Giemsa stain, (f) Rapi-Diff stain; original magnification X1000.)

Examination of leucocytes

A differential white cell count is performed by counting leucocytes at both the edges and in the middle of the smear in the examination area; larger cells tend to be pushed to the edges of the smear, and smaller cells tend to be more concentrated in the middle. An example of a battlement meander method of counting is shown in Figure 3.17. A total of at least 100, preferably 200 cells, should be counted. Nucleated red cells should be included and then the corrected white cell count is calculated. The percentage of each cell type is then multiplied by the total white cell count to determine an absolute count for each cell type. White cell morphological abnormalities, such as toxic change or atypical blast cells, should be noted (see Chapter 5).

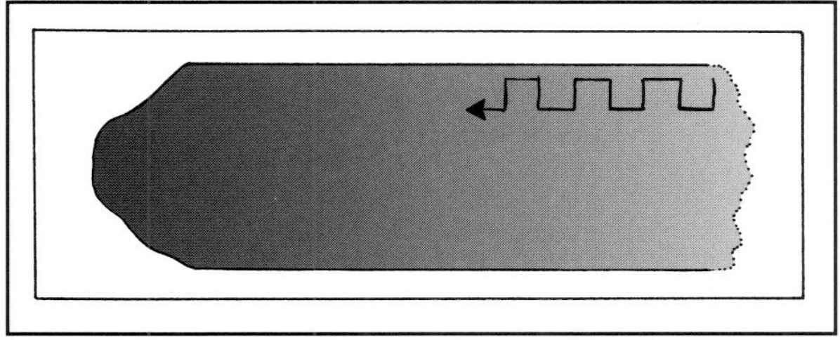

3.17 Battlement meander track for performing a white cell differential count.

Neutrophils are the predominant cell type, followed by lymphocytes. The ratio of neutrophils:lymphocytes is 3.5:1 in the dog and 2:1 in the cat. Normal animals have only small numbers of eosinophils and monocytes and only very occasional to absent basophils.

Neutrophils: These are relatively large (approximately two times the diameter of a red cell) and have an elongated, segmented nucleus with three to five lobes (Figure 3.16b). Cytoplasm is light blue–grey but the cytoplasmic granules present do not stain. Immature neutrophils, termed 'bands', are seen infrequently in health but increased numbers are present in inflammatory conditions. Band neutrophils have an elongated, often U-shaped, non-lobulated nucleus with parallel sides. Shallow indentations less than 50% of the width of the nucleus may be present. Toxic neutrophils are seen in severe inflammation, especially associated with bacterial infection and are discussed in Chapter 5.

Monocytes: These are larger than neutrophils and have abundant sky-blue cytoplasm, often containing clear discrete vacuoles and sometimes fine, pink, dust-like granules (Figure 3.16c). The shape of the nucleus is very variable and can be round, kidney bean-shaped, lobulated, U-shaped or S-shaped. Monocytes with U-shaped nuclei may be difficult to distinguish from band neutrophils, especially those showing toxic change, but several differences aid identification, as shown in Figure 3.18.

Lymphocytes: These have a round nucleus with condensed, smudged chromatin and a narrow rim of basophilic cytoplasm (Figure 3.16d). Lymphocytes vary in size: small lymphocytes predominate and are slightly larger than canine red cells and have sparse cytoplasm which is not be visible all the way round the nucleus. Medium-sized lymphocytes may approach the size of neutrophils and have more abundant cytoplasm, often completely encircling the nucleus. Reactive lymphocytes are larger still, with a nucleus approximately 1.5 times the diameter of a canine red cell and abundant deeply basophilic cytoplasm, often with a darker tinge at the periphery. Occasional reactive lymphocytes may be seen in health, but these cells usually reflect antigenic stimulation. A few lymphocytes containing several prominent magenta red/pink cytoplasmic granules on one side of the nucleus may be present. These are known as 'large granular lymphocytes'. Lymphoblasts (large cells with one or more nucleoli) are not found on blood films from healthy animals.

Monocytes with U shaped nuclei	Band neutrophils
Wider, larger nucleus with knob shaped ends	Narrow nucleus
Open, stippled chromatin	Dense, condensed chromatin
Sky-blue to deeply basophilic cytoplasm	Pale grey cytoplasm Toxic bands may be slightly basophilic, but not as dark as monocytes
Cytoplasm often contains discrete vacuoles and sometimes contains fine, pink, dust-like granules	Cytoplasm non-vacuolated Toxic bands may be foamy (not discrete vacuoles) and contain distinct granules

3.18 Factors that aid differentiation of monocytes with U-shaped nuclei from band neutrophils.

Eosinophils: These are slightly larger than neutrophils, and are characterized by numerous, prominent, pink cytoplasmic granules (Figure 3.16e). In cats these are always abundant and are rod-shaped and uniform in size. In dogs the number and size of granules are very variable. Classically there are abundant small round granules, but there may be only small numbers of larger granules. Cytoplasm between the granules is lightly basopilic and may contain clear vacuoles. Eosinophils of Greyhounds are always very vacuolated and contain few to no granules. Eosinophil nuclei are lobulated but usually only have two to three lobes.

Basophils: These are rare in blood smears from normal animals. They are a similar size to eosinophils and have an elongated 'ribbon-like' segmented nucleus and variable numbers of cytoplasmic granules. In dogs these granules are sparse and dark purple; in cats they are abundant and pale lilac, sometimes with a few dark purple granules (Figure 3.16f).

Examination of platelets

Platelets are small round structures with no nucleus. They are quarter to half the diameter of red cells with pink cytoplasm and fine granules. Platelet numbers can be estimated by counting the number of platelets seen in a X1000 field (i.e. X10 eyepiece and X100

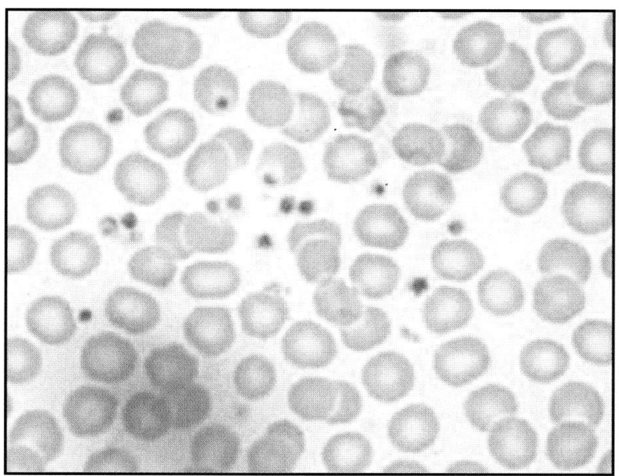

3.19 Performing an estimated platelet count. The blood film is examined using the X100 oil immersion lens in the examination area. The number of platelets per field is counted and a mean value of five fields is calculated. This value is multiplied by 15 to produce the count x 10^9/l.

objective), having first determined that no platelet clumps are present. Five fields are counted and a mean value is calculated. The normal count is 10–30 platelets per X1000 field (Figure 3.19). Each platelet per X1000 field equates to *approximately* 15 x 10^9/l. Thus if 10 platelets are seen per X1000 field, the platelet count is approximately 10 x 15 = 150 x 10^9/l. Animals with severe thrombocytopenia (<30 x 10^9/l) have only 0–3 platelets per field. The presence of large 'shift' platelets should be noted, as these may be an indicator of active thrombopoiesis, especially in dogs.

Further reading

Harvey JW (2001) Bone marrow examination. In: *Atlas of Veterinary Haematology. Blood and Bone Marrow of Domestic Animals,* ed. JW Harvey, pp. 93–123. WB Saunders, Philadelphia

Knoll JS (2000) Clinical automated haematology systems. In: *Schalms Veterinary Haematology 5th edn,* ed. BF Feldman, JG Zinkl and NC Jain, pp. 3–11. Lippincott, Williams and Wilkins, Philadelphia.

Stockham SL and Scott MA (2002) Basic haematological assays In: *Fundamentals of Veterinary Clinical Pathology, 1st edn,* ed. SL Stockham and MA Scott, pp. 31–48. Iowa State Press, Iowa.

4

Disorders of erythrocytes

Elizabeth Villiers

Introduction

Erythrocyte disorders fall into two broad groups: anaemia; and erythrocytosis (or polycythaemia). Anaemia may be due to reduced red cell production, which results in non-regenerative anaemia, or increased red cell loss, which results in regenerative anaemia. Changes in red cell parameters, such as mean corpuscular volume (MCV) and mean corpuscular haemoglobin concentration (MCHC), and morphological changes (e.g. presence or absence of polychromasia) aid in the differentiation of the cause of anaemia. To understand how these changes arise, it is necessary to review the process of erythropoiesis.

A review of erythropoiesis

Erythropoiesis takes place in the bone marrow, in islets around central macrophages known as nurse cells. These cells phagocytose debris, such as extruded nuclear material, store iron as haemosiderin and supply iron as ferritin for haem synthesis. The main regulator of erythropoiesis is erythropoietin, a glycoprotein produced in the kidney in response to renal tissue hypoxia. Other hormones, such as thyroxine, growth hormone and corticosteroids, enhance the effect of erythropoietin. Certain cytokines released during inflammation, e.g. interleukin 1 and tumour necrosis factor, inhibit erythropoiesis.

- Pluripotent stem cells develop into early erythroid precursors, known as burst-forming units-erythroid (BFU-E), under the influence of interleukin 3.
- BFU-E divide and form colony-forming units-erythroid (CFU-E), which, in turn, divide and differentiate into proerythroblasts (also known as rubriblasts) under the influence of erythropoietin.
- Proerythroblasts develop into early normoblasts (prorubricytes), which, in turn, divide into intermediate normoblasts (metarubricytes) and then late normoblasts (rubricytes) (Figures 4.1 and 4.2). As these divisions take place the cells progressively become smaller, and also accumulate increasing amounts of haemoglobin.
- Once a critical amount of haemoglobin has formed, the nucleus is extruded and a reticulocyte is formed.

The development time from BFU-E to reticulocyte is approximately 7 days. Reticulocytes remain in the bone marrow for 24–48 hours before being released into the circulation, where they reach full maturation

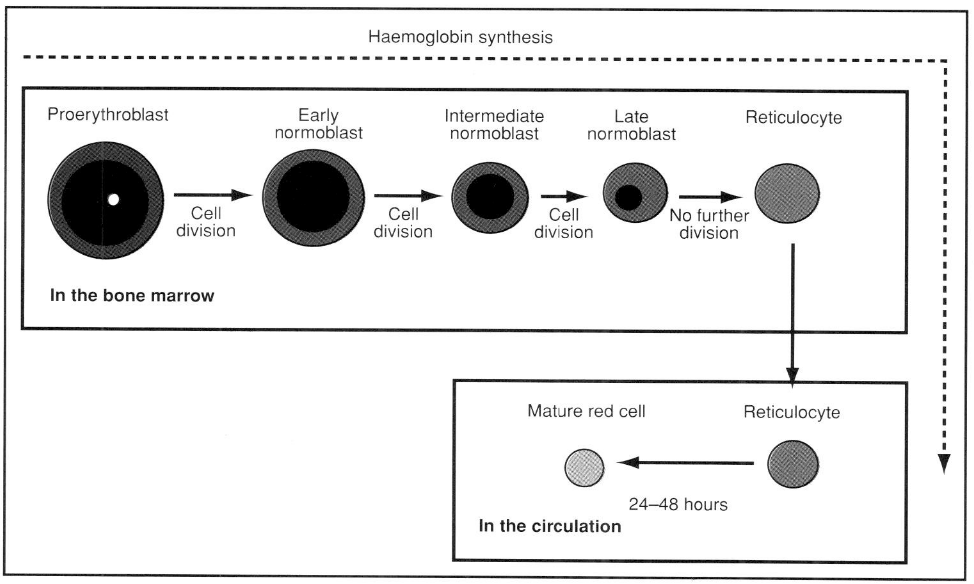

4.1 Erythropoiesis. The developing red cells become progressively smaller and accumulate haemoglobin. They are released into the circulation as reticulocytes.

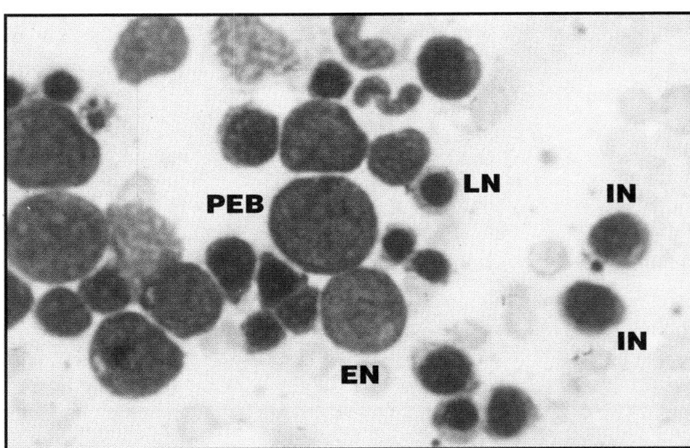

4.2 Stages of erythropoiesis shown on a bone marrow aspirate (EN, early normoblast; IN, intermediate normoblast; LN, late normoblast; PEB, proerythroblast). (May–Grünwald–Giemsa stain; original magnification X1000.)

after a further 24–48 hours. Reticulocytes are not capable of cell division but continue to synthesize haemoglobin. They develop into mature erythrocytes when haemoglobin synthesis is completed and the cell size has reduced to adult size.

Key features of reticulocytes are:

- They are larger than mature red cells
- They contain less haemoglobin than mature red cells
- They contain numerous clumps of ribosomal RNA which impart a polychromatophilic (bluish-pink) colour to the cytoplasm on Romanowsky staining (Figure 4.3) and stain as dark clumps with new methylene blue.

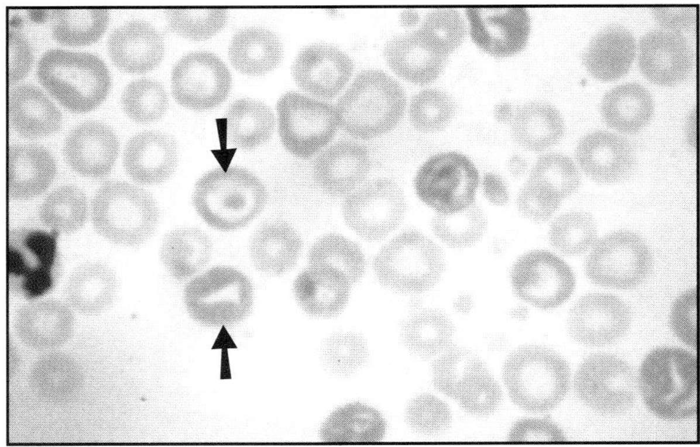

4.3 Blood film from a dog with regenerative anaemia due to blood loss. There is marked polychromasia (darker purple cells, bottom arrow). Target cells (codocytes) are present (top arrow); these have a wide area of central pallor within which there is a central circular density of haemoglobin. (May–Grünwald–Giemsa stain; original magnification X1000.)

Mature erythrocytes circulate for approximately 110 days in the dog and 70 days in the cat. Senescent red cells are lost in the liver, spleen and bone marrow. As old cells are lost, they are replaced by reticulocytes released from the marrow and thus small numbers (approximately 1%) of polychromatic cells or reticulocytes are seen on blood smears from normal dogs and cats.

Normal erythropoiesis depends on normal haemoglobin synthesis and normal DNA synthesis. Haemoglobin consists of four interlinked globin chains (constructed from amino acids), each of which has a cleft containing a haem molecule. Haem consists of a protoporphyrin ring containing a central molecule of iron (Figure 4.4). The protoporphyrin ring is synthesized from the amino acid glycine and the Krebs cycle intermediate succinyl-CoA, by a series of enzymatic reactions. Thus the basic 'ingredients' of haemoglobin are amino acids and iron, and haemoglobin synthesis is impeded if there is protein deficiency (e.g. malnutrition) or iron deficiency (due to dietary deficiency or chronic external blood loss). Defective haemoglobin synthesis may also result from lead toxicity, due to inhibition of some of the enzymatic reactions involved in protoporphyrin synthesis.

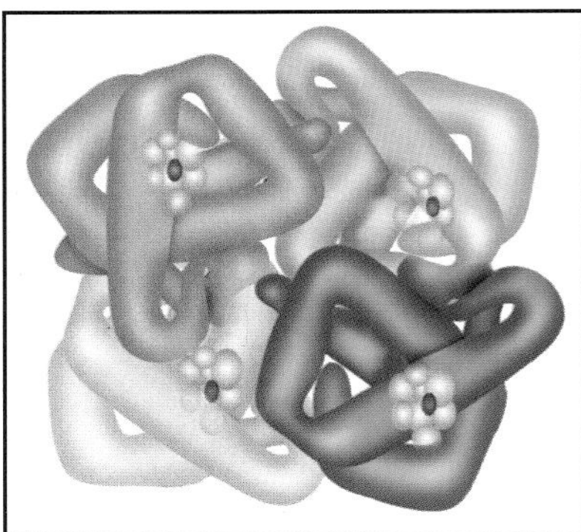

4.4 Diagrammatic representation of the structure of haemoglobin with four haem rings connected by globin chains.

The trigger for extrusion of the nucleus from the normoblast is the accumulation of a critical amount of haemoglobin. If the rate of haemoglobin synthesis is reduced, for example due to iron deficiency, the nucleus is retained within the red cell precursor for longer and additional cell divisions take place, resulting in the production of smaller (microcytic) cells.

Anaemia

Anaemia is characterized by reduced numbers of erythrocytes, which results in reduced packed cell volume (PCV) and red cell count, and reduced haemoglobin concentration. Decreased erythrocyte haemoglobin content also produces anaemia and a reduced haemoglobin concentration. There are many causes of anaemia, but these all fall into one of two groups:

- Anaemia due to reduced red cell production (leading to non-regenerative anaemia)
- Anaemia due to increased red cell loss (leading to regenerative anaemia). This may result from haemorrhage or haemolysis.

Characteristics of regenerative anaemia

The bone marrow responds to red cell loss by increasing red cell production and, after an initial lag phase of 3–5 days, increased numbers of reticulocytes are released into the circulation. Reticulocytes are released at an earlier stage than they would be in a normal animal and may be larger, or even nucleated. Thus a regenerative anaemia is characterized by numerous circulating reticulocytes ± nucleated red cells. Since reticulocytes are larger, mean corpuscular volume (MCV) is increased, and since they have less haemoglobin, mean corpuscular haemoglobin concentration (MCHC) is reduced: the anaemia is *macrocytic* and *hypochromic*. However, MCV and MCHC are *mean* values and so, in a mildly regenerative anaemia, there may not be sufficient reticulocytes present to move the mean out of the normal range. MCV and MCHC are not very sensitive markers of regeneration, and may be altered for other reasons (Figures 4.5 and 4.6). The red cell distribution width (RDW, see Chapter 3) is a more sensitive indicator, since relatively small numbers of larger cells will increase this parameter. On histogram plots produced by impedance analysers a hump of larger cells is seen on the right of the curve, representing reticulocytes (Figure 4.7).

Causes of altered MCV	Mechanism/other features
Increased MCV	
Regenerative anaemia	Increased circulating reticulocytes, which are larger
Feline leukaemia virus infection; myeloproliferative disease	During erythropoiesis there is delayed nuclear maturation alongside normal haemoglobin production, resulting in fewer cell divisions before the nucleus is extruded
Familial macrocytosis in Toy and Miniature Poodles (Schalm, 1976)	Also increased nucleated red cells and Howell–Jolly bodies. Incidental finding. Pathogenesis unknown. No anaemia or clinical signs
Hereditary stomatocytosis in Alaskan Malamutes and Miniature Schnauzers (Fletch *et al.*, 1975; Brown *et al.*, 1994)	Stomatocytes are cup-shaped red cells that form when red cells take up excess sodium and water. Miniature Schnauzers are asymptomatic. Malamutes have concurrent chondrodysplasia
Aged blood samples (>24 hours)	Red cell swelling *in vitro*
Autoagglutination	Clumps of red cells counted by analyser as one large red cell
Hyperosmolality, e.g. due to hypernatraemia	When blood is mixed with analyser diluent, water moves into red cells leading to swelling
Decreased MCV	
Iron deficiency	During erythropoiesis there is a reduced rate of haemoglobin synthesis, so the nucleus is retained for longer. Extra cell divisions occur, resulting in formation of small red cells
Liver disease; portosystemic shunts	Cause unclear but likely to be due to abnormal iron metabolism. MCHC normal or mildly reduced. May also see mild anaemia
Anaemia of chronic inflammatory disease	Usually normocytic normochromic but may become microcytic if long-standing. Likely to be due to abnormal iron metabolism
Familial microcytosis in Akitas	Incidental finding

4.5 Causes of altered mean corpuscular volume and their mechanisms.

Cause of altered MCHC	Mechanism
Increased MCHC	
Intravascular haemolysis; haemolysis *in vitro*	Free haemoglobin (Hb) as well as Hb from cells is measured and this affects calculation of MCHC
Lipaemia; numerous Heinz bodies	Interference with spectrophotometric Hb assay
Reduced MCHC	
Regenerative anaemia	Increased circulating reticulocytes, which have less haemoglobin. Not all regenerative anaemias have low MCHC
Iron deficiency	Reduced production of haemoglobin
Aged blood samples (>24 hours)	Red cell swelling *in vitro* leads to increased HCT and consequent decreased calculated MCHC

4.6 Causes of altered mean corpuscular haemoglobin concentration and their mechanisms.

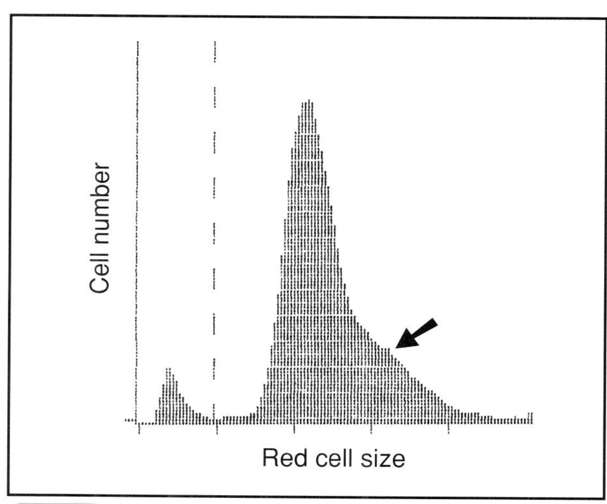

4.7 A histogram showing red cell size on the X axis and cell number (n) the Y axis, from a dog with regenerative anaemia. There is a 'hump' to the right of the main peak (arrow) indicating increased numbers of large red cells.

On a blood film stained with a routine Romanowsky or rapid (e.g. Diff-Quik) stain, the regenerative response manifests as polychromasia (increased numbers of polychromatic cells) and anisocytosis (variation in cell size) with macrocytosis (see Figure 4.3). The number of polychromatic cells and macrocytes per high power field should be assessed to gauge the regenerative response, as shown in Figure 4.8. In cats, reticulocytes tend to remain in the marrow until they are only weakly polychromatophilic and so the degree of polychromasia seen in a regenerative anaemia is less marked than for the dog.

Other blood film features of regeneration include:

- Howell–Jolly bodies (remnants of nuclear material, most often seen in cats) (Figure 4.9a)
- Target cells (see Figure 4.3) are frequently seen, but are not specific for regeneration. They may also be seen in renal and hepatic disorders, and hypochromic target cells are seen in iron deficiency (see below)
- Basophilic stippling (due to aggregated ribosomes, appearing as small punctuate inclusions; Figure 4.9b) is occasionally seen in regeneration in small animals but is more often associated with lead poisoning
- Nucleated red cells (Figure 4.9c).

Circulating nucleated red cells in the absence of polychromasia are not indicative of a regenerative response and may be seen with bone marrow disease (e.g. myeloproliferative disease) and with splenic disease (e.g. neoplasia), as well as in lead poisoning.

Characteristics of non-regenerative anaemia

In non-regenerative anaemia there is no increased release of reticulocytes from the bone marrow and the anaemia is normocytic and normochromic, with no increase in RDW. On a blood film, the red cells are uniform in size and polychromatic cells are rare (<1.5% of red cells or <1 per high power 100X field). Immediately following red cell loss, anaemia appears non-regenerative, and an increase in circulating reticulocytes is not seen for 3–4 days.

Distinguishing regenerative from non-regenerative anaemia

Evaluation of the MCV, MCHC and the presence or absence of polychromasia and anisocytosis help to distinguish regenerative and non-regenerative anaemia, but the most accurate way of evaluating the bone marrow's response is by measuring the circulating reticulocyte count.

Reticulocyte counts

Reticulocytes can be identified using supravital stains (stain living cells), such as new methylene blue and brilliant cresyl green, which stain the reticulum network of aggregated ribosomes, mitochondria and organelles present in immature cells. This reticulum network is lost as the red cell matures and so reticulocyte counts should be performed on fresh samples (preferably < 6 hours old).

To perform a reticulocyte count:

1. Mix equal parts of blood (in EDTA) and a 0.5% solution of new methylene blue in normal saline.

Grade	Polychromasia in dogs	Polychromasia in cats	Macrocytosis (dogs and cats)
Occasional	<1 cell/hpf	<1 cell every other hpf	Slightly larger cells, <1 cell/hpf
1+	1–2 cells/hpf	<1 cell/hpf	Slightly larger cells, 1–2 cells/hpf
2+	2–3 cells/hpf	1–2 cells/hpf	Slightly larger and larger still cells present, 3–5 cells/hpf
3+	4–8 cells/hpf	3–5 cells/hpf	Large cells present, 5–10/hpf
4+	>8 cells/hpf	>5 cells/hpf	Large cells present, >10/hpf

4.8 A grading system for polychromasia and macrocytosis in dogs and cats. Occasional indicates no regeneration, 1+ and 2+ indicate mild regeneration, 3+ and 4+ indicate moderate and marked regeneration. This grading is subjective and will also depend on the thickness of the smear and the total number of cells per high power (100X) field (hpf). Grading systems may vary slightly between different laboratories.

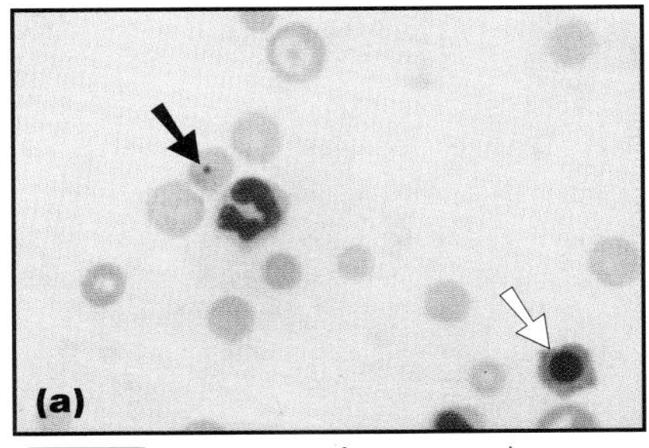

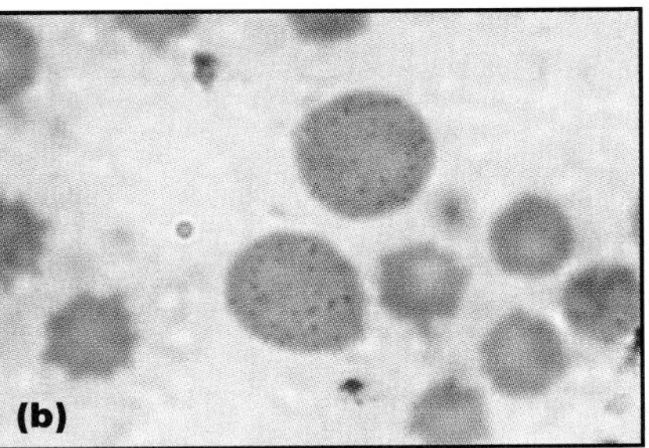

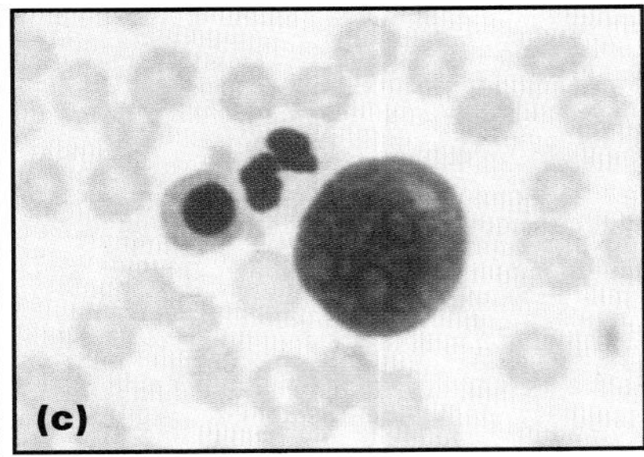

4.9 Features of regenerative anaemia. (a) Howell–Jolly bodies in red cells are prominent dark circular inclusions of varying size (black arrow). A nucleated red blood cell is also present (white arrow). (b) Basophilic stippling. Numerous tiny inclusions are seen across the cell surface. (c) A late normoblast with a small dark nucleus and polychromatic cytoplasm (left) and proerythoblast with a larger nucleus and relatively less cytoplasm (right), with a neutrophil between the two. (May–Grünwald–Giemsa stain; original magnification X1000.)

2. Leave to stand at room temperature for 15–20 minutes.
3. Mix again.
4. Make a blood smear (see Chapter 3).
5. Scan the smear at low power first to check for even distribution of reticulocytes. Occasionally, the reticulocytes are unevenly distributed and are preferentially pushed to the tail.
6. Evaluate the smear at high power (100X) in the monolayer region (examination area, see Chapter 3).

In dogs, all reticulocytes are aggregate forms: these are larger than mature red cells and contain large clumps of aggregated ribosomes (Figure 4.10a). In cats there are two forms of reticulocyte: punctuate and aggregate. Punctate reticulocytes are more mature than aggregate reticulocytes, are similar in size to mature red cells, and contain two to six fine dots of residual RNA (Figure 4.10b). Only the aggregate forms should be included in the count (punctate reticulocytes are counted as mature red cells). Because there is a transition from the aggregate to the punctuate stage, some cells may be difficult to classify.

To perform the count at least 300 cells, but preferably 1000 cells (mature red cells and aggregate reticulocytes), are counted and the percentage of reticulocytes is calculated.

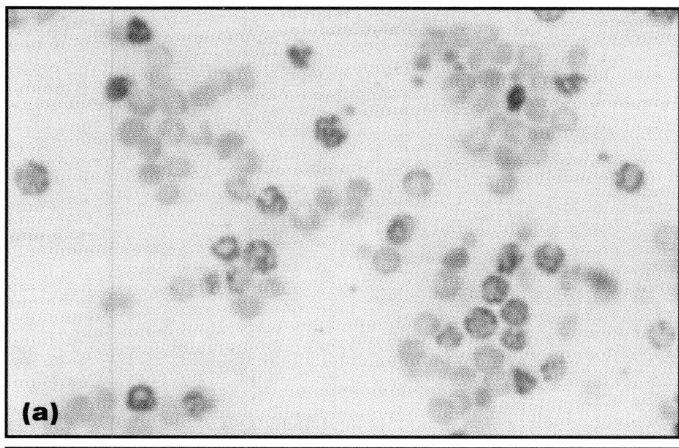

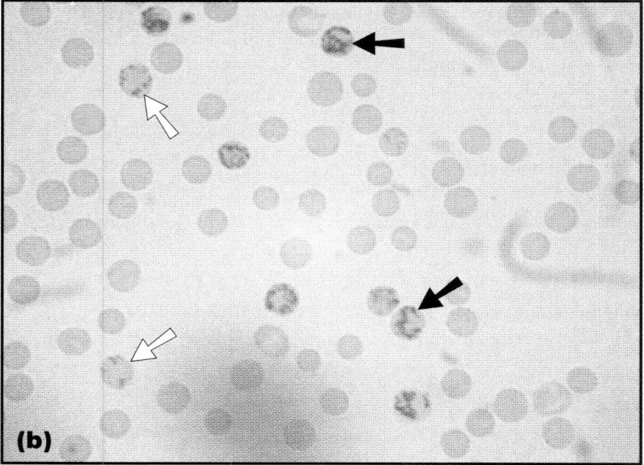

4.10 Reticulocytes. (a) In the dog, reticulocytes have numerous dark-staining aggregates of ribosomes. (b) In the cat, aggregate reticulocytes have large clumps of ribosomes (black arrow), whilst punctuate reticulocytes have a few small inclusions (white arrow). (New methylene blue stain; original magnification X1000.)

Reticulocytes are absent or present only in small numbers (<1.5%) in normal blood. Following acute haemorrhage or haemolysis, increased numbers of reticulocytes are not evident for at least 48 hours, with maximal production by 4–7 days. In regenerative anaemias, with a normal functioning bone marrow, the magnitude of the reticulocyte response should match the severity of the anaemia. For example, in a dog, mild anaemia and a PCV of 30% should lead to a slight increase in reticulocyte count (e.g. 2%), whilst severe anaemia and a PCV of 15% should lead to a much higher reticulocyte count (e.g. 20–50%). Haemolytic anaemias generally result in a more marked reticulocytosis than do haemorrhagic anaemias.

The reticulocyte count must be interpreted in the light of the degree of anaemia. It is preferable to use the absolute reticulocyte count, as this is not affected by variation in red cell number in the way that reticulocyte percentage is, as shown in Figure 4.11.

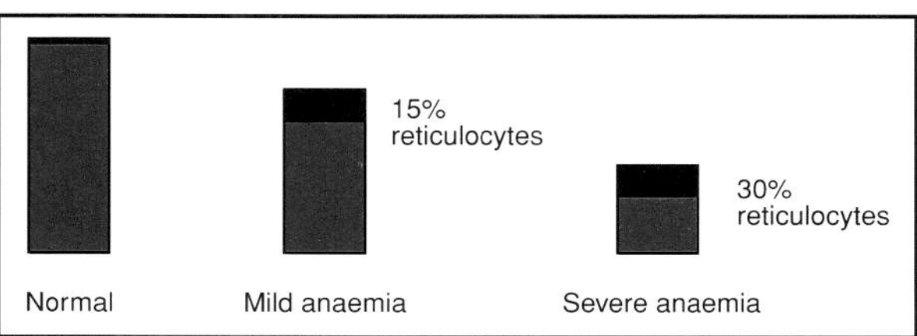

4.11 The effect of degree of anaemia on uncorrected reticulocyte percentage. The proportions of mature red cells and reticulocytes are shown schematically in red and black, respectively. The normal animal on the left has a low percentage of reticulocytes. In the animals with mild and severe anaemia, the same absolute number of reticulocytes is circulating, but the reticulocyte percentage is higher in severe anaemia because there are fewer mature cells. This gives the false impression that the severe anaemia is more regenerative than the mild anaemia.

$$\text{Absolute reticulocyte count } (\times 10^9/\text{l}) = \text{Observed \% reticulocytes} \times \text{RBC } (\times 10^{12}/\text{l}) \times 10$$

Guidelines for the degree of reticulocyte response are shown in Figure 4.12.

Alternatively, the corrected reticulocyte percentage (CRP) can be used.

$$\text{CRP (\%)} = \frac{\text{Reticulocyte percentage} \times \text{Patient's PCV}}{\text{Average PCV for patient (45\% in dog, 37\% in cat)}}$$

A third correction, the reticulocyte production index (RPI), is sometimes used in dogs. With increasing severity of anaemia, reticulocytes spend less time maturing in the bone marrow and longer in the circulation before maturing into erythrocytes. This means that CRP and absolute reticulocyte count may overestimate the degree of erythropoietic activity in the bone marrow. The RPI is calculated by dividing the CRP by the reticulocyte maturation time (RMT), which varies depending on the degree of anaemia:

$$\text{RPI} = \text{CRP/ RMT}$$

where RMT = 1 day for a PCV of 45%, 1.5 days for 35%, 2 days for 25%, and 2.5 days for 15%.

Degree of regeneration	Canine reticulocytes (x 10^9/l) (RP shown in parentheses)	Feline aggregate reticulocytes (x 10^9/l) (RP shown in parentheses)	Feline punctate reticulocytes (x 10^9/l)
None	<60 (<1.5%)	<40 (<0.5%)	<200
Slight	60–150 (1.5–4%)	41–70 (0.5–2%)	200–500
Moderate	150–300 (5–20%)	70–100 (3–4%)	500–1000
Marked	>500 (>20%)	>200 (>4%)	1000–1500

4.12 Guidelines for interpreting the reticulocyte response, based on absolute reticulocyte count. (RP, reticulocyte percentage (uncorrected).)

An RPI of <1 indicates a non-regenerative anaemia, RPI of 1–2 indicates a slight response, RPI >2 indicates a moderate response and RPI >3 indicates a marked response, as is seen in haemolysis. However, these are *human* red cell maturation times and values for anaemic dogs or cats are not known (Stockham and Scott, 2002). Thus, the RPI may not be reliable in dogs and cats and is infrequently used. The author's preference is to calculate the absolute reticulocyte count.

Feline reticulocytes

Aggregate and punctuate reticulocytes are present in feline blood (see Figure 4.10b). Aggregate reticulocytes circulate for a short time (approximately 12 hours) before developing into punctate reticulocytes, which develop into mature red cells after 10 days. Aggregate reticulocytes are polychromatic on Romanowsky stains but punctate reticulocytes are not. Normal cats may have up to 10% punctate reticulocytes. Following an episode of red cell loss, punctate reticulocytes start to increase by 1 week, peak at around 2–3 weeks and then gradually decline. Thus, increased punctate reticulocytes indicate a regenerative response 2–4 weeks earlier, whilst increased aggregate reticulocytes indicate recent bone marrow stimulation. The aggregate reticulocyte count is most useful in assessing the marrow's response to anaemia, and punctate reticulocytes are not usually counted (they are counted as mature cells). However, in mild anaemia the punctate count is useful because the marrow tends to retain the aggregate reticulocytes until they mature into punctate reticulocytes. Guidelines for interpreting the punctate reticulocyte count are shown in Figure 4.12.

Physiological response to anaemia

The release of oxygen from haemoglobin to the tissues is determined by the affinity of haemoglobin for oxygen. Lower affinity means that a higher proportion of oxygen carried by haemoglobin is released to tissues. Haemoglobin affinity is reduced in tissue hypoxia, as lactic acid released via anaerobic glycolysis leads to lowered microenvironmental pH. In addition, haemoglobin affinity is regulated by 2,3 diphosphoglycerate (2,3 DPG), a compound found in high concentrations in red cells. Increased 2,3 DPG concentration leads to lowered affinity and hence greater delivery of oxygen to the tissues. 2,3 DPG concentration increases in anaemia and in this way anaemic animals undergo a physiological adaptation to the anaemic state, maximizing the capacity of their reduced number of red cells to carry and deliver oxygen. Animals with chronic anaemia can compensate remarkably well and have relatively mild clinical signs for the degree of anaemia. In contrast, animals with acute anaemia, which have not had time to adapt physiologically, have severe clinical signs associated with a relatively mild to moderate anaemia.

Blood loss anaemia

The clinical and clinicopathological picture of acute and chronic haemorrhage differ in many respects and so are considered separately.

Acute haemorrhage

Acute haemorrhage may occur following trauma or surgery, or due to bleeding gastrointestinal ulcers or tumours, rupture of a vascular tumour (e.g. splenic haemangiosarcoma) or coagulopathy (e.g. warfarin toxicity). Acute severe blood loss (up to 30–40% of blood volume, beyond which death is likely to occur) causes hypovolaemic shock with collapse, marked mucosal pallor, tachycardia and weak pulses (contrasting with the bounding pulses seen in animals with acute haemolysis). Immediately following acute haemorrhage the plasma protein and red cell parameters (including PCV) are normal because both red cells and plasma are lost in proportion. After about 4 hours, the PCV and plasma protein start to fall as blood volume is expanded by interstitial fluid moving into the circulation. Plasma protein usually falls first because splenic contraction may offset the fall in PCV. The PCV does not indicate the full magnitude of blood loss for at least 24 hours after the onset of haemorrhage.

Following internal haemorrhage up to approximately 60% of the red cells as well as plasma protein are reabsorbed via the lymphatics over a few days, resulting in a rapid increase in PCV and plasma protein. Red cells may be damaged during this process, resulting in the formation of acanthocytes; these should be distinguished from echinocytes (Figure 4.13). The remaining red cells are phagocytosed by macrophages and their iron is recycled. The anaemia resolves due to a combination of red cell reabsorption and bone marrow regeneration. The magnitude of the regenerative response may not be very marked if a large proportion of cells is reabsorbed.

Following external haemorrhage, protein and red cells (and hence iron) are lost from the body and so recovery from anaemia depends totally on the bone marrow's response. This regenerative response is usually apparent in the peripheral blood after 3–4 days. The PCV rises quite rapidly and is usually low normal within 2–3 weeks of a single haemorrhagic episode. Plasma protein should return to normal after 5–7 days: persistently low protein beyond this time is suggestive of ongoing external blood loss.

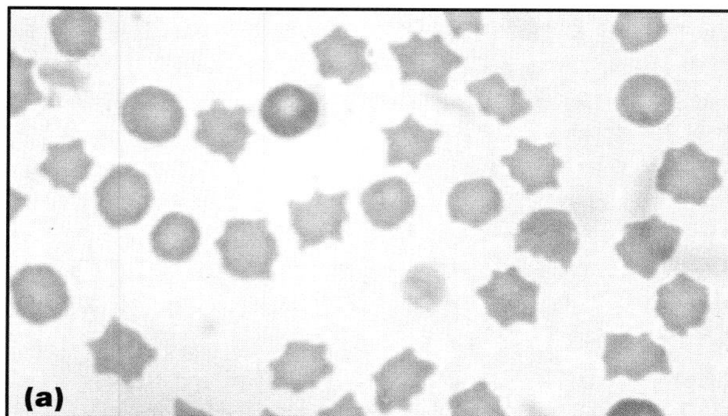

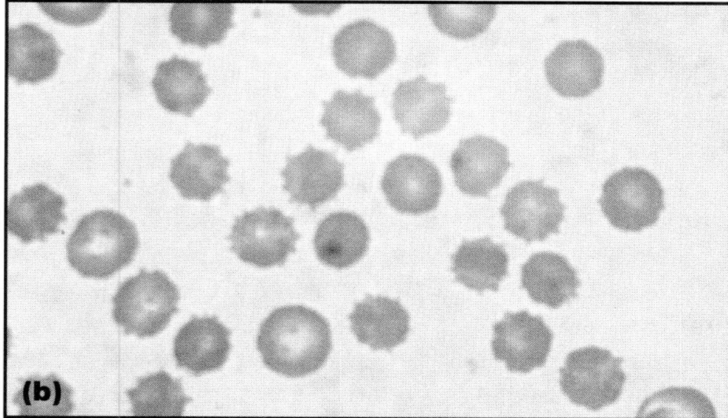

4.13 (a) Acanthocytes ('spur cells') have rounded projections of variable length and reflect membrane damage, which may occur with reabsorption of red cells following internal haemorrhage, or fragmentation as red cells pass through tumours, such as haemangiosarcoma and lymphoma, or clots in disseminated intravascular coagulation. (b) Crenated red cells/echinocytes have numerous short, evenly spaced surface projections of uniform dimensions and are usually an artefactual change in thick smears; red cells shrink when the smear dries or with excess EDTA. Echinocytes may sometimes be seen in uraemia. (May–Grünwald–Giemsa stain; original magnification X1000.)

Acute blood loss is usually associated with a neutrophilic leucocytosis with increased numbers of band neutrophils, especially following haemorrhage into a body cavity. The presence of immature red cells and granulocytic precursors in the circulation is known as a leucoerythroblastic response and may also be seen in immune-mediated haemolytic anaemia (see Figure 5.6). Immediately following haemorrhage there will be a mild to moderate thrombocytopenia, reflecting increased consumption of platelets; this is usually rapidly followed by a rebound thrombocytosis with the production of large 'shift' platelets.

In summary, the clinicopathological features of acute haemorrhage are:

- Anaemia: initially non-regenerative, after 3–4 days becomes regenerative. Acanthocytes may be seen with internal haemorrhage
- Low plasma proteins, returning to normal more quickly with internal haemorrhage
- Neutrophilia with left shift
- Thrombocytopenia then rebound thrombocytosis.

The cause or source of the haemorrhage may be obvious on clinical examination, or further investigations may be required. Depending on the clinical signs, coagulation tests (see Chapter 6), radiography, ultrasonography, and urine and faecal analysis may be indicated.

Chronic haemorrhage and iron-deficiency anaemia
Chronic haemorrhage results in an insidious onset, chronic anaemia. The animal is able to adapt to the anaemic state and so shows relatively mild signs for the degree of anaemia. Chronic external haemorrhage initially leads to a regenerative anaemia, but, as iron deficiency develops, the anaemia progressively becomes non-regenerative. Most body iron is found in haemoglobin (65%), and only small amounts of iron are found in myoglobin and enzymes or attached to the transporter molecule, transferrin (5%). The remainder is stored in various tissues as haemosiderin and ferritin: a small amount of ferritin is present in the plasma. Chronic external blood loss results in loss of haem iron. In response to the blood loss, iron stores are mobilized and utilized for erythropoiesis, but when these stores become depleted iron deficiency develops. Young animals become iron deficient following blood loss more quickly then adults because they have low iron stores, and the bone marrow has less capacity to increase the rate of haematopoiesis, as it is very actively producing red cells to match growth rate.

Iron deficiency results in inadequate haemoglobinization of red cells and the release of microcytic hypochromic red cells into the circulation, with resultant low MCV and MCHC. MCV falls first; as iron becomes progressively depleted, MCHC then falls. The combination of microcytic and normocytic (present from prior to the onset of iron deficiency) red cells leads to increased RDW. Persistent thrombocytosis is a common feature of chronic haemorrhage. Plasma proteins are lost along with red cells and, if blood loss is substantial, there is hypoproteinaemia with proportionately low albumin and globulin.

On the blood film the red cells do not always have a smaller diameter but are thin (flat), pale-staining cells termed leptocytes, which have a large area of central pallor and a thin rim of haemoglobin (Figure 4.14). Target cells (codocytes) and folded or fragmented red cells (schistocytes, see Figure 4.25) may be present.

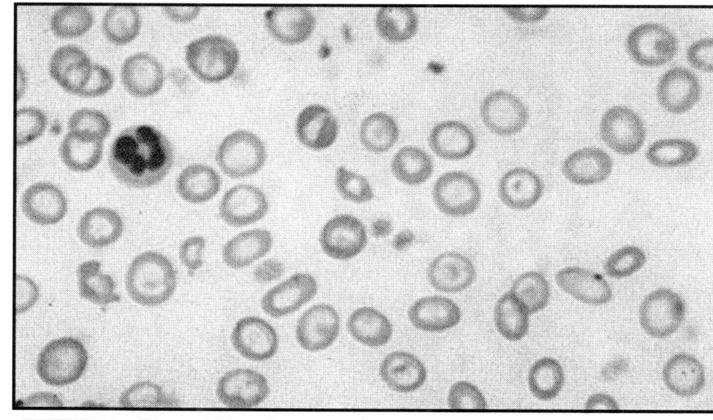

4.14 Blood film from a dog with severe iron-deficiency anaemia with numerous leptocytes. These are very pale, with a wide area of central pallor and a thin rim of haemoglobin but do not appear to have a reduced diameter (they have reduced mean cell volume because they are thin/flat). (May–Grünwald Giemsa stain; original magnification X1000.)

In summary, the clinicopathological features of chronic blood loss/iron-deficiency anaemia are:

- Microcytic hypochromic anaemia with hypochromic leptocytes seen on blood film
- Low plasma protein with severe blood loss
- Thrombocytosis
- Reticulocyte count increased initially, then falls as animal becomes iron-deficient.

These findings should prompt a search for external blood loss. Chronic external blood loss may result from blood loss into the gastrointestinal (GI), urogenital or respiratory tract, or from the skin surface (e.g. in severe flea infestation). GI bleeding is the most common cause of iron-deficiency anaemia in dogs and may be due to ulceration, parasitism, neoplasia or inflammatory bowel disease (Ristic and Stidworthy, 2002). Urogenital bleeding may be due to neoplasia, chronic infections/inflammatory conditions or idiopathic renal haemorrhage. Respiratory tract bleeding may be due to nasal or pulmonary haemorrhage, most often caused by neoplasia. Blood can be coughed up and swallowed, thus mimicking GI haemorrhage. The source of bleeding may be evident from the clinical history (e.g. melaena, haematuria, lice or flea infestation). Otherwise, urinalysis and faecal occult blood tests should be carried out. The patient should be on a meat-free diet for at least 3 days before performing the faecal occult blood test, since myoglobin (present in meat) cross reacts with haemoglobin in the test. Faecal analysis for endoparasitism, and/or imaging (ultrasonography and contrast radiography) of the GI or urogenital tract may be useful in determining the site of blood loss.

Anaemia of chronic inflammatory disease (AID, see later) usually leads to a mild to moderate normocytic normochromic non-regenerative anaemia, but occasionally leads to microcytic normochromic or microcytic hypochromic anaemia due to reduced iron availability. This can be confused with iron-deficiency anaemia. A severe microcytic hypochromic anaemia (PCV <20%) is almost certainly due to iron deficiency, but, if the anaemia is mild or moderate, evaluation of iron stores is useful to distinguish iron-deficiency anaemia and AID (Figure 4.15). Iron stores may be assessed by measuring serum iron, serum ferritin, total iron binding capacity (TIBC), percentage transferrin saturation and bone marrow haemosiderin stores.

PCV	Iron stores	Type of anaemia
<20%: severe anaemia		Iron-deficiency anaemia
>20%: mild to moderate anaemia	Low serum iron Low total iron-binding capacity High bone marrow iron High percentage transferrin saturation	Anaemia of inflammatory disease
>20%: mild to moderate anaemia	Low serum iron Normal or high total iron-binding capacity Low bone marrow iron Low percentage transferrin saturation	Iron-deficiency anaemia

4.15 Role of iron stores in microcytic hypochromic anaemia in distinguishing anaemia of chronic inflammatory disease from iron-deficiency anaemia.

Serum iron: Serum iron measures the total amount of iron bound to both transferrin and ferritin. However, the amount of ferritin–iron in serum is very small unless ferritin is markedly increased (e.g. occasionally in hepatic damage or malignant histiocytosis (Newlands *et al.*, 1994)), so serum iron generally reflects iron bound to transferrin. Iron within haemoglobin is not detected by this test.

Serum iron concentration is low in iron-deficiency anaemia, AID and with acute and chronic inflammatory reactions (due to sequestration of iron within macrophages in the liver, spleen and marrow) and in dogs with portosystemic shunts.

Ferritin: Ferritin concentrations in the serum correlate well with body iron stores and so are low in iron-deficiency anaemia and normal in AID. However, ferritin is an acute phase protein reactant, and so can increase with acute inflammation. Ferritin is measured using immunoassays, which are unfortunately not routinely available for use in the dog and cat.

Total iron-binding capacity: TIBC is an indirect measurement of transferrin. The patient's serum sample is flooded with excess iron, which binds to all the available binding sites on transferrin. The unbound iron is then removed by chemical methods and the iron concentration in the remaining sample is evaluated. The amount of iron measured is proportional to the amount of transferrin present. TIBC is low in AID and also with severe liver disease (due to reduced production of transferrin), but it is normal in dogs and cats with iron-deficiency anaemia (it is elevated in most other species with iron deficiency).

Percentage transferrin saturation: This is calculated by dividing the serum iron concentration by the TIBC and is an indicator of the percentage of transferrin binding sites which are occupied by iron. In normal animals this is approximately 33%; it is reduced in iron-deficiency anaemia and increased in AID.

Bone marrow haemosiderin stores: Haemosiderin stores can be assessed by staining a bone marrow aspirate with Prussian blue. Haemosiderin in seen as blue aggregates within macrophages. This is the most accurate method of assessing body iron stores in dogs, but is an invasive procedure. If there is stainable iron in the bone marrow, this rules out iron deficiency as a cause for anaemia (Stone and Freden, 1990). Stainable iron is not present in normal cat bone marrow (Harvey, 2001).

Haemolytic anaemia

There are many causes of haemolysis, but the most important in dogs and cats are:

- Immune-mediated haemolytic anaemia (IMHA) (primary or secondary)

- Heinz body/eccentrocyte anaemia due to oxidative damage
- Microangiopathic haemolytic anaemia, e.g. associated with haemangiosarcoma
- Feline leukaemia virus (FeLV) infection
- *Mycoplasma haemofelis* (*Haemobartonella felis*) infection
- *Babesia canis* infection
- Malignant histiocytosis (discussed later in non-regenerative anaemia)
- Inherited red cell defects
- Severe hypophosphataemia.

Haemolytic anaemia results in regenerative anaemia, and the response is usually more marked than that seen following haemorrhage because iron is more readily utilizable. Depending on the cause, the red cells may be destroyed intravascularly or extravascularly, or both.

In extravascular haemolysis, damaged red cells are phagocytosed by macrophages, mainly in the spleen, and to some extent in the liver and bone marrow. The anaemia usually has an insidious onset (days to weeks) and may be mild or severe.

In intravascular haemolysis, red cells are lysed within the circulation as a consequence of direct membrane damage. The anaemia is acute in onset (hours to days) and is severe. Free intravascular haemoglobin from lysed red cells immediately forms a complex with haptoglobin; this complex is cleared from the circulation by hepatocytes and macrophages, and within these cells haemoglobin is broken down to bilirubin. Accumulating haemoglobin/haptoglobin complexes result in haemoglobinaemia (pink plasma). When the supply of haptoglobin becomes saturated, free haemoglobin accumulates in the plasma and haemoglobinaemia worsens. Free haemoglobin is able to pass through the glomerular barrier resulting in haemoglobinuria and associated renal tubular damage.

Jaundice may be seen with both forms of haemolysis, if it is acute and/or severe. Haemoglobin is broken down within macrophages (and hepatocytes following intravascular haemolysis) to form unconjugated bilirubin, iron and amino acids. Iron and amino acids are recycled for future erythropoiesis. Unconjugated bilirubin is released from the macrophages and transported to the liver where it is taken up, conjugated and excreted in the bile. The rate-limiting step in this process is the excretion of conjugated bilirubin into bile. If this limit is exceeded, conjugated bilirubin backs up in hepatocytes and spills out into the circulation where it competes with unconjugated bilirubin for uptake by hepatocytes. Thus both forms of bilirubin are increased in the plasma. Initially unconjugated bilirubin predominates but, with time, the proportion of conjugated bilirubin increases, and may become the predominant form, especially if there is concurrent liver damage (e.g. due to hypoxia). The renal threshold for bilirubin excretion is low, especially in dogs, and so relatively minor increases in plasma bilirubin result in bilirubinuria. Thus bilirubinuria is generally detected before tissue jaundice.

Immune-mediated haemolytic anaemia

Immune-mediated haemolytic anaemia (IMHA) is a common cause of haemolytic anaemia in dogs (especially bitches) but is less common in cats. Cocker Spaniels, English Springer Spaniels, Poodles, Old English Sheepdogs and Collie breeds are predisposed. The absence of dog erythrocyte antigen 7 has been reported to be associated with an increased risk of IMHA in Cocker Spaniels (Miller *et al.*, 2004). In dogs, 60–75% cases are primary (idiopathic) and are sometimes termed autoimmune haemolytic anaemia. IMHA may also be secondary to certain drugs (e.g. potentiated sulphonamides, cephalosporins, non-steroidal anti-inflammatory drugs), neoplasia (Mellanby *et al.,* 2004), systemic lupus erythematosus and infections, such as babesiosis, ehrlichiosis or localized bacterial infections (e.g. subacute endocarditis). There are conflicting reports regarding the association of IMHA with vaccination (Duval and Giger, 1996). Primary IMHA is much less common in the cat but secondary IMHA may be induced by haemotrophic *Mycoplasma* (formerly *Haemobartonella*) infections, FeLV infection, lymphoproliferative diseases, transfusion with blood of inappropriate blood group, and certain drugs.

Pathophysiology and laboratory findings: In IMHA the animal produces antibodies (most commonly IgG but sometimes IgM or occasionally IgA) directed against its own red cells. In severe cases, high levels of complement-fixing antibody (usually IgM) are present on the red cell surface, leading to severe membrane damage; extracellular water leaks into the cell leading to swelling and rupture within the circulation (Figure 4.16). The result is intravascular haemolysis and the anaemia is acute and severe.

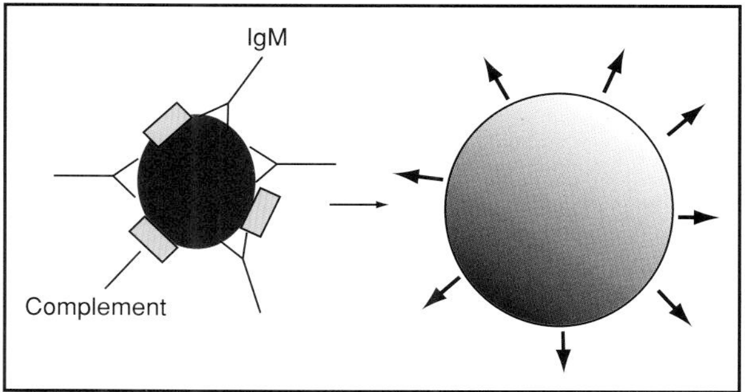

4.16 Intravascular haemolysis. Large amounts of antibody on the red cell surface lead to complement fixation, damage to the red cell membrane and movement of water into the cell, causing swelling and lysis.

Erythrogram changes: Erythrocyte ghosts may be seen on the blood film as pale-staining 'empty' cells. In less severe cases the surface antibody (usually IgG) is recognized by the Fc receptor on macrophages in the spleen (and to a lesser extent in the liver), and the entire cell is phagocytosed, resulting in extravascular haemolysis (Figure 4.17). Sometimes only part of the cell membrane is phagocytosed and the remaining cell contents are squeezed within a smaller surface area leading to spherocyte formation.

Spherocytes are spherical in shape, and on blood films they appear smaller than normal red cells with darker/denser cytoplasm lacking central pallor (Figure 4.18). Care should be taken to look in the examination area monolayer and avoid looking at the tail of the smears where cells are flattened and lose their normal central pallor, giving the false impression of spherocytes. Spherocytes are difficult to see in cat blood because normal feline red cells have minimal or no central pallor. Spherocytes are less flexible than normal red cells and so become sequestered in the liver or spleen leading to accelerated erythrophagocytosis. They are regarded as diagnostic for IMHA in dogs, and often very large numbers are seen (30–40% or more). Small numbers of spherocytes may be seen with zinc toxicosis, oxidative damage and neoplasia.

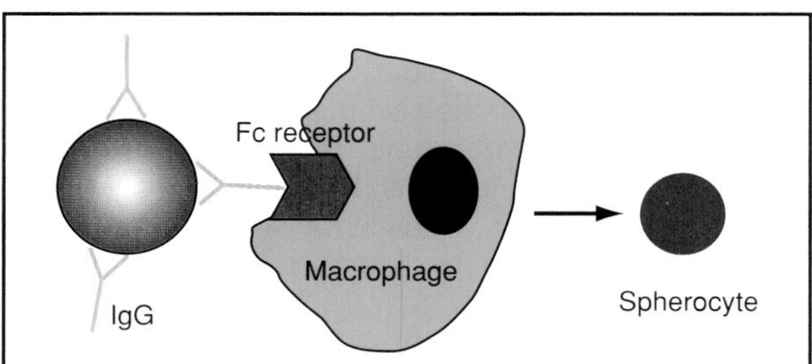

4.17 Extravascular haemolysis. Antibody Fc receptors on macrophages bind to the antibody on the red cell surface, leading to phagocytosis of the red cell. Phagocytosis of a portion of the red cell membrane leads to formation of spherocytes.

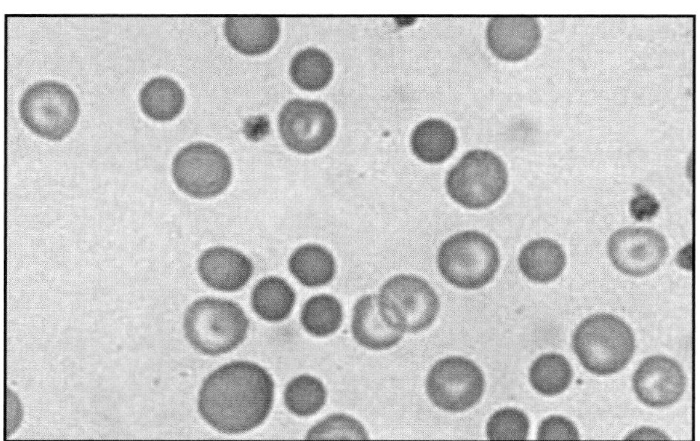

4.18 Blood film from a 4-year-old female Cocker Spaniel with IMHA. Numerous spherocytes are seen, which are smaller and denser than normal red cells and lack central pallor. (May–Grünwald–Giemsa; original magnification X1000.)

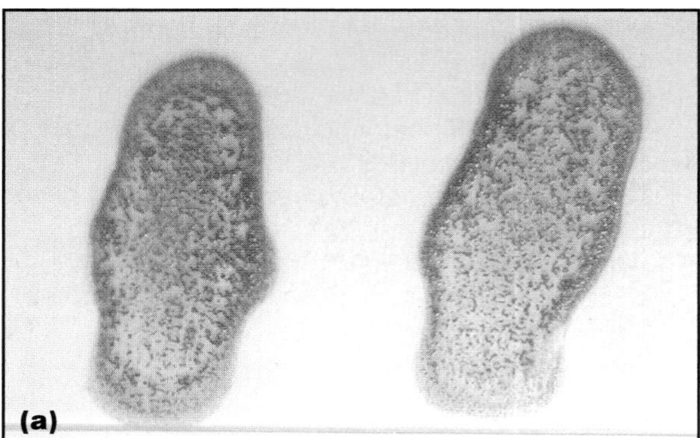

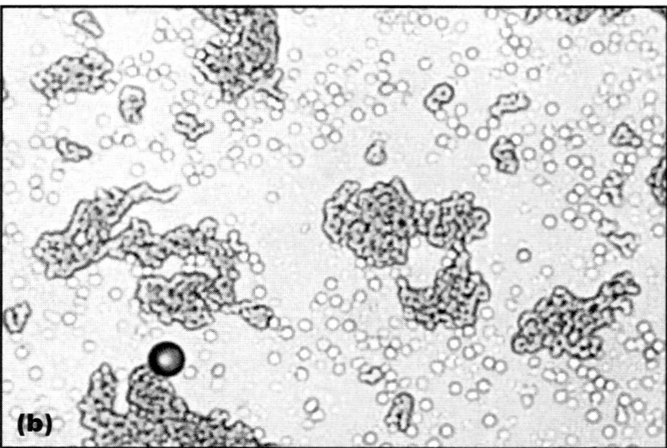

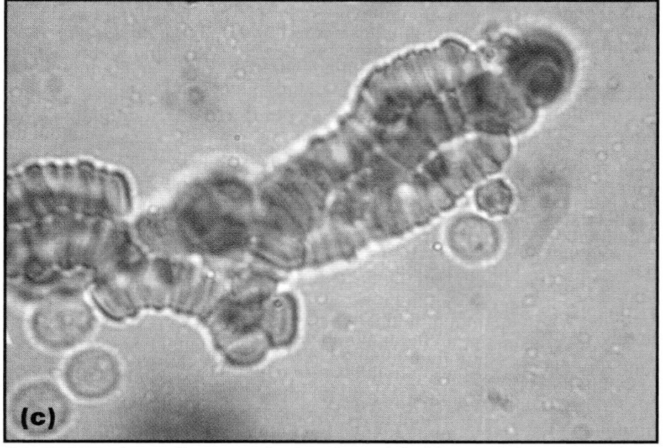

4.19 In-saline agglutination. (a) After mixing equal volumes of blood and saline on a slide, large clumps of red cells are seen. This should be confirmed by examining microscopically (b), since occasionally saline fails to break up rouleaux. Agglutination leads to formation of large irregular clumps of red cells. Rouleaux (c) are long chains or stacks of red cells. The unstained slide is examined using the 20X or 40X objective, with the condenser lowered.

Autoagglutination: If very high levels of antibody are present, individual antibodies can bind to more than one red cell, causing cells to clump together: this is autoagglutination. Cell clumps sequester in the spleen and liver, leading to accelerated removal and so a higher rate of haemolysis. Autoagglutination may be seen grossly within the sample tube, but is best detected by placing a few drops of blood on a glass slide and adding an equal (or greater) volume of saline. The slide is rocked gently and after 1–2 minutes is examined grossly before a coverslip is added and it is examined microscopically (Figure 4.19).

The addition of saline distinguishes true agglutination from rouleaux formation (stacking of red cells in chains); rouleaux are broken up following the addition of saline. Rouleaux may form in normal animals, especially cats, and often form if there is inflammation and/or hyperglobulinaemia. Some authors advocate serial washing of red cells (up to four times) before assessing for autoagglutination, but this may wash off sufficient erythrocyte-bound antibody to render the test falsely negative and is not recommended (Scott-Moncrieff *et al.*, 2001). Autoagglutination is regarded as being diagnostic for IMHA.

In dogs, most cases of IMHA show extravascular haemolysis leading to a subacute or insidious onset anaemia, which is mild to severe. Spherocytosis is common but autoagglutination is not. The regenerative response is not seen for 2–5 days after the onset but then may be marked. Sometimes this form may present as a persistently non-regenerative anaemia because red cell precursors are phagocytosed before they are released from the bone marrow. IMHA with intravascular haemolysis is much less common, and leads to acute onset, severe anaemia, often with autoagglutination. The prognosis is much more guarded. Haemoglobinaemia and haemoglobinuria are seen only in severe cases and are often transient. Due to the acute onset, animals often present when the anaemia is non-regenerative ('pre-regenerative'). With both extravascular and intravascular forms jaundice is seen only in severe cases, although hyperbilirubinuria is common. Marked or persistent jaundice usually indicates concurrent hepatobiliary disease and has been shown to be a poor prognostic indicator (Klag *et al.*, 1993).

Leucogram changes: In dogs with both forms of IMHA, a moderate to severe neutrophilia (may exceed 50 x 10^9/l) and monocytosis are common. There may be a marked left shift and toxic changes in the neutrophils and bands (see Chapter 5). The mechanism of this leucocytosis is unclear, but may be a consequence of non-specific stimulation of the bone marrow, or secondary to the effects of complement which is increased due to the immune-mediated disease. Leucocytosis may be much more significant, occurring secondary to tissue necrosis arising due to anaemic hypoxia (most frequently hepatic necrosis) or due to infarction caused by thromboembolism. There appears to be an association between the magnitude of the leucocytosis and the severity of necrosis (McManus and Craig, 2001). Necrosis results in release of various cytokines which stimulate granulopoiesis and release of neutrophils from the marrow.

Coagulation abnormalities: Thrombocytopenia occurs in about 65% of cases of IMHA. In less than 20% of patients it is severe (<50 x 10^9/l), with associated clinical signs such as petechial haemorrhages, epistaxis and melaena. This usually reflects concurrent immune-mediated thrombocytopenia (Evans syndrome) (McCullough, 2003). Dogs with IMHA are frequently in a hypercoagulable state at the time of diagnosis and are at risk of developing disseminated intravascular coagulation (DIC) (McCullough, 2003). Coagulation test abnormalities (elevations in activated partial thromboplastin time, prothrombin time, fibrin(ogen) degradation products or D-dimers and reductions in antithrombin III) are also common (Scott-Moncrieff *et al.*, 2001). DIC is recognized in 12–45% of dogs with IMHA and thromboembolism is a common cause of death (Klag et al., 1993; Scott-Moncrieff *et al.*, 2001). Schistocytes may be seen in DIC due to red cell fragmentation (see Figure 4.25).

Biochemical changes: Elevated liver enzymes may reflect hypoxic damage, as discussed above. Azotaemia may be prerenal, or may reflect haemoglobin-induced damage. Fibrinogen is frequently increased and hyperglobulinaemia is not uncommon.

Summary: The clinicopathological features of IMHA are:

- Moderate to severe anaemia, which is initially non-regenerative ('pre-regenerative')
- After 2–3 days becomes regenerative: macrocytic hypochromic with marked polychromasia (3+ or 4+) reflecting marked reticulocytosis. Often the reticulocyte count is >25% and the absolute reticulocyte count is >350 x 10^9/l. The reticulocyte index is generally >3. (Occasionally remains non-regenerative due to intramedullary destruction of reticulocytes)
- Marked anisocytosis due to the presence of large reticulocytes and small spherocytes
- Spherocytes are usually seen (not always). These are difficult to see in the cat
- Autoagglutination in severe cases
- Mild, moderate or severe neutrophilia with left shift and sometimes toxic change
- Plasma proteins normal to slightly increased
- Bilirubin and liver enzymes may be elevated. Bilirubinuria is almost invariably present
- Haemoglobinaemia and haemoglobinuria may be present with intravascular haemolysis.

Confirmatory testing

Coombs' test: The Coombs' test, or direct antibody test (DAT), is used to detect the presence of antibody and/or complement on the surface of red cells. Serial dilutions of Coombs' reagent, which contains species-specific antiglobulin directed against IgM, IgG and complement, is incubated with the patient's washed red cells. The antiglobulin binds with the antibodies/complement on the red cells, resulting in agglutination, which may be seen grossly as small specks of clumped cells suspended in the test well (Figure 4.20). A small amount of the suspension is placed on a microscope slide and examined at low power to confirm agglutination. The maximal dilution at which agglutination takes place is the recorded result. There is no clear association between the titre and disease severity, although low titre results are more commonly due to secondary rather than primary IMHA (Day, 2000). The test is performed at 37°C, but should also be performed at 4°C, since occasionally IgM antibody causing acute onset intravascular haemolysis is detected at 4°C but not (or at a lower titre) at 37°C (Day, 1996 and 2000). However, non-pathogenic cold agglutinins may cause a false positive result (generally at a low titre).

The Coombs' test has rather poor sensitivity, and false negative results have been reported to occur in 10–40% of cases. This may be due to:

- The inherently poor sensitivity of the test (low amounts of antibody on the red cell surface may not be detectable)
- Problems with laboratory technique:
  - Inadequate dilution of the antiglobulin which may lead to the prozone effect (excess antiglobulin in relation to the amount of antibody present inhibits agglutination)
  - Poor antiglobulin storage
  - Performing the test at incorrect temperatures.

False positive results (generally a low titre) may occur due to:

- Non-specific adsorption of antibody on to the red cell surface
- The presence of antibodies attached to organisms or drugs on the red cell surface
- Previous blood transfusion
- The presence of low titres of non-pathogenic cold agglutinins which may be present in healthy dogs and cats.

Therefore, titres < 1:16 should be interpreted with caution. A positive Coombs' test provides supportive evidence for IMHA in animals with appropriate clinical signs and laboratory results, but a positive result should not be used to make a diagnosis by itself. A negative result should not exclude IMHA if signs and laboratory results are consistent with the disease.

Because of the problem of false negative results, other immunological tests have been developed. A direct flow cytometric immunofluorescence assay was found to be highly sensitive and specific and had the additional advantage of being quick and easy to perform (Quigley *et al.*, 2000); however, this test is not commercially available. A cell-enzyme-linked immunosorbent assay (an ELISA-based method) has also been described; this test has good sensitivity but is very time-consuming and, again, is not commercially available (Barker *et al.*, 1993).

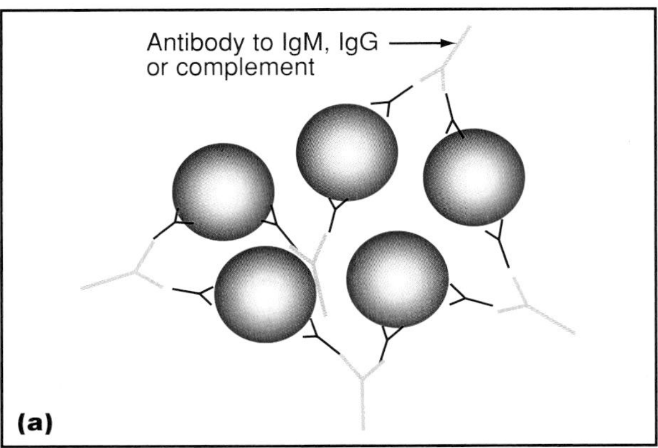

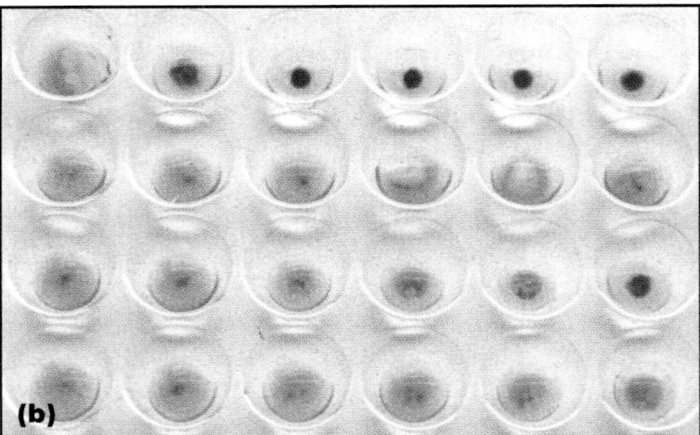

4.20 Coombs' test. (a) Antibody directed against IgM, IgG and complement is incubated with the patient's washed red cells. The antiglobulin binds with the antibodies/complement on the red cells, resulting in agglutination. (b) The test is performed on a microtitre plate, with progressively more dilute antiglobulin. In a positive test, small clumps of red cells remain suspended in the well, whilst in a negative test the red cells sink to the bottom of the well, forming a button.

Other investigations: Since IMHA may be secondary to underlying neoplastic or infectious disease, investigations should be performed to exclude or confirm the presence of an underlying cause. These tests should be tailored to the individual, since blanket testing may be expensive and unrewarding.

In cats, FeLV testing and examination of smears for *Mycoplasma haemofelis* (*Haemobartonella felis*), as well as PCR testing (of EDTA samples) is useful. In dogs, blood film examination and PCR testing may be used to check for babesiosis and ehrlichiosis if there is a history of foreign travel to an endemic area.

Screening radiographs may be useful to screen for underlying neoplasia. The antinuclear antibody (ANA) test is indicated if there are signs of multisystem involvement (e.g. glomerulonephritis, polyarthritis, polymyositis, immune-mediated skin disease) and systemic lupus erythematosus is suspected, but this is very rare. Bone marrow analysis is useful if the anaemia is persistently non-regenerative, or where there is a suspicion of underlying lymphoproliferative disease.

Haemolytic anaemia associated with infections

Important causes of haemolysis in cats are FeLV and *Mycoplasma haemofelis* infections and in dogs, *Babesia canis*. FeLV is discussed under non-regenerative anaemia.

Feline infectious anaemia: This may occur as a primary disease or in combination with another disease process, such as FeLV infection, feline immunodeficiency virus (FIV) infection, feline infectious peritonitis or toxoplasmosis. The causative organism of feline infectious anaemia, formerly called *Haemobartonella felis*, has recently been reclassified following DNA analysis. Two distinct genotypes have been identified: the large form, *Mycoplasma haemofelis*, and the small form, *Candidatus* Mycoplasma haemominutum. *M. haemofelis* is known to be more pathogenic than *M. haemominutum*. Following acute infection the former may cause a severe haemolytic anaemia; the latter results in minimal clinical signs and negligible haematological changes unless there is co-infection with FeLV, when it leads to anaemia and may induce myeloproliferative disease (Foley *et al.*, 1998; George *et al.*, 2002).

These organisms attach themselves to the external surface of the red cell rather than passing into the cytoplasm. Infection with *M. haemofelis* leads to direct red cell membrane damage resulting in mainly extravascular haemolysis, although intravascular haemolysis may also occur. Attachment may also trigger formation of anti-erythrocyte antibodies resulting in secondary IMHA. Following infection, cyclic episodes of parasitaemia, lasting 1–2 days, occur at roughly 6-day intervals. During parasitaemia organisms may be seen in a high proportion of red cells (90% or more), but between episodes parasites are not detectable on blood films. The haematocrit (HCT) fluctuates with the parasitaemia; it may fall sharply to 0.15 l/l or lower with peak parasitaemia, and then rise rapidly, although not to baseline levels. This rise in HCT is not simply due to a regenerative bone marrow response, but also reflects release of red cells from the spleen after removal of parasites from their surface by macrophages (a process known as pitting). Episodes of parasitaemia result in a progressively worsening anaemia. Following recovery, cats remain chronically infected for undetermined period, during which time there is no detectable parasitaemia, although PCR testing is positive. Reactivation of infection may cause clinical disease (Foley *et al.*, 1998).

Laboratory findings: The anaemia is usually highly regenerative (macrocytic and hypochromic with marked reticulocytosis), but may be non-regenerative, reflecting concurrent disease (commonly FeLV infection, which may result in macrocytic normochromic anaemia). Nucleated red cells are commonly seen. Leucocyte counts are variable, and platelets are usually normal. Reticulocyte counts are likely to be unreliable if performed during parasitaemic episodes, since the supravital stains used also stain the organisms. There may be autoagglutination and/or a positive Coombs' test if there is secondary IMHA.

Provided that samples are obtained during an episode of parasitaemia, organisms may be identified using the Romanowsky stains (Giemsa, May–Grünwald Giemsa, Wright's) or with acridine orange. The latter is most sensitive, but requires a fluorescent microscope: the organisms stain bright orange but false positive results may occur due to non-specific fluorescence or staining of Howell–Jolly bodies. The organisms stain blue–grey to pale purple with Romanowsky stains and appear as small cocci, singly or in chains (Figure 4.21).

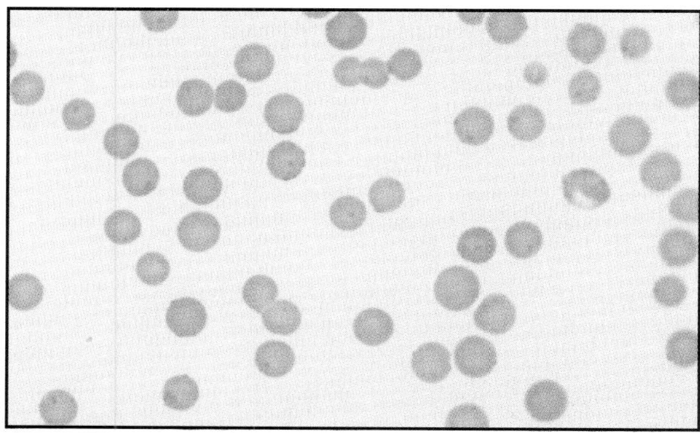

4.21 Blood film from a 5-year-old female Domestic Shorthair cat with anaemia. Single *Mycoplasma* (*Haemobartonella*) organisms are seen at the periphery of many cells. (May–Grünwald–Giemsa stain; original magnification X1000.)

Stain precipitate may be confused with organisms and so stain should be carefully filtered before use. Stain precipitate generally appears as clumps or dots of irregular size and shape, seen both within red cells and between cells. Experimentally, it has been shown that EDTA dislodges parasites from red cells, although the concentration of EDTA used was far greater than that present in EDTA collection tubes (Harvey and Gaskin, 1977). It is prudent either to make smears immediately after sampling with no anticoagulant, or to ensure blood has been in EDTA for no more than 30 minutes prior to making smears. Because of the episodic parasitaemia and the lack of sensitivity of examination, a negative blood film does not exclude FIA and serial films can be examined over a few days. PCR provides a better alternative method of detection and has the added advantage of being able to distinguish *M. haemofelis* and *M. haemominutum* (see Chapter 27). Real-time PCR, which can quantify organism DNA, is now commercially available (Tasker *et al.*, 2003). PCR is positive from 3 days post-infection, becomes negative whilst on antibiotic treatment, and may become positive 3–5 weeks after finishing antibiotic treatment. Following recovery cats remain positive for at least 6 months.

Babesiosis: The causative organisms of babesiosis in dogs are *Babesia canis* and *B. gibsoni*. There are three subtypes of *B. canis*:

- *B. canis* var. *rossi*, which occurs in South Africa and is highly pathogenic, causing severe disease
- *B. canis* var. *canis*, which occurs in Europe and is moderately severe
- *B. canis* var. *vogeli*, which occurs worldwide and is mildly pathogenic.

Babesiosis is not endemic in the UK. It is a tick-borne infection, and the tick vectors are not endemic, but small numbers have been identified close to quarantine kennels. *Babesia* is an intracytoplasmic protozoan parasite that replicates by budding in the red cells. It causes both intravascular and extravascular haemolysis (and thus a regenerative anaemia) and, depending on the strain, can lead to moderate anaemia or marked anaemia with haemoglobinuria, haemoglobinaemia and jaundice. In addition, secondary complications, such as renal, hepatic, respiratory or CNS dysfunction, can arise as a result of an excessive systemic inflammatory response. Thrombocytopenia is very common, arising either due to secondary immune-mediated thrombocytopenia or to DIC. Secondary IMHA may also develop. Dogs are sometimes co-infected with *Ehrlichia*.

In the acute phase of infection, organisms may be seen on the blood film using Romanowsky stains. *B. canis* appears as large pear-shaped organisms, usually in pairs (Figure 4.22). *B. gibsoni* organisms are much smaller, circular bodies. Organisms are more often seen in capillary blood (e.g. from an ear prick) or on smears made from red cells just below buffy coat after centrifugation of a microhaematocrit tube. Organisms are not always visualized, and serology or PCR are more sensitive methods for diagnosis (see Chapter 27).

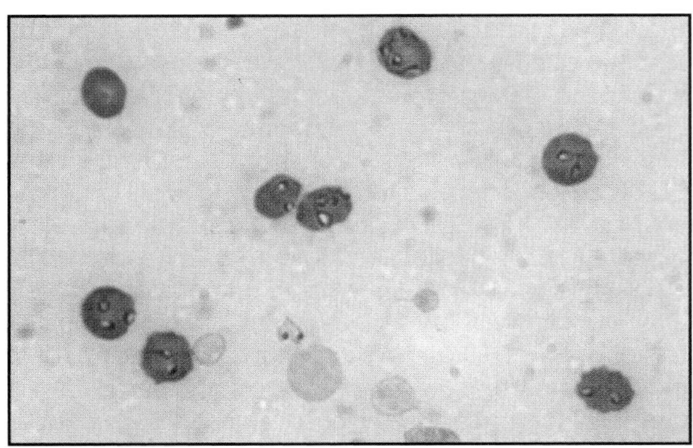

4.22 Blood film from a dog with babesiosis. Budding *Babesia canis* organisms are seen in several red cells. (May–Grünwald Giemsa stain; original magnification X1000.)

Haemolysis caused by oxidative damage

Oxygen is a potent oxidant because it can give rise to highly reactive derivatives, such as hydrogen peroxide and superoxide free radicals. Due to the presence of oxygen within red cells, there is a constant low level of oxidant production. Oxidant damage within the cells is limited by several protective enzymes, such as reduced glutathione, superoxide dismutase and methaemoglobin reductase. When animals are exposed to oxidative toxins, these protective enzymes become overwhelmed and oxidative injury occurs. Oxidants can damage haemoglobin or red cells in three ways:

- Oxidation of the sulphydryl (–SH) groups on the globin chains in haemoglobin results in the formation of Heinz bodies (HBs), aggregates of precipitated haemoglobin attached to the inner erythrocyte membrane. Cats are more susceptible to HB formation because they have eight weak –SH groups on their haemoglobin compared with two in other species
- Direct damage to the red cell membrane results in haemolysis and the formation of eccentrocytes
- Oxidation of the ferrous iron (Fe^{2+}) to ferric iron (Fe^{3+}) in haem molecules results in the formation of methaemoglobin (metHb).

There are numerous substances reported to have caused oxidative damage in dogs and cats, including paracetamol (acetaminophen), onions and zinc. Oxidants may cause all three types of injury or one type may predominate. For example, paracetamol leads to metHb and HB formation but not eccentrocytes. Onions in dogs lead to the formation of HBs and eccentrocytes but not metHb. The reason for these differences is not known.

Heinz body haemolytic anaemia: HB formation has been associated with onion toxicity in both dogs and cats. Onions may be raw, cooked or dried. Onion powder in baby food is the most common source of onion in cats. Other causes of HB haemolytic anaemia include ingested paracetamol, zinc, garlic and naphthalene, application of benzocaine spray or cream to inflamed skin and injection of vitamin K (vitamin K3 and occasionally vitamin K1).

HBs damage red cells by reducing their deformability, leading to entrapment in the sinusoids of the spleen and subsequent extravascular haemolysis. In addition, depletion of SH groups leads to altered membrane permeability, which can result in osmotic swelling of red cells and intravascular haemolysis (Solter and Scott, 1987). Thus HB haemolytic anaemia is characterized by extravascular and sometimes intravascular haemolysis. There is a regenerative anaemia and often a neutrophilia and monocytosis. HBs are seen in a large proportion of the red cells as non-staining round bodies, usually protruding from the surface of the cell (Figure 4.23). HBs may interfere with the spectrophotometric assay for haemoglobin, resulting in an incongruously high Hb (and hence MCHC), with low HCT and RBC reflecting the true severity of the anaemia.

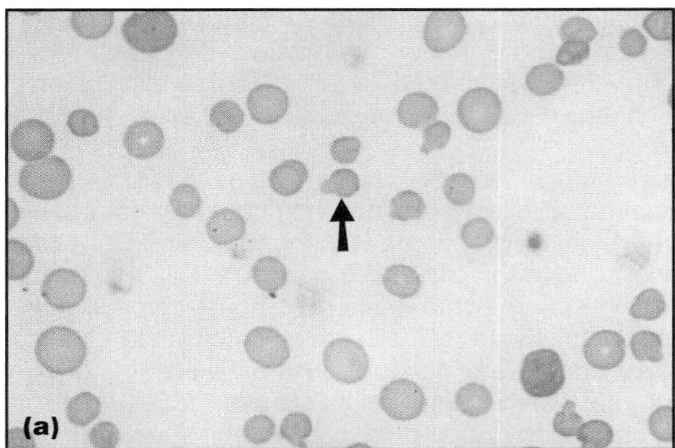

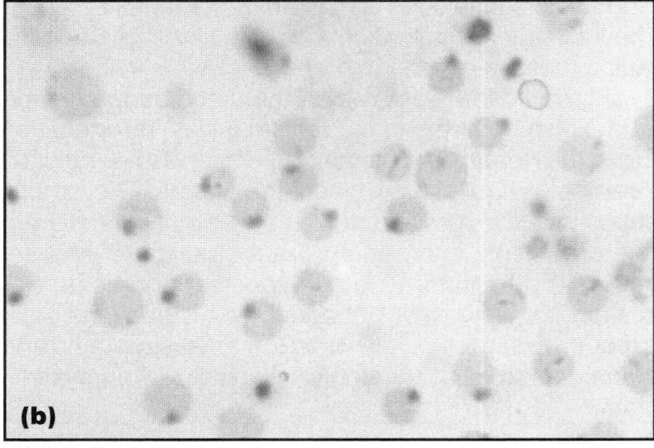

4.23 Blood films from a cat with Heinz body haemolytic anaemia. (a) Using May–Grünwald Giemsa stain, non-staining bodies are seen protruding from the cell membrane (arrowed). (b) On a smear stained with new methylene blue, the Heinz bodies are obvious dark-staining round bodies. (Original magnification X1000.)

In cats HB formation is not always associated with anaemia and low to moderate numbers of HBs may be seen in cats with diabetes mellitus, hyperthyroidism and lymphoma, and after propofol administration. HB formation occurs more readily in cats due to the structure of globin (eight –SH groups) and HBs are seen more frequently because the feline spleen does not contain sinusoids and so is not efficient at removing HBs from the red cell surface.

Oxidative injury leading to direct membrane damage: Zinc and naphthalene (in mothballs) can cause membrane damage and intravascular haemolysis, with minimal or absent Heinz body or MetHb formation, although zinc can also lead to HB formation. Membrane damage may lead to the formation of eccentrocytes, which are red cells in which haemoglobin is displaced to one side of the cell leaving a pale 'empty' area on the other side (Figure 4.24). Again these are less deformable than normal red cells and become entrapped in the spleen and removed by extravascular haemolysis. They are an indicator of severe oxidative injury.

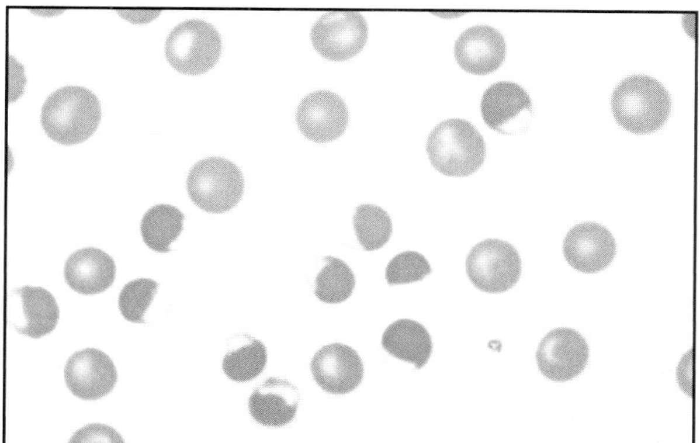

4.24 Blood film from a dog with zinc toxicity, showing large numbers of eccentrocytes with haemoglobin shifted to one side of the cell, leaving the other side clear. (Wright's stain; original magnification X1000.) (Courtesy of Dennis DeNicola.)

Oxidative injury leading to formation of methaemoglobin: In small animals, this is most commonly caused by paracetamol, especially in cats where the toxic dose is very low (usually 50–60 mg/kg). This toxin leads to the formation of metHb and HBs. HB formation leads to haemolysis, but the overriding clinical feature of paracetamol toxicity in cats is the hypoxia associated with metHb, which cannot take up oxygen. Blood appears chocolate-brown when 30–40% of total haemoglobin is in the form of metHb; death occurs when this level exceeds 80%. Methaemoglobinaemia can be readily detected by placing a drop of venous blood on white blotting paper: the spot of blood stays brown whereas normal venous blood would become oxygenated on exposure to air and the spot would turn red.

Haemolysis caused by mechanical damage: microangiopathic haemolytic anaemia

Red cells may become damaged as they pass through abnormal vessels within vascular neoplasms, such as haemangiosarcoma, or when passing through fibrin clots in the circulation in DIC. This mechanical damage results in the formation of schistocytes and/or acanthocytes which are subsequently phagocytosed in spleen, leading to anaemia (Figure 4.25). The anaemia is usually mild, unless there is concurrent haemorrhage (e.g. from a neoplasm). Schistocytes are commonly found in association with splenic lesions, classically with haemangiosarcoma, but also with benign lesions, such as haemangiomas and haematomas; the presence of

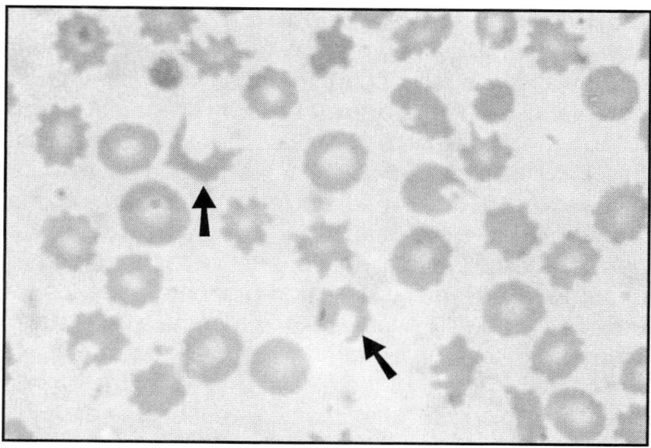

4.25 Blood smear from an 8-year-old German Shepherd Dog with a splenic mass, showing schistocytes (arrowed). (May–Grünwald Giemsa stain; original magnification X1000.)

schistocytes or anaemia should not be used as a predictor of malignancy when splenic lesions are detected (Elders and Blackwood, 2003).

Inherited red cell defects

Inherent metabolic defects, most frequently red cell enzyme deficiencies, have been reported in certain breeds. The defect leads to membrane damage with consequent extravascular haemolysis and anaemia.

Red cell pyruvate kinase deficiency occurs in Basenjis, West Highland White Terriers, Cairn Terriers, Miniature Poodles and Abyssinian, Somali and Domestic Shorthair cats. In dogs the anaemia is highly regenerative and moderate to severe and there is progressive development of myelofibrosis and osteosclerosis, leading to death between 1 and 5 years of age. Affected cats have a mild to moderate (sometimes intermittent) anaemia and may live to an advanced age.

Red cell phosphofructokinase (PFK) deficiency occurs in English Springer Spaniels. The defect leads to energy depletion in red cells, causing low-grade red cell loss. There is a marked regenerative response which may completely compensate for red cell loss, maintaining the PCV within the normal range. The defect also causes red cells to have marked alkaline fragility. Hyperventilation during strenuous exercise or excessive barking can lead to alkalosis and consequent intravascular haemolysis: a haemolytic crisis associated with severe anaemia, jaundice and haemoglobinuria may ensue. PFK-deficient dogs may have a normal lifespan if alkalosis-inducing situations are avoided.

Both these diseases can be identified using a PCR-based DNA test.

Hypophosphataemia

Hypophosphataemia may arise in small animals following commencement of insulin therapy for diabetes mellitus and following tube feeding of anorexic cats with hepatic lipidosis ('refeeding syndrome'). Low phosphate concentrations cause depletion of adenosine triphosphate (ATP), increased red cell rigidity and haemolysis.

Non-regenerative anaemia

Non-regenerative anaemia may be due to primary bone marrow disease, secondary to underlying inflammatory or metabolic disease or may be 'pre-regenerative', due to acute red cell loss before the regenerative response has become established. The pre-regenerative anaemia will have developed acutely and so the animal shows marked clinical signs, such as tachycardia, weakness and exercise intolerance, relative to the degree of anaemia. Conversely, truly non-regenerative anaemia develops gradually over weeks to months as a result of progressive loss of the already circulating red cells as they reach the end of their lifespan. The animal undergoes physiological adaptation to anaemia and shows relatively mild clinical signs for the degree of anaemia. Primary bone marrow disorders lead to moderate to severe anaemia, whilst anaemia of chronic disease leads to mild to moderate anaemia (PCV generally not less than 24% in dogs and 20% in cats).

Primary bone marrow disorders

Important causes of primary bone marrow disease are aplastic pancytopenia (aplastic anaemia), leukaemia, myelophthisis, pure red cell aplasia, myelofibrosis, myelodysplastic syndrome (MDS) and FeLV infection. In addition to the sometimes severe anaemia, there may be depression of other cell lines and, depending on the cause, atypical circulating cells. Severe iron deficiency leads to non-regenerative anaemia and is discussed above.

Aplastic pancytopenia (aplastic anaemia): Aplastic pancytopenia results from damage to stem cells or marrow microenvironment leading to bone marrow failure. The frequently used term, aplastic anaemia, is confusing since all cells lines are affected, not just the red cells. Marrow damage may be caused by infections, drugs, toxins or by immune-mediated mechanisms, or may be idiopathic. In the acute form of the disease, destruction of progenitor and dividing cells leads to leucopenia/neutropenia and thrombocytopenia within 5 days and 8–10 days, respectively. Anaemia develops more gradually due to the long red cell lifespan. Bone marrow aspiration reveals a mix of necrotic lysing cells, macrophages and stromal cells. Depending on the cause, the bone marrow may recover and be repopulated, usually within 3 weeks of the original marrow injury, or the disease may progress to the chronic form. In the chronic form the stem cell damage is irreversible, and the red marrow is replaced by fat, leading to neutropenia, thrombocytopenia and moderate to severe anaemia. Causes of aplastic anaemia are summarized in Figure 4.26.

Infections
Canine and feline parvovirus (R) *Ehrlichia canis* (R/I) FIV (I) FeLV (I)
Drugs
Oestrogens (R/I) Meclofenamic acid (I) Griseofulvin (R) Chemotherapy (R) Phenylbutazone (I) Trimethoprim/sulphonamide (R)
Idiopathic (I)
Immune-mediated (R/I)
Endogenous oestrogen (R/I)

4.26 Causes of aplastic anaemia. R, may be reversible; I, irreversible.

Oestrogen toxicity: The dog is very susceptible to the myelotoxic effects of oestrogen, either when given for urinary incontinence or as misalliance therapy, or when released from a testicular tumour, although there is wide individual variation. Toxicity can be due to an overdose of administered oestrogen, but may also occur as an idiosyncratic reaction to a therapeutic dose. In the early stages there is a neutrophilia, which may be marked, with a left shift and a thrombocytopenia. The latter may lead to spontaneous bleeding and associated anaemia. Within 2–3 weeks there is a neutropenia, continuing thrombocytopenia and a non-regenerative anaemia develops. Clinical signs relate to thrombocytopenia (petechial haemorrhages, melaena etc.) and neutropenia (pyrexia and sepsis), as well as the anaemia (lethargy and pallor).

Pure red cell aplasia and non-regenerative IMHA: These conditions are both characterized by immune-mediated destruction of red cell precursors in the bone marrow leading to severe non-regenerative anaemia. Other cell lines are unaffected. In primary pure red cell aplasia (PRCA) there is depletion of the entire red cell series due to selective destruction of the early erythroid precursors. Bone marrow aspiration reveals a complete absence of erythroid cells, or very small numbers of proerythroblasts and early normoblasts (the earliest precursors). Granulocytic, monocytic and platelet precursors are present in normal to increased numbers. Plasma cells and small lymphocytes may be increased, especially in cats, where lymphocytes constitute up to 45% of total marrow cells (Stokol, 1999). In non-regenerative IMHA, red cell destruction takes place at a later stage, commonly at the late normoblast stage or reticulocyte stage. There are normal to increased erythroid cells in the bone marrow, but with a maturation arrest at the intermediate or late normoblast stage (i.e. cells appear to mature normally to the intermediate or late normoblast stage, but late normoblasts or and/or polychromatic red cells (reticulocytes), respectively, are absent or reduced in number). In some cases there are numerous marrow macrophages containing haemosiderin or phagocytosed red cells/normoblasts reflecting intramedullary destruction (Figure 4.27). Marrow plasma cells and lymphocytes may be increased. In both diseases spherocytes are occasionally seen, although the Coombs' test is less commonly positive (Weiss, 2002). Iron stores are normal to increased. Immunosuppressive therapy (as for IMHA) is often effective.

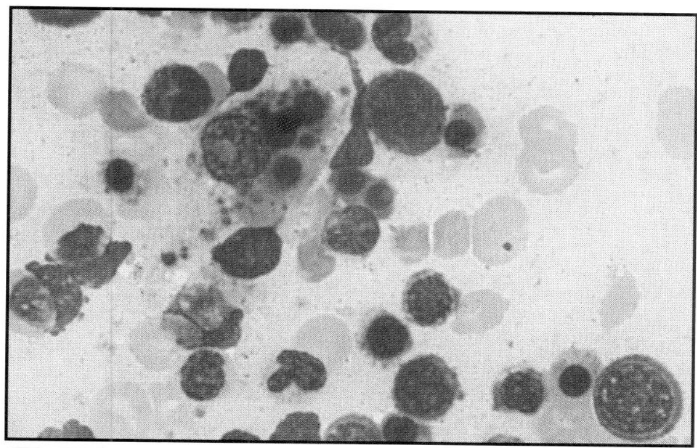

4.27 Bone marrow aspirate from a dog with non-regenerative IMHA. There are numerous red cell precursors and a macrophage containing haemosiderin and phagocytosed normoblasts. (May–Grünwald–Giemsa stain; original magnification X1000.)

Secondary PRCA occurs in association with human recombinant erythropoietin therapy, parvovirus infection and in cats infected with FeLV subgroup-C. FeLV-induced PRCA is progressive, invariably fatal, and does not lead to increased numbers of lymphocytes in the bone marrow.

Leukaemia/myelophthisis: Leukaemia is characterized by neoplastic transformation of haemopoietic precursor cells of one cell line in the bone marrow, leading to clonal expansion of the affected cell line and, usually, release of large numbers of neoplastic cells into the circulation (see Chapter 5). The bone marrow becomes crowded out by the neoplastic cells, leading to suppression of normal haemopoiesis (Figure 4.28). The neoplastic cells compete for nutrients and also may release inhibitory substances, all adding to the suppression. The result is anaemia, neutropenia and thrombocytopenia, together with circulating atypical (leukaemic) cells. In acute leukaemia, in which the cells do not undergo differentiation but remain at a primitive blast stage, the neoplastic infiltrate develops rapidly and those cell lines with the shortest circulating time (neutrophils and platelets) become depleted first. Anaemia develops more slowly, and may not have developed at the time of first presentation in very acute cases. In chronic leukaemia the neoplastic cells undergo differentiation within the bone marrow and the neoplastic infiltrate develops more slowly. Bone marrow suppression is much less marked and may be confined to a mild to moderate, non-regenerative anaemia, sometimes with a mild thrombocytopenia.

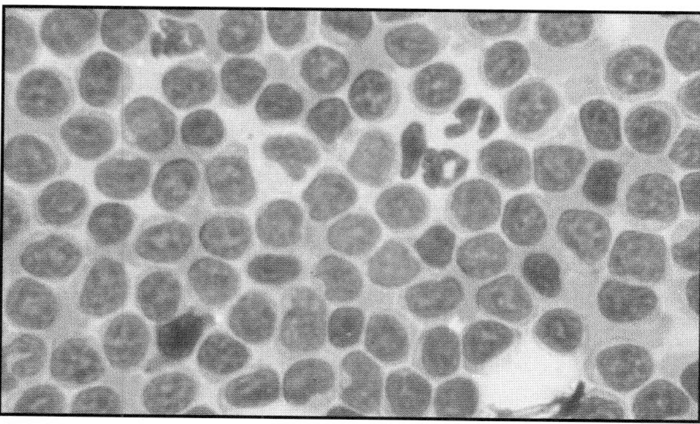

4.28 Bone marrow aspirate from a dog with acute lymphoid leukaemia. The marrow is effaced by lymphoblasts. (May–Grünwald–Giemsa stain; original magnification X1000.)

Myelophthisis refers to an infiltration of the bone marrow with non-haemopoietic neoplastic cells, for example metastasis of carcinoma/adenocarcinoma or, less commonly, sarcoma. As with leukaemia, a pancytopenia may develop.

Malignant histiocytosis and erythrophagocytic disorders: A less common neoplastic cause of anaemia is malignant histiocytosis (MH) which occurs in dogs, especially Bernese Mountain Dogs and Golden Retrievers; it is rare in cats (Kraje *et al.*, 2001). MH is a systemic, neoplastic proliferation of histiocytic cells. These are antigen-presenting cells, which arise in the bone marrow and, in health, are found in the skin, mucosal surfaces, various organs and lymph nodes. The neoplastic histiocytes may infiltrate the spleen, liver, lung, lymph nodes, skin and bone marrow. The latter leads to anaemia and sometimes depression of other cell lines, most commonly platelets. The anaemia may be regenerative or non-regenerative and is not simply due to bone marrow crowding, but also due to erythrophagocytosis by the histiocytic cells. Leucophagia occurs much less commonly. The cells are found in clusters or sheets and are large with moderate abundant foamy or vacuolated cytoplasm, and large round pleomorphic nuclei containing coarse chromatin and pale nucleoli (Figure 4.29). Binucleate or multinucleate cells may be present (Moore and Rosin, 1986; Dunn *et al.*, 1995).

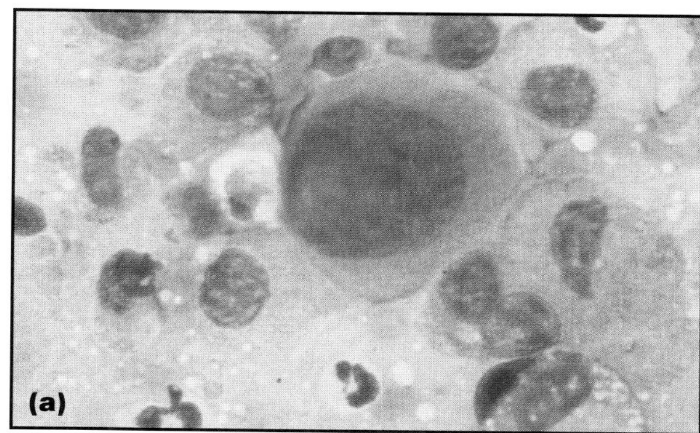

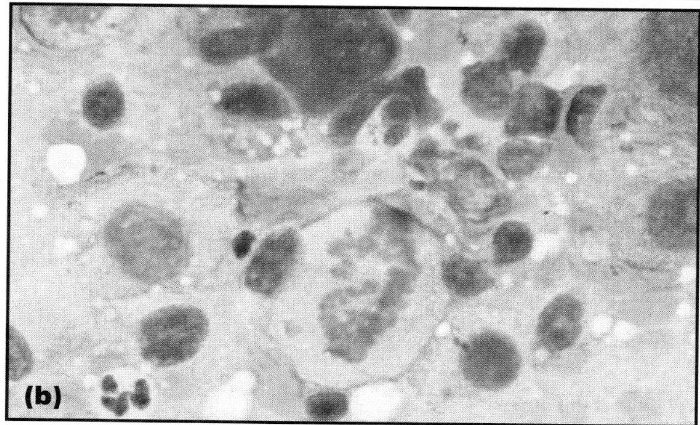

4.29 Bone marrow aspirate from a Bernese Mountain Dog with malignant histiocytosis. (a) There are large atypical histiocytic cells showing marked anisocytosis. (b) An atypical mitotic figure is seen. (May–Grünwald–Giemsa stain; original magnification X1000.)

Increased numbers of erythrophagocytic macrophages may be seen in non-regenerative IMHA (see above). These macrophages resemble the histiocytic cells in MH, but are less pleomorphic, and are present in smaller numbers as either single cells or in small clusters. In addition, MH involves multiple organs whilst the macrophages in non-regenerative IMHA are confined to the bone marrow, thus the two diseases can be differentiated. The prognosis for MH is very poor.

A third disease leading to erythrophagocytic macrophages in the bone marrow is haemophagocytic syndrome (haemophagic histiocytosis). This is a benign proliferation of histiocytes, occurring secondary to infectious, neoplastic or metabolic diseases, resulting in cytopenias of at least two cell lines: anaemia and thrombocytopenia, anaemia and neutropenia or pancytopenia may occur (Walton *et al.*, 1996). Although the cytopenias are potentially reversible if the underlying disease is treated, generally the prognosis is poor.

Myelofibrosis: In this disease the normal haemopoietic tissue is replaced with proliferating fibroblasts and associated reticulin and collagen fibres. Fibroblast proliferation may be due to a primary myeloproliferative disease, but more commonly is secondary to an underlying cause, such as IMHA, pure red cell aplasia, neoplasia (within or outside the bone marrow), toxic marrow damage and the inherited red cell defect, pyruvate kinase deficiency (see above). Deposition of fibrous tissue results in reduced haemopoiesis, especially reduced erythropoiesis. The result is severe non-regenerative anaemia, sometimes thrombocytopenia, but rarely leucopenia. Bone marrow aspiration results in a 'dry tap' and a core biopsy is required to make a diagnosis (Figure 4.30).

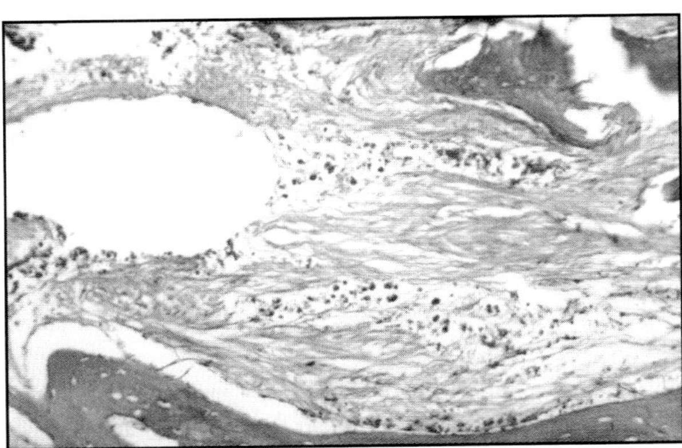

4.30 Bone marrow core biopsy stained with reticulin from a dog with myelofibrosis. There are numerous black-staining collagen fibres replacing the normal haemopoietic tissue. (Reticulin stain; original magnification X200.)

Myelodysplastic syndrome (MDS): This comprises a heterogenous group of diseases, characterized by abnormal development of haemopoietic precursors, leading to atypical (dysplastic) changes in erythroid, granulocytic or megakaryocytic cell lines and peripheral cytopenias (Figure 4.31) (see also Chapter 5). There is usually a bicytopenia or pancytopenia, although only anaemia is seen in one form of MDS, MDS-refractory anaemia. In MDS-refractory anaemia, dysplastic changes are confined to the erythroid line and this condition appears to have a fair prognosis; other forms of MDS appear refectory to therapy and are associated with short survival times. MDS may progress to acute myeloid leukaemia. Most cats with MDS are infected with FeLV. Secondary MDS may occur in association with an underlying cause, such as lymphoma, IMHA, immune-mediated thrombocytopenia, myelofibrosis and drugs, including cephalosporins and vincristine; it may be reversible once the underlying cause is removed (Weiss and Aird, 2001).

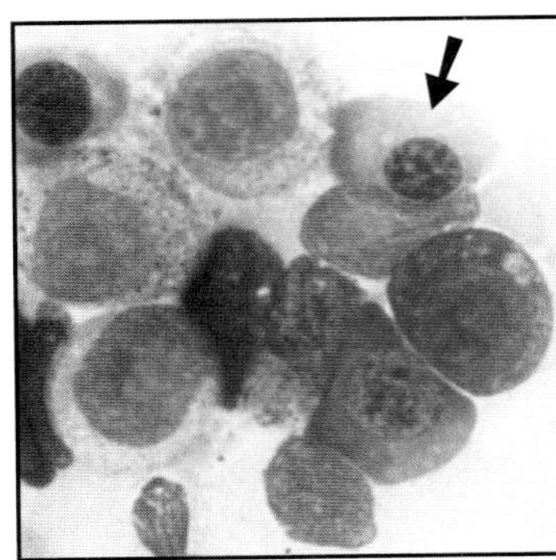

4.31 Bone marrow aspirate from a cat showing megaloblastic change of the red cell precursors. The normoblasts have immature nuclei with abundant, mature cytoplasm (arrowed). (Courtesy of JK Dunn.) (May–Grünwald–Giemsa; original magnification X1000.)

Anaemia and feline leukaemia virus

FeLV may cause anaemia due to several mechanisms:

- Macrocytic non-regenerative anaemia, probably due to a direct myelodysplastic effect of the virus. Nuclear maturation is depressed and so is out of step with haemoglobinization of the cytoplasm, and haemoglobinization is complete before nucleus is mature. The nucleus is extruded before the cell has undergone the usual number of mitotic divisions, resulting in a macrocytic red cell
- Aplastic pancytopenia
- Secondary pure red cell aplasia
- Leukaemia and MDS typically cause anaemia as well as leucopenia and thrombocytopenia
- FeLV-related immunosuppression may lead to infectious or inflammatory diseases which, in turn, may lead to anaemia of chronic disease
- FeLV may also induce haemolytic anaemia by inducing the formation of antibodies directed against virus antigen on the red cell surface.

Anaemia due to nutritional deficiencies

Iron deficiency is the most common nutritional deficiency and is discussed above in chronic blood loss. Severe malnutrition may also cause anaemia, due to combined deficiency of protein, energy, B vitamins and minerals. Folate or cobalamin (Vitamin B12) deficiency may cause anaemia because these vitamins are required for DNA synthesis. The effect of deficiency on erythropoiesis is that nuclear maturation lags behind cytoplasmic maturation and the red cell precursor divides fewer times than usual before the critical amount of haemoglobin accumulates to trigger extrusion of the nucleus. The result is the formation of large red blood cells which contain a normal amount of haemoglobin (macrocytic, normochromic).

Deficiencies of these vitamins are unusual in dogs and cats, but cobalamin deficiency occurs in as an autosomal recessive disorder in Giant Schnauzers due to defective ileal absorption. Affected puppies are stunted, have moderate non-regenerative anaemia (normocytic but with increased RDW and some macrocytic cells present on the blood film) and also neutropenia (again due to defective DNA synthesis). Platelet numbers are usually normal. All these abnormalities resolve following parenteral supplementation with cobalamin. Cobalamin deficiency may occur in cats with exocrine pancreatic insufficiency and severe ileal disease, although does not always lead to anaemia. Folate-deficiency anaemia is very uncommon, despite widespread use of drugs that cause folate depletion, such as phenobarbital.

Anaemia secondary to inflammatory or metabolic disease

Non-regenerative anaemia commonly results from a disease outside the bone marrow. Such diseases can be broadly categorized into anaemia of inflammatory disease (AID), anaemia secondary to endocrine disease and anaemia of chronic renal failure.

Anaemia of inflammatory disease: This is often termed anaemia of chronic (inflammatory) disease, although anaemia may develop quite quickly (within 10 days) in association with many inflammatory disorders, e.g. due to chronic infection, tissue trauma or tissue necrosis associated with malignant neoplasms. The anaemia is mild to moderate (PCV approximately 25–36% in the dog, 19–26 % in the cat) and is rarely clinically significant; clinical signs relate to the underlying cause. There are several mechanisms involved in the development of AID:

- Decreased iron delivery from storage sites to red cell precursors results in a relative iron deficiency
- Shortened red cell survival, possibly due to increased oxidative damage or binding of immunoglobulin to red cell membranes leading to increased clearance by macrophages
- Blunted release of and response to erythropoietin, probably due to the effect of cytokines, such as interleukin 1 and tumour necrosis factor, which are released in inflammation.

The anaemia is usually normocytic and normochromic, although occasionally it is microcytic and hypochromic (due to relative iron deficiency), in which case evaluation of iron stores is useful to distinguish this from true iron deficiency (see Figure 4.15). There is often an inflammatory leucogram and acute phase proteins (such as fibrinogen) as well as globulins may be elevated.

Anaemia secondary to renal failure: Chronic renal failure leads to decreased production of erythropoietin, leading to decreased erythropoiesis, resulting in normocytic, normochromic, non-regenerative anaemia. Other factors contributing to the anaemia include haemorrhage, due to gastric ulceration, and reduction in red cell lifespan, due to uraemic toxins. Unlike other secondary anaemias, the anaemia of renal failure can be severe and cause significant clinical signs. Treatment with recombinant human erythropoietin (rhRPO) increases PCV and improves well-being, but eventually leads to the development of anti-erythropoietin antibodies which block the effects of, not only the administered rhRPO, but also the animal's endogenous erythropoietin. This leads to secondary pure red cell aplasia and severe anaemia. Recombinant canine erythropoietin has recently become available.

Anaemia secondary to endocrine disease: Both cortisol and thyroxine enhance the effects of erythropoietin, so deficiencies in these hormones lead to anaemia. Mild anaemia is often seen in hypothyroidism, and can be considered a physiological adaptation to lowered metabolic rate. Mild to moderate anaemia frequently occurs in dogs with hypoadrenocorticism, although this may be masked by haemoconcentration. GI haemorrhage may occur, in which case a more severe anaemia is seen.

Evaluating non-regenerative anaemia

Bone marrow sampling is indicated in animals with non-regenerative anaemia, once it has been established that the anaemia is truly non-regenerative rather than pre-regenerative, and when underlying causes of secondary anaemia have been ruled out. Renal failure is the main secondary cause of severe non-regenerative anaemia (PCV <20% in dogs, <18% in cats) whilst AID and endocrine disease are unlikely to cause such severe anaemia. Bone marrow may be sampled either by performing a bone marrow aspirate or a core biopsy. Aspirates provide superior cellular detail whilst core biopsies allow evaluation of cellularity and for the presence of fibrous tissue. Often an aspirate and core sample are taken simultaneously as the samples provide complementary information. Other indications for bone marrow sampling are given in Chapter 5.

Bone marrow aspiration: The aspirate is obtained using a 10–20 ml syringe and a Klima needle which has an interlocking stylet. Klima needles are designed for repeated use but must be sharpened regularly. Alternatively, disposable needles can be used several times before they are discarded (these cannot be steam sterilized so require chemical or ethylene oxide sterilization). The needle and syringe can be primed with EDTA solution (obtained by adding 2–3 ml of saline to a 10 ml EDTA tube) prior to sampling.

Sampling sites include the iliac crest, the greater tubercle of the humerus, the tibial crest and the trochanteric fossa of the femur. The usual site for aspiration in the dog is the iliac crest and this is described below. In small dogs and cats the iliac crest is rather narrow and the proximal humerus or the trochanteric fossa of the femur are the preferred sites. Samples from dogs are usually obtained under sedation, whilst general anaesthesia may be preferred in cats.

To obtain a sample from the iliac crest:

1. The dog is positioned in sternal recumbency with the hind legs tucked up alongside the trunk.
2. The skin over the iliac crest is aseptically prepared.
3. A small amount of local anaesthetic is infiltrated into the skin and subcutis over the iliac crest and the needle is then advanced onto the bone which feels hard. Mild pressure is applied to the needle and further local anaesthetic is infiltrated into the periosteum.
4. A small stab incision is made in the skin and the Klima needle is introduced through the subcutis and onto the iliac crest which is stabilized between finger and thumb (Figure 4.32a).
5. The needle is directed ventrally and slightly medially and advanced into the bone cortex by rotating it to and fro whilst applying firm pressure. Once the needle is through the bone cortex it will be firmly lodged in the bone (moving the needle from side to side will move the dog from side to side).
6. The stylet is removed and a 10 or 20 ml syringe is attached to the needle. The marrow is then aspirated by several quite forceful withdrawals of the plunger. (There may be a transient pain response as the marrow is aspirated from conscious animals.)
7. The plunger is released as soon as marrow appears in the syringe and the needle and syringe are removed quickly, as one unit.

A drop of marrow is placed at the top end of several slides which are positioned at a near vertical angle (Figure 4.32b). Blood runs down to the bottom of the slide, whilst the marrow spicules remain on the slide. A smear is made by placing a second slide flat over the first slide at right angles to it. This has the effect of crushing the marrow spicules. The second slide is then drawn across the first slide in a horizontal plane and the smear is produced on the lower surface of the second slide (Figure 4.32c). Smears should be made quickly as the marrow clots rapidly. The smears are allowed to air dry.

If the needle is not completely through the cortex or if has been pushed in too far and is lodged against the far cortex, aspiration will be unsuccessful. The stylet should be replaced and the needle moved accordingly before re-aspirating. If aspiration if still unsuccessful the needle should be withdrawn and a second attempt made, directing the needle in a slightly different direction, e.g. slightly obliquely, or at an alternative site, such as the proximal shaft of humerus. If aspiration is still unsuccessful a bone marrow core biopsy should be performed. Repeated 'dry taps' may be due to myelofibrosis or packing out of the bone marrow by tumour infiltrate.

Evaluation is generally carried out by a clinical pathologist since it requires training and experience. However the clinician should check the quality of the sample by staining one or two smears (e.g. with a rapid dunking stain kit). A good smear contains marrow flecks (spicules) of haemopoietic cells which have spread out to form a monolayer (Figure 4.33). Excessive haemodilution results in poor cell morphology. If no intact spicules are present interpretation is difficult or impossible.

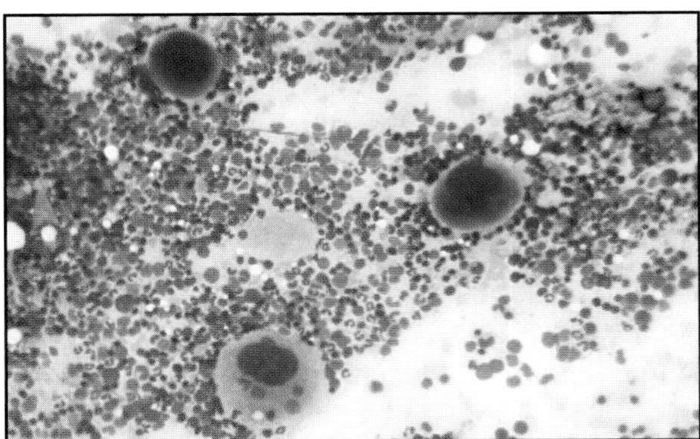

4.33 A good quality bone marrow aspirate. The smear is very cellular and cells have spread into a monolayer without clotting. Three large megakaryocytes are present with large multilobulated nuclei. (May–Grünwald–Giemsa stain; original magnification X1000.)

In normal bone marrow approximately two to six megakaryocytes are seen in a marrow fleck, which occupies most of a low power (X20) field. The myeloid (granulocytic) and erythroid series are examined under high power. The ratio of myeloid:erythroid cells is 0.75–1.5, and there should be a pyramidal arrangement with small numbers of early precursors and larger numbers of maturing cells. The bone marrow of normal dogs contains <15% lymphoid cells (<20% in cats), which are mostly small lymphocytes, and <2% plasma cells. Small numbers of macrophages are present, which may contain phagocytosed cellular debris. Bone marrow cytology is beyond the scope of this chapter but is well described by Harvey (2001).

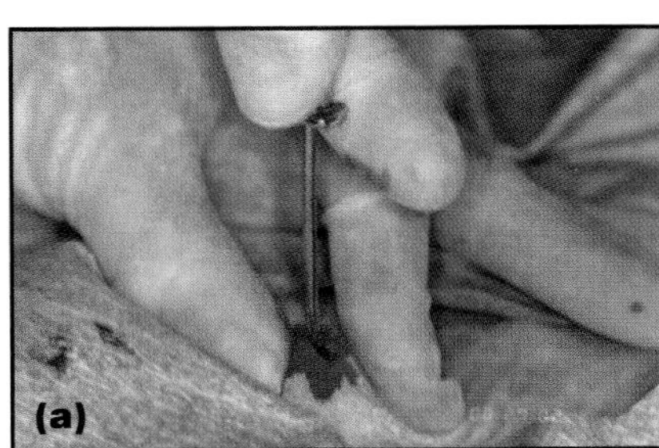

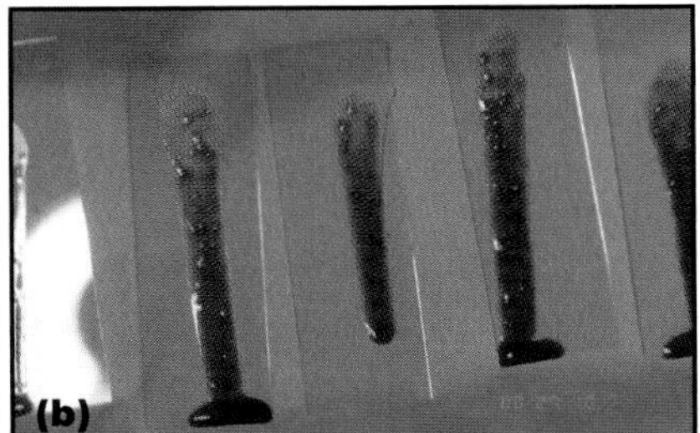

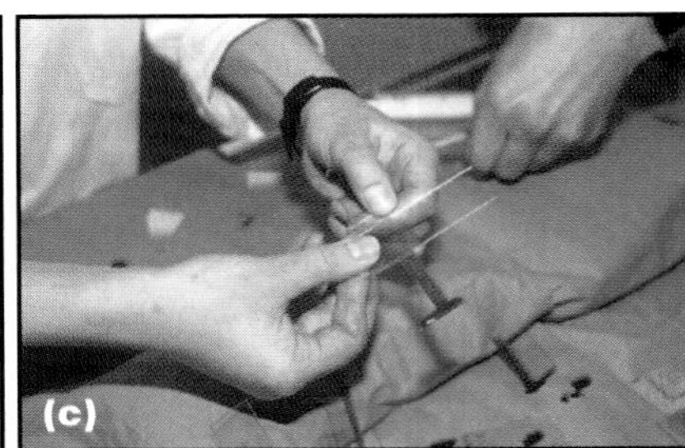

4.32 Bone marrow aspiration. (a) The Klima needle is introduced through the subcutis and on to the iliac crest, which is stabilized between finger and thumb. (b) Drops of marrow are placed at the top of a tilted slide, allowing blood to run off the bottom of the slide but retaining the spicules.(c) Smears are made by placing a second slide over the first slide, thus spreading the spicules, and then smoothly drawing the slides apart.

Bone marrow core biopsy: A Jamshidi needle is used and again the site of choice is the iliac crest in medium to large dogs and usually the trochanteric fossa in cats and small dogs.

1. The needle is inserted through the cortex as described for the aspirate.
2. The stylet is removed and the needle is advanced a further 1–2 cm into the marrow cavity.
3. The needle is then rotated vigorously in one direction to ensure the biopsy sample is sectioned at its base.
4. The needle is removed from the bone and the core is expelled from the top of needle using a blunt probe.
5. The core should be fixed in buffered formalin. The sample must be decalcified prior to sectioning and staining, and this process may take several days.

A core biopsy has the advantage that the architecture of the marrow can be evaluated and cellularity can be accurately assessed. The core biopsy is particularly useful in the diagnosis of aplastic pancytopenia and myelofibrosis.

Erythrocytosis

Erythrocytosis is characterized by an increase in the red cell count, haemoglobin concentration and PCV. It can be classified as relative or absolute. Absolute erythrocytosis is classified as primary (true) or secondary. *Relative erythrocytosis* is caused by disturbances in fluid balance resulting in dehydration. The total red cell mass remains normal but the decrease in plasma volume result is in an increase in the total plasma protein concentration. The term polycythaemia is frequently used to describe increased red cell count, but this implies an increase of several cell lines, not just red cells, and so its use is discouraged.

Primary erythrocytosis

Primary erythrocytosis, also known as polycythaemia rubra vera, is a chronic myeloproliferative disease characterized by clonal proliferation of erythroid precursor cells with maturation and differentiation into morphologically normal red blood cells. This proliferation is not controlled by normal feedback mechanisms and is not driven by erythropoietin. Indeed erythropoietin levels are usually low or undetectable.

Secondary erythrocytosis

This occurs in response to increased erythropoietin secretion, which may be an appropriate compensatory response to chronic hypoxia due to:

- Chronic pulmonary disease
- Right to left cardiovascular shunting, e.g. patent ductus arteriosus, tetralogy of Fallot
- Animals living at high altitude.

Alternatively, the increased levels of erythropoietin may be present without systemic hypoxia, termed inappropriate secondary erythrocytosis. This has been reported in conjunction with renal tumours (carcinoma, adenocarcinoma, fibrosarcoma and lymphoma) and is thought to be the result of local hypoxia within the kidney or secretion of erythropoietin by the tumour. Benign renal cysts and hydronephrosis have also been suggested as causes of inappropriate secondary erythrocytosis. Extra-renal neoplasia is uncommonly associated with erythrocytosis but one case report documented erythrocytosis in a dog with a nasal fibrosarcoma in which the tumour was found to secrete erythropoietin (Couto *et al.*, 1989). In the cat most cases of erythrocytosis are primary, and secondary erythrocytosis is very uncommon, only occurring occasionally in response to hypoxia (Watson *et al.*, 1994). Mild erythrocytosis may occure in association with hyperthyroidism but does not cause clinical signs.

Differentiating causes of erythrocytosis

In relative erythrocytosis clinical examination usually reveals signs of dehydration. In addition, total protein, urea and creatinine are usually elevated. The PCV returns to normal once the dehydration is corrected.

If relative erythrocytosis can be ruled out causes of secondary erythrocytosis should be investigated. Thoracic radiographs and echocardiography are used to assess the cardiopulmonary systems. Arterial blood gases are useful in assessing for hypoxia. The normal partial pressure of oxygen (P_aO_2) is 85–100 mmHg, whilst in cases of physiologically appropriate erythrocytosis the P_aO_2 is significantly reduced (e.g. <60 mmHg). Renal ultrasonography or an intravenous excretory urogram are used to assess for renal neoplasia.

If no secondary cause is identified a presumptive diagnosis of primary erythrocytosis is made. Bone marrow aspiration is not helpful in distinguishing primary and secondary erythrocytosis since in both cases erythroid hyperplasia is present, but the red cells and their precursors are morphologically normal. Measurement of erythropoietin is helpful: erythropoietin is low or low normal in primary erythrocytosis and is usually elevated in secondary erythrocytosis, in particular in animals with renal tumours. However, erythropoietin is not always elevated in secondary erythrocytosis and may be normal in animals with primary erythrocytosis, thus erythropoietin concentrations should never replace a thorough clinical and laboratory evaluation.

Blood typing

Rapid in-house tests are available for blood typing of canine and feline blood. These tests are used prior to blood transfusion and in cats can be used prior to mating to prevent neonatal isoerythrolysis.

In cats there are 3 blood types: A, B and AB. Type A is dominant over AB and B and type AB is dominant over B. Type A is common in the Domestic Shorthair. Type B is common in the British Shorthair and to a lesser extent the Cornish and Devon Rex and Birman breeds. Type AB is very rare. All type B cats have high titre of naturally occurring anti-A isoantibodies. If a type B cat receives a type A blood transfusion a severe life-threatening or fatal transfusion reaction will take place. A proportion of type A cats have naturally occurring anti-B isoantibodies, these lead to mild/delayed transfusion reaction when such a cat is given type B blood. Transfusion reactions can be prevented by ensuring donor and recipient are of the same blood type using in-house test cards (Rapid Vet-H (feline)) which identify blood group using an agglutinating reaction.

In dogs six blood groups, termed dog erythrocyte antigens (DEA), are described: DEA 1.1, 1.2, 3, 4, 5 and 7. More than one DEA may be present in an individual, although if DEA type 1 is present, it is either DEA 1.1 or DEA 1.2. DEA 1.1 is the most potent stimulator of isoantibody production. There are no naturally occurring isoantibodies to DEA 1.1 and so acute transfusion reactions are not seen following a first transfusion, but will occur following subsequent transfusions. There is a low prevalence of naturally occurring isoantibodies to DEA 3, 5 and 7, which can lead to mild, delayed, but not acute transfusions reactions. DEA 4 is present in most dogs and naturally occurring isoantibodies do not occur. Rapid in-house tests cards are available for identifying DEA1.1 (Rapid Vet-H (canine)), but not for other canine blood types. Blood typing and transfusion are discussed in detail in the *BSAVA Manual of Small Animal Haematology and Transfusion Medicine* (2000).

Case examples

Case 1

Signalment

6-year-old, neutered female Labrador.

History and clinical findings

The dog had a history of lethargy, anorexia and depression over the previous 4 days. She had been treated with immunosuppressive doses of prednisolone on the assumption that IMHA was the cause of the clinical signs. The dog's condition had deteriorated and so she was referred to a second clinic. Clinical examination revealed jaundice and mucosal pallor, palpable splenomegaly, tachycardia and tachypnoea.

Clinical pathology data

Haematology	Result	Reference interval
RBC (x 10^{12}/l)	1.46	5.5–8.5
Hb (g/dl)	3.5	12–18
HCT (l/l)	0.105	0.37–0.55
MCV (fl)	72	60–77
MCHC (g/dl)	32	30–36
RDW (%)	22	13–17
Uncorrected reticulocyte percentage (%)	15.8	<1
Absolute reticulocyte count (x 10^9/l)	24	<50
Platelets (x 10^9/l)	175	200–500
Plasma proteins (g/l)	86	60–80
WBC (x 10^9/l)	26.9	6.0–15.0
Neutrophils (band) (x 10^9/l)	2.6	<1.0
Neutrophils (segmented) (x 10^9/l)	22.4	3.0–11.5
Lymphocytes (x 10^9/l)	0.8	1–4.8
Monocytes (x 10^9/l)	1.1	0.2–1.5
Eosinophils (x 10^9/l)	0.0	0.05–0.8

Film comments

Red cells: 2+ anisocytosis 3+ polychromasia. Large numbers of Heinz bodies. Occasional nucleated red cell and Howell-Jolly body.

Leucocytes: Neutrophil cytoplasm often basophilic. Some neutrophils contain Döhle bodies.

Platelets: Numbers seen appear consistent with count. Some anisocytosis.

Biochemistry	Result	Reference interval
Sodium (mmol/l)	145.3	135.0–155.0
Potassium (mmol/l)	3.02	3.5–5.8
Glucose (mmol/l)	7.3	3.3–5.8
Urea (mmol/l)	8.6	2.5–6.7
Creatinine (µmol/l)	48	45–150
Calcium (mmol/l)	2.49	2.3–2.8
Inorganic phosphate (mmol/l)	0.97	0.78–1.41
TP (g/l)	61	60.0–80.0
Albumin (g/l)	29	25–40
Globulin (g/l)	32	20–45
ALT (IU/l)	33	5.0–60.0
ALP (IU/l)	1078	<130
GGT (IU/l)	8	0.1–9.0
Cholesterol (mmol/l)	3.9	2.5–5.9
Bile acids (µmol/l)	5	0–10
Bilirubin (µmol/ml)	42	2–17

Sample comment: plasma is icteric.

What are the significant abnormalities and what are the possible causes?

There is a severe anaemia which is normocytic, normochromic. However the polychromasia, anisocytosis and elevated reticulocyte count indicate this is a regenerative anaemia (illustrating that evaluation of numerical red cell parameters alone is an insensitive method of detecting regeneration). Given the jaundice the anaemia is likely to be due to haemolysis. The Heinz bodies are highly significant and suggest the haemolysis is due to oxidative damage. Plasma protein measured by refractometer (haematology results) is elevated, whilst serum protein measured biochemically is within the reference interval. The plasma protein is erroneously high due to the icterus, which does not interfere with the biochemical assay. The leucogram shows a neutrophilia and left shift reflecting an inflammatory response. The basophilic cytoplasm and Döhle inclusions noted in the neutrophils indicate a degree of toxic change, which may be severe inflammatory responses and is not specific for bacterial infection (see Chapter 5). The lymphopenia may be due to stress and/or the effects of steroid therapy.

On biochemistry ALP is markedly elevated whilst GGT and ALT are within the reference interval. This pattern is consistent with steroid

Case 1 continues ▶

Case 1 continued

induction. The elevated bilirubin in association with anaemia and normal bile acids is consistent with prehepatic jaundice. The normal bile acids mean hepatic or posthepatic jaundice is very unlikely. The mild hyperglycaemia may be due to stress or the effects of steroid therapy, causing insulin resistance. The hypokalaemia is likely to be due to the combination of vomiting and inappetance.

The overall findings are of haemolytic anaemia caused by oxidative red cell injury. Possible causes include onions, garlic, paracetamol, benzocaine, naphthalene, copper and zinc.

What further investigations should be performed?

Further investigations should include careful questioning of the owner regarding possible access to any of these toxins. Abdominal radiography may be useful to check for metallic foreign bodies, such as pennies, nuts and bolts, which may contain zinc.

Case outcome

Following questioning the owner volunteered that the dog had vomited a child's toy 2 days prior to referral. The vomited toy was approximately half the weight of a newly purchased identical toy, indicating that substantial corrosion had taken place within the stomach. This toy could have been a source of zinc, and so serum zinc was evaluated: it was markedly elevated at 257 μmol/l (reference interval 30–61 μmol/l), confirming that the cause of the haemolysis was zinc toxicity. The dog made an uneventful recovery.

(Case 1 courtesy of Nicholas Bexfield, University of Cambridge)

Case 2

Signalment

7-year-old male Cocker Spaniel.

History

Sudden collapse, dark red urine, jaundice for the previous 2 days. Clinical examination revealed pyrexia, pallor and icterus.

Clinical pathology data

Haematology	Result	Reference interval
RBC (x 10^{12}/l)	0.75	5.5–8.5
Hb (g/dl)	4.53	12–18
PCV (%)	10	37–55
MCV (fl)	77	60–77
MCHC (g/dl)	79	30–36
WBC (x 10^9/l)	9.3	6.0–15.0
Metamyelocytes (x 10^9/l)	1.4	–
Neutrophils (band) (x 10^9/l)	3.6	<1.0
Neutrophils (segmented) (x 10^9/l)	13.7	3.0–11.5
Lymphocytes (x 10^9/l)	0.8	1–4.8
Monocytes (x 10^9/l)	0.6	0.2–1.5
Eosinophils (x 10^9/l)	0.0	0.05–0.8
Platelets (x 10^9/l)	100	200–500
Plasma proteins (g/l)	86	60–80

Film comments

White cells: Neutrophils show mild toxic change with occasional Döhle body.
Red cells: 2+ polychromasia. Moderate numbers of spherocytes and numerous ghost red cells seen.
Platelets: Some small clumps and some macroplatelets. Numbers seen appear higher than count.

Biochemistry	Result	Reference interval
Sodium (mmol/l)	146.2	135.0–155.0
Potassium (mmol/l)	3.5	3.5–5.8
Glucose (mmol/l)	3.9	3.3–5.8
Urea (mmol/l)	22.8	2.5–6.7
Creatinine (μmol/l)	49	45–150
Calcium (mmol/l)	2.6	2.3–2.8
Inorganic phosphate (mmol/l)	1.1	0.78–1.41
TP (g/l)	64.8	60.0–80.0
Albumin (g/l)	32.0	25–40
Globulin (g/l)	32.8	20–45
ALT (IU/l)	2773	5.0–60.0
ALP (IU/l)	455	<130
Bilirubin (μmol/ml)	141	2–17

Sample comment: EDTA and serum samples grossly haemolysed.

Urine analysis	
Gross appearance	Red–brown
SG	1.037
Dipstick	Sample too strongly coloured to read accurately. Possibly 4+ blood/Hb and 4+ bilirubin.
Sediment examination	Red cells <5/hpf; white cells <5/hpf

What abnormalities are present and what is the likely cause?

There is a severe anaemia, based on the manual PCV. The presence of numerous spherocytes and ghost cells coupled with the icterus/elevated bilirubin and haemolysed plasma is strongly suggestive of immune-mediated haemolytic anaemia with intravascular haemolysis. There is a neutrophilia and marked left shift, which is commonly seen in this disease.

There is a discrepancy between the PCV, which is approximately a quarter of the lower reference interval, the RBC count, which is less than 1/5th of the lower reference interval and the haemoglobin, which is approximately 1/3rd of the lower reference interval. In addition the MCHC is extremely high. These discrepancies suggest laboratory error. Further inspection of the sample revealed marked autoagglutination. Clumps of red cells were not counted by the analyser, falsely lowering the RBC, whilst the manual PCV accurately reflects the degree of anaemia. The haemoglobin gives a falsely high indication of red cell mass, because free haemoglobin present as a result of *in vivo* haemolysis has been measured along with haemoglobin liberated from the red cells within the analyser. This also explains the elevated MCHC, which is calculated by

Case 2 continues ▶

Case 2 continued

dividing the haemoglobin by the PCV. Haemolysis has resulted in a falsely high plasma protein (read on a refractometer) whilst the biochemical protein measurement is unaffected. The MCV is likely to be inaccurate because some small clumps of red cells may have been counted as single large red cells. Thus of the red cell values, only the manual PCV is accurate in this case. The blood film shows only moderate polychromasia, which may reflect the acute presentation, before the regenerative response has become fully established.

There is a marked elevation in ALT and AST as well as a moderate elevation in ALP. This indicates hepatic damage, which may be due to hypoxia or thrombus formation leading to ischaemic damage. The elevated bilirubin may be in part prehepatic, due to haemolysis, and partly hepatic due to reduced uptake, conjugation and excretion of bilirubin. The elevated urea with normal creatinine may reflect increased protein breakdown due to the high rate of haemolysis, or possibly gastrointestinal haemorrhage.

Urine dipstick analysis shows a marked reaction for blood/haemoglobin. The lack of red cells on the sediment suggest true haemoglobinuria rather than haematuria, although red cells can lyse *in vitro*, especially in dilute urine. Haemoglobinuria indicates intravascular haemolysis. Bilirubinuria is almost invariably detected in animals with haemolytic anaemia, due to the low renal threshold for bilirubin.

What other tests would you do?

Autoagglutination should be confirmed by performing a saline agglutination test and examining microscopically. A Coombs' test could be performed if autoagglutination were not present. A coagulation profile could be performed to investigate the possibility of DIC.

Other investigations aimed at detecting an underlying disease (e.g. neoplasia, infection) should be considered, although primary IMHA is seen commonly in this breed.

Case 3

Signalment

10-month-old female neutered Domestic Shorthair.

History and clinical examination

Gradual onset of dullness and lethargy over the preceding 3 weeks. Clinical signs have deteriorated over the last few days and the cat is now anorexic, very weak and depressed. Clinical examination reveals very pale mucous membranes and moderate tachycardia but no other abnormalities.

Clinical pathology data

Haematology	Results	Reference interval
RBC (x 10^{12}/l)	1.23	5.0–10.0
Hb (g/dl)	1.8	8–15
HCT (l/l)	0.052	0.26–0.45
MCV (fl)	42	39–55
MCHC (g/dl)	36	30–36
Reticulocytes (x 10^{9}/l)	42	<50
WBC (x 10^{9}/l)	12.9	5.5–19.5
Neutrophils (x 10^{9}/l)	6.7	3.0–11.5
Lymphocytes (x 10^{9}/l)	6.1	1.5–4.8
Monocytes (x 10^{9}/l)	0.1	0.2–1.5
Eosinophils (x 10^{9}/l)	0.0	0.05–0.8
Platelets (x 10^{9}/l)	209	200–800
Plasma proteins (g/l)	74	60–80

Film comments

Red cells are normocytic normochromic with marked rouleaux formation. Leucocyte morphology is unremarkable.

Classify this anaemia. What are the potential causes for this?

This is a very severe normocytic, normochromic, non-regenerative anaemia. The chronic history and the fact that the cat is still alive with this very severe anaemia indicate the disease must have had a gradual onset, with time for the cat to adapt physiologically. Possible causes are primary bone marrow diseases, such as pure red cell aplasia and non-regenerative IMHA, myelodysplasia, myelo/lymphoproliferative diseases, myelophthisis and FeLV-related anaemia. The anaemia is too severe to be secondary to inflammatory disease or renal failure, and in addition there are no clinical signs suggesting renal failure.

What other abnormalities are present and what is their significance?

The marked rouleaux formation may suggest an increase in globulins. There is a mild lymphocytosis but this is significant in a sick/stressed animal in which lymphopenia or low normal lymphocyte count is expected. This may suggest a lymphoproliferative disease, although the lymphocyte morphology is normal and could also suggest chronic immune stimulation.

What further tests would you do?

Further tests should include FeLV and FIV testing, biochemical screening, in particular to assess renal and liver parameters, and bone marrow aspiration. Screening for *Mycoplasma haemofelis/haemominutem* should also be performed since this infection could contribute to the anaemia.

Further data

In-house FeLV and FIV and *Mycoplasma* PCR tests were negative. Biochemical screening revealed mildly elevated liver enzymes consistent with hypoxic damage. Bone marrow aspiration revealed a normal myeloid series but markedly depleted erythroid series with only occasional proerythroblasts seen. There were increased numbers of small lymphocytes which accounted for 28% of the total nucleated cells. These findings indicate pure red cell aplasia. The cat received a blood transfusion and high-dose prednisolone and made a good recovery.

References and further reading

Barker RN, Gruffydd-Jones TJ and Elson CJ (1993) Red cell-bound immunoglobulins and complement measured by an enzyme-linked antiglobulin test in dogs with autoimmune haemolysis or other anaemias. *Research in Veterinary Science* **54,** 170–178

Brown DE, Weiser MG and Thrall MA (1994) Erythrocytic indices and volume distribution in a dog with stomatocytosis. *Veterinary Pathology* **31,** 247–250

Couto CG, Boudrieau RJ and Zanjani ED (1989) Tumour associated erythrophagocytosis in a dog with nasal fibrosarcoma. *Journal of Veterinary Internal Medicine* **3,** 183–185

Day MJ (1996) Serial monitoring of clinical, haematological and immunological parameters in canine autoimmune haemolytic anaemia. *Journal of Small Animal Practice* **37,** 523–534

Day MJ (2000) Immune-mediated haemolytic anaemia In: *Schalms Veterinary Haematology, 5th edn*, ed. BF Feldman, JG Zinkl and NC Jain, pp. 799–806. Lippincott, Williams and Wilkins, Philadelphia

Day M, Littlewood J and Mackin A (2000) *BSAVA Manual of Small Animal Haematology and Transfusion Medicine.* BSAVA Publications, Gloucester

Dunn JK, Jefferies AR and Villiers EJ (1995) Anaemia associated with intramedullary erythrophagocytosis in the dog: A spectrum of diseases. Abstract *Proceedings, 5th European Society of Veterinary Internal Medicine Congress*, 72–73.

Duval D and Giger U (1996) Vaccine associated immune-mediated haemolytic anaemia in the dog. *Journal of Veterinary Internal Medicine* **10,** 290–295

Elders R and Blackwood L (2003) Haematological parameters in benign and malignant canine splenic diseases. *Proceedings, American College of Veterinary Internal Medicine 2003,* p.932 [Abstract]

Fletch SM, Pinkerton PH and Bruecker PJ (1975) The Alaskan malamute chondrodysplasia (dwarfism-anaemia) syndrome in review. *Journal of the American Animal Hospital Association* **11,** 353–361

Foley JE, Harrus S and Poland A (1998). Molecular, clinical and pathologic comparison of two distinct strains of *Haemobartonella felis* in domestic cats. *American Journal of Veterinary Research* **59,** 151–158

George JW, Rideout BA, Griffey SM, Pedersen NC (2002) Effect or pre-existing FeLV infection or FeLV and feline immunodeficiency virus co-infection on pathogenicity of the small variant of *Haemobartonella felis* in cats. *American Journal of Veterinary Research* **63,** 1172–1178

Harvey JW and Gaskin JM (1977) Experimental feline haemobartonellosis. *Journal of the American Animal Hospital Association* **13,** 28–38

Harvey JW (2001) Bone marrow evaluation. In: *Atlas of Veterinary Haematology. Blood and Bone Marrow of Domestic Animals, 1st edn,* ed. JW Harvey, pp 121–123. WB Saunders, Philadelphia

Klag AR, Giger U and Shofer FS (1993) Idiopathic immune-mediated haemolytic anaemia in dogs: 42 cases (1986–1990). *Journal of the American Veterinary Medical Association* **202,** 783–788

Kraje AC, Patton CS and Edwards DF (2001). Malignant histiocytosis in 3 cats. *Journal of Veterinary Internal Medicine* **15,** 252–256

Mellanby RJ, Holloway A, Chantrey J, Herrtage ME and Dobson JM (2004) Immune-mediated haemolytic anaemia with a sarcoma in a flat-coated retriever. *Journal of Small Animal Practice* **45,** 21–24

Miller SA, Hohenhaus AE and Hale AS (2004) Case controlled study of blood-type, breed, sex and bacteremia in dogs with immune-mediated haemolytic anaemia. *Journal of the American Veterinary Medical* Association **224,** 232–235

McManus P and Craig LE (2001) Correlation between leucocytosis and necropsy findngs in dogs with immune-mediated haemolytic anaemia: 34 cases (1994–1999). *Journal of the American Veterinary Medical* Association **218,** 1308–1313

McCullough S (2003) Immune-mediated haemolytic anaemia: understanding the nemesis. *Veterinary Clinics of North America Small Animal Practice* **33,** 1295–1315

Moore PF and Rosin A (1986) Malignant histiocytosis in Bernese Mountain Dogs. *Veterinary Pathology* **23,** 1–10

Newlands CE, Houston DM and Vasconelos DY (1994) Hyperferritinaemia associated with malignant histiocytosis in a dog *Journal of the American Veterinary Medical Association* **205,** 849–851

Quigley KA, Chelack BJ, Haines DM and Jackson ML (2000). Application of a direct flow cytometric erythrocyte immunofluorescence assay in dogs with immune-mediated haemolytic anaemia and a comparison to the direct antiglobulin test. *Journal of Veterinary Diagnostic Investigation* **13,** 297–300

Ristic JME and Stidworthy MF (2002) Two cases of severe iron deficiency anaemia due to inflammatory bowel disease in the dog. *Journal of Small Animal Practice* **43,** 80–83

Schalm OJ (1976) Erthrocytic macrocytosis in miniature and toy poodles. *Canine Practice* **3,** 55–57

Scott-Moncrieff JC, Treadwell NG, McCullough SM and Brooks MB (2001) Haemostatic abnormalities in dogs with primary immune-mediated haemolytic anaemia. *Journal of the American Animal Hospital Association* **37,** 220–227

Solter P and Scott R (1987) Onion ingestion and subsequent Heinz body anaemia in a dog: A case report. *Journal of the American Animal Hospital Association* **23,** 544–546

Stockham SL and Scott MA (2002) Basic haematological assays In: *Fundamentals of Veterinary Clinical Pathology, 1st edn,* ed. SL Stockham and MA Scott, pp. 44–45. Iowa State Press, Iowa

Stokol T and Blue J (1999) Pure red cell aplasia in cats: 9 cases (1989–1997). *Journal of the American Veterinary Medical Association* **214,** 75–79

Stone MS and Freden GO (1990) Differentiation of anaemia of inflammatory disease from anaemia of iron deficiency. *Compendium of Continuing Education for the Practicing Veterinarian* **12,** 963–966

Tasker S, Helps CR and Day MJ (2003) Use of real-time PCR to detect and quantify *Mycoplasma haemofelis* and '*Candidatus* Mycoplasma haemominutum' DNA. *Journal of Clinical Mircobiology* **41,** 439–441

Walton RM, Modiano JF, Thrall MA and Wheeler SL (1996) Bone marrow cytological findings in 4 dogs and a cat with haemophagocytic syndrome. *Journal of Veterinary Internal Medicine* **10,** 7–14

Watson ADJ, Moore AS and Hefland SC (1994) Primary erythrocytosis in the cat: treatment with hydroxyurea. *Journal of Small Animal Practice,* **25,** 320–325

Weiss DJ and Aird B (2001) Cytological evaluation of primary and secondary myelodysplastic syndromes in the dog. *Veterinary Clinical Pathology* **30,** 67–75

Weiss DJ (2002) Primary pure red cell aplasia in dogs: 13 cases (1996–2000). *Journal of the American Veterinary Medical Association* **221,** 93–95

5

Disorders of leucocytes

Laura Blackwood

Introduction

Leucocytes (white blood cells) include both granulocytes (neutrophils, eosinophils and basophils) and mononuclear cells (monocytes and lymphocytes). Leucocytes are vital for host defence, and for initiation and control of inflammation and immunity. Neutrophils, macrophages and natural killer (NK) cells (specialized lymphoid cells) provide the innate immune response, which is the first line of defence against an invading pathogen and does not involve immunological memory. Lymphoid cells orchestrate the adaptive or acquired immune response, activated by the inflammation induced by any pathogen that gets past the innate response. The adaptive immune response develops immunological memory.

In addition to being effector cells (cells that carry out functions), white blood cells play important regulatory roles in haemopoiesis and immune function. Although generally protective or supportive of the host tissue, leucocytes are also involved in host-harmful allergic and immune-mediated disease.

Normal leucocyte morphology is illustrated in Figure 3.16 and an overview of haemopoiesis is given in Chapter 4. The haemopoietic cells in the bone marrow can be divided into three groups: pluripotent stem cells; differentiating progenitor cells; and fully functional mature blood cells. Pluripotent stem cells are capable of self-renewal. As cells become committed to a certain cell lineage, their ability to proliferate is reduced and eventually lost. Thus, the marrow has a pyramidal structure, in which one stem cell gives rise to many daughter cells (Figure 5.1). Specific information concerning production of all cell lines in dogs and cats is lacking, so the descriptions in this chapter also draw

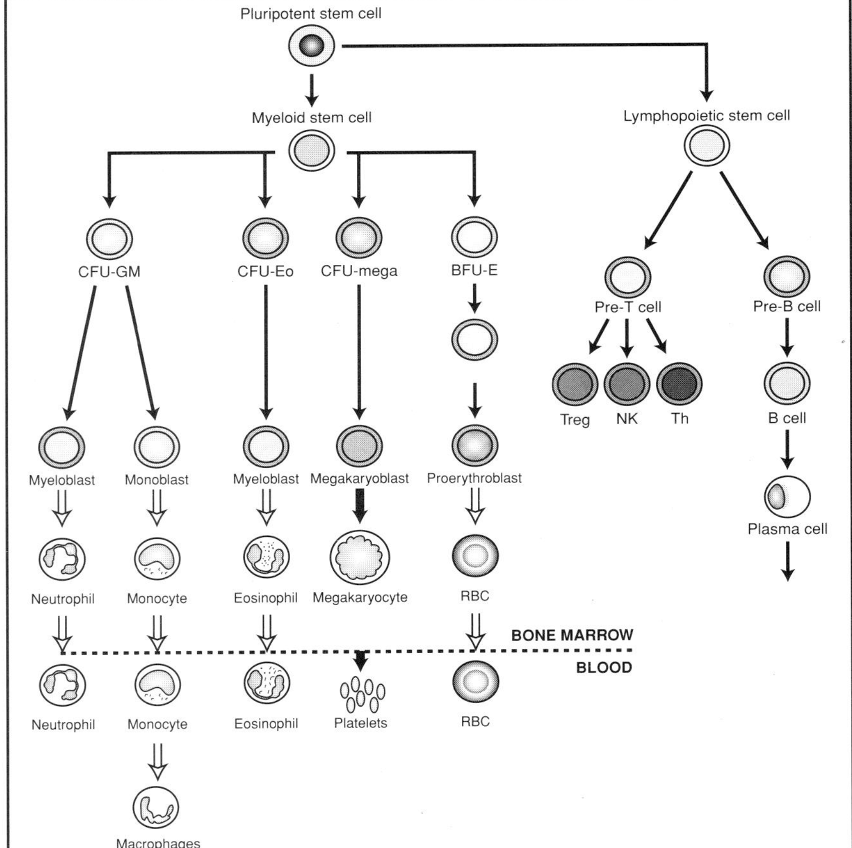

5.1 Haemopoiesis.

from available information in other mammalian studies. The factors controlling granulopoiesis are less well defined than those controlling erythropoiesis.

Assessment of leucocytes

Assessment of white blood cells requires total and differential white cell counts (determined using blood samples taken into EDTA) and blood smear examination (see Chapters 2 and 3). A fresh blood smear should be submitted to the laboratory with every EDTA blood sample, as artefactual changes in cells occur within hours of sampling. Most in-house analysers produce reliable total WBC counts but differential and platelet counts are generally less reliable (Bienzle *et al.*, 2000; Papasouliotis, 2002; Dewhurst *et al.*, 2003). All machine-generated differential counts should be verified by a manual 200-cell differential count, and in every case a blood smear should be evaluated for morphological abnormalities. Automated analysers count normoblasts as white blood cells because they are nucleated, and these must be identified on smears. Lastly, platelet counts should be verified by smear examination, and automated analysers do not always provide accurate platelet counts for cats (see Chapter 4).

Buffy coat smears (where a smear is made of the buffy coat only, after centrifugation) can be examined. There are no red blood cells, and very large numbers of white blood cells can be examined rapidly. Buffy coat smears are rarely used but may be useful in identifying low numbers of aberrant cells or intracellular organisms where only a small proportion of cells are affected.

Reference intervals

Reference intervals are derived from available 'normal' populations and are seldom truly demographically appropriate for the individual patient. Ideally age-, breed- and sex-matched animals with similar backgrounds and environment and from the same geographical area should be used (see Chapter 2) but this is clearly impractical. The reference interval provided by the laboratory carrying out the analyses should be used.

Age- and breed-related changes

Leucocyte counts in infant and juvenile cats and dogs vary from those in adults, and this reflects the new challenges they face. Changes are also apparent in dams: total WBC counts are increased during pregnancy and lactation, and return to normal after weaning. Kittens have a normal leucogram at birth, but, by 3–4 months of age, neutrophil and lymphocyte counts considerably exceed the adult range. These return to the adult range by 5–6 months of age.

Much of the initial data for dogs are based on laboratory Beagles; in these dogs band neutrophils may be above the reference range for the first few days of life but are within the adult range by 7–10 days (Shafrine *et al.*, 1973). Lymphocytosis is a common finding, and dogs less than 6 months of age typically have lymphocyte counts between 2 and 10 x 10^9/l. Total WBC counts have also been assessed in a group of Beagles and Labrador Retrievers from pet stock held by a nutrition company. Total leucocyte counts were higher at 3–8 weeks of age than at any later life stage, and remained elevated above adult values until 4 months of age (Harper *et al.*, 2003). In this group, total WBC counts tended to decrease from 2 years of age, and WBC counts in dogs under 5 years old were significantly greater than for those over 5 years (Harper *et al.*, 2003). For the young (< 1 year) and the old (> 8 years) there were also significant differences in total count between the two breeds, with Beagles having higher counts, especially as puppies. Thus, juvenile ranges based on laboratory Beagles may not reflect normality in other breeds.

Other breed-related physiological (rather than pathological) leucocyte abnormalities have been identified. Sighthounds tend to have lower WBC counts than other breeds. Belgian Tervueren dogs in the USA have been documented to have lower neutrophil, monocyte and lymphocyte counts than other dogs (Greenfield *et al.*, 2000), although a recent study failed to show such physiological leucopenia in Terveurens in their home country (Gommeren *et al.*, 2004). The latter study also supported a decrease in total WBC count with ageing, as found in Labradors and Beagles.

Morphological variations in leucocytes are also breed-related. For example, Greyhounds have abnormal eosinophils, which lack distinct granules and contain numerous clear cytoplasmic vacuoles, but these dogs have no related disease problems. Similarly, Birman cats show atypical neutrophil granulation that is not associated with neutrophil dysfunction.

Granulocytes

Granulopoiesis is the process by which granulocytes are produced. The CFU-C (so called because it was first described in colony-forming units in culture) is the multipotent stem cell for the granulocyte series. These stem cells are morphologically similar to small lymphocytes. In the presence of colony-stimulating factors (CSFs) they proliferate and differentiate into the cells of the granulocyte–monocyte lineages. The CFU-GM (granulocyte– monocyte colony-forming unit) has been identified as the particular CFU-C progenitor that gives rise to both granulocytes and monocytes.

G-CSF (granulocyte colony-stimulating factor) and GM-CSF (granulocyte–monocyte colony-stimulating factor) are the specific CSFs involved in granulopoiesis. There are most likely colony-stimulating factors (CSFs) for each cell lineage. In addition to CSFs, macrophages, activated lymphocytes and endothelial cells produce local factors (mainly cytokines) that stimulate granulopoiesis. Regulation of production is partly achieved by a negative feedback effect mediated by inhibitory substances from mature neutrophils and prostaglandin E from macrophages, unless there is continued stimulation for granulocyte release.

The first morphologically recognizable granulocyte is the myeloblast. These cells differentiate through progranulocyte, myelocyte, metamyelocyte and band forms to become mature granulocytes (Figure 5.2). The capacity for cell division is lost at the metamyelocyte stage, by which time 16–32 myelocytes have arisen from each myeloblast.

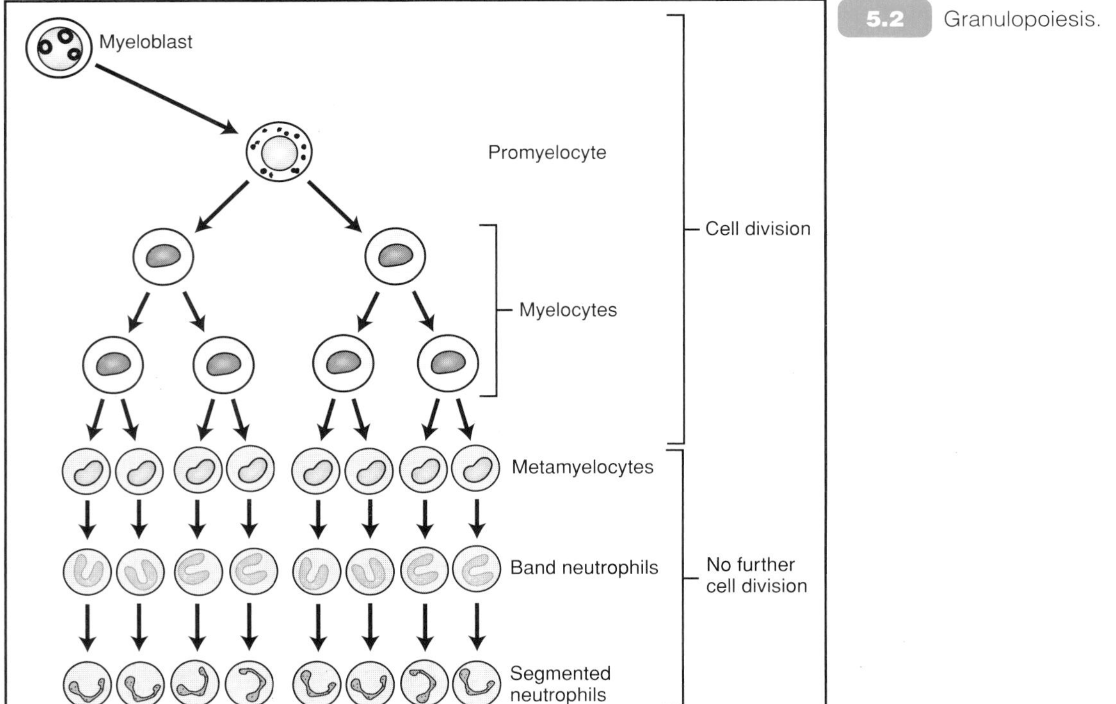

5.2 Granulopoiesis.

Neutrophils

The neutrophil, or polymorphonuclear (PMN) leucocyte (Figure 5.3), is approximately 10–15 μm in diameter (about 1.5–2 canine red cells) and has a nucleus divided into three to five lobes by indentations. The nucleus has dark purple-staining clumped chromatin. The cytoplasm contains microbicidal and enzymatic granules important to its function, but these are either indiscernible or only faintly visible as eosinophilic granules against the pale pink cytoplasm on Romanowsky stains. Barr bodies (see Figure 3.16bii) are protrusions of the nucleus present in bitches and in up to 11% of queens, and are of no clinical significance.

Neutrophils play a vital role in the defence of the organism against pathogens, and can:

- Kill or inactivate bacteria, yeasts, fungi or parasites
- Modulate the immune response
- Eliminate infected and, in some cases, transformed cells.

Neutrophils exist in the body in three major pools: the bone marrow, blood and tissue pools (Figure 5.4). The bone marrow pool consists of the mitotic (dividing) pool, the maturation pool and the storage pool. In the normal animals the storage pool of mature neutrophils harbours 5–7 days' worth of neutrophils. It is only when the demand is great and this pool is depleted that neutrophils are released from the maturation pool and immature forms (band forms or more immature cells, Figure 5.3) are released into the circulation. In the circulation, the neutrophils form two pools, the circulating (CNP) and marginating (MNP) pools. The MNP consists of cells stuck to or rolling along the endothelium of small blood vessels. Blood samples only harvest cells from the CNP, and movement of cells between the MNP and CNP pools can affect counts. In dogs roughly half the neutrophils exist in each pool, but in cats the marginating pool is three times greater than the circulating pool.

The circulating half-life of neutrophils in dogs and cats is only 6–12 hours, and counts can change rapidly in disease states. Even in the normal animal, the total neutrophil pool is replaced 1–2.5 times daily. Neutrophils leaving the circulation are lost across mucosal surfaces or phagocytosed in the liver and spleen. In the normal animal, there is no appreciable tissue pool, although large numbers of neutrophils may accumulate in tissues in disease. Neutrophils in normal tissues survive only 1–4 days, and survival is shortened in disease.

Neutrophil shifts

Circulating neutrophils may show left and right shifts. These terms arise from the side of the cell counter/page on which the neutrophils are recorded: band neutrophils are recorded to the left of mature neutrophils, so an increased number of immature cells is described as a left shift.

Left shift: This occurs when the storage pool is depleted and there is continued demand for neutrophils, which is met by the release of immature neutrophils (predominantly band forms) from the maturation pool. If disease is severe or protracted, metamyelocytes and earlier precursors may also appear. Band neutrophils are of similar size to mature cells but have a minimally indented (suggested < 50% of the width) U-shaped nucleus with almost parallel sides (Figure 5.3b,c,d). Clinical pathologists are variably

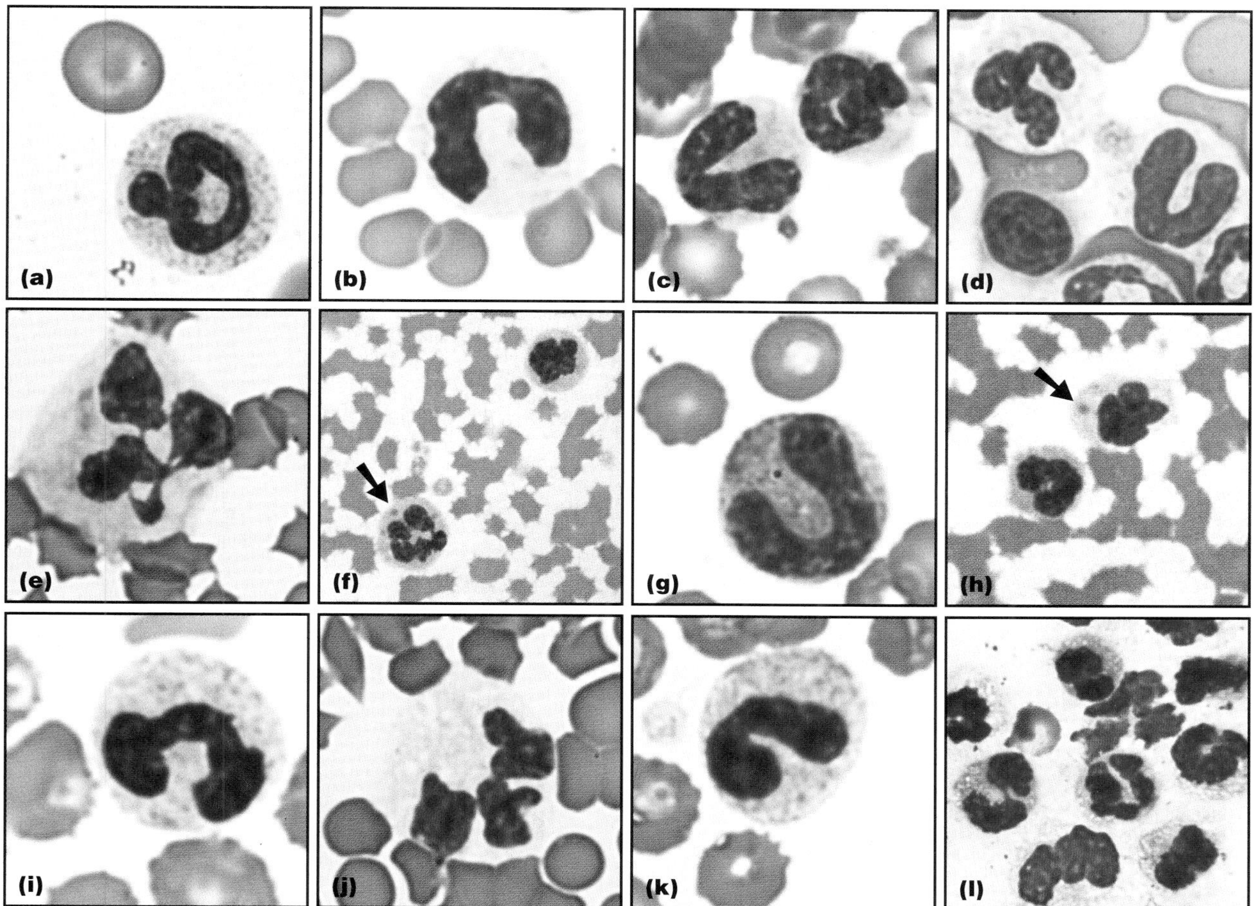

5.3 Neutrophils, characterized by a segmented nucleus with three to five lobes. **(a)** Normal neutrophil from a dog. **(b, c, d)** Band neutrophils, with U-shaped nuclei lacking segmentation. In (c) the band cell is to the left of a poorly preserved segmented neutrophil. **(e, f)** Hypersegmented neutrophils (feline). There is also pyknotic change. In (f) the neutrophil on the right has a condensed nucleus while the one on the left is hypersegmented; blue Döhle bodies are also evident (arrowed). In both (e) and (f) there is red cell crenation, supporting *in vitro* change due to an aged sample. These changes make appreciation of toxic change difficult. **(g, h, i, j, k)** Toxic changes in band and mature neutrophils. In (g) there is nuclear swelling, chromatin clumping, cytoplasmic basophilia, and faint granulation. In (h) there is nuclear swelling, cytoplasmic basophilia and a Döhle body (arrowed). In (j) there is a swollen nucleus, with slightly clumped chromatin, and faint vacuolation. In (k) nuclear swelling, chromatin clumping and cytoplasmic basophila are seen. **(l)** Degenerate neutrophils, with nuclear swelling, eosinophilia and lysis. Degenerative changes occur in neutrophils in the tissues and these changes are almost never seen in the circulation. (May–Grünwald–Giemsa stain (except (b, l) Rapi-Diff II); original magnification X1000 (except (f, h) X400).)

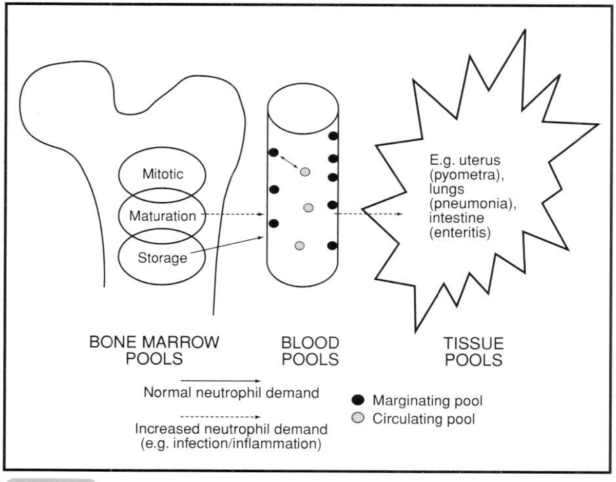

5.4 The major neutrophil pools of the body.

strict in their definition of a band neutrophil and argue as to how deep the indentations can be before the neutrophil is mature, and this results in different normal reference intervals for band forms. The nuclei of band forms stain less heavily than those of mature neutrophils, as the chromatin is less condensed.

Left shifts may be either regenerative or degenerative:

- In a *regenerative* left shift, there are increased band neutrophils and there is a neutrophilia in which mature neutrophils exceed bands
- In a *degenerative* left shift, there is a low or normal leucocyte count and band cells exceed mature neutrophils. This is inappropriate and suggests that the bone marrow is unable to maintain adequate neutrophil numbers to meet the increased demand.

There is no universally accepted value for what constitutes a significant left shift, but > 1 x 10^9/l band neutrophils is often used. An increase in band neutrophils reflects an active inflammatory response, which could be due to infection, immune-mediated disease, tissue damage/necrosis or neoplasia; band cells are not pathognomonic for bacterial infection (see below). In animals with Pelger–Huët anomaly, band neutrophils are released into the circulation and left shift is not indicative of an increased inflammatory response.

A neutrophilia with a declining left shift may reflect declining tissue demand or accelerated bone marrow production meeting demand, and can be a good prognostic indicator. A degenerative left shift is a poor prognostic indicator.

Right shift: This occurs when there is reduced egress from the circulation, most often mediated by endogenous cortisol or exogenous corticosteroids. A mature neutrophilia results, though this may be indistinguishable from other types of mature neutrophilia unless morphological changes occur. Hypersegmentation and pyknosis represent normal ageing change but neutrophils usually exit the circulation before these changes are evident: these changes may be seen in a right shift. Both changes may also occur *in vitro*, and are common artefacts (Figure 5.3e,f). However, the presence of such cells in a fresh blood smear suggests extended neutrophil transit time. Hypersegmented neutrophils have more than five lobes in the nucleus.

Neutrophilia

The most common causes of neutrophilia are summarized in Figure 5.5.

Physiological neutrophilia: This is especially common in cats. Emotional distress or fear results in release of adrenaline (epinephrine), and neutrophils redistribute from the marginating to the circulating pools. There is no left shift. Vigorous exercise also produces a similar response, most commonly in young dogs. Physiological neutrophilia may be accompanied by lymphocytosis (which is often greater in magnitude than the neutrophilia in cats) and/or hyperglycaemia, and is transient (20 minutes).

Stress/steroid-induced neutrophilia: Endogenous cortisol or exogenous corticosteroids produce a mature neutrophilia, mainly as a result of increased release of neutrophils from the storage pool, and also, to a lesser extent, shift of cells from the marginating to the circulating pool, and reduced endothelial adherence resulting in prolonged circulation time (a true right shift). There is usually no left shift. Counts in dogs tend to be in the range 15–25 x 10^9/l but may occasionally be as high as 40 x 10^9/l. Increases in cats are less marked and the total WBC count does not usually exceed 20 x 10^9/l (but may occasionally be as high as 30 x 10^9/l). Other steroid-associated abnormalities may be present: in dogs, monocytosis, lymphopenia and eosinopenia, and biochemical changes (markedly elevated alkaline phosphatase with moderately elevated alanine transaminase) are typical; in cats, monocytosis is not common and lymphopenia and eosinopenia may be the only other abnormalities, as there is no steroid-induced alkaline phosphatase.

Acute inflammatory response: Neutrophilia due to inflammation is seen in a wide range of disease processes, and may feature a left shift. The left shift may be regenerative or degenerative, depending on the demand for neutrophils and the marrow's ability to produce these. In the face of increased demand, marrow transit time may be reduced and the neutrophils (mature and immature) may show toxic change (see below). Although bacterial infections may be the most

Cause	Associated conditions	Mechanism of neutrophilia	Recognition factors
Physiological neutrophilia	Emotional distress; fear; vigorous exercise	Redistribution of neutrophils from marginating to circulating pools	No left shift Concurrent abnormalities: • Lymphocytosis • Hyperglycaemia
Stress/steroid response	Hyperadrenocorticism; exogenous corticosteroids	Increased release of neutrophils from storage pool. Shift from marginating to circulating pool. Prolonged circulation time	No left shift Concurrent abnormalities (dogs): • Monocytosis • Lymphopenia • Eosinopenia • Elevated alkaline phosphatase Concurrent abnormalities (cats): • Lymphopenia • Eosinopenia
Acute inflammatory response	Bacterial infections; other infections; immune-mediated disease; neoplasia; tissue necrosis	Increased demand in response to pathogens and inflammation	May feature: • Left shift • Toxic change Superimposed stress haemogram
Others (rare)	Chronic granulocytic leukaemia; neutrophil dysfunction	See Figure 5.7	See Figure 5.7

5.5 Causes of neutrophilia in dogs and cats.

common cause of an acute inflammatory response in practice, immune-mediated diseases and neoplasia are also frequent causes. In immune-mediated haemolytic anaemia (IMHA), a marked neutrophilia with a left shift is common. This is thought to be due to non-specific effects of marrow hyperactivity in response to the anaemia, endogenous steroid production and, in some cases, systemic inflammatory response secondary to tissue hypoxia and thrombosis. If the left shift is profound and accompanied by a strongly regenerative anaemia with circulating nucleated red blood cells (normoblastosis), this is called a leucoerythroblastic blood picture (Figure 5.6; see also Chapter 4). In many animals with an acute inflammatory response there is a superimposed stress haemogram, and eosinopenia and lymphopenia are common.

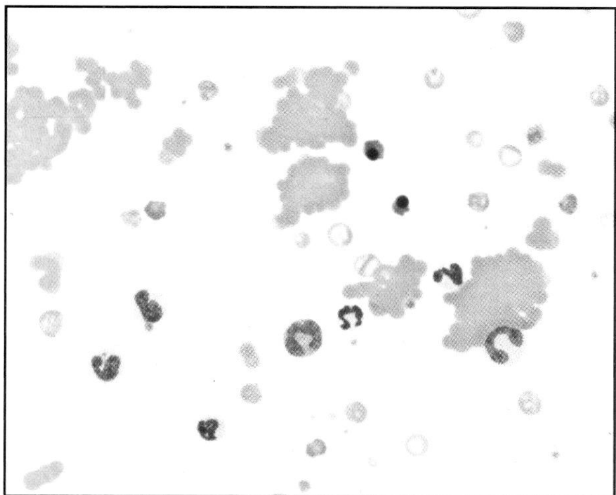

5.6 A leucoerythroblastic blood picture in a dog with IMHA. There is red cell agglutination, and most of the red cells that have agglutinated are spherocytes. There is a strongly regenerative red cell response, with reticulocytes and normoblasts, and a similarly regenerative myeloid response, with band neutrophils and also band-like monocytes. (May–Grünwald–Giemsa stain; original magnification X400.)

Toxic change

Toxic change refers to the morphological abnormalities (Figure 5.3g–k) seen in neutrophils in severe inflammatory disease, especially severe bacterial infections, and in IMHA. These changes occur in the bone marrow prior to release and are associated with enhanced neutrophil turnover and reduced maturation time, as a result of intense stimulation of granulopoiesis. Some drugs and toxins can cause similar morphological changes. Toxic changes include:

- Increased cytoplasmic basophilia, as a result of increased residual cytoplasmic RNA
- Cytoplasmic vacuolation due to loss of granule and membrane integrity during disturbed maturation
- Döhle bodies: these are grey–blue intracytoplasmic inclusions representing aggregates of cytoplasmic reticulum. Döhle bodies are found in normal cats and are not considered to reflect toxic change unless they are frequent and prominent
- Toxic granulation due to retention of acid mucopolysaccharides in primary granules (which stain with Romanowsky stains, unlike the secondary granules usually present in normal neutrophils)
- Giant neutrophils
- Nuclear swelling
- Doughnut nuclei.

Degenerative changes

Degenerative changes occur in neutrophils in the tissues rather than in the circulation, as a result of endotoxin exposure; they include nuclear swelling, chromatin dissociation and nuclear eosinophilia (Figure 5.3l). These changes are more often appreciated in tissue and fluid samples, and are only rarely seen in the circulation in bacteraemia/septicaemia.

Extreme neutrophilia

Markedly elevated neutrophil counts are again seen in a wide variety of disease situations, and have been associated with poor prognosis in both dogs and cats. Extreme neutrophilias where there is a marked left shift have been described as leukaemoid reactions, because of the presence of immature cells. This term is misleading, and either extreme neutrophilia or extreme neutrophilic leucocytosis is preferred. The absolute numbers that constitute an extreme neutrophilia are controversial, but a total WBC count > 50 x 10^9/l, with > 50% neutrophils, has been suggested for dogs and cats (Lucroy and Madewell, 1999, 2001). The causes of extreme neutrophilia are summarized in Figure 5.7. All diseases that can cause extreme neutrophilias can also cause less marked neutrophilia.

Neutropenia

Neutropenia is generally a result of:

- Overwhelming demand and increased migration from circulation to tissues
- Decreased survival of cells
- Reduced or ineffective granulopoiesis.

Cause	Examples of disease processes	Mechanism of neutrophilia	Recognition factors
Severe localized pyogenic infections	Pyometra; pyothorax; peritonitis; abscess	Extreme demand for neutrophils as disease process not controlled	Compatible clinical signs. Toxic change in neutrophils. Significant left shift
Other infectious diseases	Parasitic (e.g. *Dirofilaria*); Rickettsial (*Ehrlichia*); *Hepatozoon*; Fungal	Extreme demand for neutrophils as disease process not controlled	Compatible clinical signs. Radiographic, cytological and polymerase chain reaction (PCR) findings

5.7 Causes of extreme neutrophilia in dogs and cats. (continues) ▶

Cause	Examples of disease processes	Mechanism of neutrophilia	Recognition factors
Immune-mediated disease	Immune-mediated haemolytic anaemia (IMHA); immune-mediated thrombocytopenia (IMTP); immune-mediated polyarthritis (IMPA)	Non-specific stimulation of granulopoiesis (IMHA, IMTP). Response to inflammation. Tissue necrosis due to hypoxia (IMHA), thrombosis	Compatible clinical signs: • IMHA: markedly regenerative anaemia, spherocytosis, possibly autoagglutination • IMTP: profound thrombocytopenia, flow cytometry anti-platelet antibody positive (see Chapter 6) • IMPA: appropriate joint fluid cytology (see Chapter 22)
Neoplasia	Any solid tumour	Tissue necrosis in large mass lesions. Possible production of colony-stimulating factors by the tumour	Compatible clinical signs (mass lesion)
Tissue necrosis	Trauma; infection; neoplasia; vascular occlusion (torsions, thrombosis, tumour emboli)	Response to inflammation at site of necrosis	Clinical signs of the primary disease
Chronic granulocytic leukaemia		Neoplastic transformation of committed mature granulocyte	Left shift. Aberrant cells. Thrombocytopenia. Myeloid extramedullary haematopoiesis in multiple sites
Neutrophil dysfunction	Leucocyte adhesion deficiency (Irish Setters)	Continued demand for neutrophils as pathogens not eliminated due to neutrophil dysfuntion	Breed. Demonstrable neutrophil dysfunction

5.7 (continued) Causes of extreme neutrophilia in dogs and cats.

Overwhelming demand is most common in severe bacterial infections, such as pyometra, peritonitis or pyothorax. In these cases, toxic change and a degenerative left shift are common, and there are compatible clinical signs. Reduced granulopoiesis is due either to bone marrow disease or to drug toxicity (cytotoxic drug-related myelosuppression or idiosyncratic drug reactions), and other cell lines may be affected. There is also a fourth, less common, type of neutropenia caused by shift from the circulating to marginating pool. This is a transient cause of neutropenia in the first minutes to hours of endotoxic or anaphylactic shock. The causes of neutropenia and features that help differentiate them, are summarized in Figure 5.8.

Cause	Examples of disease process	Mechanism of neutropenia(s)	Recognition factors
Peracute bacterial infections	Endotoxic or septic shock; peritonitis; pyometra; aspiration pneumonia; acute salmonellosis	Overwhelming demand/decreased survival	Left shift (may be degenerative). Toxic change. Appropriate clinical signs
Extreme pyrexia	Heat stroke; septic shock	Overwhelming demand/decreased survival due to systemic inflammatory response	Appropriate clinical signs
Initial period of endotoxic or anaphylactic shock		Shift from CNP to MNP	Transient (minutes to hours). May resolve or neutropenia may persist due to increased demand if endotoxaemic
Retroviral infection	Feline leukaemia virus (FeLV); feline immunodeficiency virus (FIV)	Reduced or ineffective granulopoiesis. FeLV: maturation arrest, possible immune-mediated aetiology in some cases, myelodysplastic syndromes and leukaemias. FIV: disturbance of myeloid progenitor growth	Appropriate virological results (see Chapter 26). FeLV: other haematological abnormalities common, especially anaemia (non-regenerative, possibly macrocytic), occasional pancytopenia. Neutropenia may be transient, persistent or cyclic. FIV: non-regenerative anaemia, lymphopenia common. Neutropenia often mild and transient in clinical cases
Parvoviral infection	Feline panleucopenia virus; canine parvovirus	Increased consumption (endotoxaemia, gastrointestinal disease). Viral cytotoxicity to haemopoietic stem cells. Ineffective neutrophil production	Compatible history and clinical signs. Profound degenerative left shift with early and aberrant precursors

5.8 Causes of neutropenia in dogs and cats. (continues) ▶

Cause	Examples of disease process	Mechanism of neutropenia(s)	Recognition factors
Myelodysplastic disease	Myelodysplastic syndrome; refractory cytopenia	Ineffective granulopoiesis	Non-specific clinical signs. Other cytopenias (often anaemia, especially cats). Morphological evidence of disturbed maturation in granulocyte, and other cell lines. Diagnosis requires bone marrow evaluation. May progress to myeloid leukaemia. May be associated with FeLV infection
Leukaemia	Acute lymphoblastic leukaemia; acute myeloid leukaemia (less severe neutropenia with chronic leukaemias)	Reduced/ineffective granulopoiesis due to marrow infiltration by tumour cells	Non-specific clinical signs: pyrexia, sepsis, petechial haemorrhages, disseminated intravascular coagulation (DIC), paraneoplastic syndromes. Thrombocytopenia. Mild anaemia. Circulating abnormal cells. Bone marrow required for diagnosis
Myelophthisis/ myelofibrosis	Leukaemia (see above); metastatic neoplasia; myelofibrosis/osteopetrosis; occasionally granulomatous disease	Reduced/ineffective granulopoiesis due to marrow infiltration by non-haemopoietic cells	Signs of underlying disease. Non-specific clinical signs. Other cytopenias. Bone marrow required for diagnosis. N.B. Myelofibrosis in dogs is characterized by a non-regenerative anaemia, and significant other cytopenias are uncommon. Myelofibrosis in cats is often associated with FeLV infection, and neutropenia is also common
Cytotoxic drug therapy	Virtually all cytotoxic agents (L-asparaginase not myelosuppressive, and vincristine mildly)	Targeting of cytotoxic effect to rapidly dividing cells in the marrow	History of recent cytotoxic drug administration. Pyrexia, clinical signs of sepsis. Possibly thrombocytopenia. Left shift and toxic change as recover. Usually occurs 5–7 days after drug administration, and resolves in 24–72 hours
Idiosyncratic drug reactions	Oestrogen; chloramphenicol; phenylbutazone; cephalosporins; many others	Toxicity to progenitor and committed cells at any level. Immune-mediated component suspected for many drugs	Oestrogen toxicity produces initial neutrophilia, then neutropenia, thrombocytopenia and anaemia. Others may affect only neutrophils or cause pancytopenia (aplastic anaemia). May be reversible or irreversible
Chédiak–Higashi syndrome (rare)	Autosomal recessive disorder in Persian cats	Impaired release of neutrophils from the marrow. Other factors	Breed. Hypopigmentation of skin, hair, eyes. Increased susceptibility to bacterial infections (neutrophil dysfunction)
Cyclic haemopoiesis in grey Collies (rare)	Autosomal recessive, grey Collies	Possible defect in G-CSF post-receptor signal transduction	Other white cell, platelet and reticulocyte counts may also fluctuate cyclically. Rebound neutrophilia after 2–4 days of neutropenia
Immune-mediated neutropenia (rare)		Idiosyncratic drug reaction. Primary immune-mediated destruction. Secondary immune-mediated destruction	No other cytopenias. Demonstrable antineutrophil antibodies (flow cytometry). (Response to steroids)
Hereditary neutropenia (rare)	Reported in Giant Schnauzers and Collies (both autosomal recessive)	Giant Schnauzers: selective malabsorption of vitamin B12	Age and breed; family history. Giant Schnauzers: concurrent anaemia

5.8 (continued) Causes of neutropenia in dogs and cats.

Neutrophil dysfunction

Neutrophil dysfunction may be hereditary or acquired. Hereditary neutrophil dysfunction has been reported in Irish Setters (leucocyte adhesion deficiency, LAD), Weimeraners (oxidative metabolic disorder) and Dobermanns (defect in bacterial cell killing). These diseases can be confirmed on the basis of neutrophil function tests (with appropriate controls) and, in the case of LAD, by the absence of CD11b and CD18 expression.

Chédiak–Higashi syndrome is an inherited autosomal recessive disorder of the microtubules and granules in leucocytes and other cells, reported in smoke-blue Persian cats with yellow–green irises. Haematologically, abnormally large eosinophilic granules are seen in neutrophils and eosinophils. Affected cats have bleeding tendencies due to platelet dysfunction. They have low to normal neutrophil counts, and the neutrophils show impaired chemotaxis and bacterial cell killing.

Acquired neutrophil dysfunction is probably quite commonly seen in small animals but is largely unrecognized. The most studied occurrence is in diabetes mellitus in dogs, where reduced neutrophil bactericidal activity and impaired adhesion, migration and phagocytosis occur. The degree of adhesion correlates inversely with glucose levels, so the more poorly controlled the diabetes, the less able the neutrophils are to function. Reduced adherence capacity has not yet been demonstrated in diabetic cats. Defective chemotaxis and reduced bacterial killing have been reported in cats with feline leukaemia virus (FeLV) infection, and defective chemotaxis in feline infectious peritonitis. Neoplasia is also a recognized cause of neutrophil dysfunction in humans, but this has not been studied in dogs and cats. Lastly, glucocorticoids result in impaired neutrophil function in humans but, again, this has not been documented in small animals.

Other hereditary neutrophil abnormalities

Pelger–Huët anomaly is an autosomal dominant inherited disorder reported in Domestic Shorthair cats and in dogs. The homozygous form is lethal, and in heterozygotes granulocytes fail to lobulate from band to segmented forms, so there is a persistent left shift. These unsegmented neutrophils appear to have normal function. Megakaryocytes are also hyposegmented. Cyclic haemopoiesis, leucocyte adhesion deficiency and Birman cat neutrophil granulation are other hereditary abnormalities.

Cytoplasmic inclusions

The cytoplasm of neutrophils may contain abnormal granules, vacuoles, organisms and various other inclusions, not of all which are associated with disease states.

Döhle bodies and toxic granulation are associated with toxic change (see above and Figure 5.3). The neutrophils of Birman cats may contain similar granules, which are more azurophilic, but are normal in this breed. Both dogs and cats with genetic defects in mucopolysaccharide metabolism resulting in lysosomal storage diseases may have coarse red granules in their neutrophils (and large abnormal basophil granules).

Cytoplasmic vacuolation may develop in neutrophils in EDTA; these vacuoles are clear and few in number, and are not as pronounced or 'foamy' as those seen in toxic change (see Figure 5.3). Vacuolation has been associated with high doses of chloramphenicol and phenylbutazone, and subtle vacuolation may be seen in cholesteryl ester storage disease.

Infectious agents are sometimes seen within neutrophils: these include *Ehrlichia canis, E. ewingii, Histoplasma capsulatum, Hepatozoon canis* and *Leishmania donovani* (see Chapter 27). However, the sensitivity of microscopic detection for diagnosis is generally low. It is very unusual to see bacteria within circulating neutrophils, except in a septicaemic crisis.

Canine distemper inclusions may be seen in dogs either following vaccination or after natural infection: these are homogenously pink–magenta roundish structures.

Haemosiderin granules have been observed in the neutrophils of dogs following blood transfusion: their significance is unknown.

Eosinophils

The eosinophil is a striking cell, slightly larger than a neutrophil, with a segmented nucleus with only two or three lobes, and coarse eosinophilic cytoplasmic granules. In the dog, these granules are round and variably sized, and numbers are very variable: occasionally, only one or two very large granules are seen within a cell (Figure 5.9). In the cat, the small rod-shaped orangey pink granules are very numerous and uniform (Figure 5.9). These granules contain an arsenal of preformed toxins. Background cytoplasm is lightly basophilic.

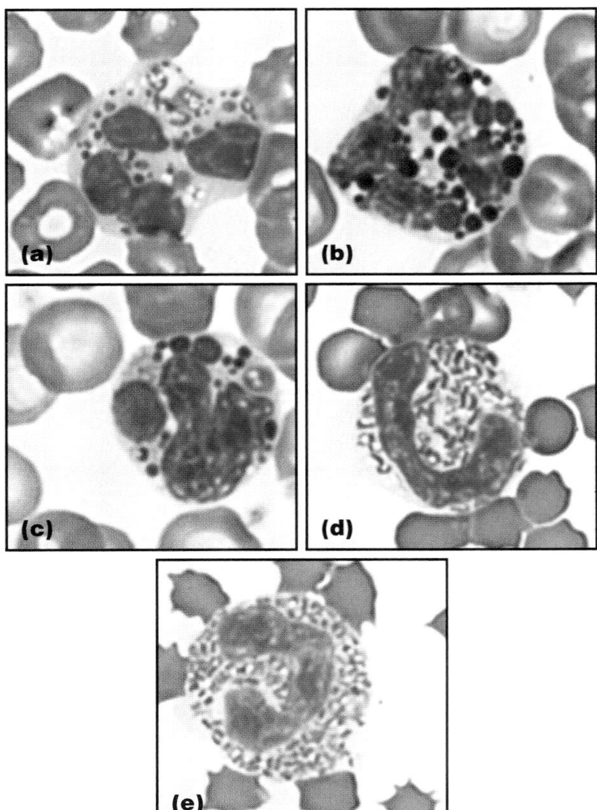

5.9 Eosinophils have a segmented nucleus with only two or three lobes, and coarse eosinophilic cytoplasmic granules. **(a, b, c)** Canine eosinophils have widely varying numbers of round variably sized granules. **(d, e)** Feline eosinophils have small rod-shaped orangy pink granules, which are very numerous and uniform. (May–Grünwald–Giemsa; original magnification X1000.)

Eosinophils are important defenders against parasites, particularly helminths, and mediate inflammatory reactions. Additionally, they are often the effector cell of host tissue damage in allergic disease. Like neutrophils, they have a marrow storage pool and a short circulating half-life, but, unlike neutrophils, there is a large tissue pool of eosinophils in normal animals. They congregate in the loose connective tissues of organs vulnerable to entry by pathogens: the skin, the respiratory tract and the gastrointestinal tract. Because eosinophils normally represent only a small percentage of the circulating granulocytes, a 500-cell differential count is recommended for accurate determination of numbers.

Eosinophilia

There are very many potential causes of eosinophilia, particularly in cats: these are summarized in Figure 5.10. As eosinophils are really tissue cells, local eosinophilic inflammation is not always accompanied by circulating eosinophilia. In addition, the degree of eosinophilia is variable, and is not indicative of the disease process. Paraneoplastic eosinophilias are particularly

Disease process
Parasitic
Ectoparasites*: pulmonary (*Aelurostronglyus, Angiostrongylus*); heartworm (*Dirofilaria*); enteric (*Giardia*, coccidia, ascarids)
Allergic
Feline asthma* Eosinophilic bronchopenumonopathy (dogs)* Flea allergy dermatitis* Eosinophilic granuloma complex (cats)* Atopy (dogs)* Food hypersensitivity*
Inflammatory
Inflammatory bowel disease (eosinophilic enteritis)* Eosinophilic myositis* Panosteitis Focal inflammation Lower urinary tract disease (cats) Rhinitis/sinusitis Eosinophilic granuloma complex (cats) Steatitis
Neoplastic
Mast cell tumour (disseminated/intestinal)* Lymphoma Myeloproliferative disease (eosinophilic leukaemia, hypereosinophilic syndrome (cats)) Miscellaneous tumours
Infectious
Feline panleucopenia virus Feline infectious peritonitis Toxoplasmosis Upper respiratory tract infection Pyometra
Miscellaneous
Hypoadrenocorticism (dogs)* Chronic renal failure (cats) Cardiac disease (cats) Immune-mediated skin disease Others

5.10 Causes of eosinophilia in cats and dogs. The more frequent causes are asterisked.

common in cats, and may be associated with many tumours, including lymphoma. In some diseases, there may be tissue infiltration as well as eosinophilia, and a resultant hypereosinophilic syndrome. This is reported in feline (and human) intestinal T-cell lymphomas, and is mediated by excessive production of the cytokine interleukin 5 by the neoplastic T cells (Barrs *et al.*, 2002; Cave *et al.*, 2004).

Hypereosinophilic syndrome (HES) is characterized by a persistent, marked, predominantly mature eosinophilia, eosinophilic infiltration of multiple tissues. Most cases are idiopathic, with no underlying cause, and idiopathic HES is uncommon in cats and extremely rare in dogs. In cats, bone marrow, lymph node and small intestine are major sites of infiltration. Diagnosis relies upon exclusion of the causes of secondary eosinophilia. Differentiation of idiopathic HES in cats from chronic eosinophilic leukaemia (CEL) is difficult, if not impossible, as both are characterized by eosinophilic hyperplasia in the bone marrow and eosinophilic infiltration of other organs. It has been suggested that abnormal eosinophil precursor morphology and concurrent anaemia suggest CEL. In any case, the prognosis is similarly grim for both, and they may represent variants of the same disease. It is controversial whether eosinophilic leukaemia occurs in the dog.

Eosinopenia

Eosinopenia is a relative term as many reference intervals extend to zero, but it may be seen in acute infections, in response to corticosteroids and as part of the stress leucogram. Corticosteroids inhibit eosinophil release from bone marrow and also promote sequestration of eosinophils in tissues.

Basophils

The basophil is larger than the neutrophil (similar to eosinophil and monocyte) with a long, mildly lobulated, ribbon-like nucleus. In the dog, unevenly scattered dark purplish cytoplasmic granules are seen against a pale grey–blue cytoplasm (Figure 5.11). In the cat, the round to oval granules are much denser and tend to pack the cell: these stain less intensely with Romanowsky stains and appear pale grey–lavender with a pink to orange tint (Figure 5.11).

Basophils are involved in allergic disease and in the immune response to some parasites. Basophils also participate with eosinophils in inflammatory

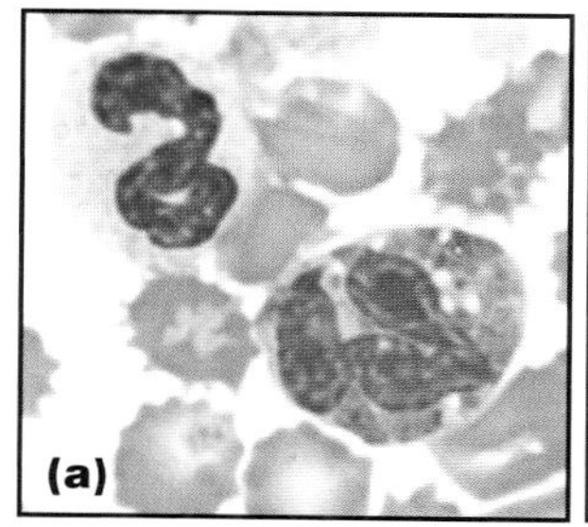

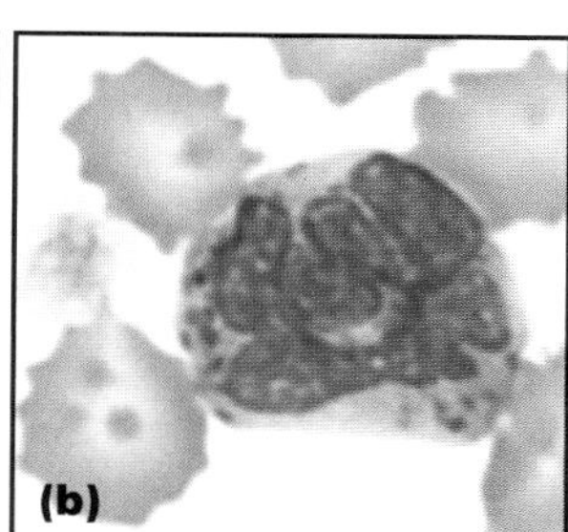

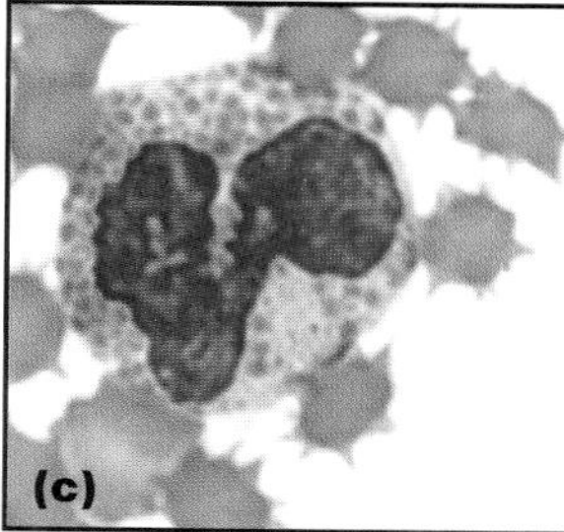

5.11 Basophils. (a) Canine basophil and neutrophil. The basophil (on the right) is larger than the neutrophil and has a long mildly lobulated ribbon-like nucleus. (b) Canine basophil with unevenly scattered dark purplish cytoplasmic granules against a pale grey–blue cytoplasm. (c) Feline basophil, showing much more densely packed oval grey–lavender granules. (May–Grünwald–Giemsa; original magnification X1000.)

reactions, and they may also have roles in delayed hypersensitivity, haemostasis and lipolysis. Like neutrophils and eosinophils, they have a marrow storage pool and a short circulating half-life. In tissues, they may survive up to 2 weeks. Because basophils normally represent only a tiny percentage of the granulocytes, accurate counts can only be determined by counting thousands of cells or by using direct counting methods (haemocytometer, see Chapter 3) and special stains (toluidine blue or histamine immunocytochemical stains).

Basophilia tends to echo eosinophilia, and is most often due to allergic disease or parasitism; it is occasionally seen in inflammatory haemograms. *Dirofilaria immitis* infection is an important cause in North America. Basophilia may also be seen in animals with mast cell neoplasia, and is a common finding in humans with leukaemia and myeloproliferative disorders. Basophilic leukaemia has been reported in cats and dogs, and may be associated with hyperhistaminaemia.

Basopenia is rarely appreciated, but can be caused by corticosteroids.

Mast cells

Mast cells are not seen in the circulation in healthy animals but may be seen infrequently in inflammatory or neoplastic conditions. They are round cells with a central round to oval nucleus, which may stain pale blue, but is often at least partially obscured by the variably sized, red-to-purple granules in the cytoplasm (Figure 5.12). Mast cells are essentially tissue cells, and have important roles in allergic and other inflammatory responses, where they interact with other leucocytes. If present in the circulation, mast cells on a blood smear tend to accumulate at the feathered edge, as they are large cells.

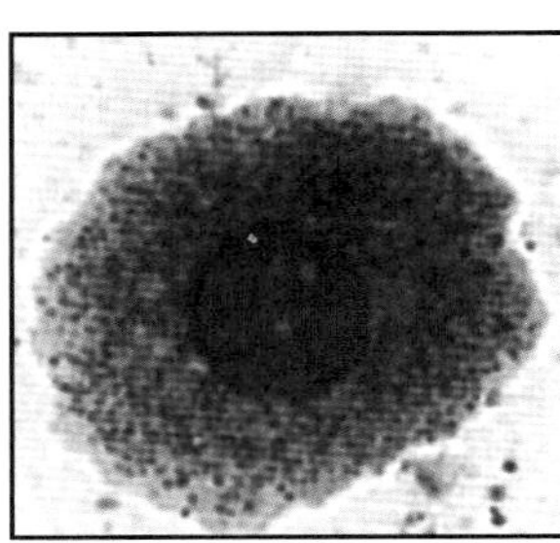

5.12 Canine mast cell. This is a round cell with a central round-to-oval nucleus, partially obscured by the variably sized red-to-lilac and purple granules in the cytoplasm. (Rapi-Diff II; original magnification x1000.)

Mast cells may be seen in the circulation in a variety of non-neoplastic and neoplastic conditions, and are often found in inflammatory conditions, accompanying an inflammatory leucogram. Non-neoplastic and neoplastic mast cells cannot be readily differentiated morphologically. The examination of a buffy coat smear as part of clinical staging of dogs with cutaneous mast cell tumours is not recommended, as the presence of mast cells has not been shown to correlate with stage or prognosis, and very high numbers of mast cells may be seen in non-neoplastic disorders. Circulating mast cell numbers high enough to cause an overall leucocytosis merit further investigation and bone marrow sampling.

Mononuclear cells

Monocytes

The monocyte appears larger than a neutrophil; although the cells are similar in size, in a smear the monocyte adheres more to the glass and becomes more flattened. It has a variably shaped nucleus (round, oval, bean to dumbbell, bi- or multilobed) with reticular or lacy chromatin. Cytoplasm is relatively abundant and blue–grey in colour with a ground glass appearance and occasional fine pink/magenta granules (canine are more granular than feline monocytes) (Figure 5.13). Vacuolation in blood samples is usually an *in vitro* change but can also reflect increased phagocytic activity. Cells may have rather irregular cytoplasmic boundaries and appear round or slightly angular, or even have little projections or pseudopodia. It can be difficult to differentiate a toxic band neutrophil from a monocyte: monocytes that have band-shaped nuclei usually have rounded, knob- or dumbbell-shaped ends (Figure 5.13h).

The monocyte is the circulating precursor of the macrophage, and circulates for only a short time (approximately 8 hours in the cat) before migrating into the tissues. There is no storage pool of monocytes, but in the dog there are probably marginating and circulating pools. The tissue pool is sizeable, and resident macrophages in normal tissue have a very long lifespan (up to years), while those recruited in inflammation and disease are much shorter lived. Macrophages, along with neutrophils and natural killer cells, are the first line of defence in the innate immune response. They present antigen to lymphocytes to initiate the adaptive immune response, and secrete cytokines and chemical mediators of inflammation. Monocytes/macrophages also phagocytose pathogens, dead or infected cells, cells coated with antibodies, and foreign material. Macrophages within the bone marrow provide an essential supporting role for haemopoiesis. Monocytes/macrophages are essential for life, and, together with specialized macrophages in some tissues, form the mononuclear phagocyte system (MPS).

Monocytosis is traditionally associated with chronic inflammation and may accompany neutrophilia in these cases. However, monocytosis may also be seen in acute inflammatory responses and overall is an inconsistent finding in inflammatory diseases. It is common in immune-mediated disease and in disease processes where there is tissue necrosis, e.g. where there is a large solid tumour or tumours with areas that have outgrown the blood supply. Occasionally, monocytosis may be seen in neutropenic animals, when it is believed to be a 'compensatory' response, and a rebound monocytosis is common in animals recovering from neutropenia. Monocytosis is also part of a stress leucogram, but is not always present in dogs and is not generally observed in cats. Finally, monocytosis may be seen in monocytic or myelomonocytic leukaemias, where counts are likely greatly to exceed the normal range.

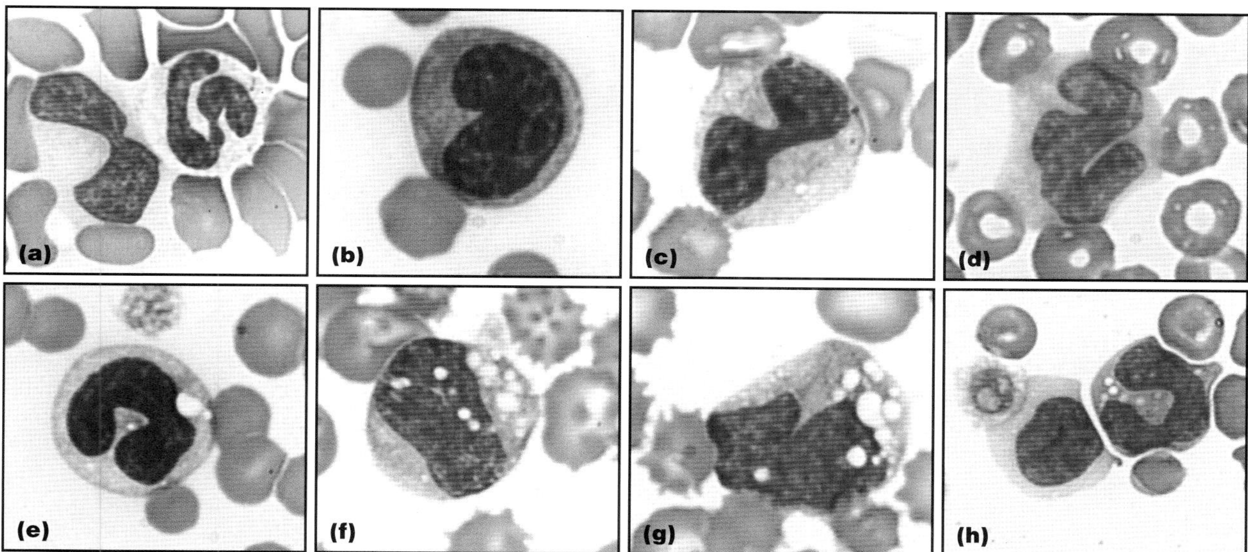

5.13 Monocytes. The nucleus varies in shape and the chromatin appears reticular or lacy. chromatin. In (a), the monocyte (left) appears larger than the neutrophil. (e–h) Vacuolation in blood samples is usually an *in vitro* change but can also reflect increased phagocytic activity. In (h) a medium-sized lymphocyte (left) is beside a monocyte with a band-shaped nucleus with rounded ends. ((a,c,f,g) Rapi Diff II, (b,d,e,h) May–Grünwald–Giemsa; original magnification X1000.)

Lymphocytes

Lymphopoiesis

Most lymphopoiesis occurs in the peripheral lymphoid tissues in response to antigenic stimulation: there are no lymphoid germinal centres in normal marrow, and lymphoid cells make up only 5% or less of the marrow haematopoietic cells. Primitive lymphocytes (pre-T cells) migrate from the bone marrow and undergo development in the thymic cortex (and some other peripheral lymphoid sites) into T cells. Pre-B cells develop into B cells in the marrow, then migrate to the peripheral lymphoid tissues. Immunologically, T cells are defined by the surface expression of a T cell receptor complex called CD3, while B cells express a B cell receptor complex called CD79a. These two complexes, and other cell surface expressed markers, are used to identify T and B cell tumours by immunohistochemistry and flow cytometry (see below).

Both T and B lymphocytes become activated on exposure to appropriately presented antigens. Various subsets of T cells have been identified:

- T helper cells (Th, $CD4^+$) mediate cell-mediated immunity and humoral immunity. Th cells are vital to the process by which activated B lymphocytes undergo transformation to lymphoblasts, then plasma cells, which produce antigen-specific immunoglobulin
- Regulatory T cells (Treg, $CD25^+$; another group of $CD4^+$ cells) are generally immunosuppressive T cells required for maintenance of self-tolerance and control of immune function. Activation of these cells is thought to be part of pathogenesis during feline immunodeficiency virus infection (Valenkamp *et al*., 2004)
- Cytotoxic T cells ($CD8^+$ cells) and natural killer (NK) cells (morphologically large granular lymphocytes) mediate cell killing.

The pathways of cell activation and regulation are highly coordinated, and activated T cells orchestrate the antigen-specific immune response through a complex web of intercellular signals and interactions. Much of lymphocyte production occurs in the periphery in response to these signals.

Distribution

Most of the lymphocytes in the circulation are small lymphocytes. These cells have densely staining, round to slightly oval/indented nuclei and very scant, pale blue cytoplasm, which appears to extend only part way round the nucleus (Figure 5.14). The nuclei have smudged chromatin and no nucleoli. A few slightly larger (up to about the size of a neutrophil) medium lymphocytes, with more cytoplasm, are also a normal finding, and occasionally cells containing a few reddish granules are seen. Reactive lymphocytes may be larger and have increased amounts of intensely basophilic cytoplasm. Atypical and malignant lymphoblasts may be seen in lymphoproliferative diseases: features of malignancy are discussed in Chapter 20 and illustrated in Figure 5.14.

Blood acts as a transport system for lymphocyte redistribution and recirculation, but only 5% of the total body lymphocyte pool is circulating in the blood. This does not mean that lymphocytes are static cells in the tissues, and unlike other cells they re-enter the circulation after migrating into the peripheral lymphoid tissues: there is a continuous recirculation of lymphoid cells throughout the body. Lymphoid cells drain from tissues (via afferent lymphatics) to the regional lymph nodes, then (via efferent lymphatics) enter the thoracic duct. The lymphoid cells enter the circulation via the thoracic duct, and leave the circulation in response to adhesion factors expressed in vascular endothelium. This recirculation, and a continued ability to mitose, are unique features of lymphoid cells. The circulating lymphocytes consist of various populations but, in normal animals, most are long-lived recirculating memory T cells.

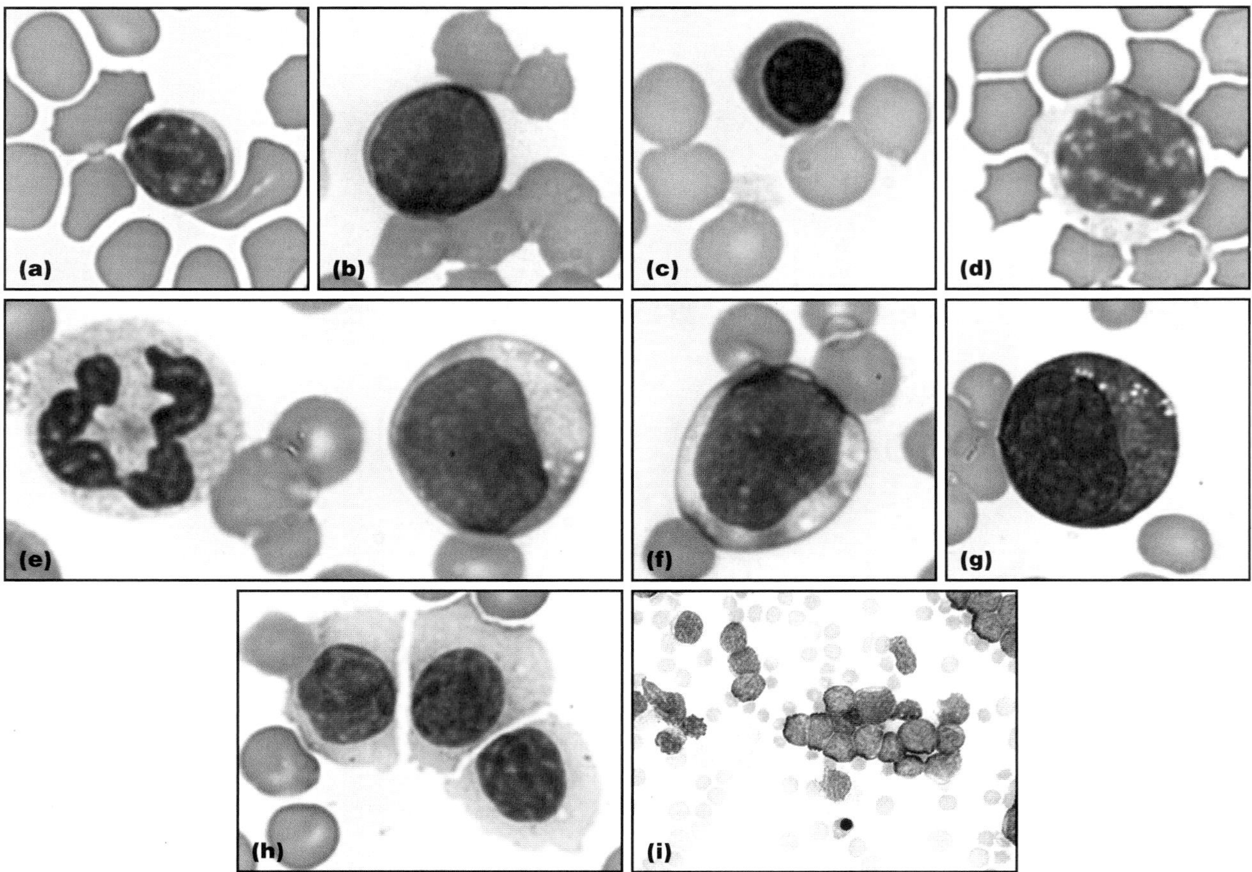

5.14 Lymphocytes. **(a)** Normal canine small lymphocyte, with very scant blue cytoplasm that appears to extend only part way round the nucleus. **(b)** Normal feline small lymphocyte, larger relative to red blood cells. Note the absence of nucleoli. **(c)** Late normoblast (nucleated red blood cell). This is NOT lymphoid and is smaller, with an eccentrically placed nucleus and clumped chromatin. **(d,e,f)** Medium lymphocytes may be up to about the size of a neutrophil; occasionally cells contain a few reddish granules. **(g)** Large reactive lymphocyte with increased amounts of intensely basophilic cytoplasm. **(h)** Large atypical neoplastic cells from a case of lymphoid leukaemia. **(i)** Large lymphoblasts showing features of malignancy: cytoplasmic basophilia, course nuclear chromatin, prominent nucleoli and nuclear moulding. (May–Grünwald–Giemsa; original magnification (a-f, h) X1000, (g) X400.)

Lymphocytosis

Lymphocytosis may be physiological, mediated by adrenaline release (especially in cats); counts may be >20 x 10^9/l. Young dogs and cats tend to have higher lymphocyte counts than adult animals. Lymphocytosis may also occur transiently after vaccination or prolonged immune stimulation. Mild lymphocytosis, or a normal lymphocyte count despite medical stress, is a common finding in hypoadrenocorticism. In lymphoproliferative diseases, either lymphocytosis or lymphopenia may be seen; in lymphoma, lymphopenia is more common.

Lymphopenia

Lymphopenia is most commonly seen as a result of exogenous or endogenous corticosteroids, which cause a shift of lymphocytes from the circulation, and also lymphocytolysis. This is a common feature of the stress haemogram. However, in acute inflammation, lymphopenia may not simply be a 'stress' response but may result from increased margination of lymphocytes to the site of inflammation and to lymph nodes, coupled with reduced migration out of lymph nodes. Lymphopenia is also a feature of the acute phase of many viral infections, and may be seen in sepsis or endotoxaemia. Loss of lymph, e.g. in chylothorax or lymphangiectasia, can depress circulating lymphocyte numbers. More canine and feline lymphoma patients show lymphopenia than show lymphocytosis; this may reflect either stress or blockage of normal lymphatic flow and failure of cells to reach the circulation. Immunosuppressive drug therapy reduces circulating lymphocyte numbers. Rarely, animals with primary immunodeficiencies may be lymphopenic (but counts may also be normal).

Reactive lymphocytes

Reactive lymphocytes are antigenically stimulated lymphocytes that are occasionally seen in the circulation in a very wide range of conditions. They may be large, and nuclei have clumped chromatin (but no prominent nucleoli) and a scalloped outline. These cells have increased amounts of intensely basophilic cytoplasm and may have a perinuclear Golgi zone (Figure 5.14f).

Abnormal lymphocytes

The presence of circulating abnormal cells is much more suggestive of lymphoproliferative disease than any change in lymphocyte count. The features associated with malignancy are discussed in Chapter 20 and illustrated in Figure 5.14. In lymphoproliferative diseases, abnormal lymphoid cells on blood smear examination may either reflect escape from cells from neoplastic peripheral lymphoid tissue into the circulation (so called 'overspill'), or bone marrow involvement. Some clinical pathologists use the term 'overspill leukaemia' whenever they see increased or aberrant lymphoid cells in the circulation of patients with lymphoma: this is a misleading term as the circulating cells may reflect marrow involvement, especially where counts are high.

Leukaemias

Lymphoproliferative disorders include lymphoma, lymphoid leukaemias and plasma cell myeloma, while myeloproliferative disorders encompass myeloid, monocytic, megakaryocytic and erythroid leukaemias (i.e. all non-lymphoid leukaemias) and myelodysplastic syndromes. Leukaemia is a neoplastic condition of the bone marrow, in which neoplastic cells arising from either lymphoid or non-lymphoid haematopoietic stem cells or their progeny undergo clonal expansion, with or without cellular differentiation. Frequently, the leukaemic cells are released into the peripheral blood, often in large numbers, and may also infiltrate other organs, such as the liver, spleen and peripheral lymph nodes. Leukaemia causes clinical signs by four main mechanisms:

- Failure of normal haemopoiesis
- Organ dysfunction due to infiltration by leukaemic cells
- Hyperviscosity due to very high circulating numbers of aberrant cells
- Paraneoplastic syndromes, such as hypercalcaemia or immune-mediated disease.

Leukaemia may be acute or chronic. Acute leukaemias occur when neoplastic transformation occurs at the stem cell/committed blast stage, and the malignant cells have little differentiation potential. The neoplastic cells are poorly differentiated, and proliferate rapidly and in an uncontrolled manner, with arrested or defective maturation. The clinical course is rapid, and clinical signs are severe. Marrow infiltration due to uncontrolled proliferation of tumour cells results in crowding of normal marrow elements, competition for nutrients, failure of marrow to elaborate stimulatory factors and the build up of inhibitory factors released by the neoplastic cells. As a result of this, normal blood cell production is reduced. The first manifestation of this is usually neutropenia, because neutrophils have a half-life of hours in the circulation, and a storage pool in the marrow which will provide a supply for about 5 days. Platelets are also short-lived, so concurrent thrombocytopenia is common, and some patients show thrombocytopenia first. Red cells have a long circulating lifespan, so anaemia develops much later as pre-existing cells maintain levels for longer. The haemopoietic consequences of leukaemia, and clinical consequences of these, are summarized in Figure 5.15.

Features suggestive of leukaemia	Clinical manifestations
Neutropenia	Sepsis
Thrombocytopenia	Petechial and ecchymotic haemorrhages, melaena, epistaxis
Leucocytosis	Possibly hyperviscosity syndrome: bleeding diatheses; ocular changes; neurological signs; polyuria/polydipsia; thromboembolic disease

5.15 Haematological features of leukaemia, and the clinical consequences of these abnormalities.

Chronic leukaemias occur when the neoplastic transformation occurs in either a stem cell or later cell but progeny retain a strong tendency to differentiate. Although proliferation is uncontrolled, the cells are morphologically well differentiated (but often are functionally abnormal). These conditions generally have an insidious onset of less severe clinical signs, and less profound cytopenias, but may still present acutely.

Acute leukaemia

Acute lymphoblastic leukaemia (ALL) is more common than acute myeloid leukaemia (AML) in both the dog and cat. In either type, animals present with acute onset lethargy, malaise, anorexia and weakness. Clinical signs include pallor, hepatosplenomegaly, mild lymphadenopathy, pyrexia, shifting lameness and, occasionally, central nervous system signs. Marked neutropenia and thrombocytopenia are common and there are usually abnormal cells in circulation: if counts are very high hyperviscosity may result. Bone marrow aspirates have >30% neoplastic blast cells (>40% for lymphoblasts) and often the marrow is virtually ablated by tumour cells, resulting in depletion of megakaryoctes, and both erythroid and myeloid series (including the storage pool) (Figure 5.16).

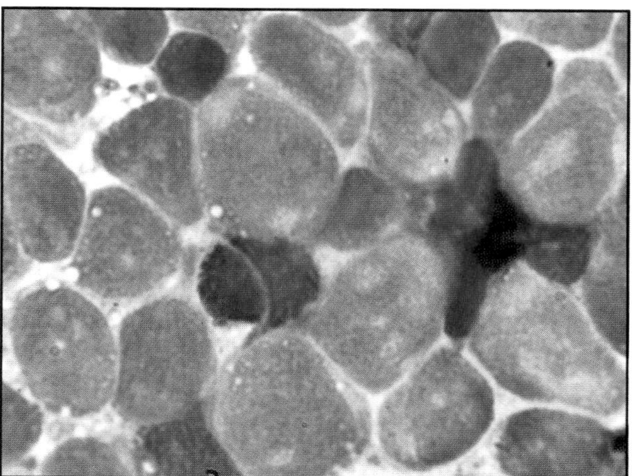

5.16 Bone marrow aspirate from a dog with acute lymphoblastic leukaemia. The marrow has been ablated by tumour cells, and virtually no normal haemopoietic cells are seen. In this field, there are densely packed large neoplastic blast cells. These cells show features of malignancy (course chromatin, pleomorphic nucleoli, cytoplasmic basophilia, nuclear moulding).

The diagnosis of leukaemia is generally straightforward when concurrent haematology and bone marrow are examined, although typing is difficult. The main cytological differential diagnosis for acute leukaemia is bone marrow in the acute stages of repopulation, for example after chemotherapeutic drug administration or parvovirus infection. Generally the clinical history in these cases would ensure against confusion with leukaemia, and bone marrow sampling is seldom indicated in these cases. It can be difficult to differentiate ALL from stage V lymphoma with bone marrow involvement: criteria are summarized in Figure 5.17.

Lymphoma with bone marrow involvement	Acute lymphoblastic leukaemia
<40% blasts in marrow	>40% blasts in marrow
Lower number of circulating blasts	Higher number of circulating blasts
Mild or absent cytopenias	Severe cytopenias
Massive lymphadenopathy	Mild to moderate lymphadenopathy
May not be systemically ill	Usually systemically ill

5.17 Selected criteria to assist differentiation of lymphoma with bone marrow involvement from acute lymphoblastic leukaemia.

Immunophenotyping can be carried out by flow cytometry (blood or marrow in EDTA) or by immunocytochemistry (marrow smears or biopsy specimens) to identify whether the tumour is myeloid or lymphoid, and to further subtype the cell of origin in some cases.

The biochemical changes seen in acute leukaemias may reflect organ infiltration (e.g. raised liver enzymes), hyperviscosity (azotaemia) and paraneoplastic syndromes (hypercalcaemia or hypergammaglobulinaemia in lymphoid leukaemias).

Chronic leukaemia

Chronic lymphocytic leukaemia

Chronic lymphocytic leukaemia (CLL) usually affects middle-aged to old dogs, with a male predisposition. It is very rare in cats. Animals present vaguely, and signs may wax and wane; anorexia, lethargy, polyuria and polydipsia, mild hepatosplenomegaly, lymphadenopathy, pallor and pyrexia are common. Lymphocytosis (6 to >100 x 10^9/l) is seen, with a population of morphologically normal mature lymphocytes, and mild cytopenias.

Diagnosis requires exclusion of other causes of lymphocytosis, haematology and aspiration or biopsy of bone marrow, though in a small proportion of these cases (especially large granular leukaemias) disease may originate in the spleen. Bone marrow examination must be carried out as the circulating population may appear more mature than that in the marrow, and disease requiring more aggressive management than CLL must be identified, as inappropriate treatment will provoke resistance. Bone marrow aspiration demonstrates increased numbers of small lymphocytes (>30% of nucleated cells in the bone marrow) and either apparently normal or mildly decreased erythroid and myeloid activity.

Chronic granulocytic leukaemia

Chronic granulocytic leukaemia (CGL) is rare and difficult to diagnose. Clinical signs are vague, with lethargy, inappetence and weight loss over an insidious course. There may be hepatosplenomegaly. Haematology shows a massive mature neutrophilia, and bone marrow aspirates show marked myeloid hyperplasia. In CGL (and other chronic myeloid leukaemias), bone marrow evaluation shows <30% blast cells, and blast counts may even be normal. Mild dysplastic changes, with morphologically abnormal granulocyte precursors, may be seen in the bone marrow; marrow more typically shows only hypercellularity due to myeloid hyperplasia, with no obvious atypical features, and so does not differentiate CGL from a reactive neutrophilia. The mature neutrophils may be hypersegmented, but otherwise appear normal, and diagnosis relies on elimination of other causes of neutrophilia.

Myelodysplastic syndromes

Myelodysplastic syndromes (MDS) are challenging to diagnose, and rely on examination of a bone marrow aspirate, and concurrent haematology, by an experienced clinical pathologist. The hallmark of MDS is ineffective haemopoiesis with disturbed maturation, resulting in haematological and bone marrow abnormalities. These are a heterogeneous group of conditions and in some circumstances may represent a preleukaemic state. Haematological features include non-regenerative anaemia (which is occasionally macrocytic), neutropenia, thrombocytopenia and occasionally monocytosis. On bone marrow examination there are less than 30% blast cells, and dysplastic change is seen, often affecting more than one cell line. Cells are morphologically abnormal and maturation may appear disorderly.

Myelofibrosis

Myelofibrosis is an increase in collagen and other fibrous elements in the marrow matrix (see Figure 4.30). It is thought to be a reactive marrow response that can be associated with many diseases but often the initiating cause is unknown. In humans, megakaryocytic disorders are a common cause of myelofibrosis; where these cells are not involved, activated monocytes and macrophages have been implicated. The aetiopathogenesis is poorly understood in small animals.

Dogs with myelofibrosis usually present with non-regenerative anaemia, and it is thought that in many cases there is an immune-mediated mechanism. They present when the anaemia becomes severe, weeks to months after the initiating insult, which is seldom identified. Myelofibrosis is also associated with some myeloid leukaemias, and is common in cats with MDS or AML, where the primary disease dominates presentation. FeLV infection or exposure may play a role. Idiosyncratic drug reactions may also initiate myelofibrosis in both species.

Beyond the haemogram: other evaluations of leucocytes

Bone marrow aspiration

Bone marrow evaluation is required to diagnose and subtype myelodysplastic and leukaemic diseases, and is very useful in many disease situations (Figure 5.18).

Neutropenia
Thrombocytopenia
Pancytopenia
Abnormal/immature lymphocytes or granulocytes in the circulation
Inexplicably high numbers of any cell line in the circulation
Non-regenerative anaemia
Lymphoma
Hyperproteinaemia
Hypercalcaemia of unknown origin
Pyrexia of unknown origin
Suspected systemic infections with *Ehrlichia*, *Leishmania* or fungi
Detection of FeLV in discordant cats

5.18 Indications for bone marrow sampling in cats and dogs.

In normal marrow, the myeloid to erythroid ratio is approximately 0.75–1.5:1 in dogs, and 1–4:1 in cats. Myeloid hyperplasia, and an increase in this ratio, will be seen in any inflammatory response. Where there is an ongoing demand for neutrophils, depletion of the storage pool may be evident, and there may be toxic change.

Sampling of bone marrow and sample handling are discussed in Chapter 4.

Immunophenotyping of leucocytes

Immunophenotyping is the determination of cell type by the identification of cell surface markers using antibodies. In canine lymphoma, immunophenotyping is of prognostic significance, as, in general, T cell tumours carry a poorer prognosis. Morphological subtype, based on cytological evaluation, may also prove to be of prognostic relevance (Ponce *et al.*, 2004), and there are also established clinical prognostic indicators. Immunophenotyping also has a role in prognostication and treatment selection in leukaemias: morphological differentiation of acute lymphoid and myeloid leukaemias is often difficult or impossible, and cytochemical stains established in human medicine have not proved useful in cats and dogs (see below). Immunophenotyping gives not only a cell lineage, but also, in some cases, can suggest stage of maturation arrest and clonal expansion, because some cell surface markers are expressed during restricted phases of cell development.

Immunophenotyping of haemolymphatic cells relies on detection of cell surface markers usually assigned CD (clusters of differentiation) numbers. There are more than 150 CDs assigned in human medicine, but only relatively few currently have defined roles in leucocyte disorders in small animals: selected important CDs are summarized in Figure 5.19. In many laboratories, samples are initially screened for CD3 and CD79a to confirm lymphoid origin and identify T or

Antigen detected or clone	Cellular specificity
Canine	
CD3	All T cells
CD4	T helper cells, neutrophils
CD5	All T cells
CD8	Cytotoxic T cells, NK cells
CD11/18	All leucocytes
CD11b/CD11c	Granulocytes, monocytes
CD11d	NK cells, cytotoxic T large granular lymphocytes
CD18	All leucocytes
CD14	Monocytes, macrophages
CD18	All leucocytes
CD21	B cells
CD25	B and T cells, monocytes
CD34	Haemopoietic progenitor cells
CD41	Platelets, megakaryocytes
CD41/CD61	Platelets, megakaryoctyes
CD45	All leucocytes
CD45RA	B cells, T cell subset, primitive blasts of other lineages
CD62	Activated platelets
CD79a	B cells
MHC class II	Monocytes, macrophages, B cells
Thy-1	Monocytes, macrophages, T cells, some B cells
MAC387	Monocytes, macrophages, neutrophils and their precursors
MPO	Neutrophils and their precursors
Feline	
CD3	All T cells
CD4	Helper T cells
CD8	NK cells, T cells
CD5	All T cells
CD11b	Granulocytes, monocytes
CD18	All leucocytes
CD21-like	B cells
CD41/CD61	Platelets, megakaryocytes
CD45	All leucocytes
MHC class II	Monocytes, macrophages, B cells
CL2A	Platelets
CF2555A	T cells
CF26A	T and B cells
FeMy	Mature granulocytes and monocytes, mature myeloid precursor cells
FeEr1, FeEr2	Immature erythroid precursors (60%), mature erythroid precursors
K-1, Q-3	Immature erythroid precursors
K-7	Immature erythroid precursors

5.19 Selected markers used for immunophenotyping canine and feline blood and bone marrow cells. (Data from Weiss (2003); sources of monoclonal antibodies are available in the reference.)

B cell lineage. However, some lymphoid tumours are negative for CD3 and CD79a; the use of a panel of antibodies will allow identification of further cases of lymphoproliferative disease and also myeloproliferative disease. Some lymphoid tumours are dually positive for CD3 and CD79a; in these cases, the use of a panel can help determine the cell of origin.

Immunophenotyping may be carried out by immunocytology or immunohistology (Figure 5.20) or by flow cytometry (Figure 5.21). Immunochemical techniques often work best on unfixed tissues/smears but some antibodies detect epitopes resistant to the effects of fixation and can be used on routine formalin-fixed tissue, for example CD3 (CD3-12 (Serotec) or #A452 (Dako)) and CD79a for typing canine lymphoma.

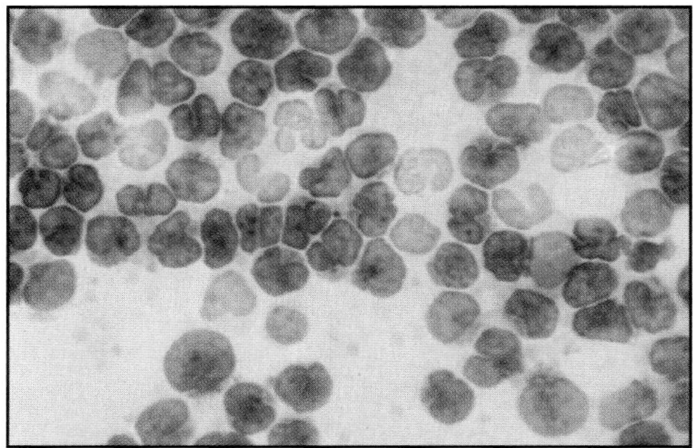

5.20 Immunophenotyping leukaemia. This is a buffy coat smear, from a dog with leukaemia, stained with anti-CD3 antibodies. The brown staining is a positive result, indicating that this is a tumour of T cell origin. (Courtesy of E. Villiers.)

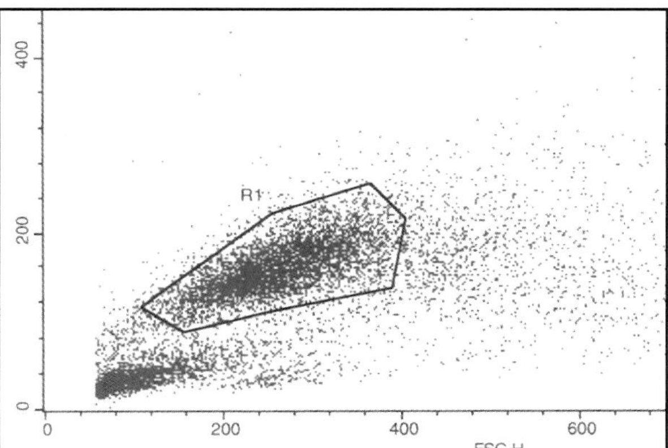

5.21 Flow cytometry results (dot plot) from a blood sample, from a dog with acute myeloid leukaemia. The concentrated dots in the boxed off area (known as the gate) represent blast cells of myeloid origin. The small cluster in the lower left corner are lymphoid. (Courtesy of E. Villiers.)

Flow cytometry

Flow cytometry is a generic technology that counts and measures multiple characteristics of individual particles in a flow stream: this technology is used by many automated haematology analysers (see Chapter 3). In immunological flow cytometry (FC), the cells to be investigated are labelled with one or more fluorochrome-labelled antibodies (fluorochromes are coloured dyes that accept light energy at a given wavelength and re-emit it at a higher wavelength). A stream of labelled cells is then directed through a laser beam and the amount of fluorescence and light scatter patterns are recorded and analysed by a computer to produce histograms and dot plots from which the cell types present can be identified. Further information can be found at www.hmds.org.uk/cytometry.htlm and http://flowcyt.salk.edu/. FC can be used in a variety of clinical situations:

- To immunophenotype lympho- and myeloproliferative diseases, where it detects specific marked antigens on the surface of the cells
- To confirm immune-mediated disease (especially immune-mediated thrombocytopenia), where it detects antibodies bound to target cells
- For the detection of minimal residual disease in human leukaemia patients (not available for small animals).

FC is available at the University of Cambridge: 5–10 ml of EDTA–blood should be submitted together with an unstained air-dried blood smear. FC will confirm the cell of origin in a leukaemic patient, but cytological bone marrow evaluation is also required for accurate diagnosis, treatment planning and prognostication, and bone marrow samples should be submitted at the same time. FC can also be carried out on marrow aspirates in either EDTA or citrate anticoagulant.

Polymerase chain reaction

PCR tests for infectious organisms (see Chapter 27) may be useful in cases where arthropod-borne infections are suspected. In addition, PCR from EDTA-treated blood samples is used to detect microscopic residual disease in human leukaemia and lymphoma patients, where particular genetic derangements specific to neoplastic cells are detected. This technique has recently been reported in canine lymphoma patients, although its value in detecting residual disease and relapse has not been determined (Keller *et al.*, 2004).

Cytochemical tests

Neoplastic cells often contain the same enzymes and cellular product as their normal counterparts, and techniques which stain for these may help identify the cell of origin. However, abnormal cells may have also metabolic abnormalities that alter their staining characteristics, and a negative result does not exclude a particular lineage. In addition, some of the molecules stained for are common to cells of different lineages. To overcome these difficulties, a panel of stains must be used (Figure 5.22).

Cytochemical analysis has been widely used for identification of origin of human haemopoietic tumours, but was never well established in small animals. In both humans and small animals, usefulness has been limited due to the lack of specific stains for lymphoid cells; while many myeloid tumours can be identified,

Cytochemical stain	Lymphoid leukaemia	Myeloid leukaemia	Monocytic leukaemia
Peroxidase	Negative	Positive (usually strongly, may be negative in cats)	Negative or weakly positive in dogs; negative in cats
Alkaline phosphatase	Negative	Positive (some cells)	Negative
Lipase	Negative	Negative	Positive
Chloroacetate esterase (CAE) (specific esterase)	Usually negative	Positive	Negative
Alpha naphthyl butyrate esterase (NBE) (non-specific esterase)	Negative (or focal staining)	Negative	Positive
Sudan black	Negative	Positive	Positive in dogs; negative in cats

5.22 Cytochemical tests for leukaemia, with guidelines as to typical staining characteristics. Lymphoid cells generally do not stain with cytochemical stains (though are occasionally positive with alkaline phosphatase or alpha naphthyl butyrate esterase), but negative staining does *not* indicate a lymphoid neoplasm, as myeloid neoplasms may also stain negatively. Results can be difficult to interpret, and the use of a screening panel makes successful identification more likely, for example by picking up markers of both myeloid and monocytic cells in myelomonocytic leukaemia. For further details see Grindem (2000) and Raskin and Valenciano (2000).

negative staining with myeloid stains does not imply lymphoid origin. In addition, there is often discordance between cytochemical and immunological diagnoses (Kheiri *et al.*, 1998) and immunochemistry is, as a single procedure, superior. In human medicine, classification of leukaemia integrates clinical information, cell morphology, cytochemistry, immunophenotyping, cytogenetic and molecular genetic diagnostic techniques. In animals, often only clinical information, cell morphology and immunophenotyping are used.

Functional tests

B cell function can be assessed to some extent by quantifying IgG, IgA and IgM, but it is important to have age-matched reference ranges or controls. Deficiencies in T cell responses can be identified by assessing response to stimulation in a lymphocyte stimulation (or blastogenesis) test.

Neutrophil dysfunction may involve abnormalities in any of the steps in neutrophil activity (adherence, chemotaxis and migration, phagocytosis, cytotoxicity), and ideally all steps should be assessed by carrying out a panel of tests. Most assays are species-specific, and require rigorous optimization and quality control, and there are currently no commercially available tests of neutrophil function for small animals. However, a variety of assays have been carried out, including neutrophil adherence, chemotaxis, migration and bacterial cell killing test in dogs with diabetes mellitus, and in dogs and cats with morphologically abnormal white blood cells or suspected immunodeficiency syndromes (Andreasen and Roth, 2000).

Platelets

The platelet is a small anucleate cytoplasmic fragment. In dogs, platelets are generally about 25–50% of the diameter of a red cell, with occasional larger cells. The cytoplasm is clear and pale grey with numerous pink–purple granules (Figure 5.23). Feline platelets are morphologically similar, but there is considerable overlap with red cell size (see Chapter 3). Activated platelets may have small pseudopodia and may form aggregates, which tend to be dragged to the feathered edge of the blood smear. Feline platelets are especially prone to aggregation *in vitro*.

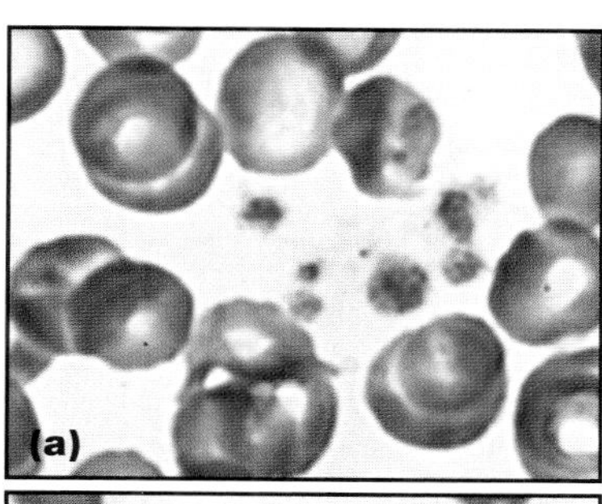

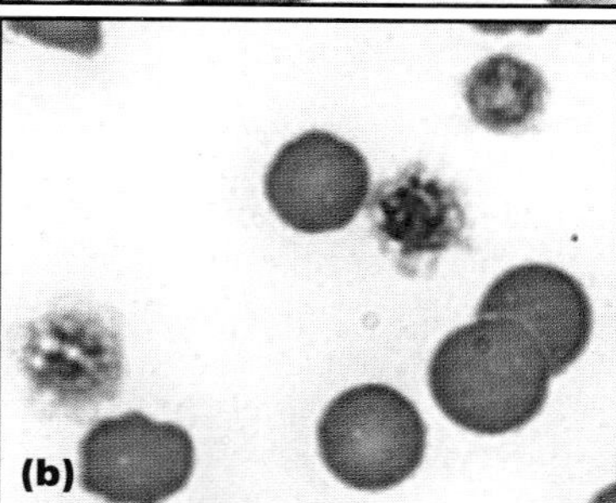

5.23 Platelets. (a) Canine platelets are considerably smaller than red blood cells. They are anucleate fragments containing purplish granules. (b) Feline platelets overlap in size with red blood cells. Pseudopodia are just visible. (May–Grünwald–Giemsa; original magnification X1000.)

Platelets have a critical role in haemostasis and maintenance of vascular integrity (see Chapter 6) but are also essential for inflammation and wound healing. These effects are mediated by complex cell-to-cell interactions and release of many soluble mediators from activated platelets (Gentry, 2000).

Platelets are produced from megakaryocytes, mainly within the bone marrow, but also within the pulmonary and splenic parenchyma. The regulation of thrombopoiesis is fairly well characterized, but the mechanism by which platelets are formed remains unclear. Platelets have a short circulating half-life and there is no tissue pool. If production fails, thrombocytopenia develops within 5 days in dogs and less in cats, where the half-life may be as short as 36 hours. Platelets are phagocytosed by macrophages, mainly in the spleen.

Platelet counts from automated analysers should always be verified by manual smear examination (see Chapters 3 and 6). Mean platelet volume (MPV) is reported by some analysers and may be useful in dogs, although the presence of large immature shift platelets is a better indicator of increased thrombopoiesis than is an overall increase in MPV. In cats, platelet size is very variable and large platelets are not a reliable indicator of increased thrombopoiesis.

Thrombocytopenia

Thrombocytopenia is discussed in Chapter 6, and causes are summarized in Figure 6.18.

Thrombocytosis

There are three main types of thyrombocytosis:

- Physiological thrombocytosis can occur due to mobilization of platelets from the splenic and pulmonary pools due to epinephrine release or exercise
- Reactive thrombocytosis is most often a transient, reactive response to another primary disease process, and is the commonest type of thrombocytosis
- Essential thrombocythaemia (primary thrombocytosis, thromboasthenia, idiopathic thrombocythaemia) is a rare myeloproliferative disorder.

Reactive thrombocytosis

This is associated with many conditions; in particular, conditions associated with peripheral loss of platelets (haemorrhage, destruction) often produce a 'rebound' thrombocytosis. Increased thrombopoiesis is also associated with acute and chronic inflammatory conditions (of infectious or immune-mediated cause), neoplasia, drug therapy and splenectomy. In dogs and cats, reported neoplastic associations include lymphoma, leukaemia, mast cell tumours and a variety of other solid tumours. Of the inflammatory conditions, gastrointestinal diseases predominate, and thrombocytosis may, in part, be a response to blood loss in some cases, as well as a secondary effect of the inflammatory process. It is thought cytokines mediate thrombocytosis in most reactive causes, but this has not been investigated in small animals.

Thrombocytosis has also been associated with some endocrine disorders, including hyperadrenocorticism, where high levels of endogenous glucocorticoids may decrease platelet phagocytosis by macrophages. Exogenous corticosteroids and other drugs, including vincristine, can cause thrombocytosis. Splenectomy causes thrombocytosis by decreasing platelet phagocytosis by macrophages. Most cases of reactive thrombocytosis in dogs have counts $<1000 \times 10^9$/l. In cats, counts are more variable, and in this species the presence of microcytic red cells can also result in an artefactually vastly increased platelet count.

Essential thrombocythaemia

This is a myeloproliferative disorder where there is megakaryocyte proliferation in the bone marrow and excessive, autonomous production of structurally and functionally abnormal platelets. It is rare in small animals, and poorly characterized, but it is well documented in people, where there are clearly defined criteria for diagnosis. Features reported in animals include a marked thrombocytosis, anaemia (which may be regenerative or non-regenerative) and haemorrhage or haemolysis. Splenomegaly, due to extramedullary haematopoiesis, is common. Bone marrow aspirates show megakaryoblast and megakaryocyte hyperplasia, increased platelet budding with sheets of platelets, erythroid hypoplasia and myeloid hyperplasia. Diagnosis depends upon meeting defined criteria and an experienced clinical pathologist should be consulted. Thrombocytosis secondary to other causes should be excluded.

Platelet dysfunction

Thrombopathia (or thrombocytopathy) should be suspected in animals with bleeding tendencies, but normal (or slightly increased) platelet counts, coagulation test results and von Willebrand factor antigen. Diagnosis is discussed in Chapter 6. Thrombocytopathias may be inherited or acquired, and causes are summarized in Figure 5.24.

Inherited
Cats: Chédiak–Higashi syndrome
Dogs: Breed-associated in Otterhound, Great Pyrenees, American Cocker Spaniel, Basset, Spitz, grey Collies (associated with cyclic neutropenia)
Acquired
Azotaemia
Disseminated intravascular coagulation
Drug-associated: non-steroidal anti-inflammatory drugs
Dysproteinaemia
Ehrlichial infection
Hepatopathy
Immune-mediated thrombocytopenia

5.24 Examples of causes of platelet dysfunction in the dog and cat.

Case examples

Case 1

Signalment
10-year-old male neutered Collie cross.

History
Presumptive diagnosis of immune-mediated skin disease had been made several months previously; treated with prednisolone and azathioprine. Recent history of slowing down and poor exercise tolerance. Clinical examination revealed tachycardia (168 bpm), a tapping pulse, pale mucous membranes, and petechiae on the gums.

Clinical pathology data

Haematology	Result	Reference interval
RBC (x 10^{12}/l)	1.78	5.4–8.0
Hb (g/dl)	4.9	12.00–18.00
HCT (l/l)	0.13	0.35–0.55
MCV (fl)	73.0	65.0–75.0
MCHC (g/dl)	37.4	32.0–37.0
Reticulocytes (%)	<0.1	0.0–1
WBC (x 10^9/l)	2.6	6.0–18.0
Neutrophils (segmented) (x 10^9/l)	1.89	3.0–12.0
Neutrophils (band) (x 10^9/l)	0.20	0.0–0.3
Lymphocytes (x 10^9/l)	0.47	1.0–3.8
Monocytes (x 10^9/l)	0.03	0–1.20
Eosinophils (x 10^9/l)	<0.01	0.1–1.30
Basophils (x 10^9/l)	<0.01	Rare
Platelets (x 10^9/l)	8	150–400

Film comment
Red blood cells normocytic, normochromic. No platelet aggregates seen: count appears genuine.

Biochemistry	Result	Reference interval
Sodium (mmol/l)	150	140–153
Potassium (mmol/l)	4.24	3.80–5.30
Chloride (mmol/l)	119	99–115
Glucose (mmol/l)	6.5	3.5–5.5
Urea (mmol/l)	5.0	3.5–6.0
Creatinine (µmol/l)	59.0	20–110
Calcium (mmol/l)	2.38	2.20–2.70
Inorganic phosphate (mmol/l)	1.33	0.80–2.0
TP (g/l)	43.0	57.0 –78.0
Albumin (g/l)	23.0	23.0 –31.0
Globulin (g/l)	20.0	27.0–40.0
ALT (IU/l)	230	7–50
ALP (IU/l)	1090	0–100
Cholesterol (mmol/l)	3.9	3.2–6.5
Bile acids (µmol/l)	29.4	0–15
Bilirubin (µmol/l)	0.8	0–20

What abnormalities are present?

Haematology
- Severe, non-regenerative anaemia
- Profound thrombocytopenia
- Moderate neutropenia
- Lymphopenia
- Monocytopenia

Biochemistry
- Hypoproteinaemia: bottom of reference range albumin; low globulin
- Markedly elevated (10x) ALP
- Moderately to markedly elevated (5x) ALT
- Mildly elevated preprandial bile acids
- Very mildly elevated glucose

How would you interpret these results and what are the likely differential diagnoses?
There is a pancytopenia (anaemia, thrombocytopenia, leucopenia), suggesting failure of bone marrow to produce sufficient blood cells. Given the dog's history, this is most probably due to drug-induced myelosuppression. The main differential is emergence of an underlying cause of the immune-mediated disease, such as lymphoproliferative disease, affecting the bone marrow. The degree of anaemia is very profound for recent myelosuppression (as red blood cells are long lived), and may in part be due to blood loss due to the thrombocytopenia. This is supported by the hypoproteinaemia. (Immune-mediated destruction is less likely, as there is no evidence of regeneration, no spherocytosis, and no increase in bilirubin.)

The very elevated ALP and moderately elevated ALT most likely reflect previous corticosteroid administration, although hypoxia due to anaemia may be contributing the elevation in ALT. The mildly elevated preprandial bile acid concentration is in the 'grey' area (Chapter 12), and may be due to mild steroid-induced hepatopathy or non-specific elevation.

The mildly elevated glucose is most likely due to stress or corticosteroids.

What further tests would you recommend?
- Bone marrow aspiration (if cell counts do not rapidly improve)
- Possibly Coombs' test and anti-platelet antibody
- Biopsy of skin lesions

Case outcome
In view of the history, drug-induced myelosuppression was suspected. Azathioprine treatment was stopped and the haematology was monitored. The cytopenias persisted and there was no evidence of red cell regeneration. After 10 days, bone marrow aspiration, Coombs' test and anti-platelet antibody tests were carried out. Coombs' and anti-platelet antibody tests were negative. Bone marrow aspirates were consistent with recovering haemopoiesis, and there was no evidence of neoplastic infiltrate. Within 3 weeks, neutrophils and platelet numbers were normal; red cell parameters normalized within 5 weeks. It transpired the dog had been given twice the recommended dose of azathioprine for 5 weeks prior to presentation. Biopsy of the skin lesions confirmed immune-mediated disease, and this was managed with ciclosporin.

Case 2 follows ▶

Case 2

Signalment

Young adult (rescued) male crossbred dog.

History and clinical findings

Three-week history of a dry hacking cough, precipitated by exercise or excitement. No history of travel outside the UK. On clinical examination, the dog was obese. On thoracic auscultation, breath sounds were dull in the mid-dorsal thorax, especially on the right. The dog tended to pant, but at rest the respiratory pattern returned to normal.

Clinical pathology data

Haematology	Result	Reference interval
RBC (x 10^{12}/l)	6.46	5.4–8.0
Hb (g/dl)	17.1	12.00–18.00
HCT (l/l)	0.44	0.35–0.55
MCV (fl)	68.0	65.0–75.0
MCHC (g/dl)	37.8	32.0–37.0
Reticulocytes (%)	0.7	0.0–1
WBC (x 10^9/l)	40.4	6.0–18.0
Neutrophils (segmented) (x 10^9/l)	14.4	3.0–12.0
Neutrophils (band) (x 10^9/l)	0.94	0.0–0.3
Lymphocytes (x 10^9/l)	1.51	1.0–3.8
Monocytes (x 10^9/l)	0.18	0–1.20
Eosinophils (x 10^9/l)	22.0	0.1–1.30
Basophils (x 10^9/l)	1.32	Rare
Platelets (x 10^9/l)	367	150–400

Film comment

Eosinophils are morphologically normal.

Biochemistry

No abnormalities.

What abnormalities are present?

Haematology

- Moderate mature neutrophilia
- Slight left shift
- Eosinophilia
- Basophilia

How would you interpret these results and what are the likely differential diagnoses?

There is a neutrophilia with a slight left shift, most likely reflecting an acute inflammatory response. The marked eosinophilia could have a number of causes (see Figure 5.10) but the most likely, considering the dog's history and clinical signs, are:

- Pulmonary parasites (*Angiostrongylus vasorum*)
- Heartworm (*Dirofilaria immitis*: not UK, and the eosinophilia is very marked)
- Eosinophilic bronchopneumonopathy (previously known as pulmonary infiltrate with eosinophils).

Hypereosinophilic syndrome is also a possibility, though evidence of other organ infiltration should be sought. Finally, the dog may have eosinophilia for a reason unrelated to its respiratory signs.
The mildly elevated albumin may reflect dehydration, due to being starved prior to travelling to the surgery.

What further tests would you recommend?

- Thoracic radiography
- Bronchoscopy
- Bronchoalveolar lavages
- Faecal parasitology (for lung worm larvae)
- Coagulation screen (as coagulopathies may occur secondary to *Angiostrongylus*)
- Further investigations to rule out infiltration of other organs (abdominal ultrasonography, FNA as indicated, bone marrow aspiration)

Results of further tests

Thoracic radiographs revealed tracheobronchial lymph node enlargement, and several ill-defined radio-opacities and diffuse areas of mixed alveolar and interstitial pattern. Bronchoscopy revealed slight reddening of the trachea, and excess mucoid material in both trachea and bronchi. Abdominal ultrasonography was unremarkable. Faecal parasitology was negative.

Bronchoalveolar lavage fluid	
RBC (x 10^{12}/l)	0.003
WBC (x 10^9/l)	7.39
Neutrophils (x 10^9/l)	1.18
Lymphocytes (x 10^9/l)	0.07
Macrophages (x 10^9/l)	0.07
Eosinophils (x 10^9/l)	6.06

Cytology

Occasional mast cells and basophils seen. No evidence of parasites or bacteria.

How would you interpret these results and what are the likely differential diagnoses?

These findings of an eosinophilic infiltrate on BAL are supportive of an allergic process. Basophils are also associated with hypersensitivity reactions and, like mast cells, are often found where there is an eosinophilic infiltrate. A diagnosis of eosinophilic bronchopneumonopathy was made on the basis of these findings and the radiographic appearance. A parasitic cause has not been entirely ruled out.

Case outcome

The dog received a 5-day course of fenbendazole at lungworm doses (in case of undiagnosed parasitism) and was then treated with immunosuppressive doses of corticosteroids. He responded dramatically and was weaned off therapy gradually over 4 months.

Case 3

Signalment

11-year-old male crossbred dog.

History and clinical findings

Two-week history of malaise, lethargy and polyuria/polydipsia. On clinical examination the dog was quiet. The mucous membranes were pale. There was mild generalized lymphadenopathy and hepatosplenomegaly.

Clinical pathology data

Haematology	Result	Reference interval
RBC (x 10^{12}/l)	2.38	5.4–8.0
Hb (g/dl)	9.8	12.00–18.00 ▶

Case 3 continues ▶

Case 3 continued

Haematology *(continued)*	Result	Reference interval
HCT (l/l)	0.21	0.35–0.55
MCV (fl)	87.8	65.0–75.0
MCHC (g/dl)	37.8	32.0–37.0
Reticulocytes (%)	2.0	0.0–1
WBC (x 10^9/l)	156.0	6.0–18.0
Neutrophils (segmented) (x 10^9/l)	4.20	3.0–12.0
Neutrophils (band) (x 10^9/l)	0.24	0.0–0.3
Lymphocytes (x 10^9/l)	149.0	1.0–3.8
Monocytes (x 10^9/l)	0.70	0–1.20
Eosinophils (x 10^9/l)	0.50	0.1–1.30
Basophils (x 10^9/l)	0	Rare
Normoblasts (x10^9/l)	0.20	0–0.1
Platelets (x 10^9/l)	57	150–400

Film comment

The lymphocytes are approximately the same size as neutrophils and have abundant pale to deep blue (basophilic) cytoplasm. Some of the cells show cytoplasmic blebbing and small red intracytoplasmic granules, and a few cells have reniform (kidney- or bean-shaped) nuclei. Few other nucleated cells seen.

Biochemistry	Result	Reference interval
TP (g/l)	54.0	57.0–78.0
Albumin (g/l)	21.0	23.0–31.0
ALT (IU/l)	110	7–50

All other biochemical parameters normal.

What abnormalities are present?

Haematology

- Moderate macrocytic but normochromic anaemia
  - Inappropriately poor regeneration
  - Absolute reticulocyte count 47 x 10^9/l
  - Macrocytosis
- Low normal neutrophil count
- Lymphocytosis, composed of atypical lymphoid cells
- Slight increase in normoblasts
- Moderate thrombocytopenia

Biochemistry

- Mild hypoproteinaemia: albumin just below reference range; normal globulin
- Moderately elevated (2x) ALT

How would you interpret these results and what are the likely differential diagnoses?

The very high lymphocyte count and the atypical features of these cells described by the clinical pathologist are suggestive of leukaemia. The degree of increase in cell numbers is very unlikely to be due to a reactive process. Bone marrow disease (infiltrate) is supported by the thrombocytopenia, low normal neutrophil count (for a sick dog), and anaemia. The presence of normoblasts (disproportionate to the regenerative response) is also supportive of bone marrow disease.

The low albumin may be a result of reduced hepatic synthesis, or of protein loss in urine or from the intestine secondary to tumour infiltrate. The elevated ALT most likely reflects hypoxic damage to the hepatocytes (as a result of the anaemia) but may be due to tumour infiltrate in the liver.

What further tests would you recommend?

- Bone marrow aspiration
- Flow cytometry
- Ultrasonography (for tumour staging)
- Urinalysis (to rule out urinary protein loss)

Results of further tests

Bone marrow aspiration

Aspirate cellular, with flecks/spicules present. No megakaryocytes or iron stores. The majority of the cells (85–95%) on the smears are large lymphocytes around the same size as, or slightly smaller than, a neutrophil. Extremely low numbers of erythroid and myeloid series cells were present, but these showed orderly maturation.

Flow cytometry

The lymphoid cells expressed CD3 (expressed by T cells), CD5 (T cells and a subset of B cells), CD8 (cytotoxic T cells), CD11d (NK cells/cytotoxic T large granular lymphocytes), Thy-1 (T cells, a subset of B cells and some antigen-presenting cells), CD11a (all leucocytes), CD45 (all haemopoietic cells) and CD45RA (B cells and a subset of T cells). They did not express CD34 (stem cells). These findings confirmed a leukaemia of large granular lymphocytes.

Case outcome

The prognosis was guarded due to the severity of marrow infiltration. The dog was treated with combination chemotherapy, and achieved partial remission. He enjoyed an excellent quality of life for 10 months, after which time disease progression occurred and euthanasia was performed.

Case 4

Signalment

7-year-old neutered crossbred bitch.

History and clinical findings

History of being subdued and lethargic for several months: stopped wanting to exercise, and had difficulty sitting down comfortably. Slight improvement on anti-inflammatory doses of steroids approximately 3 weeks ago. Recent reduction in appetite. Periarticular soft tissue swelling around stifles, hocks, elbows and carpi, with mild distal limb oedema. Joints painful on manipulation. Pyrexia (39.9 °C).

Clinical pathology data

Haematology	Result	Reference interval
RBC (x 10^{12}/l)	6.07	5.4–8.0
Hb (g/dl)	14.6	12.00–18.00 ▶
HCT (l/l)	0.41	0.35–0.55
MCV (fl)	67.0	65.0–75.0
MCHC (g/dl)	35.5	32.0–37.0
Reticulocytes (%)	2.6	0.0–1
WBC (x 10^9/l)	21.0	6.0–18.0
Neutrophils (segmented) (x 10^9/l)	16.6	3.0–12.0
Neutrophils (band) (x 10^9/l)	2.56	0.0–0.3
Lymphocytes (x 10^9/l)	1.20	1.0–3.8 ▶

Case 4 continues ▶

Case 4 continued

Haematology *(continued)*	Result	Reference interval
Monocytes (x 10^9/l)	0.22	0–1.20
Eosinophils (x 10^9/l)	0.37	0.1–1.30
Basophils (x 10^9/l)	0	Rare
Platelets (x 10^9/l)	378	150–400

Film comments

Neutrophils show a left shift. Occasional Döhle bodies.

Biochemistry	Result	Reference interval
Sodium (mmol/l)	150	140–153
Potassium (mmol/l)	4.49	3.80–5.30
Chloride (mmol/l)	112	99–115
Glucose (mmol/l)	7.9	3.5–5.5
Urea (mmol/l)	5.5	3.5–6.0
Creatinine (μmol/l)	62.0	20–110
Calcium (mmol/l)	2.46	2.20–2.70
Inorganic phosphate (mmol/l)	1.77	0.80–2.0
TP (g/l)	71.0	57.0–78.0
Albumin (g/l)	28.0	23.0–31.0
Globulin (g/l)	43.0	27.0–40.0
ALT (IU/l)	63	7–50
ALP (IU/l)	961	0–100
Cholesterol (mmol/l)	9.0	3.2–6.5

What abnormalities are present?

Haematology

- Moderate mature neutrophilia
- Left shift

Biochemistry

- Slightly elevated globulin
- Markedly elevated ALP (x9)
- Slightly elevated ALT (<x2)
- Hypercholesterolaemia

How would you interpret these results and what are the likely differential diagnoses?

There is a neutrophilia with significant left shift, most likely reflecting an acute inflammatory response. The elevated globulin also supports an ongoing inflammatory condition. The markedly elevated ALP and mildly elevated ALT may be a result of previous steroid therapy (as ALP is typically elevated to a much greater degree than ALT by corticosteroids, and also has a much shorter half-life). Endogenous hyperadrenocorticism is not excluded, but is not suggested by the history and clinical findings. Non-specific elevation secondary to systemic inflammatory disease may also contribute. The elevated cholesterol is a non-specific finding that may reflect inadequate fasting prior to sampling, endocrinopathies (including hyperadrenocorticism), pancreatitis, cholestasis, protein-losing nephropathy or primary hyperlipidaemia. The clinical presentation suggests polyarthritis (with associated periarticular soft tissue swelling) is the most likely cause.

What further tests would you recommend?

- Arthrocentesis
- Investigation for comorbidity
  - Urinalysis
  - Radiography and ultrasonography of the thorax and abdomen
- Synovial fluid culture
- (Biopsy of periarticular soft tissue to rule out vasculitis)
- (Serology for RF and ANA – may help classify the disease but unlikely to change clinical decision-making)

Case outcome

Cytology of joint samples was consistent with immune-mediated polyarthritis; cultures were negative. The dog was treated with prednisolone and azathioprine and responded well.

Case 5

Signalment

4-year-old female neutered Cocker Spaniel.

History and clinical findings

Two day history of generalized and progressive cutaneous erythema; marked peripheral and facial oedema, and malaise. The patient was tachycardic (180bpm) and had tacky, hyperaemic mucous membranes and a slow capillary refill time. She was hyperpnoeic. There was generalized cutaneous erythema.

Clinical pathology data

Haematology	Result	Reference interval
RBC (x 10^{12}/l)	8.24	5.5–8.5
Hb (g/dl)	19.5	12.00–18.00
HCT (l/l)	0.60	0.37–0.55
MCV (fl)	73.0	60.0–77.0
MCH (pg)	23.7	19.5–24.5
MCHC (g/dl)	32	32.0–37.0 ▶
Haematology *(continues)*	**Result**	**Reference interval**
WBC (x 10^9/l)	1.23	6.0–17.0
Neutrophils (segmented) (x 10^9/l)	0.37	3.0–11.5
Neutrophils (band) (x 10^9/l)	0.63	0.0–0.3
Lymphocytes (x 10^9/l)	0.2	1.0–4.8
Monocytes (x 10^9/l)	0.1	0.2–1.50
Eosinophils (x 10^9/l)	0	0.1–1.30
Basophils (x 10^9/l)	0	0.0–0.5
Platelets (x 10^9/l)	146	150–400

Film comments

Neutropenia with left shift. Cells show toxic change (foamy basophilic cytoplasm and occasional Döhle bodies). Platelet clumps seen on film.

Case 5 continues ▶

Case 5 continued

Biochemistry	Result	Reference interval
Sodium (mmol/l)	136	140–153
Potassium (mmol/l)	4.78	3.80–5.30
Glucose (mmol/l)	4.5	3.5–5.5
Urea (mmol/l)	6.2	3.5–6.0
Creatinine (μmol/l)	54.0	20–110
Calcium (mmol/l)	1.91	2.20–2.70
Inorganic phosphate (mmol/l)	0.64	0.80–2.0
TP (g/l)	55.0	57.0–78.0
Albumin (g/l)	28.0	23.0–31.0
Globulin (g/l)	27.0	27.0–40.0
ALT (IU/l)	29	7–50
ALP (IU/l)	470	0–100
Cholesterol (mmol/l)	6.6	3.2–6.5

What abnormalities are present?

Haematology

- Raised haematocrit
- Leucopenia
- Neutropenia with left shift and toxic change
- Borderline thrombocytopenia but clumps seen on smear; probably normal

Biochemistry

- Slightly low total protein
- Moderately elevated ALP (4x)
- Hyponatraemia
- Hypocalcaemia
- Borderline cholesterol

How would you interpret these results and what are the likely differential diagnoses?

The raised haematocrit most likely reflects hypovolaemia, as this is supported by the clinical findings. There is a severe neutropenia, with a left shift and toxic change. This represents a degenerative left shift, as band cells exceed mature neutrophils. This suggests that the bone marrow is unable to maintain adequate neutrophil numbers to meet the increased demand. Toxic change reflects reduced maturation time as a result of intense stimulation of granulopoiesis. Degenerative left shift with toxic change suggests a very severe inflammatory process (often associated with bacterial infection) and a degenerative left shift is a poor prognostic indicator. Lymphopenia may be due to stress, or may reflect loss into the oedema fluid (third-space loss).

The slightly low total protein may also be a result of third-space loss, though usually albumin loss exceeds globulin loss. As the dog is hypovolaemic, a more significant hypoproteinaemia may be unmasked by correction of fluid deficits.

The elevated ALP may reflect secondary effects of the underlying disease, for example, cholestasis secondary to the release of inflammatory mediators and cytokines in sepsis. ALT is normal, which suggests there is not significant hepatocellular damage, but this could reflect also end-stage liver disease and enzyme exhaustion. This may be less likely, as albumin remains within the normal range, but again hypoalbuminaemia may be unmasked by rehydration.

Hyponatraemia may be caused by hypoadrenocorticism, third-space loss of fluid, volume overload associated with congestive heart failure, liver disease, or nephrotic syndrome. Diabetes mellitus is excluded by the normal blood glucose. The sodium: potassium ratio is 28.45, and the history and presentation are not typical of hypoadrenocorticism. Third-space loss of sodium into the oedema fluid seems the most likely cause.

What further tests would you recommend?

Investigations should be directed at identifying the underlying inflammatory disease:

- Biopsy and culture of the cutaneous lesions
- Imaging (radiography and ultrasonography to identify inflammatory foci and effusions).

Case outcome

Skin biopsy revealed a massive infiltrate of neutrophils into the skin and subcutis, with many bacteria evident. The skin/subcutis was the only focus of infection/inflammation identified. This may have been either primary or secondary, and may have developed secondary to impaired vascular integrity or immune-mediated vasculitis. The dog was treated with aggressive supportive therapy (for hypovolaemic/endotoxic shock and metabolic acidosis) and broad-spectrum (four-quadrant) antibiotics, but deteriorated precipitously and was euthanased. Post-mortem examination was declined.

(Case 5: primary clinician was Sophia Tzannes.)

References and further reading

Andreasen CB and Roth JA (2000) Neutrophil function abnormalities. In: *Schalm's Veterinary Hematology,* ed. BF Feldman *et al.*, pp. 356–365. Lippincott Williams & Wilkins, Baltimore

Barrs VR, Beatty JA, McCandlish IA and Kipar A (2002) Hypereosinophilic paraneoplastic syndrome in a cat with intestinal T cell lymphosarcoma. *Journal of Small Animal Practice* **43,** 401–405

Bienzle D, Stanton JB, Embry JM, Bush SE and Mahaffey EA (2000) Evaluation of an in-house centrifugal haematology analyzer for use in veterinary practice. *Journal of the American Veterinary Medical Association* **217,** 1195–1200

Cave TA, Gault EA and Argyle DJ (2004) Feline epitheliotroohic T-cell lymphoma with paraneoplastic eosinophilia – immunochemotherapy with vinblastine and human recombinant interferon α2b. *Veterinary and Comparative Oncology* **2,** 91–97

Day MJ (2000) Biology of lymphocytes and plasma cells. In: *Schalm's Veterinary Hematology,* ed. BF Feldman *et al.*, pp. 240–246. Lippincott Williams & Wilkins, Baltimore

Dewhurst EC, Crawford C, Cue S, Dodkin S, German AJ and Papasouliotis K (2003) Analysis of canine and feline haemograms using the VetScan HMT analyser. *Journal of Small Animal Practice* **44,** 443–448

Gentry PA (2000) Platelet biology In: *Schalm's Veterinary Hematology,* ed. BF Feldman *et al.*, pp. 459–466. Lippincott Williams & Wilkins, Baltimore

Gommeren KWG, Daminet S, Vanholen L, Vandenberghe A and Duchateau L (2004) Prevalence of physiologic leucopenia in the Tervuren and the Groenendael in Flanders. Scientific Proceedings, BSAVA 47th Annual Congress, Birmingham, 566

Greenfield CL, Messick JB, Solter PF and Schaeffer DJ (2000) Results of hematologic analyses and prevalence of physiologic leukopenia in Belgian Tervuren. *Journal of the American Veterinary Medical Association* **216,** 866–871

Grindem CB (2000) Acute myeloid leukaemia. In: *Schalm's Veterinary Hematology,* ed. BF Feldman *et al.*, pp. 717–726. Lippincott Williams & Wilkins, Baltimore

Hammer AS (1999) Thrombocytosis in dogs and cats; a retrospective study. *Comparative Haematology International* **1,** 181–186

Harper EJ, Hackett RM, Wikinson J and Heaton PR (2003) Age-related variations in hematologic and plasma biochemical test results in Beagles and Labrador Retrievers. *Journal of the American Veterinary Medical Association* **223,** 1436–1442

Jones RF and Paris R (1963) The Greyhound eosinophil. *Journal of Small Animal Practice* **4(Supp),** 29–33

Keller RL, Avery AC, Burnett RC, Walton JA and Olver CS (2004) Detection of neoplastic lymphocytes in peripheral blood of dogs with lymphoma by polymerase chain reaction for antigen receptor gene rearrangement. *Veterinary Clinical Pathology* **3,** 144–149

Kheiri SA, MacKerrell T, Bonagural VR, Fuchs A and Billett HH (1998) Flow cytometry with or without cytochemistry for the diagnosis of acute leukaemias. *Cytometry* **34,** 82–86

Lucroy MD and Madewell BR (1999) Clinical outcome and associated diseases in dogs with leukocytosis and neutrophilia: 118 cases (1996–1998). *Journal of the American Veterinary Medical Association* **214,** 805–807

Lucroy MD and Madewell BR (2001) Clinical outcome and diseases associated with extreme neutrophilic leukocytosis in cats: 104 cases (1991–1999) *Journal of the American Veterinary Medical Association* **218,** 736–739

Messick JB (2003) Hematology. *Veterinary Clinics of North America: Small Animal Practice* **33**

Papasouliotis K (2002) In-house haematology analysers – knowing their limits. Scientific Proceedings, BSAVA 45th Annual Congress, Birmingham, 294–297

Ponce F, Magnol JP, Ledieu D, Marchal T, Turinelli V, Chalvet-Monfray K and Fournel-Fleury C (2004) Prognostic significance of morphological subtypes in canine malignant lymphomas during chemotherapy *The Veterinary Journal* **167,** 158–166

Raskin RE and Valenciano A (2000) Cytochemical tests for diagnosis of leukaemia. In: *Schalm's Veterinary Hematology,* ed. BF Feldman *et al.*, pp.755–763. Lippincott Williams & Wilkins, Baltimore

Shafrine M, Munn SL, Rosenblatt LS, Bulgin MS and Wilson FD (1973) Hematologic changes to 60 days of age in clinically normal beagles. *Laboratory Animal Science* **23,** 894–898

Vahlenkamp TW, Tompkins MB, and Tompkins WA (2004) Feline immunodeficiency virus infection phenotypically and functionally activates immunosuppressive CD4+CD25+ T regulatory cells. *Journal of Immunology* **172,** 4752–4761

Weiss DJ (2003) Immunophenotyping hematopoietic neoplasia. *Scientific Proceedings, European Society of Veterinary Clinical Pathology, Uppsala, Sweden,* A14

6

Disorders of haemostasis

Tracy Stokol

Introduction

The haemostatic system consists of a complex array of cells, enzymes, cofactors and inhibitors that function in an integrated fashion to facilitate repair of injured blood vessels (see also *BSAVA Manual of Canine and Feline Haematology and Transfusion Medicine*). Formation of a stable thrombus is essential to prevent life-threatening haemorrhage, and its dissolution restores vessel patency. Excessive haemorrhage and/or thrombosis occur when components of haemostasis are defective.

Overview of haemostasis

Haemostasis is initiated when the endothelium is disrupted, exposing the thrombogenic subendothelial matrix to platelets and haemostatic proteins. A complex series of events then occurs, ultimately producing a thrombus. It is useful to divide haemostasis into primary, secondary and tertiary pathways. However, this distinction is artificial; all the pathways probably occur simultaneously *in vivo*, rather than in a sequential fashion. The outcome of these pathways is an intricate balance of activation offset by inhibition. Initially, coagulation is favoured, permitting formation of a stable thrombus. Fibrinolysis then dominates, promoting thrombus dissolution and restoration of vessel patency.

Primary haemostasis

Primary haemostasis is the formation of the platelet plug, the initiating event in haemostasis. It involves platelet adhesion, via von Willebrand factor (vWf), to the subendothelial matrix, with subsequent activation and aggregation to form a primary platelet plug (Figure 6.1). This plug is weak and readily removed by re-established blood flow; it must, therefore, be further stabilized by fibrin. An important consequence of platelet activation is phosphatidylserine (PS) exposure on the outer platelet membrane. PS, also called platelet procoagulant activity or platelet factor 3, provides the surface upon which coagulation factors assemble, permitting the coagulation cascade to proceed (Figure 6.2). PS exposure on activated platelets provides an essential link between primary and secondary haemostasis (Heemskerk *et al.*, 2002).

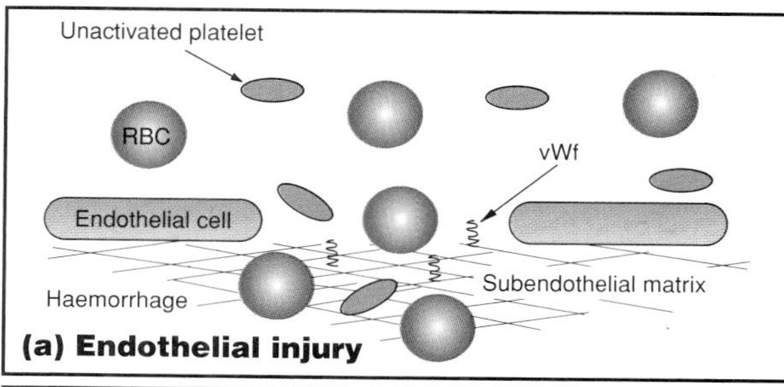

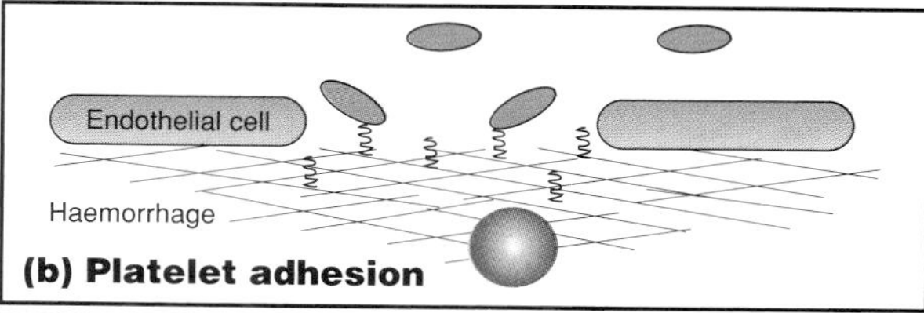

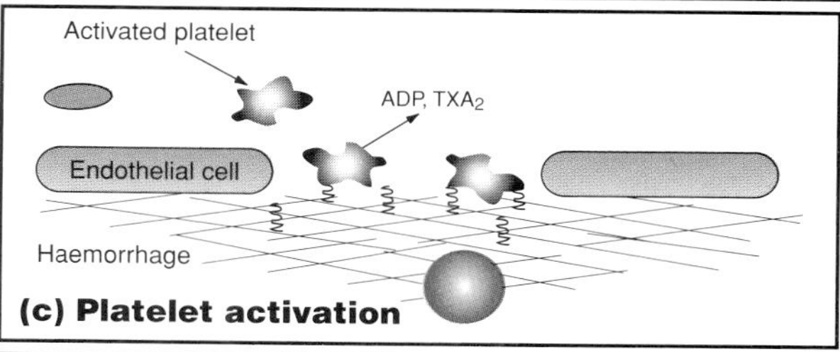

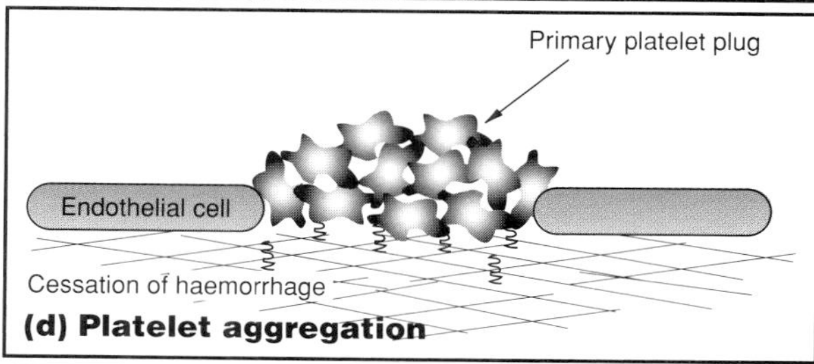

6.1 Primary haemostasis: (a) The subendothelial matrix, containing tissue factor–bearing cells and von Willebrand factor, is exposed on vessel injury. (b) Platelets adhere. vWf acts as a bridge between matrix components and platelet glycoprotein (GP) receptors, specifically GPIb-V-IX. (c) Once adherent, platelets activate, undergo shape change, release storage granules (e.g. ADP), produce lipid mediators (e.g. thromboxane A_2, TXA_2), upregulate fibrinogen receptors (GPIIb/IIIa), and expose PS (illustrated by darker platelet exteriors). The release of lipid mediators and granule contents activates and recruits more platelets. (d) Platelets aggregate, mediated by fibrinogen binding to GPIIb/IIIa, thus forming a platelet plug. vWf can also participate in platelet aggregation by binding to GPIIb/IIIa. The plug is stabilized when fibrin binds to aggregated platelets.

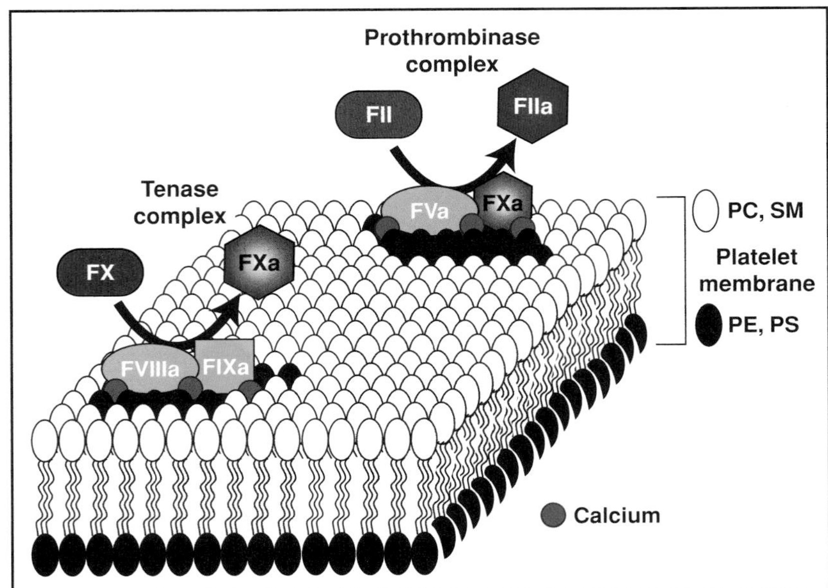

6.2 The link between primary and secondary haemostasis. Platelet activation provides the essential link. Coagulation proceeds on the negatively charged phospholipid surface of activated platelets. The platelet membrane is an asymmetrical phospholipid bilayer, enriched in phosphatidylcholine (PC) and sphingomyelin (SM) on the outer surface and phosphatidylethanolamine (PE) and phosphatidylserine (PS) on the inner surface. This asymmetry is lost on platelet activation. PS is exposed on the outer surface and is a crucial binding component for coagulation factors. The tenase (FIXa, FVIIIa, calcium) and prothrombinase (FXa, FVa, calcium) complexes assemble on the PS surface, are protected from inhibitors and activate FX and prothrombin (FII), respectively.

Secondary haemostasis

Secondary haemostasis is the formation of fibrin. The traditional separation of the coagulation cascade into intrinsic, extrinsic and common pathways is useful for understanding test abnormalities, but haemostasis does not occur as such *in vivo*. Coagulation is initiated by the extrinsic pathway, specifically by tissue factor (TF), and amplified by the intrinsic pathway (Figure 6.3) (Hoffman and Monroe, 2001; Morrissey, 2001). The cascade is initiated and proceeds on a PS-containing cell surface, particularly on platelets and, possibly, leucocytes. Coagulation proteases (coagulation factors) and cofactors bind as supramolecular complexes to PS (see Figure 6.2); this localizes coagulation factors, protects them from inactivation and enhances their activity (Hoffman and Monroe, 2001; Heemskerk *et al.*, 2002). Factors historically thought to activate coagulation, such as contact pathway factors (factor

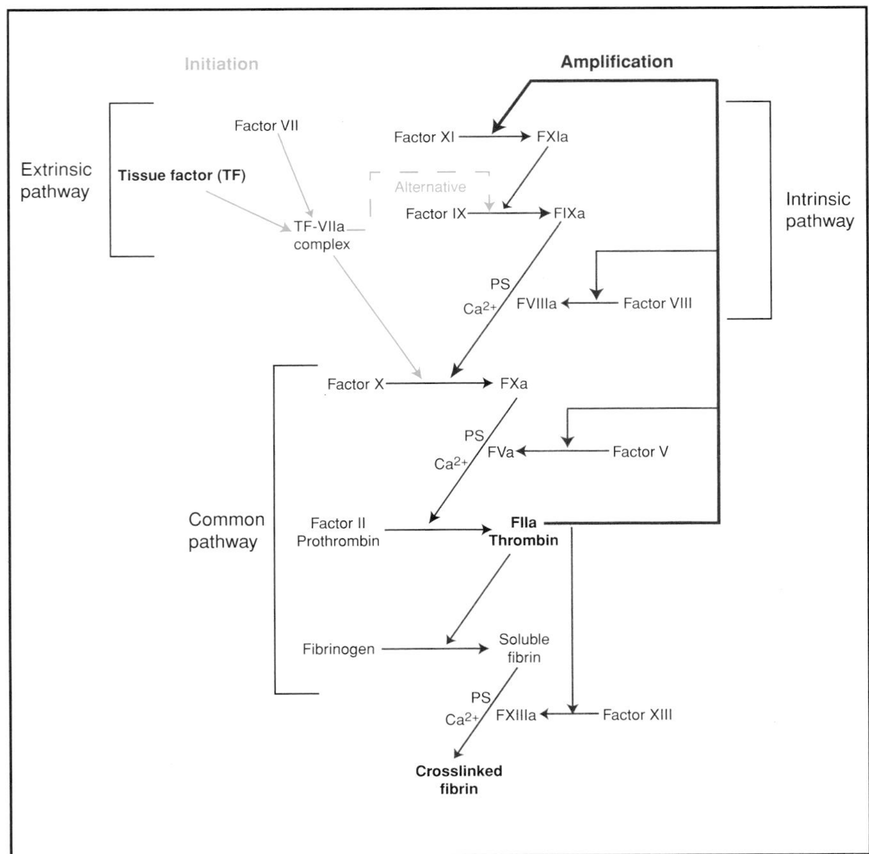

6.3 Secondary haemostasis: the coagulation cascade. The cascade is **initiated** (blue arrows) by the extrinsic pathway and **amplified** (red arrows) by the intrinsic pathway. Tissue factor (TF), expressed by subendothelial matrix cells, binds and activates FVII. This complex initiates coagulation by activating FX, which cleaves prothrombin to thrombin. The small amount of thrombin generated activates platelets (exposing PS) and FXI, FVIII and FV. FXIa, bound to PS on activated platelets, rapidly activates FIX. FIXa and FXa, as part of the tenase and prothrombinase complexes, respectively (see Figure 6.2), produce an explosive localized burst of thrombin. This thrombin burst converts fibrinogen to soluble fibrin and inhibits fibrinolysis. Thus, the intrinsic pathway amplifies thrombin generation. Soluble fibrin rapidly polymerizes and is crosslinked by thrombin-activated FXIIIa. Crosslinked fibrin incorporates into the platelet plug, forming a stable thrombus. The TF-FVIIa complex can directly activate FIX (alternative pathway – dotted blue lines), but FX is its preferred substrate. Contact factors are not illustrated, because they do not participate in fibrin formation.

XII, prekallikrein and high molecular weight kininogen (HMWK)), are now known to have no role in fibrin formation, explaining why animals with contact factor deficiencies do not bleed excessively. Although contact factors are important in clotting tests *in vitro*, their significance in coagulation *in vivo* is doubtful. The end product of secondary haemostasis is crosslinked fibrin, which binds to and stabilizes the platelet plug.

Once again, there are essential links between pathways. Platelets, which are activated by thrombin, provide the PS surface for the cascade. Thrombin also inhibits fibrinolysis and activated coagulation factors (see Figure 6.5).

Tertiary haemostasis

Tertiary haemostasis is fibrinolysis or breakdown of the fibrin clot. Plasminogen is converted to plasmin by tissue plasminogen activator (tPA). Plasmin cleaves fibrin or fibrinogen, releasing fibrin(ogen) degradation products (FDPs). D-dimer is also released by plasmin-mediated lysis of crosslinked fibrin (Figure 6.4). Again, haemostatic pathways are inextricably linked. Contact pathway activation produces bradykinin, which induces tPA release and cleaves plasminogen directly, thus promoting fibrinolysis. Thrombin inhibits fibrinolysis, preventing dissolution of the clot as it is being formed.

Inhibitors

There are naturally occurring inhibitors for every aspect of haemostasis (Figure 6.5). Most are effective at binding 'fluid-phase' factors, whereas their activity is limited when factors are PS- or fibrin-bound. This restricts haemostasis to sites of injury and limits the extent of thrombus formation and/or fibrinolysis (Hoffman and Monroe, 2001). Excessive thrombosis is the usual consequence of inadequate inhibition.

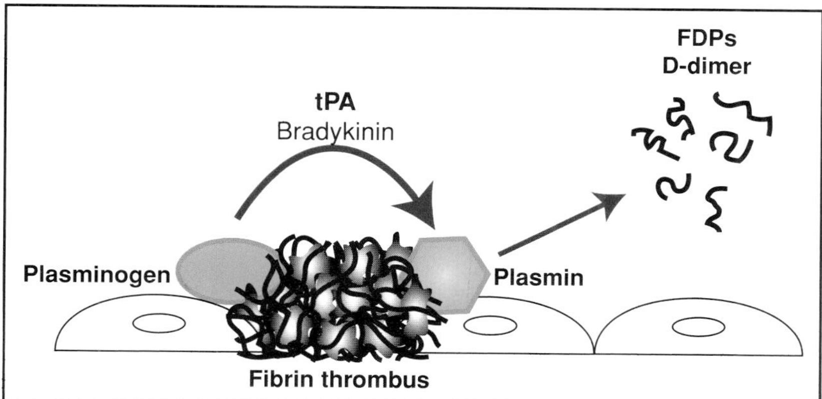

6.4 Fibrinolysis. Tissue plasminogen activator (tPA), released by endothelial cells, converts plasminogen to plasmin. Plasmin lyses fibrinogen and fibrin within the clot, releasing fibrin(ogen) degradation products (FDPs), including D-dimer. Bradykinin, produced by FXIIa/kallikrein-mediated cleavage of HMWK, induces tPA release and can directly activate plasminogen. Thus, contact pathway factors are involved in fibrinolysis, not coagulation.

Inhibitor	Mechanism of action
General inhibitors	
Endothelium	Physical barrier Receptors for inhibitors, e.g. thrombomodulin binds thrombin and activates protein C Heparin-like glycosaminoglycans (GAGs): enhance antithrombin, tissue factor pathway inhibitor activity Secrete platelet antagonists, e.g. prostacyclin, nitric oxide, ADPase Secrete fibrinolytic inhibitors, e.g. plasminogen activator inhibitor
Plasma proteins	Non-specific inhibitors of enzymes in fluid phase, e.g. α_2-macroglobulin, α_1-antitrypsin
Coagulation cascade inhibitors	
Tissue factor pathway inhibitor	Inhibits TF-FVIIa complex – activity enhanced by heparin-like GAGs
Antithrombin	Inhibits thrombin, TF-VIIa, FXIIa, FXIa, FXa and FIXa – activity enhanced by heparin and heparin-like GAGs
Thrombin	Inhibits FVIIIa and FVa by activating protein C and protein S after binding to thrombomodulin
Protein C	Inactivate FVa and VIIIa – activated by thrombin binding to thrombomodulin
Protein S	Cofactor for activated protein C
Fibrinolytic pathway inhibitors	
Thrombin-activatable fibrinolytic inhibitor	Binds fibrin, preventing plasminogen binding and activation; activated by burst of thrombin generated by the intrinsic pathway
Plasminogen activator inhibitors (PAI)	Bind and inactivate tissue plasminogen activator
Antiplasmin	Binds and inactivates plasmin

6.5 Inhibitors of haemostasis.

Clinical signs associated with haemostatic disorders

Clinical signs are excessive haemorrhage or thrombosis, depending on the disorder. Clues to the underlying disorder can be obtained from a thorough clinical examination and complete history (Figure 6.6), because abnormalities in each pathway produce characteristic clinical signs.

Signalment
Age, breed, sex
Details of haemorrhage
Site
Frequency
Severity
Initiating factors (e.g. trauma)
Age at first episode
Family history – signs in siblings, parents, progeny?
Access to toxins
E.g. anticoagulant rodenticides
Drug history
E.g. non-steroidal anti-inflammatory drugs
Travel history
Infectious diseases

6.6 Pertinent history details for investigating haemostatic disorders.

With all disorders, depending on disease severity, haemorrhage can be spontaneous or induced by surgery or trauma.

- Primary haemostatic disorders usually result in spontaneous bleeding from mucosal surfaces, e.g. epistaxis or haematuria. Petechiae are symptomatic of thrombocytopenia (Figure 6.7) or vasculitis, but not von Willebrand's disease (vWD)
- Secondary haemostatic disorders usually cause more severe bleeding into body cavities (e.g. joints) or subcutaneous tissue, with ecchymoses (bruising), but not petechiae (Figure 6.8). Delayed bleeding or rebleeding often occurs due to lack of platelet plug stabilization
- Tertiary haemostatic disorders cause thrombosis. Ischaemia due to vessel or microvessel thrombosis causes end-organ (e.g. liver, lung) dysfunction or failure. Because resulting signs are not specific (e.g. dyspnoea from pulmonary thromboembolism), thrombosis can be difficult or impossible to diagnose, even on post-mortem examination (thrombi can lyse after death).

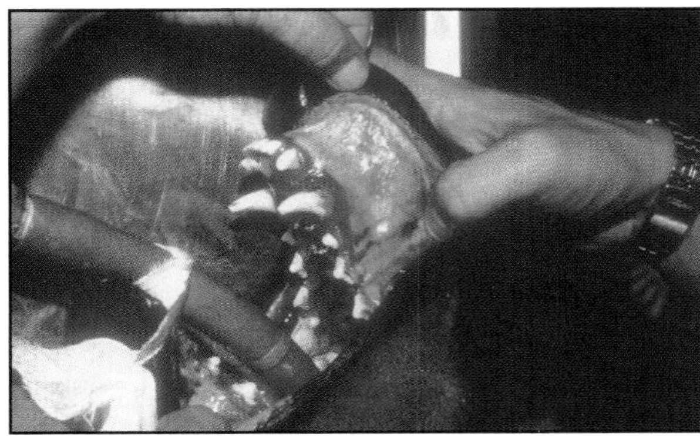

6.7 Clinical signs of primary haemostatic disorders. Petechiae and ecchymoses, with gingival haemorrhage, are evident in the oral mucosa of a young Dobermann with immune-mediated thrombocytopenia. (Courtesy of S Barr)

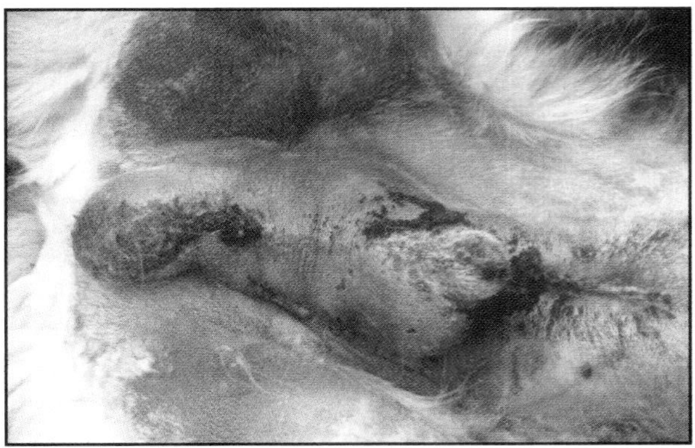

6.8 Clinical signs of secondary haemostatic disorders. Severe and extensive bruising occurred in the inguinal area after neutering in a male German Shepherd Dog with haemophilia A (FVIII deficiency).

Tests for the diagnosis of haemostatic disorders

Tests can be separated along haemostatic pathways (Figure 6.9). Only those tests readily available to the practitioner will be discussed in detail. Blood should be collected into two tubes:

- EDTA (platelet count, D-dimer and von Willebrand factor antigen (vWf:Ag), genetic testing)
- Citrate (coagulation testing, FDPs, D-dimer, specific factors, antithrombin (AT), vWf:Ag).

It cannot be overemphasized that blood must be collected and handled properly to ensure accurate test results (Figure 6.10). Coagulation factors are readily activated by venepuncture and are unstable in stored samples. Whenever possible, blood should be collected from a resting, quiet animal. Known stresses, such as surgical trauma or drugs, can influence test results, hindering interpretation. For example, increases in D-dimer and fibrinogen can occur as a consequence of surgery-induced fibrinolysis and inflammation, respectively. If an animal bleeds excessively during a

Primary haemostasis
Platelet count [a] Clot retraction [a] vWD: vWf:Ag, genetic testing [a] Buccal mucosal bleeding time [a] Biopsy – vascular disorders [a] Platelet function testing – adhesion, aggregation, procoagulant activity
Secondary haemostasis
Whole blood clotting time (WBCT) [a] Activated coagulation time (ACT) [a] Prothrombin time (PT) [a] Activated partial thromboplastin time (aPTT) [a] Fibrinogen concentration or thrombin clot time [a] Proteins induced by vitamin K absence or antagonism ('PIVKA test') Specific factor assays [a] Thrombin/antithrombin complexes – indicates thrombin activation (thrombosis)
Tertiary haemostasis
Fibrin(ogen) degradation products (FDPs), D-dimer [a] Plasminogen Tissue plasminogen activator (TPA) Plasmin Plasmin/antiplasmin complexes – indicates plasmin activation (fibrinolysis)
Inhibitors
Antithrombin [a] Protein C and protein S

6.9 Tests for the diagnosis of haemostatic disorders. [a] Test available to the veterinary practitioner, either in-house or through referral laboratories.

- Clean venipuncture, preferably from a large peripheral vein. If venipuncture is clean, the first ml of blood does not need to be discarded.
- Constant steady blood flow during venipuncture.
- Correct filling of citrate tube: under- or over-filling can prolong or shorten coagulation times (especially under-filling). A ratio of 1 part citrate to 9 parts blood should be maintained.
- Minimize frothing, shearing, haemolysis; do not force blood through needles.
- Ideally, draw citrate anticoagulant into a syringe and draw blood (through a butterfly catheter) into the syringe, e.g. to collect 5 ml blood, draw up 0.5 ml citrate and collect 4.5 ml of blood. Remove the catheter/needle, and gently syringe the blood into a non-anticoagulant tube.
- Centrifuge tube promptly and separate plasma.
- Ship cooled plasma (ideally on ice) to reach laboratory within 24 hours.
- If there is to be delay in submission >24 hours, freeze sample and submit on dry ice.

6.10 Correct sample collection and handling of citrate tubes for haemostatic assays.

surgical procedure, however, perioperative sample collection will be necessary. In such cases, abnormal results of screening assays, such as prothrombin time (PT) and activated partial thromboplastin time (aPTT), should reflect the cause of haemorrhage rather than being a consequence of surgery.

Primary haemostasis

Platelet count

This is mandatory in every patient presenting with signs attributable to a haemostatic disorder. Counts can be estimated from blood smears (Figure 6.11), but accurate enumeration is usually achieved with automated or in-house analysers. In-house analysers are

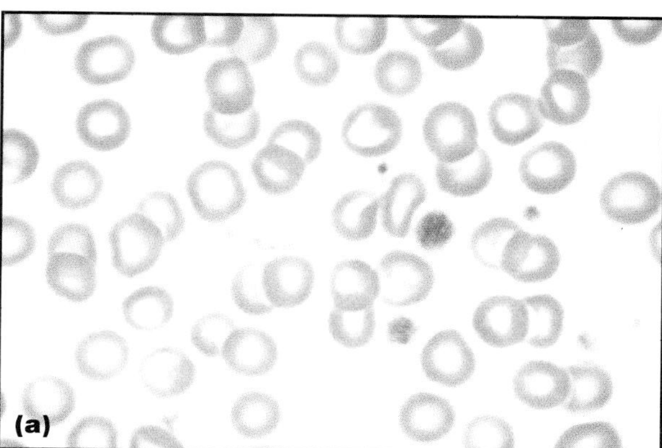

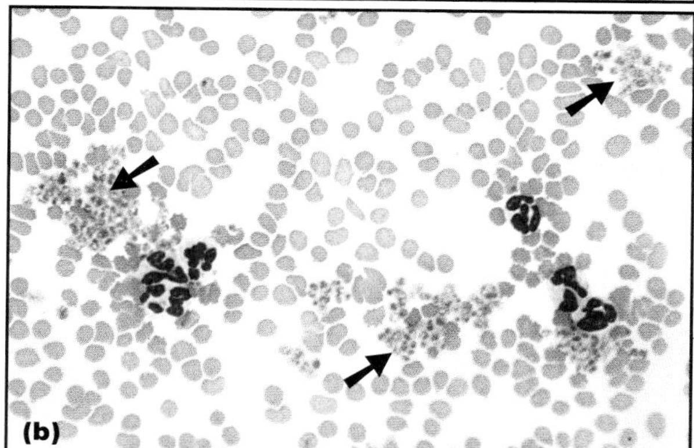

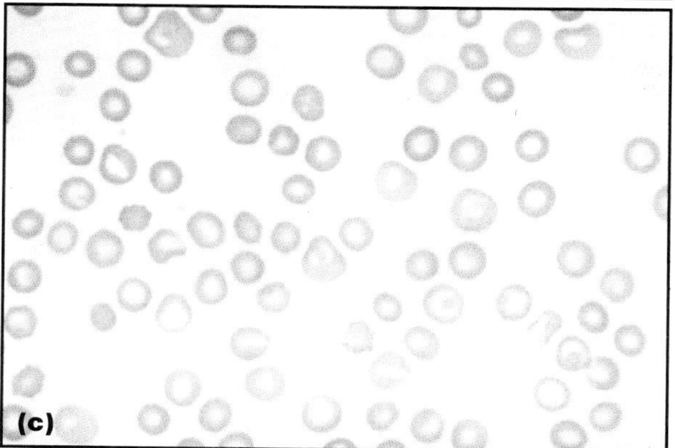

6.11 Estimation of platelet counts from blood smears. (a) Platelet numbers can be estimated from the monolayer of a good quality blood smear. Approximately, 1 platelet/100x oil immersion field (OIF) = 15×10^9/l in dogs and 15–20 x 10^9/l in cats. Healthy dogs and cats typically have >10 platelets/OIF (>150 x 10^9/l). (b) Platelet clumps (arrowed), often located at the feathered edge, invalidate platelet counts obtained by any method. These are usually a consequence of poor venipuncture technique in dogs, but are often unavoidable in cats. (c) Blood smear from a dog with severe immune-mediated thrombocytopenia; no platelets are seen. (Wright's stain; original magnification (a,c) X250; (b) X100)

usually based on quantitative buffy coat analysis (Bienzle *et al.*, 2000) or electronic counting methods. In general, their accuracy is lower than that of automated analysers at veterinary laboratories, some of which flag platelet clumps. In general, platelet clumps decrease the count and increase the mean platelet volume (clumps are 'seen' as single large platelets). They may also artefactually increase the leucocyte count (clumped platelets are 'seen' by the machines as leucocytes). These artefacts are analyser-dependent; clumps may actually increase the platelet count in buffy coat analysers, for example. Platelets clump readily during blood collection in cats for unknown reasons, making it difficult to obtain accurate platelet counts in this species. Sampling into citrate may reduce the clumping tendency. However, if citrate is used for platelet counts, it is essential to fill the tube to the appropriate volume. Even with appropriate filling, the count may be slightly lower than that in EDTA due to dilutional effects. All counts should be verified by smear examination, because clumping will decrease and even invalidate the count. A general rule of thumb is that, in the presence of clumps, the platelet count should be considered a minimum number and the 'real' count is likely to be much higher. Spontaneous haemorrhage typically occurs with platelet counts <30 x 10^9/l, whereas surgery- or trauma-induced haemorrhage can occur with counts <50 x 10^9/l. If platelet function is concurrently impaired (e.g. aspirin therapy), bleeding may occur at higher counts (<150 x 10^9/l). It also must be emphasized that, for unknown reasons, not all animals with severe thrombocytopenia (<30 x 10^9/l) will bleed excessively.

Platelet function

Thrombopathia (or thrombocytopathy) should be suspected in animals with bleeding tendencies, but normal platelet counts and coagulation test results. Specific diagnosis requires specialized platelet function tests, such as evaluation of platelet aggregation, which are not readily available and may only be offered by referral laboratories. Rudimentary platelet function tests that can be performed in veterinary practice include buccal mucosal bleeding time (BMBT), cuticle bleeding time and clot retraction; only the former of these is still used for this purpose.

Buccal mucosal bleeding time: This is a global test of primary haemostasis but is not specific for a particular disorder. A shallow cut is made in the buccal mucosa and the time required for cessation of bleeding is recorded (Figure 6.12). The cut is shallow enough to be sealed by the primary platelet plug and does not require fibrin (secondary haemostasis). Therefore, it specifically tests primary haemostasis. In healthy dogs, BMBT is 1.7–3.3 minutes and can be mildly prolonged (to 4.2 minutes) in anaesthetized or sedated dogs. BMBT of healthy anaesthetized cats is <3.3 minutes. BMBT can be prolonged with thrombocytopenia (<75 x 10^9/l), thrombopathias (e.g. aspirin) and vWD. BMBT is insensitive; it will only be prolonged with relatively severe defects (e.g. vWf:Ag <20%). It is useful for the following:

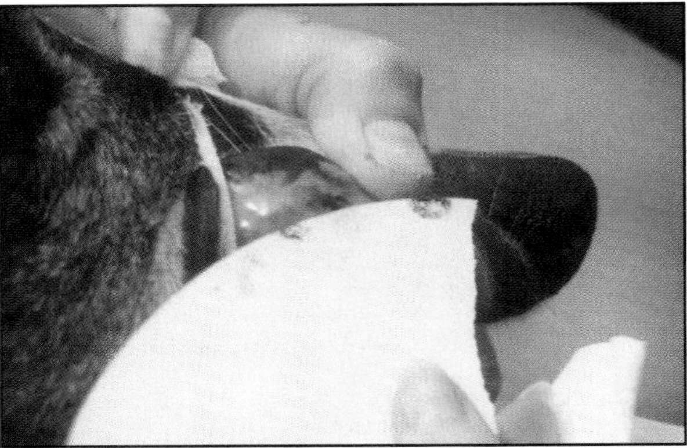

6.12 Buccal mucosal bleeding time. This procedure can be performed in awake or sedated dogs; however, cats require sedation (e.g. diazepam and ketamine). The upper lip is tied back with gauze. This must be firm enough to hold the lip in place, but not cause vascular engorgement, which can prolong the bleeding time. A standardized incision (5 mm long by 1 mm wide) is then made in the buccal mucosa using a specialized device. The wound is blotted with filter paper (taking care not to touch the actual incision, which can disturb the forming platelet plugs). BMBT is the time taken from creating the incision to cessation of bleeding.

- Detection of a primary haemostatic defect in bleeding animals. BMBT is indicated if results of routine haemostatic testing (platelet count, coagulation assays) are within reference intervals in an animal with excessive bleeding, particularly that associated with primary haemostatic defects, e.g. mucosal bleeding
- Presurgical screen to identify Dobermanns (particularly those with unknown vWf:Ag values) 'at risk' of haemorrhage due to vWD. If presurgical BMBT is prolonged in a Dobermann, elective surgery should be delayed and the dog should be tested for vWD. Alternatively, surgery could proceed, but appropriate prophylactic treatment should be provided, particularly with invasive procedures where surgical haemostasis may be difficult
- BMBT has been used anecdotally as a routine screening test of haemostasis before invasive biopsy or aspiration procedures in animals, e.g. liver biopsy. The use of the test for this purpose is controversial in human patients, however, and no controlled studies have been performed in animals to verify that BMBT is predictive of haemorrhage (other than in dogs with vWD) in this setting.

Cuticle bleeding time: This has been used historically to identify vWD in dogs. The tip of a dog's nail is removed using guillotine-type nail clippers and the duration of bleeding is timed. However, this test suffers from lack of reproducibility (lack of standardization of cut depth). The depth of the cut requires both platelet plug and fibrin formation to seal the defect, thus it will be prolonged in disorders of secondary, as well as primary, haemostasis. Therefore, it is less specific than BMBT for primary haemostasis and is no longer recommended for this purpose.

Clot retraction: After a clot has formed in a glass or non-anticoagulant tube, the clot retracts, condenses and separates from serum. Clot retraction is mediated by contractile proteins in platelets and thus requires normal platelet number and function. Maximal retraction takes about 1–2 hours, after which the clot lyses. However, this is a crude and insensitive test; interpretation is subjective and difficult. Furthermore, it is not specific; the retraction time will be abnormal with anaemia and defects in fibrin formation, such as hypofibrinogenaemia.

von Willebrand's disease

von Willebrand's disease (vWD) is due to a deficiency or abnormality in von Willebrand factor (vWf), a large multimeric glycoprotein, which circulates as a non-covalent complex with factor VIII (FVIII). vWf used to be called FVIII-related antigen, but this term is confusing and should no longer be used. vWf is esssential for primary haemostasis by acting as a 'glue', binding platelets to the subendothelial matrix and to each other (see Figure 6.1). vWD is usually diagnosed by measuring vWf (vWf antigen or vWf:Ag) using antibodies against vWf in enzyme-linked immunosorbent assay (ELISA) or immunoelectrophoresis assays. The results of individual patients are expressed as a unit value or percentage of a species-specific standard plasma pool, which is designated as 100% or 100 U/dl. vWD is diagnosed when vWf:Ag values are <50% (50 U/dl), whereas values >70% are considered normal. Values between these ranges are 'equivocal': the animal could be a carrier of vWD or could be normal. In symptomatic dogs, it is important to obtain a vWf:Ag value, because this is diagnostic (values <50% are compatible with vWD) and correlates to clinical signs (clinical bleeding is seen with values <35% in dogs). BMBT is prolonged in vWD, but cannot be used for diagnosis, as it is not specific or sensitive for this disorder (BMBT will only be prolonged if vWf:Ag is <20%). Tests for the specific vWf gene mutation are available for select breeds, e.g. Scottish Terrier, Manchester Terrier (see www.vetgen.com) and Dutch Kooiker dogs. DNA samples are stable for airmail shipping. Genetic tests are best used for carrier detection (due to the overlap of vWf:Ag values in dogs that are carriers or normal) and management of breeding programs. Genetic tests do not provide information about vWf:Ag values (which can be predictive of clinical bleeding), and are more expensive and less available than vWf:Ag assays.

Secondary haemostasis

The coagulation cascade is evaluated by global screening assays. When these tests are abnormally prolonged, individual factor assays are used to identify the specific factors involved.

Coagulation screening assays

Prothrombin time (PT), activated partial thromboplastin time (aPTT) and thrombin clot time: PT (also called one-stage prothrombin time), aPTT and thrombin clot time (TCT or fibrinogen concentration) are used to detect coagulation cascade abnormalities. PT tests the extrinsic and common pathways, aPTT tests the intrinsic and common pathways (Figure 6.13) and TCT primarily tests the fibrinogen component of the common pathway. These tests are performed on citrated plasma, using specific reagents that activate clotting *in vitro*, with the formation of fibrin being the end point. Results are expressed as the time taken for a fibrin clot to form. For PT and aPTT, the test reagents include a specific activator of the coagulation pathway (tissue factor or thromboplastin for PT and a contact activator, such as kaolin, for aPTT), an exogenous source of phospholipid, and calcium (which must be provided as it is chelated by the citrate anticoagulant). These assays do not rely on the patient's platelets to provide phospholipid for fibrin formation and are unaffected by thrombocytopenia or thrombopathia, including Scott syndrome (see below).

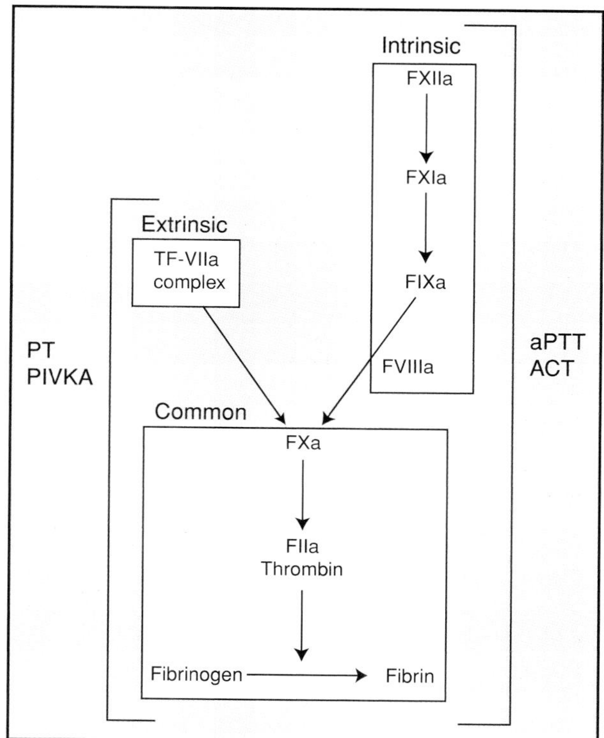

6.13 Coagulation assays. The coagulation cascade can be divided into three pathways: intrinsic (FXII, FXI, FIX, FVIII), extrinsic (FVII, TF) and common (FX, FII, and fibrinogen). Prothrombin time (PT) and PIVKA test (FVII, FX and FII) evaluate extrinsic and common pathway factors. Activated partial thromboplastin time (aPTT) and activated coagulation time (ACT) measure intrinsic and common pathway activities. These tests can be used to identify specific factors potentially responsible for prolonged results.

Abnormal results are best interpreted using the 'waterfall' model of the coagulation cascade (Figures 6.13 and 6.14). Results from different coagulation analysers (and laboratories) are not directly comparable, due to different reagents and methods for clot detection. Animals have more rapid coagulation times than humans. Therefore, species-specific reference intervals should be established and provided by each laboratory and testing should, ideally, be performed by

Assay result			Associated defects
PT	*aPTT*	*TCT*	
↑	N	N	Extrinsic pathway: FVII
N	↑	N	Intrinsic pathway: FXII, FXI, FIX, FVIII
N	N	↑	Hypofibrinogenaemia, heparin therapy
↑	↑	N	Common pathway defects: FX, FII Multiple defects in combined pathways, e.g. vitamin K deficiency, DIC
↑	↑	↑	Severe hypofibrinogenaemia (<0.05 g/l), heparin therapy Multiple defects in combined pathways, e.g. liver disease, DIC

6.14 Abnormalities in coagulation assay results and associated defects. (DIC = disseminated intravascular coagulation; N = normal.)

a veterinary laboratory. Newer analysers allow these tests to be performed in-house. Reference intervals should still be established and/or samples from control animals tested with patients to verify results; control data can then be used to establish intervals. These analysers may not be sensitive to mild factor deficiencies; if results do not match clinical signs, sample referral to a specialized testing laboratory is advised.

For TCT, a standard concentration of thrombin is added to the patient's plasma; this converts fibrinogen to fibrin. TCT will be prolonged by deficient (hypofibrinogenaemia) or abnormal fibrinogen (dysfibrinogenaemia), defective fibrin formation (e.g. inhibition of polymerization due to FDPs) or thrombin inhibitors (e.g. heparin). The time can be converted to a fibrinogen concentration (g/l) by comparing the patient's clotting time to that of a standard curve derived from purified fibrinogen. Once again, reference intervals should be established for this assay and, wherever possible, species-specific fibrinogen should be used to derive the standard curve. The use of human fibrinogen for this purpose decreases assay sensitivity. Fibrinogen concentration can also be measured in EDTA-anticoagulated blood by heat precipitation (Schalm's fibrinogen). With this technique, the fibrinogen concentration is equivalent to the difference in plasma protein (as measured by a refractometer) before and after heating plasma to 56°C (which precipitates fibrinogen). The test is only sensitive to changes in fibrinogen of 1.0 g/l (which is also the lowest measurable value) and, therefore, should not be relied upon for identifying decreased fibrinogen concentrations in dogs with bleeding disorders. Schalm's fibrinogen can be used for detecting high fibrinogen concentrations in animals with inflammatory disease (fibrinogen is an acute phase reactant protein) or hypercoagulable states (e.g. immune-mediated haemolytic anaemia, IMHA). Mild changes will be missed, however.

Whole blood clotting time: Whole blood clotting time (WBCT) is a simple, but crude, screening test for the intrinsic pathway of coagulation. Reported reference intervals are 3–13 minutes for dogs and 8 minutes for cats. However, the test is insensitive to factor deficiencies (it will only be prolonged if factors are <5% of normal) and is influenced by other variables, including the volume of blood, haematocrit, tube size and tube coating (clotting times are longer, e.g. 9–20 minutes, in dogs where plastic or silicone tubes are used for samples, so glass must be used). Furthermore, WBCT is not specific for intrinsic pathway defects. Platelet phospholipid is required for clot formation, therefore the WBCT will be prolonged with severe thrombocytopenia. Due to these considerations, this test is not recommended for routine use, with the activated coagulation time (ACT) being the preferred test. In emergency situations or if ACT tubes are unavailable, WBCT may be used. A prolonged WBCT suggests a severe coagulopathy, for example due to anticoagulant rodenticide toxicosis, particularly in those animals with a high clinical index of suspicion of this disorder. If WBCT is within reference intervals, however, a haemostatic disorder may still be present and blood should always be collected into citrate for more specific coagulation testing.

Activated coagulation time: This is a modified aPTT that is less sensitive to factor deficiencies (<10%) than aPTT (<30%). Whole blood without anticoagulant is added to a special tube containing diatomaceous earth as a contact (factor XII) activator, and the tube is gently inverted at specific intervals until a clot is detected. To minimize variability in results due to temperature, the tube should be prewarmed and kept at 37°C during testing, preferably in a heating block (the armpit can serve as a heater). Unlike the aPTT test, in which an exogenous source of phospholipid is provided, the ACT test relies on the patient's platelets for phospholipid to support the reaction. Therefore, severe thrombocytopenia (<10 x 10^9/l) will mildly prolong ACT. ACT is a useful in-house screening test for severe defects and will be prolonged with anticoagulant rodenticide intoxication and disseminated intravascular coagulation (DIC). It can also be used to monitor heparin therapy (desirable therapeutic target is 1.2 x baseline). Reported reference intervals are 60–90 seconds in dogs and <165 seconds in cats.

PIVKA test: PIVKAs refer to inactive proteins induced by vitamin K absence or antagonism. However, the PIVKA test does not directly test for these inactive precursors but is a modified PT performed on diluted plasma, which is sensitive to deficiencies in FX, FVII and FII. Although the most severe prolongations (>63 s; reference 15–18 s) are seen with anticoagulant rodenticide intoxication, the PIVKA test is not specific for this. Prolonged values are also seen with other vitamin K-responsive disorders, e.g. cholestatic liver disease, inflammatory bowel disease, and non-vitamin K-responsive disorders, e.g. DIC, acute liver disease/failure, heparin therapy, FVII deficiency. Routine use of this test cannot be recommended due to limited availability and lack of clear superiority over PT and aPTT assays for disease diagnosis.

Specific factor assays

Individual factor assays are performed to determine the underlying defect responsible for abnormal screening coagulation tests. These are modifications of the screening assays, where the ability of patient plasma to correct the prolonged clotting times of specific factor-deficient plasma is determined. Results are expressed as a percent coagulant activity of a standard plasma pool, assigned a value of 100%. An inability to correct the prolonged time indicates a deficiency of that factor. Typically, single factor deficiencies of <30% cause haemorrhage, but if multiple factor deficiencies exist, milder reductions (<50%) may yield clinical signs.

Tertiary haemostasis

Tests for fibrinolysis are generally restricted to FDPs and D-dimer, because other assays, such as plasminogen, tPA and plasminogen activator inhibitor (PAI), are not readily available.

Fibrin(ogen) degradation products

Plasmin cleaves fibrinogen and soluble fibrin similarly, yielding degradation fragments (Figure 6.15), which are detected with latex agglutination-based immunological assays. Traditional FDP assays contain polyclonal antibodies which crossreact with intact fibrinogen and require specialized collection tubes for its removal. However, monoclonal antibodies in newer assays permit measurement of FDPs in plasma (Figure 6.16), allowing all coagulation assays to be performed on a single (citrate) tube. Plasma FDP assays appear to be sensitive for detecting FDPs in dogs and are preferred over older serum assays for this purpose. However, they may not work in cats (Stokol, 2003). FDPs are not specific for DIC; increased values may be seen with other thromboembolic diseases and internal haemorrhage.

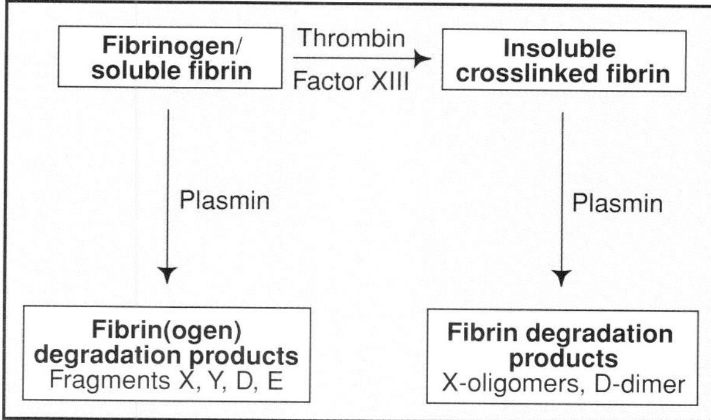

6.15 Fibrin(ogen) degradation products and D-dimer. Fibrinogen is converted to soluble fibrin by thrombin. Thrombin also activates FXIII, which crosslinks fibrin. Plasmin cleaves fibrinogen and soluble fibrin similarly, yielding fibrin(ogen) degradation products (FDPs), fragments X, Y, D and E. In contrast, plasmin degradation of crosslinked fibrin yields specific crosslinked fragments of varying molecular weight, called X-oligomers. D-dimer is a neo-epitope produced by crosslinking and is the smallest X-linked fragment. It is rarely found as an individual entity *in vivo*, but occurs within X-oligomers. D-dimer is thus specific for fibrinolysis and indicates thrombin and plasmin activation, whereas FDPs indicate plasmin activation only.

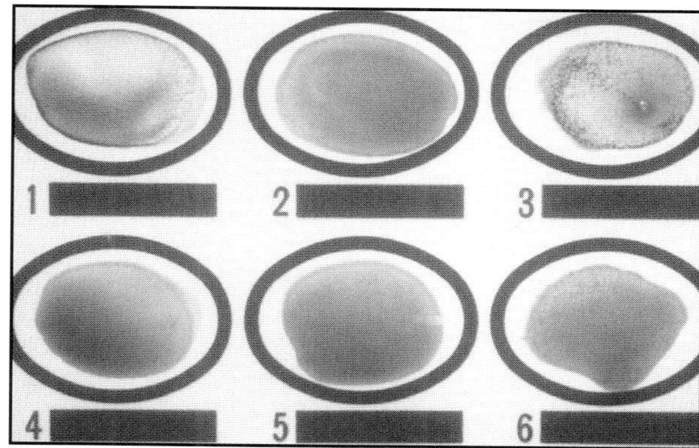

6.16 Latex agglutination plasma FDP assays. The assay contains red latex beads coated with monoclonal antibodies against FDPs (fragments X, Y, D or E). Well 1 = positive control. Well 2 = negative control. Wells 3–6 = patient samples, diluted as indicated before adding latex beads: well 3 = patient 1, diluted 1:2; well 4 = patient 1, diluted 1:8; well 5 = patient 2, diluted 1:2; well 6 = patient 2, diluted 1:8. The absence of agglutination at both dilutions indicates a negative reaction, i.e. FDPs <5 μg/ml (patient 2). Healthy dogs have FDPs <5 μg/ml. An agglutination reaction indicates a positive reaction with FDPs >5 μg/ml, which is semi-quantified by the dilutions, i.e. FDPs are >20 μg/ml if both dilutions are positive, whereas FDPs are 5–20 μg/ml (patient 1) if only the 1:2 dilution is positive.

D-dimer

The use of D-dimer tests for diagnosis of haemostatic disorders in dogs has been recently reviewed (Stokol, 2003). D-dimer is a new antigen (neo-epitope) created on fibrin when it is crosslinked by FXIIIa. Plasmin cleavage of crosslinked fibrin (but not fibrinogen) exposes the D-dimer epitope within crosslinked fragments, called X-oligomers (Figure 6.15). D-dimer can then be detected using immunological assays, particularly latex agglutination. D-dimer values are <0.25 μg/ml in healthy dogs. D-dimer tests appear to be sensitive for detecting thrombosis in dogs with DIC, but values may be increased with any fibrinolytic condition, e.g. postsurgical wound healing or internal haemorrhage. Quantitative D-dimer results should be provided, because the highest values appear to occur with thromboembolism (TE). In most laboratories, D-dimer has replaced FDP testing for the detection of fibrinolysis in dogs.

Inhibitors

Currently, antithrombin III (AT) is the only available inhibitor test. AT is measured using tests based on its ability to inhibit thrombin or activated factor X (factor Xa) activity. The activity of these factors is detected using chromogenic substrates specific for each factor. The AT concentration is inversely proportional to factor activity (i.e. high factor Xa activity indicates low AT concentration). The result is expressed as a percentage of a species-specific standard pool, designated as 100%. Healthy animals have AT values >80%; values <50% are associated with a risk for thrombosis. AT levels are decreased in DIC, protein-losing disorders (enteropathy, nephropathy) and with certain drugs, e.g. L-asparaginase. Newer tests which measure heparin concentrations are being developed for monitoring prophylactic heparin therapy.

Disorders of haemostasis

Haemostatic disorders can be inherited (Figure 6.17) or acquired. Inherited defects should be suspected in young animals, especially those with recurrent bleeding episodes or a known family history. Most inherited diseases cause excessive haemorrhage; animals generally do not suffer from inherited fibrinolytic disorders, which predispose humans to thrombosis. Acquired disorders affect animals of any age, but are common in older animals, due to underlying diseases which affect haemostasis.

Inherited disorders

Primary haemostasis

Inherited primary haemostatic defects are uncommon, with the exception of vWD, which is the most common inherited disorder of haemostasis.

von Willebrand's disease: This has been diagnosed in many breeds of dogs and, rarely, in cats (Brooks, 2000).

- Type I is characterized by decreased vWf of normal multimeric structure. This is the most common type and is found in high prevalence in Dobermanns (60%), Manchester Terriers, Airedale Terriers and Rottweilers. The genetic mutation appears to be a splice site defect in breeds tested to date and it is inherited as an autosomal recessive trait. Bleeding can occur if vWf:Ag values are <35%
- Type II vWD results in more severe bleeding than type I, as vWf is defective in amount and structure, with a relative lack of higher molecular weight multimers (which are more effective in haemostasis). This type has been diagnosed in German Wirehair and Shorthair Pointers
- Type III vWD is the most severe type, with an absolute vWf deficiency (vWf:Ag <1%). This is inherited as an autosomal recessive trait and has been diagnosed in Scottish Terriers, Shetland Sheepdogs, Chesapeake Bay Retrievers and Dutch Kooiker dogs.

Defect	Cause	Breeds	Diagnostic tests
Primary haemostasis			
Inherited thrombocytopenia	? – dogs are asymptomatic	Cavalier King Charles Spaniel	Platelet count (usually 30–150 x 10^9/l)
Glanzman's thrombasthenia	GPIIb/IIIa deficiency	Great Pyrenees, Otterhound	BMBT, platelet function tests, flow cytometry for platelet GP receptors
Bassett Hound thrombopathia	? cAMP defect	Bassett Hound	BMBT, platelet function tests
Unknown thrombopathia	? signalling defects	Boxer, Spitz, mixed-breed	
Storage pool deficiency	? dense granule defect	American Cocker Spaniel	
Chediak–Higashi syndrome	Dense granule defect	Persian cat	
Scott syndrome	Defective platelet PS exposure	German Shepherd Dog	Specific tests for platelet procoagulant activity
vWD	Deficiency (type I or III) or abnormality (type II) in vWf	Type I: many Type II: German Wirehaired pointer, German Shorthair pointer Type III: Scottish terrier, Dutch Kooiker, Shetland Sheepdog	vWf:Ag, BMBT, genetic tests
Secondary haemostasis			
Haemophilia A	FVIII deficiency, sex-linked	Many dogs and cats	aPTT, FVIII:C
Haemophilia B	FIX deficiency, sex-linked	Many dogs, British Shorthair, Siamese, Domestic Shorthair (DSH)	aPTT, FIX:C, genetic tests
Haemophilia C	FXI deficiency, autosomal	German Shepherd Dog, Kerry Blue Terrier, Pyrenean Mountain Dog	aPTT, FXI:C
Factor X deficiency	Autosomal	Boxer, American Cocker Spaniel, Jack Russell Terrier, DSH	PT, aPTT, FX:C
Factor VII deficiency	Autosomal	Beagle, Alaskan Malamute	PT, VII:C
Hageman trait	FXII deficiency	Cats, Poodles	aPTT, FXII:C
Vitamin K-dependent factors (FII, FVII, FIX, FX)	Carboxylase enzyme abnormality	Devon Rex	PT, aAPTT, PIVKA

6.17 Inherited disorders of haemostasis. (F:C = factor coagulant activity.)

Thrombocytopenia: Up to 50% of Greyhounds, and perhaps other sight hounds, have platelet counts that are lower (80–148 x 10^9/l) than reference intervals established for mixed breeds of dogs (150–400 x 10^9/l) (Sullivan *et al.*, 1994). An inherited thrombocytopenia occurs in Cavalier King Charles Spaniels (Pedersen *et al.*, 2002). These dogs have low platelet counts (30–150 x 10^9/l), and many platelets are large and may not be included in the platelet count with some analysers. These dogs are typically asymptomatic.

Thrombopathia: Inherited thrombopathias have been recognized in several breeds of dogs and cats (Figure 6.17) and should be suspected in a young animal displaying bleeding attributable to a defect in primary haemostasis, but with platelet counts and screening coagulation assays within reference intervals. BMBT is typically prolonged and platelet function tests, e.g. aggregation, are abnormal. Flow cytometric-based immunological tests for platelet glycoprotein receptors have permitted the accurate diagnosis of Glanzmann's thrombasthenia or GPIIb/IIIa deficiency. The mutation in the GPIIb/IIIa gene has also been identified in certain dog breeds with this disorder. Scott syndrome is a newly recognized, inherited platelet defect in German Shepherd Dogs. Dogs present with moderate to severe spontaneous (e.g. epistaxis or hyphaema) or surgery-induced haemorrhage. They have defective platelet PS exposure, therefore fibrin formation, but not platelet aggregation, is defective. Diagnosis remained elusive because routine and specialized assay results, e.g. BMBT and platelet aggregation, were normal. The advent of assays specific for platelet procoagulant activity, such as flow cytometric-measured platelet PS exposure, enabled accurate diagnosis of this unusual disorder (Brooks *et al.*, 2002). This disease highlights the importance of PS-expressing cells in the haemostatic process.

Secondary haemostasis

Inherited deficiencies of all coagulation factors have been reported in animals, with the exception of tissue factor (see Figure 6.17). FVIII (haemophilia A) and FIX (haemophilia B) deficiency are most common. Factor deficiencies are identified when screening tests (PT, aPTT, TCT) are prolonged; the combination of assay abnormalities provides clues as to the underlying defect (see Figure 6.14). Associated clinical signs depend on the underlying defect (e.g. FXII deficiency is asymptomatic) and the degree of factor deficiency.

Haemophilia A and B: Haemophilia A (FVIII deficiency) is the most common inherited defect of secondary haemostasis. It has been diagnosed in many breeds of dogs, including mixed breeds, but is particularly prevalent in German Shepherd Dogs. Haemophilia A has also been detected in cats. Dogs typically present with excessive haemorrhage at a young age, including haematomas, bleeding after surgery and recurring joint lameness from haemarthrosis. Clinical signs correlate to the degree of FVIII deficiency. The worst symptoms are seen in dogs with severe deficiencies (<1% FVIII coagulant activity, FVIII:C); dogs with moderate (1–5% FVIII:C) or mild (5–25% FVIII:C) deficiencies may show subtle clinical signs. Indeed, the widespread dissemination of haemophilia A in German Shepherd Dogs has been attributed to a single prolific sire with mild FVIII:C deficiency. Haemophilia A and B (FIX deficiency) are sex-linked disorders, with expression being restricted to males (dams being obligate carriers). Breed-specific defects have been identified in the FIX gene (Mauser *et al.*, 1996; Gu *et al.*, 1999). A FVIII gene inversion has been described in several dog breeds with severe haemophilia A, i.e. <1% FVIII:C (Hough *et al.*, 2002; Lozier *et al.*, 2002; Brooks, personal communication).

These diseases cause prolonged aPTT and require specific factor analysis to identify the precise defect in the intrinsic pathway (see Figures 6.13 and 6.14). Assay reagents and procedures differ in their sensitivity to factor deficiencies, with aPTT being more prolonged with haemophilia B than haemophilia A. The degree of prolongation in aPTT with haemophilia A may be mild and the disease may be missed if insensitive aPTT assays are used for screening patients. ACT and WBCT may be prolonged with severe deficiencies of both factors. However, due to their poor sensitivities and lack of specificity (both are affected by thrombocytopenia), they should not be used as screening tests for inherited factor deficiencies.

Factor XII deficiency: Haemophilia A and B have been reported in cats, but the most common cause for prolonged aPTT in this species is FXII (Hageman factor) deficiency. This factor has no role in fibrin formation, so these animals are asymptomatic and the disease is most often diagnosed when prolonged aPTT is detected on presurgical or other screening assays.

Vitamin K-dependent factors: A hereditary vitamin-K responsive coagulopathy has been reported in Devon Rex cats. Cats of both sexes suffer from haematomas, conjunctival haemorrhage, haemarthrosis and massive bleeding into body cavities. They have prolonged PTs and aPTTs, with normal fibrinogen and platelet counts. All vitamin K-dependent factors (FII, FVII, FIX and FX) are decreased. The abnormal coagulation times and bleeding symptoms are responsive to vitamin K1 therapy. The defect is due to an abnormal gamma-glutamyl carboxylase enzyme, which activates the vitamin K-dependent coagulation factors.

Acquired disorders

Primary haemostasis

Thrombocytopenia: Thrombocytopenia is the most common acquired haemostatic disorder and is due to decreased bone marrow production, destruction, consumption, sequestration and loss of platelets (Figure 6.18). Severe thrombocytopenias (<50 x 10^9/l) are due to decreased production, destruction or consumption. It is rare to see platelet counts <100 x 10^9/l due to haemorrhage or sequestration alone. Therefore, a severe thrombocytopenia (<50 x 10^9/l) is usually the cause, rather than a consequence, of haemorrhage. Also, sequestration (in the liver, spleen or pulmonary circulation) is the least likely cause of thrombocytopenia.

Decreased bone marrow production
Immune-mediated (more common in dogs than cats)
Infectious, e.g. *Ehrlichia canis*, feline leukaemia virus
Drug reactions – can be due to direct cytotoxicity or immune-mediated effects
Neoplasia, e.g. acute leukaemia, myelodysplastic syndrome, myelophthisis
Increased destruction
Primary immune-mediated
Secondary immune-mediated, e.g. infectious diseases, neoplasia, systemic lupus erythematosus (rare)
Increased consumption
Disseminated intravascular coagulation, e.g. *Dirofilaria immitis*, *Angiostrongylus vasorum*, pancreatitis, neoplasia, immune-mediated haemolytic anaemia
Localized intravascular coagulation, e.g. haemangiosarcoma
Vasculitis
Increased loss
Haemorrhage, e.g. secondary to anticoagulant rodenticide toxicity, neoplasia
Sequestration
Splenomegaly, hepatomegaly
Pulmonary circulation – secondary to sepsis, endotoxaemia or hypoxia

6.18 Causes of acquired thrombocytopenia.

Immune-mediated thrombocytopenia (ITP) is a common cause of acquired thrombocytopenias in dogs and cats and can be primary or secondary to infectious diseases (e.g. rickettsial or viral infections), immune-mediated diseases (e.g. lupus) or neoplasia. A high prevalence of primary ITP is found in Cocker Spaniels, Miniature and Toy Poodles, German Shepherd Dogs and Old English Sheepdogs, suggesting a genetic predisposition to ITP in these breeds. Animals typically present with mucosal haemorrhage, petechiae and ecchymoses. Platelet counts are usually <30 x 10^9/l. Routine coagulation screening tests (PT, aPTT, TCT) are within reference intervals, although ACT and WBCT may be prolonged, because both rely on platelet phospholipid for clot formation. Platelet-bound IgG antibodies can be detected using ELISA or flow cytometric assays. These antibodies confirm that the thrombocytopenia is immune-mediated (completely or in part), but does not differentiate between primary and secondary causes. For instance, dogs with neoplasia and infectious diseases, such as ehrlichiosis and heartworm infection, can have anti-platelet IgG, indicating that the thrombocytopenia is, at least in part, immune-mediated; treatment of the underlying disease is required, however, to resolve clinical signs (Lewis *et al.*, 1995, Scott *et al.*, 2002). Values of anti-platelet IgG increase in stored samples; samples should be tested for antibody within 24 hours of collection to minimize false-positive results.

Acquired von Willebrand's disease: This has been associated with hypothyroidism in some dog breeds. However, proof for a definitive association is lacking and thyroid supplementation is not recommended as treatment for dogs with vWD, unless the dog is proven to be concurrently hypothyroid.

Acquired thrombopathias: These occur with neoplasia, renal and hepatic disease, infectious diseases (e.g. feline infectious peritonitis virus), DIC (due to the anti-platelet effect of FDPs) and drugs. Drugs known to interfere with platelet function, such as aspirin, should be avoided in animals with proven or suspected haemostatic defects. Aspirin irreversibly inhibits platelet cyclo-oxygenase, causing platelet function abnormalities that persist for the lifespan of the platelet (7–10 days). However, haemorrhage is rarely induced by aspirin administration alone; a concurrent haemostatic abnormality (e.g. thrombocytopenia) must usually be present to induce bleeding.

Secondary haemostasis

Vitamin K deficiency or antagonism: Vitamin K is an essential cofactor for the enzyme gamma-glutamyl carboxylase, which catalyses the conversion of glutamic acid to gamma-carboxyglutamic acid in specific coagulation factors (FII, FVII, FIX, FX) and inhibitors (proteins C and S). This carboxylation is required for the calcium-dependent binding of these factors to PS. In the absence of vitamin K, these factors accumulate as inactive precursors, resulting in functional deficiencies which manifest as prolonged PT, aPTT, PIVKA and ACT/WBCT (the latter with severe deficiencies). FVII has the shortest half-life of all factors (approximately 6 hours), so PT and PIVKA tests will be prolonged before aPTT; thus these tests are more sensitive to vitamin K deficiency and are preferred for diagnosis or monitoring response to therapy. Vitamin K deficiency occurs with anticoagulant rodenticide toxicosis, cholestatic liver disease (vitamin K is fat soluble), malabsorption (e.g. exocrine pancreatic insufficiency) and administration of some drugs (e.g. sulphaquinoxolone). Excessive haemorrhage is typically seen with anticoagulant rodenticide poisoning, but is not always evident with these other diseases, despite abnormal test results. Some dogs with anticoagulant rodenticide toxicosis may be mildly to moderately thrombocytopenic (45–153 x 10^9/l); the mechanism is unclear and may be due to blood loss or immune-mediated destruction after blood transfusions. Elevated FDPs may also be seen, probably as a result of internal haemorrhage.

Animals with vitamin K deficiency should be treated with vitamin K1. Response to treatment can be assessed by cessation of haemorrhage and normalization of coagulation tests. Most first-generation anticoagulant rodenticides, e.g. warfarin, have a short half-life (approximately 15 hours), thus treatment should be given for at least 1 week if animals are intoxicated with these compounds. However, second generation anticoagulant rodenticides, e.g. brodifacoum, or first generation indandiones, e.g. diphacinone, have longer half-lives (up to 6 days) and require vitamin K therapy for up to 6 weeks. Since in many cases the nature of the ingested compound is unknown, it is best to treat animals suspected of having rodenticide toxicosis for a minimum of 4–6 weeks. This can be expensive; if desired, therapy can be stopped after 1 week and PT (or PIVKAs) can be measured 2–3 days later to determine if the rodenticide is still in the circulation. This is not routinely recommended, however, as clinical signs can redevelop during this time.

Disseminated intravascular coagulation: DIC results from the systemic activation of haemostasis due to an underlying disease which causes severe vessel injury or excessive TF expression. In some disorders, e.g. mucinous carcinomas, DIC can be initiated by direct activation of FX. The result is systemic platelet and coagulation factor activation and fibrinolysis, causing thrombocytopenia, factor deficiencies (from plasmin-mediated cleavage), inhibitor consumption and FDP generation. FDPs can exacerbate clinical signs by inhibiting platelet function and fibrin polymerization. Many diseases can induce DIC, e.g. sepsis, pancreatitis, neoplasia and IMHA. *Angiostrongylus vasorum*, a nematode found in the pulmonary circulation, can cause DIC and haemorrhage in affected dogs. This has been attributed to the first stage larvae and immature parasites (Schelling *et al.*, 1986; Ramsey *et al.*, 1996). Clinically, animals with DIC present with excessive haemorrhage and/or thrombosis. Haemorrhage is often obvious and dramatic, but most patients have concurrent or preceding thrombosis resulting in end-organ dysfunction or failure. The consequences of thrombosis are often underestimated, but they contribute significantly to morbidity and mortality.

There is no single pathognomonic test for DIC. It is diagnosed if all of the following are present:

- Appropriate clinical signs
- An initiating disease
- Abnormalities in all haemostatic pathways
  - Thrombocytopenia
  - Prolonged coagulation times (one or more) and/or hypofibrinogenaemia
  - Increased FDPs and/or D-dimer
  - Decreased AT.

Red cell fragmentation (schistocytes, acanthocytes, keratocytes) from microthrombosis may be evident in blood smears but is not specific. The most consistently abnormal and therefore most diagnostically useful tests are AT, aPTT, platelet counts and plasma FDPs/D-dimer. Specific factor assays are of no value due to activation and cleavage of coagulation factors.

Hepatic disease: The liver is the site of factor synthesis and clearance and is a rich source of tissue factor. Bile is required for vitamin K absorption. Liver disease can result in haemostatic defects due to factor deficiencies (synthetic liver failure), DIC (acute or fulminant liver disease) or vitamin K deficiency (cholestatic diseases). Furthermore, platelet number or function may be abnormal. Many animals with liver disease have abnormal coagulation times, including PT, aPTT, PIVKAs and FDPs, which do not always correlate to clinical bleeding tendencies.

Renal disease: Renal disease can result in either haemorrhage or thrombosis. Renal failure-induced haemorrhage has been attributed to thrombopathia (defective adhesion and/or aggregation), whereas thrombosis, seen with protein-losing nephropathy, is due to AT loss, hyperfibrinogenaemia and/or platelet hyperaggregability.

Other diseases: Many other disorders are associated with haemostatic defects, including snake envenomation, infectious diseases (e.g. leptospirosis), neoplasia and immune-mediated conditions. The haemostatic problems can be due to vasculitis, thrombocytopenia or thrombopathia (enhanced or decreased function), anticoagulants (e.g. heparin from mast cell tumors), and DIC. Many drugs, including analgesics, anaesthetics and chemotherapeutics, can cause coagulation factor and platelet abnormalities.

Tertiary haemostasis

Most acquired fibrinolytic disorders are associated with DIC, which has the dual effect of promoting haemorrhage from excessive plasmin activation (cleaves coagulation factors and fibrin) and thrombosis from stimulating the secretion of fibrinolytic inhibitors.

Thrombosis

Thromboembolism (TE) encompasses all haemostatic pathways. Thrombosis can be due to:

- Endothelial cell injury, e.g. heartworm infection
- Increased platelet function or number, e.g. nephrotic syndrome, neoplasia
- Increased activity or decreased inhibition of coagulation factors, e.g. AT deficiency, hyperfibrinogenaemia
- Inhibition of fibrinolysis, e.g. DIC.

DIC is the prototypical thromboembolic disease, but other disorders, predisposing to or resulting in thrombosis, are being recognized with increased frequency. These include protein-losing diseases, immune-mediated disease, neoplasia, sepsis, cardiac disease, hyperadrenocorticism, intravenous catheterization and administration of some drugs (e.g. corticosteroids). Unfortunately, specific diagnostic tests for TE are unavailable. Diagnosis relies upon a high clinical index of suspicion (e.g. pulmonary TE should be suspected in a dog with IMHA and dyspnoea with ventilation/perfusion mismatch), and supportive laboratory evidence, including increased D-dimer and decreased AT values.

Case examples

Case 1

Signalment

2-year-old female, intact Dobermann.

History and clinical examination

10-day history of epistaxis, melaena and gingival bleeding. Epistaxis had also occurred 3 months previously and resolved without treatment. The dog collapsed just before presentation. She was weak, depressed, tachycardic and tachypnoeic, with pale mucosa, and petechial and ecchymotic haemorrhages.

Clinical pathology data

Haematology and TP	Result	Reference interval
RBC (x 10^{12}/l)	1.5	5.6–8.5
HCT (l/l)	0.09	0.39–0.57
MCV (fl)	61	64–73
MCHC (g/dl)	31	31–37
Reticulocytes (%)	18.5	0–1.5
Absolute reticulocyte count (x 10^9/l)	278	<60
Normoblasts (/100 WBC)	7	0
Normoblasts (x 10^9/l)	2.5	0
WBC (x 10^9/l)	35.0	7.5–19.9
Neutrophils (segmented) (x 10^9/l)	23.0	3.9–14.7
Neutrophils (band) (x 10^9/l)	2.8	0–0.3
Lymphocytes (x 10^9/l)	2.1	1.5–5.2
Monocytes (x 10^9/l)	5.7	0.3–2.2
Eosinophils (x 10^9/l)	1.4	0.1–1.6
Platelets (x 10^9/l)	<12 [a]	179–483
TP (g/l)	45	59–78

[a] The blood smear from this dog is shown in Figure 6.11c.

Coagulation	Result	Reference interval
PT (s)	6	6–8
aPTT (s)	18	12–21
Fibrinogen (g/l)	3.5	1.1–2.6
Plasma FDP (µg/ml)	<5	<5
vWf:Ag (%)	12	70–180

Based on the presenting clinical signs, which haemostatic pathways are involved and is this inherited or acquired?

Mucosal haemorrhage and petechiae indicate a primary haemostatic disorder, probably involving platelets (petechiae are rarely seen with vWD). The most common platelet disorders are acquired, rather than inherited. However, this dog is young, has had recurrent haemorrhage and is a Dobermann, a breed with a high prevalence of vWD. Therefore, concurrent vWD is possible.

How would you interpret the changes in the haemogram and coagulation results?

The dog has a severe microcytic, normochromic, regenerative anaemia. Regeneration is evident from the reticulocytosis (18.5%) with a high absolute reticulocyte count (278 x 10^9/l; reference interval <80 x 10^9/l). The anaemia is probably due to blood loss (low total protein), with secondary iron deficiency resulting in microcytosis. The blood loss is due to a severe thrombocytopenia (<12 x 10^9/l).

The dog also has a leucocytosis, with a neutrophilia and a left shift (no toxic change) and monocytosis. This leucogram is common in dogs with IMHA or ITP and is thought to be due to generalized bone marrow stimulation secondary to macrophage activation and/or hypoxia-induced inflammation or necrosis in organs, such as the liver.

Haemostatic screening assays are within normal limits. Fibrinogen is an acute phase protein and will increase in inflammatory states; in this dog, this may be secondary to hypoxic tissue damage. vWf:Ag is severely decreased; values this low can result in spontaneous haemorrhage.

What is your diagnosis?

Severe thrombocytopenia with secondary haemorrhagic and iron-deficiency anaemia, exacerbated by inherited vWD. The thrombocytopenia is likely to be immune-mediated, because underlying disorders were not found and the normal coagulation profile argues against DIC. The dog responded to immunosuppressive doses of corticosteroids. Note that the dog's previous bout of epistaxis could have been due to vWD or the thrombocytopenia (which was of sufficient duration to induce the severe anaemia).

Case 2

Signalment

1-year-old male, neutered Scottish Terrier.

History

Excessive haemorrhage and bruising after neutering, with repeated subcutaneous haematomas. Cautery was needed to stop haemorrhage after nail-clipping. Initial coagulation assays were performed at a local medical laboratory.

Clinical pathology data

Initial testing

Coagulation	Result	Reference interval
PT (s)	<9	11–14
aPTT (s)	22	20–31

Further evaluation

An oral mucosa swab was taken for vWD genetic testing. The dog was considered normal. A repeat coagulation panel was performed at a veterinary laboratory:

Coagulation	Result	Reference interval
Platelet count (x 10^9/l)	259	179–483
PT (s)	15	13–19
aPTT (s)	20	10–17
TCT (s)	8	5–9

The blood was referred to a specialized veterinary coagulation testing laboratory for more specific tests:

Case 2 continues ▶

Case 2 continued

Coagulation	Result	Reference interval
Factor VIII:C (%)	2	50–200
Factor IX:C (%)	81	50–150
vWf:Ag (%)	127	70–180

Based on presenting signs, is the disorder inherited or acquired and which pathway is involved?

Spontaneous and surgery-induced haemorrhage in a young dog suggests an inherited disorder. Although vWD should be suspected in a young Scottish Terrier (of either sex), the severity of the haemorrhage and occurrence of haematomas is more compatible with a disorder of secondary haemostasis. Since the dog is male, haemophilia A or B should be the primary differential diagnoses.

How would you interpret the results?

Medical laboratory

Decreased PT, normal aPTT. This argues against a coagulation cascade defect, therefore a vWD genetic test was done. This indicated that the dog did not have the vWD mutation.

Veterinary laboratory

Normal PT, normal fibrinogen (TCT) and prolonged aPTT, indicating a defect in the intrinsic pathway (FXII, FXI, FIX, FVIII) (see Figures 6.13 and 6.14).

Specific factor assays

Factor VIII:C is severely decreased, with normal FIX:C and vWf:Ag (the latter was done out of interest and was not required).

How would you explain the discrepancy in results from the medical and veterinary laboratories?

This case emphasizes that all laboratories are not equal for coagulation testing. Dogs have more rapid coagulation pathways than humans, therefore human-based reference intervals (including those provided from a medical laboratory) are longer than dog-based intervals. Therefore, the PT was shorter and the aPTT was within the provided reference intervals from the medical laboratory, which delayed the diagnosis and led to unnecessary and expensive testing (vWD genetic test).

What is your diagnosis?

The results are consistent with haemophilia A (FVIII deficiency).

Was the vWD genetic test required?

Testing for vWD was a logical step after receiving 'normal' coagulation results, but a vWf:Ag test would have been cheaper and just as diagnostic. All affected Scottish Terriers (homozygous for vWD) have undetectable vWf:Ag values (<1%).

Case 3

Signalment

8-year-old female, neutered Labrador Retriever.

History

Inguinal mass removed 7 days ago. Now, acute vomiting, infected and dehisced wound (bruising, bloody discharge), hindleg oedema. Severe dehydration, depression, fever, prolonged capillary refill times, cold extremities and oliguria.

Clinical pathology data

Haematology	Result	Reference interval
HCT (l/l)	0.45	0.39–0.57
WBC (x 10^9/l)	28.1	7.5–19.9
Neutrophils (segmented) (x 10^9/l)	19.1	3.9–14.7
Neutrophils (band) (x 10^9/l)	5.4	0–0.3
Lymphocytes (x 10^9/l)	0.8	1.5–5.2
Monocytes (x 10^9/l)	2.8	0.3–2.2
Eosinophils (x 10^9/l)	0.0	0.1–1.6
Platelets (x 10^9/l)	60	179–483

Smear comments

Red cells: moderate schistocytes, few acanthocytes
White cells: neutrophils show marked toxic change

Coagulation	Result	Reference interval
PT (s)	17	13–19
aPTT (s)	25	10–17
Fibrinogen (g/l)	0.9	1.1–2.6
Plasma FDP (µg/ml)	>20	<5
D-dimer (µg/ml)	2.0	<0.25

Urine analysis	Result (Dipstick)
Specific gravity	1.012
Protein	3+
Sediment findings	Moderate granular casts

Biochemistry	Result	Reference interval
Glucose (mmol/l)	2.4	3.3–6.7
Urea (mmol/l)	44	3–11
Creatinine (µmol/l)	370	44–124
Inorganic phosphate (mmol/l)	6.2	0.7–2.1
Bicarbonate (mmol/l)	5	16–26
Anion gap (mmol/l)	47	13–26
ALT (IU/l)	1037	13–79
AST (IU/l)	427	13–52

Cytology of wound discharge: Septic neutrophilic inflammation

How would you interpret the results?

Haemogram:

- The dog has a leucocytosis due to a neutrophilia with a left shift, with marked toxic change and monocytosis: this indicates an inflammatory leucogram
- There is a concurrent lymphopenia and eosinopenia: this can be attributed to inflammation or stress (endogenous corticosteroid release)
- There is a moderate thrombocytopenia with fragmentation injury of red blood cells (acanthocytes and schistocytes).

Case 3 continues ▶

Case 3 continued

Coagulation panel:

- Normal PT and prolonged aPTT: intrinsic pathway abnormality
- Hypofibrinogenaemia: indicates excessive consumption
- Increased FDPs and D-dimer: indicate excessive fibrinolysis.

Biochemistry:

- Severe azotaemia and hyperphosphataemia: decreased glomerular filtration rate from acute renal failure (oliguria, azotaemia with isosthenuria, granular casts, proteinuria)
- Moderate hypoglycaemia: sepsis
- Hepatocellular injury (increased ALT, AST)
- Severe high anion gap metabolic acidosis: titration acidosis (lactic acid from hypoxia and retained organic acids from renal failure)
- Isosthenuria with acute tubular injury (granular casts, proteinuria that is excessive for the USG).

What is your diagnosis?

The results indicate DIC secondary to septic shock from an infected surgical wound. There are abnormalities in all three haemostatic pathways, i.e. thrombocytopenia, prolonged aPTT, hypofibrinogenaemia, and increased FDPs/D-dimer, red cell fragmentation (from thrombosis), an initiating disease (sepsis) and evidence of haemorrhage (bruising, bloody discharge) and thrombosis (acute renal failure and liver injury, acidosis).

References and further reading

Day MJ, Littlewood J and Mackin A (2000) *BSAVA Manual of Canine and Feline Haematology and Transfusion Medicine.* BSAVA Publications, Gloucester

Bienzle D, Stanton JB, Embry JM, Bush SE and Mahaffey EA (2000) Evaluation of an in-house centrifugal hematology analyzer for use in veterinary practice. *Journal of the American Veterinary Medical Association* **217,** 1195–1200

Brooks M (2000) von Willebrand's disease. In: *Schalm's Veterinary Hematology, Vol. 4,* ed. BF Feldman *et al.*, pp. 509–515. Lippincott, Williams & Wilkins, Philadelphia

Brooks MB, Catalfamo JL, Brown HA, Ivanova P and Lovaglio J (2002) A hereditary bleeding disorder of dogs caused by a lack of platelet procoagulant activity. *Blood* **99,** 2434–2441

Gu W, Brooks M, Catalfamo J, Ray J and Ray K (1999) Two distinct mutations cause severe hemophilia B in two unrelated canine pedigrees. *Thrombosis and Haemostasis* **82,** 1270–1275

Heemskerk JW, Bevers EM and Lindhout T (2002) Platelet activation and blood coagulation. *Thrombosis and Haemostasis* **88,** 186–193

Hoffman M and Monroe DM (2001) A cell-based model of hemostasis. *Thrombosis and Haemostasis* **85,** 958–965

Hough C, Kamisue S, Cameron C, Notley C, Tinlin S, Giles A and Lillicrap D (2002) Aberrant splicing and premature termination of transcription of the FVIII gene as a cause of severe canine hemophilia A: similarities with the intron 22 inversion mutation in human hemophilia. *Thrombosis and Haemostasis* **87,** 659–665

Lewis DC, Meyers KM, Callan MB, Bucheler J and Giger U (1995) Detection of platelet-bound and serum platelet-bindable antibodies for diagnosis of idiopathic thrombocytopenic purpura in dogs. *Journal of the American Veterinary Medical Association* **206,** 47–52

Lozier JN, Dutra A, Pak E, Zhou N, Zheng Z, Nichols TC, Bellinger DA, Read M and Morgan RA (2002) The Chapel Hill hemophilia A dog colony exhibits a factor VIII gene inversion. *Proceedings of the National Academy of Sciences of the United States of America* **99,** 12991–12996

Mauser AE, Whitlark J, Whitney KM and Lothrop CD (1996) A deletion mutation causes hemophilia B in Lhasa Apso dogs. *Blood* **88,** 3451–3455

Morrissey JH (2001) Tissue factor: an enzyme cofactor and a true receptor. *Thrombosis and Haemostasis* **86,** 66–74

Pedersen HD, Haggstrom J, Olsen LH, Christensen K, Selin A, Burmeister ML and Larsen H (2002) Idiopathic asymptomatic thrombocytopenia in Cavalier King Charles Spaniels is an autosomal recessive trait. *Journal of Veterinary Internal Medicine* **16,** 169–173

Ramsey IK, Littlewood JD, Dunn JK and Herrtage ME (1996) Role of chronic disseminated intravascular coagulation in a case of canine angiostrongylosis. *Veterinary Record* **138,** 360–363

Schelling CG, Greene CE, Prestwood AK and Tsang VC (1986) Coagulation abnormalities associated with acute *Angiostrongylus vasorum* infection in dogs. *American Journal of Veterinary Research* **47,** 2669–2673

Scott MA, Kaiser L, Davis JM and Schwartz KA (2002) Development of a sensitive immunoradiometric assay for detection of platelet surface-associated immunoglobulins in thrombocytopenic dogs. *American Journal of Veterinary Research* **63,** 124–136

Stokol T (2003) Plasma D-dimer for the diagnosis of thromboembolic disorders in dogs. *Veterinary Clinics of North America: Small Animal Practice* **33**, 1419-1435.

Sullivan PS, Evans HL and McDonald TP (1994) Platelet concentration and hemoglobin function in greyhounds. *Journal of the American Veterinary Medical Association* **205,** 838–841

Editors' addendum: Methodology for whole blood clotting time

- Clean venipuncture – preferably from a large peripheral vein. (If venipuncture is clean, the first millilitre of blood does not need to be discarded).
- Place approximately 1 ml of blood in two or three plain **glass** tubes, and incubate at 37°C in either a water bath or a dry block if available: a makeshift water bath in a plastic container can be kept close to 37°C for the period of time required.
- Check one tube every 30 seconds, and replace in water bath after examining.
- WBCT can also be determined by drawing blood into (non-heparinized) capillary tubes and then breaking these at 30 s intervals: a suitable dryblock should be used if available, or alternatively the tubes can be warmed in an armpit. The capillary method is more hazardous to personnel.
- Reported reference intervals are 3–13 minutes for dogs and 8 minutes for cats.

7

Disorders of plasma proteins

Yvonne McGrotty and Kathleen Tennant

Introduction

Plasma protein abnormalities are associated with a wide variety of disease processes and are a significant biochemical finding in both dogs and cats. The *plasma* proteins are comprised of albumin, globulin and fibrinogen fractions. Measurement of *serum* proteins excludes fibrinogen, which is involved in blood clotting, so serum values are approximately 5% lower than plasma protein levels. Adult reference intervals are shown in Figure 7.1, although results should always be interpreted using a laboratory's own reference intervals. Reference intervals for juvenile animals are lower than those of adults.

Protein	Reference interval in dogs (g/l)	Reference interval in cats (g/l)
Total protein	50–78	60–85
Albumin	29–36	26–36
Globulin	28–42	27–45
Fibrinogen	2–4	2–4

7.1 Adult reference ranges from Glasgow University Diagnostic Services.

Albumin

Albumin is a large osmotically active protein with an average molecular weight of 69,000 daltons and a half-life of between 17 and 19 days. Albumin is synthesized in the liver. Almost 75% of colloid oncotic pressure is attributed to albumin. Any decrease in albumin concentration can result in a significant decrease in oncotic pressure with a resultant fluid shift from the intravascular space into the interstitium. This causes hypotension, oedema (subcutaneous, pulmonary) and body cavity effusions (pleural effusion, ascites). Increases in albumin concentration are usually a result of dehydration and haemoconcentration.

Globulin

Globulins have molecular weights ranging from 90,000 Daltons (β_1-globulin) to 156,000 daltons (γ-globulin). The α-globulins and most of the β-globulins are synthesized in the liver, while the immunoglobulins are produced following antigenic stimulation of plasma cells and B lymphocytes in lymphoid tissue. The immunoglobulins (IgG, IgM, IgA and IgE) are the main components of the globulin fraction, but globulins also provide oncotic support and are involved in drug transport. The globulin fractions can be separated by serum protein electrophoresis.

Fibrinogen

Fibrinogen is converted to insoluble fibrin during the coagulation cascade leading to the formation of a stable blood clot. Fibrinogen is synthesized in the liver. Increased levels of fibrinogen signify non-specific inflammatory disease, while reduced levels can result from severe hepatic insufficiency, disseminated intravascular coagulation or, rarely, a congenital deficiency (Factor I deficiency). The presence of a clot within the sample or the use of lithium heparin as an anticoagulant will lead to falsely reduced fibrinogen levels.

Methods of measuring protein

Total protein is measured by spectrophotometry or the Biuret method. The Biuret method uses a reagent composed of copper ions at an alkaline pH. A violet-coloured complex is formed when serum or plasma are mixed with the reagent. The intensity of the violet colour is proportional to the number of peptide bonds present and so is also proportional to the amount of total protein present. The amount of protein is then quantified using spectrophotometric methods. An estimate of protein concentration can also be obtained using a refractometer, which measures total solids (Figure 7.2). Several factors (Figure 7.3) falsely increase refractometer measurements of total solids:

- Haemolysis
- Lipaemia
- Synthetic colloids (including haemoglobin based oxygen carrying solutions)
- Severe hyperglycaemia
- Azotaemia
- Hypernatraemia
- Hyperchloraemia
- Hyperbilirubinaemia.

Thus the refractometer method can only be used for clear, non-lipaemic serum.

1. The refractometer should be calibrated to 1.000 using distilled water prior to use
2. EDTA blood or heparinized blood is centrifuged and the plasma aspirated into a syringe
3. The plasma is placed on the refractometer and the total solids value is read from the appropriate scale

Units are in g/dl (to convert to g/l, multiply by 10)

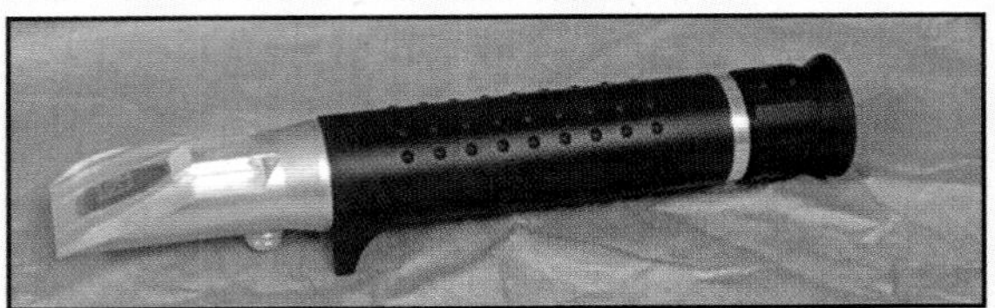

7.2 Refractometer measurement of total solids.

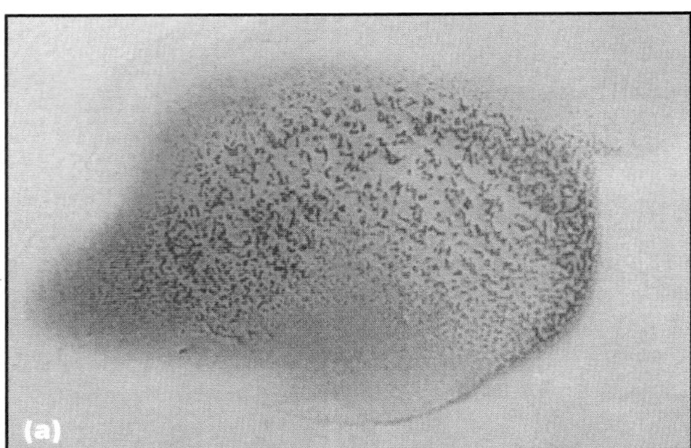

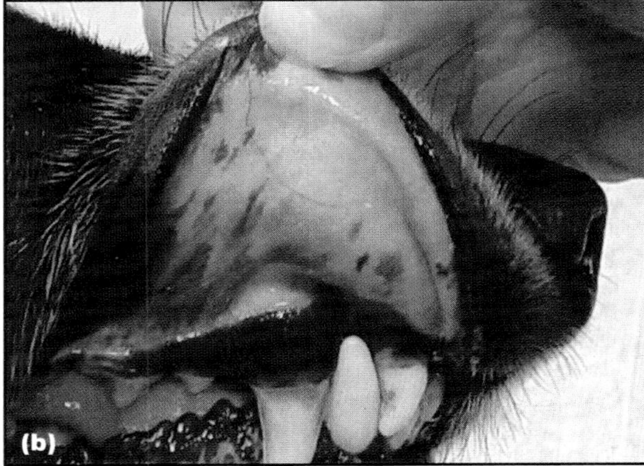

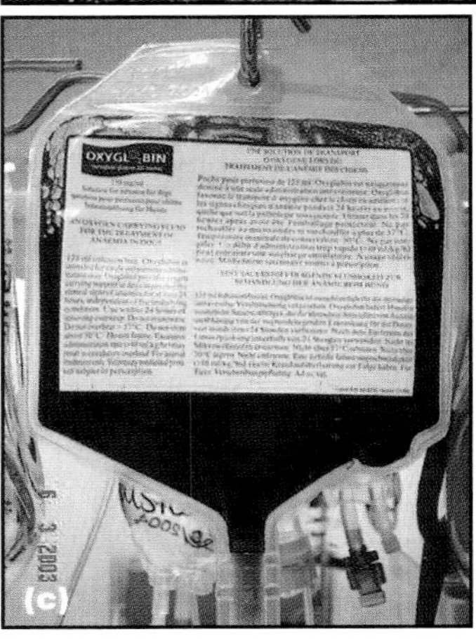

7.3 Factors that interfere with refractometer methods of measuring total solids. (a) Haemolysis. In this case, immune-mediated haemolytic anaemia has led to autoagglutination. (b) Hyperbilirubinaemia. (c) Synthetic colloids.

Spectrophotometric methods of total protein measurement will be falsely increased by hyperbilirubinaemia.

Albumin concentration can be determined by binding to bromocresol green (BCG) dye. The resulting coloured solution is then measured spectrophotometrically. Globulin concentration is then determined by subtracting the albumin concentration from the total protein measurement. A more accurate determination of the globulin fraction is obtained by electrophoresis. Fibrinogen can be measured by either heat precipitation (Figure 7.4) or the Von Clauss method, which evaluates functional fibrinogen. The Von Clauss method is not widely available. The heat precipitation method is not sufficiently accurate to detect decreased fibrinogen and so cannot be used in assessment of disseminated intravascular coagulation or fibrinogen deficiency.

1. Fill two haematocrit tubes with heparinized blood (tubes A and B)
2. Heat one tube to 56–58°C for 3 minutes (B)
3. Centrifuge tubes A and B in a microhaematocrit centrifuge
4. Measure total solids in each of the tubes using a refractometer (see Figure 7.2)
5. Calculate the amount of fibrinogen according to the following formula:

Fibrinogen measurement = Total solids of tube A (g/l) – Total solids of tube B (g/l)

7.4 Measurement of fibrinogen by heat precipitation.

Serum protein electrophoresis

Electrophoresis can be used to separate the different protein fractions. Serum or plasma, in an alkaline environment, is placed on a cellulose acetate gel in an electrical field. The individual protein fractions migrate towards the anode at different speeds depending on their size and charge and are then stained and scanned by a densitometer. The intensity of the staining is illustrated as an electrophoretic trace. Electrophoretic traces from normal animals produce a tall narrow albumin spike at one end and three globulin fractions: α-globulins, β-globulins and γ-globulins (immunoglobulins) (Figure 7.5). Canine and feline α-globulins

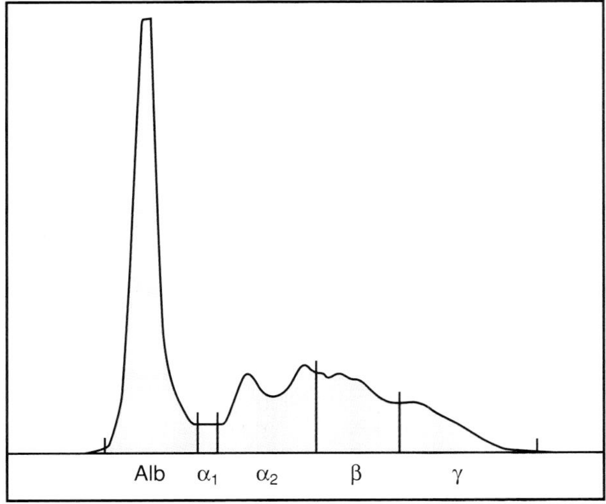

7.5 Serum protein electrophoresis from a normal dog.

and β-globulins are further subdivided into α_1, α_2, β_1 and β_2 sub-fractions. If plasma is used instead of serum, a large fibrinogen peak will be present between the β and the γ fractions, which can obscure the immunoglobulin fraction and make interpretation difficult. Figure 7.6 lists the proteins present in the three globulin fractions.

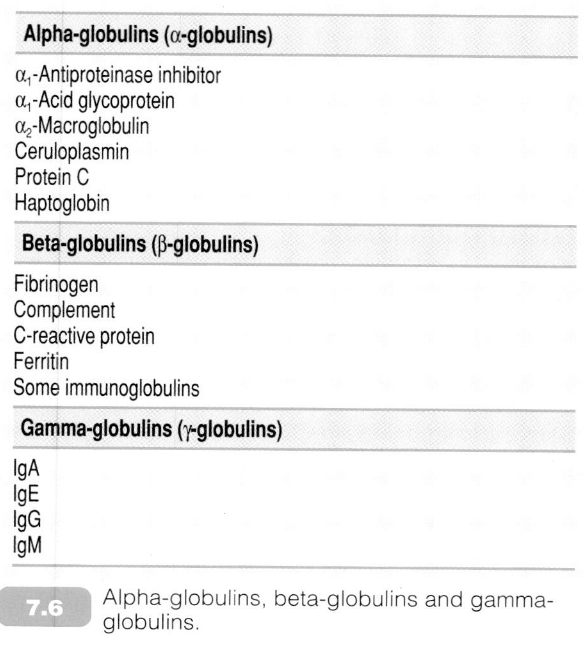

Alpha-globulins (α-globulins)
α_1-Antiproteinase inhibitor
α_1-Acid glycoprotein
α_2-Macroglobulin
Ceruloplasmin
Protein C
Haptoglobin
Beta-globulins (β-globulins)
Fibrinogen
Complement
C-reactive protein
Ferritin
Some immunoglobulins
Gamma-globulins (γ-globulins)
IgA
IgE
IgG
IgM

7.6 Alpha-globulins, beta-globulins and gamma-globulins.

Functions of plasma proteins

The plasma proteins have a wide variety of functions, including maintaining oncotic pressure, blood buffering, coagulation and transport of hormones and drugs.

- Oncotic pressure: capillary walls are relatively impermeable to the large osmotically active plasma proteins. The osmotic pressure generated by these large protein molecules encourages movement of fluid into the intravascular space. Approximately 75% of colloid oncotic pressure is attributed to albumin.
- Blood buffering: buffers donate or accept hydrogen ions in order to minimize a change in the blood pH. Bicarbonate is the most important blood buffer, but the plasma proteins provide approximately 20% of the buffering capacity (see Chapter 9). Albumin has a greater role than globulin in blood buffering.
- Hormone transport: thyroxine, reproductive hormones and a wide variety of other hormones are bound to the plasma proteins in the circulation.
- Drug transport: numerous drugs, including non-steroidal anti-inflammatory drugs, thiopentone and furosemide are highly protein-bound.
- Coagulation: secondary haemostasis involves the conversion of soluble fibrinogen to insoluble fibrin by the action of thrombin.
- Acute phase response: acute phase proteins produced by the liver in response to inflammation assist healing and limit tissue damage.

The acute phase proteins

The acute phase response is an innate defence mechanism that is designed to limit tissue damage and promote healing following trauma, infection or inflammation. Activation of granulocytes and mononuclear cells at the site of inflammation leads to release of pro-inflammatory cytokines, such as interleukin-6 (IL-6), which in turn stimulates the hepatic production of the acute phase proteins (Figure 7.7). Clinically, the acute phase response results in pyrexia and anorexia. Canine haematological changes include leucocytosis and increased erythrocyte sedimentation rate.

The acute phase proteins (APPs) produced by the liver are glycoproteins: they include haptoglobin (Hp); C-reactive protein (CRP); serum amyloid A (SAA); and α_1-acid glycoprotein (AGP). The concentration of these proteins in the bloodstream is related to the severity of the initiating disease process.

Haptoglobin, CRP, SAA, AGP, ceruloplasmin and fibrinogen increase in response to inflammation in the dog and are therefore called positive APPs. CRP is the most sensitive APP in dogs and serum concentrations increase over 100 times within 24–48 hours of stimulation. Production of albumin decreases during inflammation as the liver switches to production of those proteins described above, so albumin is a negative

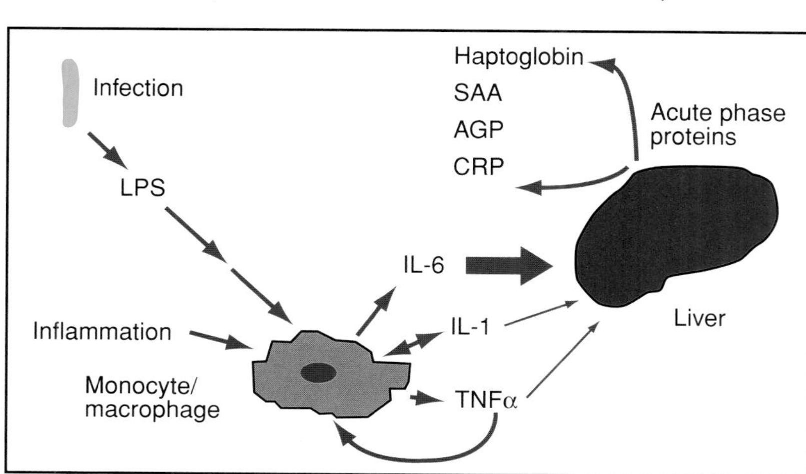

7.7 Stimulation of the acute phase response. AGP: α_1-acid glycoprotein; CRP: C-reactive protein; IL: interleukin; LPS: lipopolysaccharide; SAA: serum amyloid A; TNFα: tumour necrosis factor alpha. (Courtesy of Dr PD Eckersall.)

APP. Studies relating to the acute phase response in the dog have focused mainly on haptoglobin and CRP concentrations. Haptoglobin is measured in an automated assay based on haptoglobin–haemoglobin binding. In healthy dogs, haptoglobin is present in low concentrations, but increases following surgery, trauma or prednisolone administration. This response of haptoglobin to glucocorticoids is not documented in other species. It may be related to the canine species-specific hepatocyte induction of steroid-induced alkaline phosphatase, in response to raised glucocorticoid concentrations. A reference range for canine haptoglobin has been reported as 0–3 g/l and concentrations above 10 g/l are considered consistent with a major inflammatory response.

CRP is analysed using an enzyme-linked immunosorbent assay (ELISA) or immunoturbidimetric assay. Immunoturbidimetric assays for canine CRP measure light absorbed by the formation of an antigen–antibody complex following addition of antiserum. In humans, increased CRP concentration has been shown to predict an increased risk of myocardial infarction, and increased mortality in patients following myocardial infarction or stroke. In dogs, CRP has been shown to increase rapidly following surgery and to decrease as inflammation resolves. CRP may prove to be a useful marker of disease and response to therapy in dogs, but further research is required. In human medicine, CRP assays are used as an aid to diagnosis, prognosis and response to treatment. Studies using an ELISA assay validated for canine CRP determined that healthy animals have a CRP of <10 mg/l whilst those with an acute phase response have a CRP of >10 mg/l (Eckersall *et al.*, 1989). Although a test for CRP should provide a valuable addition to diagnostic investigations in canine medicine, it has had limited application due to current lack of availability.

In cats, AGP is the acute phase protein which has received most attention in veterinary medicine. AGP is a non-specific marker of inflammation and increases following viral, bacterial or fungal infection, as well as trauma. Serum AGP concentrations have also been documented to increase in cats with various neoplasms, including lymphosarcoma. In cases of suspected feline infectious peritonitis (FIP), raised AGP concentrations (>1500 mg/ml), in conjunction with fluid cytology or appropriate clinical signs, can help distinguish cats with FIP from cats with similar clinical signs.

Transferrin and ferritin are β-globulins involved in the transport of iron and are also APPs. Iron transported in the blood is bound to transferrin and this is measured as serum iron. Total iron binding capacity (TIBC) is an indirect measurement of the amount of iron that transferrin will bind. Decreased transferrin concentrations are associated with liver disease, while normal or increased concentrations are seen with iron deficiency. Transferrin is a negative APP and concentrations decrease during the acute phase response. Serum ferritin assays are species-specific, but provide a more accurate indication of total body iron status. Ferritin concentrations increase during the acute phase response following stimulation by interleukin-1 (IL-1). Liver disease, haemolytic disease and some neoplastic disorders also result in increased ferritin concentrations.

Hyperproteinaemia

Hyperproteinaemia is a relative or absolute increase in protein concentration and results from hyperalbuminaemia or hyperglobulinaemia, or both. Albumin and globulin concentrations should be assessed concurrently. Hyperalbuminaemia is usually relative, due to haemoconcentration, and is accompanied by other haematological and clinical indicators of hypovolaemia (e.g. increased packed cell volume, tachycardia). Hyperalbuminaemia is sometimes found in dogs with hyperadrenocorticism, although the reason for this is unclear. Artefactual hyperalbuminaemia occurs in the presence of lipaemia when spectrophotometric methods are used.

Hyperglobulinaemia

Increases in globulin concentration may occur with infectious and inflammatory diseases (e.g. canine pyoderma, feline gingivitis/stomatitis) in which a wide variety of antigens are presented to B lymphocytes. This subsequently results in numerous different clones of plasma cells, each of which produces a single antigen-specific immunoglobulin. This results in a polyclonal gammopathy characterized by broad-based peaks migrating mostly across the β and γ regions of the electrophoretic trace (Figure 7.8). IgM production dominates in the early response. Previously encountered antigens stimulate a more rapid response from memory B cells, resulting in more IgG production than the initial response. Occasionally a range of different immunoglobulin types migrate to a restricted/narrow band on the electrophoretic trace resulting in a narrow-based spike. This is known as a restricted polyclonal gammopathy or oligoclonal gammopathy, and may be seen in association with ehrlichiosis, leishmaniasis and FIP.

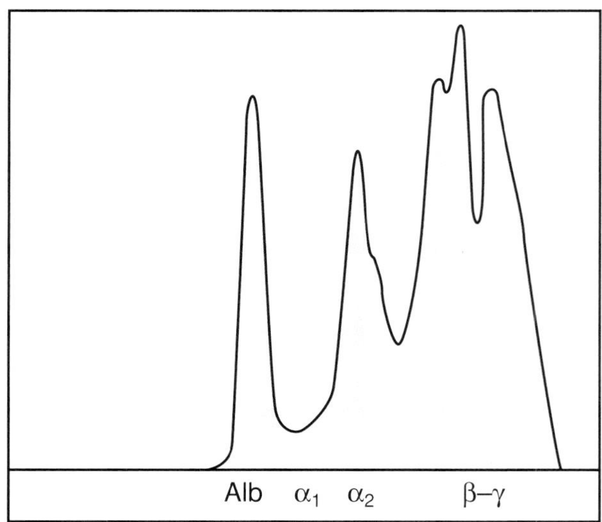

7.8 A polyclonal gammopathy with β–γ bridging in a German Shepherd Dog with chronic hepatitis.

In contrast, a monoclonal gammopathy results from production of a single type of immunoglobulin by a neoplastic proliferation of a single clone of plasma cells or B lymphocytes. It is characterized by a steeply sided, narrow-based monoclonal spike on the electrophoretogram, usually in the β or γ regions (Figure 7.9). A true monoclonal elevation is composed of a single immunoglobulin with a single heavy chain class and light chain type (Figure 7.10). Monoclonal gammopathies can be difficult to differentiate from oligoclonal gammopathies using the electrophoretic trace alone, as both may give a narrow spike. Immunoelectrophoresis can be used to identify the type of antibody present (e.g. IgG, IgM, IgA) and to distinguish monoclonal from oligoclonal gammopathy. Monoclonal gammopathy has a single light chain (either kappa or lambda), whereas oligoclonal gammopathy has both types of light chain present.

In standard immunoelectrophoresis, once electrophoresis has separated the proteins, antibody is placed in a trough alongside the zone of electrophoresis and allowed to diffuse passively through the gel. Precipitation occurs if the antibody (e.g. anti-IgM) interacts with the relevant antigen (e.g. IgM), and a precipitation arc is formed. Most commonly, antibodies against particular immunonoglobulin isotypes are are used to identify the type of antibody present.

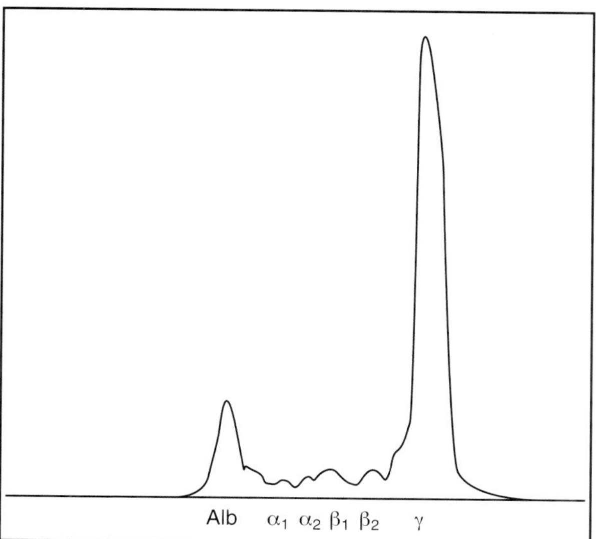

7.9 A monoclonal gammopathy in a Kerry Blue Terrier with chronic lymphocytic leukaemia.

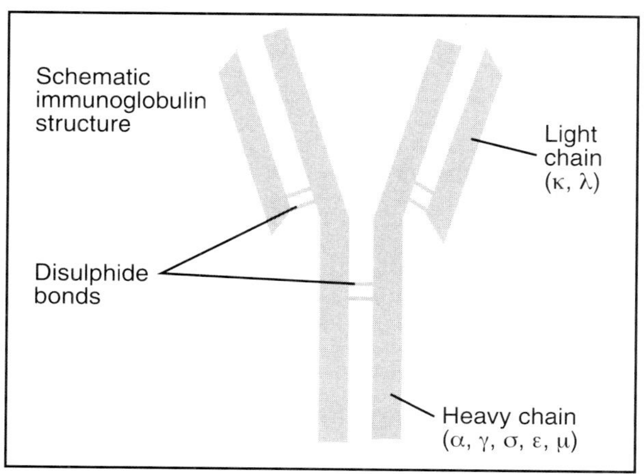

7.10 A simplified diagram showing immunoglobulin structure.

In order to determine whether there is a monoclonal or a polyclonal gammopathy, antibodies against different light chains are used. With an anti-kappa and an anti-lambda antibody, only one will form a precipitation arc if there is a monoclonal gammopathy; in an oligoclonal gammopathy both antibodies will form arcs. It is useful to run a control serum on the opposite side of the trough. Immunoelectrophoresis is illustrated in Figure 7.11.

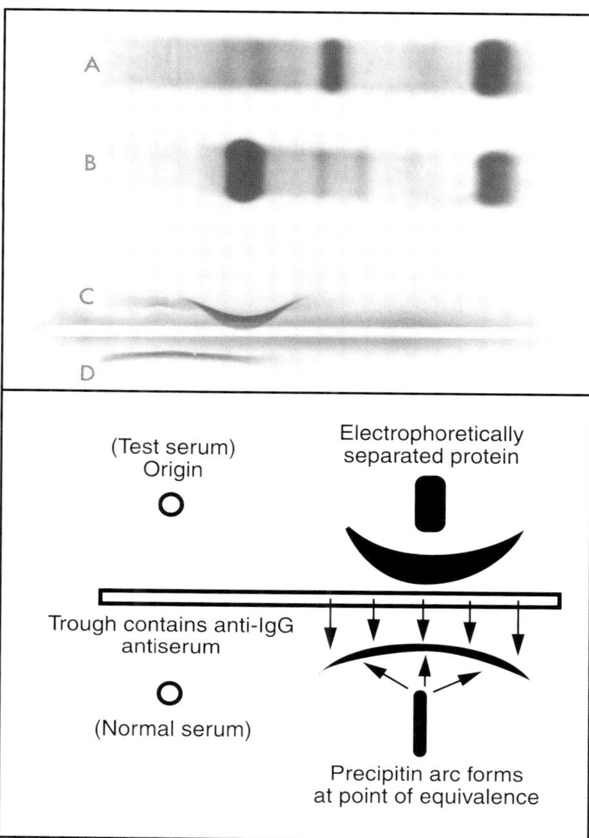

7.11 Characterization of serum paraprotein in multiple myeloma by immunoelectrophoresis (IEP). Electrophoretically separated serum from a normal dog (Lane A) and a dog with paraproteinaemia (Lane B) demonstrating a monoclonal gammopathy. Serum from this dog (Lane C) and the normal dog (Lane D) are separated, and antiserum to dog IgG loaded into a trough cut between the electrophoresed proteins. During overnight incubation, the antiserum diffuses from the trough and interacts with serum protein, forming an arc of precipitation. The nature of the precipitin arc in Lane C confirms that this is an IgG myeloma. (Courtesy of MJ Day)

Polyclonal gammopathies

Polyclonal gammopathies may occur in response to suppurative and inflammatory conditions, including pyometra, skin disease (particularly parasitism or chronic pyoderma) and viral, fungal and protozoal infections.

Immune-mediated disease, such as systemic lupus erythematosus or immune-mediated polyarthritis, may cause polyclonal gammopathies, but the increases in globulin concentrations are generally less marked than those seen in infectious disease.

Animals with *Ehrlichia* (Hoskins *et al.*,1983) or *Leishmania* infections (Font et al., 1994) (see Chapter

27) may have either a typical polyclonal gammopathy, or a monoclonal gammopathy. In some cases, notably with *Ehrlichia*, an apparently monoclonal spike is produced which, on immunoelectrophoresis, is found to be oligoclonal, with more than one subclass of heavy chain protein present in serum and both κ and λ light chains present in urine.

Chronic pyoderma (Burkhard *et al.*, 1995) and plasmacytic gastroenterocolitis (Diehl *et al.*, 1992) may also produce either polyclonal or apparent monoclonal gammopathies, although polyclonal elevations are much more frequent. Cats with FIP most often have large polyclonal gammopathies, with most of the elevation in the γ region. Chronic hepatitis in dogs may also produce polyclonal gammopathies, in some cases producing a bridge between the β and γ regions as shown in Figure 7.8. Causes of polyclonal gammopathy are shown in Figure 7.12.

Chronic infection (bacterial, viral, fungal, protozoal)
Inflammation (acute and chronic)
Immune-mediated disease (e.g. immune-mediated polyarthritis, systemic lupus erythematosus)
Neoplasia
Chronic hepatopathies
Feline infectious peritonitis
Parasites (e.g. *Sarcoptes scabiei*, *Leishmania* , *Dirofilaria*)
Ehrlichia (can be monoclonal)

7.12 Conditions associated with polyclonal gammopathies.

Monoclonal gammopathies

Monoclonal gammopathies result from the excessive synthesis of a single immunoglobulin, heavy chain or light chain (Bence–Jones protein) subunit by a single clone of B cells. The protein products of the clone may also be referred to as paraproteins or 'M-proteins'. Clinical signs associated with monoclonal gammopathies vary according to the underlying aetiology, the magnitude of the gammopathy and the class of immunoglobulin or subunit involved.

Lymphoid or plasma cell neoplasms are the most common causes (Figure 7.13) although idiopathic cases are reported (Dewhirst *et al.*, 1977). As discussed above, certain inflammatory conditions including *Ehrlichia* and *Leishmania* infections, chronic pyoderma and plasmacytic gastroenterocolitis have been reported to produce monoclonal gammopathies, although these may, in fact, have been oligoclonal gammopathies.

Multiple myeloma
Waldenström's macroglobulinaemia
Lymphoma
Extramedullary plasmacytoma
Chronic lymphocytic leukaemia
Monoclonal gammopathy of undetermined significance
Ehrlichia infection [a]
Leishmania infection [a]
Plasmacytic gastroenterocolitis [a]

7.13 Conditions associated with monoclonal gammopathies. [a] May be oligoclonal gammopathy rather than true monoclonal gammopathy.

Monoclonal gammopathies appear on the electrophoretogram as narrow steep-sided peaks, smaller in width at the base of the peak than the albumin band (see Figure 7.9). They are infrequently found in the α_2 region, the majority occurring in β or γ regions. Often there is a depression in the production of other globulins, giving a relatively flattened baseline from which the spike arises. Rarely biclonal gammopathies result in two discrete narrow spikes, in circumstances similar to those which give rise to monoclonal spikes (Jacobs *et al.*,1986). This appearance may be due to variation in the configuration of the same immunoglobulin causing differential migration, or due to a true biclonal gammopathy (Figure 7.14). As discussed above, differentiation of mono- or biclonal gammopathies from oligogammopathies can be undertaken with immunoelectrophoresis.

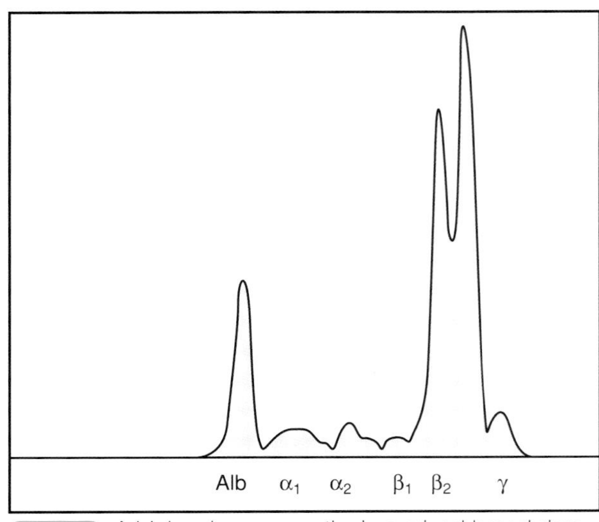

7.14 A biclonal gammopathy in a mixed breed dog with multiple myeloma.

Waldenström's macroglobulinaemia: This is a primary neoplasm of lymphocytoid plasma cells, the intermediate stage of differentiation between B lymphocytes and functional plasma cells in which the paraprotein secreted is IgM (Dimopoulous and Alexanian, 1994). Neoplastic cells are present in the bone marrow and sometimes in other tissues, but not in the peripheral blood. Bony lesions do not occur and Bence–Jones proteinuria is uncommon.

Solitary plasma cell tumours: Cutaneous, gastrointestinal and solitary osseous plasma cell tumours, along with plasma cell tumours at other extramedullary sites, may all uncommonly be associated with hyperglobulinaemia (Mandel and Esplin, 1994). Solitary osseous plasmacytoma may progress to multiple myeloma.

Monoclonal gammopathy of unknown significance (MGUS): Rarely, a monoclonal gammopathy without a detectable underlying cause occurs in dogs. (Dewhirst *et al.*, 1977). In human patients, approximately 16% of MGUS cases go on to develop multiple myeloma.

Multiple myeloma: Multiple myeloma is a common cause of monoclonal gammopathy. This plasma cell neoplasm is associated with:

- Neoplastic plasma cell infiltration of the bone marrow, usually with >30% plasma cells. Frequently the cells are atypical and are in clusters (Figure 7.15). Due to the often patchy nature of the infiltrate, single bone marrow aspirates or biopsies can miss the neoplastic cells: multiple samples may be required. Other causes for plasma cell proliferation in the bone marrow, such as *Ehrlichia* or *Leishmania* infections, should be excluded, as these may cause plasma cell counts approaching the numbers seen in multiple myeloma. In these instances, atypia of the plasma cells, the presence of a true monoclonal gammopathy and hypercalcaemia are more supportive of multiple myeloma. Neoplastic plasma cells may also be aspirated from other affected tissues, including lytic bone lesions
- Monoclonal gammopathies (commonly IgG/IgA)
- Osteolytic skeletal lesions (punched out or mottled ill defined lucencies radiographically)
- Bence–Jones proteinuria (seen in 30–40% of cases of myeloma)
- Hypercalcaemia. Although parathyroid hormone-related protein (PTHrP) production has been rarely reported in association with multiple myeloma, hypercalcaemia is present in up to 20% of dogs with the disease, partly due to increased protein-bound calcium (some calcium binds to globulins, although four times as much binds to albumin) and also due to osteolysis and release of skeletal calcium. If renal function is decreased, this may compound hypercalcaemia.

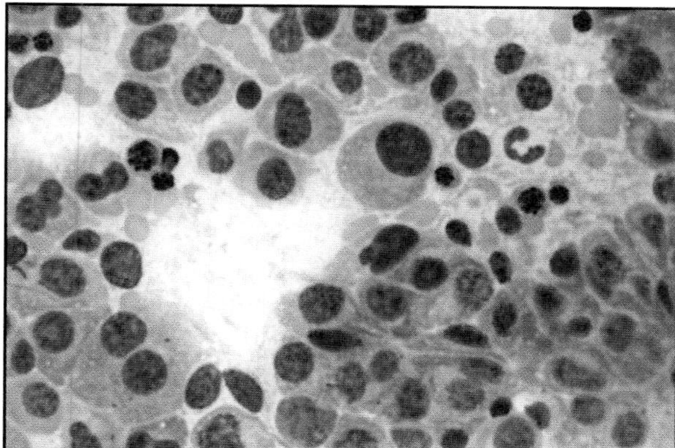

7.15 Bone marrow aspirate cytology showing plasma cell infiltration in a case of canine multiple myeloma. (Wright's stain; original magnification X1000.)

In dogs, multiple myeloma is not uncommon, comprising approximately 8% of haemopoietic tumours, with IgA and IgG gammopathies equally common (up to 40% of all cases). IgM gammopathies are less common, and skeletal lesions are found less frequently in association with IgM than IgA or IgG. Multiple myeloma occurs rarely in cats, where it is associated with a greater proportion of IgG gammopathies and rarely results in skeletal lesions (Drazner, 1982).

Multiple myeloma is associated with increased susceptibility to infection: this may be due to leucopenia occurring if the bone marrow is effaced. Thrombocytopenia and anaemia may also occur as a result of myelophthisis. In addition, the presence of a monoclonal gammopathy suppresses immunoglobulin production by normal plasma cells, so decreases the ability to mount a normal humoral response to infection.

Renal dysfunction is a common feature of multiple myeloma, due to tissue hypoxia where hyperviscosity exists, precipitation of light chains in glomeruli and tubules and the secondary effects of hypercalcaemia and dehydration.

Hyperviscosity syndrome

Hyperviscosity of the blood is seen in approximately 20% of dogs with multiple myeloma (Forrester and Relford, 1992). High levels of IgA or IgG are usually required to create this effect (total protein measurements are often >100 g/l) but where larger, high molecular weight IgM is the paraprotein (such as in Waldenström's macroglobulinaemia), hyperviscosity is common. Hyperviscosity can also be caused by marked erythrocytosis or marked leucocytosis, for example in leukaemia. These causes can be detected on routine haematology.

Clinical signs of hyperviscosity are associated with sludging of blood and consequent tissue hypoxia. The CNS and kidneys are the most susceptible organs and clinical signs include lethargy, stupor, coma or seizures as well as polydipsia/polyuria associated with renal dysfunction. Bleeding diathesis may result from coating of platelets with paraproteins and consequent platelet dysfunction or by paraproteins inhibiting or binding clotting factors, resulting in prolongations in prothrombin time (PT) and activated partial thromboplastin time (aPTT) in the presence of normal factor plasma concentrations. Gingival bleeding or epistaxis are common manifestations. Retinal haemorrhages may be present in addition to tortuous retinal vessels. Cardiovascular effects are related to increased workload; tachycardia, murmurs and refractory heart failure are reported (McBride *et al.*, 1988).

An Ostwald's viscometer can be used to measure serum viscosity, or a simplified method can be used in the practice laboratory (Forrester and Relford, 1992). The principle of the test is to compare the time taken for a given volume of serum to empty from a narrow gauge pipette or capillary tube compared to an equal volume of distilled water. The pipette or tube is filled with a standard volume of water or test serum and suspended vertically. A clamp can be used to hold the pipette or tube in the upright position to ensure there is no variation in angle between samples. The time for the standard volume of water and then test serum to drain completely from the tube is recorded. A normal serum can be timed in addition as a control.

Flow of serum (seconds)/ Flow of water (seconds) = Relative viscosity

There are many reported reference ranges for relative viscosity in the dog, but values >2 are suspicious and many animals with hyperviscosity have values >5.

Bence–Jones proteins

A monomorphic population of immunoglobulin light chains, Bence–Jones proteins, have been reported in almost all conditions which induce monoclonal gammopathies. In myeloma they are present in 40% of dogs and 17% of cats. They are filtered at the glomerulus, and when they exceed the tubular resorptive capacity, appear in urine. Standard urine analysis dipsticks are not sensitive to Bence–Jones proteins so other methods are employed for detection. The heat precipitation method relies on the Bence–Jones proteins precipitating when heated to between 40°C and 60°C, redissolving at 100°C then precipitating as cooled. Samples with low concentrations of Bence–Jones proteins may give a false negative. While rarely performed in veterinary laboratories, concentration of the urine by ultrafiltration or polyethylene glycol dialysis may yield positive precipitation results in some of these cases. This has largely been superseded by urine electrophoresis, which is more reliable (Figure 7.16). The resulting narrow-based spike on the urine electrophoretogram may be confirmed as Bence–Jones proteins by immunoelectrophoresis with antibodies directed at light chain subtypes.

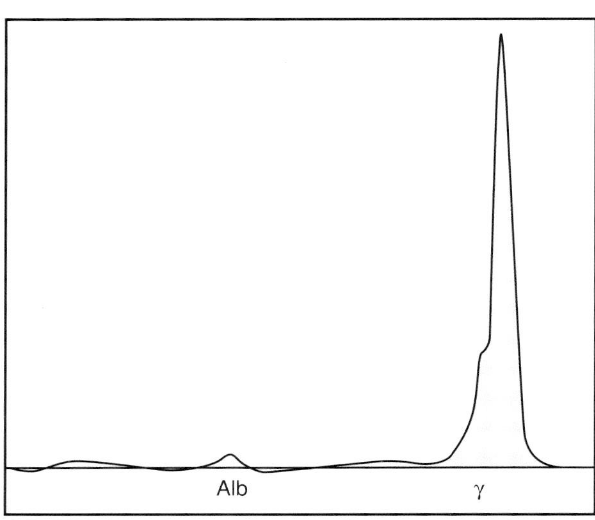

7.16 Urine electrophoresis of a concentrated urine sample, showing Bence–Jones proteinuria.

Cryoglobulins

Cryoglobulins, which precipitate out in low temperatures to resolubilize on warming, may be formed from monoclonal IgG, IgM and occasionally IgA, as well as monoclonal or polyclonal mixtures of these immunoglobulins. They may arise in lymphoproliferative disease or be associated with inflammatory disorders. On occasion there is no apparent underlying cause (Nagata *et al.*, 1998). Clinically, skin lesions or necrosis may occur, particularly at the extremities. Arthritis, glomerulonephritis and neurological signs may also be noted.

Cryoglobulins are easily overlooked, as they may precipitate out and then fall into the cell pellet during centrifugation, especially if this is carried out at low temperatures. Centrifugation should be performed at 37°C; heated centrifuges are not widely available, however, and the technique is largely confined to human hospitals. As the sample cannot be allowed to cool between sampling and processing, the patient must be taken to the laboratory and phlebotomized on site. Electrophoresis or quantification is performed on one sample maintained at 37°C and on another after precipitation of the cryoglobulins by refrigeration at 4°C. This difficult technique is rarely employed in veterinary patients.

Hypoproteinaemia

Simultaneous decreases in both albumin and globulin may be due to equal dilution of the plasma, non-selective/discriminatory external losses, or failure of protein absorption, assimilation or production. Selective decreases of albumin or globulin may occur due to failure of production in their different tissues of origin, or due to selective losses that are determined by their different physical qualities.

Dilutional hypoproteinaemia

Dilutional hypoproteinaemia occurs when the total amount of protein in the plasma is static but the plasma volume expands, giving an equal dilution of albumin and globulin. This may be seen as a sequel to vigorous fluid therapy, especially with concurrent renal disease, in congestive heart failure and liver disease, or in water retention due to excessive antidiuretic hormone secretion. Certain erythrocyte parameters (packed cell volume (PCV), red blood cell count (RBC) and haemoglobin) and biochemical parameters, such as sodium, may also be relatively decreased.

Protein loss

Whole blood loss

In the peracute stage of blood loss the PCV and total protein will be unchanged, but as extravascular fluid moves intravascularly to compensate, a dilutional effect takes place. Albumin and globulins decrease in proportion along with PCV, RBC and haemoglobin. Recovery of protein levels following haemorrhage may occur more quickly in internal haemorrhage, with the reabsorption of plasma proteins and other blood constituents, compared with external haemorrhage where *de novo* synthesis is required to replace lost plasma proteins.

Protein-losing nephropathy

Glomerulonephritis or amyloidosis can lead to disruption of the selective permeability of the glomerular basement membrane, allowing normally retained proteins, including albumin and antithrombin III, to escape into the filtrate. The ability of the tubules to reabsorb these proteins is limited and losses into urine occur. The relatively large size of most globulins means that most are retained. Hypercholesterolaemia may develop in nephrotic syndrome, as hepatic production of very low density lipoproteins (VLDL) increases and defective lipolysis of lipoproteins in plasma occurs. It has been suggested that proteins needed for the activation of lipoprotein lipase or for low density lipoproteins (LDL) binding to endothelial cells are lost along with other small proteins, contributing to the development of hypercholesterolaemia through failure of lipolysis rather than upregulated synthesis (Orth and Ritz, 1998).

Quantification of renal protein loss may be achieved using the urine protein:creatinine ratio; this essentially corrects protein loss to allow for variation in concentration of the urine, by relating the protein loss to the creatinine loss, which should be constant (see Chapter 10). In addition to glomerular disease, the protein:creatinine ratio is also elevated where there is significant inflammation, for example due to urinary tract infection, so urine sediment examination should be performed first to rule this out. Time of day and feeding do not significantly alter results, but the test does rely on a constant rate of creatinine excretion and may not be suitable for animals in acute renal failure.

Urine protein electrophoresis may be employed to demonstrate that the protein lost is albumin.

Mild to moderate hypoproteinaemia may occur in Fanconi's syndrome, where a renal tubular defect results in the inability to reabsorb normally filtered amino acids and glucose (see Chapter 11).

Dermal protein loss

Widespread skin disease or damage with exudation, particularly burns, may result in non-specific hypoproteinaemia during the early stages. Inflammation may mask the losses as the disease progresses, with APPs and globulins rising. Widespread burns may induce a hypermetabolic state that worsens the negative protein balance.

Malabsorption, maldigestion and protein-losing enteropathies

Digestion and absorption are intimately related anatomically and physiologically, so disturbances in one often lead to abnormalities in the other, and hypoproteinaemias can result from failure in either mechanism in a variety of disease states. For example, exocrine pancreatic insufficiency (EPI) can cause enteropathy, and has both direct (failure to produce proteases) and indirect (maldigestion of carbohydrates and lipids, creating a negative energy balance) effects on albumin levels. There are marked decreases in pepsin, chymotrypsin, carboxypeptidases, elastase and collagenase activity, with much dietary protein lost in faeces. Serum trypsin-like immunoreactivity (TLI) levels are low (see Chapter 14). Undigested muscle fibres and lipid droplets may be demonstrated on faecal examination.

Despite the multiple derangements in protein digestion, some animals with EPI demonstrate normal protein levels while others develop hypoalbuminaemia. Where there is concurrent enteropathy, loss of both albumin and globulins is possible.

Protein-losing gastroenteropathies may result from a number of pathological processes, including ulceration, inflammation, lymphatic or vascular disorders, with many possible underlying aetiologies, such as neoplasia, idiopathic enteropathies, hypersensitivities, lymphangiectasia or infectious (viral, parasitic, fungal) enteropathies. Many processes may contribute to hypoproteinaemia in enteropathies, but the luminal loss of both globulins and albumin is most important. These proteins are derived from the mucosal vasculature and interstitial space. Breakdown of the mucosal barrier leads to indiscriminate protein loss into the lumen. In addition, lymphatic obstruction or dysfunction allows losses of protein-rich lymph into the gut via ruptured lymphatics, and, in most cases, panhypoproteinaemia results. Reduced peptidase and amino acid transport activity at the brush border, and reduction of absorptive surface area where there is villous destruction, may also contribute to hypoproteinaemia.

Recently validated tests for protein-losing enteropathy include faecal α_1-proteinase inhibitor (see Chapter 13). This protein is normally found in plasma, lymph and interstitial fluid but not in the gastrointestinal tract. The amount in faeces has been shown to correlate with histological abnormalities of the gastrointestinal tract but may not always correlate to serum albumin in the dog, making it a more useful screening test for possible early protein-losing enteropathy before significant protein loss has occurred.

Rarely, protein-losing enteropathy may be associated with hyperglobulinaemia; this has been reported in a small number of Basenjis with lymphangiectasia or eosinophilic enteritis (Breitschwerdt *et al.*, 1980).

Failure of production

Hepatic insufficiency

Albumin is synthesized exclusively in the liver and so reduced hepatic function can lead to hypoalbuminaemia. The liver is capable of approximately doubling albumin production in response to losses and the functional reserve is large, so that normal albumin production is maintained even in the face of widespread hepatic disease. Only when function is markedly compromised, as in end-stage liver disease or with portosystemic shunting, is hypoalbuminaemia noted. Clotting factors may also be affected, with resultant prolongations of clotting times (potentially both PT and aPTT). APP production may decline. It is unusual for globulins to decrease significantly due to the other tissues of origin: more frequently there is an increase in globulins with hepatic inflammatory disorders giving an elevation in the β and γ fractions of the electrophoretogram (β–γ bridging) (see Figure 7.8).

Hepatic function tests may reveal elevated resting and stimulated serum bile acids (see Chapter 12). Liver enzymes are often elevated, although they may be within reference ranges in portosytemic shunts and chronic hepatic diseases, such as cirrhosis. Other markers for decreased hepatic function include decreases in urea (the ornithine cycle taking place predominantly in the liver) and glucose.

Cachexia

Cachexia is one of the most common paraneoplastic syndromes in veterinary and human patients, although it may be associated with other disease states, and a major feature is weight loss in the face of normal intake. Anorexia may compound the effects. Derangements in carbohydrate and lipid metabolism occur in addition to alterations in nitrogen balance and amino acid profiles (Vail *et al.*, 1990). A shift toward inefficient anaerobic respiration, and the predilection of tumour tissue for amino acid derived gluconeogenesis can result in marked loss of muscle tissue and total body nitrogen. Although total liver protein synthesis tends to increase, this does not match breakdown and, in some animals, hypoalbuminaemia may eventually result.

Hypoglobulinaemia

Hypoglobulinaemia is most commonly seen in puppies that are not yet fully immunocompetent, as their maternal immunity wanes from approximately 12 weeks of age. Most have achieved adult levels of immunoglobulins by 6 months of age, but, until that time, they may be predisposed to upper respiratory infections. Lower reference values for retired Greyhounds compared to standard reference ranges have been reported (Steiss *et al.*, 2000) and breed-related variations in IgA concentrations have been documented (McNeil and Spit, 2002).

Several specific genetically based immunodeficiencies with resultant decreases in globulin production have been identified in the dog and cat (Figure 7.17). Identification relies on quantification of specific immunoglobulins and on a demonstrated deficiency compared to normal animals of the same age.

Hereditary immunodeficiencies	Breeds affected
IgA deficiency	German Shepherd Dog, Shar-Pei, Beagle, Irish Wolfhound, English Cocker Spaniel
IgG (± IgA ± IgM) deficiency and neutrophil dysfunction	Weimeraner
Lethal acrodermatitis	English Bull Terrier
X-linked SCID	Cardigan Corgi, Bassett Hound
Autosomal recessive SCID	Jack Russell Terrier
IgM deficiency	Dobermann

7.17 Hereditary immunodeficiencies resulting in reduced immunoglobulins. SCID: severe combined immunodeficiency.

Immunoglobulins can be individually quantified using a radial immunodiffusion technique similar to that used for the identification of specific immunoglobulins on an electrophoretogram. An agarose gel, impregnated evenly with an antibody raised against the immunoglobulin of interest, has wells cut into it. Test serum and known concentrations of the target immunoglobulin are added to the wells. After incubation and diffusion of the immunoglobulin out into the gel, a ring of precipitation formed by antigen–antibody complexes forms where the immunoglobulin and antibody concentration is optimal (Figure 7.18). The radius of the ring is dependent on the concentration of the target immunoglobulin in the well. The radius of the rings of precipitiation formed by different standards is plotted against the concentration of immunoglobulin used, to give a standard curve.The radius of the test serum is compared to the standard curve to allow calculation of immunoglobulin concentration. The assay is not currently performed in UK veterinary laboratories, but quantitiative immunoglobulins may be measured at the Department of Small Animal Medicine and Surgery, School of Veterinary Medicine, Hanover, Germany, or at many US or Canadian laboratories. Individual laboratories should be contacted for confirmation of tests performed and sample requirements.

IgA deficiency has been recognized in several breeds, including German Shepherd Dogs, where it is responsible for decreased skin and mucosal immunity. Some healthy Shar-Peis have relatively low IgA concentrations. Clinically significant decreases in either IgA or IgM have also been reported in this breed along with decreased lymphocyte response to mitogens: clinically this may affect older dogs (mean age 3 years) than those affected by other primary immunodeficiencies (Rivas *et al.*, 1995).

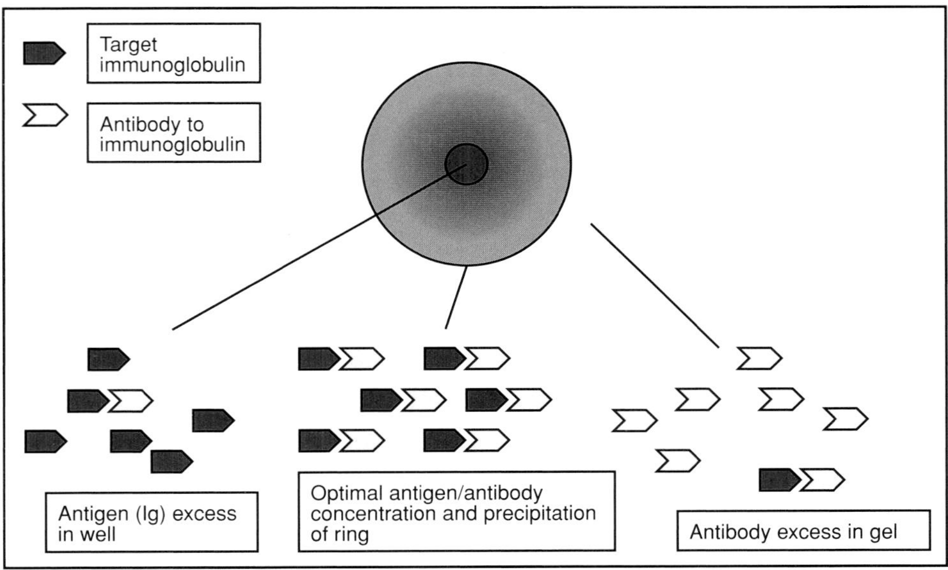

7.18 Radial immunodiffusion technique for quantifying immunoglobulins.

IgG deficiency has been demonstrated in Weimeraners, in individuals with recurrent bacterial infections or infections refractory to treatment (Couto *et al.*,1989; Day *et al.*,1997). These dogs may also have decreased IgM and/or IgA concentrations. Neutrophil dysfunction may also be present. Selective IgM deficiency has been documented in the Dobermann (Plechner, 1979).

Lethal acrodermatitis of Bull Terriers, which follows an autosomal recessive mode of inheritance, results in decreased IgA in addition to a domed palate, progressive hyperkeratotic skin lesions and decreased zinc levels in peripheral blood.

X-linked severe combined immunodeficiency (X-SCID), which results in low lymphocyte counts and low to absent IgG and IgA, has been reported in the Bassett Hound and the Cardigan Corgi (Pullen *et al.*,1997). IgM may be unaffected. Autosomal SCID has been recorded in the Jack Russell Terrier (Bell *et al.*, 2002) in multiple litters from the same dam and sire; these dogs had undetectable IgM, reduced IgG and leucopenia and lymphopenia compared with unaffected littermates.

There are many immunodeficiencies that do not affect immunoglobulin levels or function, and a normal immunoglobulin panel is no guarantee of immunocompetence.

Case examples

Case 1

Signalment

10-year-old male Boxer dog.

History

Recurrent unilateral epistaxis, lethargy for 2 weeks. Clinical examination was unremarkable.

Clinical pathology data

Haematology	Result	Reference interval
RBC (x 10^{12}/l)	4.25	5.5–8.5
Hb (g/dl)	9.6	12.0–18.0
HCT (l/l)	0.30	0.37–0.55
MCV (fl)	70.5	60–77
MCH (pg)	22.5	19.5–24.5
MCHC (g/dl)	32.1	31.0–37.0
Reticulocytes (%)	0	0–0.5
WBC (x 10^9/l)	4.38	6–17.1
Neutrophils (x 10^9/l)	2.98	3–11.5
Lymphocytes (x 10^9/l)	0.90	1–4.8
Monocytes (x 10^9/l)	0.5	0.15–1.5
Eosinophils (x 10^9/l)	0.00	0–1.3
Basophils (x 10^9/l)	0.00	0–0.2
Platelets (x 10^9/l)	112	150–900

Film comment

Erythrocytes normochromic, normocytic. Neutrophils mature and unremarkable morphology. Platelet numbers appear slightly reduced with no clumps noted. Two plasma cells noted in the feathered edge.

Biochemistry	Result	Reference interval
Sodium (mmol/l)	151	146 – 155
Potassium (mmol/l)	4.1	4.1 – 5.3
Chloride (mmol/l)	112	107 – 115
Glucose (mmol/l)	4.7	3.4 – 5.3
Urea (mmol/l)	6.6	3 – 9.1
Creatinine (µmol/l)	132	98 – 163
Calcium (mmol/l)	2.81	2.13 – 2.7 ▶

Biochemistry *(continued)*	Result	Reference interval
Inorganic phosphate (mmol/l)	1.09	0.8 – 2.0
TP (g/l)	104.1	49 – 71
Albumin (g/l)	23.3	28 – 39
Globulin (g/l)	80.3	21 – 41
ALT (IU/l)	23	13 – 88
ALP (IU/l)	280	19 – 285
CK (IU/l)	129	61 – 395
Total bilirubin (µmol/l)	0.8	0 – 2.4

What abnormalities are present?

Haematology

- Moderate leucopenia, due to mild neutropenia and lymphopenia
- Mild normochromic, normocytic non-regenerative anaemia
- Mild thrombocytopenia.

Biochemistry

- Moderate to marked hyperproteinaemia due to marked hyperglobulinaemia
- Mild hypoalbuminaemia
- Mild hypercalcaemia.

How would you interpret these results and what are the likely differential diagnoses?

Haematology

The haematology shows a mild pancytopenia with no evidence of regenerative attempts by the erythroid line (lack of reticulocytes) or granulocytes (no evidence of left shift in neutrophils). There is no film comment concerning shift (immature) platelets, although this is an unreliable indicator of platelet production. The degree of thrombocytopenia is insufficient alone to cause the epistaxis seen clinically. The anaemia is in part at least due to the epistaxis, although a regenerative response would be expected if this was the sole cause. The pancytopenia is suggestive of widespread bone marrow compromise, such as myelopthisis, myelofibrosis, toxicity or aplastic anaemia. The presence of plasma cells in peripheral blood is extremely unusual, even in plasma cell neoplasia.

Biochemistry

The biochemistry shows a marked increase in globulins. This may be due to inflammation or neoplastic production, e.g. in multiple myeloma, B cell

Case 1 continues ▶

Case 1 continued

lymphoma. The former is unlikely, considering the haematology findings. Increases due to haemoconcentration or dehydration are possible, but albumin and sodium have not increased in step and both urea and creatinine fail to show azotaemia.

The mild decrease in albumin is likely to be compensatory to the hyperglobulinaemia, although decreases due to haemorrhage, poor liver function, effusions or protein-losing nephropathy are possible.

The hypercalcaemia measured is mild, but, when combined with the hypoalbuminaemia, becomes more significant since decreased albumin leads to decreased total calcium. However, calcium also binds to globulins (four times less than to albumin) and the marked increase in globulin here may be sufficient to offset the reduction in albumin. Thus the mild hypercalcaemia may be due to increased protein binding. Other possible causes to consider in this case are hypercalcaemia of malignancy, and hypercalcaemia due to bone lysis which may occur in multiple myeloma.

What further tests would you recommend?

- **Bone marrow aspiration:** this could be justified on the basis of the pancytopenia alone, but the presence of plasma cells in circulation, hypercalcaemia and lytic lesions make this the single most important further test to pursue a diagnosis of multiple myeloma
- **Serum protein electrophoresis** to define the hyperglobulinaemia and distinguish an inflammatory wide-based response (which may be expected with osteomyelitis) from a monoclonal response (from multiple myeloma)
- **Skeletal survey radiographs** to look for lytic bone lesions seen in multiple myeloma
- **Urine analysis** including both protein:creatinine ratio, to exclude renal loss of albumin, and assay for Bence–Jones proteins. Specific gravity may be used to confirm that haemoconcentration is not a contributer to the hyperproteinaemia
- **Clotting profiles:** with normal platelet numbers, prothrombin time and activated partial thromboplastin time will help to eliminate secondary haemostatic disorders as a cause of epistaxis. With the presence of such high globulins, platelet function disorders should be suspected; buccal mucosal bleeding times will help investigate this cause.

Results of further tests

Radiography showed mottled lucencies on several dorsal spinous processes. Bone marrow aspiration showed hypercellularity despite erythroid and myeloid hypoplasia, due to effacement with plasma cells. These comprised 45% of all nucleated cells, present in broad sheets and clusters, showing mild variation in size and some morphological abnormalities including binucleated examples and increased nuclear to cytoplasmic ratio in a few. Serum protein electrophoresis demonstrated a single monoclonal spike in the γ region and confirmed the hypoalbuminaemia. These findings are consistent with multiple myeloma.

Bence–Jones proteins were absent from urine. These are found inconsistently in multiple myeloma.

Case outcome

Owners declined treatment. At post-mortem examination plasma cell infiltration was demonstrated in the skeletal lytic lesions.

Case 2

Signalment

8-year-old female neutered Jack Russell Terrier.

History

Three-week history of vomiting, diarrhoea, lethargy, anorexia and weight loss.

Clinical pathology data

Haematology	Result	Reference interval
RBC (x 10^{12}/l)	4.4	5.500–8.500
Hb (g/dl)	105	12.0–18.0
HCT (l/l)	0.31	0.39–0.55
MCV (f/l)	71.1	60.0–77.0
MCHC (g/dl)	33.5	32.0–36.0
Reticulocytes (%)	0.0	0.0–0.5
WBC (x 10^9/l)	28.5	6.00–15.00
Neutrophils (segmented) (x 10^9/l)	20.52	3.600–12.000
Neutrophils (band) (x 10^9/l)	0.57	0.00–0.04
Lymphocytes (x 10^9/l)	2.85	0.70–4.80
Monocytes (x 10^9/l)	1.71	0.000–1.500
Eosinophils (x 10^9/l)	0.0	0.0–1.0
Basophils (x 10^9/l)	0.0	0.0–0.2
Atypical mononuclear cells (x 10^9/l)	2.57	
Metamyelocytes (x 10^9/l)	0.29	
Platelets (x 10^9/l)	126	200–500

Film comments

Red cell morphology: red cells normocytic normochromic with minimal polychromasia.
White cells: left shift. Atypical cells appear lymphoid in origin, possibly reactive, although some have nucleoli.
Platelets: appear consistent with count given.

Biochemistry	Result	Reference interval
Sodium (mmol/l)	146.1	139–154
Potassium (mmol/l)	2.9	3.60–5.60
Glucose (mmol/l)	3.8	3.0–5.0
Urea (mmol/l)	6.1	1.7–7.4
Creatinine (μmol/l)	37.5	30–90
Calcium (mmol/l)	1.71	2.30–3.00
Inorganic phosphate (mmol/l)	1.31	0.90–1.20
TP (g/l)	30.2	58.0–73.0
Albumin (g/l)	12.4	26.0–35.0
Globulin (g/l)	17.8	28.0–42.0
ALT (IU/l)	59.0	15–60
ALP (IU/l)	47.8	20–60

What abnormalities are present?

Haematology

- Mild normocytic, normochromic non-regenerative anaemia
- Leucocytosis, which is due to a neutrophilia with a mild left shift
- Mild monocytosis
- Mild thrombocytopenia
- Atypical mononuclear cells.

Case 2 continues ▶

Case 2 continued

Biochemistry

- Severe hypoalbuminaemia
- Hypoglobulinaemia
- Hypocalcaemia
- Hypokalaemia.

How would you interpret these results and what are the likely differential diagnoses?

The haematology shows a neutrophilia with a left shift. These changes may reflect inflammation, possibly due to infection. Mild non-regenerative anaemia may result from any chronic disease, bone marrow disease or acute blood loss (with insufficient time for the bone marrow to respond). Mild thrombocytopenia may be due to decreased production (bone marrow disease), increased consumption (thrombus formation, disseminated intravascular coagulation), loss (blood loss), or possibly increased destruction (immune-mediated thrombocytopenia, although this usually results in much more severe thrombocytopenia).

A mild monocytosis in conjunction with left shifted neutrophilia is consistent with on-going inflammation. The presence of atypical mononuclear cells is suspicious of an underlying neoplastic disorder, but may also be a response to a severe inflammatory process.

The biochemical changes are dominated by severe panhypoproteinaemia. Hypoalbuminaemia may be due to:

- Protein loss: protein-losing enteropathy (PLE) (globulins are also decreased); protein-losing nephropathy (globulin concentration usually normal); haemorrhage (PCV and globulins also decreased); effusions
- Decreased production of protein: severe liver insufficiency; malabsorption; maldigestion; starvation.

Hypoglobulinaemia results from blood loss or protein-losing enteropathy.

Calcium is highly protein-bound; therefore, hypoalbuminaemia will result in decreased serum calcium concentration. A corrected calcium concentration can be calculated to determine the significance of the hypocalcaemia. An ionized calcium concentration will determine whether the biologically active calcium fraction is decreased.

Hypokalaemia occurs due to decreased intake (e.g. anorexia) or increased losses (e.g. renal failure, diarrhoea). Severe hypokalaemia can cause profound weakness, paralytic intestinal ileus and cardiac arrhythmias.

The biochemical and haematological abnormalities are suggestive of a PLE, and this correlates with clinical signs. Severe inflammatory bowel disease, alimentary lymphosarcoma and lymphangiectasia are all possible differential diagnoses.

What further tests would you recommend?

- **Urinalysis:** to exclude protein loss via the urine (including urine protein:creatinine ratio and sediment examination)
- **Bile acid function test:** to exclude severe hepatic insufficiency as the cause of hypoproteinaemia
- **Abdominal ultrasonography:** to assess gastrointestinal wall thickness and architecture. Mesenteric lymph node size can also be assessed. If enlarged, fine needle aspirates can be obtained
- **Thoracocentesis/abdominocentesis:** if clinical signs indicated the presence of a body cavity effusion, centesis should be performed to determine protein content and cytology of the fluid
- **Faecal α_1-protease inhibitor:** to detect protein loss via the gastrointestinal tract. This test is useful in the early stages of PLE when few clinical signs are present
- **Gastrointestinal biopsy:** endoscopic or full-thickness gut biopsies are necessary to confirm a diagnosis of PLE. Severe hypoalbuminaemia may impair wound healing and increase the risk of surgical wound dehiscence following full-thickness gut biopsies. Endoscopic gut biopsies are safer in such cases, but only superficial tissue is obtained and so pathological changes in deeper layers of the intestinal wall may be missed.

Further results

- Thickened intestinal loops were identified using ultrasound
- Upper gastrointestinal endoscopy was performed to obtain intestinal biopsies. The duodenal mucosa was grossly abnormal with a cobblestone appearance and was very friable. An increased number of lymphocytes and plasma cells were present in the lamina propria consistent with a diagnosis of lymphocytic plasmacytic enteritis.

Outcome and post-mortem findings

The dog responded poorly to treatment and was euthanased 4 weeks later. A post-mortem examination was performed and confirmed the presence of lymphoma, which unfortunately may be misdiagnosed as inflammatory bowel disease on endoscopy due to the superficial nature of the tissues specimens obtained. This may explain the presence of atypical mononuclear cells in the blood.

References and further reading

Baker R and Valli V (1986) A review of feline protein electrophoresis. *Veterinary Clinical Pathology* **15,** 20–25

Bell T, Butler K, Sill H, Stickle J, Ramos-Vara J and Dark M (2002) Autosomal recessive severe combined immunodeficiency of Jack Russell Terrier. *Journal of Veterinary Diagnostic Investigation* **14,** 194–204

Breitschwerdt E, Halliwell W, Foley C, Stark D and Corwin L (1980) A hereditary diarrhetic syndrome in the Basenji characterised by malabsorption, protein losing enteropathy and hypergammaglobulinemia. *Journal of the American Animal Hospital Association* **16,** 551–560

Burkhard M, Meyer D, Rosychuk R, O'Neil S and Schultheiss P (1995) Monoclonal gammopathy in a dog with chronic pyoderma. *Journal of Veterinary Internal Medicine* **9,** 357–360

Bush BM (1991) *Interpretation of Laboratory Results for Small Animal Clinicians, 1st edn.* Blackwell Science Ltd, Oxford

Couto C, Krakowka S, Johnson G, Ciekot P, Hill L, Lafrado L and Kociba G (1989) In vitro immunological features of Weimaraner dogs with neutrophil abnormalities and recurrent infections. *Veterinary Immunology and Immunopathology* **23,** 103–112

Day M (1999) Immunodeficiency disease. In: *Clinical Immunology of the Dog and Cat,* ed. M Day, pp. 197–215. Manson Publishing Limited, London

Day M, Power C, Oleshko J and Rose M (1997) Low serum immunoglobulin concentrations in related Weimeraner dogs. *Journal of Small Animal Practice* **38,** 311– 315

Dewhirst M, Stamp G and Hurwitz A (1977) Idiopathic monocolonal (IgA) gammopathy in a dog. *Journal of the American Veterinary Medical Association* **170,** 1313–1316

Diehl K, Lappin M, Jones R and Cayatte S (1992) Monoclonal gammopathy in a dog with plasmacytic gastroenterocolitis. *Journal of the American Veterinary Medical Association* **201,** 1233–1236

Dimopoulous M and Alexanian R (1994) Waldenstrom's macroglobulinaemia. *Blood* **83,** 1452–1459

Drazner F (1982) Multiple myeloma in the cat. *Journal of the American Animal Hospital Association* **4,** 200–214

Eckersall PD, Connor JG and Parton H (1989) An enzyme-linked immunosorbent assay for canine C-reactive protein. *Veterinary Record* **124,** 490–491

Eckersall PD, Duthie S, Safi S, Moffatt D, Horadagoda, NU, Doyle S, Parton R, Bennett D and Fitzpatrick JL (1999) An automated assay for haptoglobin: prevention of interference from albumin. *Comparative Haematology International* **9,** 117–124

Felsburg P (1992) Overview of the immune system and immunodeficiency disease. *Veterinary Clinics of North America: Small Animal Practice* **24,** 629– 653

Font A, Closa J and Mascort J (1994) Monoclonal gammopathy in a dog with visceral leishmaniasis. *Journal of Veterinary Internal Medicine* **8,** 233–235

Forrester S and Relford R (1992) Serum hyperviscosity syndrome: its diagnosis and treatment. *Veterinary Medicine* **87,** 48–54

Giraudel J, Pages J-P and Guelfi J-F (2002) Monoclonal gammopathies in the dog: a retrospective study of 18 cases (1986–1999) and literature review. *Journal of the American Animal Hospital Association* **38,** 135–147

Hoskins J, Barta O and Rothschmitt J (1983) Serum hyperviscosity syndrome associated with *Ehrlichia canis* infection in a dog.

Journal of the American Veterinary Medical Association **183,** 1011–1012

Jacobs R (1982) The qualitative analysis of canine immunoglobulins and myeloma proteins by immunofixation. *Veterinary Clinical Pathology* **11,** 7–10

Jacobs R, Couto C and Wellman M (1986) Biclonal gammopathy in a dog with myeloma and and cutaneous lymphoma. *Veterinary Pathology* **23,** 211–213

Kaneko J (1997) Serum proteins and the dysproteinaemias. In: *Clinical Biochemistry of Domestic Animals, 5th edn*, ed Kaneko J, Harvey J, Bruss M pp 117–138. Academic Press, London

Kyle R and Rajkumar S (2003) Monoclonal gammopathies of undetermined significance: a review. *Immunological Reviews* **194,** 112–139

Mandel N and Esplin D (1994) A retroperitoneal extramedullary plasmacytoma in a cat with monoclonal gammopathy. *Journal of the Americal Animal Hospital Association* **30,** 603–608

McBride W, Jackman J, Bammon R and Willerson J (1986) High output cardiac failure in patients with multiple myeloma. *New England Journal of Medicine* **319,** 1651–1653

McGrotty YL and Knottenbelt CM (2002) Significance of plasma protein abnormalities in dogs and cats. *In Practice* **24(9),** 512–517

McNeil L and Spit L (2002) The effects and importance of age and breed on haematological measurements in the dog. *Waltham Focus* **12,** 38–41

Nagata M, Nanko H, Hashimoto K, Ogawa M and Sakashita E (1998) Cryoglobulinaemia and cryofibrinogenaemia: a comparison of canine and human cases. *Veterinary Dermatology* **9,** 277–281

Orth S and Ritz E (1998) The nephrotic syndrome. *New England Journal of Medicine* **338,** 1202–1211

Peterson E and Meininger A (1997) Immunoglobulin A and immunoglobulin G biclonal gammopathy in a dog with multiple myeloma. *Journal of the American Animal Hospital Association* **33,** 45–47

Plechner A (1979) IgM deficiency in two dobermann pinschers. *Modern Veterinary Practice* **60,** 150

Pullen R, Somberg R, Felsburg P and Herthorn P (1997) X-linked severe combined immunodeficiency in a family of Cardigan Welsh corgis. *Journal of the American Animal Hospital Association* **33,** 494–499

Ramaiah S, Seguin M, Carwile H and Raskin R (2002) Biclonal gammopathy associated with Immunoglobulin A in a dog with multiple myeloma. *Veterinary Clinical Pathology* **31,** 83–89

Rivas A, Tintle L, Argentieri D, Kimball E, Goodman M, Anderson D, Capetola R, and Quimby F (1995) A primary immunodeficiency syndrome in Shar–Pei dogs. *Clinical Immunology and Immunopathology* **74,** 243–251

Steiss J, Brewer W, Welles E and Wright J (2002) Haematological and serum biochemical reference values in retired greyhounds. *Compendium of Continuing Education for the Practicing Veterinarian* **22,** 243–248

Stockham S and Scott M (2002) Proteins. In: *Fundamentals of Veterinary Clinical Pathology*, pp. 251–276. Iowa State Press, Iowa

Vail D (2000) Hematopoietic tumors. In: *Textbook of Veterinary Internal Medicine: Diseases of the Dog and Cat, 5th edn,* ed. SJ Ettinger and EC Feldman, pp. 516– 520. WB Saunders, London

Vail D, Ogilvie G and Wheeler S (1990) Metabolic alterations in patients with cancer cachexia. *Compendium of Continuing Education for the Practicing Veterinarian* **12,** 381–387

Willard MD, Tvedten H and Turnwald GH (1994) *Small Animal Clinical Diagnosis by Laboratory Methods, 2nd edn.* WB Saunders, Philadelphia

8

Electrolyte imbalances

Barbara Skelly and Richard Mellanby

Introduction

The maintenance of normal electrolyte concentrations is fundamental to health. Derangements affect many organs, including the nervous system and cardiac and skeletal muscle. Major imbalances can cause severe clinical signs and death. Levels of the major electrolytes (potassium, sodium, calcium and magnesium) are closely controlled by the action of multiple hormones and by the kidneys.

Disorders of potassium homeostasis

Measurement of potassium in serum and plasma

Potassium can be measured by flame emission spectrophotometry or, more commonly, by using direct or indirect ion-selective electrodes. Only direct ion-sensitive electrodes are unaffected by lipaemia or marked hyperproteinaemia, which artefactually raise potassium concentration when other methods are used.

Distribution of potassium in the body

Potassium is primarily located within cells and is maintained in this compartment by the sodium/potassium ATPase pump. The result of this pumping mechanism is that the serum concentration of potassium is low (3.5–5.8 mmol/l in dogs and 3.6–4.5 mmol/l in cats), while the intracellular potassium concentration is high (140–150 mmol/l in both species).

Both hyper- and hypokalaemia have profound effects on the heart. Hyperkalaemia leads to bradycardia, atrial standstill and ventricular escape, while hypokalaemia can predispose to tachyarrhythmias.

How is potassium balance maintained?

Potassium enters the body in food.The main route for excretion is renal, and a small amount is lost in sweat and faeces (Figure 8.1). Alterations in aldosterone and serum potassium concentrations control the loss of potassium in the distal nephron.

Hyperkalaemia

Hyperkalaemia may be due to laboratory error, failure of renal excretion, redistribution of potassium out of cells into the extracellular fluid (ECF) or exogenous sources (Figure 8.2).

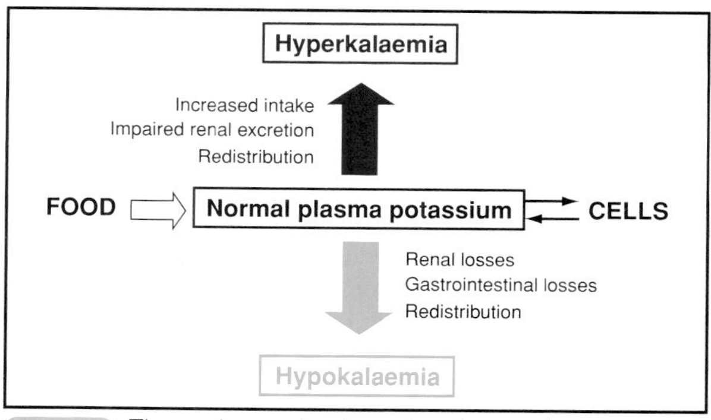

8.1 The main mechanisms leading to the development of hyper- or hypokalaemia.

Laboratory or interpretive error	
Haemolysed blood sample	
Thrombocytosis	
Massive leucocytosis	
Akita dogs	
Increased potassium from exogenous sources	
Intravenous fluid therapy containing potassium salts	
Increased dietary intake or supplementation	
Reduced potassium excretion	
Anuric or oliguric renal failure	
Urinary outflow obstruction	
Urinary bladder rupture	
Hypoadrenocorticism	
Primary hypoaldosteronism	
Drug therapy	Potassium-sparing diuretics, e.g. spironolactone
	Angiotensin converting enzyme inhibitors
	Non-steroidal anti-inflammatory agents
Potassium redistribution – movement from cells into extracellular fluid	
Metabolic acidosis – caused by an inorganic acid	
Hyperosmolality	
Pseudohypoadrenocorticism	Whipworms
	Hypovolaemia caused by severe vomiting/diarrhoea
	Effective circulating volume depletion due to pleural, peritoneal or pericardial effusion
Massive tissue destruction, e.g. tumour lysis syndrome	
Beta-adrenergic blockade	
Digitalis toxicity	
Miscellaneous causes	
Drug therapy – ACE-inhibitors	
EDTA contamination of blood samples	
Late gestation pregnancy	

8.2 Differential diagnosis of hyperkalaemia. The most common differentials are shown in italics.

Laboratory or interpretive error

Elevated numbers of platelets and leucocytes can release their intracellular potassium *in vitro*, especially in clotted serum samples, with resultant hyperkalaemia. A haemolysed blood sample may have an increased potassium concentration although, since red cells have a low intracellular potassium concentration, the increase observed may reflect the lysis of other cell lines. The red cells of Akita have unusually high intracellular potassium; haemolysis thus produces a more dramatic effect (Degen, 1987).

Failure of renal excretion

Failure of renal excretion is usually due to either renal failure or urinary tract obstruction. Hypoadrenocorticism is a less common cause.

Renal failure as a cause for hyperkalaemia: Serum potassium rises because a fall in the glomerular filtration rate (GFR) reduces distal tubular flow and, as a consequence, reduces potassium excretion. For renal failure to cause hyperkalaemia there must be a significant reduction in urine production (either anuria or oliguria), usually due to acute renal failure or end-stage chronic renal failure.

Urinary tract obstruction: If there is complete obstruction to urine outflow then potassium concentrations rise rapidly and dramatically due to a sudden marked reduction in GFR. Metabolic acidosis also develops and exacerbates the hyperkalaemia due to a shift of potassium out of cells into the interstitium and plasma. Azotaemia, hyperphosphataemia and hypocalcaemia are commonly present.

Urinary tract rupture: In uroabdomen, urine is not voided and the whole body potassium load rises, with a subsequent rise in plasma potassium. High levels of creatinine in abdominal fluid suggests that urinary tract rupture has occurred (Chapter 21).

Hypoadrenocorticism: In hypoadrenocorticism (Chapter 18) low levels of aldosterone lead to decreased sodium resorption and reduced potassium excretion in the distal nephron. This usually results in a marked elevation in serum potassium, coupled with hyponatraemia and a marked reduction in the sodium:potassium ratio (<24). A small proportion of cases do not have electrolyte abnormalities (Sadek and Schaer, 1996). An ACTH stimulation test provides the definitive diagnosis, with cortisol levels usually being undetectable pre and post ACTH (see Chapter 18).

Potassium redistribution

Factors affecting potassium redistribution are summarized in Figure 8.3.

Acid–base disturbances: Hydrogen ions from strong acids, such as hydrochloric acid, are able to displace potassium from cells, resulting in hyperkalaemia (see Chapter 9). This occurs because chloride (the major extracellular anion) cannot follow hydrogen ions into cells, and so when hydrogen ions enter cells, potassium enters the ECF to preserve electroneutrality. Organic acids, such as lactic acid or ketoacids, do not provoke this movement of potassium or do so to a limited extent, presumably since their associated anions are able to follow them to an intracellular location more easily. The hyperkalaemia of diabetic ketoacidosis occurs via a different mechanism (solvent drag) whereby water movement out of cells draws potassium into the ECF. Respiratory acidosis does not appear to provoke potassium redistribution; the reasons for this are unclear.

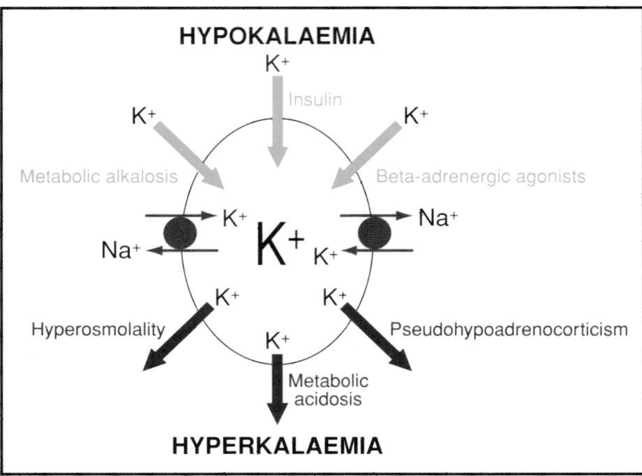

8.3 Factors affecting potassium movement into and out of the cell (represented by an oval in this diagram). The Na^+/K^+/ATPase pump mediates the movement of potassium into the cell, whereas outward movement is caused by solvent drag or by displacement of potassium by other cations.

Pseudohypoadrenocorticism: This has been described in dogs with *Trichuris vulpis* infection and other primary gastrointestinal diseases (DiBartola *et al.*, 1985; Graves *et al.*, 1994). Fluid sequestration into body cavities or into the pericardial sac (so-called third space loss) may also cause electrolyte abnormalities that mimic hypoadrenocorticism. The mechanisms for this are complex and involve:

- Hypovolaemia, inducing anti-diuretic hormone (ADH) release and water retention (lowering sodium)
- A reduction in tubular fluid flow to the distal tubule, due to decreased GFR, leading to reduced potassium excretion
- Repeated drainage of effusions, leading to total body sodium loss
- Patient thirst, leading to increased water intake (lowering sodium)
- Metabolic acidosis may develop due to alimentary loss of bicarbonate, leading to a shift of potassium out of cells.

The net result is a dilution of extracellular sodium and an increase in extracellular potassium.

Massive tissue breakdown: This results in hyperkalaemia due to release of massive amounts of intracellular potassium into the circulation. Causes include:

- Tumour lysis syndrome following chemotherapy in the face of a large chemosensitive tumour burden, e.g. lymphoma
- Reperfusion injury following aortic thromboembolic disease in cats
- Severe trauma.

Miscellaneous causes of hyperkalaemia

Drug therapy: Angiotensin converting enzyme (ACE) inhibitors cause hyperkalaemia by inhibition of angiotensin-mediated aldosterone release. As they are frequently used in conjunction with loop diuretics, which increase renal potassium loss, this effect is often insignificant.

EDTA contamination of blood samples: If the syringe tip touches the inside of an EDTA tube it may become contaminated with potassium EDTA, so that when the remaining sample is expelled into the serum/heparin tube, it becomes contaminated. This results in marked hyperkalaemia, hypocalcaemia (calcium chelated by the EDTA) and also low alkaline phosphatase.

Hypokalaemia

The causes of hypokalaemia are summarized in Figure 8.4 and the most common causes are discussed below.

Decreased intake	
Anorexia	
Fluid therapy using K^+-free fluids	
Increased loss	
Gastrointestinal losses	
Vomiting and/or diarrhoea	
Urinary losses	
Chronic renal failure	
Post-obstructive diuresis	
Polyuria	
Renal tubular acidosis	
Hyperadrenocorticism	
Hyperaldosteronism (Conn's syndrome)	
Hypomagnesaemia	
Metabolic acidosis	
Drug therapy:	Penicillin
	Loop and thiazide diuretics
	Mineralocorticoid excess
Potassium redistribution – increased entry into cells	
Alkalaemia	
Elevated insulin levels	
Beta-adrenergic agonist administration	
Hypothermia	
Hypokalaemic myopathy of Burmese cats	
Miscellaneous causes	
Hyperthyroidism	

8.4 Differential diagnosis of hypokalaemia. The most common differentials are shown in italics.

Decreased intake

Anorexia: This is probably the most common cause of hypokalaemia in small animal practice.

Iatrogenic causes: Fluid therapy using potassium-free fluids (0.9% NaCl) or low-potassium fluids (Hartmann's solution) can lead to hypokalaemia, particularly in anorexic animals. Fluids containing glucose, or insulin therapy, will cause the serum/plasma potassium concentration to drop as potassium moves into cells from the ECF (see Figure 8.3).

Increased loss of potassium

Gastrointestinal disease: Vomiting and diarrhoea, or the two combined, can lead to clinically significant hypokalaemia by the following mechanisms:

- Potassium loss into the gastrointestinal (GI) tract
- Volume contraction stimulates aldosterone release and retention of sodium with concurrent potassium loss
- Vomiting of gastric contents may result in metabolic alkalosis, promoting movement of potassium into cells from the ECF.

Reduced intake due to anorexia or inappetence may compound these effects.

Chronic renal failure: Cats with chronic renal failure are much more likely to be hypokalaemic than dogs and may develop muscle weakness associated with potassium depletion. The mechanism behind the hypokalaemia is probably multifactorial (increased urinary and GI losses and reduced absorption). An improvement in renal function occurs following potassium supplementation, and supplementation has been recommended in all cats with chronic renal failure (Dow and Fettman, 1992).

Drug-associated hypokalaemia: Loop diuretics (e.g. furosemide) and thiazide diuretics commonly cause hypokalaemia. Spironolactone, a potassium-sparing diuretic, is often used in combination with furosemide to offset the hypokalaemia. Dogs and cats receiving digoxin must be monitored particularly closely, since hypokalaemia potentiates digoxin toxicity and predisposes to development of dysrhythmias.

Hyperadrenocorticism and hyperaldosteronism: Hypokalaemia due to endocrine disease is rare in dogs and cats. Hypokalaemia develops in hyperaldosteronism due to excessive urinary excretion of potassium, and this has been reported in cats (Conn's syndrome) (Bruyette, 2001) and, more rarely, in dogs (Rijnberk *et al.*, 2001). Diagnosis relies on demonstrating an elevated aldosterone concentration in the face of low or normal renin concentrations. Hypokalaemia can also occur in hyperadrenocorticism when excess cortisol acts as an agonist for the aldosterone receptor. This effect is usually blocked by the rapid conversion of cortisol to cortisone in the kidney but can be seen when adrenal tumours produce excessive amounts of cortisol that exceed the maximum rate of this conversion.

Hypokalaemia caused by potassium shift into cells

Just as metabolic acidosis causes potassium to move out of cells, alkalaemia can cause potassium to move into cells (Figure 8.3). This effect is slight, however, and rarely causes clinically significant hypokalaemia. (See also section below on Diabetes mellitus.)

Hypokalaemic myopathy of Burmese cats: Burmese cats have been reported to suffer from intermittent, spontaneously improving weakness that has an age of onset of 2–6 months (Figure 8.5). Serum potassium is usually <3.0 mmol/l and creatine kinase is often elevated. Diagnosis is by exclusion of other known causes and by proving that the fractional excretion of potassium is normal, i.e. appropriately decreased (<5%) in a potassium-depleted animal (see Chapter 11).

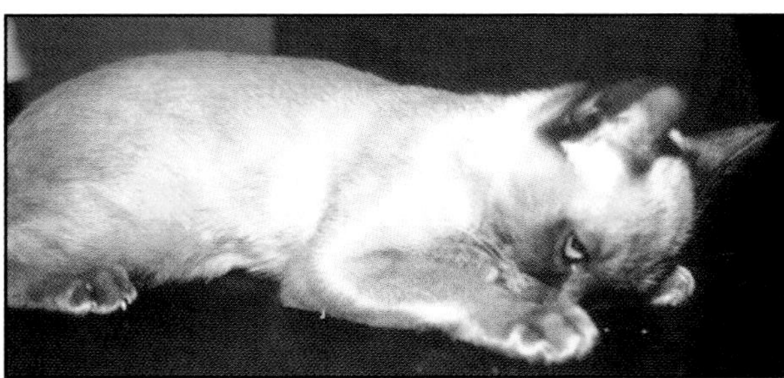

8.5 Young Burmese cat showing generalized weakness and cervical ventroflexion due to hypokalaemic myopathy. (Courtesy of ME Herrtage, University of Cambridge.)

Hyperthyroidism: Hypokalaemia is a rare consequence of hyperthyroidism in cats and is speculated to be secondary either to polyuria causing potassium wasting or to potassium shift into cells (Nemzek *et al.*, 1994).

Diabetes mellitus – a cause of both hyper- and hypokalaemia

Uncontrolled or ketoacidotic diabetic patients may present with normal potassium levels or may be hyperkalaemic, although most have whole-body potassium depletion due to polyuria (osmotic diuresis). Several mechanisms are involved, including serum hyperosmolality and insulin deficiency. In addition, ketones, such as acetoacetate and β-hydroxybutyrate, act as non-absorbable anions in the urine, trapping cations so that potassium excretion is enhanced. When insulin therapy is started, potassium rapidly returns to an intracellular location leaving the animal hypokalaemic and the whole-body potassium deficit becomes apparent. Once fluid therapy for management of a ketoacidotic crisis is underway, potassium monitoring is vital in order to avoid severe hypokalaemia.

Disorders of sodium homeostasis

Measurement of sodium in serum and plasma

Sodium can be measured by flame emission spectrophotometry or, more commonly, by using direct or indirect ion-selective electrodes. Only direct ion-sensitive electrodes are unaffected by lipaemia or marked hyperproteinaemia, which artefactually increase sodium (to a greater extent than potassium) concentration when other methods are used.

The role of sodium in the body

Sodium is primarily responsible for providing the means with which water is retained or lost through the action of the kidneys. Under normal conditions, the sodium and, therefore, the water content of the body is maintained within a narrow range. This balance is upset by either:

- Loss of sodium and water (volume depletion)
- Loss of water alone (dehydration)
- Gain of water (volume overload).

In cats and dogs normal serum sodium concentrations range between 135 and 155 mmol/l.

Sodium is the major cation present in the ECF and is responsible for the preservation of electroneutrality. Each sodium ion is balanced with an appropriate anion; chloride makes up two thirds of the total concentration of anions in the ECF, with bicarbonate the next most prevalent.

Regulation of plasma sodium

Plasma sodium levels are controlled by the regulation of blood volume and plasma osmolality via the following mechanisms:

- Activation of the renin–angiotensin–aldosterone system (RAAS)
- Release of ADH.

Reduced blood volume results in activation of the RAAS, leading to formation of angiotensin II and release of aldosterone (Figure 8.6). Angiotensin II causes increased sympathetic tone and so increased blood pressure and increased absorption of sodium, chloride and water in the proximal tubule of the kidney. Aldosterone causes increased resorption of sodium in exchange for potassium in the distal tubule.

Volume reduction and *effective* volume reduction, as found in congestive heart failure, also trigger release of ADH via stimulation of carotid sinus baroreceptors (Figure 8.6). However, these volume receptors are much less sensitive and, unlike the RAAS, are activated only after a substantial decrease in circulating volume.

These changes are reversed if there is an expansion of circulating volume.

Plasma osmolality

Plasma osmolality is a reflection of the number of osmotically active particles of solute, measured in mosmol/kg. It is regulated by ADH and the thirst mechanism (Figure 8.7). Changes in plasma osmolality, principally caused by changes in sodium concentration, are detected by osmoreceptors in the hypothalamus. Increased osmolality leads to activation of the thirst mechanism and ADH release from the neurohypophysis of the pituitary gland. ADH acts at the renal collecting ducts to increase the reabsorption of water.

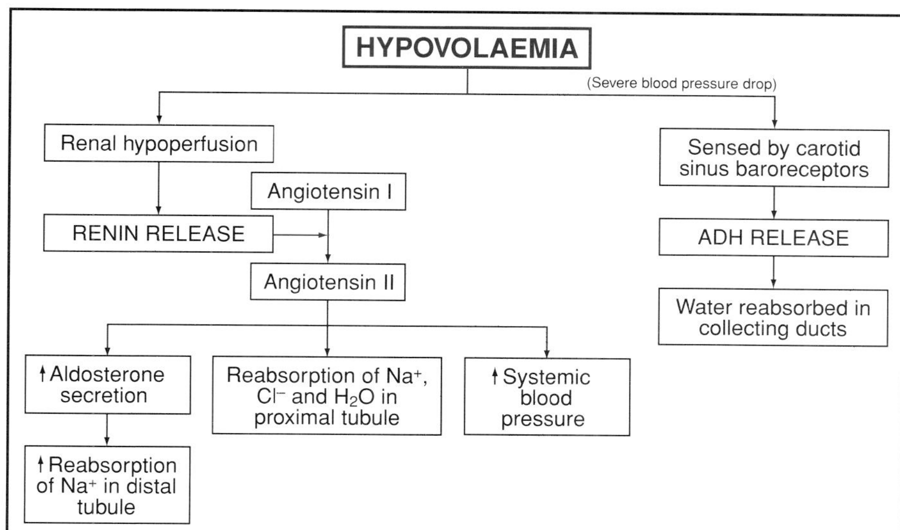

8.6 Activation of the renin–angiotensin system leading to aldosterone secretion and an increase in systemic blood pressure. When there is a significant drop in blood pressure, ADH release is also stimulated.

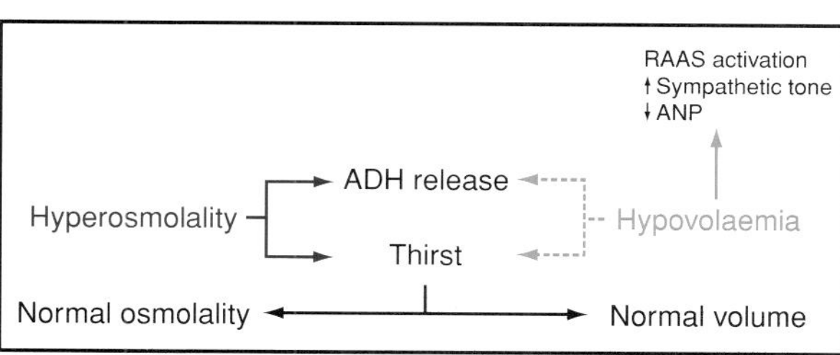

8.7 The relationship between osmoregulation and volume regulation. Although hyperosmolality is the primary stimulus for ADH release and increase in thirst, severe hypovolaemia can also stimulate the same mechanisms. (ANP, atrial natriuretic peptide)

The maintenance of normal osmolality involves the gain or loss of *water* while the maintenance of circulating volume involves the gain or loss of *sodium*. When volume depletion is severe, even if osmolality is low, ADH release and the thirst mechanism are activated leading to dilutional hyponatraemia.

Hypernatraemia

In animals where the hypernatraemia is secondary to volume depletion, the early clinical signs reflect hypovolaemia. When the plasma sodium concentration increases, plasma osmolality increases. This creates an osmotic gradient, that favours water movement out of cells, and cellular dehydration, which leads to rupture of cerebral vessels and focal haemorrhage in the nervous system. Clinical signs include lethargy, weakness, vocalization, muscle rigidity, twitching, seizures and coma, signs similar to those associated with hyponatraemia. The severity of the clinical signs depends on the rate at which the hypernatraemia develops as well as the magnitude of the sodium concentration.

The differential diagnoses of hypernatraemia are listed in Figure 8.8. For an animal to become hypernatraemic it must either:

- Lose water in excess of sodium
- Have an increased sodium intake either orally or through parenteral routes, e.g. intravenous fluid therapy.

Hypernatraemia with water loss in excess of sodium
Hypotonic fluid loss
Gastrointestinal disease – vomiting and/or diarrhoea
Renal failure
Diabetes mellitus
Diuretic therapy
Loss of pure water
Nephrogenic diabetes insipidus
Central diabetes insipidus
Primary adipsia
Heatstroke
Pyrexia
Burns or extensive degloving injury
Water deprivation
Hypernatraemia caused by excessive sodium gain
Increased salt ingestion
Hypertonic intravenous fluid therapy
Intravenous sodium bicarbonate
Hyperaldosteronism
Hyperadrenocorticism

8.8 The differential diagnosis of hypernatraemia. The most common differentials are shown in italics.

Hypernatraemia with water loss in excess of sodium

Hypotonic fluid loss: Hypovolaemia due to hypotonic fluid loss is the most common cause of hypernatraemia because the diseases underlying the electrolyte imbalance are so frequently encountered. When water is lost in excess of sodium, for example through vomiting or diarrhoea, then hypovolaemia and whole body sodium depletion may occur in the face of hypernatraemia. Movement of hypotonic fluid into a body cavity (ascites or pleural effusion) or other third spaces can similarly lead to hypernatraemia. Renal hypotonic losses can occur secondary to the use of diuretics, osmotic diuresis (e.g. glucosuria) or post-obstructive diuresis.

Heatstroke, pyrexia, burns or extensive degloving injury: This group of conditions is characterized by free water loss through the skin due to skin deficits, or to the increase in water evaporation from the skin and respiratory tract as an animal attempts to lower its body temperature.

Water deprivation: Animals that are either unable or unwilling to drink water, such as disorientated geriatric patients or those with neurological disease, may become water deprived and should be assisted to drink.

Central diabetes insipidus: Central diabetes insipidus is an uncommon condition in which there is a complete or partial absence of the production and release of ADH in response to increased plasma osmolality or to volume depletion. It can be congenital (Post *et al.*, 1989) or acquired secondary to trauma (Authement *et al.*, 1989), neoplasia, pituitary cysts, inflammation or pituitary malformation (Harb *et al.*, 1996). Affected animals are unable to concentrate their urine and produce large quantities of very dilute urine (urine specific gravity typically <1.005). Polydipsia occurs secondarily to try to maintain adequate water balance. Hypernatraemia results when pure water loss exceeds intake. Diagnosis is by the water deprivation test or modified water deprivation test and response to exogenously administered synthetic ADH (1-desamino-8-D-arginine vasopressin or DDAVP) (see Chapter 10).

Nephrogenic diabetes insipidus: Congenital nephrogenic diabetes insipidus is extremely rare (Takemura, 1998; Luzius *et al.*, 1992), while acquired nephrogenic diabetes insipidus is a relatively common consequence of many systemic diseases, e.g. hyperadrenocorticism, hypoadrenocorticism, hepatic disease, hypercalcaemia and diseases in which there is a septic focus, such as pyometra. Although ADH is produced and released in response to hyperosmolality, the kidney is unable to respond adequately. The congenital form of this disease is difficult to confirm and is a diagnosis of exclusion (Luzius *et al.*, 1992).

Primary adipsia (essential hypernatraemia): Primary adipsia is a rare condition defined by a defect in the central thirst mechanism caused by malfunction of the osmoreceptors of the hypothalamus. Consequently, ADH secretion from the hypothalamus fails to occur in response to increased plasma osmolality but can occur when volume is depleted (Crawford *et al.*, 1984; Dow *et al.*, 1987; Jeffery *et al.*, 2003). This condition is usually congenital but there have been reports of acquired forms in older animals secondary to inflammatory disease (Mackay and Curtis, 1999). Plasma sodium levels are typically >170 mmol/l and overt neurological signs are often present, although animals are not volume depleted.

Hypernatraemia caused by excessive sodium gain

Increased salt ingestion, hypertonic intravenous fluid therapy, intravenous sodium bicarbonate: Hypernatraemia as a result of excessive salt intake is uncommon (Khanna *et al.*, 1997) but it can occur due to the ingestion of sea water, use of sodium phosphate enemas and as a consequence of intravenous hypertonic saline fluid therapy or large doses of sodium bicarbonate.

Hyperaldosteronism and hyperadrenocorticism: Hypernatraemia can occur secondary to aldosterone or cortisol excess from secretory tumours of the adrenal gland. This is discussed in more detail in the section on hypokalaemia.

Hyponatraemia

Clinical signs of hyponatraemia are generally not observed at all until the plasma sodium concentration falls below 125 mmol/l. If hyponatraemia develops gradually then the clinical signs are few and less severe: the brain is protected from becoming oedematous by the movement of organic, osmotically active molecules (osmolytes) and potassium ions out of the cells, thus ensuring that the intracellular osmolality decreases with the extracellular osmolality. If, however, there is a rapid decrease in sodium and of plasma osmolality then water can move into the brain rapidly and cerebral oedema develops (Figure 8.9), resulting in lethargy, weakness, nausea, vomiting, incoordination and seizures.

Hyponatraemia may be due to excess loss of sodium or gain of water or a combination of both (Figure 8.10).

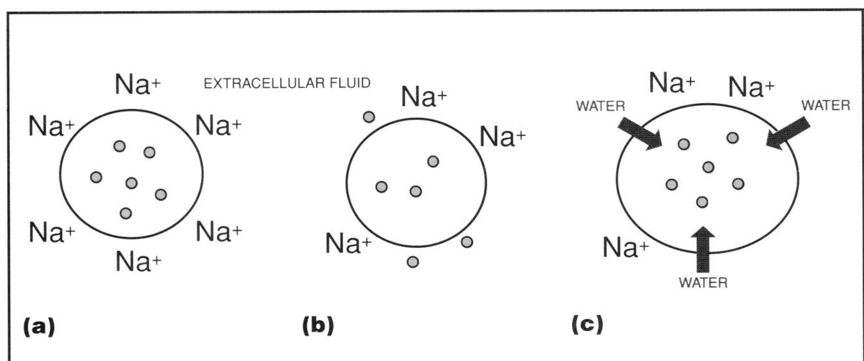

8.9 The cellular adaptation to hyponatraemia in the nervous system. (a) Cells within the nervous system are protected from dehydration by the presence of idiogenic, organic osmoles (●). (b) When hyponatraemia develops slowly a re-equilibration can occur and osmotic balance is maintained. However, when hyponatraemia develops rapidly, the intracellular space is hyperosmolar with respect to the extracellular fluid, water moves into the cells and cerebral oedema develops (c).

Sodium loss
Hypoadrenocorticism
Gastrointestinal loss, e.g. vomiting and/or diarrhoea
Third-spacing of fluid
Pleural effusion, e.g. chylothorax or lung lobe torsion
Peritoneal effusion, e.g. septic or non-septic peritonitis, ruptured bladder
Diuretic administration
Volume overload
Congestive heart failure
Nephrotic syndrome
Liver disease
Advanced renal disease
Hyponatraemia with normovolaemia
Psychogenic polydipsia
Inappropriate fluid therapy, e.g. administration of hypotonic fluids
Inappropriate ADH secretion
Hypothyroid myxoedematous coma
Exercise-associated hyponatraemia
Hyponatraemia due to increase in plasma osmolality
Diabetes mellitus
Mannitol administration
Pseudohyponatraemia
Hyperlipidaemia
Hyperproteinaemia

8.10 The differential diagnoses of hyponatraemia. The most common differentials are shown in italics.

Hyponatraemia due to sodium loss

Hypoadrenocorticism: The most common cause of hyponatraemia due to sodium loss is hypoadrenocorticism. Aldosterone mediates sodium uptake and potassium loss in the distal tubule (see Figure 8.7) so the combination of hyponatraemia with hyperkalaemia provides the classic electrolyte profile for hypoadrenocorticism. In this case, although there is volume depletion, the urine specific gravity and osmolality are inappropriately low. An ACTH-stimulation test would provide confirmation.

Sodium loss with volume depletion due to GI, renal or third space loss: Animals may become hyponatraemic when electrolytes and water are lost concurrently through the GI tract or when fluid moves into a third space, e.g. the pleural or peritoneal cavity, or when renal losses have occurred (Figure 8.11). Although fluid losses, particularly through the GI tract, are usually hypotonic in nature, the subsequent physiological responses (increase in ADH release, increase in thirst, decrease in renal water excretion) serve to dilute the plasma via an increase in water intake and water retention. In volume-depleted animals the urinary specific gravity will be appropriately increased.

Diuretic administration: Animals receiving thiazide and, to a lesser extent, loop diuretics are commonly mildly hyponatraemic. Severe hyponatraemia is unusual, although idiosyncratic reactions can occur. Thiazide diuretics can produce a situation whereby sodium and potassium are lost in excess of water. Electrolyte monitoring is important in animals receiving chronic diuretic therapy.

Hyponatraemia due to volume overload

Congestive heart failure, hepatic failure, nephrotic syndrome and end-stage renal failure: The common feature in these conditions is volume expansion in the face of a perceived, but not true, hypovolaemia. Hyponatraemia results from decreased sodium concentration in an expanded volume. Total body stores of sodium are generally increased.

In congestive heart failure (CHF), as cardiac output falls, renal perfusion and, consequently, GFR decrease. This increases the proximal tubule's ability to reabsorb sodium and water and decreases the tubular flow to more distal sites where tubular fluid would then be diluted to allow water to be excreted. The renin–angiotensin system is rapidly activated and ADH release is precipitated through the stimulation of baroreceptors in the arterial circulation. Volume overload on the venous side of the circulation, though sensed by baroreceptors in the left atrium, fails to prevent ADH release. What is perceived is a volume deficit, although what has really occurred

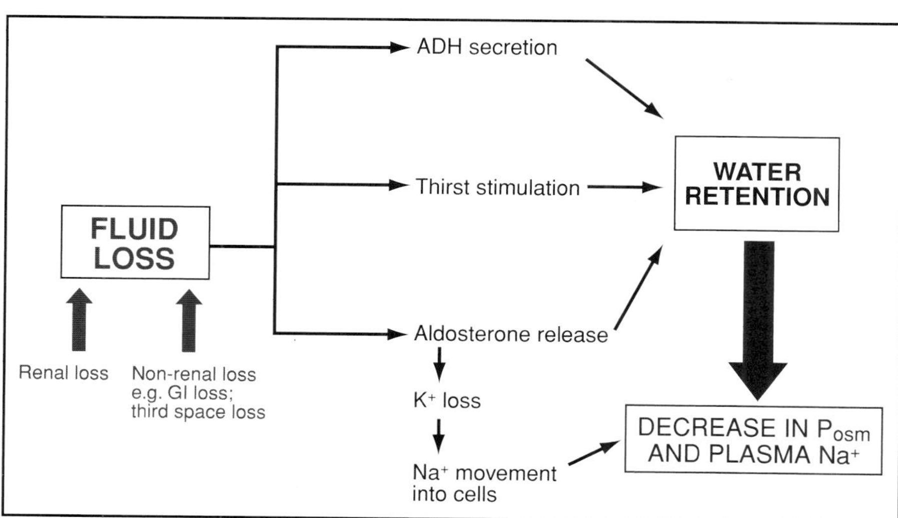

8.11 The mechanism of the development of hyponatraemia through volume depletion via renal and non-renal routes. (P_{osm} = plasma osmolality)

is a redistribution of volume and a decrease in effective volume (i.e. the volume effectively involved in tissue perfusion).

In nephrotic syndrome or where there is hepatic cirrhosis, similar volume redistribution occurs. Reduced plasma protein levels result in reduced plasma oncotic pressure so that water moves into extravascular locations and volume depletion leads again to ADH release. Other mechanisms also contribute to a reduction in circulating volume. In hepatic disease portal hypertension leads to the development of ascites, while arteriovenous shunting reduces the perceived circulating volume. Nephrotic syndrome presents a complex picture in which volume expansion and oedema develop due to sodium retention that is governed by mechanisms other than the renin–angiotensin system (Brown *et al.*, 1982).

In advanced renal failure polydipsia can lead to an excessive water load that the poorly functioning kidneys find difficult to excrete. This results in volume expansion and dilutional hyponatraemia.

Syndrome of inappropriate ADH secretion: Inappropriate ADH release, or potentiation of the effects of ADH, is rarely identified in veterinary patients, although it is widely recognized in human medicine. A recent report describes the syndrome in conjunction with granulomatous meningoencephalitis in a dog (Brofman *et al.*, 2003). When ADH is secreted inappropriately, water is retained and body fluids are, therefore, diluted and expand. This leads to hyponatraemia and hypo-osmolality and also upregulation of the excretion of sodium and water through the activation of volume receptors. This latter effect means that oedema does not occur and that hyponatraemia is the major net result.

Psychogenic polydipsia: Psychogenic polydipsia is usually described in large-breed dogs and is classified as a behavioural problem as there is no deficiency of ADH synthesis, release and function, but the normal control of thirst is overruled (Houpt, 1991). As the daily water consumption increases, water excretion also increases along with renal sodium excretion. Thus both the plasma and urine osmolalities are low. A water deprivation test or modified water deprivation test (designed to correct medullary washout) can identify most cases and can differentiate between psychogenic polydipsia and the ADH deficiency present in central diabetes insipidus (see Chapter 10).

Hypothyroid myxoedematous coma: Both cardiac output and glomerular filtration rate are reduced in hypothyroid animals. In hypothyroid myxoedema this may be pronounced, leading to ADH release and a reduction in flow in the distal tubule of the kidney, stimulating further ADH release. In addition there is movement of water from the intravascular compartment into the interstitium. Hyponatraemia results from a dilutional effect while normal volume is maintained.

Hypotonic fluid administration: Hypotonic fluids are classified as those that result in a net water gain, such as 5% dextrose. When 5% dextrose is infused, the sugar is rapidly taken up by cells leaving an addition of water to the circulation. Much of the water is also redistributed between body compartments so that the circulation is not appreciably expanded. The net result is that the induction of *natriuresis* leads to hyponatraemia in the face of normovolaemia.

Causes of sodium:potassium ratio abnormalities

Although hypoadrenocorticism is the most obvious cause for a reduced sodium:potassium ratio, there are several other commonly encountered causes (Figure 8.12).

Hypoadrenocorticism
Primary gastrointestinal disease including *Trichuris vulpis* infestation and *Toxocara canis* infestation
Pleural, peritoneal or pericardial effusion
Renal failure
Heart failure
Pancreatitis
Diabetic ketoacidosis
Urinary tract rupture
Urinary bladder obstruction
Pyometra
Neoplastic disease
Late gestation pregnancy (Schaer *et al.*, 2001)

8.12 Differential diagnosis of low sodium:potassium ratio.

Disorders of chloride homeostasis

Measuring chloride concentrations

Chloride can be measured in serum or plasma samples using spectrophotometric and colorimetric methods and by using ion-selective electrodes, and should be measured on samples promptly separated from cells.

Lipaemia, hyperbilirubinaemia and haemoglobinaemia can artificially raise the chloride concentration when colorimetric methods are used. Ion-specific electrodes are prone to interference from bromide ions in animals being treated with potassium bromide.

Sodium is the major cation present in the ECF and, for the preservation of electroneutrality, each sodium ion must be balanced with an appropriate anion. Chloride makes up two thirds of the total concentration of anions in the ECF, with bicarbonate the next most prevalent. Thus changes in chloride concentration tend to follow changes in either sodium or bicarbonate concentration, in order to maintain electroneutrality.

Hyperchloraemia

Hyperchloraemia may occur in association with hypernatraemia where there is water loss in excess of sodium loss or excess gain of sodium. Hyperchloraemia without hypernatraemia is generally due to increased loss of bicarbonate into the gut in diarrhoea, or into the kidney in renal tubular acidosis. Both of these situations lead to a non-anion gap (hyperchloraemic) metabolic acidosis (see Chapter 9). Hyperchloraemia may also occur due to increased intake, either iatrogenic (fluid therapy, chloride-containing drugs) or accidental (salt poisoning, see section on hypernatraemia).

Hypochloraemia

Hypochloraemia may occur in association with hyponatraemia as discussed above. In the absence of hyponatraemia, hypochloraemia usually suggests the presence of alkalosis (excess bicarbonate results in a reduction in chloride to maintain electroneutrality) and the clinical signs are secondary to the acid–base disturbance. The most common cause of a metabolic alkalosis and hypochloraemia in small animal practice is the vomiting of stomach contents. Other causes of hypochloraemia include:

- The use of diuretics such as thiazides or loop diuretics (furosemide)
- The administration of any drugs or fluid therapy that contain proportionately more sodium than chloride, e.g. penicillins and sodium bicarbonate; this effect is rarely seen at commonly used dosages
- Hyperadrenocorticism, as steroid hormones increase sodium reabsorption and renal chloride loss
- High anion gap metabolic acidosis (see Chapter 9). Accumulation of unmeasured anions, such as ketones in diabetic ketoacidosis, or in ethylene glycol toxicity, leads to a fall in the measured anions (chloride and bicarbonate) in order to maintain electroneutrality.

Disorders of magnesium homeostasis

Measuring serum magnesium

Only about 1% of total body magnesium is present in serum. Like calcium, the physiologically active form of magnesium is the ionized form that makes up about 70% of the total. Few laboratories offer ionized magnesium measurement so usually total serum levels are used. The drawbacks to this include:

- Variation in total magnesium levels with hyper- and hypoalbuminaemia (compare calcium)
- Poor representation of total body magnesium status through serum measurement
- The occurrence of normal serum magnesium in the face of whole body hypomagnesaemia.

The normal range for total magnesium concentration is 0.59–0.86 mmol/l for dogs and 0.74–1.20 mmol/l for cats (Clinical Pathology Laboratory, Cambridge Veterinary School): published values for both total and ionized magnesium are variable and one should refer to the reference range for the laboratory used.

The importance of magnesium in the body and the consequences of imbalances

Magnesium exists in the body in an intracellular location and, after potassium, is the second most abundant intracellular cation. Magnesium is a critical co-factor for the functioning of the sodium/potassium ATPase pump and thus has an important role in the partitioning of sodium and potassium into their extra- and intracellular compartments respectively. Magnesium is absorbed through the gut and is excreted by the kidneys but no hormone has been found to have a role in regulating the concentration of magnesium in the blood.

The clinical signs of magnesium imbalance have a major impact on the cardiovascular system and the neuromuscular system.

There is little published data or experience in the management of magnesium disorders in veterinary patients, though there is considerable interest in this electrolyte in critical care patients.

Hypermagnesaemia

Hypermagnesaemia is a rare disorder and the primary cause in veterinary medicine is renal failure where the rate of magnesium excretion falls in parallel with the decline in GFR. Other less common causes of hypermagnesaemia include iatrogenic overdose and the endocrinopathies hypoadrenocorticism, hypothyroidism and hyperparathyroidism.

Clinical signs of hypermagnesaemia are not obvious unless the serum concentration is severely elevated. Electrocardiographic changes include prolongation of the PR interval and widening of the QRS complex. This can progress to complete atrioventricular block and asystole. Neuromuscular signs include myotactic hyporeflexia and, in extreme cases, muscle paralysis (Martin, 1998).

Hypomagnesaemia

Many of the conditions that result in hypokalaemia will also cause hypomagnesaemia.

Causes of hypomagnesaemia include:

- GI loss
- Anorexia
- Renal tubular disease
- Hypercalcaemia
- Glucosuria
- Drug administration (diuretics, digoxin, cisplatin and ciclosporin)
- Endocrine disease (hyperthyroidism, hypoparathyroidism)
- Redistribution induced by insulin or catecholamines.

Hypomagnesaemia can cause cardiac arrhythmias and can increase the sensitivity of the heart to digoxin-induced arrhythmias. These arrhythmias may be difficult to control without magnesium as well as potassium supplementation. Neuromuscular signs also occur when there is concurrent hypokalaemia or hypocalcaemia and include muscle weakness, muscle fasciculations, ataxia or seizures.

In metabolic disorders, such as diabetic ketoacidosis, magnesium depletion may cause hypokalaemia that is refractory to potassium supplementation unless magnesium is administered simultaneously (Dhupa and Proulx, 1998). Similarly, in human critical care patients, hypomagnesaemia was identified frequently as either a primary electrolyte disorder or as part of a complex disorder alongside hypokalaemia.

Disorders of calcium homeostasis

Disorders of calcium metabolism are relatively common in small animal practice. As well as causing significant clinical signs which may require urgent treatment, altered plasma calcium concentrations can help refine the differential diagnoses in an animal showing vague clinical signs and can direct subsequent diagnostic evaluation.

Review of calcium metabolism

Calcium is found in three forms within plasma (Ganong, 2001) :

- Physiologically active ionized form (approximately 50%)
- Chelated form complexed with lactate, citrate and bicarbonate (approximately 10%)
- Protein-bound form (approximately 40%). Four times more calcium binds to albumin than to globulin.

The percentage of calcium in each form is variable and depends on albumin and other protein levels, acid–base balance and concentrations of administered potential chelators, such as citrate (Dhupa and Proulx, 1998). An animal's calcium concentration should always be interpreted alongside the albumin concentration. Hypoalbuminaemia can result in a spurious hypocalcaemia (i.e. low total but normal ionized calcium) or mask hypercalcaemia. A correction formula has been described for dogs which adjusts the total calcium concentration to the albumin concentration:

$$\text{Corrected calcium (mg/dl)} = \text{Measured calcium (mg/dl)} - \text{Albumin (g/dl)} + 3.5$$

To use this calculation SI units must first be converted to non-SI units:

- Ca (mmol/l) x 4 = Ca (mg/dl)
- Albumin (g/l) ÷ 10 = Albumin (g/dl)

It is now widely accepted that this formula has limitations and it is not commonly used (Meuten *et al.*, 1982).

Changes in blood pH lead to alterations in the negative charges on protein molecules which, in turn, lead to alterations in the amount of calcium bound to protein. In acidosis, there is a decrease in negative charge on albumin molecules which results in a decreased protein-bound fraction and an increased ionized fraction of calcium, whilst the total calcium is unchanged. The converse is true of alkalosis.

The main hormones involved in the regulation of calcium metabolism in healthy animals are parathyroid hormone (PTH), 1,25 dihydroxyvitamin D (1,25(OH)$_2$D3) and calcitonin (Figure 8.13).

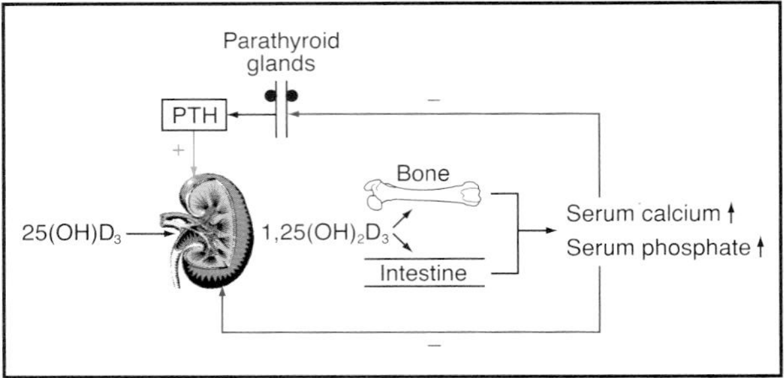

8.13 Feedback control of the formation of 1,25 dihydroxyvitamin D3 (1,25(OH)$_2$D3) from 25 hydroxvitamin D3 (25(OH)D3).

- Parathyroid hormone is secreted by the chief cells in the parathyroid glands and causes plasma calcium concentrations to increase by mobilizing calcium from bone, increasing calcium reabsorption in the distal tubule of the nephron and increasing urinary phosphate excretion. Circulating ionized calcium acts directly on the parathyroid glands in a negative feedback fashion to regulate the secretion of PTH. Increased plasma phosphate concentration stimulates PTH secretion by lowering plasma calcium concentration and inhibiting the formation of 1,25(OH)$_2$D3
- Vitamin D is first metabolized in the liver to 25 hydroxyvitamin D which is then metabolized to 1,25(OH)$_2$D3 in the kidneys. 1,25(OH)$_2$D3 raises serum calcium concentrations by increasing intestinal absorption of calcium, mobilizing calcium from bone and causing calcium reabsorption in the kidney. The formation of 1,25 (OH)$_2$D3 is catalysed by 1α hydroxylase and is regulated by calcium, phosphate and PTH concentrations. 1,25(OH)$_2$D3 formation is facilitated by PTH and inhibited by hyperphosphataemia (Figure 18.13). The less active 24,25 dihydroxyvitamin D is also formed in the kidneys
- Calcitonin is secreted by C cells of the thyroid gland and reduces calcium resorption from the bone thereby lowering plasma calcium concentrations.

A fourth hormone, parathyroid hormone related protein (PTHrP), plays an important role in calcium metabolism, particularly in malignant conditions in humans and dogs (Rosol *et al.*, 1992). PTHrP has a similar structure and function to parathyroid hormone and causes hypercalcaemia by increasing bone resorption and renal tubular resorption of calcium.

Assays used in the investigation of calcium disorders

The pathogenesis of calcium metabolism disorders varies between diseases and has become better understood with the development and validation of hormone assays and routine measurement of ionized calcium concentrations (Refsal *et al.*, 2001).

Total calcium

Total calcium is measured by spectrophotometric methods using serum (preferable) or heparin plasma. Calcium cannot be measured in EDTA, citrate or oxalate plasma as these anticoagulants chelate calcium.

Haemolysis and lipaemia usually result in a false increase, although the effect depends on the assay system being used. Total calcium may be falsely reduced in samples more than 24 hours old. Reference ranges for serum are lower than for plasma because calcium is utilized in clot formation.

Ionized calcium

Ionized calcium concentrations can be measured by an ion-specific electrode (e.g. in a laboratory or patient-side analyser). Ionized calcium concentrations can be altered by *in vitro* changes in sample pH: red cell metabolism results in lactic acid formation, reduced pH and, thus, increased ionized calcium; conversely evaporation of carbon dioxide (CO_2) from the sample results in increased pH and, thus, decreased ionized calcium. Ionized calcium should be measured immediately after collection. Alternatively, sample into a heparin vacutainer, immediately separate the plasma and then place in a closed tube with no space above the sample, preventing CO_2 evaporation. Serum gel tubes should not be used as the gel contains calcium. Some laboratories process standard serum or heparin and then correct for the altered pH using a chemical formula. This assumes that the patient's pH is normal and so can be misleading: if the patient was acidotic or alkalotic the adjusted ionized calcium will not be a true reflection of the plasma concentration in the animal.

Parathyroid hormone assays

A two-site immunoradiometric PTH assay has been validated for both the dog and cat (Torrance and Nachreiner, 1989; Barber *et al.*, 1993). PTH is a labile protein and care has to be taken in the transportation of the sample to the laboratory; it is advisable to discuss specific requirements with the laboratory. Usually, the sample is collected into EDTA, the plasma separated immediately and stored frozen (–20°C is adequate for short-term shortage). The plasma should be delivered to the laboratory frozen in special freezer packs (usually supplied by the laboratory; see Chapter 18). PTH tends to be markedly elevated in primary hyperparathyroidism and chronic renal failure. PTH is also elevated in hyperadrenocorticism, probably due to increased urinary excretion of calcium; however, ionized and total calcium concentrations are normally within the reference ranges (Ramsey and Herrtage, 2001).

Parathyroid hormone-related protein

Recent studies have clinically validated a two-site immunoradiometric assay for parathyroid hormone-related protein (PTHrP) in both dogs and cats (Bolliger *et al.*, 2002; Mellanby *et al.*, 2003a). The assay uses two different antibodies to human PTHrP which are specific for different, well defined regions of the PTHrP molecule. The two-site assays are generally considered to be superior to assays which only detect one region of the PTHrP molecule since the two-site assays are more likely to measure intact PTHrP rather than PTHrP fragments. A radioimmunoassay has also been validated in the dog, although this assay is not currently commercially available (Rosol *et al.*, 1992). PTHrP is also a labile protein and should be handled in the same careful fashion as PTH. The majority of hypercalcaemic dogs with an underlying malignancy have an elevated PTHrP concentration. In contrast, dogs with hypercalcaemia associated with chronic renal failure or primary hyperparathyroidism due to a parathyroid adenoma do not have an elevated PTHrP concentrations (Mellanby *et al.*, 2003a). There is no correlation between PTHrP concentration and the degree of hypercalcaemia (either ionized or total calcium).

Vitamin D

The measurement of serum 25 hydroxyvitamin D concentration by high performance liquid chromatography and 1,25$(OH)_2$D3 concentrations by radioimmunoassay has recently been described in dogs (Rumbeiha *et al.*, 1999; Gerber *et al.*, 2003; Mellanby *et al.*, 2003b). Separated serum is sent overnight to The Supraregional Assay Service Vitamin D Laboratory, University Department of Medicine, Manchester Royal Infirmary, Oxford Road, Manchester, M13 9WL. Based on a small number of clinically normal adult dogs, the provisional reference ranges for 25(OH)D3 and 1,25$(OH)_2$D3 are 19.3–43.6 ng/ml and 16.0–40.0 pg/ml, respectively.

Calcitonin

A radioimmunoassay has been developed for canine calcitonin, but is not currently available. Disorders of altered calcitonin secretion in small animals have not been described (Rosol *et al.*, 1995).

Hypercalcaemia

Hypercalcaemia in dogs

The clinical signs of hypercalcaemia vary depending on the underlying cause, although neuromuscular, GI, renal and cardiac systems are most commonly affected (Nelson, 2003). One of the most important effects of hypercalcaemia is the inhibition of ADH which leads to an inability to concentrate urine and causes polyuria and polydipsia. Urine specific gravity may be isosthenuric or hyposthenuric. If the animal fails to drink enough water to compensate for the increased urinary water loss, dehydration will develop with resultant prerenal azotaemia. Long-standing or severe hypercalcaemia, especially if accompanied by hyperphosphataemia, may result in renal tubular damage and an intrinsic renal azotaemia. Consequently, it is difficult to distinguish prerenal and renal azotaemia in animals with hypercalcaemia, since the urine specific gravity will be lowered in both situations. Other clinical signs can include lethargy, muscle weakness, seizures, inappetance, vomiting, constipation, diarrhoea and cardiac arrhythmias. Clinical signs maybe mild, especially in cases of primary hyperparathyroidism when the hypercalcaemia may be first detected accidentally, often when biochemistry panels are performed for unrelated reasons (Nelson, 2003).

The most common causes of hypercalcaemia in the dog are malignancy, hypoadrenocorticism, primary hyperparathyroidism and renal failure (Figure 8.14). These four disorders accounted for 95% of dogs in a series of 40 cases of hypercalcaemia (Elliott *et al.*, 1991). Lymphoma and anal sac adenocarcinomas are

Disease	Pathophysiological mechanism	Comments
Malignancy	Frequently, but not invariably, due to ectopic production of PTHrp	Total and ionized hypercalcaemia tends to be marked. PTH concentration is usually suppressed
Primary hyperparathyroidism	Due to excessive production of PTH by a parathyroid tumour (usually adenoma). PTHrp concentration is usually within reference range	Hypercalcaemia tends to be marked and ionized calcium is elevated. Phosphate concentration tends to be low or low normal
Chronic renal failure	Precise mechanism is poorly understood – maybe due to autonomous production of PTH or altered calcium set point	Hypercalcaemia tends to be mild and ionized calcium is usually within the reference range. 1,25 $(OH)_2D3$ concentration is often low. PTH is elevated
Hypoadrenocorticism	Precise mechanism is poorly understood	Hypercalcaemia is found in approximately one third of all cases. Urea, phosphate and creatinine are commonly elevated. Ionized calcium can be elevated or normal
Young animal	Bone remodelling	Hypercalcaemia tends to be mild and associated with mild elevations in phosphate and alkaline phosphatase
Less common causes		
Hypervitaminosis D	Elevated vitamin D metabolites cause hypercalcaemia and frequently hyperphosphataemia. Ionized calcium is elevated and PTH is usually suppressed	Can occur due to rodenticide poisoning or in management of hypoparathyroidism. Hypercalcaemia can be marked and animals are frequently at risk of soft tissue mineralization due to concurrent elevated phosphate
Granulomatous diseases	Commonly observed in humans – hypercalcaemia considered to be due to dysregulated production of 1,25 $(OH)_2D3$ by macrophages in granulomatous lesions; limited data supports this mechanism in both dogs and cats. PTH usually suppressed	Reported in only a handful of cases. Elevated PTHrp concentrations have been associated with two hypercalcaemic dogs with granulomatous diseases (Fradkin *et al.*, 2001)

8.14 Causes and pathophysiology of hypercalcaemia in dogs.

two of the most common causes of malignancy-related hypercalcaemia. Other, less commonly recognized causes of hypercalcaemia include hypervitaminosis D, granulomatous diseases, non-malignant skeletal disease, dehydration, juvenile animals and laboratory error (Nelson, 2003).

Malignancy: Lymphoma is one of the most common canine neoplasms and is the most common cause of malignancy-related hypercalcaemia (Figure 8.15). Hypercalcaemic dogs with lymphoma tend to have elevated concentrations of PTHrP, in contrast to normocalcaemic dogs with lymphoma, which have low or undetectable concentrations of PTHrP (Figure 8.16) (Mellanby *et al.*, 2003a). PTH concentrations tend to be suppressed. However, not all hypercalcaemic dogs have elevated PTHrP concentrations and elevated concentrations of 1,25$(OH)_2$D3 and prostaglandins have been implicated in the pathogenesis of malignancy-related hypercalcaemia in humans. Hypercalcaemia is also associated with other lymphoproliferative diseases, such as multiple myeloma and leukaemia.

Anal sac adenocarcinoma are arguably the second most common cause of malignancy-related hypercalcaemia and typically affect older dogs. The reported incidence of hypercalcaemia varies between 25 and 90% of all cases and, in some instances, the tumour is not detected until hypercalcaemia-related problems develop (Bennett *et al.*, 2002; Williams *et al.*, 2003). Again, ectopic production of PTHrP by the tumour appears to be the cause of the hypercalcaemia in most cases.

A large number of other tumours have been associated with hypercalcaemia. These included thymoma, pulmonary carcinoma, nasal carcinoma, malignant melanoma, multiple myeloma and leukaemia (Matus *et al.*, 1986; Rosol *et al.*, 1992; Foley *et al.*, 2000; Kleiter *et al.*, 2001; Pressler *et al.*, 2002).

Since hypercalcaemia of malignancy is largely PTHrp driven, both total and ionized calcium are elevated whilst phosphate is usually low or low normal.

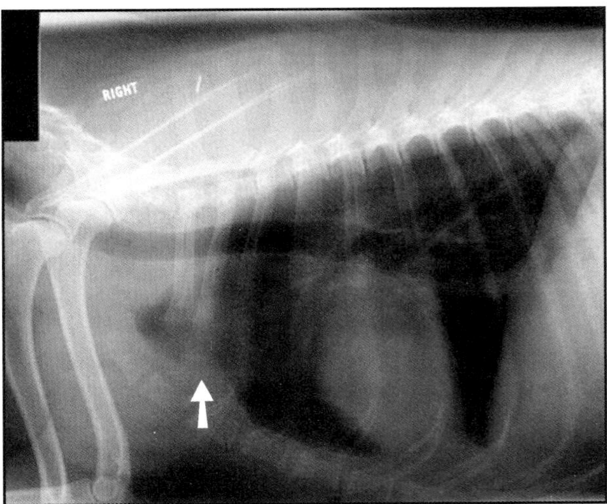

8.15 Right lateral radiograph showing a soft tissue mass in the cranial thorax (arrowed). Fine needle aspirates were obtained and a cytological diagnosis of lymphoma was made.

	Primary hyperparathyroidism	Malignancy-associated hypercalcaemia	Hypervitaminosis D	Chronic renal failure
Total calcium	↑	↑	↑	↑ or N or ↓
Ionized calcium	↑	↑	↑	↓ or N
Phosphate	N or ↓ (May be elevated if there is azotaemia secondary to hypercalcaemia)	N or ↓ (May be elevated if there is azotaemia secondary to hypercalcaemia)	N or ↑	↑
Urea/creatinine	N or ↑	N or ↑	N or ↑	↑
	(May be elevated with hypercalcaemia of any cause due to dehydration and in severe, prolonged hypercalcaemia due to renal tubular damage)			
PTH	↑	↓	↓	↑
PTHrp	N	↑ (usually)	N	N
1,25 $(OH)_2D3$	n/a	n/a	↑ or N or ↓ (depends on nature of vitamin D toxin)	↓
25 (OH)D	n/a	n/a	N or ↑ (depends on nature of vitamin D toxin)	N or ↑

8.16 Typical biochemical and hormonal changes in common causes of hypercalcaemia (↑, increased; ↓, decreased; N, normal; n/a, no data) (Bruyette and Feldman, 1988; Barber and Elliot, 1998; Gerber *et al.*, 2003; Mellanby *et al.*, 2003a,b).

Primary hyperparathyroidism: Primary hyperparathyroidism is a well recognized cause of hypercalcaemia in dogs (Figure 8.17). Hypercalcaemia is often found incidentally when the dog has a biochemistry profile for another reason. Most dogs are middle-aged to elderly and the Keeshond is over-represented. In the majority of cases the disease is caused by a single parathyroid adenoma, although parathyroid gland carcinomas have also been recognized. When present, clinical signs include polyuria, polydipsia, listlessness and muscle weakness (Berger and Feldman, 1987). As well as a moderate to marked hypercalcaemia, most dogs with primary hyperparathyroidism have low or low normal phosphate concentrations and a moderate to marked elevation in PTH (Figure 8.16). The presentation of dogs with primary hyperparathyroidism can be biochemically very similar to dogs with secondary hyperparathyroidism due to chronic renal failure; both conditions may have elevated total plasma calcium, urea, creatinine and PTH concentrations and produce urine which is isosthenuric. In these cases measurement of ionized calcium is advisable, as it is elevated in dogs with primary hyperparathyroidism whereas it is frequently normal in dogs with chronic renal failure. Also, in chronic renal failure phosphate is elevated, whilst in primary hyperparathyroidism phosphate is expected to be low, although this may be offset by reduced renal excretion of phosphate due to renal damage caused by the hypercalcaemia. Thus normal or even elevated phosphate concentrations may be seen in azotaemic dogs with primary hyperparathyroidism.

Ultrasonography of the ventral neck can be very helpful in the detection of an enlarged parathyroid gland (Wisner *et al.*, 1993). Because the autonomous parathyroid adenoma causes suppression of the other three parathyroid glands, hypocalcaemia is a common postoperative complication. Vitamin D supplementation is therefore usually given a few days before surgery and continued after surgery, and plasma calcium concentration should be closely monitored.

Chronic renal failure: Chronic renal failure is usually associated with normocalcaemia or hypocalcaemia, Typically, renal dysfunction leads to serum phosphate retention due to decreased glomerular filtration. This leads to a fall in ionized calcium since the blood ionized

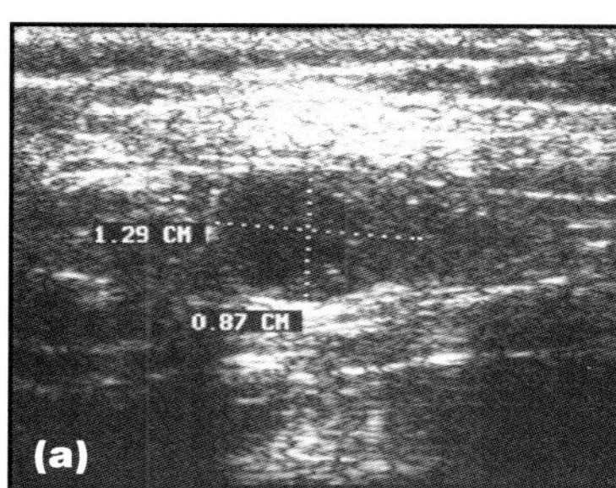

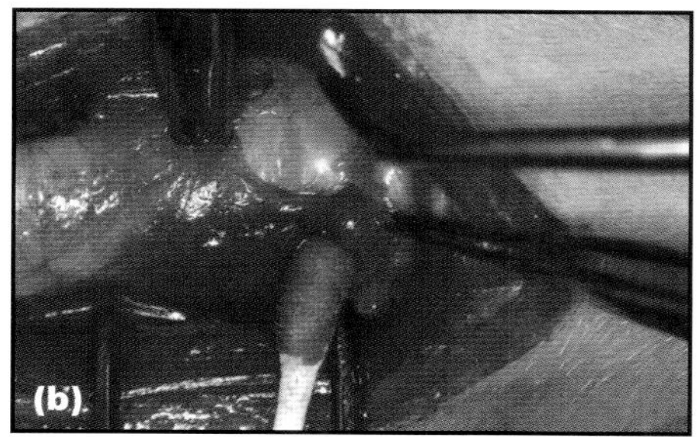

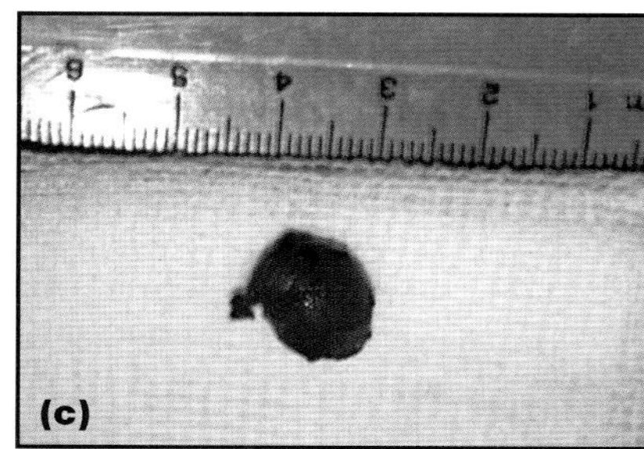

8.17 (a) Ultrasonography of the thyroid gland frequently detects parathyroid nodules in dogs with primary hyperparathyroidism. (b) Appearance of parathyroid adenoma during surgery. (Courtesy of N. Bacon.) (c) Parathyroid gland adenoma following surgical excision.

calcium x phosphate product must remain constant. Elevated phosphate inhibits 1α hydroxylase resulting in reduced formation of $1,25(OH)_2D3$. In addition the failing kidney has a reduced capacity to produce 1α hydroxylase, further contributing to lowered $1,25 (OH)_2D3$, which leads to reduced absorption of calcium from the intestine. These factors result in a decrease in plasma calcium concentration and an increase in parathyroid hormone. This initially results in a return of calcium to normal but, as renal dysfunction worsens, this negative feedback may become insufficient to maintain plasma calcium concentrations and hypocalcaemia develops. Thus the hallmarks of chronic renal failure are azotaemia, hyperphosphataemia, mild hypocalcaemia and isosthenuria.

Although chronic renal failure is typically associated with normocalcaemia or hypocalcaemia, in a small proportion of cases the patient becomes hypercalcaemic. The aetiology of hypercalcaemia associated with chronic renal failure, however, is poorly understood; it may be due to autonomous secretion of PTH, a raised set point for calcium autoregulation or increased binding of calcium to retained anions, such as citrate or phosphate. As discussed above, ionized calcium is usually normal in renal failure, although on occasion it may be elevated.

Hypoadrenocorticism: Hypoadrenocorticism was the second most common cause of hypercalcaemia in one large series of hypercalcaemic dogs and approximately 30% of dogs with hypoadrenocorticism present with hypercalcaemia (Elliot *et al.*, 1991; Peterson *et al.*, 1996). The hypercalcaemia tends to be mild and the aetiology is unclear.

Miscellaneous causes: Young animals often have a mild hypercalcaemia and hyperphosphataemia. Hypercalcaemia is also associated with vitamin D intoxication. This can develop following ingestion of vitamin D-containing rodenticides, or may be iatrogenic due to overzealous dietary supplementation, treatment of hypoparathyroidism or following ingestion of topical preparations for the treatment of psoriasis. The principal effect of excessive consumption of vitamin D is increased GI absorption of calcium and phosphate leading to hypercalcaemia and hyperphosphataemia. Ionized calcium concentrations will be elevated and PTH concentration should be suppressed. Hypercalcaemia is occasionally associated with granulomatous diseases, such as blastomycosis and schistosomiasis (Dow *et al.*, 1986; Fradkin *et al.*, 2001; Mellanby *et al.*, 2003b). The precise mechanism of the hypercalcaemia associated with granulomatous diseases in small animals is ill defined but may be due to excessive production of $1,25(OH)_2D3$ by macrophages. The hypercalcaemia is often mild and should resolve with appropriate treatment of the underlying disease. Again, ionized calcium concentration is elevated and PTH is suppressed.

Hypercalcaemia in cats

There are many similarities in the causes of hypercalcaemia between cats and dogs but there are also some important differences. The most frequently recorded clinical signs are anorexia and lethargy, with polydipsia and polyuria being less commonly noted (Figure 8.18) (Elliott *et al.*, 1991; Savary *et al.*, 2000).

Clinical sign	Noted frequency (%) in hypercalcaemic dogs	Noted frequency (%) in hypercalcaemic cats
Anorexia	88	70
Polydipsia/ polyuria	68	24
Vomiting	53	18
Muscular weakness or twitching	23	0

8.18 Clinical signs noted in hypercalcaemic dogs and cats (Elliot *et al.*, 1991; Savary *et al.*, 2000).

In cats, malignancy and renal failure appear to be the most common causes of hypercalcaemia (Savary *et al.*, 2000). Squamous cell carcinoma is associated with hypercalcaemia as frequently as lymphoma, in contrast to dogs, where lymphoma is the most common cause of malignancy-related hypercalcaemia. Anal sac adenocarcinomas are very infrequently diagnosed in cats and there are no published reports of hypercalcaemia associated with these tumours. Hypercalcaemia has also been associated with a wide range of other neoplastic disorders including multiple myeloma, leukaemia, bronchogenic carcinoma and various sarcomas (Savary *et al.*, 2000).

As in dogs, hypercalcaemia is occasionally observed in cats with chronic renal failure and the underlying mechanism for hypercalcaemia is poorly understood. There are only a very small number of reported cases of hypercalcaemia associated with feline hypoadrenocorticism (Peterson *et al.*, 1989). Primary hyperparathyroidism has been reported in small numbers of Domestic Shorthair and Siamese cats, and, as in dogs, is characterized by autonomous secretion of PTH by a parathyroid adenoma: these animals have a normal or high PTH in the face of hypercalcaemia (Kallet *et al.*, 1991). Dietary factors may contribute to hypercalcaemia: for example, long-term use of phosphate-restricted diets in animals without renal disease often results in hypophosphataemia and compensatory mild hypercalcaemia.

Idiopathic hypercalcaemia is emerging as an important differential of hypercalcaemia in cats (Midkiff *et al.*, 2000). It is a diagnosis reserved for cats where the underlying cause of the hypercalcaemia cannot be identified despite extensive diagnostic evaluation and long-term follow-up. Affected cats tend to be young to middle-aged and longhaired cats may be predisposed. Both total and ionized calcium are moderately increased and plasma PTH concentrations are normal or low, with normal PTHrP concentrations. Feline idiopathic hypercalcaemia has also been associated with calcium oxalate urolithiasis. An association between acidifying diets and hypercalcaemia has also been noted. It is important to rule out known causes of hypercalcaemia in suspected cases of idiopathic hypercalcaemia prior to symptomatic treatment. Prednisolone may reduce plasma calcium concentrations, although the long-term prognosis remains guarded.

Diagnostic approach to hypercalcaemia

There is no well defined, universally accepted strategy for the evaluation of small animals with hypercalcaemia, but the following evaluations are often included:

- Thorough history
- Careful clinical examination
- Serum/plasma biochemistry
- Imaging techniques to identify neoplasia (or granulomatous lesions), including ultrasonography of the ventral neck if primary hyperparathyroidism is suspected.

Ultimately PTH, PTHrP and vitamin D metabolite assays will not only allow the clinician to understand the pathogenesis of the hypercalcaemia in individual cases, but, in many cases, will be required before a firm diagnosis can be made (see Figure 8.16). Elevated PTH concentrations in a generally well dog with marked hypercalcaemia, normal urea and creatinine, low phosphate and a single parathyroid nodule on ultrasonography are indicative of primary hyperparathyroidism. Elevated PTHrP and low PTH concentrations are highly suggestive of an underlying neoplasia. Hypervitaminosis D can be confirmed as the cause of hypercalcaemia if vitamin D metabolites are elevated and the PTH concentration is suppressed. Figure 8.16 summarizes the biochemical and hormonal changes seen in common causes of hypercalcaemia and Figure 8.19 outlines a suggested approach to hypercalcaemia, although the investigations depend on the initial clinical findings and biochemistry results.

Hypocalcaemia

Clinical signs

The clinical signs of hypocalcaemia vary, depending on the underlying cause. Animals can be asymptomatic, although many animals predominantly show signs of neurological dysfunction, directly attributable to a hypocalcaemia-induced increase in neuronal excitability. These include nervousness, behavioural changes, focal muscle twitching (especially ear and facial muscles), facial rubbing, muscle cramps, stiff gait, tetany and

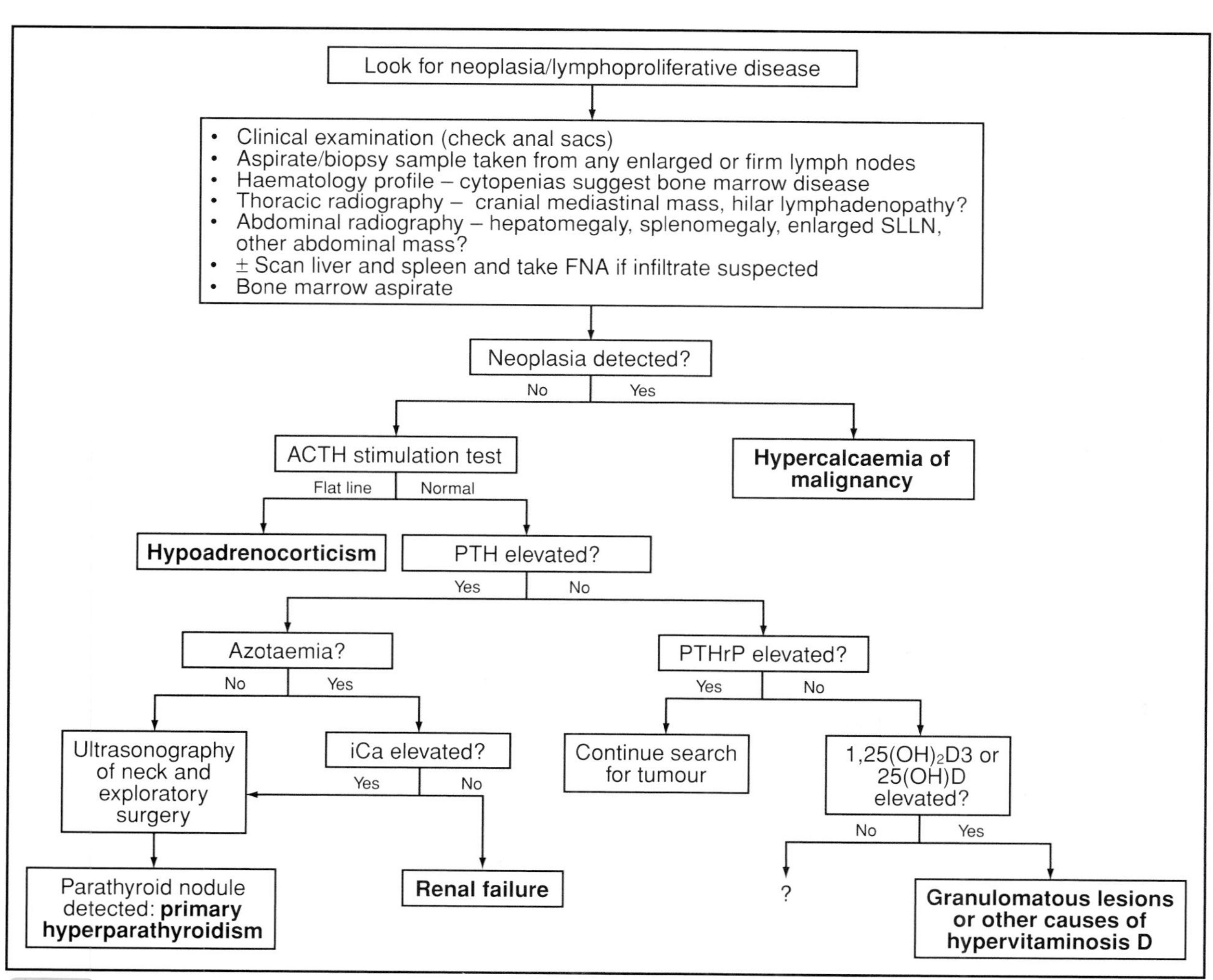

8.19 Diagnostic approach to hypercalcaemia.

seizures. Exercise, excitement and stress may induce or worsen clinical signs. Additional clinical signs may include fever, cataracts and cardiac abnormalities, such as tachyarrhythmias (Nelson, 2003).

Causes of hypocalcaemia

Hypocalcaemia has been reported in a variety of clinical conditions and occurs when there is either impaired PTH secretion or action, impaired vitamin D synthesis or action, or in cases of calcium precipitation or chelation (Figure 8.20) (Dhupa and Proulx, 1998).

Hypoalbuminaemia: This is a common cause of hypocalcaemia; the hypocalcaemia is normally not of clinical significance as ionized calcium is not decreased.

Impaired PTH secretion: Idiopathic primary hypoparathyroidism can result in severe hypocalcaemia (Bruyette and Feldmann, 1988). Primary hypoparathyroidism is rare, but iatrogenic hypoparathyroidism may occur in cats due to damage of the parathyroid gland during thyroidectomy. Again this may cause severe hypocalcaemia.

Increased calcium loss: Eclampsia occurs most commonly in young, small dogs although any age or breed may be affected. The syndrome is relatively rare in cats. Clinical signs are usually seen 2 weeks post whelping (i.e. at peak lactation) due to a combination of massive calcium loss through lactation and fetal drain of calcium during fetal skeleton ossification. Other speculated causative factors include parathyroid gland atrophy and poor dietary supply of calcium (Drobatz and Casey, 2000).

Vitamin D deficiency: Inadequate dietary vitamin D is a rare cause of hypocalcaemia. Chronic renal failure in both dogs and cats may lead to mild hypocalcaemia, usually with normal ionized calcium (Barber and Elliott, 1998), due to reduced 1,25(OH)$_2$D3 (see above).

Reduced intestinal absorption of Vitamin D (a fat-soluble vitamin) in dogs and cats with a protein-losing enteropathy or exocrine pancreatic insufficiency, may lead to mild hypocalcaemia (Mellanby *et al.*, 2003b). Hypoalbuminaemia contributes to the hypocalcaemia.

Precipitation or chelation of calcium: Causes of precipitation or chelation of calcium are listed below.

- **Ethylene glycol toxicity:** calcium binding to oxalic acid in the renal tubules leads to calcium oxalate crystalluria and increased renal loss of calcium.
- **Acute renal failure:** rapidly rising phosphate complexes with calcium leading to hypocalcaemia. Increased renal tubular loss of calcium exacerbates hypocalcaemia.
- **Urinary tract obstruction:** mild to moderate hypocalcaemia may be due to increased binding of calcium to phosphate.
- **Phosphate enemas:** have been reported to cause hypocalcaemia in cats due to rapidly rising serum phosphate levels.
- **Acute tumour lysis syndrome:** hypocalcaemia may result from phosphate (released from lysed cells) binding calcium.

Disease	Pathophysiological mechanism	Comments
Acute renal failure Chronic renal failure	Rapidly rising phosphate complexes with calcium leading to hypocalcaemia. Increased renal tubular loss of calcium exacerbates hypocalcaemia Reduced 1,25 (OH)$_2$D3 production	Azotaemia, elevated phosphate
Hypoparathyroidism	Reduced PTH production by parathyroid gland	Both ionized and total calcium reduced. Phosphate concentration tends to be elevated, PTH concentration inappropriately low for hypocalcaemic condition
Pancreatitis	Precise mechanism ill defined but maybe due to sequestration of calcium in peripancreatic fat, as a result of saponification, or in soft tissues	Increasing severity of ionized hypocalcaemia has been correlated with poorer prognosis (Kimmel *et al*,. 2001)
Hypoalbuminaemia	Since 40% per cent of total calcium is albumin bound, hypoalbuminemia leads to a reduced total calcium concentration	Ionized calcium is normal
Eclampsia	Speculated causes include parathyroid gland atrophy, poor dietary sources of calcium, massive calcium loss through lactation and fetal drain of calcium during fetal skeleton ossification	Occurs most commonly in young, small dogs 2 weeks post whelping
Protein-losing enteropathies	Hypocalcaemia maybe due to hypoalbuminaemia alone; however, many cases of lymphangiectasia have low ionized calcium concentrations. This maybe due to vitamin D malabsorption or to hypomagnesaemia leading to impaired PTH secretion or altered PTH action	

8.20 Causes and pathophysiology of hypocalcaemia in dogs.

- **Pancreatitis:** hypocalcaemia may result from sequestration of calcium in peripancreatic fat or in soft tissues as a result of saponification. Increasing severity of ionized hypocalcaemia has been correlated with poorer prognosis in cats with acute pancreatitis (Kimmel *et al.*, 2001).
- **Blood transfusion:** citrate chelation of calcium may lead to hypocalcaemia (Juktowitz *et al.*, 2002). This is only likely to occur if several units are transfused or if blood collection bags are underfilled, resulting in citrate excess (this most commonly occurs when inappropriate volumes of blood are collected into the full volume of anticoagulant and subsequently administered to a small patient).

Spurious hypocalcaemia can be seen with sample contamination by EDTA when the tip of the syringe becomes contaminated with potassium EDTA as it touches the inside of the tube. The rest of the sample is then injected into the serum or plasma tube along with the potassium EDTA. This causes a combination of low calcium, low alkaline phosphatase and high potassium. Total calcium may fall in samples which have been stored for over 24 hours before analysis.

Diagnostic approach to hypocalcaemia

The list of the common differentials for hypocalcaemia is relatively short and the history, physical examination findings, haematology, biochemistry and urinalysis are often very helpful in establishing the cause of the hypocalcaemia (Figure 8.21). Bile acids may be helpful in evaluating liver function in cases of hypoalbuminaemia (see Chapter 12). Trypsin-like immunoreactivity and/or canine pancreatic lipase are useful if pancreatic disease is suspected (see Chapter 14). Abdominal imaging maybe helpful to evaluate the patient for GI, liver and renal diseases and pancreatitis. PTH is required definitively to confirm cases of primary hypoparathyroidism. Primary hypoparathyroidism is the most likely diagnosis in a non-lactating, non-azotaemic, hyperphosphataemic dog with clinical signs of hypocalcaemia (Nelson, 2003).

Disease process	Total calcium (tCa)	Ionized calcium(iCa)	Other laboratory abnormalities
Hypoalbuminaemia	↓	N	Low albumin
Hypoparathyroidism	↓	↓	↑ Phosphate, low normal to low PTH
Chronic renal failure	↓	N	↑ Phosphate, urea, creatinine Non-regenerative anaemia
Protein-losing enteropathy	↓	N or ↓	↓ Albumin, globulin, N or ↓ Cholesterol
Exocrine pancreatic insufficiency	↓	N or ↓	↓ Albumin Low trypsin-like immunoreactivity
Ethylene glycol toxicity	↓	↓	↑ Urea, creatinine, phosphate ↓ Glucose, pH Calcium oxalate crystalluria
Acute renal failure	↓	N or ↓	↑ Urea, creatinine, phosphate oliguria or anuria
Pancreatitis	↓	↓	↑ Amylase, lipase ± ↑ Urea, creatinine, phosphate Inflammatory leucogram

8.21 Biochemical changes in selected causes of hypocalcaemia (↑, increased; ↓, decreased; N, normal).

Case examples

Case 1

Signalment

9-year-old male, neutered Lhasa Apso.

History

Polyuria, polydipsia and weight loss. More recently he has become dull and depressed and inappetent. He is now vomiting and collapsed.

Clinical pathology data

Biochemistry	Result	Reference interval
pH	7.195	7.38–7.43
P_vCO_2 (mmHg)	27.1	35–45 ▶

Biochemistry *(continued)*	Result	Reference interval
Sodium (mmol/l)	132.4	135–155
Potassium (mmol/l)	4.0	3.5–5.8
Glucose (mmol/l)	32.0	3.4–5.3
Ionized calcium (mmol/l)	1.40	1.18–1.40
Bicarbonate (mmol/l)	14.3	20–24

Case 1 continues ▶

Case 1 continued

Urine analysis

Dipstick: 4+ ketones, 4+ glucose, no other abnormalities

What abnormalities are present?

- Acidaemia
- Low bicarbonate
- Low P_vCO_2
- Hyponatraemia
- Hyperglycaemia
- Glucosuria
- Ketonuria.

How would you interpret these results and what is the most likely diagnosis?

Acidaemia with a low bicarbonate concentration indicates that there is a metabolic acidosis. If this were the case then a reduced P_vCO_2 would be predicted, caused by hyperventilation to get rid of the excess CO_2 and allow respiratory compensation for the metabolic acidosis to occur.

Hyponatraemia is caused by a combination of urinary loss due to polyuria and dilutional hyponatraemia, whereby an expansion of the extracellular fluid occurs through water movement out of cells. This water movement is provoked by the high extracellular glucose concentration. In this case the polyuria is likely to be an osmotic diuresis caused by the high glucose concentration.

Urine analysis reveals glucosuria, which is unsurprising given the blood glucose concentration, and also ketonuria.

The most likely diagnosis is that this dog has diabetic ketoacidosis (DKA).

What further tests would you recommend?

- Measure urea and creatinine to assess renal function
- Measure phosphate concentration
- Assess other major organ function, e.g. liver, pancreas
- Look for a focus of infection/inflammation that may have precipitated the DKA crisis:
  - Haematology profile
  - Urine culture
  - Blood culture
  - ± Radiography and ultrasonography depending on the body system involved.

Continue to monitor glucose, electrolytes and blood gas parameters to assess ongoing treatment.

Treatment and further tests

Therapy was initiated using 0.2 IU/kg soluble insulin and 0.9% NaCl. Two hours after the start of treatment venous blood gas measurement was repeated:

Biochemistry	Result	Reference interval
pH	7.225	7.38–7.43
P_vCO_2 (mmHg)	24.9	35–45
Sodium (mmol/l)	143.3	135–155
Potassium (mmol/l)	3.2	3.5–5.8
Glucose (mmol/l)	21.6	3.4–5.3
Ionized calcium (mmol/l)	1.40	1.18–1.40
Bicarbonate (mmol/l)	16.2	20–24

After treatment, what abnormalities are present?

- Acidaemia
- Low bicarbonate
- Low P_vCO_2
- Hypokalaemia
- Hyperglycaemia.

What has caused these abnormalities?

The blood gas abnormalities are still present, although they have improved in comparison to the original blood gas picture. The pCO_2 has fallen still lower as respiratory compensation becomes more marked.

The blood glucose has dropped markedly after insulin administration.

Hypokalaemia has now developed after the onset of treatment while the hyponatraemia has resolved. Hypokalaemia in this setting is due to the intracellular movement of potassium stimulated by insulin. Partial resolution of the hyperglycaemia will also contribute, as there will be less solvent drag to encourage potassium movement out of the cells. As potassium has now been redistributed, a potassium deficit has been unmasked and the dog is hypokalaemic.

Case summary

Hypokalaemia could have been avoided in this case if potassium had been added to the fluid therapy used initially. Diabetic animals are usually normokalaemic or hypokalaemic when initially assessed but frequently become severely hypokalaemic once fluids and insulin are given. By supplementing potassium in the intravenous fluids from the beginning, severe hypokalaemia can be avoided. It must be remembered that electrolytes are constantly in flux and can change rapidly. Close monitoring of electrolytes in DKA patients is advisable, as hypokalaemia can result in severe weakness, gut stasis and can predispose to cardiac arrhythmias. Hypophosphataemia, due to the intracellular movement of phosphorus, can also be precipitated once treatment has begun and generally occurs on the second day of treatment. The signs of hypophosphataemia include muscle weakness, gut stasis, anorexia and vomiting. Red blood cell fragility is increased by a lack of adenosine triphosphate (ATP) within the erythrocyte and, in severe cases, haemolysis can occur.

Case 2

Signalment

2-year-old male, neutered Cairn Terrier.

History

Reported to have had some neurological problems (bizarre behaviour, head pressing) as a puppy. Several week history of vomiting and diarrhoea, peculiar behaviour and a reluctance to drink. Clinical examination shows him to be thin but very bright and with minimal signs of dehydration.

Clinical pathology data

Haematological parameters were unremarkable.

Biochemistry	Result	Reference interval
Sodium (mmol/l)	187.2	135–155
Potassium (mmol/l)	4.25	3.50–5.80
Chloride (mmol/l)	149	105–120
Glucose (mmol/l)	6.0	3.0–5.0
Urea (mmol/l)	9.4	3.3–8.0 ▶

Case 2 continues ▶

Case 2 continued

Biochemistry *(continued)*	Result	Reference interval
Creatinine (μmol/l)	135	45–150
Calcium (mmol/l)	2.80	2.30–2.80
Inorganic phosphate (mmol/l)	1.27	0.60–1.30
TP (g/l)	67.2	60.0–80.0
Albumin (g/l)	40.0	25.0–40.0
Globulin (g/l)	27.2	20.0–45.0
ALT (IU/l)	29	21–59
ALP (IU/l)	323	3–142

Urine analysis

Urine specific gravity >1.050
Dipstick: unremarkable

What abnormalities are present?

- Marked hypernatraemia
- Hyperchloraemia
- Mild elevation in urea.

How would you interpret these results and what are the likely differential diagnoses?

Hypernatraemia with few or no signs of dehydration can be caused by:

- Increased sodium intake (sea water and salt ingestion or via inappropriate fluid therapy)
- Primary adipsia or essential hypernatraemia
- Diabetes insipidus.

In this case, the absence of thirst and reluctance to drink had been remarked upon by the owner, even after bouts of vomiting and diarrhoea that would be assumed would make the dog still more hypernatraemic and dehydrated. This dog can concentrate its urine, evidenced by the fact that the urine specific gravity is high. The concurrent gastrointestinal disease seemed to be the precipitating problem that led the owner to seek veterinary help. This dog had displayed similar neurological signs at a young age but these had not persisted and had not been investigated further. Given this history and the severe hypernatraemia coupled to a lack of thirst, it seems most likely that this dog has primary adipsia or essential hypernatraemia.

What further tests would you recommend?

- Brain magnetic resonance imaging (MRI)
- Cerebrospinal fluid (CSF) analysis.

Case summary

Primary adipsia is caused by dysfunction of the osmoreceptors of the hypothalamus such that they do not respond appropriately to an increase in plasma osmolality. This can be an inherited or congenital defect or can be precipitated by conditions that involve the appropriate areas of the hypothalamus, e.g. granulomatous meningoencephalitis. In this dog it seems likely that there is a congenital defect as the same neurological signs were observed when the dog was a few months of age. An MRI was performed that confirmed that there were structural abnormalities in the brain that could explain the dog's clinical signs.

The management of this condition involves cautious fluid therapy to restore normal sodium balance followed by regulated water intake in the form of food made into a gruel or encouraging the dog to drink by using flavoured water or a mixture of milk and water.

Case 3

Signalment

5-year old, female Old English Sheepdog.

History and physical examination

2-week history of lethargy, inappetance and weight loss. On clinical examination the dog was depressed, slightly dehydrated and in poor body condition. The heart rate was 120 beats/minute. Peripheral lymph nodes and anal sacs were palpably normal.

Clinical pathology data

Haematology	Result	Reference interval
RBC (x 10^{12}/l)	6.94	5.5–8.5
Hb (g/dl)	17.2	12.0–18.0
HCT (l/l)	0.497	0.37–0.55
MCV (fl)	71.6	60–77
MCH (pg)	24.8	19.5–24.5
MCHC (g/dl)	34.7	30.0–37.0
WBC (x 10^9/l)	23.9	6.0–17.5
Neutrophils (x 10^9/l)	18.6	2.5–11.5
Lymphocytes (x 10^9/l)	3.52	0.5–4.8
Monocytes (x 10^9/l)	0.45	0.2–1.5
Basophils (x 10^9/l)	0.034	0.0–0.50
Eosinophils (x 10^9/l)	1.26	0.05–1.3
Platelets (x 10^9/l)	244	150–500

Biochemistry	Result	Reference interval
Sodium (mmol/l)	139.5	135–155
Potassium (mmol/l)	5.73	3.5–5.8
Sodium:potassium ratio	24.3	>27
Chloride (mmol/l)	115	105–120
Urea (mmol/l)	7.9	3.3–8.0
Creatinine (μmol/l)	139	45–150
Calcium (mmol/l)	3.56	2.2–2.7
Inorganic phosphate (mmol/l)	2.03	0.6–1.3
TP (g/l)	58.5	60–80
Albumin (g/l)	30.4	25–40
ALT (IU/l)	70	21–59
ALP (IU/l)	179	3–142

What are the abnormalities?

The most significant abnormality is the moderate hypercalcaemia. The sodium:potassium ratio is low, although sodium and potassium concentrations are within the reference range. Phosphate is mildly elevated, which is not typical of malignancy-associated hypercalcaemia or primary hyperparathyroidism. The mild elevation in liver enzymes is a non-specific change and could be secondary to a variety of extra-hepatic causes as well as any hepatopathy. There is a mild neutrophilia which could reflect inflammation or a stress response. The lymphocyte count is towards the top of the reference range, which is unusual in a sick animal.

Case 3 continues ▶

Case 3 continued

What are the differential diagnoses in this case?

The most likely differential diagnoses are hypoadrenocorticism, malignancy and primary hyperparathyroidism. The absence of azotaemia rules out chronic renal failure. Less common differential diagnoses include granulomatous disease and hypervitaminosis D.

How would you investigate this case further?

An adrenocorticotrophin (ACTH) stimulation test should be performed to assess for hypoadrenocorticism, especially given the low sodium:potassium ratio. The dog can be assessed for an underlying malignancy with diagnostic imaging including thoracic and abdominal radiography and ultrasonography. If no cause is found, ultrasonography of the thyroid gland and measurement of PTH would be useful to evaluate the dog for hyperparathyroidism.

An ACTH stimulation revealed undetectable concentrations of cortisol pre and post administration of ACTH hormone resulting in a diagnosis of hypoadrenocorticism. Dogs with hypoadrenocorticism do not always have abnormal sodium and potassium concentrations (Peterson *et al.*, 1996) or the classical leucogram findings (see Chapter 18), although the lack of lymphopenia in this sick dog was significant.

Case 4

Signalment

10-year old male, neutered crossbreed dog.

History

3-week history of lethargy, inappetance and weight loss. Clinical examination revealed that the dog was depressed and slightly dehydrated. On palpation, peripheral lymph nodes and anal sacs were normal.

Clinical pathology data

Haematology	Result	Reference interval
RBC (x 10^{12}/l)	7.49	5.5–8.5
Hb (g/dl)	17.1	12.0–18.0
HCT (l/l)	0.50	0.37–0.55
MCV (fl)	67.2	60–77
MCH (pg)	22.9	19.5–24.5
MCHC (g/dl)	34.0	32.0–37.0
WBC (x 10^9/l)	7.52	6.0–17.5
Neutrophils (x 10^9/l)	5.31	3–11.5
Lymphocytes (x 10^9/l)	0.96	1.0–4.8
Monocytes (x 10^9/l)	1.16	0.2–1.5
Eosinophils (x 10^9/l)	0.024	0.05–1.3
Basophils (x 10^9/l)	0.067	0.0–0.5
Platelets (x 10^9/l)	219	150–500

Biochemistry	Result	Reference interval
Sodium (mmol/l)	143.5	135–155
Potassium (mmo/l)	3.80	3.5–5.8
Sodium: potassium ratio	37.8	>27
Chloride (mmo/l)	107.2	105–120
Urea (mmol/l)	7.9	3.3–8.0
Creatinine (μmol/l)	118	45–150
Calcium (mmol/l)	3.96	2.3–2.8 ▶
Biochemistry *(continued)*	**Result**	**Reference interval**
Ionized calcium (mmo/l)	2.12	1.18–1.40
Inorganic phosphate (mmol/l)	0.98	0.78–1.41
TP (g/l)	72.8	60–80
Albumin (g/l)	33.3	25–45

What are the abnormalities and what are the differential diagnoses in this case?

The most significant abnormality is the moderate to marked total and ionized hypercalcaemia. The most likely differential diagnoses are malignancy and primary hyperparathyroidism. Hypoadrenocorticism is unlikely given the normal sodium and potassium concentrations, normal sodium:potassium ratio and the lymphopenia. The normal creatinine and phosphate concentrations rule out chronic renal failure.

How would you investigate this case further?

Because malignancy is considered to be the most likely cause of the hypercalcaemia, further diagnostic imaging is advisable. PTHrp and PTH could be measured to investigate the pathogenesis of the hypercalcaemia further. Ultrasonography of the thyroid gland would be helpful in assessing the dog for a primary hyperparathyroidism. If these tests do not identify the cause of the hypercalcaemia then an ACTH stimulation test should be considered as the normal electrolyte concentrations and ratios do not eliminate hypoadrenocorticism as a differential diagnosis.

In this case thoracic radiography revealed a cranial mediastinal mass. An ultrasound guided fine needle aspirate of the mediastinal mass revealed that the predominant cells were lymphoblasts leading to a diagnosis of lymphoma.

The absence of peripheral lymphadenopathy does not rule out lymphoma and in dogs which have suspected malignancy-related hypercalcaemia, thoracic and abdominal radiography and ultrasonography should be performed. However, many other disease processes can cause a mass in the mediastinum, e.g. thymomas, cysts, lipomas, heart base tumours, ectopic thyroid tumours. Thymomas are also associated with hypercalcaemia: the presence of hypercalcaemia and a cranial mediastinal mass does not necessarily mean that the dog has lymphoma.

See also Chapter 16, Case 1.

References

Authement JM, Boudrieau RJ and Kaplan PM (1989) Transient, traumatically induced, central diabetes insipidus in a dog. *Journal of the American Veterinary Medical Association* **194,** 683–685

Barber PJ, Elliott J and Torrance AG (1993) Measurement of feline intact parathyroid hormone: assay validation and sample handling studies. *Journal of Small Animal Practice* **34,** 614–620

Barber PJ and Elliott J (1998) Feline chronic renal failure: calcium homeostasis in 80 cases diagnosed between 1992 and 1995. *Journal of Small Animal Practice* **39,** 108–116

Bennett PF, DeNicola DB, Bonney P, Glickman NW and Knapp DW (2002) Canine anal sac adenocarcinomas: clinical presentation and response to therapy. *Journal of Veterinary Internal Medicine* **16,** 100–104

Berger B and Feldman EC (1987) Primary hyperparathyroidism in dogs: 21 cases (1976–1986). *Journal of American Veterinary Medical Association* **191,** 350–356

Bolliger AP, Graham PA, Richard V, Rosol RJ, Nachreiner RF and

Refsal KR (2002) Detection of parathyroid hormone-related protein in cats with humoral hypercalcemia of malignancy. *Veterinary Clinical Pathology* **31,** 3–8

Brofman PJ, Knostman KA and DiBartola SP (2003) Granulomatous amebic meningoencephalitis causing the syndrome of inappropriate secretion of antidiuretic hormone in a dog. *Journal of Veterinary Internal Medicine* **17,** 230–234

Brown EA, Markandu ND, Roulston JE, Jones BE, Squires M and MacGregor GA (1982) Is the renin-angiotensin-aldosterone system involved in the sodium retention in the nephrotic syndrome. *Nephron* **32,** 102–107

Bruyette DS (2001) Feline endocrinology update. *Veterinary Clinics of North America Small Animal Practice* **31,**1063–1081

Bruyette DS and Feldman EC (1988) Primary hypoparathyroidism in the dog. *Journal of Veterinary Internal Medicine* **2,** 7–14

Crawford MA, Kittleson MD and Fink GD (1984) Hypernatremia and adipsia in a dog. *Journal of the American Veterinary Medical Association* **184,** 818–821

Degen M (1987) Pseudohyperkalaemia in Akitas. *Journal of the American Veterinary Medical Association* **190,** 541–543

Dhupa N and Proulx J (1998) Hypocalcaemia and hypomagnesaemia. *Veterinary Clinics of North America: Small Animal Practice* **28,** 587–608

DiBartola SP, Johnson SE, Davenport DJ, Prueter JC, Chew DJ and Sherding RG (1985) Clinicopathologic findings resembling hypoadrenocorticism in dogs with primary gastrointestinal disease. *Journal of the American Veterinary Medical Association* **187,** 60–63

Dow S and Fettman M (1992) Renal disease in cats: the potassium connection. In: *Current Veterinary Therapy XI*, ed. R Kirk and J Bonagura, pp. 820–822. WB Saunders, Philadelphia

Dow SW, Fettman MJ, Lecouteur RA and Allen TA (1987) Hypodipsic hypernatraemia and associated myopathy in a hydrocephalic cat with transient hypopituitarism. *Journal of the American Veterinary Medical Association* **191,** 217

Dow SW, Legendre AM, Stiff M and Greene C (1986) Hypercalcaemia associated with blastomycosis in dogs. *Journal of American Veterinary Medical Association* **188,** 706–709

Drobatz KJ and Casey KK (2000) Eclampsia in dogs: 31 cases (1995–1998). *Journal of American Veterinary Medical Association* **217,** 216–219

Elliott J, Dobson JM, Dunn JK, Herrtage ME and Jackson KF (1991) Hypercalcaemia in the dog: a study of 40 cases. *Journal of Small Animal Practice* **32,** 564–571

Foley P, Shaw D, Runyon C, McConkey S and Ikede B (2000) Serum parathyroid hormone-related protein concentration in a dog with a thymoma and persistent hypercalcemia. *Canadian Veterinary Journal* **41,** 867–870

Fradkin JM, Braniecki AM, Craig TM, Ramiro-Ibanez F, Rogers KS and Zoran DL (2001) Elevated parathyroid hormone-related protein and hypercalemia in two dogs with schistosomiasis. *Journal of American Animal Hospital Association* **37,** 349–355

Ganong WF (2001) Hormonal control of calcium metabolism and physiology of bone. In: *Review of Medical Physiology, 20th edn,* ed. WF Ganing, pp. 369–382. Lange Medical Books/McGraw-Hill, New York

Gerber B, Hassig M and Reusch CE (2003) Serum concentration of 1,25-dihydroxycholecalciferol and 25-hydroxycholecalciferol in clinically normal dogs and dogs with acute and chronic renal failure. *American Journal of Veterinary Research* **64,** 1161–1166

Graves TK, Schall WD, Refsal K and Nachreiner RF (1994) Basal and ACTH-stimulated plasma aldosterone concentrations are normal or increased in dogs with *Trichuris*-associated pseudohypoadrenocorticism. *Journal of Veterinary Internal Medicine* **8,** 287–289

Harb MF, Nelson RW, Feldman EC, Scott-Moncrieff JC and Griffey SM (1996) Central diabetes insipidus in dogs: 20 cases (1986–1995) *Journal of the American Veterinary Medical Association* **209,** 1884–1888

Houpt KA (1991) Feeding and drinking behavior problems. *Veterinary Clinics of North America: Small Animal Practice* **21,** 281–298

Jeffery ND, Watson PJ, Abramson C, Notenboom A (2003) Brain malformations associated with primary adipsia identified using magnetic resonance imaging. *Veterinary Record* **152,** 436–438

Jutkowitz LA, Rozanski EA, Moreau JA and Rush JE (2002) Massive transfusion in dogs: 15 cases (1997–2001). *Journal of American Veterinary Medical Association* **220,** 1664–1669

Kallet AJ, Richter KP, Feldman EC and Brum DE (1991) Primary hyperparathyroidism in cats: seven cases (1984–1989). *Journal of American Veterinary Medical Association* **199,** 1767–1771

Khanna C, Boermans HJ and Wilcock B (1997) Fatal hypernatraemia in a dog from salt ingestion. *Journal of the American Animal Hospital Association* **33,** 113–117

Kimmel SE, Washabau RJ and Drobatz KJ (2001) Incidence and prognostic value of low plasma ionized calcium concentration in cats with acute pancreatitis. *Journal of American Veterinary Medical Association* **219,** 1105–1109

Kleiter M, Hirt R, Kirtz G and Day MJ (2001) Hypercalcaemia associated with chronic lymphocytic leukaemia in a Giant Schnauzer. *Australian Veterinary Journal* **79,** 335–338

Luzius H, Jans DA, Grunbaum EG, Moritz A, Rascher W and Fahrenholz F (1992) A low affinity vasopressin V2-receptor in inherited nephrogenic diabetes insipidus. *Journal of Receptor Research* **12,** 351–368

Mackay BM and Curtis N (1999) Adipsia and hypernatraemia in a dog with focal hypothalamic granulomatous meningoencephalitis. *Australian Veterinary Journal* **77,** 14–17

Martin L (1998) Hypercalcaemia and hypermagnesaemia. *Veterinary Clinics of North America: Small Animal Practice* **28,** 565–585

Matus RE, Leifer CE, MacEwen EG and Hurvitz AI (1986) Prognostic factors for multiple myeloma in the dog. *Journal of American Veterinary Medical Association* **188,** 1288–1292

Mellanby RJ, Craig R, Evans H and Herrtage ME (2003a) Parathyroid hormone related protein concentrations in dogs with lymphoma, primary hyperparathyroidism, anal sac adenocarcinoma and chronic renal failure. *Proceedings of the 13th ECVIM Congress,* p.162

Mellanby RJ, Friend EJ, Mellor PJ, Herrtage ME, Mee A and Berry J (2003b) Vitamin D metabolite concentrations in dogs with unusual calcium metabolism disorders. *Proceedings of the 13th ECVIM Congress* p.178

Meuten DJ, Chew DJ, Capen CC and Kociba GJ (1982) Relationship of serum total calcium to albumin and total protein in dogs. *Journal of American Veterinary Medical Association* **180,** 63–67

Midkiff AM, Chew DJ, Randolph JF, Center SA and DiBartola SP (2000) Idiopathic hypercalcaemia in cats. *Journal of Veterinary Internal Medicine* **14,** 619–626

Nelson RW (2003) Electrolyte imbalances. In: *Small Animal Internal Medicine, 3rd edn,* ed. RW Nelson and CG Couto, pp. 828–846. Mosby Publishing, St Louis

Nemzek JA, Kruger JM, Walshaw R and Hauptman JG (1994) Acute onset of hypokalaemia and muscular weakness in four hyperthyroid cats. *Journal of the American Veterinary Medical Association* **105,** 65–68

Peterson ME, Greco DS and Orth DN (1989) Primary hypoadrenocorticism in ten cats. *Journal of Veterinary Internal Medicine* **3,** 55–58

Peterson ME, Kintzer PP and Kass PH (1996) Pretreatment clinical and laboratory findings in dogs with hypoadrenocorticism: 225 cases (1979–1993). *Journal of American Veterinary Medical Association* **208,** 85–91

Post K, Mcneill JR, Clark EG, Dignean MA and Olynyk GP (1989) Congenital diabetes insipidus in two sibling Afghan Hound pups. *Journal of the American Veterinary Medical Association* **194,** 1086–1088

Pressler BM, Rotstein DS, Law JM, Rosol TJ, LeRoy B, Keene BW and Jackson MW (2002) Hypercalcemia and high parathyroid hormone related protein concentration associated with malignant melanoma in a dog. *Journal of American Veterinary Medical Association* **221,** 263–240

Ramsey IK and Herrtage ME (2001) Increased parathyroid hormone concentrations in dogs with hyperadrenocorticism. *Journal of Veterinary Internal Medicine* **14,** 298

Refsal KR, Provencher-Bolliger AL, Graham PA and Nachreiner RF (2001) Update on the diagnosis and treatment of disorders of calcium regulation. *Veterinary Clinics of North America: Small Animal Practice* **31,** 1043–1062

Rijnberk A, Kooistra HS, van Vonderen IK, Mol JA, Voorhout G, Vansluijs FJ, Ijzer J, van den Ingh TSGAM, Boer P and Boer WH (2001) Aldosteronoma in a dog with polyuria as the leading symptom. *Domestic Animal Endocrinology* **20,** 227–240

Rosol TJ, Nagode LA, Couto CG, Hammer AS, Chew DJ, Peterson JL, Ayl RD, Steinmeyer CL and Capen CC (1992) Parathyroid hormone (PTH)-related protein, PTH, and 1,25-dihydroxyvitamin D in dogs with cancer-associated hypercalcemia. *Endocrinology* **131,** 1157–1164

Rosol TJ, Chew DJ, Nagode LA and Capen CC (1995) Pathophysiology of calcium metabolism. *Veterinary Clinical Pathology* **24,** 49–63

Rumbeiha WK, Kruger JM, Fitzgerald SF, Nachreiner RF, Kaneene JB, Braselton WE and Chiapuzio CL (1999) Use of pamidronate to reverse vitamin D_3-induced toxicosis in dogs. *American Journal of Veterinary Research* **60,** 1092–1097

Sadek D and Schaer M (1996) Atypical Addison's disease in the dog: a retrospective survey of 14 cases. *Journal of the American Animal Hospital Association* **32,** 159–163

Savary KC, Price GS and Vaden SL (2000) Hypercalcemia in cats: a retrospective study of 71 cases (1991–1997). *Journal of Veterinary Internal Medicine* **14,** 184–189

Schaer M, Halling KB, Collins KE and Grant DC (2001) Combined hyponatraemia and hypokalaemia mimicking acute hypoadrenocorticism in three pregnant dogs. *Journal of the American Veterinary Medical Association* **218,** 897–899

Takemura N (1998) Successful long-term treatment of congenital nephrogenic diabetes insipidus in a dog. *Journal of Small Animal Practice* **39,** 592–594

Torrance AG and Nachreiner R (1989) Human-parathormone assay for use in dogs: validation, sample handling studies, and parathyroid function testing. *American Journal of Veterinary Research* **50,** 1123–1127

Willard MD, Fossum TW, Torrance A and Lippert A (1991) Hyponatraemia and hyperkalaemia associated with idiopathic or experimentally induced chylothorax in four dogs. *Journal of the American Veterinary Medical Association* **199,** 353–358

Williams LE, Gliatto JM, Dodge RK, Johnson JL, Gamblin RM, Thamm DH, Lana SE, Szymkowski M and Moore AS (2003) Carcinoma of the apocrine glands of the anal sac in dogs: 113 cases (1985–1995). *Journal of American Veterinary Medical Association* **223,** 825–831

Wisner ER, Nyland TG, Feldman EC, Nelson RW and Griffey SM (1993) Ultrasonographic evaluation of the parathyroid glands in hypercalcemic dogs. *Veterinary Radiology and Ultrasound* **34,** 108–111

Further reading

DiBartola SP (2000) *Fluid Therapy in Small Animal Practice, 2nd edition.* WB Saunders, Philadelphia

Hodson S (1998) Feline hypokalaemia. *In Practice* **20,** 135–144

Jones BR (2000) Hypokalaemic myopathy in cats. In: *Kirk's Current Veterinary Therapy XIII,* ed. J Bonagura, pp. 985–987. WB Saunders, Philadelphia

Ross LA (1990) Disorders of serum sodium concentration: diagnosis and therapy. *Compendium of Continuing Education for the Practicing Veterinarian* **12,** 1277

Rubin SI (1995) Management of fluid and electrolyte disorders in uraemia. In: *Kirk's Current Veterinary Therapy XIII,* ed. J Bonagura, pp. 951–955. WB Saunders, Philadelphia

9

Blood gas analysis and acid–base disorders

Derek Flaherty and Laura Blackwood

Introduction

Acid–base disturbances are common, and can significantly impact on case morbidity and mortality if unrecognized or treated inappropriately. While blood gas analysis can identify the presence of these disturbances, a reasonable understanding of the underlying pathophysiology is required to manage the case adequately. Unfortunately, much of the published work on blood gas analysis is based on human sampling. The differences between normal values in small animals and humans also mean that some of the definitions used in human medicine fit awkwardly when applied to animals. For example, acidaemia is often defined as a blood pH <7.35, but many reference intervals for cats extend into this range. However, the principles applied in human medicine have been applied to small animals for decades now and, while it is likely that some of the detailed data reported in the literature are unsuitable for direct transfer to animal patients, the principles of interpretation provide useful guidelines. As for any other analyte, the reference interval should be established for each system.

This chapter will give an overview and basic guidance on blood gas analysis, but it is only with regular assessment of blood gas samples that the clinician is likely to become competent in their interpretation. Complex acid–base disorders will not be covered in detail in this chapter; the interested reader is referred to Further Reading. The abbreviations and terminology used in the chapter are summarized in Figure 9.1.

Term (units)	Definition
A	Alveolar
a	Arterial
A^- (mmol/l)	Anion (of a weak acid buffer pair)
AG (mmol/l)	Anion gap
BE	Base excess. Amount of acid, in mmol/l, required to return 1 litre of blood to a pH of 7.4 at a P_aCO_2 of 40 mmHg (5.3 kPa)
F_iO_2 (% or decimal of 1)	Fraction of inspired oxygen; e.g. room air has a F_iO_2 of 21% or 0.21
H^+	Hydrogen ion
$[H^+]$ (nmol/l)	Hydrogen ion concentration
HA	Weak acid
HCO_3^-	Bicarbonate ion
H_2CO_3	Carbonic acid
kPa	Kilo Pascal: SI unit of pressure: 1 kPa = 7.52 mmHg
mEq/l	Milliequivalents per litre
mmHg	Millimetres of mercury; commonly used unit of pressure
P or *p*	Pressure (or partial pressure: the term partial pressure refers to the fact that the total pressure is due to a combination of gases)
$P_{(A-a)}O_2$ (mmHg or kPa)	Alveolar arterial oxygen gradient, i.e. difference between calculated alveolar PO_2 and measured arterial P_aO_2
P_aCO_2 (mmHg or kPa)	Partial pressure of carbon dioxide in arterial blood
P_aO_2 (mmHg or kPa)	Partial pressure of oxygen in arterial blood
P_B (mmHg or kPa)	Barometric pressure
PH_2O (mmHg or kPa)	Saturated vapour pressure of water
pK	Negative log of the dissociation constant; pH at which the concentrations of the ionized $[A^-]$ and unionized forms [HA] are the same
P_vCO_2 (mmHg or kPa)	Partial pressure of carbon dioxide in venous blood
P_vO_2 (mmHg or kPa)	Partial pressure of oxygen in venous blood
RQ	Respiratory quotient (ratio of O_2 uptake to CO_2 exhaled). Nominal value = 0.8
S_aO_2 (%)	Saturation of haemoglobin with oxygen in arterial blood
S_pO_2 (%)	Saturation of haemoglobin with oxygen in arterial blood measured by pulse oximetry
V/Q	Ventilation–perfusion

9.1 Abbreviations and terminology used in blood gas analysis.

pH scale

The concentration of hydrogen ions ($[H^+]$) in the body is tightly controlled within a relatively narrow range of approximately 35–45 nmol/l. These tiny concentrations are awkward to work with clinically and it is more common to discuss the negative logarithm (base 10) of the H^+ concentration, i.e. the pH.

- $pH = -\log_{10}[H^+]$
- pH changes in the opposite direction to $[H^+]$: reductions in $[H^+]$ lead to an increase in pH and *vice versa*.
- Because of the logarithmic scale, the changes in $[H^+]$ required to produce any given numerical change in pH vary at different pH values. For

example, twice as many H^+ ions are needed to change the pH from 7.5 to 7.4 as are needed to change it from 7.8 to 7.7. This means that changes in pH in acidaemic (usually defined as blood pH <7.35) animals can reflect large deviations from normal $[H^+]$. Around the normal range a change of 1 nmol/l of H^+ equates to 0.01 pH unit.

Buffering

Chemical reactions within the body produce hydrogen ions that would rapidly lead to alterations in pH incompatible with life if they were allowed to accumulate. The rate of production of H^+ is too rapid for elimination from the body to keep pace, and *buffering* must come in to play. *Buffers* are combinations of weak acids with their 'conjugate bases'. If $[H^+]$ in the body starts to rise, the conjugate base can 'mop up' this excess, limiting the effect on pH. Similarly, if $[H^+]$ starts to drop, more weak acid can dissociate to raise the $[H^+]$ back towards normal.

Many different buffers exist within the body, in the intracellular (ICF) and extracellular fluid (ECF) and in bone. Acutely, buffering in the ECF is most important, as it takes hours for the H^+ load to be distributed throughout the body and for intracellular buffers to be activated. The most important buffering system is the carbonic acid (H_2CO_3)–bicarbonate (HCO_3^-) system in the ECF:

$$CO_2 + H_2O \rightleftharpoons H_2CO_3 \rightleftharpoons H^+ + HCO_3^-$$

The significance of this particular system lies in the fact that, unlike most other buffers, saturation does not occur because the end products (CO_2, water, H^+ and HCO_3^-) are dissipated by pulmonary (CO_2) or renal routes. The pulmonary capacity to excrete CO_2 is enormous. In addition, virtually total resorption or massive excretion of HCO_3^- can occur in the kidney in response to alterations in plasma HCO_3^-. For both these reasons, the buffering potential is huge compared with that of other weak acids found in the ECF and ICF.

The H_2CO_3–HCO_3^- system links the respiratory and renal responses to changes in H^+, which are vital for buffering purposes:

- Respiratory response: increased free H^+ ions, reduced ECF pH, hypercapnia (an increase in PCO_2, also called hypercarbia) and hypoxaemia all stimulate ventilation. Healthy patients can excrete a great deal of CO_2. In normal lungs, the limit to CO_2 excretion is the availability of HCO_3^-
- Renal response: the kidney excretes H^+, and also effectively regenerates the HCO_3^- supply, so allows buffering to continue. Renal control of plasma HCO_3^- is mediated by control of HCO_3^- resorption, and titratable acid and ammonium excretion.

The respiratory and renal responses are effectively yoked together in a continuum. If CO_2 levels within the body increase, the equation above will push to the right and the excess H^+ (and HCO_3^-) produced can then be eliminated by the kidneys. If H^+ concentrations rise, the equation will move to the left, generating extra CO_2, which can be eliminated via the lungs. This reaction is not limited by HCO_3^- because of the large quantities of HCO_3^- in the ECF, and also the tremendous capacity of the kidney to reabsorb and regenerate HCO_3^- as required. This is an oversimplification of what occurs *in vivo*, but gives some idea of the importance of the H_2CO_3–HCO_3^- system.

The Henderson–Hasselbalch equation relates pH, H_2CO_3 and HCO_3^- for the H_2CO_3–HCO_3^- system. The derivation of this equation (Figure 9.2) illustrates one of the most important points in acid–base physiology: provided the *ratio* of HCO_3^- to CO_2 remains at its usual value of approximately 20:1, the pH will be normal regardless of any deviation from normal in the *individual* HCO_3^- and CO_2 values. This concept is important when trying to calculate the appropriate compensatory responses for an acid–base disturbance (see later).

Derivation of the Henderson–Hasselbalch equation

- $pH = -\log_{10}[H^+]$
- For any weak acid, the ionization equilibrium can be expressed as: $HA \rightleftharpoons H^+ + A^-$
- K is the equilibrium constant (or ionization constant) for this reaction and is defined as: $K = [H^+][A^-] / [HA]$
- Rearranging this equation gives: $[H^+] = K [HA] / [A^-]$
- If we express this in log form: $-\log_{10}[H^+] = -\log_{10}K + \log_{10}([A^-] / [HA])$
- $-\log_{10} K = pK_a$ (the pH at which the concentrations of the ionized $[A^-]$ and unionized forms [HA] are the same, i.e. when the reaction is evenly balanced)
- Thus: $pH = pK_a + \log_{10}([A^-]/[HA])$. This is the *Henderson–Hasselbalch equation.*

For carbonic acid in the bicarbonate buffering system:

$pH = pK_a + \log_{10}([HCO_3^-] / [H_2CO_3])$	(pK_a of carbonic acid = 6.1)
$pH = 6.1 + \log_{10}\{[HCO_3^-] / (0.225 \times P_aCO_2)\}$	The concentration of H_2CO_3 depends upon the dissolved CO_2, which depends upon the pCO_2. Most carbonic acid in the body exists as dissolved CO_2, and 0.225 is the solubility coefficient of CO_2 in blood in ml/kPa
$pH = 6.1 + \log_{10}\{24 / (0.225 \times 5.3)\}$	Mean $[HCO_3^-]$ in arterial blood is 24 mmol/l, while mean P_aCO_2 is 5.3 kPa
$pH = 6.1 + \log_{10}(24 / 1.1925)$	
$pH = 6.1 + 1.3$	
$pH = 7.4$	7.4 is the midpoint of the normal pH range of body fluids

9.2 Derivation of the Henderson–Hasselbalch equation.

Blood gas analysis

A blood gas analyser will directly measure pH, PCO_2 (partial pressure of CO_2) and PO_2 (partial pressure of oxygen) in the sample, and will derive values for HCO_3^- and base excess, based on standard normograms. Hand-held analysers are becoming more widely available in veterinary practice, and are useful for measurement of blood gases and also ionized calcium. These units also offer a range of other biochemical analyses, but have not been fully validated in small animals for these tests.

Arterial samples are essential for assessment of respiratory function, but either venous or arterial samples can provide useful information of the animal's metabolic status. Arterial samples may be drawn from the dorsal pedal arteries (Figure 9.3) or femoral artery in dogs, and from the femoral artery in cats. After sampling, pressure must be applied for an adequate period of time (5 minutes) to prevent haematoma formation. Heparin is the standard anticoagulant for blood gas analysis. Heparin sodium (1000 IU/ml) can be aspirated from a vial in a sterile manner, using a 23 or 25 G needle, until the syringe barrel is filled, then the excess expelled; this preloaded 1 or 2 ml syringe is used to collect the sample. The syringe should be 50–100% full after sampling. Too much heparin can cause a drop in P_aCO_2 (and in calculated HCO_3^-). Alternatively, pre-heparinized blood-gas syringes can be purchased, which ensures there is no anticoagulant excess.

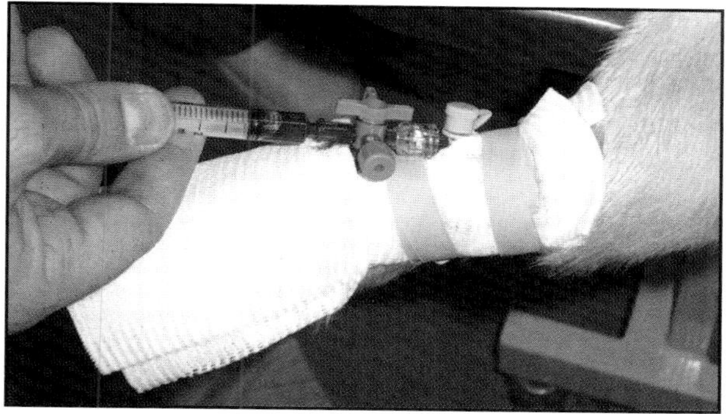

9.3 Sampling for blood gas analysis from the dorsal pedal artery.

Samples for blood gas analysis must be stored aerobically, with no air/vacuum space adjacent to the blood sample into which CO_2 could evaporate. Commonly, samples are obtained in an anticoagulant-treated syringe and, after sampling, the syringe is capped with a rubber bung or plastic cap. Alternatively, the needle may be bent over to form a seal, but this is less effective and more dangerous. The sample is introduced to the blood gas analyser directly from the syringe. Transferring blood to a tube will alter gas pressures, and exchange will occur between the blood and air trapped in the tube with it. Samples should be processed within 15 minutes, and placed on ice until analysis, to minimize changes in blood gas concentrations as a result of continued cell metabolism. Less than 200 µl of fresh whole blood or heparinized whole blood is required for hand-held analysers, and traditional analysers also require only small volumes of blood.

Blood gas analysers routinely analyse samples at 37°C, but some units have facilities for entry of the actual patient temperature and correction of output to allow for deviations from 37°C. Patient temperature has an effect on both P_aO_2 and P_aCO_2. However, it is thought that more errors are made by correcting for patient temperature than by ignoring temperature, so correction is not recommended. Reference values for pyrexic and hypothermic states are unknown.

Reported normal values for arterial and venous blood gases are summarized in Figure 9.4.

pH

The normal pH value of blood is approximately 7.35–7.45, although reference intervals for small animals sometimes include values slightly outside this range (Figure 9.4).

- **Acidaemia** refers to a pH value <7.35 (7.36 in some texts)
- **Alkalaemia** refers to a pH >7.45 (7.44 in some texts)
- The terms **acidosis** and **alkalosis** refer to the processes that occur at a cellular level, which may give rise to an acidaemia or alkalaemia if left uncompensated.

Parameter	Dogs		Cats	
	Arterial blood	*Venous blood*	*Arterial blood*	*Venous blood*
pH	7.35–7.46	7.35–7.44	7.31–7.46	7.28–7.41
PCO_2	30.8–42.8 mmHg 4.10–5.69 kPa	33.6–41.2 mmHg 4.47–5.48 kPa	25.2–36.8 mmHg 3.35–4.89 kPa	32.7–44.7 mmHg 4.35–5.94 kPa
PO_2 (room air)	80.9–103.3 mmHg 10.76–13.74 kPa	47.9–56.3 mmHg 6.37–7.49 kPa	95.4–118.2 mmHg 12.69–15.72 kPa	27–50 mmHg 3.59–6.65 kPa
HCO_3^-	18.8–25.6 mmol/l	20.8–24.2 mmol/l	14.4–21.6 mmol/l	18.0–23.2 mmol/l
Base excess	0 ± 4	0 ± 4	0 ± 4	0 ± 4

9.4 Approximate normal arterial and venous blood gas values for dogs and cats. (Data from Zweens *et al.* (1977), Rodkey *et al.* (1978), Haskins (1983) and Senior (1995).) The accepted SI unit for gas pressure is the kilopascal, but many clinicians still use the older units of mmHg. 1 kPa = 7.52 mmHg.

As a general rule, pH values of ≤7.0 and ≥7.65 are immediately life-threatening. Specific treatment of the acid–base disorder may be required if the pH is <7.2 or >7.6, but treatment of the underlying disease is most important for correction of acid–base disturbances.

P_aCO_2

P_aCO_2 values (subscript 'a' signifies arterial sample; 'v' signifies venous) indicate the ability of alveolar ventilation to remove the CO_2 produced by the body. P_aCO_2 is directly proportional to the rate of CO_2 production, and inversely proportional to alveolar ventilation; i.e. if alveolar minute ventilation were to decrease by 50% without any change in CO_2 production, the P_aCO_2 would double. Measurement of P_aCO_2 is considered the 'gold standard' for assessing adequacy of ventilation in any patient. Many clinicians use a working range of 35–45 mmHg in dogs, and, using these parameters, P_aCO_2 values < 35 mmHg (< 4.65 kPa) indicate *hyperventilation*, while values > 45 mmHg (> 5.98 kPa) indicate *hypoventilation*. However, reported normal ranges are lower than this (30.8–42.8 mmHg, 4.10–5.69 kPa), and cats tend to have lower values again (25.2–36.8 mmHg, 3.35–4.89 kPa) (see Figure 9.4).

Normal P_vCO_2 is higher than P_aCO_2, and values are approximately 33–41 mmHg (4.47–5.48 kPa) in dogs and 33–45 mmHg (4.35–5.94 kPa) in cats. The capacity of venous blood to carry CO_2 is greater than that of arterial blood because of the ability of deoxyhaemoglobin to buffer more H^+.

P_aO_2

P_aO_2 values indicate the ability of the lungs to oxygenate blood. However, the P_aO_2 can only be interpreted in light of the P_AO_2 (alveolar partial pressure of oxygen), which, in turn, is based on the fraction of oxygen in the inspired air, according to the alveolar gas equation:

$$P_AO_2 = F_iO_2\,(P_B - P_{H_2O}) - \frac{P_aCO_2}{0.8}$$

where:

- FiO_2 is the fractional inspired oxygen concentration (e.g. FiO_2 is 0.21 for room air (21% O_2) or 1.0 for 100% O_2)
- P_B is barometric pressure
- P_{H_2O} is the saturated vapour pressure of water (47 mmHg (~6.25 kPa) at normal body temperature)
- 0.8 is the respiratory quotient (RQ). The RQ is the ratio of O_2 uptake to CO_2 exhaled, and is assumed to be 0.8. (Some variation in RQ occurs depending on diet, as a consequence of nitrogen excretion, but this is generally not clinically significant.)

Once the P_AO_2 has been calculated from the above equation, it can then be compared with the P_aO_2 value from the arterial blood sample. The arithmetic difference between the two is known as the alveolar–arterial oxygen difference or gradient, and is signified by $P_{(A\text{-}a)}O_2$. In normal patients breathing room air, the upper limit of normality for the $P_{(A\text{-}a)}O_2$ is approximately 25 mmHg (3.3 kPa), although this can rise to around 120 mmHg (16.0 kPa) in patients breathing 100% oxygen. Calculation of the alveolar–arterial oxygen gradient can be used to help assess the contribution of hypoventilation or ventilation perfusion mismatch to hypoxaemia.

P_aO_2 for dogs breathing room air is approximately 80–104 mmHg (10.76–13.74 kPa), and for cats is 95–118 mmHg (12.69–15.72 kPa). P_vO_2 is lower than P_aO_2, and venous samples should not be used to assess adequacy of oxygenation. Normal P_vO_2 values (breathing room air) are approximately 48–56 mmHg (6.37–7.49 kPa) in dogs and as varied as 27 to 50 mmHg (3.59–6.65 kPa) in cats.

Bicarbonate

HCO_3^- may be measured directly by the blood gas analyser but, more commonly, it is a derived value based on the PCO_2 and pH values. Some analysers give a result for only one form of HCO_3^- (usually 'actual' bicarbonate), while others provide information on two forms: 'actual' and 'standard' bicarbonate. If the analyser just gives a *single* bicarbonate value, it is most likely to be *actual* bicarbonate, though this should be confirmed with the manufacturer. For example, the i-STAT provides a calculated actual bicarbonate value.

Actual bicarbonate

Actual bicarbonate ($HCO_3^-{}_a$) is the HCO_3^- concentration in the blood that results from both metabolic *and* respiratory effects. The H_2CO_3–HCO_3^- equation is as follows:

$$CO_2 + H_2O \rightleftharpoons H_2CO_3 \rightleftharpoons H^+ + HCO_3^-$$

Thus, although HCO_3^- concentration can change directly as a result of a metabolic disorder (loss or gain of HCO_3^-), from the equation, it can also be seen that alterations in CO_2 levels in the blood will influence the HCO_3^- levels; an increase in CO_2 causes a shift of the equation to the right, increasing HCO_3^- production, and *vice versa*. Consequently, $HCO_3^-{}_a$ values as reported by blood gas analysers will be abnormal with either a respiratory or a metabolic disturbance.

Standard bicarbonate

Many analysers can titrate the CO_2 back to a value of 40 mmHg (5.3 kPa), and can then calculate what the HCO_3^- value would be at this CO_2 concentration. This is reported as the standard bicarbonate ($HCO_3^-{}_s$) value, which estimates the HCO_3^- concentration in the blood which arises solely due to metabolic factors, but ignores the change in HCO_3^- which is brought about by altered CO_2 concentrations; i.e. $HCO_3^-{}_s$ only deviates from normal when there is a primary metabolic disorder or where there is metabolic compensation for a respiratory disorder.

Total CO_2

Total CO_2 (TCO_2) represents the total amount of CO_2 that can be recovered from the sample under anaerobic conditions, and encompasses CO_2 from both HCO_3^- and H_2CO_3. As the HCO_3^- to H_2CO_3 ratio is 20:1, TCO_2 gives a good index of total HCO_3^- activity. TCO_2 will be about 5% higher than plasma HCO_3^- concentration, and a difference between TCO_2 and HCO_3^- of more than 5% suggests the patient probably has an acidosis. However, by itself, TCO_2 offers little information, and as a general rule, TCO_2 is typically ignored when HCO_3^- results are concomitantly presented. The plasma HCO_3^-, $PaCO_2$ and pH are more useful in evaluating acid–base status. TCO_2 gives no direct information about respiratory function.

Base excess/base deficit

The base excess (BE) value is a parameter derived by the blood gas analyser. Like the HCO_3^- measurement it provides an indication of the degree of metabolic dysfunction, but with slightly greater accuracy, since it takes into account all the buffering systems within the body, not just the contribution from the H_2CO_3–HCO_3^- buffer. It is defined as the amount of acid, in mmol/l, required to return 1 litre of blood to a pH of 7.4 at a P_aCO_2 of 40 mmHg (5.3 kPa). Like the HCO_3^- value, BE only deviates from normal when there is a primary metabolic disturbance, or metabolic compensation for a respiratory disorder. While some analysers report a BE result, others report a *base deficit* result, one simply being the negative of the other, i.e. a base excess of 6 mmol/l is the same as a base deficit of –6 mmol/l. The situation is confused by the fact that either can have a positive or negative value: normal base excess is 0 ± 4 mmol/l, and negative BE values are often reported. To avoid confusion, it is recommended that BE is used.

Simple acid–base disorders

There are four primary (or simple) acid–base disturbances: metabolic acidosis; metabolic alkalosis; respiratory acidosis; and respiratory alkalosis. Metabolic acidosis is the most common clinically significant acid–base disturbance.

- Metabolic disturbances affect primarily HCO_3^- concentration, and there is usually a compensatory change in P_aCO_2 (Figure 9.5)
- Respiratory disturbances affect primarily CO_2 partial pressure, and there is usually a compensatory change in HCO_3^- (Figure 9.5).

pH is determined by the ratio of HCO_3^- to CO_2 (Henderson–Hasslebalch equation), which is normally maintained at approximately 20:1. Remembering this allows one always to determine the appropriate bodily response to a primary acid–base disturbance.

Metabolic acidosis

Metabolic acidosis implies a primary reduction in HCO_3^- concentration. This may arise due to:

- Loss of HCO_3^-, e.g. as a result of severe diarrhoea
- Failure to excrete H^+, e.g. in renal failure or renal tubular acidosis
- Accumulation of acid, which is 'mopped up' by the HCO_3^-. For example, in shock the acid that accumulates is lactic acid, and in diabetic ketoacidosis, ketoacids. Lactic acidosis is a common pathway in many disease processes, and lactate levels may correlate with prognosis (high and persistently high levels being associated with a poor prognosis).

In metabolic acidosis, the body attempts to compensate for the disturbance by lowering CO_2 levels through hyperventilation to maintain the $HCO_3^-:CO_2$ ratio.

Anion gap

The anion gap (AG) is a useful measurement when attempting to determine the cause of a metabolic acidosis. It represents the difference between the commonly measured cations (positive ions) in plasma and commonly measured anions (negative ions). To maintain electroneutrality, the number of cations and anions in the plasma must be equal (Equation 9.1), but a proportion of circulating anions and cations are not measured routinely by laboratory tests. The unmeasured anions (e.g. negatively charged proteins, phosphate, lactate) are present in larger quantities than unmeasured cations (e.g. calcium, magnesium, globulins) so there are fewer measured anions. This means that when the measured anions are subtracted from the measured cations the answer is not zero, and this is the calculated anion gap (Equation 2).

Equation 9.1 $(Na^+ + K^+ + UC^+) - (Cl^- + HCO_3^- + UA^-) = 0$

where UC = unmeasured cations; UA = unmeasured anions.

Equation 9.2 $AG = (Na^+ + K^+) - (Cl^- + HCO_3^-)$

(K^+ is omitted by some authors from the equation as it contributes little to the overall charge difference).

Disorder	Uncompensated			Compensated			
	pH	*HCO_3^-*	*PCO_2*	*pH*	*HCO_3^-*	*PCO_2*	*Compensatory response*
Metabolic acidosis	↓↓	↓	Normal	↓	↓	↓	Hyperventilation to ↓ P_aCO_2
Metabolic alkalosis	↑↑	↑	Normal	↑	↑	↑	Hypoventilation to ↑ P_aCO_2
Respiratory acidosis	↓↓	Normal	↑	↓	↑	↑	HCO_3^- retention by kidneys
Respiratory alkalosis	↑↑	Normal	↓	↑	↓	↓	Increased HCO_3^- elimination by kidneys

9.5 Simple acid–base disorders and their compensatory responses.

From Equation 9.1, to maintain electroneutrality, a decrease in HCO_3^- (metabolic acidosis) has to be balanced by an increase in either chloride or unmeasured anions. If the chloride replaces the HCO_3^- (as usually occurs with direct HCO_3^- loss from the body), it can be seen from Equation 9.2 that the AG will be normal (hyperchloraemic metabolic acidosis). However, if the reduction in HCO_3^- is due to accumulation of unmeasured anions (such as lactate, beta-hydroxybutyrate or acetoacetate) and the chloride concentration remains normal (normochloraemic metabolic acidosis), it can be seen from Equation 9.2 that the AG will be high. Thus, the AG is used to determine whether metabolic acidosis is due to primary HCO_3^- loss (normal AG), or to accumulation of organic acids within the body (high AG).

Normal AG values have been reported to be in the range of 12–25 mmol/l in dogs and 13–27 mmol/l in cats.

Causes of metabolic acidosis and the associated AG are summarized in Figure 9.6. Changes in AG do not imply metabolic acidosis, though increased anion gap is most often associated with acidosis. AG is usually used to categorize an already diagnosed acidosis.

Cause of altered anion gap	Disease state	Mechanism
High anion gap acidosis		
Azotaemia or uraemia	Advanced renal failure	Accumulation of organic acids due to failure of renal excretion (elevation in AG may not be very marked)
Lactic acidosis	Shock, hypovolaemia, poor tissue perfusion	Lactate accumulation
Ketoacidosis	Diabetic ketoacidosis	Increased hepatic production of ketoacids (acetoacetate and beta-hydroxybutyrate) Volume contraction and acidaemia causes lactic acidosis
Hyperosmolar non-ketotic diabetes mellitus	Diabetes mellitus	Accumulation of measured cations, especially sodium N.B. Will only be acidotic if volume contraction causes lactic acidosis
Toxicity	Ethylene glycol, aspirin, methanol or paraldehyde toxicosis	Accumulation of metabolic products (acids)
Normal anion gap (hyperchloraemic) acidosis		
Diarrhoea	Many GI diseases: diarrhoea must be severe	Loss of HCO_3^-
Early renal failure	Early renal failure	Reduced excretion of ammonia, with subsequent retention of H^+ and failure to regenerate HCO_3^-
Renal tubular acidosis	Proximal (Fanconi syndrome) or distal renal tubular defects	Defective renal acid processing, with failure to excrete normal quantities of metabolically produced acid
Carbonic anhydrase inhibitors		Inhibition of carbonic anhydrase conversion of H_2CO_3 to HCO_3^-
Acidifying agents		Exogenous acid load
Hyperalimentation (in parenteral nutrition)		Acid load as a consequence of metabolism of nutrients (especially amino acids)
Very rapid intravenous rehydration		Rapid dilution of plasma bicarbonate
Ketoacidosis with renal ketone loss	Diabetes mellitus	Renal excretion of ketoacids sufficient to prevent a high anion gap developing
Low anion gap *(often occurs in absence of metabolic acidosis)*		
Retained non-sodium cations • Paraneoplastic hyperproteinaemia (increased cations) • Hypercalcaemia • Hypermagnesaemia • Lithium toxicity		Where there are increased cations, ECF sodium is reduced to maintain electroneutrality, so measured cations fall. The calculated anion gap is therefore low
Hypoalbuminaemia, dilution		Reduced concentration of unmeasured anions (by dilution), with compensatory increase in measured anions to maintain electroneutrality. Sodium and potassium, which are physiologically maintained in a narrow range, are not greatly altered

9.6 Types of metabolic acidosis and causes of altered anion gap. (Low anion gap conditions are not well characterized in small animals and some of the causes are extrapolated from humans.)

High anion gap acidosis: This occurs due to accumulation of acids in the ECF. If the ion that accumulates is readily excreted (by the kidney), then the concentration of the acid is limited and a high AG does not develop. High AG acidosis is seen in impaired tissue perfusion (e.g. hypovolaemic shock), advanced renal failure (see below), toxicosis (ethylene glycol and salicylate) and diabetic ketoacidosis. In ethylene glycol toxicity, the high AG is due to accumulations of metabolites (organic acids) of the compound, exacerbated by lactic acidosis and acute renal failure. Further examples are given in Figure 9.6.

Normal anion gap (hyperchloraemic) metabolic acidosis: This occurs in any clinical situation where the kidney is able to excrete the accumulating acid, and reduced HCO_3^- is balanced by increased chloride, or where there is HCO_3^- loss with subsequent chloride retention. Classic examples are shown in Figure 9.6. In the early stages of ketoacidosis, or early or mild lactic acidosis, this type of acidosis will also develop but will become a high AG acidosis as the acids accumulate.

Low anion gap: This arises less commonly, and is poorly characterized in small animals. A low AG is most often seen where there are increased unmeasured cations (globulins, calcium and magnesium), as ECF sodium is reduced to maintain electroneutrality, so measured cations fall. The calculated AG is therefore low. Low AG often occurs in the absence of acidosis.

Diabetes mellitus

Metabolic acidosis in ketoacidotic diabetics may be characterized by a normal or high AG, depending on the balance between production, metabolism and excretion of ketone anions. Ketones are filtered and resorbed by the kidneys.

In high AG ketosis, ketones produced by the liver exceed renal excretion. This is the common clinical situation, as volume contraction associated with polyuria drives renal sodium resorption, and enhanced tubular resorption of sodium is associated with enhanced resorption of accompanying anions, including the ketoacids. In addition, lactic acidosis (due to poor perfusion in volume-contracted patients) can contribute to the high AG, and result in a much more severe metabolic acidosis than diabetic ketoacidosis alone.

In animals with less severe hypovolaemia, renal excretion of ketoacids may be sufficient to prevent a high AG developing. These animals are acidotic, but with normal AG.

Rarely, patients develop hyperosmolar non-ketotic diabetes mellitus (HNDM), which is characterized by severe hyperglycaemia (>35 mmol/l), hyperosmolality (>350 mOsm/kg) and dehydration without ketosis or acidosis (unless there is lactic acidosis). HNDM may result in high AG due to increases in both sodium and potassium, which are measured cations, as part of the hyperosmolar state. Not all cases of HNDM are initially acidotic (though all have high AG), but most cases rapidly develop severe hypovolaemia and lactic acidosis, further increasing the AG.

Renal failure

In early renal failure, AG is normal and there is a hyperchloraemic metabolic acidosis. This is thought to be due to reduced excretion of ammonium ions (NH_4^+) (formed by ammonia (NH_3) binding H^+ in the tubule lumen), with subsequent retention of H^+ and failure to regenerate HCO_3^-. In normal animals, renal ammonia production is one method by which the kidney excretes H^+.

In advanced renal failure, reduced glomerular filtration rate and associated retention of anions (phosphate, sulphate and, sometimes, lactate) results in a high AG acidosis.

Metabolic alkalosis

Metabolic alkalosis implies a primary increase in HCO_3^- levels. This may occur iatrogenically (e.g. over-treatment of a metabolic acidosis with $NaHCO_3$ in the intravenous fluids) or, more commonly, due to loss of acid from the body, which leaves a relative excess of HCO_3^-. The classical clinical situation is severe protracted true gastric vomiting, for example, due to pyloric outflow obstruction. Compensation is by a reduction in respiration to allow CO_2 levels to rise to maintain the all-important HCO_3^-:CO_2 ratio. However, there is a limit to respiratory compensation for metabolic alkalosis, as the reduced respiration may induce hypoxaemia, which will then stimulate respiration. (Most patients with chronic vomiting, due to causes other than true pyloric obstruction, are acidotic, as bilious vomiting tends to lead to acidosis due to loss of HCO_3^-.) The causes of metabolic alkalosis are summarized in Figure 9.7.

Respiratory acidosis

Respiratory acidosis implies a primary rise in P_aCO_2, which the body will attempt to correct by retention of HCO_3^- by the kidney, thus restoring the HCO_3^-:CO_2 ratio. Respiratory acidosis is seen most commonly with alveolar hypoventilation: causes are summarized in Figure 9.8.

Cause of alkalosis	Disease state	Mechanism
HCO_3^- overload	Iatrogenic (most common)	Excess supplementation
Severe and protracted gastric vomiting	Pyloric outflow obstruction	Loss of H^+ (in vomit), HCO_3^- accumulation, volume depletion and enhanced renal H^+ secretion in exchange for Na^+ retention maintains alkalosis
Loop or thiazide diuretics	Cardiac patients	Loss of Cl^- in amounts greater than HCO_3^- loss, and relative ECF depletion with HCO_3^- retention. Na^+ retention due to hypovolaemia maintains acidososis (as above)

9.7 Causes of metabolic alkalosis.

Respiratory acidosis	Respiratory alkalosis
Upper airway obstruction	
Pleural cavity disease: • Pleural effusion • Pneumothorax	
Pulmonary disease: • Severe pneumonia • Severe pulmonary oedema • Diffuse metastatic disease • Massive pulmonary thromboembolism	Pulmonary disease: • Pneumonia • Interstitial lung disease
Depression of central control of respiration: • Drugs • Toxins • Brainstem disease	Central stimulation of respiration: • Anxiety, fear • Excitement • Pain • Pyrexia • (Drug therapy)
Depression of neuromuscular respiratory function: • Neurological/neuromuscular disease • Toxins	
Cardiopulmonary arrest	

9.8 Causes of respiratory acidosis and respiratory alkalosis.

Respiratory alkalosis

Respiratory alkalosis implies a primary reduction in P_aCO_2 levels (hyperventilation). Compensation is by increased elimination of HCO_3^- by the kidney. The causes of respiratory alkalosis are summarized in Figure 9.8.

Responses to acid–base disturbances

Whenever an acid–base disorder occurs, the body will attempt to restore pH back towards the normal range. Intra- and extracellular buffering systems will begin working as soon as an alteration in acid–base status is detected, thus providing rapid protection against changes in pH. Over the next few minutes, the respiratory system will start to attempt to compensate for the disturbance (provided the primary disorder is metabolic and not respiratory), either by retaining or excreting extra carbon dioxide. Although respiratory compensation begins working fairly rapidly, it takes several hours to achieve maximum effect. Finally, metabolic compensation will come into play. This usually takes several hours to begin having a significant effect, and 2–5 days for these effects to become maximal. Although metabolic compensation will occur for a primary respiratory disorder, it is also possible to have metabolic compensation for a primary metabolic disorder. This will only occur if the kidney is not the underlying cause of the problem.

Although metabolic and respiratory compensation for simple acid–base disorders can help limit the effect of the disorder on pH, there is a limit to the body's ability to compensate. In simple disorders, the expected responses can be quantified (Figure 9.9) but the compensatory responses listed in the table are based on *mean* values, and some patients may lie outside the calculated compensation value. If there is marked discrepancy between the patient's blood value and expected compensatory response, however, it tends to suggest that there may be a *mixed* acid–base disorder, i.e. two or more disorders occurring simultaneously. Another way to identify mixed disorders in animals with high AG metabolic acidosis is to compare the change in AG to the change in HCO_3^-: in simple acid–base disturbances, these changes will be of similar magnitude (i.e. each 1 mmol/l increase in AG should be mirrored by a fall of [HCO_3^-] by 1 mmol/l).

Evaluation of samples

A systematic approach should be adopted when evaluating blood gas data.

1. Examine the pH

If pH is in the normal range, this may imply:

- There is no acid–base disturbance
- There is an acid–base disturbance which has been completely compensated for
- There are two opposing acid–base disturbances (a mixed disorder), which are cancelling each other out, in terms of effect on pH.

Disturbance	Primary change	Expected compensation
Acute respiratory acidosis	Each 10 mmHg (1.33 kPa) ↑ P_aCO_2	HCO_3^- ↑ by 1.5 mmol/l
Chronic respiratory acidosis	Each 10 mmHg (1.33 kPa) ↑ P_aCO_2	HCO_3^- ↑ by 3.5 mmol/l
Acute respiratory alkalosis	Each 10 mmHg (1.33 kPa) ↓ P_aCO_2	HCO_3^- ↓ by 2.5 mmol/l
Chronic respiratory alkalosis	Each 10 mmHg (1.33 kPa) ↓ P_aCO_2	HCO_3^- ↓ by 5.5 mmol/l
Metabolic acidosis	Each 1 mmol/l ↓ HCO_3^-	$PaCO_2$ ↓ by 0.7 mmHg (~0.1 kPa)
Metabolic alkalosis	Each 1 mmol/l ↑ HCO_3^-	$PaCO_2$ ↑ by 0.7 mmHg (~0.1 kPa)

9.9 Expected compensatory responses for primary acid–base disturbances. (Based on canine data from DiBartola (1992).)

If there is an acidaemia (pH <7.35), there must be an underlying metabolic or respiratory acidosis, or both. If there is an alkalaemia (pH >7.45), there must be an underlying metabolic or respiratory alkalosis, or both.

Even with maximal compensation for any disorder, the pH will tend not to return to the midpoint of the normal range (although it may lie just within the normal range), and the body does not usually overcompensate for an acid–base disturbance. If there were a primary metabolic or respiratory acidosis, even with respiratory or metabolic compensation, respectively, the pH would still be <7.4; it would lie towards the acidaemic side of the midpoint of the pH range. Similarly, if there were a primary metabolic or respiratory alkalosis, even with appropriate compensation, the pH would still be >7.4.

2. Look at the PCO_2

- If PCO_2 is elevated, there is either a primary respiratory acidosis or a compensatory response to a metabolic alkalosis.
- If PCO_2 is low, there is either a primary respiratory alkalosis or a compensatory response to a metabolic acidosis.

3. Look at the actual and standard bicarbonate values, and the base excess

In general, BE and HCO_3^- will change in a similar direction, as they are both variants on the same theme (see earlier).

- If there is purely a respiratory disturbance, $HCO_3^-{}_a$ will be altered but $HCO_3^-{}_s$ and BE will be normal
- If there is a metabolic disorder, or a metabolic compensatory response, $HCO_3^-{}_s$ and $HCO_3^-{}_a$ and BE will change.

4. Distinguish the primary disturbance from the compensatory response

In a patient with a low PCO_2 and a low HCO_3^-, for example, does the patient have:

- A primary respiratory alkalosis with metabolic compensation, *or*
- A primary metabolic acidosis with respiratory compensation?

Evaluation of the patient's history and clinical signs should help identify the primary disturbance.

It should be remembered that the pH will move in the same direction as for the primary disorder, and the body does not usually overcompensate (see above). Even with maximal compensation, if the pH returns to the normal range it usually lies at its extremes. Thus, in this case, if the pH of the sample were <7.4 (i.e. to the acidaemic side of the pH range), it would suggest that the primary problem was an acidosis, and would fit best with the second explanation, above. If the pH were >7.4 (i.e. to the alkalaemic side of the pH range), the first explanation would be most appropriate. Interpretation becomes more complex if the pH is at or close to 7.4, as it becomes difficult to determine which is the primary problem. Because complete compensation is uncommon, a pH at or close to the midpoint of the pH suggests that two opposing disorders are occurring (i.e. there is a mixed disturbance). Concurrent respiratory alkalosis and metabolic acidosis could result in a pH that is at or close to 7.4.

5. Assess whether the compensatory response is as expected

Refer to Figure 9.9. If the compensatory response is not as expected, this may suggest the presence of a mixed acid–base disorder.

6. Assess the patient's oxygenation

The patient's oxygenation is assessed on an arterial sample, using the alveolar gas equation, and calculating the alveolar–arterial oxygen difference. Unless the patient is exhibiting respiratory signs, this is seldom carried out, and, as an alternative, a rough guide to the expected P_aO_2 is to multiply the inspired O_2 concentration by a factor of 5, i.e. if the patient is breathing room air (21% O_2), the P_aO_2 should be around 100 mmHg (13.3 kPa). If breathing 100% O_2, the expected P_aO_2 would be around 500 mmHg (66.5 kPa).

Blood gas analysis in respiratory patients

Arterial samples must be used to assess respiratory patients, and P_aO_2 and P_aCO_2 are the most important parameters, as it is the animal's gas exchange capacity that is of interest. Arterial blood gas tensions are affected by hypoventilation, ventilation–perfusion mismatch (VA/Q or V/Q) and, rarely, diffusion abnormalities. Blood gas analysis may, however, be normal in mild respiratory conditions and in the early stages of more severe disease.

Normal arterial oxygen tension (P_aO_2) is approximately 80–100 mmHg (10.6–13.3 kPa) on room air, and, at these values, haemoglobin saturation approaches 97–100%. At values less than about 60 mmHg (8 kPa) there is significant hypoxaemia, and below 40–50 mmHg (5.3–6.6 kPa) cyanosis may become evident.

Many clinicians use a value for normal P_aCO_2 of 35–45 mmHg (4.65–5.98 kPa) in the dog: this is based on human data and will result in overdiagnosis of hyperventilation. Normal P_aCO_2 in dogs is 30.8–42.8 mmHg (4.10–5.69 kPa), and cats tend to have lower values of 25.2–36.8 mmHg (3.35–4.89kPa) (see Figure 9.4). Normal P_vCO_2 is higher than P_aCO_2, and values are approximately 33–41 mmHg (4.47–5.48 kPa) in dogs and 33–45 mmHg (4.35–5.94 kPa) in cats.

Hypoventilation (alveolar hypoventilation) results in hypercapnia (respiratory acidosis, see Figure 9.8) and may also lead to hypoxaemia, although this depends upon both the degree of hypercapnia, and the F_iO_2. For example, an animal under general anaesthesia breathing 100% O_2 is unlikely to exhibit hypoxaemia, even in the face of severe hypercapnia. Hypoventilation is most often caused by upper airway obstruction, pleural effusion and drugs or disorders affecting central control of respiration (e.g. general anaesthesia) or diseases affecting the neuromuscular components of the respiratory system. In animals with chronic hypercapnia, chloride may become depleted. This is because the continuous acid load which the body produces must be buffered and excreted, but CO_2 excretion is limited, so more acid must be excreted by the kidney, and this requires chloride. The plasma levels of HCO_3^- remain elevated, as compensation for the respiratory acidosis.

Ventilation–perfusion (V/Q) mismatch (or imbalance) occurs when there is either normal ventilation but inadequate perfusion (so there is insufficient blood passing the alveoli for oxygen to be taken up into the pulmonary capillaries), or inadequate ventilation but adequate perfusion (where pulmonary capillary blood reaches the alveoli in adequate quantities, but ventilation to those alveoli has been insufficient to allow optimal oxygenation). In both situations, oxygen transfer is inefficient, and, if impairment is severe enough, the result is hypoxaemia. However, although blood oxygenation is usually impaired in this situation, patients with V/Q mismatch are usually normocapnic, because CO_2 diffuses easily and exchange is not limited. Indeed, patients with V/Q mismatch severe enough to induce hypoxaemia may actually be hypocapnic since the hypoxaemia may stimulate ventilatory drive. Increasing the F_iO_2 will usually improve the hypoxaemia in patients with V/Q mismatch. V/Q mismatch is most often associated with significant lower airway and pulmonary parenchymal disease, where there is diffusion impairment, especially interstitial and alveolar diseases, such as pneumonia and pulmonary oedema. Severe chronic bronchitis, asthma or obstructive pulmonary disease can also cause mismatch. Lastly, it is commonly seen in pulmonary thromboembolism.

In clinical practice, a simplified version of the alveolar–arterial oxygen gradient equation is often used to differentiate hypoxaemia caused by alveolar hypoventilation from that caused by V/Q mismatch:

$$P_{(A\text{-}a)}O_2 = [150 - (P_aCO_2/0.8) - P_aO_2]$$

This equation assumes values for F_iO_2 (based on room air), barometric pressure, saturated vapour pressure of water and respiratory quotient (RQ: see Figure 9.1). It will be greatly affected by the patient receiving supplemental oxygen (in which case the full equation should be used), and to a lesser extent the natural variations in barometric pressure, alterations in vapour pressure with body temperature, and variations in RQ (which do occur, but are never measured). However, although it is imprecise, the alveolar–arterial oxygen gradient calculated in this way does provide useful information. In normal animals, it is <25 mmHg (3.32 kPa), and usually <10 mmHg (1.33 kPa). In hypoventilation where there is hypoxaemia, it is usually slightly elevated, but may be normal, depending on the relative changes in P_aCO_2 and P_aO_2. In V/Q mismatch the alveolar–arterial oxygen gradient is usually markedly elevated (>25 mmHg; 3.32 kPa).

The relation between S_aO_2 and PO_2 is illustrated in Figure 9.10, in a haemoglobin oxygenation curve.

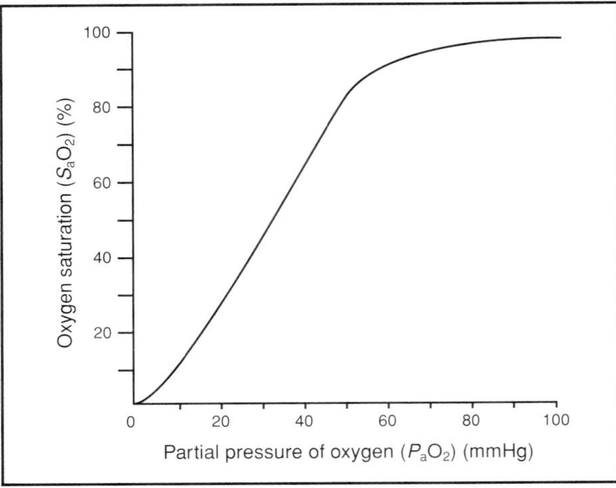

9.10 Oxygen–haemoglobin dissociation curve. Note the almost linear relation between S_aO_2 and P_aO_2 at P_aO_2 values <60 mmHg.

Some blood gas analysers will estimate the S_aO_2, the saturation of haemoglobin with oxygen in arterial gas. This value is calculated based on the P_aO_2 but does not make any allowance for other factors which affect the haemoglobin oxygenation curve, e.g. concentrations of 2,3 diphosphoglycerate in red blood cells (see Chapter 4). The S_pO_2 (haemoglobin saturation measured by pulse oximetry) is usually similar to S_aO_2 and can be used to give an indication of P_aO_2. Due to the almost linear relation between S_aO_2 or S_pO_2 and P_aO_2 at PaO_2 values <60 mmHg (7.98 kPa) (Figure 9.10), some key values are worthy of note: P_aO_2 values of 40, 50 and 60 mmHg (5.32, 6.65 and 7.98 kPa) correspond to S_aO_2 or S_pO_2 values of 70, 80 and 90%, respectively. S_pO_2 values <90% are of immediate concern.

When considering oxygenation, it should be remembered that the oxygen-carrying capacity of haemoglobin is also affected by the pH. At any given P_aO_2, haemoglobin has less affinity for oxygen if the pH drops because the oxygenation curve moves to the right. This means that oxygen is given up more readily at tissue level. However, where there is poor oxygenation, this reduced affinity also means that poorer haemoglobin saturation may be achieved, and, in hypoxaemic animals, this may actually limit the oxygen delivery to tissues.

Effects of blood gas disturbances on other analytes

Animals with acid–base disorders may have secondary abnormalities in other biochemical parameters, of which potassium is probably the most important. Chloride levels are often altered in metabolic acidosis, as described above, where there is compensatory hyperchloraemia in normal anion gap metabolic acidosis, to maintain electrical neutrality.

Potassium distribution is affected by acid–base disturbances, and potassium disorders, themselves, can exacerbate acid–base disorders. In metabolic acidosis (but not respiratory acidosis), potassium is translocated from the ICF to the ECF in exchange for

H^+; chloride cannot follow H^+ into cells, so exchange must occur. This may result in hyperkalaemia, though measured serum or plasma potassium concentration is often normal as these patients often have an overall depletion of total body potassium. Where the acid can follow the H^+ into the cell (e.g. lactate) this effect may be less profound. In metabolic alkalosis, the opposite can occur, and potassium shifts into cells, but this rarely causes a significant hypokalaemia. However, in potassium depletion, alkalosis may be exacerbated. If there is ECF volume depletion, this may limit the normal renal response to metabolic alkalosis (rapid HCO_3^- excretion) and prevent correction. The kidney prioritizes volume expansion above acid–base balance, and sodium retention occurs to expand plasma volume. Sodium is reabsorbed in the distal tubule in exchange for H^+ or potassium, and if potassium is depleted, more H^+ is exchanged. Secretion of H^+ into the tubule lumen is associated with HCO_3^- entry into the ECF, which maintains the alkalosis. Thus the alkalosis is not corrected, and there is H^+ secretion in the urine. This is called 'paradoxical aciduria', where acid urine is produced in the face of alkalosis.

Mixed acid–base disturbances

Complex or mixed acid–base disturbances should be suspected if the expected compensation for the primary disturbance fails to develop (see Figures 9.5 and 9.9), if the PCO_2 and HCO_3^- changes are not in the same direction, or if the changes in AG and HCO_3^- are not of similar magnitude. If both cause pH changes in the same direction (e.g. a combined respiratory and metabolic acidosis), life-threatening disturbances are likely and treating the immediate crises is vital. If the two conditions act disparately, the pH may be normal and treatment of one condition may unmask a second disturbance.

Case examples

Case 1

Signalment

5-year-old male Dalmatian.

History and clinical findings

Anorexia for 4–5 days, left fore lameness, previous right fore lameness. Collapsed, recumbent with congested, muddy mucous membranes and capillary refill time of <1 s. Cold extremities. Heart rate of 170 bpm and a machinery murmur (point of maximum intensity over aortic valve); temperature 40°C; respiratory rate 36 breaths per minute. Swelling, heat and pain on palpation of left elbow and right shoulder.

Clinical pathology data

Haematology	Result	Reference interval
RBC (x 10^{12}/l)	8.71	5.5–8.5
HCT (l/l)	0.565	0.37–0.55
Hb (g/dl)	18.05	12.00–18.00
MCV (fl)	66.2	60.0–77.0
MCHC (g/dl)	36.7	32.0–36.0
WBC (x 10^9/l)	33.1	6.0–12.8
Neutrophils (segmented) (x 10^9/l)	28.9	3.0–11.8
Neutrophils (band) (x 10^9/l)	1.5	0.0–0.5
Lymphocytes (x 10^9/l)	0.6	1.0–4.8
Monocytes (x 10^9/l)	2.1	0.15–1.35
Eosinophils (x 10^9/l)	0	0.1–1.25
Basophils (x 10^9/l)	0.0	Rare
Platelets (x 10^9/l)	404	200–500

Film comment

Neutrophils show toxic change.

Biochemistry	Result	Reference interval
Sodium (mmol/l)	144	135–155
Potassium (mmol/l)	4.3	3.5–5.5
Chloride (mmol/l)	118	95–115

Blood gas analysis	Result	Reference interval
pH	7.2	7.35–7.44
HCO_3^- (mmol/l)	14	20.8–24.2
P_vO_2 (mmHg)	33.9	47.9–56.3
P_vCO_2 (mmHg)	30.6	33.6–41.2
BE (mmol/l)	−11.4	0±4

What abnormalities are present?

Haematology

- Mild erythrocytosis
- Neutrophilia with mild left shirt
- Lymphopenia
- Slight monocytosis

Blood gas analysis

- Slight hyperchloraemia
- Low pH
- Reduced HCO_3^-
- Low P_vO_2
- Low P_vCO_2

How would you interpret these results and what are the likely differential diagnoses?

The increased haematocrit most likely reflects hypovolaemia. Neutrophilia with a mild left shift suggests an inflammatory response, and this may also be a cause of the monocytosis. As there is lymphopenia, there is probably a superimposed stress leucogram. The toxic change reported on smear examination suggests rapid marrow transit time due to demand for neutrophil production, suggesting there is a serious inflammatory process.

The blood gas results show the patient is acidaemic. P_vO_2 is low, but this gives no indication of arterial oxygenation and should not be used to assess respiratory function. The low HCO_3^- suggests metabolic acidosis, with the reduction in P_vCO_2 reflecting respiratory compensation. The slight hyperchloraemia has developed to maintain electroneutrality, i.e. this is a hyperchloraemic metabolic acidosis. The anion gap can be calculated:

AG = (144 + 4.3) − (118 + 14) = 16.3 (12–25 mmol/l)

Case 1 continues ▶

Case 1 continued

Given the clinical presentation (pyrexia, signs of septic shock, machinery murmur, shifting lameness consistent with infective arthritis) the most likely primary disease is bacterial endocarditis. The dog is in septic shock and has developed acidosis as a result (most likely) of lactate accumulation, but this has not exceeded renal excretion and no increase in anion gap has occurred.

What further tests would you recommend?

- Cardiac ultrasonography
- Blood and urine culture
- Arthrocentesis for cytology, culture and sensitivity testing.

Results of further tests

Cardiac ultrasonography demonstrated vegetative lesions on the aortic valve, consistent with bacterial endocarditis.

Case outcome

The dog received appropriate supportive therapy and aggressive intravenous antibiotic therapy, and made a full recovery.

Case 2

Signalment

9-year-old female Irish Setter.

History and clinical findings

2-week history of PU/PD. Now vomiting, depressed and inappetent. On clinical examination, quiet and depressed, with a respiratory rate of 42 breaths per minute. Discomfort on cranial abdominal palpation.

Clinical pathology data

Biochemistry	Result	Reference interval
Sodium (mmol/l)	128	135–155
Potassium (mmol/l)	5.5	3.60–5.60
Chloride (mmol/l)	80	100–116
Glucose (mmol/l)	35.2	3.3–5.8
Urea (mmol/l)	8.5	3.5–7.7
Creatinine (μmol/l)	62	45–150
Calcium (mmol/l)	2.14	2.40–2.90
Inorganic phosphate (mmol/l)	1.49	0.80–1.6
TP (g/l)	56.0	55.0–75.0
Albumin (g/l)	21.0	23.0–31.0
Globulin (g/l)	35.0	27.0–40.0
ALT (IU/l)	66	5.0–60.0
ALP (IU/l)	1329	0–130

Urine analysis	
SG	1.036
Protein	1+
pH	5.0
Glucose	> 3+
Ketones	3+
Bilirubin	+
Sediment examination	RBC 10 per hpf; WBC <5 per hpf

Blood gas analysis (venous)	Result	Reference interval
pH	7.187	7.35–7.44
HCO_3^- (mmol/l)	10.0	20.8–24.2
P_vO_2 (mmHg)	43	47.9–56.3
P_vCO_2 (mmHg)	25	33.6–41.2
TCO_2 (mmol/l)	10.4	20–25
BE (mmol/l)	–18.7	0 ± 4

Biochemistry

- Slightly low albumin
- Markedly elevated (10x) ALP
- Marginally elevated ALT
- Hyponatraemia
- Hypochloraemia
- Slightly low total calcium
- Slightly elevated urea
- Marked hyperglycaemia

Urine analysis

- Urine appears adequately concentrated
- Proteinuria
- Reduced pH
- Marked glucosuria
- Marked ketonuria
- Haematuria
- + bilirubin not significant

Blood gas analysis

- Acidaemia
- Low HCO_3^-
- Low P_vO_2
- Low P_vCO_2
- Low total CO_2 (consistent with low bicarbonate)
- Decreased (i.e. more negative) base excess

How would you interpret these results and what are the likely differential diagnoses?

The hyperglycaemia, glucosuria and ketonuria confirm a diagnosis of diabetic ketoacidosis (DKA). The slightly low albumin may be due to the liver producing acute phase proteins in preference to albumin, if the patient has concurrent pancreatitis. The marked elevation in ALP with much lesser elevation in ALT suggest that, in addition to secondary hepatopathy (hepatic lipid accumulation) due to the diabetes mellitus, there may also be more significant cholestasis, and this could also be explained by pancreatitis, which is a common complication of diabetes mellitus. Similarly, the low total calcium may be partly due to the low albumin, but may also be due to pancreatitis. The slightly elevated urea may reflect a degree of hypovolaemia. This would be consistent with the dog's clinical presentation.

Hyponatraemia is also likely due to the diabetes mellitus. During the development of DKA, ketone anions are excreted into urine and since electrical neutrality is always maintained, this is accompanied by an obligatory loss of sodium and potassium ions. Hyponatraemia is therefore common. Potassium is typically at the high end of the normal range in

Case 2 continues ▶

Case 2 continued

spite of this increased urine loss, as with developing acidosis there is increased uptake of hydrogen ions (into cells) in exchange for potassium ions (which move out into the ECF). Thus the serum potassium is normal despite total body depletion.

The SG of 1.036 may not, in fact, reflect adequate renal concentrating ability, as the large amount of glucose in the urine will increase the SG. The acidic nature of the urine is due to excretion of ketoacids. The haematuria is most likely due to a secondary urinary tract infection: this is not always accompanied by an inflammatory sediment.

On venous blood gas analysis, the low pH tells us the patient is acidaemic. In the absence of further data, the low bicarbonate could be due either to metabolic acidosis or to metabolic compensation for respiratory alkalosis (but this does not fit so well with the clinical picture). In addition, pH will lie in the same direction as the primary acid–base disturbance (i.e. the body does not overcompensate), so the fact that this patient is acidaemic would suggest that an acidosis must be the primary disturbance. We would therefore not expect a respiratory alkalosis to be the underlying problem. P_vO_2 is low, but this gives no indication of arterial oxygenation and should not be used to assess respiratory function. P_vCO_2 is reduced as a compensatory response to the metabolic acidosis, and the increased respiratory rate observed probably reflects respiratory compensation (though pain due to the pancreatitis may also be a contributory factor). The decreased (more negative) base excess reflects the primary metabolic disturbance (metabolic acidosis).

If we calculate the anion gap: AG = (128 + 5.5) – (80 + 10) = 43.5 (reference interval 12–25 mmol/l). This marked elevation in the anion gap is due to the accumulation of the unmeasured ketoacids (and possibly lactate accumulation).

The increase in anion gap can also be compared to the reduction in bicarbonate: in simple acid–base disturbances, these changes will be of similar magnitude (i.e. each 1 mmol/l increase in AG should be mirrored by a fall in bicarbonate concentration of 1 mmol/l). In this case, the anion gap has increased by approximately 25 mmol/l (from the mid-interval value of 18.5 mmol/l), and bicarbonate has decreased by approximately 12.5 mmol/l (from the mid reference value of 22.5). This might suggest that there is a mixed problem but most likely reflects the fact that there is incomplete compensation, as confirmed by the marked acidaemia, or the fact that these estimates of compensation are extrapolated from human data, and we are using true dog reference values for bicarbonate, which slightly reduce the appreciated drop in bicarbonate.

What further tests would you recommend?

- Urine culture and sensitivity testing
- Abdominal ultrasonography (to help confirm pancreatitis)
- cPLI, amylase, lipase ± TLI

Case 3

Signalment

10-year-old female neutered Dobermann.

History and clinical findings

Diagnosed with immune-mediated haemolytic anaemia (IMHA) and thrombocytopenia (IMTP) 3 months previously. Good response to treatment with prednisolone and azathioprine. Acute deterioration 48 hours prior to presentation, with sudden-onset poor exercise tolerance, weakness and respiratory signs. Clinical examination revealed tachypnoea, hyperpnoea and pale pink-grey to cyanotic mucous membranes. Respiratory rate and effort remained increased at rest.

Clinical pathology data

Haematology	Result	Reference interval
RBC (x 10^{12}/l)	2.47	5.50–8.00
HCT(l/l)	0.19	0.35–0.55
Hb (g/dl)	6.9	12.00–18.00
MCV (fl)	79.0	65.0–75.0
MCH (pg)	27.9	19.5–24.5
MCHC (g/dl)	35.4	32–37
RDW (%)	27.2	14–17
Reticulocytes (%)	31	<1
Normoblasts (x 10^9/l)	2.24	occasional
WBC (x 10^9/l)	21.2	6.0–18.0
Neutrophils (segmented) (x 10^9/l)	14.3	3. 0–12.0
Neutrophils (band) (x 10^9/l)	0.63	0–0.3
Lymphocytes (x 10^9/l)	2.87	1.2–3.8
Monocytes (x 10^9/l)	0.7	0.0–1.20
Eosinophils (x 10^9/l)	0.35	0.0–1.3
Basophils (x 10^9/l)	0	0.0–0.2
Platelets (x 10^9/l)	14	200–500

Biochemistry	Result	Reference interval
Sodium (mmol/l)	144	140–153
Potassium (mmol/l)	4.74	3.80–5.30
Chloride (mmol/l)	115	99–115
Urea (mmol/l)	6.1	3.5–6.0
Creatinine (μmol/l)	76	20–110
Calcium (mmol/l)	2.56	2.20–2.70
Inorganic phosphate (mmol/l)	1.46	0.80–2.0
TP (g/l)	71.0	57.0–78.0
Albumin (g/l)	24.0	23.0–31.0
Globulin (g/l)	47.0	27.0–40.0
ALP (IU/l)	931	0–100
ALT (IU/l)	122	7–50
Cholesterol (mmol/l)	3.9	3.2–6.5

Blood gas analysis (on admission; dog breathing room air)	Result	Reference interval
pH	7.403	7.35–7.44
PaO_2 (mmHg)	87	80.9–103.3
$PaCO_2$ (mmHg)	22.4	30.8–42.8
BE (mmol/l)	–11	0±4
HCO_3^- (mmol/l) (actual)	14	18.8–25.6
TCO_2 (mmol/l)	15	20–25

What abnormalities are present?

Haematology

- Moderate, intensely regenerative anaemia (see Chapter 4)
  - Macrocytic

Case 3 continues ▶

Case 3 continued

- Increased RDW
- Absolute reticulocyte count = 31/100 x 2.47 x10^{12}/l
  = 0.776 x10^{12}/l
  = 776 x 10^9/l
- Increased nucleated red blood cells (normoblasts)

- Mature neutrophilia
- Profound thrombocytopenia

Biochemistry

- Elevated globulins
- Markedly elevated (9x) ALP
- Moderately elevated (2.5x) ALT

Blood gas analysis

- Low P_aCO_2
- Decreased (more negative) base excess
- Low HCO_3^-

How would you interpret these results and what are the likely differential diagnoses?

Results suggest that the IMHA and IMTP are no longer controlled. DIC may be contributing to the thrombocytopenia. The neutrophilia may reflect non-specific bone marrow stimulation, corticosteroid therapy and/or stress. There may also be an ongoing inflammatory response.

The mildly raised globulin is most likely a result of the immune-mediated disease. The marked elevation of ALP with moderate elevation of ALT is consistent with corticosteroid therapy (see Chapter 12). ALT may also be elevated as a result of hypoxic damage to hepatocytes due to the anaemia (possibly exacerbated by suspected respiratory disease).

Blood pH falls just above the midpoint of the range. P_aO_2 is within the normal range, though the clinical signs of hyperpnoea and tachypnoea suggest this may be maintained by increased respiratory rate and effort (due to hypoxic drive if respiratory work reduced). The reduced HCO_3^- and P_aCO_2 are the most significant abnormalities. These can be explained either by a primary metabolic acidosis with respiratory compensation or by a respiratory alkalosis with metabolic compensation. As base excess deviates from normal when there is either a primary metabolic disturbance, or metabolic compensation for a respiratory disorder, this does not help discriminate. However, as the pH falls just above the midpoint of 7.4, respiratory alkalosis is the more likely primary change. Respiratory alkalosis may be due to pulmonary disease, or central stimulation of respiration (e.g. due to hypoxia, in this case). It is also possible that we have a mixed disorder, and we should determine whether the reduction in HCO_3^- is appropriate.

In respiratory alkalosis, each 10 mmHg reduction in P_aCO_2 should be accompanied by a compensatory reduction in HCO_3^- of 2.5 mmol/l if acute, or up to 5.5 mmol/l if chronic. The reduction in HCO_3^- in this case is at least 4.8 and up to 11.6 mmol/l. P_aCO_2 is reduced by approximately 8–20 mmHg, giving an expected reduction in HCO_3^- of 2–5 mmol/l if the process has occurred acutely, or 4.4–11 mmol/l if more chronic. Thus, these results could indicate a chronic respiratory alkalosis, as the HCO_3^- concentration falls within the expected compensatory range. However, it is unusual for compensation to restore the pH to exactly 7.4 and this may support a mixed disturbance, i.e. respiratory alkalosis and concurrent metabolic acidosis. The metabolic acidosis is a likely result of impaired tissue oxygenation generating lactate during anaerobic metabolism.

Another way to identify mixed disorders in animals with high AG metabolic acidosis is to compare the change in AG to the change in HCO_3^- (see above): in this case, the anion gap is normal, so does not help us in identifying a mixed disorder.

$$AG = (144 + 4.74) - (115 + 14) = 19.74 \ (12\text{–}25 \text{ mmol/l})$$

This patient has respiratory signs so we should calculate the alveolar–arterial oxygen gradient:

$$\begin{aligned} p_{(A\text{-}a)}O_2 &= [150 - (P_aCO_2/0.8) - P_aO_2] \\ &= 150 - (22.4/0.8) - 87 \\ &= 150 - 28 - 87 \\ &= 35 \text{ mmHg} \end{aligned}$$

Elevations of the alveolar–arterial oxygen gradient to > 25 mmHg in patients breathing room air are consistent with ventilation–perfusion mismatch. V/Q mismatch is most often associated with significant lower airway and pulmonary parenchymal disease (where there is diffusion impairment), especially interstitial and alveolar diseases such as pneumonia and pulmonary oedema. Severe chronic bronchitis, asthma or obstructive pulmonary disease can also cause mismatch. Lastly, it is commonly seen in pulmonary thromboembolism (PTE). The history and clinical signs in this case are consistent with PTE, and both the immune-mediated disease and the treatment are predisposing factors for thromboembolic disease: diagnosis is presumptive after exclusion of other causes. If PTE is the cause, pain associated with the disease my also be contributing to the respiratory alkalosis.

What further tests would you recommend?

- Thoracic radiography to rule out airway or pulmonary disease
- Full coagulation screen for DIC

Results of further tests

Thoracic radiographs showed only pulmonary over-inflation, with no evidence of pulmonary parenchymal disease.

Treatment and case outcome

The bitch was treated with oxygen supplementation and low molecular weight heparin. She became increasingly hypoxic if oxygen supplementation was stopped. The owners declined more aggressive immunosuppressive therapy to try to control the primary disease, and she was euthanased due to disease progression.

Further reading

Adams LG and Polzin DJ (1989) Mixed acid–base disorders. *Veterinary Clinics of North America: Small Animal Practice* **19,** 307–326

DiBartola SP (1992) Introduction to acid–base disorders. In: *Fluid Therapy in Small Animal Practice,* ed. SP DiBartola, pp. 193–215. WB Saunders, Philadelphia

DiBartola SP and De Morais HAS (1992) Respiratory acid–base disorders. In: *Fluid Therapy in Small Animal Practice,* ed. SP DiBartola, pp. 258–275. WB Saunders, Philadelphia

Driscoll P, Brown T, Gwinnutt C and Wardle T (1997) *A Simple Guide to Blood Gas Analysis.* BMJ Publishing Group, London

Haskins SC (1983) Blood gases and acid–base balance: clinical interpretation and therapeutic implications. In: *Current Veterinary Therapy, 8th edn,* ed. Kirk RW *et al.*, pp. 201–215. WB Saunders, Philadelphia

Martin L (1999) *All You Really Need to Know to Interpret Arterial Blood Gases, 2nd edn.* Lippincott, Willams and Wilkins, Philadelphia

Peterson M (1998) Endocrine emergencies. In: *BSAVA Manual of Endocrinology, 2nd edn,* ed. AG Torrance and CT Mooney, pp 163–172. BSAVA Publications, Gloucester

Polzin DJ, Stevens JB and Osborne CA (1982) Clinical application of the anion gap in evaluation of acid–base disorders in dogs. *Compendium on Continuing Education for the Practicing Veterinarian* **4,** 1021–1032

Robertson SA (1989) Simple acid–base disorders. *Veterinary Clinics of North America: Small Animal Practice* **19,** 289–306

Rodkey WG, Hannon JP, Dramise JG, White RD, Welsh DC and Persky BN (1978) Arterialized capillary blood used to determine the acid–base and blood gas status of dogs. *American Journal of Veterinary Research* **39,** 459–464

Rubush JM (2001) Metabolic acid–base disorders. *Veterinary Clinics of North America: Small Animal Practice* **31,** 1323–1354

Senior DF (1995) Fluid therapy, electrolytes and acid–base control. In: *Textbook of Veterinary Internal Medicine, 4th edn,* ed. SJ Ettinger and EC Feldman, pp. 294–312. WB Saunders, Philadelphia

Verwaerde P, Malet C, Lagente M, de la Farge F and Braun JP (2002) The accuracy of the i-STAT, portable analyser for measuring gases and pH in whole blood samples from dogs. *Research in Veterinary Science* **73,** 71–75

Zweens J, Grankena H, van Kampen EJ, Rispins P and Zijlstra WG (1977) Ionic composition of arterial and mixed venous plasma in the unanaesthetized dog. *American Journal of Physiology* **233,** F412–F415

10

Urine analysis

Joy Archer

Introduction

Urine analysis is a simple, non-invasive and cheap laboratory test that rapidly provides valuable information about the urinary tract and other body systems. A complete urine analysis (including dipstick, specific gravity (SG) and sediment examination) should be performed, even if one component part shows no abnormalities. Concurrent serum or plasma biochemical analysis is often required to gain maximum benefit from urine analysis.

Free-catch samples should be collected into a clean container with minimal contact of the voided urine with the animal's body. Ideally, new clean clear containers with tight-fitting lids should be provided. Use of containers provided by owners should be discouraged as these can contain traces of detergents, bleach, drugs, cosmetics and other compounds that can affect the tests. Aseptic collection techniques (cystocentesis, catheterization in certain circumstances) should be used if the sample is to be cultured.

Hydration status greatly affects SG and certain drugs and dietary supplements can affect results (including dipstick and sediment evaluation), so any medication or supplementation the animal has received should be noted.

Urine should be analysed as rapidly as possible after collection, ideally within 30 minutes. If this is not possible it should be refrigerated immediately and stored for preferably no more than 6–12 hours after collection. Refrigerated urine should be brought to room temperature and thoroughly mixed before analysis. Urine should not be frozen if sediment analysis is to be performed. Casts are particularly vulnerable to disintegration and will only be detected if fresh urine is examined very soon after collection. Casts may be the only laboratory abnormality present in early renal disease (prior to the development of azotaemia). During storage, other formed elements may change; there may be cellular disintegration, and urine pH may alter. These changes in urine composition are more pronounced the longer the storage time and the higher the temperature. In addition, microorganisms can continue to multiply whether they are present as infectious agents or contaminants. The common changes found in aged urine are summarized in Figure 10.1.

Gross appearance

Before beginning any analysis the urine sample should be observed in a transparent container for clarity (turbidity) and colour, and these recorded using a consistent system of semiquantitative reporting. Normal urine should be clear and yellow to straw-coloured, depending on concentration of coloured pigment molecules. The interpretation of gross findings is summarized in Figure 10.2.

Constituent	Change	Cause
Colour and clarity	Dark and turbid	RBC lysis; growth of bacteria
pH	Increase	Proliferation of urease-producing bacteria, splitting urea to ammonia
Bilirubin	Decrease	Broken down by sunlight
Casts	Disintegration	Low SG; low pH; increased temperature; vigorous shaking
Sediment	↑ Crystals and amorphous material	Storage at low temperature; evaporation; pH change
Epithelial cells	Morphological change, disintegration	Low SG and osmolality
White blood cells	Swelling, lysis, vacuolation	Low SG and osmolality
Red blood cells	Crenation, lysis	Low SG and osmolality
Bacteria	Growth	Long-term storage at high temperatures, especially voided samples and in plain (not boric acid) tubes

10.1 Changes seen in aged urine.

Appearance	Cause
Clear, very pale straw colour	Low SG (very dilute urine)
Clear to slightly turbid, deep yellow	High SG (concentrated urine)
Bright red	Fresh blood (unoxidized)
Red	Free haemoglobin/lysed RBC
Red–brown	Older (oxidized) haemoglobin/lysed RBC
Dark red–brown	Myoglobin Transfusion of haemoglobin-based oxygen-carrying solution (Oxyglobin)
Red–pink	Consumption of beetroot or red food dyes
Dark yellow/greenish	Bilirubin
Orange–yellow	Tetracycline group of drugs
Cloudy	Increases in any constituents: • Cells – WBC – RBC – Epithelial cells • Casts • Mucus • Bacteria • Amorphous material/crystals

10.2 Changes in colour and clarity of urine. RBC = red blood cells; WBC = white blood cells.

Specific gravity

The specific gravity (SG) of urine is a useful indicator of renal concentrating ability. This can be readily obtained by measuring the refractive index (RI) in a specially calibrated refractometer. The instrument measures the degree through which light is bent (refracted) when it passes through a liquid: the amount of refraction (refractive index) is a function of the amount and type of solute (particles) in that liquid. RI and SG are correlated, as the SG is defined as the ratio of the weight of the liquid to an equal volume of distilled water. The SG of a solution thus depends on the number and molecular weight (size) of particles in the solution.

Urine always has an SG greater than that of distilled water, which has an SG of 1.000. The SG of urine is increased by large amounts of glucose, protein, lipid and contrast material.

There is also a reasonably close relationship between SG and osmolality. However, urine SG varies with the type of solute present, while osmolality does not. Osmolality depends on the number of osmotically active particles in solution regardless of their size (SG depends upon both number and size) and is considered to be a more accurate assessment of renal tubular concentrating (and diluting) ability than SG. However, SG is easily measured (refractometer), while osmolality determinations require a special freeze point depression osmometer. In dogs, it is possible to calculate approximate osmolality from urine SG: multiplication of the last 2 digits of the urine SG by 36 approximates osmolality. However, this is inaccurate if the urine contains large numbers of molecules (e.g. glucose) as these have a much greater effect on urine SG than on osmolality.

Refractometers

Refractometers are calibrated to read RI, SG and plasma protein. Many refractometers compensate for changes in temperature between 15 and 37°C. Most are calibrated for use with human samples, although instruments for veterinary use are available. The latter have one calibration scale for dogs and large animal urine (which is similar to a scale for human urine) and a separate scale for cat urine. Human-based instruments will slightly overestimate the SG of cat urine. Care of the refractometer is summarized in Figure 10.3. Urine SG can be determined by some dipsticks by a chemical method but this is unreliable in veterinary patients and is not recommended.

- Rinse and dry the clear optical surface after each use
- Regularly check the zero setting with double distilled water (ddH_2O): SG 1.000
- Check accuracy of calibration with 5% NaCl solution in ddH_2O: SG 1.022
- Use it within the temperature range of calibration (15–37°C)
- Avoid scratching/damaging the optical surface

10.3 Care of the refractometer. ddH_2O = doubly distilled water.

Interpretation of results

SG in health will vary with the state of hydration and fluid intake. Under normal conditions urine SG ranges between 1.015 and 1.040 in healthy dogs and between 1.036 and 1.060 in healthy cats. Details of SG ranges and osmolality are shown in Figure 10.4.

SG should be measured in conjunction with dipstick analysis. When there is a marked increase in urine glucose or protein content, SG will be increased and this could lead to the assumption that the animal has better concentrating ability than it actually has. Interpretation of urine SG values requires knowledge of other parameters, e.g. water intake, drug therapy, clinical condition and haematological and biochemical parameters.

Condition	SG	Osmolality (mOsm)
Usual range in healthy dogs Usual range in healthy cats (May vary outside these ranges depending on fluid intake and hydration status)	1.015–1.045 1.035–1.060	
Possible range	1.001–1.080	
Hyposthenuria	<1.008	<300
Isosthenuria	1.008–1.012	Approximately 300
Hypersthenuria	>1.012	>300

10.4 Urine specific gravity and osmolality ranges.

SG is a valuable test for evaluating kidney diluting and concentrating ability, as the loss of concentrating ability is amongst the first signs of renal tubular disease.

- SG values >1.030 in the dog and >1.035 in the cat are indicative of adequate renal concentrating ability and, if found in an azotaemic animal, would indicate prerenal azotaemia.
- Isosthenuric urine in an azotaemic animal indicates intrinsic renal failure.
- SG values between 1.015 and 1.030 (dog) or 1.035 (cat) indicate that some urine concentration has occurred but do not confirm adequate renal concentrating ability and so, in an azotaemic animal, would suggest early renal failure (see Chapter 11).
- SG values persistently less than 1.020 support the presence of polyuria and consequent polydipsia.

The approach to differentiation of causes of altered urine SG is summarized in Figure 10.5.

Common causes of low urine SG and polyuria

Renal dysfunction is an important cause of polyuria leading to isosthenuria, and is discussed in Chapter 11.

Polyuria can result from:

- Osmotic diuresis
- Loss of medullary tonicity (renal medullary washout)
- Deficiency in anti-diuretic hormone (ADH)
- Resistance to ADH.

Assessment of polyuria and polydipsia by water deprivation testing is discussed at the end of the chapter.

Osmotic diuresis

This occurs in diabetes mellitus, Fanconi syndrome (see Chapter 11) and primary renal glucosuria, where an excess amount of glucose in the glomerular filtrate prevents water being reabsorbed in the distal tubule.

Loss of medullary tonicity (medullary washout)

In health, high concentrations of urea and sodium in the interstitial fluid of the renal medulla lead to an area of hypertonicity which is crucial for effective water resorption in the renal tubules. Loss of hypertonicity in the renal medulla may result from hypoadrenocorticism (loss of sodium), liver disease (reduced urea), prolonged or vigorous fluid therapy or prolonged polydipsia, e.g. due to psychogenic polydipsia (PP). SG values may be isosthenuric or hyposthenuric.

SG	Clinical findings	Other laboratory changes	Causes
>1.030 dog >1.035 cat	Dehydration	± ↑ Urea, protein, albumin, packed cell volume (PCV), Na^+	Plasma hyperosmolality causing increased water retention by the kidney
<1.030 dog <1.035 cat	Dehydration	± ↑ Urea, creatinine, protein, albumin, PCV, Na^+	Renal concentrating defect caused by renal or extrarenal disease
1.012–1.030 dog 1.012–1.035 cat	Polyuria	↑ Urea and creatinine	Early renal failure
1.020–1.030	Polyuria/ polydipsia	↑ Blood glucose	Diabetes mellitus Hyperadrenocorticism
1.008–1.012 (see also below)	Polyuria/ polydipsia	↑ Urea, creatinine ± phosphate, K^+	With oliguria: acute renal failure With polyuria: chronic renal failure, post-urinary obstruction
1.008–1.012 or <1.008	Polyuria/ polydipsia	No azotaemia with:	
		↑ Alkaline phosphatase (ALP), cholesterol, glucose	Hyperadrenocorticism, steroid therapy
		↑ Calcium	Hypercalcaemia
		↓ Na^+ and ↑ K^+	Hypoadrenocorticism
		± Inflammatory leucogram	Pyometra, pyelonephritis
		↓ Urea	Renal medullary washout post obstruction
		↓ Urea, ↑ bile acids	Hepatic insufficiency
		↑ T4	Hyperthyroidism (cats)
		None	Psychogenic polydipsia, diuretic therapy, fluid therapy Partial central diabetes insipidus
<1.008	Polyuria/ polydipsia		Central or nephrogenic diabetes insipidus

10.5 Differentiation of common causes of altered urine specific gravity.

Resistance to anti-diuretic hormone

Resistance to ADH, termed nephrogenic diabetes insipidus (NDI), occurs commonly secondary to many conditions, including hypercalcaemia, chronic liver disease, pyometra, hyperadrenocorticism and hypokalaemia. Primary NDI is rare, though it is reported as a congenital, familial disorder in Huskies. In NDI, SG values may be isosthenuric or hyposthenuric.

Deficiency in anti-diuretic hormone

Deficiency in ADH, termed central diabetes insipidus (CDI), may be idiopathic or result from intracranial trauma, neoplasia or malformations. In partial CDI suboptimal amounts of ADH are released, often only in response to very high plasma osmolality; SG values may be isosthenuric or hyposthenuric. With total ADH deficiency SG values are persistently hyposthenuric and the urine does not concentrate following water deprivation.

Dipstick chemical tests

These are a qualitative to semiquantitative method of monitoring the major chemicals of interest in urine. The dipsticks are designed for monitoring constituents in human urine; therefore, some of the tests are not suitable for use with animal urine, i.e. SG, nitrite, leucocyte esterase activity (WBC) and urobilinogen.

To ensure the most reliable results from these tests:

- Fresh, in-date sticks should be used
- The sticks should be stored in the original container tightly capped (the lid contains dessicant)
- Storage should be at the suggested temperature in a dry place
- The enclosed instructions for use should be followed carefully, i.e. tap off excess urine after dipping, and check the colour changes at the indicated times
- The test pads should not be touched with the fingers
- Test pads are read manually by comparing strip to test chart provided or by using an automated stick reader.

Practical guidelines for dipstick use are summarized in Figures 10.6 and 10.7.

Test	Reported range	Method	Comments	Interference
pH	5–9	Hydrogen ion (H^+) concentrationby colour indicator		**False pH**: contamination with acid from albumin strip, detergents. False colour due to presence of blood substitute (Oxyglobin)
Glucose	Negative 1+ (2.8 mmol/l) 2+ (5.5 mmol/l) 3+ (17 mmol/l) 4+ (55 mmol/l)	Glucose oxidase/peroxidase reaction. Calibrated to avoid interference by vitamin C (>5 mmol/l)	Not affected by ketones	**False positive**: chlorine bleach, cephalosporins, Oxyglobin **False negative**: thymol, formalin, refrigeration (since low temperature inhibits reaction)
Ketones	Negative 1+ (0.5–4 mmol/l) 2+ (4–10 mmol/l) 3+ (>10 mmol/l)	Nitroprusside reaction	Most sensitive to acetoacetate, less sensitive to acetone. Does not react with beta-hydroxybutyrate	**False positive**: pigmenturia, Oxyglobin, sulphur drugs, very concentrated urine **False negative**: old urine
Protein	Negative 1+ (0.3 g/l) 2+ (1.0 g/l) 3+ (5.0 g/l)	Tetra bromophenol blue reaction at acid pH	Most sensitive to albumin. Does not detect globulins or Bence Jones proteins	**False positive**: pigmenturia, Oxyglobin, ammonia-based disinfectants, chlorhexidine, very alkaline urine (pH >8.0)
Bilirubin	Negative 1+ 2+ 3+	Conjugated bilirubin coupled with diazodichloroaniline in acid medium		**False positive**: pigmenturia **False negative**: vitamin C, prolonged exposure to sunlight (bilirubin degraded to urobilinogen)
Blood	Negative 1+ (5–10 RBC/μl) 2+ (25 RBC/μl) 3+ (50 RBC/μl) 4+ 250 RBC/μl)	Heme peroxidases catalyse oxidation of *o*-toluidine blue	Erythrocytes result in speckles on pad but high numbers give diffuse colour	**False positive**: bleach-based detergents, bacteria or WBC peroxidases **False negative**: concentrated urine
Haemoglobin	Negative 1+, 2+, 3+, 4+ same equivalents as blood	Heme peroxidases catalyse oxidation of *o*-toluidine blue	Diffuse colour on pad with haemolysed cells, free haemomyoglobin or free myoglobin	As for blood
Urobilinogen	Negative 1+ (17 μmol/l) 2+ (70 μmol/l) 3+ (140 μmol/l) 4+ (200 μmol/l)	Specific test: diazonium salt reacts with urobilinogen		**False positive**: aspirin, transient positive when there is 3+ bilirubin present **False negative**: formalin, exposure to sunlight or aged urine (urobilinogen oxidized to urobilin)

10.6 Dipstick analysis: methods and interferences. (continues) ▶

Test	Reported range	Method	Comments	Interference
Nitrites	Negative or positive	Bacteria (e.g. *Escherichia coli*) convert nitrate to nitrite in the bladder. Nitrite reacts with napthylethylene to produce colour change	Require bacteria in urine in bladder for 4–8 hours for enough conversion of nitrate to nitrite to be detectable. Unreliable in dogs and cats	**False positive**: old voided (i.e. non-sterile collection) urine **False negative**: vitamin C, antibiotics
Leucocyte esterase	Negative or positive	Leucocytes release esterase into urine, forming indoxyl, which reacts with a diazonium salt to give a colour change	Unreliable in dogs and cats	**False negative**: common, cause unknown

10.6 (continued) Dipstick analysis: methods and interferences.

Test	Normal value	Altered value	Possible causes
pH	6.0–7.5	Increase	Urease-containing bacteria (e.g. *Staphlococcus, Proteus*) Old urine sample Transient following a meal Renal tubular acidosis Metabolic alkalosis
		Decrease	Metabolic acidosis Hypochloraemic metabolic alkalosis (uncommon) Renal tubular acidosis Hypokalaemia
Glucose	Negative or trace	1+ or greater	Hyperglycaemia exceeding renal theshold: • Diabetes mellitus • Stress hyperglycaemia in cats • Hyperadrenocorticism Normal serum glucose: • Renal tubular disease • Primary renal glucosuria • Fanconi syndrome
Ketones	Negative or trace	1+ or greater	Diabetic ketoacidosis Starvation Very young animals
Protein	Negative or trace	2+ or more >1+ in dilute urine	Pyuria (infection) Glomerulonephritis or amyloidosis leading to protein-losing nephropathy Haemorrhage (see text) Genital tract secretions
Bilirubin	Negative in cats; trace or 1+ in dogs with SG >1.025; 2+ in dogs with SG >1.040	Trace/1+ or above in cats 2+ or more in dogs	Haemolytic anaemia Hepatobiliary disease (especially cats)
Blood	Negative	Positive	Haematuria (see Figure 10.15)
Haemoglobin	Negative	Positive	Intravascular haemolysis (e.g. immune-mediated haemolytic anaemia) Myoglobinuria (due to muscle damage)
Urobilinogen	Negative	Positive	Not clinically helpful in haematological or hepatobiliary disease in dogs and cats. Bilirubin more useful
Nitrites	Negative	–	Not reliable in animals due to uncontrollable urine retention time in the bladder with frequent false negatives
Leucocyte esterase	Negative	–	Not sensitive enough to detect inflammation (urinary tract infection (UTI)) in animals. Need to check urine sediment for leucocytes

10.7 Interpretation of dipstick analysis.

Urine pH

Urine pH does not necessarily reflect the body's pH and is also influenced by diet, recent feeding, bacterial infection and storage time. Urine is usually acidic in dogs and cats. Studies have shown that dipstick measurements of pH are inherently inaccurate when compared to those taken using a pH meter, so when an accurate measurement of urine pH is critical for clinical decision making, for example when evaluating cases of urolithiasis, the measurement should be made with a pH meter (Heuter *et al.*, 1998; Raskin *et al.*, 2002).

Causes of alkaline urine include:

- Feeding: this results in transiently alkaline urine as a result of the postprandial alkaline tide which occurs when secretion of gastric acid causes a relative alkalosis
- Urinary tract infection with urease-producing bacteria, such as *Proteus* or *Staphylococcus*; these break down urea to ammonia, resulting in alkaline urine
- Metabolic and respiratory alkalosis; these result in reduced hydrogen ion (H^+) excretion into urine (see Chapter 9)
- Urinary retention (e.g. due to obstruction); this may result in decomposition of urea to ammonia
- Contamination by detergents or disinfectants.

If urine is persistently alkaline and artefacts have been ruled out, urine culture and sediment examination should be performed.

Causes of decreased pH, i.e. acidic urine, include:

- Metabolic and respiratory acidosis, leading to increased H^+ excretion
- Vomiting: paradoxical aciduria with metabolic alkalosis may occur in hypochloraemic vomiting animals. Vomiting results in loss of hydrochloric acid (HCl) and also potassium (K^+). In the kidney sodium (Na^+) is resorbed in the tubules where it is usually exchanged for K^+, which is excreted. Na^+ may be reabsorbed with chloride (Cl^-) or bicarbonate (HCO_3^-). Since both K^+ and Cl^- are in short supply due to the vomiting, Na^+ is resorbed with HCO_3^-, resulting in more acidic urine
- Hypokalaemia: increased renal resorption of K^+ is accompanied by increased excretion of H^+.

Glucosuria

Glucose is freely filtered then reabsorbed in the proximal tubule, but resorptive capacity is limited. Glucosuria occurs when blood glucose exceeds this renal threshold, for example in diabetes mellitus or as a result of stress in cats (fructosamine is useful to distinguish stress and diabetes, see Chapter 16). The renal threshold in dogs is 10 mmol/l and is slightly higher in cats (14–17 mmol/l).

Glucosuria in the absence of hyperglycaemia reflects a tubular resorption defect in which the renal tubules fail to reabsorb glucose from the glomerular filtrate. Fanconi syndrome and primary renal glucosuria are examples of tubular transport defects that occur in dogs (see Chapter 11).

Ketonuria

In small animals ketonuria is usually associated with diabetic ketoacidosis (DKA), although it may also be seen in starvation. It is important to note that dipsticks detect acetoacetate and, to a lesser extent, acetone, but do not detect betahydroxybutyrate (BHB). During the initial stages of insulin therapy for DKA there is increased conversion of BHB to acetoacetate and so the degree of ketonuria may initially appear to increase.

Proteinuria

A small amount of protein may be normal but the dipstick result should be interpreted with knowledge of the urine SG, as the significance of the result is related to the concentration of the urine. For example, a 3+ protein dipstick result in urine of SG 1.008 indicates a much greater protein loss than the same 3+ protein in urine of SG 1.045. Proteinuria may result from glomerulonephropathy, tubular transport defects, or inflammation or infection within the urinary tract. Haemorrhage must be marked (macroscopic rather than microscopic) before it causes significant proteinuria (Vaden *et al.*, 2004). Thus sediment examination is important in the evaluation of proteinuria.

Urine protein:creatinine ratio

If there is no evidence of inflammation in the sediment or no gross haematuria, the urine protein:creatinine ratio (UPC) can be used to quantify proteinuria (Figure 10.8). The quantity of protein lost is related to the amount of creatinine in the urine to correct for variation in urine SG. This is possible because the excretion of creatinine is relatively stable for an individual and there is essentially no tubular reabsorption in dogs and cats. Urine total protein and creatinine are measured on the same sample by automated chemical methods, reported in the same units and a ratio obtained:

$$\text{Urine protein:creatinine ratio (UPC)} = \frac{\text{Urine protein (mg/dl)}}{\text{Urine creatinine (mg/dl)}}$$

Units may need to be converted from SI units to perform the calculation:

Protein (g/l) x 100 = Protein (mg/dl)
Creatinine (mmol/l) x 1000/88.4 = Creatinine (mg/dl)

UPC	Significance
<0.5	Normal
0.5–1.0	Grey zone, questionable significance
>2.0	Significant proteinuria
>5.0	Indicative of glomerular disease especially glomerulonephritis and glomerular basement membrane damage/protein-losing nephropathy
>8.0–12.0	Frequently associated with amyloidosis

10.8 Interpretation of urine protein:creatinine ratio. This should not be measured in urine when inflammation or gross haematuria is present in the sediment.

The type of glomerular disease present cannot be determined from the UPC and biopsy and histology are required for a definitive diagnosis and prognosis. (See Chapter 11 for further discussion on proteinuria.)

UPC should not be measured or interpreted in urine that contains >100 white blood cells in the sediment or if there is evidence of gross haematuria, since these may cause an increase in the urine total protein and give a falsely elevated UPC. This can be above the range that indicates the presence of glomerular loss.

N.B. Microscopic haematuria has little impact on the UPC, and only gross haematuria leads to significant alteration of the ratio (Vaden *et al.*, 2004).

Albumin and globulin

The dipstick mainly detects albumin and is insensitive to globulin or Bence Jones proteins (light chain fragments of immunoglobulin which may be present in urine of animals with multiple myeloma (see Chapter 7)). Albumin, globulin and Bence Jones proteins are all detected using the sulphasalicylic acid (SSA) method: when SSA is added to urine, proteins are denatured and form a precipitate which makes the sample turbid. The turbidity can be assessed visually or more accurately using spectrophotometry, comparing the sample turbidity with that of a set of standards. The SSA method is not widely used in commercial laboratories.

Microalbuminuria

Persistent microalbuminuria (MA) is an indicator of glomerular damage associated with early progressive renal disease in humans. Such low level albumin loss is not detected by routine dipstick analysis. Recently new, very sensitive, separate dipsticks for urine microalbumin have become available for use in dogs and cats. These are immunological tests using a monoclonal antibody specific for canine or feline albumin. Studies have shown that 20–25% of healthy dogs and 13% of healthy cats have MA, whilst approximately 40% of dogs and cats with a medical condition have MA (Jensen 2001; Wisnewski *et al.*, 2004). The prevalence of MA increases with age (Radecki *et al.*, 2003). Diseases that have been associated with MA include cardiovascular disease, urogenital disease, dental disease, airway disease, pyoderma, inflammatory bowel disease, hyperthyroidism, hyperadrenocorticism, diabetes mellitus, infectious diseases and neoplasia (Grauer *et al.*, 2001; Vaden *et al.*, 2001; Pressler *et al.*, 2003; Wisnewski *et al.*, 2004). Prednisolone therapy may also lead to MA. Thus it appears that a significant proportion of normal animals and animals with diseases unrelated to the renal system may have MA. It is not clear at this time what proportion of animals with MA will develop renal disease or protein-losing nephropathy. Animals with end-stage renal disease may test negative for MA. The diagnostic usefulness of this test is still under evaluation.

Bilirubinuria

There is a low renal threshold for bilirubin and even small increases in plasma bilirubin can lead to bilirubinuria. Thus bilirubinuria is detected prior to hyperbilirubinaemia or jaundice. Bilirubin in urine is in the form of conjugated bilirubin, since unconjugated bilirubin is bound to albumin, which does not usually pass through the glomerular barrier in significant amounts unless glomerular disease is present. Bilirubinuria is not seen in healthy cats but a small amount of bilirubin may be found in the urine of normal dogs (see Figure 10.7). This is in part because they have a very low renal threshold, and in part because canine renal tubular cells are able to catabolize haemoglobin to unconjugated bilirubin, conjugate it and then secrete it into the urine. Increased bilirubinuria may be caused by cholestasis or haemolytic anaemia.

Haematuria, haemoglobinuria and myoglobinuria

The dipstick pads for blood and haemoglobin both use the same chemical method, but a speckled appearance to the dipstick pad is indicative of haematuria, whilst a diffuse colour change suggests haemoglobinuria (or myoglobinuria). However, a diffuse colour change may also be seen with severe haematuria and the pads do not reliably differentiate haematuria and haemoglobinuria. Sediment examination is useful for making the distinction, although red cells may lyse *in vitro*, especially in dilute urine, resulting in the false impression of haemoglobinuria rather than haematuria. True haemoglobinuria results from intravascular haemolysis (e.g. due to immune-mediated haemolytic anaemia) and is accompanied by haemoglobinaemia and anaemia. Haemoglobinaemia can be identified by centrifuging a blood sample and examining the plasma (which is pink/red). Myoglobinuria is seen uncommonly in small animals, but may result from severe muscle damage due to trauma or ischaemia (e.g. associated with aortic thromboembolism in cats). The muscle enzymes creatine kinase (CK) and aspartate transaminase (AST) are usually markedly elevated in serum/plasma. Myoglobin is a small protein which is rapidly cleared from the circulation, so myoglobinuria is not accompanied by pigmented plasma.

Urine sediment analysis

The third and perhaps most important component of a complete routine urinalysis is the microscopic examination of the sediment. A consistent volume of urine should be used for preparing the sediment for analysis. Laboratories use volumes that vary (10 ml, 5 ml, 3 ml) to produce a semiquantitative result. Larger laboratories also use disposable microscope slides, with a grid, which hold a set volume of sediment (usually 0.5 ml).

Experienced microscopists use unstained sediment and a phase contrast microscope. Less confident persons may elect to stain the sediment before microscopy to facilitate cell identification. A regular microscope with the condenser lowered can be used to identify cells in unstained sediment if phase contrast is not available. The microscope should be kept clean and in good working order, with lens and condenser alignment maintained for the best possible visible field and resolution. If an oil immersion (100X) objective is used for identifying bacteria or assessing cell morphology, the lens should be wiped clean after each use to prevent oil dripping into the condenser and seeping into the objective. It is also advisable to place a coverslip on the sample to protect the objective lens from damage.

A suggested method for preparation and analysis is as follows:

1. Fresh urine or warmed previously refrigerated urine should be used.
2. The sample is mixed well but gently to prevent cast destruction.
3. A constant volume (10, 5 or 3 ml, often 3 ml is used for cat urine), is placed in a conical centrifuge tube.

4. The urine is centrifuged gently (suggested 1,000 rpm for 5 minutes; this will vary with the type of centrifuge used). If a smaller volume of urine (i.e. <3 ml) is used with high speed centrifugation the amount of sediment obtained may be too small especially if the urine is very dilute. The high speed may also damage cells and destroy casts.
5. The supernatant is decanted (this can be used in the refractometer for SG or for dipstick analysis, especially if only a small volume of urine is available).
6. A few drops of liquid will remain in the tube. Sediment is mixed in this to resuspend it, either by gently tapping the tube or pipetting up and down.
7. If a specialized urine stain, such as Sedistain, is being used, 1 drop is added to the sediment and mixed. (N.B. Stain will develop precipitate with time and needs to be discarded or filtered before use because stain precipitate can be mistaken for bacteria).
8. A drop of sediment is placed on a clean glass slide and a coverslip is placed on it avoiding air bubbles.
9. The slide is placed on the microscope stage and the whole area is scanned on low power (10X objective). If unstained sediment is being used, the condenser should be lowered until there is good resolution.
10. The presence of crystals is reported at this magnification. A consistent scheme is used, i.e. 1+, 2+, 3+ or light, moderate, heavy. Identification of crystal types should be attempted.
11. The objective is changed to high power (40X) and the area is rescanned. The numbers of erythrocytes, leucocytes and epithelial cells, casts, crystals and bacteria seen per high power field are counted and recorded (Figure 10.9). It is advisable to count in 5–10 different fields and then average the numbers unless there are very large numbers seen.
12. Other constituents are reported, e.g. sperm, mucus strands, yeast, fungi, nematode eggs, fat droplets.
13. For further identification of cell types or to differentiate bacteria from particles the 100X oil immersion objective can be used.
14. Fat and air bubbles can usually be distinguished by fine focusing and moving the condenser.
15. Brownian motion of particles can usually be distinguished from motile bacteria at 100X power.

Urine sediment results should be interpreted with a knowledge of how the sample was collected, its chemical composition (dipstick analysis) and its SG. Most importantly the clinical condition of the animal and any haematology and biochemistry results (if available) should also be taken into account. The presence of increased leucocytes and bacteria in a cystocentesis sample from an animal with urinary frequency and an inflammatory leucogram would confirm the need for culture and sensitivity and appropriate antibiotic therapy, whereas a similar free-catch sample from a bitch during oestrus would not elicit the same response. Similarly, cells with an abnormal appearance in urine from an animal with painless haematuria would suggest further cytological analysis and investigation, unless it were known that the animal had received drugs known to be toxic/irritant to urinary bladder cells. Likewise further investigation of proteinuria after positive dipstick protein is not indicated where sediment contains large numbers of red and white blood cells and bacteria. If large numbers of epithelial cells and/or cells with abnormal morphology are found during routine sediment analysis further cytology is advisable, especially if there is a history of haematuria and a suspicion of neoplasia in the urinary tract (see Cytology, below).

Casts

Casts are formed in the renal tubules from Tamm–Horsfall mucoprotein secreted by renal tubular epithelial cells. These condense to form hyaline casts (Figure 10.10a). The hyaline casts may then acquire cellular debris and become granular casts (Figure 10.10b) or

Element	Look-alike	Distinguishing feature of look-alike
Red blood cells (RBCs)	Fat droplets	Variable size, refractile, out of plane of focus (float)
	Yeast	Usually oval or budding
White blood cells (WBCs)	RBCs (unstained)	Smaller than WBCs, often crenated, if stained no nuclear structure
	Transitional cells	Usually larger than WBCs and have small round nucleus
Bacteria	Fat droplets	Refractile
	Fine amorphous material	Brownian motion
	Yeast	Usually oval or budding
	Stain precipitate	Variable sizes
	Starch granules	Larger with central cross
Crystals	Glass fragments	Variable size (difficult to distinguish)
Casts	Muscle fibres	Internal striations
	Cotton fibres	Internal striations coarse, cells usually attached to surface and not incorporated as in a true cast
	Aggregates of amorphous material	Difficult to distinguish but usually scant in fresh urine

10.9 Distinguishing features of formed elements and cells in urine sediment.

trap lipid droplets to become fatty casts. When these casts age and/or deteriorate and solidify in the tubules they form waxy casts (Figure 10.10c). Normal urine may contain a few hyaline or granular casts, but increased numbers reflect renal pathology, usually acute tubular disease (Figure 10.11). Inflammation or haemorrhage in the kidney may lead to the formation of white or red cell casts, respectively (Figure 10.10d), whilst epithelial cell casts (Figure 10.10e) occur due to severe damage to the renal tubule leading to sloughing of cells. Casts may be flushed into the bladder urine intermittently, and they also disintegrate rapidly in alkaline or old urine, so the absence of casts does not exclude renal tubular disease.

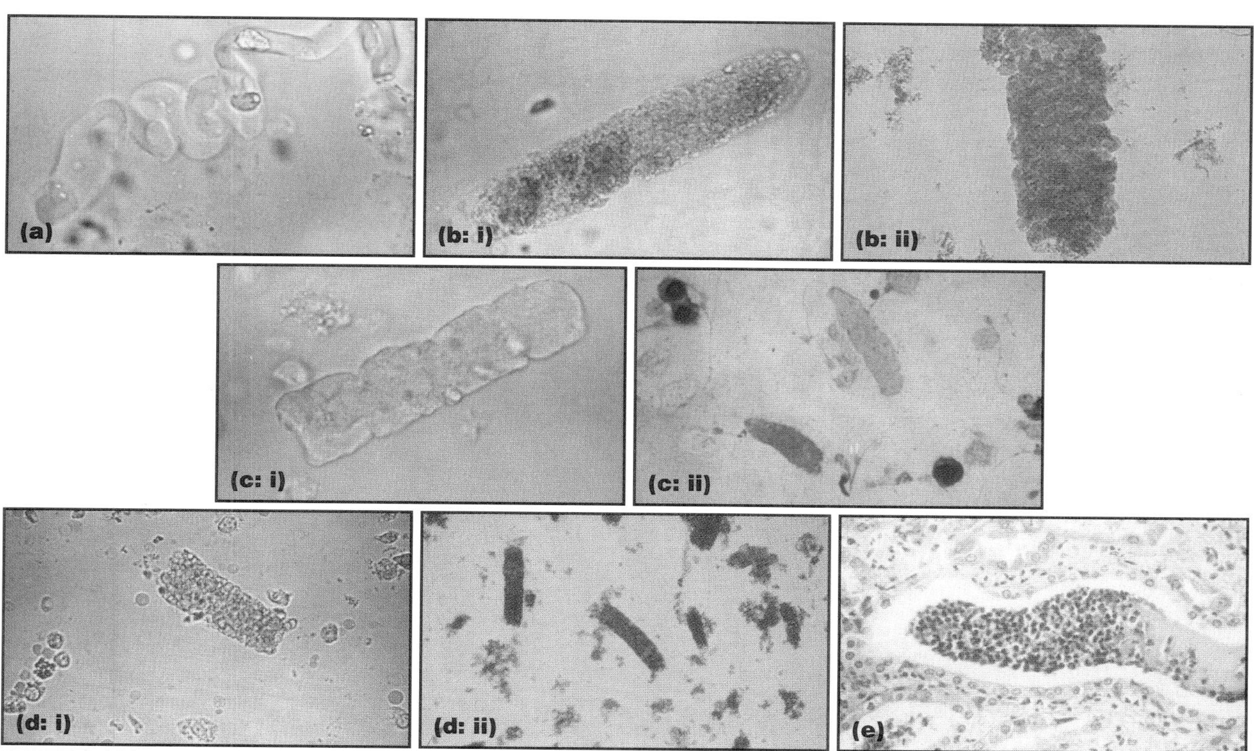

10.10 Urine sediment casts. **(a)** Hyaline cast with little structure and a faint light appearance. An occasional hyaline cast may be found in normal urine. These are the earliest casts formed in renal disease. They are very fragile and easily destroyed in urine. (Unstained sediment.) **(b)** Granular casts (i) unstained and (ii) stained with Sedistain. These casts can be seen with toxic injury to the renal tubules, and with haemoglobinuria (as well as red cell casts) and myoglobinuria. **(c)** Waxy casts (i) unstained and (ii) stained with Sedistain. These develop from the disintegration and consolidation in casts as they mature in the damaged tubules. When found in urine they indicate chronicity of the renal condition. **(d)** Mixed cellular casts (i) unstained and (ii) stained with Sedistain. These casts can be found with acute renal damage, trauma and in inflammation of the kidney. They are very fragile and readily disintegrate with rough handling and storage of urine. **(e)** Histology section from a kidney, stained with H&E, showing a large mixed cellular and waxy cast within a renal tubule. (Original magnification X400.)

Type of cast	Normal findings	Significance of abnormal findings
Hyaline	None or rare	Common in glomerular proteinuria and amyloidosis
Granular (fine or coarse)	None or rare	Tubular damage due to: • Nephrotoxins (e.g. aminoglycosides) • Haemoglobinuria- or myoglobinuria-induced nephropathy • Renal ischaemia
White cell and epithelial casts	None	Acute damage with inflammation or sloughing of cells in kidney
Red blood cell	None	Acute renal haemorrhage, e.g. due to trauma, idiopathic renal haemorrhage
Fatty	None	In cats with tubular damage In dogs with diabetes mellitus
Granular/waxy Waxy	None	These develop from degenerating granular or cellular casts and indicate duration/chronicity of disease
Haemoglobin Myoglobin	None	Develop with haemoglobinuria/myoglobinuria, respectively

10.11 Interpretation of urine sediment analysis: casts.

Crystals

The presence of crystals in urine (Figure 10.12) can be of no clinical significance in health, but in animals with histories of urolithiasis or relevant clinical signs they may be significant (Figure 10.13). A knowledge of underlying causes or predisposing factors to the formation of various crystals can help direct further investigations. Both struvite and calcium oxalate crystals may be present in healthy dogs and cats and are the most common types of crystals found. Struvite crystals (Figure 10.12a) form in alkaline urine, which may arise due to the presence of urease-producing bacteria in urinary tract infection. Calcium phosphate and, occasionally, calcium oxalate crystals may form in association with hypercalcaemia (Figures 10.12b–10.12d). Uric acid and ammonium biurate crystals (Figures 10.12e–10.12f) can be found in urine of dogs and cats with severe hepatic dysfunction and portosystemic shunting; they are also seen in the urine of Dalmatians due to a metabolic defect (discussed in Urolith section). Cystine crystals (Figure 10.12g) form due to a rare tubular resorptive defect, reported in English Bulldogs

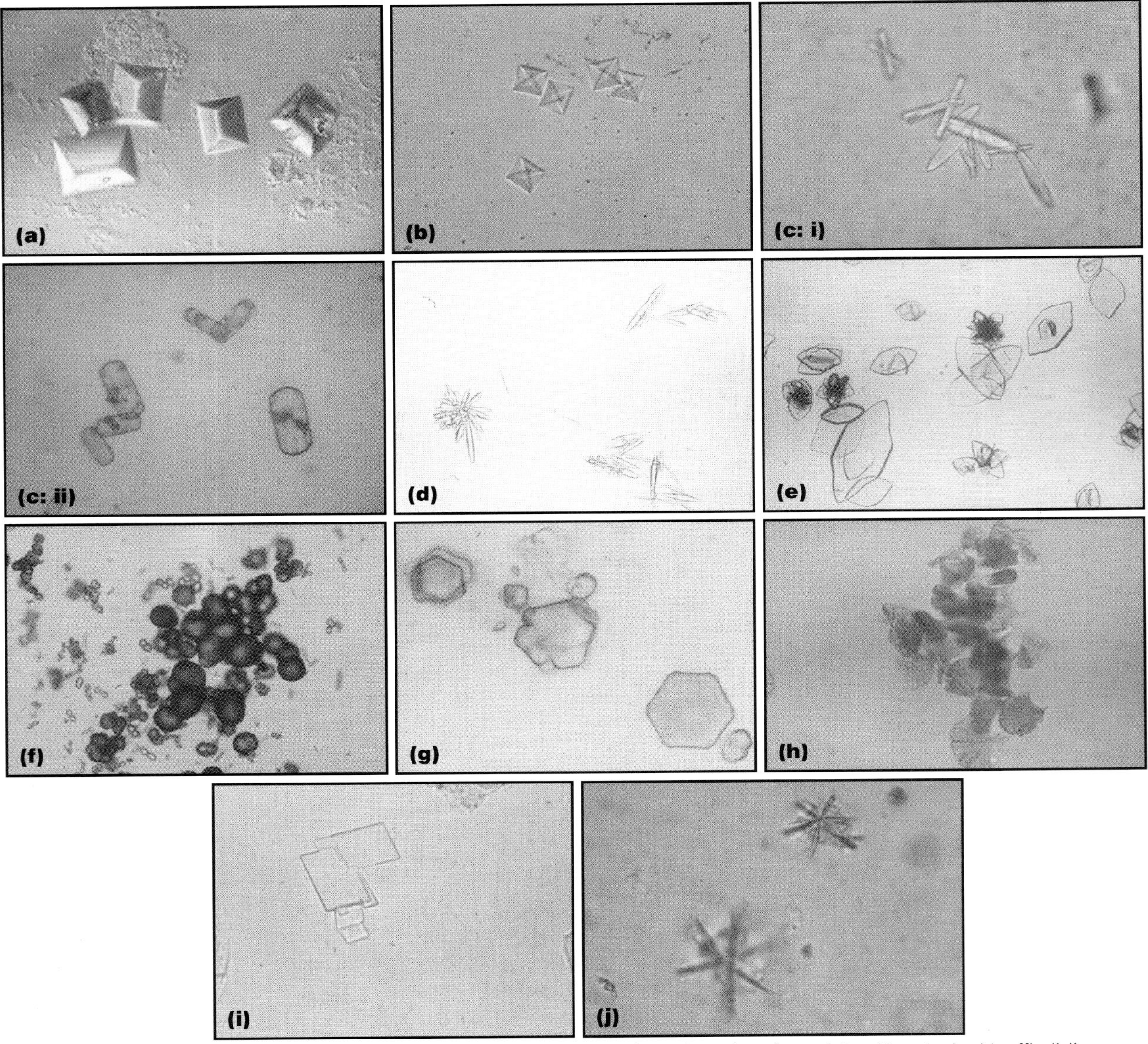

10.12 Urine sediment crystals. **(a)** Struvite (magnesium ammonium phosphate) crystals with a typical 'coffin lid' structure. These crystals can have various structures depending on conditions during formation and growth. **(b)** Calcium oxalate dihydrate crystals are the most common form of calcium oxalate crystal found. They have a typical 'Maltese cross' structure. **(c)** Calcium oxalate monohydrate crystals. Large quantities are frequently associated with ethylene glycol toxicity. The structure is distinctive and different: (i) in dogs they are elongated and needle shaped; (ii) in cats they have rounded ends and internal structure. **(d)** Calcium phosphate crystals are small, needle shaped and may form clusters. **(e)** Uric acid crystals are most commonly 'diamond' shaped but can take other forms and are clear or pale yellow. **(f)** Ammonium biurate crystals are usually pale yellow to brown and may aggregate to form clusters; the typical 'thorn apple' appearance. **(g)** Cystine crystals have a typical hexagonal shape. **(h)** Drug-associated crystals. Many drugs and their metabolites may crystallize in urine. This is an example of crystal formation from sulphonamide drugs and their metabolites in urine, which is not uncommon. **(i)** Cholesterol crystals are very thin, flat and rectangular. **(j)** Bilirubin crystals usually are in the form of yellow to red fine needles. (Unstained sediment; original magnification X400.)

Type of crystals	Normal findings	Significance of abnormal findings
Struvite (magnesium ammonium phosphate)	May be seen in normal dogs and cats with alkaline urine. Variable incidence depending on pH, SG and storage of sample	Form in alkaline urine UTI with urease-producing bacteria May lead to struvite calculi **BUT** not a reliable indicator of presence of struvite calculi as common in normal animals with urine pH >6.5
Calcium oxalate monohydrate	Very occasionally present in normal dogs and cats	Ethylene glycol poisoning Consumption of toxic plants in cats
Calcium oxalate dihydrate	May be present in normal dogs and cats	Form in acid or neutral or weakly alkaline urine May lead to calcium oxalate calculi May be present in ethylene glycol poisoning (but more commonly see monohydrate form)
Calcium phosphate	May be present in normal dogs	Form in weak acid to alkaline urine May lead to urolithiasis Hypercalcaemia is predisposing factor
Ammonium urate/biurate Uric acid	Common in Dalmatians and English Bulldogs	Uric acid crystals form in acid urine Urate/biurate crystals form in alkaline urine Form in hepatic disease/portosystemic shunts Form due to metabolic defect in Dalmatians May lead to urate calculi
Bilirubin	May be present in normal dogs with concentrated urine	Form in hepatobiliary disease especially cats Form in acid urine
Cystine	Absent in normal animal's urine	Form in acid urine Form due to a defect in tubular resorption of cystine in Bull Mastiff, English Bulldog, Dachshund, Chihuahua
Leucine/tyrosine	Absent in normal animal's urine	Form in acid urine Form due to metabolic disease/inherited tubular disease
Cholesterol	May be present in normal dogs and cats	Form in acid to neutral urine May form in chronic protein-losing nephropathy
Amorphous material (variable content)	Common in concentrated urine	–

10.13 Interpretation of urine sediment analysis: crystals.

and some other breeds. Large numbers of crystals in dilute urine, persistent crystalluria and large crystals have greater significance in relation to stone formation.

If large numbers of calcium oxalate monohydrate along with dihydrate crystals are found in urine, ingestion of toxic substances, particularly ethylene glycol (antifreeze) and certain toxic plants, should be suspected. High concentrations of these substances can be metabolized to produce oxalates, which precipitate in the renal tubules as calcium oxalates and can cause irreversible renal failure (see Chapter 11).

Unusual crystals may be formed if large quantities of drug or drug metabolites concentrate in urine, e.g. sulphonamide drugs frequently form crystals (Figure 10.12h). Unusual, difficult to identify crystals can often be drug-derived. Cholesterol crystals (Figure 10.12i) may be seen in normal animals or in nephrotic syndrome. Bilirubin crystals (Figure 10.12j) may be seen when there is marked bilirubinuria, due to cholestasis or haemolytic anaemia, and may occasionally be seen in concentrated urine from normal dogs (especially males).

Cells

Red and white blood cells may be seen in low numbers in normal urine. Red cells (Figure 10.14a) may be confused with fat droplets or yeast (Figure 10.9). White cells (usually neutrophils) are larger than red cells, and are round with granular cytoplasm and often an indistinct nucleus (Figure 10.14b). Normal urine sediment contains small numbers of transitional epithelial cells from the bladder; increased numbers are seen secondary to bladder inflammation/irritation. Transitional cells are large and round to oval, with a central round nucleus and abundant cytoplasm (Figure 10.14c). Voided urine may also contain squamous epithelial cells from the urethra and vagina which are also large but have an angular polyhedral shape and a small round nucleus (Figure 10.14d). A rare renal and ureteral epithelial cell may also be found. These are small with a relatively large round nucleus and less cytoplasm (Figure 10.14e). The significance of increased numbers of red and white blood cells and epithelial cells is summarized in Figure 10.15.

Miscellaneous findings

Bacteria may reflect contamination or infection; an associated inflammatory response would support the latter (Figure 10.16a), but is not always present. Other organisms, such as nematodes, yeast and fungi, may occasionally be identified (Figures 10.16b–e) and their significance is summarized in Figure 10.17. Sperm, mucus strands and cotton fibre contaminants are shown in Figure 10.16(f–h).

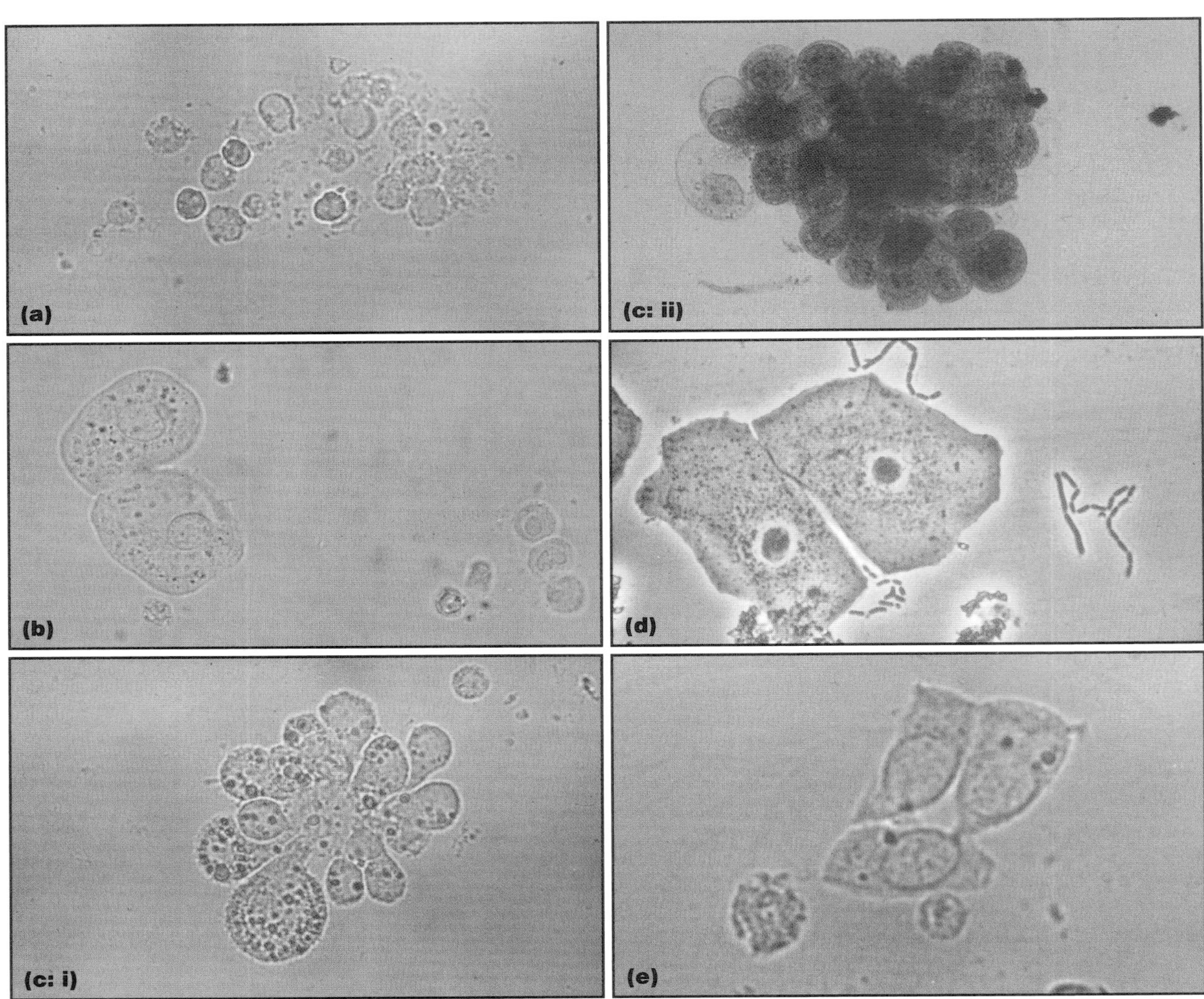

10.14 **(a)** Red cells in urine sediment showing crenation, giving them an irregular slightly spiky appearance. Crenation is common when cells are in urine for a prolonged period. (Unstained sediment.) **(b)** RBC, WBC and bladder epithelial cells in sediment. Two large epithelial cells are seen on the left, three neutrophils on the right. Just to the left of the neutrophils there are two crenated RBCs. (Unstained sediment.) **(c)** Cluster of bladder epithelial cells (i) unstained and (ii) stained with Sedistain. Bladder mucosa cells will exfoliate forming clusters and rafts in urine with inflammation/irritation. **(d)** Unstained preparation mature squamous epithelial cells and bacteria which could be contaminants from the distal urethra/genital tract. **(e)** Unstained preparation of urothelial cells. Elongated pear shaped cells are believed to originate from the ureters and renal pelvis. (Original magnification X400.)

Cell type	Normal findings	Significance of abnormal findings
RBCs	<5 per high power field (hpf)	Cystocentesis may lead to small increase Moderate numbers in free catch urine in intact females Microscopic or macroscopic haematuria in: • Renal or urinary tract disease, obstruction, trauma, neoplasia • Thrombocytopenia • Vasculitis
WBCs	<5/hpf Usually neutrophils, occasionally eosinophils	Small numbers in free catch urine Moderate to large numbers in inflammation or infection of the kidney or urinary tract
Epithelial cells	0–2/hpf Small cells from kidney/upper tract Large cells from bladder or urethra	Small numbers in free catch urine Increased numbers of small cells in upper tract inflammation or infection Sheets of uniform large cells in bladder or lower tract inflammation or infection Squamous cells in bladder and lower urinary tract inflammation or infection Increased numbers/clusters with variable morphology in neoplasia, dysplasia or hyperplasia

10.15 Interpretation of urine sediment analysis: cells.

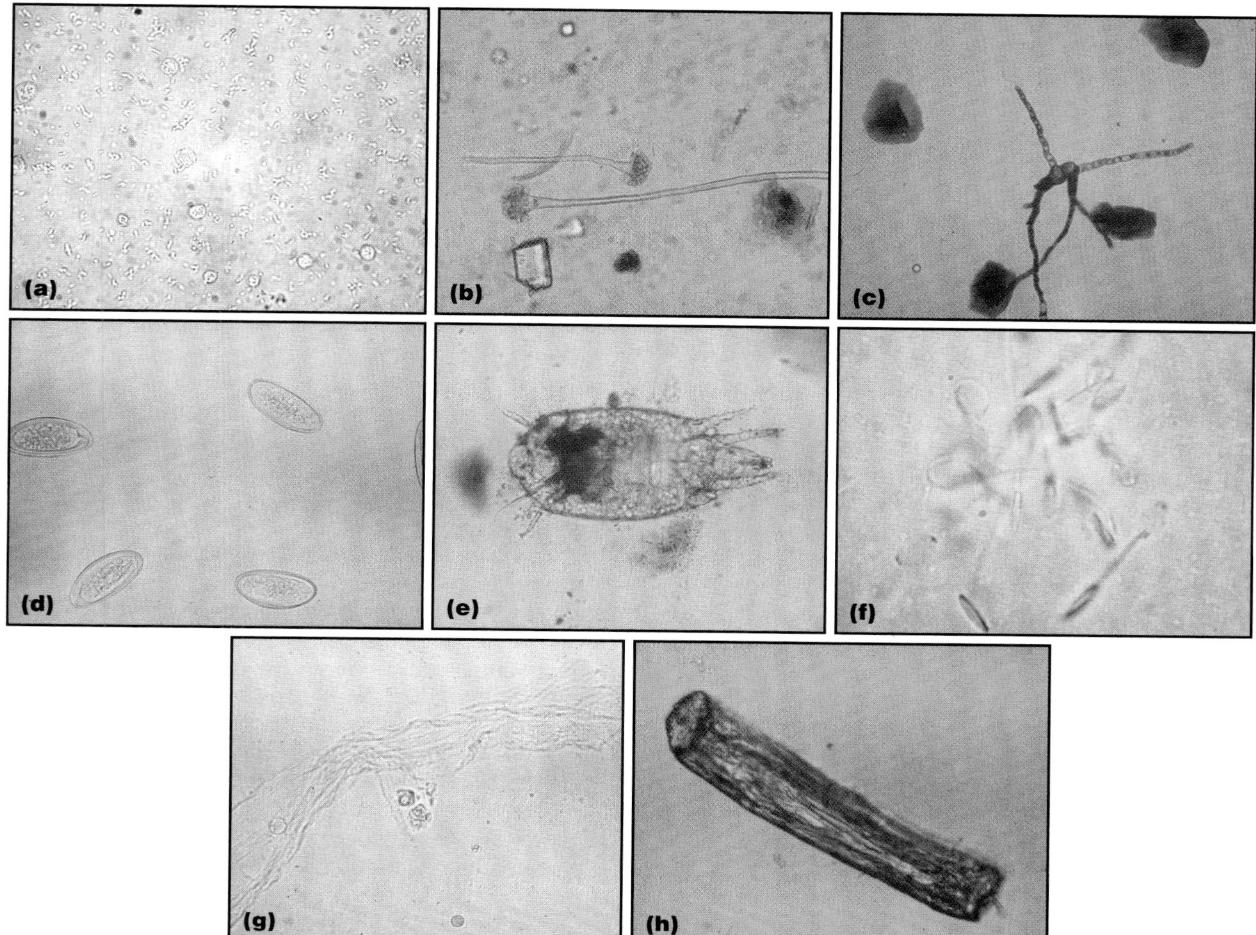

10.16 Urine sediment: miscellaneous. **(a)** Sediment containing degenerate neutrophils and numerous bacteria consistent with urinary tract infection. (Unstained.) **(b)** *Aspergillus* spp. Fungal contamination, especially in free-catch and old urine, is common. (Sedistain.) **(c)** *Alternaria* spp, a contaminant especially in free-catch urine. (Sedistain.) **(d)** Parasite eggs can be found if there is faecal contamination of the sample or, rarely, when organisms are present in the kidney itself. (Sedistain.) **(e)** Mites are rare contaminants in free-catch urine. (Sedistain.) **(f)** Sperm are found in entire male dog urine. (Sedistain.) **(g)** Mucus strands. Variable amounts of fine material float on the surface of urine preparations and are normal. (Sedistain.) **(h)** Cotton fibre common contaminant, not to be confused with casts (Sedistain.) (Original magnification (a) X1000, (b,c,d,e) X200, (f,g,h) X400.)

Component	Normal findings	Significance of abnormal findings
Bacteria: $>1–3x10^4$/ml rods or $>1x10^5$/ml cocci must be present to be detectable in urine sediment	None	If present in cystocentesis sample indicate significant infection If present in a free-catch sample may be contaminants which have proliferated
Mucin	Small amount may be present	
Fat droplets	Normal in cats	
Sperm	Normal in males	
Yeasts	None	In free-catch urine may be contaminants, thus infection should be confirmed on cystocentesis sample Infection usually occurs only in immunosuppressed animals
Fungi	None	*Aspergillus* infection usually occurs only in immunosuppressed animals
Nematodes	None	Rare infection with *Dioctophyma renale* or *Capillaria plica*. Faecal contamination
Starch granules Pollen grains	None	Contaminants

10.17 Urine sediment analysis interpretation: miscellaneous.

Urine cytology

When abnormal or increased numbers of epithelial cells are seen on a standard sediment examination, cytological examination of a stained smear should be performed. A fresh sample of urine should be concentrated (preferably using a slower centifugation speed to minimize cell damage) and the sediment placed on a slide precoated with serum (to ensure attachment of cells). The cells should be gently spread into a monolayer and the preparation air dried before staining with a Romanowsky type stain (Wright's Giemsa or a related rapid stain).

The pH, SG and ageing of urine has a profound effect on cell morphology and causes swelling and loss of internal morphological detail, so urine for special cytological analysis should be as fresh as possible. If a delay in making smears is anticipated, boric acid may help preserve cellular morphology. However, if samples are to be mailed out to an external laboratory, centrifuged smears should be prepared in house whenever possible, air dried or wet fixed with a spray fixative and mailed along with a urine sample. Smears made from 24-hour-old urine are often impossible to interpret due to cell deterioration.

Normal urine sediment contains small numbers of epithelial cells (described above) seen singly or in small clusters. Chronic infection or inflammation related to urolithiasis and certain drugs can cause increased exfoliation of lining epithelial cells into the urine. There may be marked morphological hyperplastic or dysplastic changes of these cells which can exfoliate in large numbers in rafts and clusters. There can also be metaplastic changes in the cytoplasm due to the chronicity of the condition (Figure 10.18a), and in some instances nuclear changes can be very similar to those seen with neoplasia. Guidance from a cytologist is advisable in these situations. Numerous neutrophils may be seen in inflammatory or infectious conditions: these may be very degenerate, sometimes show loss of normal segmented nuclear morphology and may be confused with small epithelial cells (Figure 10.18b).

Neoplastic disease of the urinary system is usually malignant and frequently causes haematuria. The most common tumour is the transitional cell carcinoma. Cells from this are large and can exhibit marked anisocytosis and anisokaryosis as well as many other criteria of malignancy (see Chapter 20) (Figures 10.18c–d). Less common tumours are urothelial carcinoma or adenocarcinoma, in which cells are usually smaller with deeply staining cytoplasm (Figure 10.18e), and squamous cell carcinoma, in which exfoliated cells are large and have cytoplasmic characteristics of keratinization, cytoplasmic vacuolation and nuclear changes characteristic of malignancy (Figure 10.18f). Cells from primary tumours of the kidney epithelial cells (carcinoma) are infrequently shed into the urine. These are usually small cells with clear cytoplasm and a central round nucleus.

Rhabdomyosarcoma (botyroid) bladder tumours are rare, but can occur in young dogs of large breeds. Leiomyomas/sarcomas may also occur in the urinary system but cells from these rarely exfoliate into the

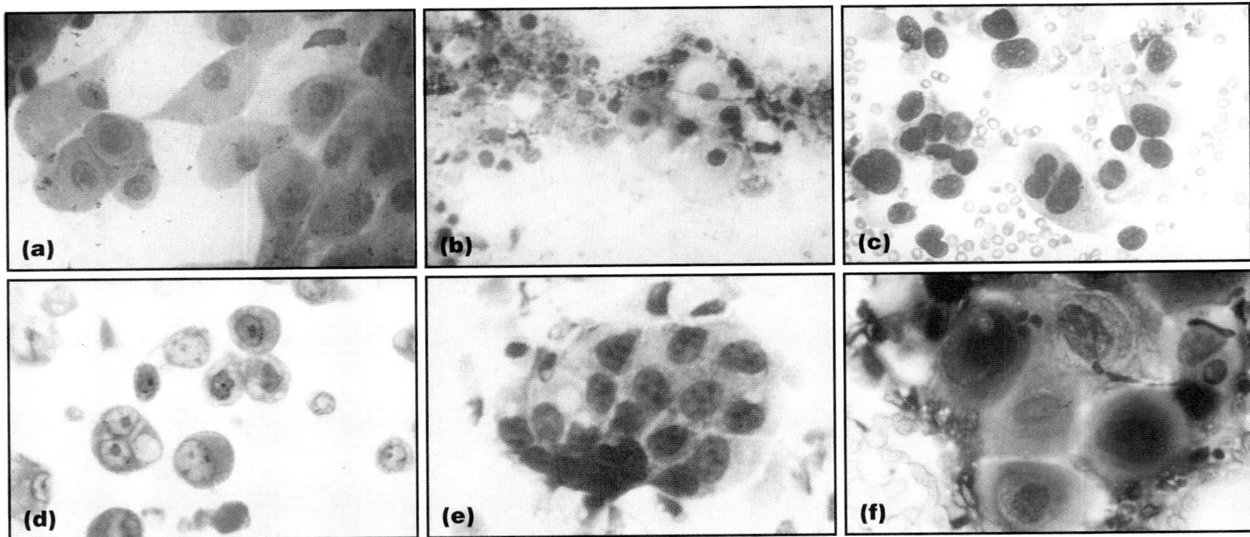

10.18 Urine sediment cytology. **(a)** Clusters of epithelial cells showing squamous metaplasia which can occur in chronic conditions with irritation/inflammation. (Wright's Giemsa stain.) **(b)** Sediment containing a mixture of bladder epithelial cells, neutrophils, erythrocytes and bacteria. If the sample was aseptically collected this would indicate pyuria urinary tract infection (UTI). This kind of sediment is some times referred to as 'active sediment'. (Giemsa stain.) **(c)** Transitional cell carcinoma of the bladder. The cells exhibit many criteria of malignancy: variation in cell and nuclear size, multinucleated cells, coarse nuclear chromatin and high nuclear:cytoplasmic ratio. (Wright's Giemsa stain.) **(d)** Transitional cell carcinoma of the bladder. Cells are stained with Papanicolaou stain which highlights nuclei and particularly size and shape of nucleoli. (Papanicolaou stain.) **(e)** A cluster of cells from an urothelial carcinoma. The cells are smaller than those in the transitional cell carcinoma with foamy cytoplasm and large nuclei with multiple nucleoli. (Giemsa stain.) **(f)** Raft of cells from a squamous cell carcinoma of the bladder. These cells are large with an angular outline and sparse cytoplasmic vacuoles around the nucleus. (Wright's Giemsa stain.) (Original magnification (a,c,e,f) X1000, (b,d) X500.)

urine. Renal or bladder lymphoma can result in exfoliation of large numbers of often abnormal lymphocytes into the urine.

Cytological diagnosis of bladder tumours is particularly difficult as polyps and epithelial hyperplasia may exfoliate similar cells. If a cytological diagnosis of malignant tumour is made, follow-up biopsy and histology are advisable, particularly in the case of bladder mucosal tumours, to confirm malignancy and the degree of invasiveness of the tumour.

Uroliths (calculi/stones)

Uroliths (the preferred term) or crystals can be analysed for mineral content using semiquantitative chemical analysis kits. The following constituents can be measured:

- Calcium
- Oxalate
- Phosphate
- Magnesium
- Ammonium
- Uric acid
- Cystine.

Uroliths can also be analysed using X-ray crystallography, polarized light microscopy and infrared (IR) spectroscopy. These methods are preferable to chemical semiquantitative mineral ion analysis. Identification of crystal types and/or mineral content is essential for successful therapy in animals with related urolithiasis.

Uroliths are believed to form more readily in supersaturated urine. However, other factors play a part:

- The presence of a nucleation centre or nidus (e.g. bacteria, mucin plug)
- Urine pH
- Duration of urine supersaturation
- Absence of crystallization inhibitors normally produced by bladder mucosal cells
- Possibly genetic factors.

Risk factor analysis for urolith formation can be performed and expressed as the relative supersaturation (RSS) index. The RSS is obtained by complex computer-based analysis of urine volume, pH and content of calcium, oxalate, magnesium, uric acid, mucin, citrate and pyrophosphate. RSS were developed and are used by food manufacturers for the formulation of diets suitable for treatment and prevention of struvite, calcium oxalate and calcium phosphate urolithiasis in both dogs and cats. Several studies have suggested that RSS can be used to predict the risk of formation of these uroliths. In practice, analysing urine pH and the amounts and types of crystals present can be used as a guide to which type of calculus may be likely to form, or has formed and is present. Such analysis can also be used to monitor the effectiveness of therapy.

Struvite and calcium oxalate are the most common uroliths identified in dogs and cats but over the last 20 years there has been a change in the relative proportion of these uroliths, with a increase in incidence of calcium oxalate urolithisis and a decrease in struvite (Ling *et al.*, 2003). This is likely to be related to the widespread use of manufactured urinary acidifying diets with restricted magnesium content. In one study in dogs analysing urolith submissions, approximately 44% were struvite and 42% were calcium oxalate (Houston *et al.*, 2004). Struvite were most common in female dogs and calcium oxalate in male dogs. In cats 50% of urolith submissions were calcium oxalate and 44% were struvite, while the majority of urethral plugs (81%) were struvite (Houston *et al.*, 2003).

Clues to the type of urolith present are the breed, urine pH, urolith radiodensity (calcium oxalate, calcium phosphate, cystine and struvite uroliths are radiodense, whilst urates are radiolucent) and the type of crystals seen in urine sediment. However the type of crystal present is not always the same as the type of urolith. All types of uroliths in the bladder may lead to a secondary urinary tract infection, and, if the organism produces urease, urine pH increases leading to struvite crystal formation.

Struvite uroliths

Struvite uroliths (Figure 10.19) may form in sterile urine that contains high concentrations of magnesium, phosphorus and ammonium ions and is of neutral to alkaline pH. In dogs, they are formed more frequently, and more rapidly, when there is also a co-existing infection, particularly with urease-producing bacteria (*Staphylococcus* and *Proteus*). This enzyme can split urea (abundant in urine) to produce ammonium ions and CO_2, which forms bicarbonate and increases urine pH. The ammonium ions become part of the struvite crystals. Increased concentrations of these ions are also reported to affect the mucins glycosaminoglycans produced by the bladder mucosal lining cells, reducing their protective ability. Struvite calculi are most common in young female dogs and in the following breeds: mixed breeds, Miniature Schnauzers, Shih Tzu and Bichon Frise.

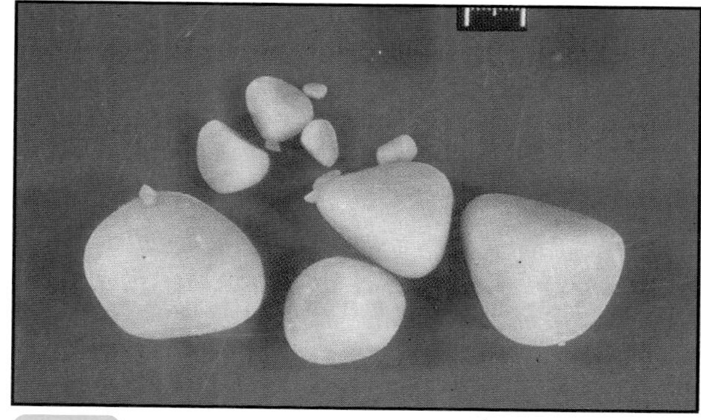

10.19 Struvite stones from the bladder of a dog.

In cats, struvite calculi formation is most common in sterile conditions in older female cats and is less commonly associated with infection (where there is no age or sex predilection). In cats, struvite is also a common component of many urethral plugs which occur almost exclusively in male neutered cats with or without urinary tract infection (UTI). High-magnesium dry diets, alkaline urine and a reduction in urine glycosaminoglycans have been implicated in the development of both struvite stones and struvite-rich plugs.

Calcium oxalate uroliths

Calcium oxalate uroliths form in acid to neutral urine, usually in the absence of UTI. In dogs, they occur more commonly in older male animals. A breed predisposition for Lhasa Apso, Shih Tzu, Bichon Frise, Miniature Poodles, Miniature Schnauzers and Yorkshire Terriers is reported. In cats, calcium oxalate uroliths are more common in males, with no age restriction. Burmese, Himalayan and Persian cats are reported to be more often affected. Risk factors for their formation are a high-protein diet, increased dietary calcium, oxalate, sodium and vitamin C. The acidifying diets for preventing struvite formation may also be contributory in some cases, as they have reduced magnesium and produce acid urine. A possible inherited mechanism which minimizes the production of mucins glycosaminoglycans and other compounds capable of inhibiting calcium oxalate crystal growth has also been implicated in both cats and dogs. These inhibitory compounds include Tamm–Horsfall protein, nephrocalcin and prothrombin fragments, which increase the solubility of calcium oxalate and prevent crystal aggregation.

Calcium phosphate uroliths

Calcium phosphate crystals form much less frequently than either struvite or calcium oxalate in both cats and dogs. Growth and aggregation can lead to stone formation which has been associated with hypercalcaemia and high urine calcium concentrations. They form most easily in alkaline urine. There are different types of calcium phosphate uroliths, including hydroxyapatite, carbonateapatite and brushite (tricalcium phosphate). They have been associated with increased dietary calcium, phosphorus and vitamin D; renal tubular acidosis; and hypercalcaemia associated with hyperparathyroidism, but not paraneoplastic syndromes. They can form at any urine pH. In dogs there is an increased incidence in males but no age association. They are more common in Cocker Spaniels, Yorkshire Terriers and Miniature Schnauzers. They are uncommon in cats but occur most frequently in middle-aged female cats, with no breed predilection.

Ammonium urate and uric acid uroliths

These form in acid to neutral pH urine. They are uncommon in both dogs and cats with the exception of the Dalmatian; in this breed there is an inherited reduced ability to oxidize uric acid to allantoin, causing accumulation of uric acid in plasma and urine, which can lead to urolith formation. There is also an increased incidence of these uroliths in other breeds, including English Bulldog, Yorkshire Terrier, Miniature Schnauzer and Shih Tzu. These uroliths can also occur in dogs and cats with severe hepatic dysfunction and portosystemic shunts.

Cystine uroliths

These form due to an inborn error of amino acid metabolism which leads to reduced tubular resorption of cystine and consequent increased urinary cystine accumulation. This results in cystine crystalluria and, in some cases, urolith formation. The condition is rare but is reported usually in young male dogs of the English Bulldog, Dachshund and Bassett Hound breeds. It is rarely reported in cats.

Silica uroliths

These are rare but their formation in acid to neutral urine, in association with acidifying diets, has been reported. Many of these diets contain large amounts of plant gluten, soya bean and maize hulls which are high in silica. They have been found in middle-aged male dogs of the German Shepherd Dog, Golden Retriever and Labrador Retriever breeds.

Urinary tests for tubular damage

Urine gamma-glutamyl transferase:creatinine ratio

If acute severe renal tubular damage or necrosis is suspected (e.g. following aminoglycoside treatment) a urinary test for tubular damage can be performed. Gamma-glutamyl transferase (γ-glutamyl transpeptidase, GGT) is synthesized by renal tubular epithelial cells, and when they are injured or sloughed, it is lost into the urine in large amounts (although plasma GGT is not increased). Creatinine is not reabsorbed by the tubules, so urine GGT can be related to urine creatinine to correct for variation in urine SG. GGT and creatinine are measured by automatic methods in the same sample of urine and a ratio obtained:

$$\frac{\text{Urine GGT (IU/l)}}{\text{Urine creatinine (mg/dl)}}$$

Units may need to be converted from SI units to perform the calculation:

$$\text{Creatinine (mmol/l)} \times 1000/88.4 = \text{Creatinine (mg/dl)}$$

A normal urine GGT:creatinine ratio of 0.14 ± 0.10 has been reported for adult dogs (Gossett *et al.*, 1987), whilst a study of 6-month-old male Beagles reported a higher value of 0.34 ± 0.53 (Grauer *et al.*, 1995). The ratio is increased with tubular damage, e.g. following gentamycin-induced nephrotoxicosis.

Assessment of polyuria/polydipsia by water deprivation testing

Water deprivation tests (WDT) are used in patients with hyposthenuria (i.e. SG <1.007) to differentiate between central diabetes insipidus (CDI), nephrogenic diabetes insipidus (NDI) and psychogenic polydipsia (PP). However, animals with hypercalcaemia, hyperadrenocorticism, hypoadrenocorticism, pyometra and urinary tract infections may occasionally have hyposthenuria, and

WDT is dangerous or contraindicated in these patients. This test is also contraindicated in polyuric animals that are dehydrated and/or azotaemic. Polyuria and polydipsia (PU/PD) are frequently reported in dogs and cats, but CDI, NDI and PP are relatively rare and it is essential to attempt to rule out all other causes of polyuria and polydipsia before performing a WDT. The test is designed to determine whether ADH is released in response to dehydration (increased plasma osmolality), and whether the kidney can respond to ADH. When the test is performed correctly CDI, NDI, and PP can be differentiated from each other in the majority of cases (Figure 10.20). Serum and urine osmolality can be measured to monitor the response to water deprivation but freeze point depression osmometers are not widely available to veterinary practitioners. Therefore the monitoring methods of choice are measuring urine SG and recording bodyweight. When performing the test the same balance/scales must be used for each weighing and the same refractometer must be used for measuring urine SG throughout.

It is important to rule out hyperadrenocorticism (Cushing's disease) as a cause of PU/PD before performing a WDT. Although some animals with this condition can concentrate urine normally following water deprivation, many are able to concentrate urine to SG >1.008, but not to >1.025, because of ADH antagonism. When desmopressin (DDAVP, a synthetic ADH analogue) is administered, concentrating ability returns, thus mimicking CDI.

If the animal is markedly polyuric, water deprivation should be done with extreme caution because such animals may become rapidly dehydrated, as a result of pre-existing medullary washout. In these animals it is better to restrict water intake partially for 5 days beforehand (120 ml/kg per day on days –5, –4 and –3, 90 ml/kg on day –2 and 60 ml/kg on the day before the test). Salt can be added to the food from day –5 to help correct medullary washout.

Protocol

Partial water restriction for 2–3 days prior to the test is recommended, to correct medullary washout. About 100 ml/kg is allowed on the first day, reducing by 10–15% per day for 2 further days. On the fourth day complete water deprivation is commenced as follows:

1. Empty bladder (catheter) measure urine S.G.
2. Weigh animal
3. Deprive the animal of food and water

At 1–2 hourly intervals:

1. Empty the bladder and measure urine S.G.
2. Weigh the animal
3. Measure serum/plasma urea and creatinine (optional)

Discontinue the test when:

- The urine S.G. is >1.025
- Or there has been >5% loss of body weight
- Or the animal becomes azotaemic or depressed

Interpretation

PP can be identified at this stage because the SG will become >1.025
CDI and **NDI** will fail to concentrate above 1.010 even when there is >5% loss of body weight
Values between 1.010 and 1.020 are equivocal and indicate submaximal concentration suggesting partial central DI.
To distinguish between CDI and NDI the **desmopressin response test** is performed (preferably immediately after the WDT):

1. Empty the bladder and measure urine SG
2. Inject desmopressin intravenously or intramuscularly (2.0 µg for small dogs <15 kg, 4.0 µg for dogs >15kg)
3. Measure urine SG every 2 hours for 6–10 hours, then at 12 and 24 hours
4. Provide small amounts of water (3 ml/kg/hour) during and following the test to prevent cerebral oedema

Intrepretation of desmopressin response test

- Urine SG values >1.015 indicative **CDI**
- Failure to concentrate above 1.010 is indicative of **NDI**
- Urine SG values between 1.010 and 1.015 are equivocal and could reflect medullary washout

10.20 Water deprivation test and its interpretation.

Tests used in conjunction with water deprivation testing

Endogenous plasma ADH levels are used to distinguish between CDI, NDI and PP in humans as part of the WDT. ADH measurement is available on a limited basis for veterinary patients in human hospital laboratories but it is expensive and has a long turnaround time, and, therefore, is impractical in most clinic cases.

The Hickey–Hare test is sometimes used if the WDT is non-diagnostic. This test measures renal tubular and pituitary responses to hyperosmolality (intravenous hypertonic saline administration) by assessing the output, SG and, if possible, osmolality of urine. In normal animals and animals with PP, the urine output progressively decreases and urine SG and osmolality increase following hypertonic saline administration, whilst there is no response in animals with CDI and NDI. However there is a significant risk of inducing marked hypertonicity (hyperosmolality), especially in severely polyuric animals. The test requires close monitoring and is probably best performed in referral hospitals.

A closely monitored trial of the ADH analogue desmopressin (DDAVP) administration over 5–7 days is often a safer alternative when WDT is non-diagnostic. Desmopressin administration should cause a >50% decrease in water intake in CDI, but will have no effect in NDI.

Case examples

Case 1

Signalment

2-year-old entire female Boxer

History

2-month history of PD/PU with a sudden onset. Cystitis had been diagnosed and treated but the PD/PU persisted. The dog was drinking 180–280 ml of water/kg/day, but was otherwise bright and well. There were no abnormalities detected on clinical examination.

Case 1 continues ▶

Case 1 continued

Clinical pathology data

Haematology	Result	Reference interval
RBC (x 10^{12}/l)	7.7	5.5–8.5
Hb (g/dl)	17.2	12–18
HCT (l/l)	0.53	0.37–0.55
MCV (fl)	69.8	60–77
MCH (pg)	22.3	19.5–24.5
MCHC (g/dl)	32.0	31–37
WBC (x 10^9/l)	6.2	6–17.1
Neutrophils (x 10^9/l)	4.4	3–11.5
Lymphocytes (x 10^9/l)	1.2	1–4.8
Monocytes (x 10^9/l)	0.2	0.15–1.5
Eosinophils (x 10^9/l)	0.37	0–1.3
Basophils (x 10^9/l)	0.00	0–0.2
Platelets (x 10^9/l)	212	150–900

Biochemistry	Result	Reference interval
Sodium (mmol/l)	149.6	136–155
Potassium (mmol/l)	4.07	3.5–5.8
Chloride (mmol/l)	116	107–120
Glucose (mmol/l)	5.6	3.4–5.3
Urea (mmol/l)	4.5	3.3–8.0
Creatinine (µmol/l)	103	45–150
Calcium (mmol/l)	2.73	2.2–2.9
Inorganic phosphate (mmol/l)	1.46	0.8–2.0
TP (g/l)	62.3	60–80
Albumin (g/l)	31.5	25–45
Globulin (g/l)	30.8	21–41
ALT (IU/l)	17	21–59
ALP (IU/l)	83	3–142
Bile acids (µmol/l)	2	<10

Urine analysis	
Gross appearance	Very pale yellow, clear
SG	1.002
Dipstick results	pH 5.0; negative for protein, ketones, bilirubin, urobilinogen
Sediment examination	1–2 WBC per hpf; no casts or crystals seen

What abnormalities are present and what are the differential diagnoses?

Haematology and biochemistry results are all within reference intervals. This rules out several important causes of PD/PU, such as renal failure, diabetes mellitus, liver disease, hypoadrenocorticism and hypercalcaemia. Hyperadrenocorticism (HAC) cannot be completely excluded but most cases would have at least one of the following: elevated cholesterol, elevated ALP, or stress leucogram; these are not seen in this case. Other than PD/PU there were no clinical findings suggestive of HAC and so this was excluded from the differential diagnosis list. The urine analysis shows a marked hyposthenuria with no evidence of inflammation. These findings are suggestive of diabetes insipidus or psychogenic polydipsia.

What further tests would you perform?

A water deprivation test should be performed.

Results of further tests

Gradual water deprivation over 48 h was followed by a water deprivation test. The water intake was reduced to 100 ml/kg/day and then the dog was abruptly deprived of water. Body weight, urine SG, and urine and plasma osmolality were recorded. Plasma urea and creatinine were 3.76 mmol/l and 81 µmol/l at time 0 and 4.62 mmol/l and 86 µmol/l at T + 12 h.

Time	Body weight (% reduction)	Urine SG	Urine osmolality	Plasma osmolality
T = 0 h	23.8 kg	1.002	100 mmol/kg	282 mmol/kg
T + 4 h	23.6 kg (0.8%)	1.004	132 mmol/kg	312 mmol/kg
T + 10 h	23.2 kg (2.5%)	1.005	165 mmol/kg	326 mmol/kg
T + 12 h	22.8 kg (4.2%)	1.004	–	–
T + 13 h	22.5 kg (5.4%)	1.004	–	–
T = 13.1 h Water was offered in 100 ml aliquots every 45 min for following 4 h then in 200 ml aliquots for 2 h then unrestricted				
T + 16 h 4µg DDAVP injected i.m.				
T + 18 h	–	1.026	772 mmol/kg	321 mmol/kg

How would you interpret these results?

The results show a failure to concentrate urine after 13 h of water deprivation in the face of dehydration (indicated by weight loss >5% of original body weight and increasing plasma osmolality). This excludes psychogenic polydipsia and is consistent with nephrogenic or central diabetes insipidus (CDI). Urine became more concentrated following administration of DDAVP, indicating CDI. In the absence of other neurological signs or history of trauma, the CDI was considered idiopathic, although underlying causes such as neoplasia were not investigated further.

Case outcome

The clinical signs were well controlled with DDAVP drops administered into the conjunctival sac. The dog was lost to follow-up after 6 months.

(Case 1 courtesy of E Villiers.)

Case 2

Signalment

13-year-old female Bearded Collie.

History and clinical findings

5-month history of haematuria. Increased frequency of urination; dysuria and nocturia. Multiple courses of antibiotics. Possible discomfort on sitting down. Very tense on abdominal palpation. No other significant clinical findings.

Case 2 continues ▶

Case 2 continued

Clinical pathology data

Urine analysis	
SG (refractometer)	1.024
Dipstick results	pH 6.5; protein + to ++; blood +++; negative for glucose, ketones, urobilinogen, bilirubin, haemoglobin
Sediment examination	See Figure 10.21

10.21 Cytological appearance of the urine sediment, showing various areas of the smear. (Wright's stain; original magnification X1000.)

What abnormalities are present?

Urinalysis

- Mild to moderate proteinuria
- Marked haematuria: this may account for the proteinuria as the dog has gross haematuria
- SG in keeping with polyuria, or early renal failure.

Urine cytology

- Mixed population of cells, consisting of neutrophils and epithelial cells
- Neutrophils are degenerate and show karyolysis. Intracellular bacteria are seen. Both rods (likely to be *Escherichia coli* in this site) and cocci are present
- Epithelial cells are pleomorphic, with some very large cells with high nuclear:cytoplasmic ratio and open chromatin. Binucleate cells are also seen. Cytoplasm is variably basophilic but in some cells shows increased basophilia, and vacuolation is also apparent
- Numerous background RBCs and free bacteria.

How would you interpret these results and what are the likely differential diagnoses?

The cytological findings confirm that the dog has bacterial cystitis. The transitional epithelial cells show features suggestive of malignancy but, in the presence of a florid inflammatory response (and with the very long history of urinary tract disease), these changes must be interpreted with caution, as dysplastic cells may mimic neoplasia.

What further tests would you recommend?

- Culture and sensitivity testing
- Imaging to identify any mass lesion, and suction biopsy via catheter if indicated, or cystoscopy and biopsy.

Results of further tests

A pneumocystogram and double-contrast cystogram (Figures 10.22 and 10.23) showed an ill-defined mass extending from the apex of the bladder along the dorsal wall almost to the trigone. The outline is irregular, with a 'moth-eaten' appearance suggesting mucosal disruption. The bladder wall appears thickened craniodorsally: on the pneumocystogram, this may be a result of insufficient inflation, but on the double-contrast study this is a genuine finding. This extensive ill-defined irregular mass, which has caused mucosal disruption, is most likely neoplastic, and most likely a transitional cell carcinoma. This should be confirmed by suction biopsy (declined by the owner on grounds of cost).

These findings are consistent with a bladder tumour with secondary urinary tract infection. Great care should be taken in diagnosing neoplasia on urine cytology, especially if there is concurrent inflammation, as in this case. The atypical cellular features could have been due to tissue dysplasia, caused by the severe inflammation present; and further diagnostic investigations should always be performed when neoplasia is suspected cytologically.

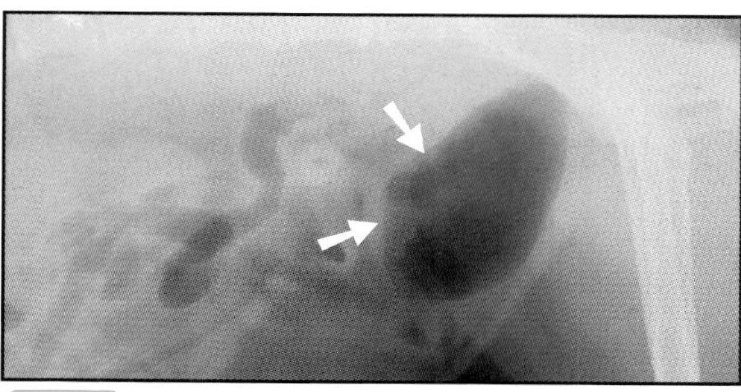

10.22 Pneumocystogram.

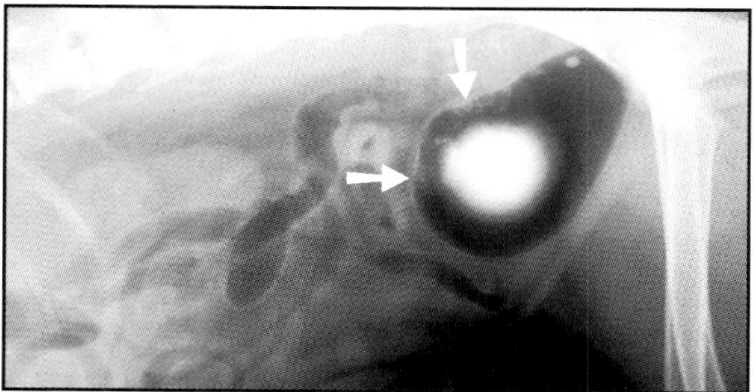

10.23 Double contrast cystogram.

Case outcome

The dog was treated palliatively with piroxicam, and survived for a further 6 months.

(Case 2 courtesy of L Blackwood.)

References and further reading

Gossett KA, Turnwald GH, Kearney MT *et al.* (1987). Evaluation of gamma-glutamyl transpetidase - to - creatinine ratio from spot urine samples of urine supernatant as an indicator of urinaryy enzyme excretion in dogs. *American Journal of Veterinary Research* **48**, 455–457

Grauer GF, Greco DS, Behrend EN *et al.* (1995)Estimation of quantitative enzymuria in dogs with gentamycin-induced nephrotoxicosis using enzyme/creatinine ratios from spot urine samples. *Journal of Veterinary Internal Medicine* **9**, 323–327

Grauer GF, Oberhauser EB, Basaraba RJ, Lappin MR, Simpson DF and Jensen DF (2002). Development of microalbuminuria in dogs with heartworm disease. *Journal of Veterinary Internal Medicine* **16**, 352 (abstract)

Heuter KJ, Buffington CA and Chew DJ (1998) Agreement between two methods for measuring urine pH in cats and dogs. *Journal of the American Veterinary Medical Association* **213**, 996–998

Houston DM, Moore AE, Favrin MG and Hof B (2004) Canine urolithiasis: a look at over 16,000 urolith submissions to the Canadian Veterinary Urolith Centre from February 1998 to April 2003. *Canadian Veterinary Journal* **45**, 225–230

Houston DM, Moore AE, Favrin MG and Hoff B (2003) Feline urethral plugs and bladder uroliths: a review of 5,484 submissions 1998–2003. *Canadian Veterinary Journal* **44**, 974–977

Jensen WA, Grauer GF, Andrews J and Simpson DF (2001) Prevalence of microalbuminuria in dogs. *Journal of Veterinary Internal Medicine* **15**, 300 (abstract)

Latimer KS, Mahaffey EA and Prasse KW (2003) Urinary System. In: *Duncan and Prasse's Veterinary Laboratory Medicine Clinical Pathology, 4th edn,* ed. CR Gregory, pp. 231–259. Iowa State Press, Iowa

Ling GV, Thurmond MC, Choi YK, Franti CE, Ruby AL, Johnson DL (2003) Changes in proportion of canine urinary calculi composed of calcium oxalate or struvite in specimens analyzed from 1981 through 2001. *Journal of Veterinary Internal Medicine* **17**, 817–823

Osborne CA and Stevens JB (1999) *Handbook of Canine and Feline Urinalysis.* Bayer Scientific, Leverkusen, Germany

Pressler BM, Proulx DA, Williams LE, Jensen WA and Vaden SL (2003) Urine albumin concentration is increased in dogs with lymphoma or osteosarcoma. *Journal of Veterinary Internal Medicine* **17**, 404 (abstract)

Radecki S, Donnelly R, Jensen WA and Stinchcomb DT (2003) Effect of age and breed on the prevalence of microalbuminuria in dogs. *Journal of Veterinary Internal Medicine* **17**, 406 (abstract)

Raskin RE, Murray KA and Levy JK (2002) Comparison of home monitoring methods for feline urine pH measurement. *Veterinary Clinical Pathology* **31**, 51–55

Vaden SL, Jensen WA and Simpson D (2001) Prevalence of microalbuminuria in dogs evaluated at a referral veterinary hospital. *Journal of Veterinary Internal Medicine* **15**, 300 (abstract)

Vaden S L, Barrak M P, Lappin M R and Jensen W A (2004) Effects of urinary tract inflammation and sample blood contamination on urine albumin and total protein concentrations in canine urine samples. *Veterinary Clinical Pathology* **33**, 14–19

Wisnewski N, Clarke KB, Powell TD and Sellins KS (2004) Prevalence of microalbuminuria in cats. www.heska.com/erd/erd_datacat.asp

11

Laboratory evaluation of renal disorders

Richard A. Squires

Introduction

Diagnostic investigation of suspected renal disease begins with a consideration of the signalment, history and physical examination findings. Thereafter, if renal disease is still suspected, laboratory investigations are carried out. The most useful laboratory tests at this stage of the investigation are a serum biochemistry profile and complete urine analysis. There is relatively little to be gained by doing one without the other, since accurate diagnosis of most renal disorders requires integration of information gained from urine and serum biochemical analyses.

Laboratory investigation of the various categories of renal failure, protein-losing nephropathy and renal tubular disorders will be described in this chapter. Urine analysis is discussed in Chapter 10.

Renal failure

Overview and definitions

A variety of adverse influences (e.g. toxins, overdosed drugs, infectious agents, ischaemic insults) can damage the kidneys, either reversibly or permanently, to produce renal disease. When renal disease is severe enough to render 66–75% of the nephrons non-functional, urine concentrating ability is compromised and the animal becomes polydipsic, polyuric and unable to produce maximally concentrated urine. This extent of renal disease is sometimes termed *renal insufficiency*. When more than 75% of the nephrons are rendered non-functional, excretory function is compromised to the extent that non-protein nitrogenous waste substances, such as creatinine and urea, begin to accumulate in the blood. This accumulation is termed *azotaemia* and renal disease severe enough to cause azotaemia in a well hydrated animal is termed *renal failure*. Advanced renal failure and other causes of severe azotaemia may be associated with a set of unpleasant clinical features termed *uraemia*. Uraemia arises principally as a consequence of accumulation of a wide variety of toxic substances, collectively termed *uraemic toxins*. Typical clinical features of uraemia include lethargy, depression, anorexia, vomiting, diarrhoea, anaemia and oral and gastric ulceration. Some common terms are defined in Figure 11.1.

Intrinsic renal failure may be categorized as acute, subacute or chronic. Acute renal failure (ARF) develops over a short period of time (typically less than a

Term	Definitions
Anion gap (serum)	Calculated by subtracting the typically measured serum anions (chloride and bicarbonate) from the typically measured cations (sodium and potassium). The normal anion gap (consisting mostly of unmeasured anions like plasma proteins) is 12–24 mmol/l in dogs and 13–27 mmol/l in cats. (See Chapter 9)
Azotaemia	An abnormal increase in the concentration of non-protein nitrogenous wastes (such as creatinine and urea nitrogen) in blood
Glomerular filtration rate (GFR)	The total volume of fluid filtered by all of the glomeruli in both kidneys per unit time. The GFR is directly proportional to the remaining functional renal mass
Isosthenuria	A state in which the kidneys cannot form urine with a higher or a lower specific gravity than that of protein-free plasma; urine specific gravity becomes fixed around 1.010 (1.007–1.013). (See Chapter 10)
Osmolality	The concentration of osmotically active particles in a solution expressed in terms of the number of osmoles of solute per kilogram of solvent. Osmolality is directly proportional to boiling point elevation, freezing point depression and decline in vapour pressure. (See Chapter 10)
Renal disease	Damage or functional impairment of the kidneys. Can vary in severity from very mild, to severe enough to cause uraemia
Renal insufficiency	Renal functional impairment not severe enough to cause azotaemia, but sufficient to cause loss of renal reserve. These patients have a reduced ability to compensate for dehydration. Their urine concentrating ability is usually diminished
Renal failure	Renal functional impairment sufficient to cause azotaemia. Urine concentrating ability is usually impaired
Uraemia	The constellation of adverse clinical signs caused by advanced renal failure, or (occasionally) other causes of severe azotaemia

11.1 Definition of some terms commonly used in discussion of renal disorders.

week) whereas chronic failure usually take months to develop. Subacute failure is an intermediate category and may be caused, for example, by some aggressive renal bacterial infections (e.g. leptospirosis). It can sometimes be a challenge for the clinician to distinguish acute from chronic renal failure (CRF). Although patients with ARF are usually extremely ill (because they have been abruptly exposed to uraemic toxins), their renal pathology may be reversible if they can be supported through their crisis. Conversely, CRF is usually a consequence of incremental, irreversible renal pathology. Patients with mild to moderate CRF may appear remarkably well for a given degree of azotaemia, because their bodies have had time to adapt to exposure to uraemic toxins. However, patients with advanced, or end-stage renal failure feel very unwell, regardless of how long their disease has been developing. History, physical examination, laboratory tests and imaging studies can help distinguish between acute, subacute and chronic forms of renal failure.

Severe intrinsic renal disease is not the only cause of azotaemia, which may also be caused by prerenal and postrenal factors. Prerenal azotaemia arises as a consequence of renal blood perfusion being inadequate to allow clearance of the nitrogenous wastes being produced in the body. Prerenal azotaemia may thus arise as a consequence of either:

- Lower than normal renal blood perfusion, e.g. severe dehydration, hypovolaemia, congestive heart failure
- Higher than normal production of nitrogenous wastes, e.g. high-protein diet, gastrointestinal haemorrhage, endogenous protein catabolism.

Postrenal azotaemia develops as a consequence of:

- Urinary tract rupture
- Obstruction of the urinary tract distal to the kidneys.

Bilateral obstruction or avulsion of the ureters, rupture of the urinary bladder and urethral obstruction are examples of causes of postrenal azotaemia. Severe renal trauma, with urine leakage, produces an equivalent pathophysiological effect. Laboratory tests can help to distinguish prerenal and postrenal azotaemia from primary, intrinsic renal azotaemia.

Components of azotaemia

Urea and creatinine accumulate in the bodies of patients with failing kidneys. The blood, plasma or serum concentrations of these substances are useful indicators of the extent of retention of nitrogenous waste products and hence the degree of renal failure. In order to interpret renal function tests accurately, a basic understanding of the origins, metabolism and excretion of urea and creatinine is necessary.

Urea

Urea is the major nitrogenous waste product of mammals and is ultimately excreted almost exclusively in urine. It is synthesized in the liver from carbon dioxide and ammonia via the urea cycle. Hepatic synthesis of urea is an energy-requiring process that permits excretion of excess ammonia, most of which is formed during deamination of amino acids. Although urea is classified as a uraemic toxin, it is considerably less toxic than its progenitor, ammonia. Urea is a small, uncharged molecule (relative molecular mass 60 daltons) that is not protein-bound. It diffuses rapidly throughout all body fluid compartments and is freely filtered at the glomerular basement membrane. When the overall glomerular filtration rate (GFR) of a dog or cat declines below about 25% of normal, serum urea concentration exceeds the upper limit of the reference range.

Most of the ammonia incorporated into urea comes from protein breakdown. Thus, the rate of urea formation is highly dependent on dietary protein content and the rate of endogenous protein catabolism. High-protein diets, particularly those that contain much protein of low biological value, and gastrointestinal haemorrhage increase the serum urea concentration somewhat, even in animals with normal renal function. The increased serum urea caused by feeding a high-protein diet is of no clinical significance to a healthy animal, but patients with renal insufficiency have a more substantial increase in serum urea as a consequence of eating such foods than do normal animals. Because of the complicating effects of recent meals, blood samples for measurement of serum urea should ideally be drawn after the animal has undergone a 12-hour fast.

Anything that increases endogenous protein catabolism can increase serum urea concentration, independent of diet and renal excretory function. Some specific causes of increased endogenous protein catabolism include:

- Fever
- Starvation
- Vigorous, prolonged exercise
- Recent glucocorticoid administration
- Burns
- Sepsis.

Conversely, the following will tend to reduce serum urea:

- Anabolic steroids
- Severe hepatic dysfunction
- Feeding of a protein-restricted, high-quality protein diet that meets calorific needs.

As well as being freely filtered at the glomerular basement membrane, urea is reabsorbed in the tubules and collecting ducts. During intense diuresis, approximately 60% of filtered urea is cleared by the kidneys, with 40% being reabsorbed. However, when the flow of fluid through the renal tubules is relatively sluggish, much more urea is reabsorbed and retained. This may be of advantage to a normal animal, since retention of urea in the renal medullary interstitium is one of the mechanisms by which the kidneys are able to concentrate urine. A healthy animal with declining urine output (e.g. because of restricted access to drinking water) becomes increasingly able to concentrate its urine. From a diagnostic point of view, serum urea will tend to underestimate GFR in dehydrated animals (i.e. the situation will look worse than it really is) and overestimate renal excretory function in well hydrated polydipsic animals or those receiving vigorous intravenous fluid therapy. An 'artificial' improvement in renal function (as assessed by a decrease in serum urea concentration) is frequently seen in hospitalized CRF patients that have been receiving 2–3 times maintenance intravenous fluid therapy for several days. In this situation, the serum creatinine is a more reliable indicator of GFR than the serum urea.

Most laboratory methods for quantitation of urea rely upon the enzyme urease to hydrolyse urea to ammonia and carbon dioxide. The ammonia can then be detected using a colour indicator and sometimes a second enzyme. This method is highly specific because urease targets urea. Most available dipsticks for semi-quantitation of blood urea are inaccurate and should only be used as a preliminary diagnostic tool in emergency settings.

In many American textbooks, the concentration of urea in blood is expressed in terms of the amount of urea *nitrogen* rather than the entire urea molecule (hence the term *blood urea nitrogen*, BUN, is commonly encountered). BUN (mg/dl) can be converted to serum urea (mmol/l; SI unit) by multiplying by 0.357.

Creatinine

Small quantities of creatinine are ingested by dogs and cats in the animal tissues they eat, but the vast majority is produced from their own skeletal muscle by breakdown of creatine. Approximately 1.6–2.0% of total body creatine is converted to creatinine each day in a rather constant, non-enzymatic, irreversible process. The amount of creatinine formed daily therefore depends upon the total body creatine, which, in turn, is determined by dietary intake, rate of synthesis and, most importantly, total skeletal muscle mass. 'Muscular' dogs or cats would be expected to have a somewhat higher serum creatinine concentration than less muscular ones, other factors (such as renal function) being equal.

Like urea, creatinine is a relatively small molecule (113 daltons) that is not protein-bound and is freely filtered at the glomerular basement membrane. Unlike urea, creatinine is not reabsorbed by the renal tubules or collecting ducts. In male dogs, a very small amount of creatinine is actively secreted into the tubular filtrate by the proximal renal tubules. Such secretion does not occur in bitches or cats of either sex and is of little clinical significance, even in male dogs.

More significantly, creatinine diffuses into the gastrointestinal lumen and is subsequently metabolized by intestinal bacteria. This represents a substantial and probably underemphasized pathway for creatinine removal, particularly in azotaemic animals. Although some of the creatinine broken down by intestinal bacteria may be recycled to produce more creatinine, most that is metabolized in this way is permanently removed from the body. Intestinal bacterial catabolism of creatinine becomes increasingly significant in severely azotaemic animals; in some patients, serum creatinine concentrations somewhat underestimate the severity of renal failure in late-stage disease.

Most laboratories measure serum creatinine using a method that involves the Jaffe reaction, in which creatinine and picrate react together under alkaline conditions to produce a detectable coloured complex. Unfortunately, a number of non-creatinine substances also react with alkaline picrate to produce coloured substances, so the method is not very specific. These *non-creatinine chromogens* adversely affect the accuracy of serum creatinine estimation, particularly when renal failure is mild and serum creatinine is relatively low. Non-creatinine chromogens are present in serum but are not usually found in urine. Therefore, diagnostic methods (such as clearance tests) that compare the serum creatinine concentration with that in urine are particularly affected by the fairly modest inaccuracies caused by these substances. Enzymatic methods for quantitation of serum creatinine exist, but are not in wide use, presumably because of their high cost.

Serum creatinine concentrations are usually provided in mg/dl in American textbooks. To convert creatinine reported in mg/dl to SI units (μmol/l), multiply by 88.4. (See also Appendix 3.)

Diagnostic value of serum creatinine and serum urea

Both serum urea and serum creatinine are insensitive measures of renal excretory dysfunction. Up to 75% of total renal filtering capacity can be lost without these blood parameters exceeding their reference ranges. This means that many renal failure patients have lost more than 90% of their nephrons, because their remnant nephrons become hypertrophied and hyperfunctional. Creatinine is not reabsorbed by the renal tubules, whereas urea is, so one would predict that serum creatinine concentration would be a more reliable indicator of GFR than serum urea. This prediction is widely accepted and has been confirmed by research (Finco *et al.*, 1995). However, serum creatinine concentration does not increase precisely in proportion to a decrease in GFR. A modest deviation occurs as a consequence of extrarenal (i.e. gastrointestinal) creatinine losses increasing in a non-linear and unpredictable fashion as azotaemia worsens.

Although serum creatinine concentration is generally held to be a superior measure of GFR in dogs and cats than serum urea, at least one study of human renal failure patients has indicated that serum urea correlates somewhat more directly with symptoms of uraemia than serum creatinine concentration does (Kassirer, 1971). Equivalent studies have not been carried out in dogs and cats, but it is clear that neither serum urea nor serum creatinine should be relied upon to predict precisely when signs of uraemia will develop in an individual patient.

Figure 11.2 summarizes important clinically relevant information about serum urea and serum creatinine. Figure 11.3 represents the relationship between GFR, serum creatinine, serum urea and key milestones in disease progression.

Feature	Urea	Creatinine
Typical serum concentration reference range of dogs	3.1–10.9 mmol/l	60–128 μmol/l
Typical serum concentration reference range of cats	4.8–11.6 mmol/l	60–163 μmol/l
Origin within the body	Exogenous or endogenous protein catabolism, via the urea cycle	Non-enzymatic hydrolysis of skeletal muscle creatine
Rate of production	Variable, depending on diet and endogenous protein metabolism	Much more constant daily production
Handling by the kidney	Freely filtered with substantial tubular reabsorption	Freely filtered and not reabsorbed by the tubules. Insignificant tubular secretion occurs in male dogs
Extrarenal clearance mechanisms	None of significance. Urea metabolized by gut bacteria is converted back to urea in a 'futile' cycle and is eventually cleared by the kidneys	Significant and variable catabolism by gut bacteria. In azotaemic humans, up to 66% of all creatinine formed may be cleared by extrarenal routes
Prediction of glomerular filtration rate	Insensitive; fair in advanced disease	Insensitive; good in advanced disease
Correlation with uraemia	Very good	Not as good (in humans)

11.2 Important features of serum urea and serum creatinine. (Reference intervals should be those provided by the specific laboratory.)

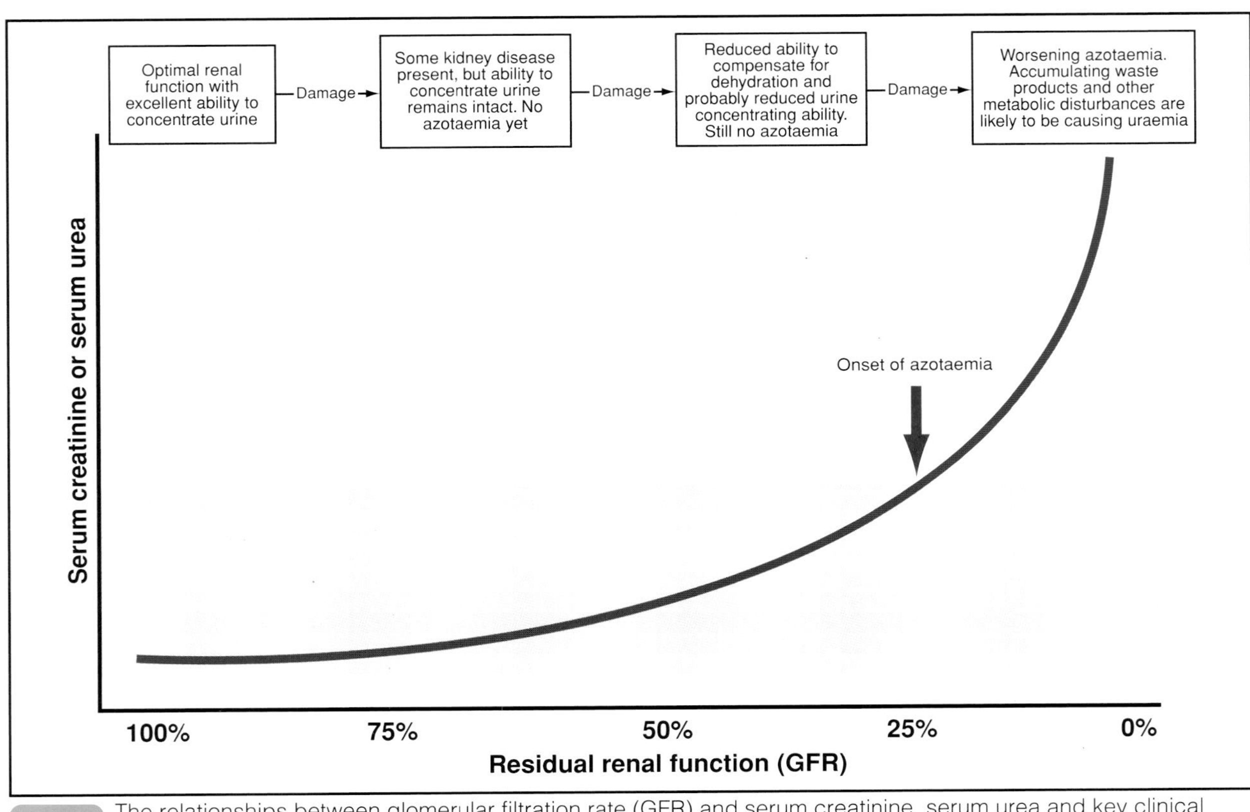

11.3 The relationships between glomerular filtration rate (GFR) and serum creatinine, serum urea and key clinical milestones. The blue panel indicates the normal range (reference interval).

The serum urea:serum creatinine ratio

When serum urea and serum creatinine concentrations have been measured simultaneously in a patient, the ratio of one to the other is easily estimated. Efforts have been made to use this ratio diagnostically, with much more success having been achieved in human medicine than in canine and feline medicine. Although the serum urea:serum creatinine ratio was found not to help in distinguishing prerenal from renal and postrenal causes of azotaemia in dogs (Finco and Duncan, 1976), an increased ratio in non-azotaemic or very mildly azotaemic animals suspected to have gastrointestinal haemorrhage is used by some clinicians to support that suspicion. Dehydration bordering on prerenal azotaemia in animals with normal renal function can also increase the serum urea:serum creatinine ratio. Given that its clinical value is rather limited, routine precise calculation and reporting of the serum urea:serum creatinine ratio is unwarranted.

Serum electrolyte disturbances in renal failure

As well as being the major organs for excretion of excess nitrogenous waste products, the kidneys play a crucial homeostatic role in controlling the plasma concentrations of several electrolytes within tight limits (see Chapter 8). These include sodium, potassium, chloride, phosphate and magnesium ions. The gastrointestinal tract has limited ability to discriminate when absorbing electrolytes. In contrast, the kidneys are able to excrete or reabsorb variable amounts of each electrolyte in response to the body's needs. For example, more than 99% of the filtered sodium is reabsorbed by healthy kidneys under normal circumstances. The handling of a particular electrolyte by the kidney is usually calculated and expressed as its *fractional excretion (FE)*, as compared with creatinine (fractional clearance is a synonym for FE). Creatinine is a useful yardstick, since it is freely filtered and not reabsorbed by the renal tubules. In other words, 100% of the filtered load of creatinine is excreted. By contrast, a much lesser proportion of the filtered load of most electrolytes is excreted. The fractional excretion of sodium, chloride and calcium is normally <1%. In contrast, the fractional excretion of potassium and phosphorus is relatively high, reaching 23.9% and 73%, respectively, in cats. Fractional excretion of electrolytes should be determined after a period of fasting (usually 12–15 hours) because ingested electrolytes surplus to requirements are excreted postprandially. However, even after fasting, the diet ingested in the days and weeks preceding the fast will influence the FE of predominantly intracellular electrolytes, such as potassium, phosphorus and magnesium; so some authorities recommend feeding a standardized diet for several days to a week before conducting a FE test. Figure 11.4 shows how FEs are calculated and lists some clinical situations in which they are useful.

In normal health, renal homeostatic mechanisms maintain plasma electrolyte concentrations within tight limits. However, when GFR reaches a very low level, plasma electrolyte homeostasis may fail. Plasma sodium, for example, usually remains normal until the very terminal stages of renal failure, when it may decrease or (sometimes) increase. In dogs, plasma potassium typically remains normal during the polyuric stages of renal failure but is increased during oliguria or anuria of terminal CRF or ARF. It also typically increases in severe postrenal azotaemic states. When cats with renal failure were fed a diet containing a marginally low potassium concentration (0.35% on a dry matter basis), renal losses of potassium were sufficient to cause total body potassium depletion and hypokalaemia. Hypokalaemic polymyopathy ensued, manifested as muscle weakness, particularly of the neck muscles (Dow *et al.*, 1987).

Hyperphosphataemia is the most consistent electrolyte disturbance in patients with renal failure. It develops as a direct consequence of decreased GFR,

Fractional excretion (%) of any solute (So) can be calculated from this formula:

$$[(Urine_{So} / Serum_{So}) / (Urine_{Cr} / Serum_{Cr})] \times 100$$

which is mathematically identical to:

$$[(Urine_{So} \times Serum_{Cr}) / (Urine_{Cr} \times Serum_{So})] \times 100$$

$Urine_{So}$ = concentration of the solute in the patient's urine
$Serum_{So}$ = concentration of the solute in the patient's serum
$Urine_{Cr}$ = concentration of creatinine in the patient's urine
$Serum_{Cr}$ = concentration of creatinine in the patient's serum

Situations in which FE determination may be useful:

- Investigation of patients with suspected renal tubular disorders, such as Fanconi syndrome. FE of electrolytes (sodium, chloride, calcium, phosphorus, magnesium), amino acids and glucose may be calculated
- FE of electrolytes can be monitored daily in animals receiving potentially nephrotoxic drugs. In this setting, FE elevation is a more sensitive indicator of renal damage than azotaemia
- FE of sodium (FE_{Na}) is occasionally used as an aid to distinguish prerenal azotaemia from acute intrinsic renal failure. Classically, FE_{Na} is <1% in cases with prerenal azotaemia and >2% in acute intrinsic renal failure. However, there are many exceptions to this rule.

11.4 Fractional excretion (FE): method of calculation and usefulness.

at about the same stage of renal disease as azotaemia. It is thought that imperceptibly mild hyperphosphataemia develops earlier in renal disease, causing marginal ionized hypocalcaemia and a consequent increase in secretion of parathyroid hormone (PTH) by the parathyroid glands. Increased plasma PTH induces enhanced phosphaturia by the kidneys, returning plasma phosphate and calcium levels towards normal, but at the expense of a persistently elevated plasma PTH.

As renal failure advances, plasma PTH increases further, but eventually is insufficient to prevent hyperphosphataemia. Hypocalcaemia may develop, perhaps in part as a consequence of precipitation of calcium phosphate from blood (because of the hyperphosphataemia). Evolving resistance of the skeleton to the calcium-mobilizing effects of PTH is another possible explanation. Hypocalcaemia may also be caused in part by impaired intestinal absorption of calcium, in turn a consequence of calcitriol deficiency. Calcitriol (1,25-dihydroxycholecalciferol; active vitamin D) is a hormone important in gastrointestinal calcium absorption, synthesis of which is normally completed by the kidneys. Synthesis is impaired in failing kidneys. The relationships between plasma calcium, plasma phosphate, PTH and calcitriol are summarized in Figure 11.5.

Some canine and feline patients with renal disease have hypercalcaemia (defined here as an increase in the plasma or serum total calcium). This may be due merely to an increase in the amount of biologically inactive complexed calcium bound to phosphates, oxalates and various other anions in their blood. However, in some hypercalcaemic renal failure patients the biologically active ionized calcium is shown to be

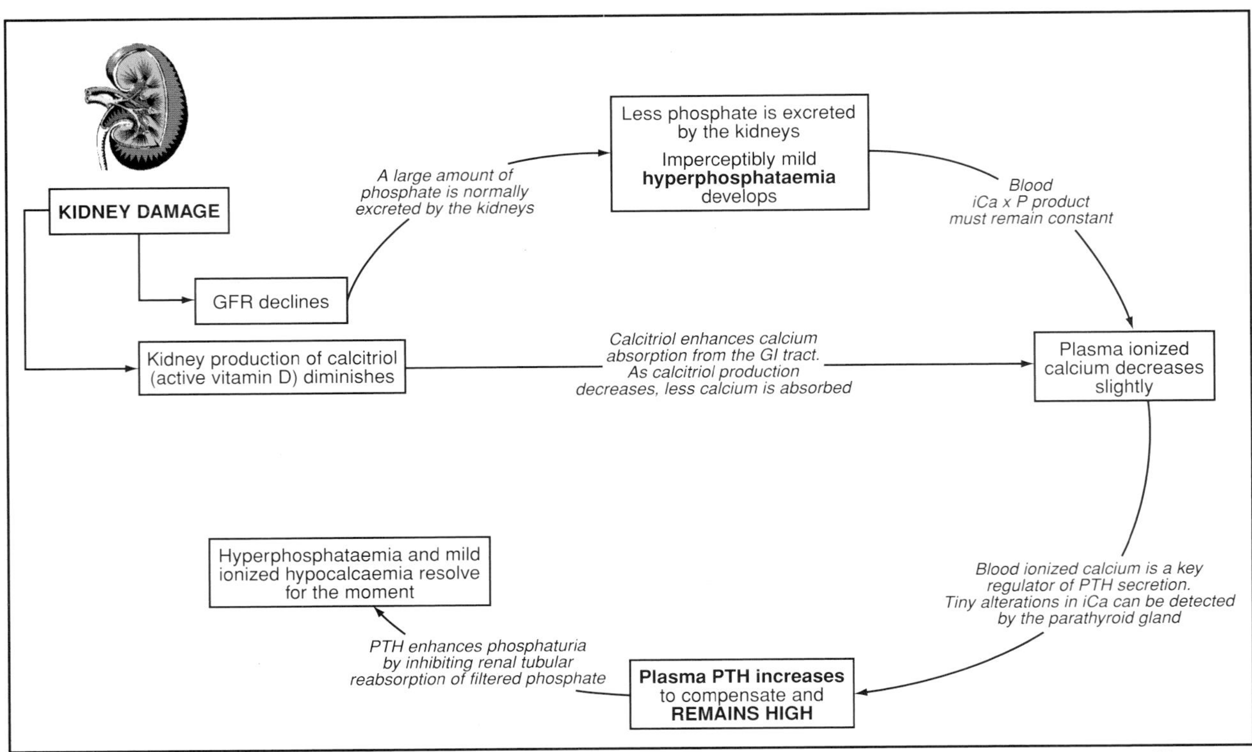

11.5 Relationships between plasma calcium, phosphate, PTH and calcitriol. (GFR: glomerular filtration rate; iCa: plasma ionized calcium concentration; P: plasma total phosphate concentration; PTH: parathyroid hormone)

elevated, even when corrected for blood pH. It has been suggested that sometimes the hyperplastic parathyroid glands found in renal failure patients have an altered set-point for detection and response to blood ionized calcium. A level of blood ionized calcium that would normally be high enough to switch off PTH secretion may fail to do so in the setting of advanced renal failure and parathyroid hyperplasia. This situation is sometimes described as *tertiary hyperparathyroidism* (where primary hyperparathyroidism refers to excessive production of PTH by a hyperplastic or neoplastic parathyroid gland, and renal secondary hyperparathyroidism refers to increased PTH production in response to renal functional impairment as described above).

Categorizing azotaemia as prerenal, renal or postrenal

Whenever azotaemia is identified, it is essential to categorize it as prerenal, renal or postrenal in origin (Figure 11.6). This should be done as early as possible in the diagnostic investigation. In most cases it is relatively straightforward to make the distinction on the basis of history, physical examination and urine analysis findings. The urine specific gravity, measured before fluid administration, can be particularly helpful in identifying prerenal azotaemia. Ultrasonography or contrast radiography may help with anatomical localization in the investigation of postrenal causes of azotaemia.

Clinical features	Prerenal	Acute intrinsic renal	Postrenal
History of pollakiuria/stranguria? Grossly enlarged bladder on physical examination? Difficult or impossible urethral catheterization?	Maybe a component of the overall azotaemia, but is not the primary cause	Unlikely unless the situation has been prolonged	Urethral obstruction causing postrenal azotaemia. Seen more commonly in males than females
Localized subcutaneous fluid accumulation around the perineum or the caudal ventral abdomen?	Maybe a component of the overall azotaemia, but not the primary cause	Unlikely	A feature of some ruptures of the lower urinary tract. A consequence of urine leakage
Peritoneal effusion found on physical examination/abdominal imaging/ abdominocentesis?	Usually no peritoneal fluid is seen. If fluid is found and analysed it will have roughly the same creatinine concentration as that found in serum		If urine is leaking into the peritoneal cavity, fluid will be found and it will have a higher creatinine concentration than serum

11.6 Features helpful for distinguishing prerenal, acute renal and postrenal causes of azotaemia ($Serum_{Cr}$: serum creatinine concentration; $Serum_{Na}$: serum sodium concentration; $Urine_{Cr}$: urine creatinine concentration; $Urine_{Na}$: urine sodium concentration). (continues)

Clinical features	Prerenal	Acute intrinsic renal	Postrenal
Hyperkalaemia concurrent with the azotaemia?	Usually absent or very mildly elevated due to dehydration. An exception is Addison's disease	Sometimes present, particularly if the patient is oliguric or anuric	Likely to be present if the post-renal problem has been present for long enough
Urine specific gravity before fluid therapy is started?	Usually hypersthenuric (>1.030 in dogs, >1.035 in cats), but some drugs and non-renal illnesses can cause dehydration and prerenal azotaemia in the face of dilute urine	Usually isosthenuric, but in peracute situations the bladder may contain concentrated urine that was formed before the onset of renal failure. Freshly formed urine should be analysed	Variable and unhelpful in making the diagnosis
Urine sediment microscopic finding before fluid therapy is started?	Benign or quiet sediment. Casts may be seen after rehydration has commenced	Active sediment with many tubular casts and (perhaps) red and white blood cells	Variable, perhaps marked haematuria if the urinary tract has recently been traumatized
Response to 12–24 hours' intravenous fluid therapy? (rehydrate over 6–8 hours then provide 1.5–2.0 x maintenance requirement, if this is judged safe on the basis of a full clinical evaluation)	Complete resolution of the azotaemia if it was entirely prerenal	Initially, some improvement if there was a prerenal component to the overall azotaemia	Minimal benefit if the lower urinary tract continues to leak undetected
Fractional excretion of sodium (%) $[(Urine_{Na} \times Serum_{Cr}) / (Urine_{Cr} \times Serum_{Na})] \times 100$	Usually <1%, as long as the patient is not receiving natriuretic diuretic therapy	Usually >2%, but there are many exceptions	Unhelpful in the diagnosis of post-renal problems
$Urine_{Cr}$:$Serum_{Cr}$ ratio	>20	<10	Unhelpful in making the diagnosis

11.6 (continued) Features helpful for distinguishing prerenal, acute renal and postrenal causes of azotaemia ($Serum_{Cr}$: serum creatinine concentration; $Serum_{Na}$: serum sodium concentration; $Urine_{Cr}$: urine creatinine concentration; $Urine_{Na}$: urine sodium concentration).

Readers will occasionally encounter an azotaemic patient with non-renal illness(es), or unknown or unconsidered drug exposure, that presents a greater diagnostic challenge than usual. In particular, drugs and non-renal illnesses that can cause isosthenuria in the face of dehydration may mislead the unwary clinician into diagnosing intrinsic renal failure when the problem is, in fact, prerenal. Examples of such situations include:

- A dehydrated, azotaemic cat with isosthenuric urine may be misdiagnosed as having renal failure when, in fact, it has been rendered dehydrated and isosthenuric by an overdose of a potent diuretic such as furosemide. If the diuretic is being used to treat cardiomyopathy, the prerenal azotaemia may be exacerbated by poor cardiac output
- A mildly dehydrated, azotaemic dog with poor pulse quality has a urine specific gravity of 1.016. Serum electrolytes (Na^+ and K^+) are not measured. It is misdiagnosed as having renal failure when in fact it has hypoadrenocorticism (Addison's disease). The azotaemia is prerenal, due to hypovolaemia, and the dog has poor urine-concentrating ability because of sodium wasting, hyponatraemia and a consequently diminished concentration of sodium in the renal medullary interstitium. The sodium wasting is a consequence of hypoaldosteronism (part of Addison's disease)
- Hypercalcaemia can cause dehydration, isosthenuria and mild to moderate prerenal azotaemia that resolves completely when appropriate intravenous fluid therapy is provided. The danger here is that clinicians are aware that hypercalcaemia can sometimes cause irreversible intrinsic renal failure and may incorrectly assume its presence in *any* azotaemic hypercalcaemic patient. This false assumption may lead them to offer a prognosis far worse than is warranted. Many causes of hypercalcaemia (e.g. lymphoma, multiple myeloma, primary hyperparathyroidism) can be managed very effectively, with patients enjoying an excellent quality of life over the medium to long term.

It is important to emphasize that some non-renal illnesses and drugs can cause prerenal azotaemia combined with excessive natriuresis (renal sodium loss). Yet avid renal sodium retention (i.e. a low fractional excretion of sodium, FE_{Na}) is one of the diagnostic criteria commonly listed as useful for identifying prerenal azotaemia, where sodium retention is required for water retention. To complicate matters further, there are several forms of acute intrinsic renal failure that are associated with a low or normal, rather than high, FE_{Na}. Here are a few examples from human medicine, not all of which have been confirmed in dogs and cats:

- Radiographic contrast agent-induced nephropathy
- Acute glomerulonephritis
- Sepsis-induced acute tubular necrosis
- Obstructive uropathy.

Clinicians should therefore be careful not to accept FE_{Na} test results uncritically and should not narrow down on a diagnosis of acute intrinsic renal failure without thoroughly excluding the possibility of polyuric prerenal disease.

Fortunately, prerenal azotaemia can be distinguished from acute intrinsic renal failure in many patients simply by providing intravenous fluid therapy and monitoring to see whether the azotaemia promptly and completely resolves. If it does so in 24–48 hours, the problem was most likely prerenal. If it is inappropriate or unsafe to use 'test' fluid therapy in a particular patient (for example, one with unstable congestive heart failure) then other approaches can be taken. The urine to serum creatinine ratio should be >20 in animals with prerenal azotaemia and <10 in animals with acute intrinsic renal failure. In human medicine, the fractional excretion of urea (FE_{Urea}) has recently been found to be superior to the fractional excretion of sodium (FE_{Na}) for distinguishing patients with prerenal azotaemia who are receiving loop diuretics from those with acute intrinsic renal failure caused by tubular necrosis (Carvounis *et al.*, 2002).

Acute renal failure *versus* severe chronic failure

This is an important distinction to make, because there is a chance that the pathology in ARF will be reversible, whereas the prognosis for significant improvement in GFR in patients with severe end-stage chronic failure is extremely poor (without renal allograft). History, physical examination and, sometimes, imaging studies play a crucial role in making the distinction between acute and chronic failure (Figure 11.7). Laboratory test results usually play a lesser role. However, none of these laboratory tests provides unequivocal results, because there is some overlap in the effects of ARF and CRF on all of these laboratory parameters.

Many animals with end-stage CRF suffer a terminal acute deterioration in renal function, often accompanied by features of ARF (for example metabolic acidosis and hyperkalaemia). This situation is sometimes termed *acute on chronic failure*. Given that this is a rather common scenario, experienced clinicians might be inclined to jump to conclusions when faced with acute deterioration of a CRF patient. There is, however, another kind of transition from chronic to acute or subacute renal failure that is not necessarily terminal. An animal that has been managed successfully for CRF for many months or years may deteriorate abruptly (say, over 2–4 weeks) both clinically and in terms of a dramatically worsening serum creatinine concentration. It should not be immediately assumed that this is due to inevitable, terminal progression of its CRF. That may indeed be the case, but vigorous efforts should be made to identify an underlying cause, particularly if the animal's renal failure was not well advanced before the acute deterioration. Urine bacterial culture is one valuable test to consider under these circumstances, regardless of urine sediment findings (see Chapters 10 and 25). Clinically silent pyelonephritis can complicate CRF and cause rapid deterioration in GFR.

Parameter	Acute failure	Severe chronic failure
History	Perfectly healthy until very recently. Maybe recent anaesthesia, or exposure to a nephrotoxic drug or toxin	Usually weeks to months of polyuria/ polydipsia, low-grade vomiting (several times a week) and weight loss
Physical examination	Good body condition but extremely depressed relative to the degree of azotaemia Kidneys are usually normal in size or enlarged and may be swollen or painful	May be cachectic. Tolerating severe azotaemia rather well (like a drug addict used to the toxins) The kidneys are usually (but not invariably) small and non-painful
Packed cell volume	Anaemia is not usually present, unless acute gastrointestinal hemorrhage has occurred	Non-regenerative anaemia is often, but not always, a feature. It may be unmasked by fluid therapy
Serum electrolytes	Hyperkalaemia is often present	Hyperkalaemia is absent until terminal acute deterioration occurs
	Serum phosphate is typically elevated in both acute and chronic failure so it does NOT help in distinguishing acute from chronic failure	
Acid–base status	Metabolic acidosis often present	Metabolic acidosis absent or mild
Urine analysis	Sediment is 'active' with casts, cells, debris etc. coming from the kidneys	Sediment is usually inactive unless, for example, a urinary tract infection has complicated CRF
Urine output	Many ARF patients are anuric or oliguric. Polyuric ARF may be under-diagnosed (e.g. caused by aminoglycosides)	CRF patients are usually polyuric until the very terminal stages
	Urine specific gravity is NOT helpful in distinguishing acute from chronic failure	
Biopsy	Acute, potentially reversible pathology	Chronic, irreversible changes
Response to therapy	Acute renal failure is often reversible, if the patient can be supported through the crisis	Chronic renal failure is irreversible, although correction of any prerenal component will reduce the degree of azotaemia and prolonged fluid therapy will 'artificially' lower the serum urea

11.7 Features that help to distinguish acute renal failure (ARF) from severe chronic renal failure (CRF). (Adapted from Squires *et al.*, 1998.)

Ethylene glycol poisoning

Ethylene glycol (1,2-ethanediol) is a poisonous, colourless, sweet-tasting liquid that mixes readily with water. It is the major ingredient (approximately 95% by volume) of most commercially available antifreeze solutions, which usually also contain a yellow–green dye. Ethylene glycol is an excellent antifreeze and de-icing agent because its small molecules (62 daltons) mix readily with water, dramatically increasing the osmolality and suppressing the freezing point. Because of its sweet taste and widespread availability, ethylene glycol commonly causes poisoning in both dogs and cats. The minimum lethal dose of ethylene glycol is 1.4 ml/kg body weight for cats and about 5.5 ml/kg for dogs. The incidence of poisoning is similar in the two species but the case fatality rate is higher in cats.

Unmetabolized ethylene glycol causes gastrointestinal, central nervous sytem depressant and osmotic diuretic effects similar to those of ethanol, but its major toxicity lies in the fact that it is biotransformed in the liver to several highly toxic metabolites (glycoaldehyde, glycolic acid, glyoxalic acid and oxalic acid). These result in severe metabolic acidosis and renal tubular injury, sufficient to cause oliguric or anuric acute renal failure. The clinical signs of antifreeze poisoning (reviewed by Thrall *et al.*, 1997) reflect these underlying metabolic processes. Early signs caused by unmetabolized ethylene glycol are seen from 30 minutes to 12 hours post-ingestion, with ARF caused by metabolites developing 12–24 hours after ingestion in cats and 48–72 hours post-ingestion in dogs.

Laboratory abnormalities found in patients presented an hour or more after ethylene glycol ingestion include serum hyperosmolality and increased osmolal gap. Serum osmolality can be measured using a freezing point depression osmometer; many veterinary clinical laboratories have these. The test is available in the UK at larger laboratories. Serum hyperosmolality develops rapidly after ingestion because ethylene glycol is a small, osmotically active molecule that diffuses readily from the gastrointestinal lumen into the blood. A relatively small volume of ingested antifreeze solution provides a massive number of osmotically active particles. The osmolal gap is the difference between measured and calculated serum osmolality, when serum osmolality is calculated (in mmol/kg) using this formula:

$$\text{Calculated serum osmolality} = 2\,(\text{Serum}_{Na} + \text{Serum}_{K}) + \text{Serum}_{Glu} + \text{Serum}_{Urea}$$

where

Serum_{Na} = serum sodium concentration (mmol/l)
Serum_{K} = serum potassium concentration (mmol/l)
Serum_{Glu} = serum glucose concentration (mmol/l)
Serum_{Urea} = serum urea concentration (mmol/l)

Measured serum osmolality range is approximately 290–313 mmol/kg in healthy dogs and cats, tending to be a little higher in cats. The osmolal gap is normally 10 mmol/kg or less. The 'extra' osmoles provided by ethylene glycol in poisoned animals markedly increase the gap between measured and calculated osmolality, often to 150 mmol/kg or more. However, other less commonly ingested toxins, like methanol, also markedly increase the serum osmolality and osmolal gap. A few clinical laboratories in 'human' hospitals can measure ethylene glycol concentrations directly, rendering unnecessary the measurement of serum osmolality for diagnosis of this poisoning.

In toxicity, generation of acid metabolites by the liver is well underway within 3 hours of ingesting ethylene glycol. Plasma pH, bicarbonate and total CO_2 concentrations are decreased. Partial respiratory compensation for the developing metabolic acidosis lowers the pCO_2 in some patients. The anion gap (see Chapter 9) widens as unmeasured anionic metabolites accumulate in the blood. By this stage, the urine will be isosthenuric as a consequence of osmotic diuresis and plasma hyperosmolality-induced polydipsia. By 3 hours post-ingestion in cats, and 6 hours in dogs, calcium oxalate crystalluria may be evident, although it sometimes takes longer to appear. Calcium oxalate monohydrate crystals (six-sided prisms) are more often seen than the calcium oxalate dihydrate form (Maltese cross or envelope shape) (see Figure 10.13).

From 12 hours post-ingestion in cats, and 36 hours post-ingestion in dogs, there is a further deterioration in untreated animals that have ingested a sufficient amount of the poison, usually culminating in death. Clinically, the following changes occur:

- Fluid intake may not match the losses caused by diuresis, so haemoconcentration may develop
- Acidic metabolites of ethylene glycol cause severe renal tubular damage
- Calcium oxalate crystals form in renal tubular lumina and continue to spill into the urine (animals that survive poisoning may continue to have calcium oxalate crystalluria for up to 2 weeks after the crisis).
- Approximately half of affected animals will be hypocalcaemic, partly because calcium is chelated by oxalate
- Glomerular filtration decreases, causing worsening azotaemia and hyperphosphataemia
- The urine remains isosthenuric but polyuria may be replaced by oliguria or anuria, signalling a much worse prognosis
- Oliguria or anuria leads to hyperkalaemia
- Uraemia develops, associated with a stress leucogram and hyperglycaemia (ethylene glycol metabolites directly affect glucose metabolism and worsen the hyperglycaemia).

Early diagnosis of ethylene glycol poisoning is essential for a successful outcome. Assuming that the history or clinical signs have aroused suspicion, ready access to an osmometer or specific ethylene glycol detection kit can be extremely helpful. Failing this, detection of an increased anion gap and, particularly, calcium oxalate crystalluria in a patient with compatible clinical signs is usually sufficient to justify commencing specific treatment.

Detecting mild or early renal disease

It is occasionally useful to determine the overall GFR of an animal that is not in renal failure but may nevertheless have significant renal disease. This might be done, for example, to investigate a suspected case of familial nephropathy or further characterize the renal excretory reserve of a non-azotaemic animal with marked proteinuria. It can also help in defining the extent of repair that has occurred after an episode of ARF. In these cases, ultrasound-guided renal biopsy might be an appropriate alternative, but GFR estimations are, nevertheless, occasionally indicated.

Creatinine clearance

Endogenous creatinine clearance is probably still the most widely applied clinical method of GFR estimation in canine and feline medicine. It is inconvenient, in that it requires collection of all of the urine produced by the animal over a timed period (usually 24 hours). Having achieved this (by intermittent urethral catheterization, indwelling catheter placement or use of a makeshift 'metabolic cage') the calculation of endogenous creatinine clearance and, by extension, GFR is straightforward:

$$\text{Endogenous creatinine clearance} = \frac{\text{Urine}_{Cr} \times \text{Urine volume (ml)}}{\text{Serum}_{Cr} \times \text{Time (minutes)} \times \text{Body weight (kg)}}$$

where
Serum_{Cr} = serum creatinine concentration (μmol/l)
Urine_{Cr} = urine creatinine concentration (mmol/l).

When the commonly employed Jaffe method for creatinine quantitation is used, endogenous creatinine clearance will tend to underestimate GFR in non-azotaemic animals because of non-creatinine chromogens being present in their serum but not their urine. Addition of 'extra' creatinine (i.e. performance of an exogenous, rather than endogenous, creatinine clearance test) solves this problem. A protocol is summarized in Figure 11.8 (Watson *et al.*, 2002).

Patient details
Aged Boxer with mild clinical dehydration and urine SG 1.025. Renal insufficiency is suspected. Plasma creatinine concentration in fasted conditions is 159 μmol/l.

Plasma exogenous creatinine clearance test
Creatinine (80 mg/kg = 707 μmol/kg) is given by intravenous bolus injection.

Option I: Dynamic test
After 2 hours, 1 ml of blood is sampled.
Observed plasma creatinine concentration is 946 μmol/l, i.e. an excess of 787 μmol/l over the basal concentration.
As 787 μmol/l exceeds the 2-hour threshold value (636 μmol/l), the animal should be considered to be renally impaired.

Option 2: Glomerular filtration rate (GFR) assessment
1 ml blood samples are collected at 10 minutes and at 1, 2, 6 and 10 hours.
The following concentrations are observed:

Time (minutes)	Observed plasma creatinine (μmol/l)	Observed plasma concentration minus basal level (μmol/l)
Just before injection	159	0
10	1733	1574
60	1025	866
120	946	787
360	645	486
600	548	389

The area under the plasma curve (AUC) is calculated by the trapezoidal rule:
The AUC between 0 and 10 min (estimated as a rectangle) = 10 x 1574 = 15,740
The trapezoid between 10 and 60 min has area = (60 – 10) x (1574 + 866)/2 = 61,000
Continue until the last trapezoid: (600 – 360) x (486 + 389)/2 = 105,000
The total AUC is the sum of the trapezoids = 384,090 μmol.min/l = 384 μmol.min/ml
The plasma creatinine clearance (i.e. GFR estimate) is equal to the dose divided by the total AUC:
GFR = 707/384 = 1.84 ml/kg/min
Comparison of this GFR value with those for healthy dogs (3–4 ml/kg/min) indicates that the dog has mild renal impairment.
The GFR value determined with an 11-point sample strategy in the same dog was 1.83 ml/kg/min, which is very similar to the value determined by the limited sampling strategy.

Notes

- The dog should be fasted overnight (at least).
- Determination of the exact dose administered is critical. Weigh out anhydrous creatinine (for a nominal rate of 80 mg/kg) and add 1 ml/kg of sterile distilled water. For conversion from mg/kg to μmol/kg, divide by the relative molecular mass of creatinine (113) and multiply by 1000 (i.e. multiply the mg/kg dose by 8.84).
- Inject the creatinine through a catheter, ideally via a stopper; then flush the dead space of the catheter with saline.
- Don't be stressed by time. What is most important is to know the exact time of sampling. For example, if the sample is taken at 12 and not 10 minutes, use the exact time (12 minutes) for AUC calculation. For the dynamic test, it is important to try to collect blood at the accurate time for comparison with the threshold value.
- Blood can be sampled from the cephalic vein. If using a tourniquet, do not place it too soon as the creatinine concentration in the sample will not be representative of the systemic concentration.
- Creatinine is stable in plasma, so assays can be delayed. However, it is important to do all the assays in one batch (i.e. avoid assaying three tubes on the day of the test and two others the day after). Use the same anticoagulant (if any) for all samplings.

11.8 Practical use of exogenous creatinine clearance test in dogs. (Modified from Watson *et al.*, 2002, with permission; see also Watson *et al.*, 2003.)

Iohexol clearance

More recently, a much more convenient method for estimation of GFR has been described, which involves measuring the clearance of the radiographic contrast agent iohexol from blood (Moe and Heiene, 1995; Finco *et al.*, 2001). The method has been shown to correlate well with 'gold standard' methods for measurement of GFR, yet no urine collection is required. A 300 mg/kg body weight bolus of iohexol is injected intravenously and blood samples are collected from the patient at 2, 3 and 4 hours subsequently. Knowing the iohexol concentration in the three samples, the weight of the patient, and the precise time the iohexol was injected and the blood samples collected, the GFR can be calculated. Measurement of serum or plasma iohexol clearance is not yet being widely practised, because expensive equipment is needed for the iohexol quantitation. However, this method should prove useful in the future for detection of early or mild renal dysfunction, well below the limits of detection of serum creatinine or serum urea. Alternatively, exogenous creatinine clearance testing can be carried out as sterile creatinine is now available in the UK.

Renal scintigraphy

When it is important to determine the relative contribution of each of the two kidneys to overall GFR, quantitative renal scintigraphy can be used. This is a sophisticated imaging method involving the injection of a radionuclide and subsequent detection of the amount of that radionuclide appearing in the kidneys over time, generally by use of a gamma camera. Renal scintigraphy is particularly valuable when unilateral nephrectomy of a diseased kidney is being contemplated.

Enzyme detection

Detection of enzymes released from damaged renal epithelial cells in urine (enzymuria) has been investigated and found to show promise in some situations as a method for detecting early or mild renal disease (Grauer *et al.*, 1995; Palacio *et al.*, 1997). *N*-acetyl-β-D-glucosaminidase (NAG) and gamma-glutamyl transferase (GGT) have been studied more than other enzymes and have shown promise. 24-hour measurement of urinary enzyme excretion is considered superior to measuring enzyme concentrations in 'spot' urine samples. However, in one study, spot urine sample GGT/creatinine and NAG/creatinine ratios were significantly correlated with 24-hour GGT and NAG excretion in dogs with mild aminoglycoside-induced nephrotoxicosis, but not in those with more severe, long-standing disease (Grauer *et al.*, 1995).

Nephrotic syndrome

Glomerular disease leading to marked proteinuria is the root cause of the nephrotic syndrome. In dogs and cats it is usually caused by glomerulonephritis or (less commonly) amyloidosis. The syndrome in humans has been classically described as consisting of marked proteinuria, hypoalbuminaemia, hypercholesterolaemia, lipiduria and oedema.

Lipiduria is, however, a common finding of no clinical significance in healthy dogs and cats. Oedema is only found in a small minority of dogs and cats with heavy proteinuria and consequent hypoalbuminaemia. Therefore, only three of the five 'classical' features of the nephrotic syndrome are likely to be found in a nephrotic dog or cat:

- Marked proteinuria
- Hypoalbuminaemia
- Hypercholesterolaemia.

Proteinuria may be detected as an incidental finding or be suspected on the basis of clinical examination or serum biochemical results. Use of dipsticks and the urine protein:urine creatinine ratio (UP:UC) to evaluate the severity of proteinuria is covered in Chapter 10. UP:UC measurement is invalid in animals that have an 'active' urine sediment that reveals evidence of urinary tract inflammation, as it has been shown that bacterial urinary tract infection can sometimes raise the UP:UC well up into the 'glomerular' range. On the other hand, the presence of blood in a urine sample (in the absence of inflammation) is a much less important contraindication for carrying out UP:UC since it has been shown that gross blood contamination of urine is required to raise the UP:UC to a point where it could lead to misdiagnosis of a glomerulopathy.

Figure 11.9 offers a diagnostic approach to proteinuria from the point of dipstick detection onwards.

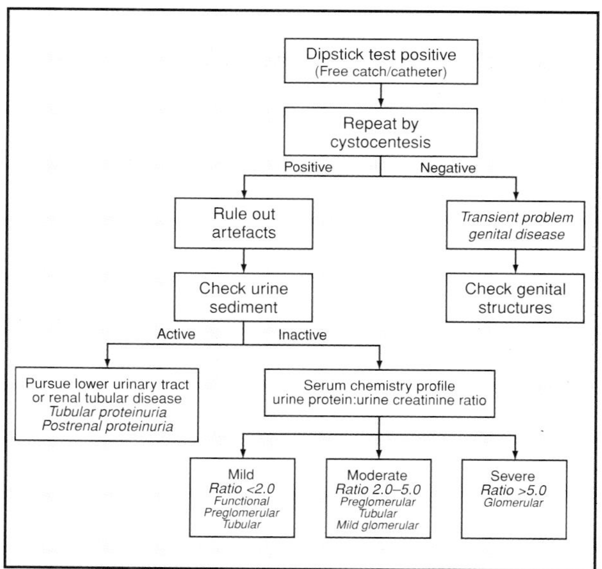

11.9 Diagnostic approach to classifying dipstick-detected proteinuria.

Renal tubular defects

Much of the discussion of renal disease to this point has emphasized glomerular dysfunction: renal excretory failure is a function of inadequate GFR and nephrotic syndrome is caused by excessive leakage of albumin through a defective or damaged glomerular basement membrane. Yet the renal tubules play a vital role in determining the final composition of urine through exquisitely selective reabsorption from the filtrate and secretion into it. They are absolutely crucial to electrolyte, water and acid–base homeostasis. The tubule cells are also responsible for synthesizing some hormones (calcitriol, erythropoietin and renin) and metabolizing others made elsewhere (e.g. peptide hormones, such as gastrin, insulin and PTH).

Although familial Fanconi syndrome of Basenjis is the best known of the renal tubular defects, not all tubulopathies are inherited. For example, heavy metals, out-of-date tetracycline and azathioprine can each cause acquired tubular disease with clinical features very similar to the familial forms of disease.

Classically, renal tubular defects cause excessive loss of substances that are normally retained by the kidneys. Depending upon which transporters are affected, the problem may be isolated to a particular substance or may be complex, involving many different substances.

An example of an isolated renal tubular defect is cystinuria, an inborn error of metabolism that affects English Bulldogs (and a number of other breeds) and strongly predisposes to cystine urolith formation. There are other isolated renal tubular defects that involve other amino acids, uric acid, carbohydrates (e.g. glucose), electrolytes (e.g. calcium, phosphate, magnesium, bicarbonate), hydrogen ions and water. Animals that have difficulty reclaiming bicarbonate from the proximal tubular filtrate or secreting acid into the collecting ducts are prone to develop metabolic acidosis. They are said to have proximal or distal *renal tubular acidosis*, respectively. Their urine is insufficiently acidic for the degree of metabolic acidosis present.

Fanconi syndrome

Fanconi syndrome is an umbrella term for a group of complex tubular disorders (familial and acquired). Excessive amounts of glucose, phosphate, amino acids, bicarbonate, calcium and potassium are lost, along with filtered proteins with a molecular weight less than 50,000 daltons. In addition, Fanconi syndrome-affected animals have renal tubular acidosis and obligatory polyuria that does not respond to exogenous antidiuretic hormone administration.

Diagnosis of renal tubular disorders

Definitive diagnosis of renal tubular disorders hinges upon detecting what substances are being 'leaked' excessively by the diseased kidneys. Glucosuria in a euglycaemic animal is often the first clue to the fact that a tubular disorder is present. A serum chemistry profile may subsequently reveal that a number of electrolytes are low or borderline low. Fractional excretion (FE) studies and quantitation of amino acids in urine are usually done next and will typically reveal excessive losses of several electrolytes and some amino acids. FE studies are relatively specialized, so it is wise to consult a clinical pathologist before submitting samples for analysis. It should be checked if the laboratory recommends any particular dietary management in the days leading up to the FE measurements. A 12–15 hour fast immediately prior to FE measurements is always recommended.

Diagnosis of renal tubular acidosis, and determining whether it is proximal or distal, is an even more specialized field that has been properly reviewed elsewhere (Bartges, 2000). In general, diagnosis requires accurate measurement of urine pH in response to orally administered acid and or alkali loads.

Case examples

Case 1

Signalment

9 year-old-male castrated mixed breed dog.

History and clinical examination

18-month history of polydipsia/polyuria, with occasional constipation. Six months of progressive lethargy, anorexia and weight loss. Another practice documented hypercalcaemia (3.75 mmol/l) one year previously. The dog was in poor body condition, and depressed. A small (~0.7 cm) nodule was palpated in the right anal sac.

Clinical pathology data

Haematology	Result	Reference interval
RBC (x 10^{12}/l)	7.03	5.5–8.5
Hb (g/dl)	16.0	12.0–18.0
HCT (l/l)	0.48	0.37–0.55
MCV (fl)	68	66–77
MCH (pg)	23	19.9–24.5
MCHC (g/dl)	33	31– 34
WBC (x 10^9/l)	12.3	6.0–17.4
Neutrophils (segmented) (x 10^9/l)	9.9	3.0–11.5

Haematology *(continued)*	Result	Reference interval
Neutrophils (band) (x 10^9/l)	0	0–0.3
Lymphocytes (x 10^9/l)	1.9	1.0–4.8
Monocytes (x 10^9/l)	0.35	0.15–1.35
Eosinophils (x 10^9/l)	0.15	0.1–1.25
Basophils (x 10^9/l)	0	Rare
Platelets (x 10^9/l)	Adequate	145– 440

Biochemistry	Result	Reference interval
Sodium (mmol/l)	153	145–158
Potassium (mmol/l)	4.4	3.6 –5.8
Chloride (mmol/l)	120	105–122
Glucose (mmol/l)	3.39	3.9–6.1
Urea (mmol/l)	33.92	3.6–7.1
Creatinine (μmol/l)	424	50–110
Inorganic phosphate (mmol/l)	2.1	0.8–1.6

Case 1 continues ▶

Case 1 continued

Biochemistry *(continued)*	Result	Reference interval
Total carbon dioxide (mmol/l)	18	18–30
Total calcium (mmol/l)	3.82	2.20–2.58
TP (g/l)	67	50–75
Albumin (g/l)	30	22–35
ALT(IU/l)	54	0–130
AST (IU/l)	12	10–50
ALP (IU/l)	188	0–200
CK (IU/l)	456	0–460
Cholesterol (mmol/l)	3.97	2.58–5.85
Total bilirubin (μmol/l)	3.42	0–6.9

Urine analysis	
Source	Cystocentesis
Volume	6 ml
Colour	Light yellow
Turbidity	Hazy
Specific gravity	1.011
pH	6.0
Protein	Negative
Glucose	Negative
Ketone	Negative
Bilirubin	1+
Blood/Hb	2+ (moderate)
Urobilinogen	1+

Urine sediment examination	
Epithelial cells	Few, transitional
Crystals	Few, amorphous
RBC	Too numerous to count (reference range <5)
WBC	15–30 per hpf (reference range <5)
Debris	Large amount
Bacteria	Many rods
Casts	None seen

What abnormalities are present?

Haematology
No significant abnormalities

Biochemistry
- Hypercalcaemia with normal serum protein and albumin
- Hyperphosphataemia
- Azotaemia

Urinalysis
- Isosthenuria
- Bilirubinuria
- Bacteruria
- Haematuria on sediment examination

How would you interpret these results?
- The concurrent presence of the anal sac mass and hypercalcaemia are suggestive of anal sac adenocarcinoma. However, the hypercalcaemia has been present for at least a year yet the mass remains small. Other likely causes of hypercalcaemia include lymphoma (although, again, the history is very long), primary hyperparathyroidism, and chronic renal failure. Uncomplicated chronic renal failure is less likely given the magnitude of the hypercalcaemia.
- Isosthenuria in this case may be due to hypercalcaemia (antagonism of ADH) or chronic renal failure, or a combination of both. The bacteruria most likely reflects urinary tract infection acquired as a consequence of the isosthenuria. A small amount of bilirubin may be found in the urine of normal dogs, or other pigments may produce a false bilirubinuria (see Chapter 10).

What further tests would you recommend?
- Urine culture and sensitivity testing
- Measurement of parathyroid hormone (PTH) and parathyroid hormone-related peptide (PTHrP)
- Measurement of blood ionized calcium

Further clinical pathology data

Urine culture and sensitivity testing
Heavy growth of *Escherichia coli* with a broad range of sensitivity.

PTH assay and ionized calcium:
PTH = 48 pmol/l (normal 2–13)
Ionized calcium = 1.53 mmol/l (reference range 1.25–1.4)
(PTHrP not measured)

What abnormalities are present?
PTH is markedly elevated in the face of markedly elevated ionized calcium. PTH is usually low in malignancy-associated hypercalcaemia, and elevations in chronic renal failure are generally of lesser magnitude. Ionized calcium is elevated.

How would you interpret these results?
These results suggest primary hyperparathyroidism is the most likely cause of the hypercalcaemia, and that the anal sac mass may not be the cause.

What further tests would you recommend?
Ultrasonography of the thyroid glands, and surgical exploration of the neck. Thoracic radiography and abdominal ultrasonography to stage for metastatic disease from the anal sac mass.

In this case, no evidence of metastatic disease was found. On surgical exploration of the neck, a solitary parathyroid nodule was resected; this was a parathyroid adenoma. The right anal sac mass was also removed; this was a low-grade apocrine gland adenocarcinoma. The azotaemia was presumed to be due to renal damage caused by the chronic hypercalcaemia. Primary hyperparathyroidism is expected to lead to low or low normal phosphate, but in this case this is offset by reduced excretion due to renal insufficiency resulting in mildly elevated phosphate.

Case 2 follows ▶

Case 2

Signalment

3-year-old male castrated Labrador Retriever.

History

A few months of polydipsia and polyuria, and a recent onset of apparent joint stiffness. Physical examination revealed no articular abnormalities, but bone pain was evident, especially over the metaphyses.

Clinical pathology data

Haemogram

Unremarkable.

Biochemistry	Result	Reference interval
Sodium (mmol/l)	146	145–158
Potassium (mmol/l)	3.5	3.6–5.8
Chloride (mmol/l)	122	105–122
Glucose (mmol/l)	4.7	3.9–6.1
Urea (mmol/l)	7.5	3.6–7.1
Creatinine (μmol/l)	127	50–110
Total carbon dioxide (mmol/l)	15.3	18–30
Total calcium (mmol/l)	2.5	2.20–2.58
Inorganic phosphate (mmol/l)	1.2	0.8–1.6
TP (g/l)	72	50–75
Albumin (g/l)	29	22–35
ALT(IU/l)	139	0–130
ALP (IU/l)	242	0–200
CK (IU/l)	455	0–460
Cholesterol (mmol/l)	5.7	2.58–5.85
Total bilirubin (μmol/l)	4.1	0–6.9

Urine analysis	
Source	Cystocentesis
Volume	5 ml
Colour	Pale yellow
Turbidity	Clear
SG	1.013
pH	6.0
Protein	2+
Glucose	4+
Ketone	Negative
Bilirubin	Negative
Haemoglobin	Negative
Urobilinogen	Negative

Sediment examination

Unremarkable.

Further tests

Repeat testing confirmed the persistence of euglycaemic glycosuria Urine protein:urine creatinine ratio = 2.3 (normal < 0.2; questionable 0.2–1.0)

What abnormalities are present?

- Euglycaemic glycosuria
- Mild azotaemia in the face of borderline isosthenuria
- Mild hypokalaemia
- Decreased total carbon dioxide
- Proteinuria.

How would you interpret these results and what are the likely differential diagnoses?

- Persistent euglycaemic glycosuria indicates that there is defective reabsorption of glucose by the renal tubules rather than supporting a diagnosis of diabetes mellitus. Defective transport of glucose by the renal tubules (so-called *renal glycosuria*) may be part of a broader disorder that also affects resorption of electrolytes and amino acids. *Fanconi syndrome* is an umbrella term for a group of conditions that are associated with defective renal tubular transport of glucose, phosphate, sodium, potassium, various amino acids and bicarbonate. Fanconi syndrome is best known as a disease of Basenjis, but it has also been reported to affect members of other breeds and may be seen as an acquired disorder in dogs of any breed that have been exposed to various nephrotoxins. Fanconi syndrome occurs occasionally in Labrador Retrievers and has been observed to cause stiffness and apparent bone or joint pain in dogs of this breed. The reason for the association of Fanconi syndrome with bone pain is uncertain, but may be related to chronic withdrawal of mineral from the bones, particularly of calcium and phosphorus, as a consequence of excessive renal losses.
- This dog's azotaemia in the face of borderline isosthenuria might be supportive of a diagnosis of early renal failure. However, the heavy glucosuria would be expected to cause an obligatory osmotic diuresis and, perhaps, obligatory isosthenuria. The azotaemia may therefore be partly or entirely prerenal, as a consequence of mild dehydration that was not detected during physical examination. The most expeditious way to establish the extent of any prerenal component is to provide generous intravenous fluid therapy and monitor to observe whether the azotaemia partly or completely resolves.
- The mild hypokalaemia was unexplained and considered relatively unimportant, given how close the observed value was to the bottom of the reference range. It could reflect excessive renal losses of potassium, but there are many other plausible explanations.
- The decreased total CO_2 is consistent with metabolic acidosis. In this case, there is a normal anion gap. (Anion gap = (146 + 3.5) – (122 + 15.3).) Normal anion gap metabolic acidosis is consistent with renal or gastrointestinal loss of bicarbonate. Total CO_2 was used to approximate bicarbonate (see Chapter 9).
- The dipstick-detected proteinuria was confirmed by urine protein:creatinine ratio determination. The magnitude of the proteinuria was relatively mild, consistent with tubular losses, or could be explained by mild glomerular disease. The absence of paraproteinaemia and abnormal urine sediment findings, respectively, make preglomerular and post renal causes of proteinuria unlikely.

What further tests would you consider?

- Venous blood gases could be analysed to determine more accurately the acid-base status of this dog.
- If prerenal azotaemia were suspected, intravenous fluid could be administered at 1.5–2.0 x maintenance overnight to determine the effect of this intervention on the overall azotaemia. Overnight fluid therapy would be expected to correct mild prerenal azotaemia in most cases.
- After completion of any intravenous fluid therapy, and after feeding a standard diet for several days, the fractional excretion of several electrolytes and amino acids could be measured to determine whether this is a case of *selective* renal glycosuria, or a case of Fanconi syndrome involving several different kinds of renal tubular transporter.

Case 2 continues ▶

Case 2 continued

- After the correction of any dehydration, endogenous creatinine clearance measurement and ultrasound-guided renal biopsy could be considered.

Further results

- Fractional excretion of sodium = 1.3% (normal 0–0.7)
- Fractional excretion of potassium = 24% (normal 0–20)
- Fractional excretion of calcium = 3.1% (normal 0–0.4)
- Fractional excretion of phosphorus = 65% (normal 3–39)
- Fractional excretion of 16 out of 23 amino acids was markedly abnormal.

These results are consistent with Fanconi syndrome.

References and further reading

Bartges JW (2000) Disorders of renal tubules. In: *Textbook of Veterinary Internal Medicine – Diseases of the Dog and Cat, 5th edn*, ed. SJ Ettinger and EC Feldman, pp. 1704–1710. WB Saunders, Philadelphia

Carvounis CP, Nisar S and Guro-Razuman S (2002) Significance of the fractional excretion of urea in the differential diagnosis of acute renal failure. *Kidney International* **62,** 2223–2229

Dow SW, LeCouteur RA, Fettman MJ and Spurgeon TL (1987) Potassium depletion in cats: hypokalemic polymyopathy. *Journal of the American Veterinary Medical Association* **191,** 1563–1568

Finco DR (1997) Kidney function. In: *Clinical Biochemistry of Domestic Animals, 5th edn*, ed. JJ Kaneko, JW Harvey and ML Bruss, pp. 441–484. Academic Press, San Diego

Finco DR, Braselton WE and Cooper TA (2001) Relationship between plasma iohexol clearance and urinary exogenous creatinine clearance in dogs. *Journal of Veterinary Internal Medicine* **15,** 368–373

Finco DR, Brown SA, Vaden SL and Ferguson DC (1995) Relationship between plasma creatinine concentration and glomerular filtration rate in dogs. *Journal of Veterinary Pharmacology and Therapeutics* **18,** 418–421

Finco DR and Duncan JR (1976) Evaluation of blood urea nitrogen and serum creatinine concentrations as indicators of renal dysfunction: a study of 111 cases and a review of related literature. *Journal of the American Veterinary Medical Association* **168,** 593–601

Grauer GF, Greco DS, Behrend EN, Indu M, Fettman MJ and Allen TA (1995) Estimation of quantitative enzymuria in dogs with gentamicin-induced nephrotoxicosis using urine enzyme/creatinine ratios from spot urine samples. *Journal of Veterinary Internal Medicine* **9,** 324–327

Kassirer JP (1971) Clinical evaluation of kidney function–glomerular function. *New England Journal of Medicine* **285,** 385–389

Moe L and Heiene R (1995) Estimation of glomerular filtration rate in dogs with 99M-Tc DTPA and iohexol. *Research in Veterinary Science* **58,** 138–143

Palacio J, Liste F and Gascon M (1997) Enzymuria as an index of renal damage in canine leishmaniasis. *Veterinary Record* **140,** 477–480

Squires RA, Elliott J and Brown S (1998) Renal failure. In: *Canine Medicine and Therapeutics, 4th edn*, ed. N Gorman, pp. 629–652. Blackwell Science Ltd, Oxford

Thrall MA, Grauer GF and Dial SM (1997) Antifreeze poisoning. In: *Kirk's Current Veterinary Therapy XII : Small Animal Practice*, eds. J Bonagura and RW Kirk, pp. 232–237. W.B. Saunders, Philadelphia

Watson AD, Lefebvre HP, German AG and Font A (2003) Early diagnosis of chronic renal failure. *Waltham Focus (Special Edition)* October 2003

Watson AD, Lefebvre HP, Concordet D, Laroute V, Ferre JP, Braun JP, Conchou F and Toutain PL (2002) Plasma exogenous creatinine clearance test in dogs: comparison with other methods and proposed limited sampling strategy. *Journal of Veterinary Internal Medicine* **16,** 22–33

12

Laboratory evaluation of hepatic disease

Edward J. Hall and Alexander J. German

Introduction

Hepatic diseases frequently present a diagnostic challenge because clinical signs are varied and often vague. Despite a range of diagnostic tests of both hepatic damage and function, there is rarely a single test that definitively identifies the problem; the many clinical signs of liver disease (Figure 12.1) are only sometimes related to specific laboratory abnormalities, such as jaundice (Figure 12.2). Furthermore, the liver has great functional reserve capacity and signs are often not apparent until significant hepatic dysfunction is present. As a result, laboratory analyses may allow early detection and characterization of early liver disease. Moreover, other systemic diseases can cause abnormal hepatic test results (Figure 12.3).

The aims of clinicopathological evaluation of hepatic disease are to:

- Identify and characterize hepatic damage and dysfunction
- Identify possible primary causes of secondary liver disease
- Differentiate causes of icterus
- Evaluate potential anaesthetic risks
- Assess prognosis
- Assess the response to xenobiotics, i.e. drugs and toxins
- Monitor response to therapy.

Depression, decreased appetite and lethargy
Stunting and weight loss
Vomiting, diarrhoea and grey acholic faeces
Polydipsia and polyuria
Ascites
Icterus
Altered liver size
Bleeding tendency
Abdominal pain (rare)
Encephalopathy

12.1 Clinical signs of hepatobiliary disease. Adapted from Sevelius and Jönsson (1996).

Function	Abnormal laboratory test result associated with liver dysfunction
Carbohydrate metabolism: Glucose homeostasis	 Hyper- or hypoglycaemia
Lipid metabolism: Cholesterol Fatty acids Lipoproteins Bile acids	 Hypo- or hypercholesterolaemia Hypertriglyceridaemia Lipaemia Elevated bile acids
Protein metabolism: Albumin Globulins Coagulation proteins	 Hypoalbuminaemia Increased acute phase proteins, immunoglobulins Coagulopathies
Vitamin metabolism	? Decreased folate, cobalamin Vitamin E, vitamin K may be reduced depending on the disease
Immunological functions	Hyperglobulinaemia Increased acute phase proteins
Detoxification	Hyperammonaemia Decreased urea Hyperbilirubinaemia

12.2 Clinicopathological abnormalities associated with disturbances of hepatobiliary function.

Acute pancreatitis
Diabetes mellitus
Exocrine pancreatic insufficiency
Extrahepatic bacterial infection
Hyperadrenocorticism
Hyperthyroidism
Hypoadrenocorticism
Hypothyroidism
Immune-mediated haemolytic anaemia
Inflammatory bowel disease
Protein-losing enteropathy
Right-sided heart failure
Septicaemia
Shock

12.3 Some of the more common extrahepatic disorders that can cause abnormal liver test results.

Diagnostic approach to liver disease

In most cases, a tentative diagnosis of liver disease can be deduced from the results of laboratory tests in conjunction with imaging techniques. However, the definitive diagnosis of primary liver disease usually depends ultimately on histological examination of liver biopsy specimens. In most cases, primary extrahepatic causes of secondary liver disease will be identified before biopsy is considered.

The age, gender and breed of the patient may assist with formulation of a differential diagnosis list; for example, chronic hepatitis is more prevalent in middle-aged female Dobermanns. Acute diseases have a sudden onset, but chronic disease may also appear to develop suddenly, as signs are only manifested once the functional reserve capacity of the liver is exhausted. Nevertheless, careful questioning of owners often elicits evidence of previous recurring low-grade illness. A history of weight loss and ascites also suggests chronic disease.

Physical examination is important in identifying underlying disorders causing secondary liver disease. For example, in hyperadrenocorticism cutaneous changes (e.g. thin skin, comedones and calcinosis cutis) may be seen in conjunction with hepatomegaly and elevated serum alkaline phosphatase. Indeed, the importance of history and physical examination cannot be overemphasized, and any test results must always be interpreted in the light of these findings.

A diagnostic approach to liver disease includes:

- Clinical history
- Physical examination
- Laboratory tests
- Examination of ascitic fluid
- Imaging
- Liver biopsy.

Minimum database

Serum biochemistry, haematology and urinalysis are performed routinely when investigating animals with suspected hepatic disease before performing more specific tests or considering liver biopsy. Biochemical findings are often the most useful in diagnosis of liver disease.

Enzyme markers of liver disease

Increased activities in serum of liver-specific enzymes are generally considered markers of liver disease as they reflect 'liver damage'. However, increased activities are common and not necessarily associated with clinically significant *primary* liver disease. Systemic disease and various drugs can cause misleading increases in serum activities (*secondary* or reactive hepatopathies) which are potentially reversible without any specific therapy for liver disease. It can be a clinical dilemma to decide whether liver enzyme elevations are significant, and whether they represent primary or secondary liver disease. It is important to interpret all results in light of the other aspects of the diagnostic investigation, in particular the history and physical examination. For example, feline hyperthyroidism causes secondary increases in liver enzymes, and so measurement of thyroid function is indicated before liver biopsy in older cats with increased enzyme activities when they have signs of polyphagia and weight loss.

Even when increased serum enzyme activities are associated with primary liver disease, it is a popular misconception that these are 'liver *function* tests'. In severe chronic hepatopathies, such as cirrhosis, and also in congenital portosystemic shunts (PSS), there may be marked hepatic dysfunction with no or minimal marker enzyme release because there is insufficient functional hepatic mass to synthesize the enzymes. These tests give little indication of the type of disease present, or the overall functional state of liver, or the reversibility of the disease. The magnitude of the increase in activity is not necessarily important, although it may correlate with the number of cells involved, especially in acute disease. Mild elevations may either be of no consequence or reflect loss of almost all hepatocytes in end-stage disease. Serum enzyme activities depend on their total hepatic activity, their intracellular location (and thus their tendency to leak from hepatocytes), their potential for induction by drugs and also their serum half-life. It has been postulated that occasional persistent elevations of liver enzymes in the absence of abnormal hepatic function and histopathology may reflect the presence of macroenzymes, which are large, antibody-bound complexes of enzymes cleared from the circulation more slowly than normal, but which have no clinical significance. However, persistently elevated liver marker enzymes usually indicate persistent, chronic disease.

Liver enzyme activities that can be measured in serum can be classified into two major types:

- The hepatocellular enzymes that are released by cell damage (leakage markers)
- The biliary enzymes whose synthesis is induced by drugs and retained bile (cholestatic markers).

A number of enzymes are available for measurement, but within each class one enzyme rarely offers greater diagnostic advantage over the others. Therefore, the routine biochemical profile usually only offers one or two enzymes within each class, with which the clinician becomes familiar. Enzyme activities are measurable in serum or heparinized plasma and are stable over several days as long as the sample is not exposed to excessive heat. The effects of haemolysis, icterus and lipaemia are variable, depending on the analyser and method being used. Reference values will vary between laboratories depending on the assay methodology, and comparison of results from different laboratories is better achieved by comparing the magnitude of any increase with respect to the upper reference range value, rather than comparing absolute numbers; e.g. an alanine aminotransferase (ALT) of 250 represents a 4-fold increase if the upper limit of the reference range is 60, but only a 2.5-fold increase if the limit is 100.

Hepatocellular/leakage enzymes

Alanine aminotransferase (ALT) (also known as serum ALT (SALT); formerly serum glutamate–pyruvate dehydrogenase (SGPT)): This is a cytosolic enzyme found in hepatocytes in concentrations 10,000-fold greater than in normal serum. Measurement of its release into serum is considered the screening test of choice for hepatocellular damage in dogs and cats because of its high sensitivity. The likelihood of false negative results, i.e. ALT within the reference range despite significant active liver damage, is very low. ALT is considered to be liver-specific in dogs and cats because, although there are other tissue sources (e.g. heart, kidney and muscle) these isoenzymes are either present in low concentrations or their serum half-life is short. However, ALT may increase in very severe muscle diseases, e.g. muscular dystrophy in dogs. In addition, ALT increases are not specific for *primary* liver damage; increases of equal magnitude may be seen in *secondary* (reactive) hepatopathies.

The serum half-life of ALT in dogs is variously reported to be between 3 hours and 4 days. The half-life is significantly shorter in cats and therefore the normal reference range is lower and smaller increases are more significant. Immediate increases in serum ALT activities are found following release either due to hepatocyte necrosis or by 'leakage' because of altered cell membrane permeability and/or altered cell metabolism. Acute hepatopathies, such as infectious canine hepatitis or liver toxins, may cause a rapid 100-fold increase in activity (Figures 12.4a, 12.5). Increases may not be as marked in chronic hepatitis, but are persistent.

The magnitude of the rise in ALT in acute liver disease is roughly proportional to the number of hepatocytes affected, but a common mistake in the interpretation of ALT is to give too much significance to the magnitude of the rise. Although at least a 2-fold increase is needed before any significance is attached, the magnitude of the rise in ALT beyond this does not directly reflect the severity of the disease, its reversibility or the prognosis, and is not an indicator of liver function or dysfunction. As mentioned above, ALT tends to increase more in acute than in chronic disease; indeed, in end-stage liver disease when there is little active damage occurring, ALT activities may be within the reference range if there are only a few hepatocytes left to leak enzyme. Yet recovery from acute hepatitis is more likely than with chronic disease, and it is the persistence of enzyme elevation that is often of more diagnostic and, particularly, prognostic importance (Figure 12.4b).

Whilst a fall in ALT activities can be a bad prognostic sign if it reflects loss of hepatocytes, a gradual decline in ALT following an acute insult usually indicates a good prognosis; in dogs activities should fall by 50% every 3–4 days, and have returned to normal in 2–3 weeks (Figure 12.4a). Activities decline more slowly than would be predicted from the enzyme's short half-life because serum ALT is derived both from leaky, damaged cells and from regenerating hepatocytes.

ALT rises immediately following acute hepatocyte injury, but increases occur more slowly in cholestatic liver disease (Figure 12.4c). Extrahepatic bile duct obstruction and consequent bile stasis lead to accumulation of toxic bile salts which cause hepatocyte damage and enzyme leakage. The rises in serum ALT activity (e.g. 2–10-fold) often do not reach the magnitude of the increase in cholestatic marker enzymes (e.g. 10–100-fold). Similarly, cholangitis in cats only causes a moderate (5–10-fold) increase in ALT.

Rises in ALT activity are also seen in some cases of primary and metastatic hepatic neoplasia if there is leakage from tumour cells or tumour-associated

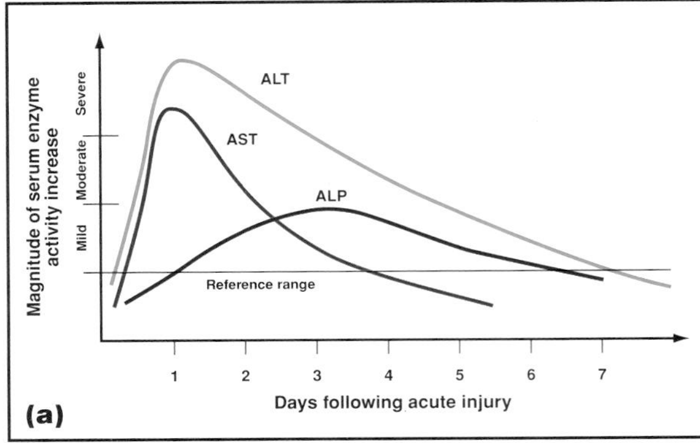

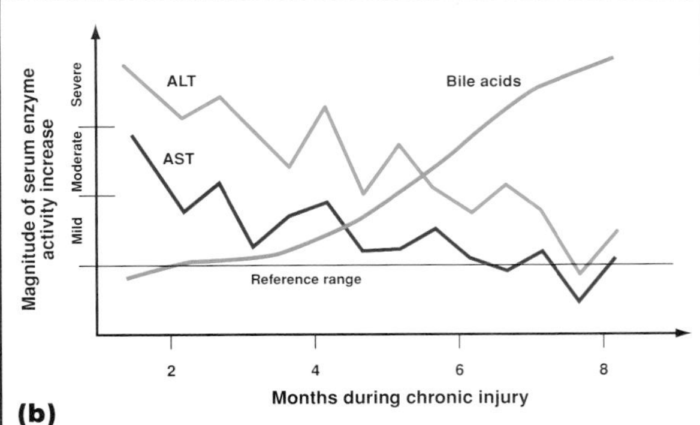

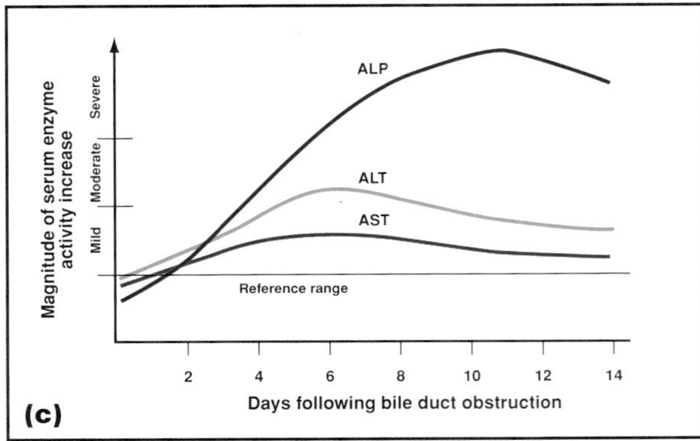

12.4 Patterns of changes in serum liver enzymes following (a) an acute injury with resolution, (b) persistent injury and (c) cholestasis. In (a) note the parallel rise in ALT and AST but longer persistence of ALT because of its longer half-life and synthesis during hepatic repair. The rise in ALP lags behind ALT, may continue for a period after resolution, and persists for longer. In (b) hepatocellular marker enzymes remain persistently elevated, although there is a general decline with disease progression as assessed by increasing bile acid concentration. In (c) note the rise and plateau in ALP with lesser increase in ALT and AST.

necrosis. However, significant infiltration with lymphoma or large primary liver tumours may cause minimal increases in ALT.

Small increases in ALT can also be caused by microsomal enzyme induction after administration of hepatotoxic drugs (Figure 12.5), and the rise in activity tends to be dose-dependent. Therapeutic doses of anticonvulsants, such as phenobarbital, usually produce a 4–5-fold increase, whereas toxic doses can cause a 50-fold rise. Idiosyncratic reactions with the development of significant liver dysfunction are likely to be associated with greater rises in ALT. Glucocorticoids can also induce ALT activity; doses of prednisolone >4 mg/kg can cause a 10-fold rise in ALT, but the increase is usually disproportionately less than the induced rise in alkaline phosphatase (ALP) (see below). Increased activity may persist for several weeks following a single dose of steroids due to enzyme induction and steroid hepatopathy.

Azathioprine
Barbiturates (including phenobarbital, primidone)
Glucocorticoids (dogs)
Griseofulvin
Halothane
Ketoconazole
Mebendazole
Paracetamol (acetaminophen)
Sulphonamides

12.5 Important hepatotoxic drugs known or suspected to cause increases in ALT.

A major problem in the interpretation of ALT activities is that the changes in activity are sensitive to secondary and clinically insignificant hepatopathies. It is not unusual to see up to 5-fold increases in ALT in dogs with primary gastrointestinal disease. Liver biopsy is not indicated in most of these cases because liver function tests (see below) are normal. If histological analysis is performed, changes are mild or absent. It is believed that release of cytokines by activated Kupffer cells results in mild, reversible hepatocyte damage.

Increased ALT can occur secondary to fatty infiltration in diabetes mellitus. ALT can also be increased secondary to hypoxic liver damage, and ALT increases in haemolytic anaemia may mislead clinicians into thinking that a primary hepatopathy is present. Given the large number of Kupffer cells in the liver, and its large blood supply, increased ALT may be seen in response to sepsis and endotoxaemia from any site. Thus, since even periodontal disease can cause mildly elevated serum ALT activities, the careful clinician usually checks at least one other liver enzyme and, if necessary, performs a liver function test before embarking on liver biopsy. However, persistent elevation of ALT over 1–2 months is indication for further investigations, such as liver biopsy, even if clinical signs are not yet apparent and liver function tests are normal (provided no primary underlying disorder can be found).

When a clinician is faced with a patient with apparently non-specific increases in ALT, found either on a routine biochemical screen or during illness, a logical approach to be taken is shown in Figure 12.6.

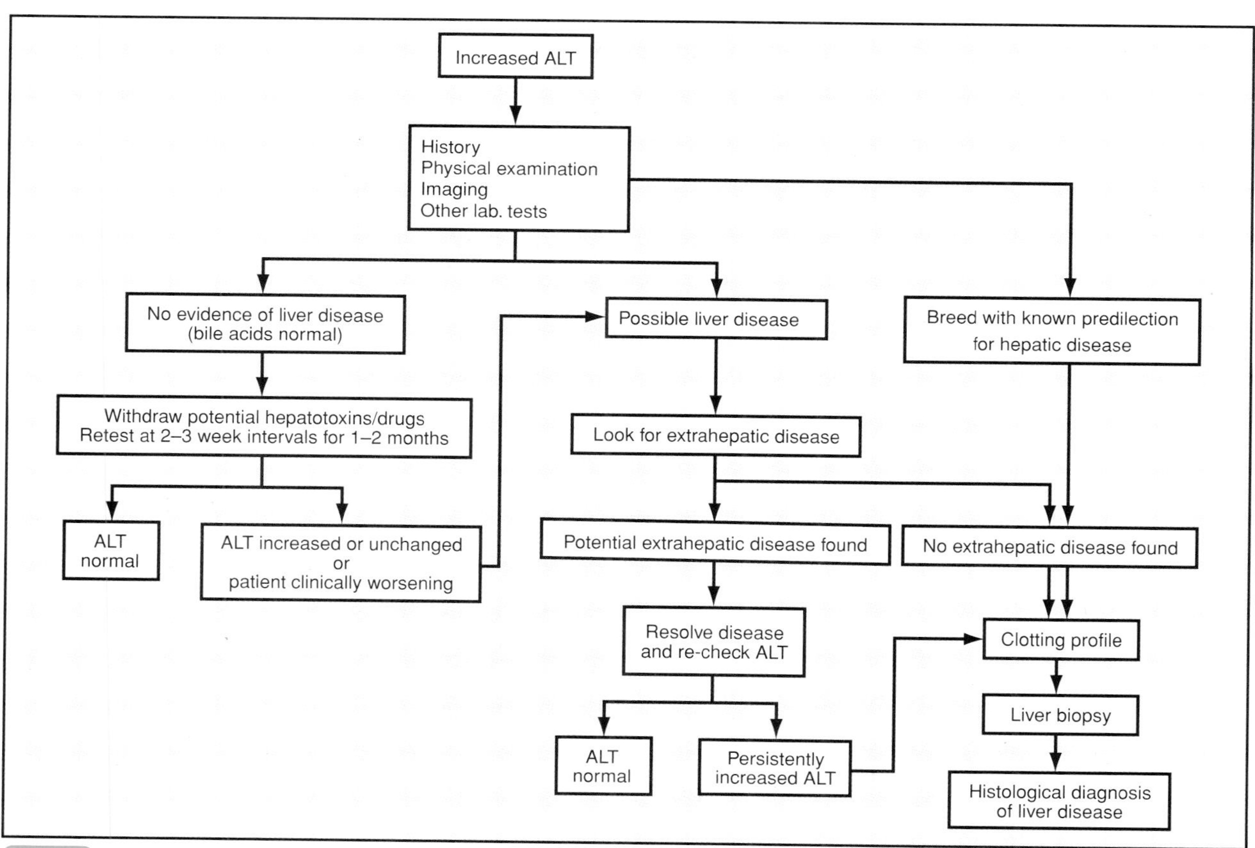

12.6 Logical approach to a patient with non-specific increase in serum ALT activity.

Aspartate aminotransferase (AST) (also known as serum AST (SAST); formerly serum glutamate-oxaloacetate transaminase (SGOT))**:** This is another hepatocellular enzyme that is released by cell damage, but, unlike ALT, it is also found in significant quantities in cardiac and skeletal muscle. However, muscle inflammation is relatively uncommon in the dog and cat, and can be identified by simultaneous measurement of a muscle-specific enzyme, e.g. creatine kinase (CK) (see Chapter 22). In liver disease, rises in AST usually parallel ALT. Thus an increase in AST and CK but not ALT probably indicates muscle damage. AST may also be increased by haemolysis and release from RBCs.

Since AST appears to have no advantage over ALT as a marker of hepatocyte damage in terms of specificity, it is of limited value. However, because some of the hepatocellular AST is mitochondrial-bound rather than all free in the cytosol, some clinicians argue that release requires more severe injury, i.e. cell necrosis rather than increased cell membrane permeability. Therefore, release of AST often lags slightly behind ALT (see Figure 12.4), but since its half-life is shorter, its presence probably indicates more profound or persistent injury than suggested by an increase in ALT alone. It may, therefore, be a more specific marker of *significant* liver damage than ALT, as it is less likely to be increased in secondary hepatopathies, e.g. glucocorticoid hepatopathy. In humans, differentiation of the cytosolic and mitochondrial isoforms of AST has prognostic implications, but this test is not currently available in veterinary medicine.

Increases in AST in acute hepatitis parallel increases in ALT, although they are rarely more than 50-fold. Although levels of AST decline over several weeks, they usually normalize before ALT; persistently elevated AST is a poor prognostic sign. Smaller increases in AST are seen in chronic hepatitis and cholestatic disease. Once again, the plasma half-life of 1 hour in cats is less than in dogs (5 hours) and therefore smaller increases are as significant; it has been suggested that AST is a more sensitive marker of *significant* liver disease in cats.

Others: In most cases ALT and AST are the only hepatocellular marker enzymes that need to be measured. However, there are a number of other candidate markers, developed primarily for ruminants, that have been proposed for use in dogs and cats. These include arginase, glutamate dehydrogenase, lactate dehydrogenase, sorbitol dehydrogenase and ornithine carbamoyltransferase. None have been shown to have any significant advantages and some, such as lactate dehydrogenase (LDH), are so ubiquitous as to be unhelpful. Arginase is perhaps potentially useful as its release tends to be less in secondary hepatopathies (as it is localized in the mitochondria), and, unlike ALT and AST, leakage ceases during recovery. Therefore, persistent increases carry a poorer prognosis.

Biliary/cholestatic marker enzymes

One or two membrane-bound enzymes that are released particularly in response to cholestasis are usually measured in a biochemistry profile in conjunction with ALT. However, their specificity for cholestatic disease is limited; increases are frequently seen in other diseases, and, in the dog, a corticosteroid-induced isoenzyme is a frequent complication.

Alkaline phosphatase (ALP) (also known as AP or serum AP (SAP))**:** In the liver, ALP is anchored in the microsomal and biliary canalicular membranes of hepatocytes and is normally secreted into bile. Hepatic ALP is released into the blood as a result of cholestasis (extra- or intrahepatic) and drug induction. The level of ALP activity cannot be used to distinguish between intra- and extrahepatic cholestasis, and the value of ALP, even as a test of cholestasis, is limited by the presence of a number of isoenzymes; this is particularly the case in dogs, where there is a steroid-induced isoenzyme (Figure 12.7). ALP has higher specificity for cholestasis in cats than in dogs as there are no steroid-induced

Primary liver disease
Cholestasis:
Intrahepatic
Extrahepatic
Hepatic inflammation:
Parenchymatous
Cholangitis
Nodular hyperplasia
Neoplasia
Extrahepatic conditions
Bone metabolism:
Growth
Osteomyelitis
Fracture repair
Osteosarcoma
Secondary renal hyperparathyroidism
Gastrointestinal disease:
Gastroenteritis
Pancreatitis
Hyperthyroidism
Pregnancy
Right-sided heart failure
Sepsis:
Systemic infections
Pyometra
Urological disease:
Nephritis
Cystic calculi
Drug-induced
Corticosteroids:
Iatrogenic
Hyperadrenocorticism
Endogenous (stress)?
Anticonvulsants:
Phenobarbital
Primidone
Phenytoin
Azathioprine

12.7 Causes of increased ALP in dogs. Cats do not produce steroid-induced ALP isoenzyme, and increased activities are less notable in extrahepatic disease.

isoenzymes (see below). In addition, the half-life of liver ALP in cats is only 6 hours compared to 3 days in dogs, and there is also a smaller total ALP activity in feline liver; therefore, lesser rises are more significant in cats than in dogs. However, ALP is not as sensitive in cats as in dogs and can be normal in jaundiced cats.

ALP is present in the liver, bone, intestine, kidney and placenta. However, renal and intestinal sources rarely contribute to increased serum levels and the key causes of increased serum ALP are cholestasis, drug/hormone induction and increased osteoblastic activity. The ALP content of intestine is actually higher than liver but, because the plasma half-life of the intestinal isoenzyme (approximately 6 minutes) is much shorter than the liver isoenzyme (3 days) and because it is largely lost into the intestinal lumen, raised serum activities of the alimentary isoenzyme are rarely seen. Increased serum ALP in primary intestinal disease is more likely to be the result of secondary hepatic damage than intestinal isoenzyme release. Similarly, renal ALP is excreted in urine and is of no significance when measuring *serum* ALP. Placental ALP is obviously only detectable in pregnancy.

Bone ALP is released in response to osteoblastic activity. In young growing dogs the normal total serum ALP range is approximately twice the adult level because of the presence of this isoenzyme. In adult dogs with active bone lesions (e.g. fractures, osteomyelitis and bone tumours) and in secondary renal hyperparathyroidism, ALP increases are seen but are rarely more than 5-fold. If there is any confusion, assay of another cholestatic marker which has no bone isoenzyme (see below) will be helpful.

Hepatic ALP is released into the blood as a result of cholestasis (extra- or intrahepatic) and drug induction. In cholestasis, the increases in serum hepatic ALP do not simply represent regurgitation from within hepatocytes, but also both solubilization of ALP from membranes by accumulated bile salts, and induction of *de novo* synthesis. Thus, after an acute hepatic insult ALP release is delayed compared with that of ALT, because of the need for induction of synthesis. In dogs, ALP begins to rise 8 hours after biliary obstruction, and increases 15-fold in 2–4 days. Peak activity 100-fold above normal is reached in 1–2 weeks, and then activity reaches a plateau at a lower level (see Figure 12.4c). ALP is also usually the last enzyme to return to the reference range after an acute insult as impairment of bile flow is usually the last functional disturbance to resolve and increased synthesis may persist beyond resolution of the injury (see Figure 12.4).

Cholestasis may be caused by a wide range of intra- or extrahepatic lesions. Extrahepatic (posthepatic) bile duct obstruction (e.g. by pancreatitis and pancreatic neoplasia) causes a rise in ALP. However, intrahepatic cholestasis is also associated with increased ALP and can be caused not only by cholangitis, but also by hepatitis with hepatocyte swelling occluding small biliary canaliculi. There is a tendency for periportal injury to cause greater increases in ALP than centrilobular damage. Similarly, primary hepatic neoplasia (hepatocellular and biliary carcinomas) has also been associated with increased ALP, presumed to be as a result of intrahepatic cholestasis. Finally, metabolic diseases, such as canine diabetes mellitus and idiopathic feline hepatic lipidosis, where there is fatty infiltration of the liver and hepatocyte swelling, also causes a rise in ALP. The level of increase in ALP does not correlate with the disease process.

Steroid-induced ALP: In dogs, interpretation of ALP is complicated by the presence of a (cortico)steroid-induced ALP isoenzyme (CIALP or SIALP). To confuse the issue further, varying proportions of SIALP may be produced in primary cholestatic liver disease. The SIALP isoenzyme can be quantified by electrophoretic separation methods, but chemical manipulations have also been described, and the levamisole inhibition assay is most useful. However, there is some controversy as to whether SIALP represents a truly novel isoenzyme; it may actually represent the intestinal isoenzyme that has undergone abnormal glycosylation, delaying its clearance from the blood by the mononuclear–phagocytic system (MPS). In this hypothesis, instead of the circulating half-life of 6 minutes of the native intestinal isoenzyme, hyperglycosylation prolongs the half-life of SIALP to 3 days (Meyer, 1996a). It is not certain whether the intestinal ALP is produced in the intestine and then glycosylated by the liver or whether it is actually synthesized by the liver, following upregulation of the normally dormant gene within hepatocytes, to produce the specific isoenzyme identical to the intestinal form but with an additional sialic acid molecule attached.

SIALP does not appear be a problem in cats, but in dogs the response to exogenous corticosteroids varies with the type of steroid, dosage, frequency and route of administration, and also between individuals, resulting in massive elevations in individual patients. Some believe that the stress-induced increases in concentrations of endogenous steroids in sick animals may be sufficient to induce ALP. Whatever its origin, SIALP complicates the interpretation of increases in total ALP, as it may be induced by endogenous and exogenous (oral, parenteral and topical) steroids. Furthermore, any increase may persist for 6 weeks after the steroid administration has ceased.

Normal dogs have <15% SIALP but, after glucocorticoid administration, this may rise to 85%, with a resultant rise in total ALP. However, increased SIALP has also been found in primary hepatobiliary disease, diabetes mellitus, hypothyroidism and pancreatitis, and synthesis can also be induced by anticonvulsants. Hyperbilirubinaemia is not a feature of steroid- (or other drug-) induced increases in ALP, although sometimes bilirubinuria and a mild increase in serum bile acid concentrations (see below) are found. The finding of increased total ALP in isolation (i.e. with no or minimal increase in ALT) is suggestive of hyperadrenocorticism but increased ALP may also be seen in benign nodular hyperplasia of the liver, and a review of the clinical signs and/or evaluation of adrenal function (see Chapter 18) should be performed to distinguish the two conditions.

Most dogs with hyperadrenocorticism have elevated SIALP and so the absence of SIALP may help rule out hyperadrenocorticism. However, induction of SIALP by steroids is unpredictable, and excessive steroid concentrations may also cause intrahepatic cholestasis and increases in the hepatic ALP isoenzyme. Equally important, SIALP may be expressed in other hepatobiliary diseases, diabetes mellitus, hypothyroidism and pancreatitis (Meyer, 1996a) and with anticonvulsant therapy. Thus measurement of the SIALP isoenzyme has fallen from favour and is not generally available in the UK.

Gamma-glutamyl transferase (GGT) (also known as γ-glutamyl transpeptidase or γ-GT): GGT is another microsomal membrane-bound glycoprotein, associated with the biliary tree, that increases in plasma in response to cholestasis. It generally parallels rises in ALP activity, but is perhaps less influenced by hepatocyte necrosis. There are GGT isoenzymes in other tissues, notably kidney, pancreas, intestine, heart, lungs, muscle and RBCs, but most circulating GGT is presumed to be of hepatic origin. There is no bone isoenzyme and therefore increased GGT is not seen in growth or bone disease. However, colostrum and milk contain GGT and may cause an increase in nursing animals up to 10 days of age. As with ALP, a steroid-induced isoenzyme is also present, but synthesis is apparently less likely to be induced by anticonvulsants.

Differences in the zonal distribution of GGT compared with that of ALP may influence the sensitivity of GGT in various diseases. GGT is also found in the lower biliary tree but, like ALP, GGT lacks complete specificity in differentiating cholestatic from hepatocellular disease. It has been suggested that measurement of ALP and GGT together increases their diagnostic value. In dogs it is probably more specific and less sensitive than ALP, but in cats the converse appears true. In cats, most cholestatic disease causes greater increases in GGT than ALP, except in idiopathic hepatic lipidosis where ALP increases may occur in the absence of a significant rise in GGT. It has been postulated that this discordance reflects either delayed clearance of ALP or excess production.

In summary, measurement of ALP in dogs is generally preferred to GGT, with the converse in cats, but, in some situations, measurement of both enzymes may provide additional information.

Other serum biochemistry parameters commonly altered in liver disease

Many biochemical tests are not specific indicators of liver disease, but do offer a crude assessment of liver status, or aid recognition of diseases that either mimic the clinical signs of liver disease or actually cause secondary liver disease.

Cholesterol

Cholesterol is derived from the diet and hepatic synthesis, and undergoes enterohepatic recycling. However, the usefulness of serum cholesterol concentration as a marker of liver disease is limited as its concentration may be decreased, normal or increased, depending on the type of liver disease and the dietary intake.

Hypercholesterolaemia may develop in major bile duct occlusion in dogs and cats, but may also be seen in diseases which secondarily affect the liver, e.g. diabetes mellitus, hyperadrenocorticism, hypothyroidism, hyperlipidaemia, pancreatitis and nephrotic syndrome. Whilst hypocholesterolaemia can be found in cases of PSS, cirrhosis and liver failure, it can also be a consequence of malabsorption.

Triglycerides

Abnormalities of lipid metabolism in hepatic disease are not well characterized. Hypertriglyceridaemia is seen in biliary obstruction, and reduced concentrations may be seen in chronic hepatitis. Lipaemia is seen in a number of metabolic diseases that secondarily affect the liver, e.g. diabetes mellitus, hyperadrenocorticism and hypothyroidism (see Chapter 15).

Glucose

Homeostatic mechanisms are so effective that significant fasting hypoglycaemia is only seen occasionally in primary liver diseases, when there is severe hepatic compromise, e.g. massive hepatic necrosis, PSS and end-stage liver disease. Congenital hepatic enzyme deficiencies, termed glycogen storage diseases, are very rare but may cause hypoglycaemia and hepatic engorgement with stored glycogen. Sepsis and large or diffuse tumours, such as hepatoma or lymphoma, may also cause hypoglycaemia through excessive glucose utilization or release of insulin-like factors (see Chapter 16).

Urea and creatinine

Low serum concentrations of urea, relative to serum creatinine, are sometimes seen in animals with PSS or severe liver dysfunction because of failure to convert ammonia to urea (see below).

Azotaemia (increased serum urea and creatinine concentrations) indicates decreased glomerular filtration, which can be a consequence of primary hepatic disease. In a fasting sample, a disproportionate increase in urea compared with creatinine can be seen with gastrointestinal haemorrhage. A combination of coagulopathy and portal hypertension in liver disease can lead to occult gastrointestinal haemorrhage that may be detected by changes in the urea:creatinine ratio in mildly azotaemic animals before haematemesis or melaena are noted.

Serum proteins

The liver is the source of all albumin and most globulins (except γ-globulins), so serum total protein and, especially, albumin concentrations can be considered crude markers of liver function. The differential diagnosis for hypoproteinaemia includes liver disease, protein-losing nephropathies (PLN) and protein-losing enteropathies (PLE). These three classes of disease can often be distinguished by their clinical signs, their relative changes in albumin and globulin concentrations, and simple confirmatory laboratory tests (Figure 12.8). A further differential diagnosis for hypoproteinaemia is blood loss, which can be assessed by concurrently measuring haematological parameters.

Cause	Albumin	Globulin	Clinical signs	Confirmatory test
Liver disease	↓	Normal or ↑	Varied (includes diarrhoea and weight loss)	Liver function test
Protein-losing enteropathy	↓	↓	Diarrhoea and weight loss	None readily available (^{51}Cr-albumin excretion, faecal α_1-PI)
Protein-losing nephropathy	↓	Normal	Nephrotic syndrome and weight loss	Proteinuria (dipstick, urine protein:creatinine ratio)

12.8 Differentiation of hypoproteinaemia.

- Albumin: mild decreases (<20%) in albumin concentration are seen in anorexia, as an acute phase response in inflammatory diseases (with the down-regulation of synthesis inversely related to the increase in serum globulin) and in ascitic animals, because of the increased volume of distribution. The half-life of albumin in dogs is reported to be between 1 and 3 weeks, so significant reductions in albumin concentration develop slowly and indicate the existence of chronic disease. Dogs and cats also have a large reserve capacity for albumin synthesis, and profound hypoalbuminaemia in liver disease is usually only seen with PSS and severe hepatocellular dysfunction. In end-stage liver disease there is both decreased albumin synthesis and dilution of serum by sodium and water retention.
- Globulins: hyperglobulinaemia is common in acquired liver disease, not just because there may be an inflammatory aetiology, but also because of acute phase responses and decreased clearance of antigen by Kupffer cells, resulting in a systemic immune response. Therefore, most globulins are increased in inflammatory diseases: α- and β-globulins include acute phase proteins and increase in inflammation in parallel with γ-globulins. The hyperglobulinaemia may be sufficient to mask hypoalbuminaemia if only total protein concentration is measured. Hyperglobulinaemia is particularly seen in cats with feline infectious peritonitis (FIP) and lymphocytic cholangiohepatitis, two conditions that can both cause jaundice and ascites.

Serum protein electrophoresis can be helpful in long-term monitoring and determining prognosis; normal to elevated haptoglobin and α_1-antitrypsin concentrations indicate a better prognosis (Figure 12.9), whilst an increase in albumin concentration (unless due to dehydration) is a good prognostic sign.

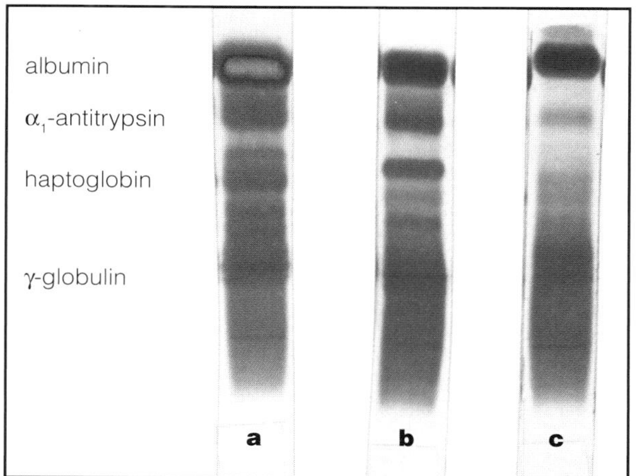

12.9 Serum protein electrophoresis from (a) one healthy dog, (b) one dog with chronic progressive hepatitis and good prognosis (note weak staining of albumin and the distinct α_1-antitrypsin and haptoglobin fractions), and (c) one dog with late stage cirrhosis and poor prognosis (note the weak staining of albumin and the almost abolished α_1-antitrypsin and haptoglobin fractions). (From *BSAVA Manual of Canine and Feline Gastroenterology*.)

Routine haematology

Red cell series

Mild to moderate anaemia (haematocrit >0.20 and <0.35 l/l in dogs, and >0.18 but <0.24 l/l in cats) is common in liver disease, and usually results from chronic illness and/or gastrointestinal bleeding and/or haemostatic disorders (see Chapter 4). Internal bleeding from hepatic tumours, such as haemangiosarcoma, generally results in moderate anaemia. More profound anaemia may result from primary haemolytic disease (with associated icterus), or from hepatic diseases that result in profuse haemorrhage, e.g. hepatic trauma, peliosis and hepatic amyloidosis (conditions that cause spontaneous hepatic rupture) or gastrointestinal bleeding secondary to portal hypertension. Microcytosis (Figure 12.10) is relatively common in dogs with congenital portosystemic shunt (PSS) and is seen occasionally in acquired liver disease; it is believed to reflect abnormal iron metabolism. Chronic blood loss with iron deficiency anaemia is the major differential diagnosis.

Variable red cell shapes (poikilocytosis) with irregularly spiculated erythrocytes (acanthocytes or spur cells) and target cells are seen in chronic liver disease (Figures 12.10 and 12.11) and are probably the result of changes in phospholipid metabolism. Microangiopathic haemolytic anaemia with the presence of RBC fragments (schistocytes) can be associated with inflammatory and benign or malignant neoplastic hepatic (and splenic) diseases (Figure 12.11b).

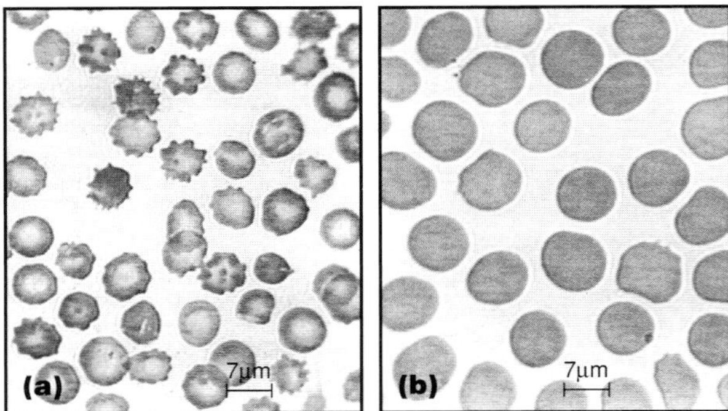

12.10 Blood smears from (a) a dog with a congenital PSS, showing anisocytosis, microcytosis, mild hypochromia, and a number of acanthocytes (spur cells); and (b) a normal dog. (Wright's Giemsa) (Courtesy of M Graham.)

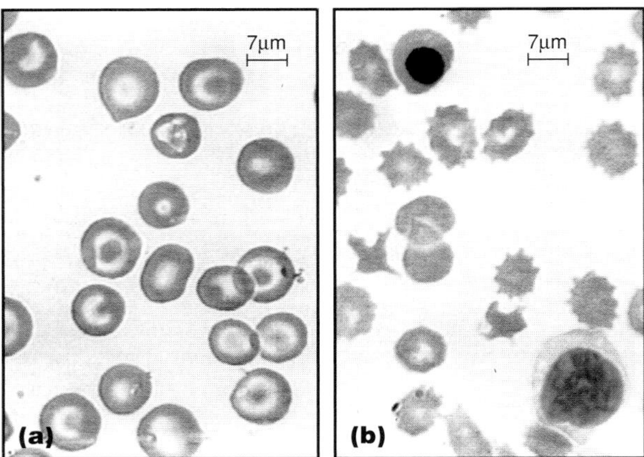

12.11 Blood smears from (a) a Cocker Spaniel with chronic hepatitis showing slight anisocytosis, hypochromia and target cells, and (b) a German Shepherd Dog with hepatic haemangiosarcoma showing large polychromatic RBCs and several acanthocytes, with a single nucleated RBC (normoblast), and two acanthocytes. A large lymphocyte is also present. (Wright's Giemsa) (Courtesy of M Graham.)

White cell series

There are no WBC changes pathognomonic for hepatic disease (see Chapter 5). The total WBC count may be increased and an inflammatory leucogram is seen in acute infectious disease (e.g. leptospirosis) and sometimes in severe chronic inflammatory hepatopathies and neoplastic liver diseases with necrosis of tumour nodules.

Platelets

Moderate reduction in platelet numbers and abnormal platelet function are non-specific changes sometimes seen in severe liver disease.

Urinalysis

Discoloured (i.e. orange) urine may be the first indication to owners that their pet is jaundiced, but further biochemical and microscopic examination of urine may provide the clinician with additional information about liver dysfunction.

Specific gravity

If polyuria/polydipsia is suspected from the history, this can be confirmed by documenting a consistently low urine specific gravity (<1.020).

Bilirubin

The normal degradation and metabolism of bilirubin is shown in Figure 12.12. Small quantities of bilirubin are common in urine samples from normal dogs, as the renal threshold is low. There are three potential sources. Firstly, a small amount of conjugated bilirubin escapes from the liver into the circulation, and readily passes through the glomeruli. Secondly, unconjugated bilirubin (bound to albumin) may be present where there is mild proteinuria, which can be found in normal dogs. Thirdly, in dogs the normal kidney may have a minor role in processing effete haemoglobin. Only a large total amount of urinary bilirubin is significant and semi-quantitative dipstick results should be interpreted in the light of the overall urine concentration. In cats, the quantity of bilirubin excreted urine is insufficient to give positive results, and bilirubinuria is almost always significant.

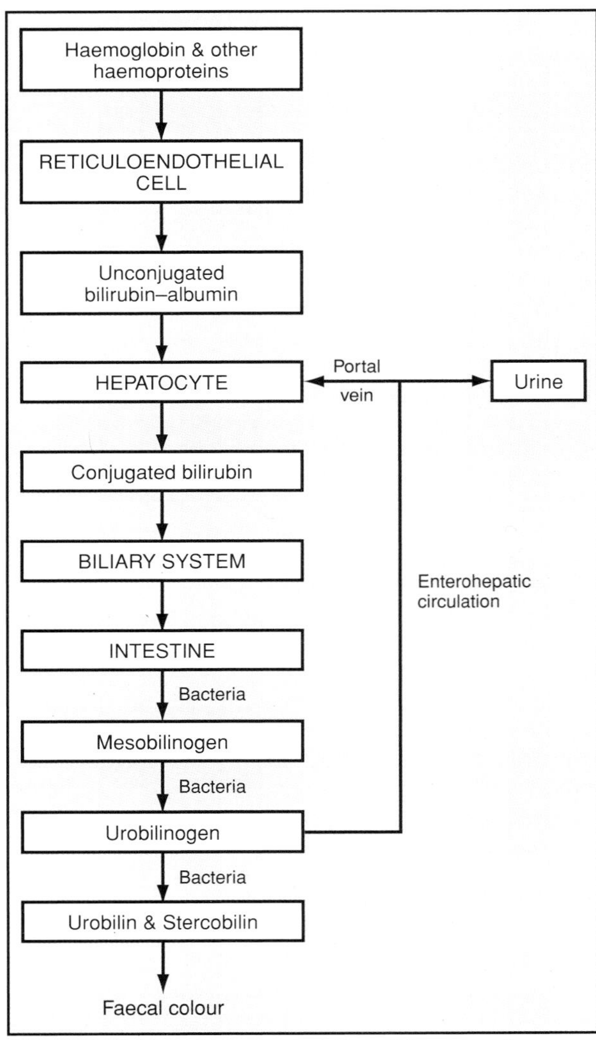

12.12 Schematic representation of the normal metabolism of bilirubin and urobilinogen.

Urobilinogen

Urobilinogen is synthesized from bile pigments by intestinal bacteria. Some is reabsorbed, most of which undergoes enterohepatic recycling and re-excretion in bile. However, about 20% passes the glomerulus. Thus, the presence of urobilinogen in urine is normal and a marker of enterohepatic recycling of bile (see Figure 12.12). Increased amounts in the urine are associated with hyperbilirubinaemia, unless complete biliary obstruction is present, when urobilinogen will be absent. Although the test is found on most 'multi-test' urine dipsticks, its usefulness is minimal.

Urate crystalluria

Abnormal uric acid metabolism and hyperammonaemia in liver disease can result in precipitation of ammonium biurate crystals in the urine. Occasionally massive crystalluria causes obvious brown turbidity (Figure 12.13a), but mostly characteristic crystals are found by microscopic examination of urine sediment. The crystals resemble mites or thorn-apples (Figure 12.13b). Urate crystals can be found on serial urinalyses in approximately two-thirds of dogs with congenital PSS.

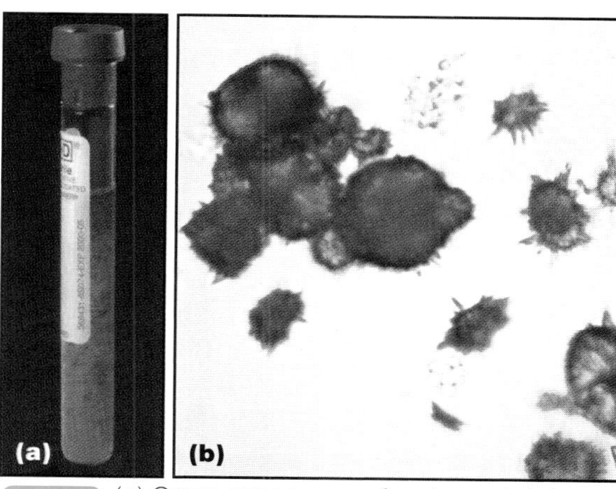

12.13 (a) Gross appearance of urate crystals in canine urine. (b) Microscopic appearance of urate crystals in urine sediment from a dog with a congenital portosystemic shunt. (Courtesy of W Millard.)

Liver function tests

Increases in liver marker enzymes do not necessarily correlate with the degree of liver damage and do not distinguish localized from diffuse disease. They, therefore, do not offer any information on overall liver function, and in cases of congenital PSS may actually be normal. In these situations specific tests are available to measure liver function.

Liver function tests may be crude markers of overall liver function (e.g. bilirubin metabolism) or they may dynamically assess certain functional pathways in the liver (e.g. enterohepatic recycling of bile acids). The former are often adequate when hepatic dysfunction is marked, whilst the latter are useful in confirming the requirement for further investigation when clinical signs are equivocal. In the presence of jaundice, many dynamic liver function tests (e.g. bile acid assay) will invariably be abnormal and do not assist in identifying the disease process. Therefore, once haemolytic (prehepatic) jaundice has been ruled out, evidence of hyperbilirubinaemia is a specific marker of hepatobiliary dysfunction and no other test of function is required to indicate liver disease and/or or biliary obstruction.

Markers of liver function

Bilirubin

Serum bilirubin concentration in dogs and cats should not normally exceed 7 μmol/l. Hyperbilirubinaemia results in jaundice (icterus), which is the yellow discoloration of tissues by accumulated bile pigments. Jaundice may be indicative of liver disease, but can be caused by other conditions (Figure 12.14) and does not occur in all hepatic disorders. For example, it is *not* seen in congenital PSS or steroid hepatopathy and is only rarely seen in metastatic disease.

Clinically, jaundice is firstly and most readily detected in the sclera when concentrations exceed 25 μmol/l, because the human eye can usually only detect the yellow colour against pink mucous membranes at about 45 μmol/l. However, hyperbilirubinaemia can be seen in separated serum at about 17 μmol/l. Chemical measurements of serum bilirubin are therefore most

Dogs	Cats
Prehepatic	
Haemolytic anaemia: Immune-mediated haemolytic anaemia *Babesia*	Haemolytic anaemia: Haemoplasmas *(Haemobartonella)* Immune-mediated haemolytic anaemia
Primary liver disease	
Acute hepatitis: Drugs, leptospirosis, infectious canine hepatitis Chronic hepatitis and cirrhosis: Copper, α_1-antitrypsin, anticonvulsants Cholangiohepatitis: Suppurative Neoplasia: Carcinoma	Acute hepatitis Chronic hepatitis and cirrhosis Cholangiohepatitis: e.g. lymphocytic–plasmacytic type Idiopathic hepatic lipidosis Neoplasia: Lymphoma
Secondary liver disease	
Septicaemia and endotoxaemia	Feline infectious peritonitis Diabetes mellitus *Toxoplasma* Paracetamol (acetaminophen) Hyperthyroidism (rarely)
Posthepatic disease	
Extrahepatic biliary disease: Common bile duct or gall bladder rupture Pancreatitis Pancreatic carcinoma Biliary carcinoma	Extrahepatic biliary disease: Chronic pancreatitis

12.14 Common causes of jaundice in dogs and cats.

sensitive. Further, because of the low renal threshold, bilirubinuria usually precedes jaundice in dogs.

In order to understand jaundice it is necessary to understand the physiology of bilirubin metabolism (Figure 12.12). Bilirubin is the major bile pigment and is a product of the degradation of haemoprotein from haemoglobin, myoglobin and haem-containing enzymes (e.g. cytochromes). The phagocytic cells of the MPS, particularly in the liver, spleen and bone marrow, engulf senescent and abnormal RBCs, and convert haemoglobin to bilirubin via biliverdin. Free bilirubin is insoluble in water and is carried in the plasma to hepatocytes reversibly bound to albumin. Here it is taken up and, along with bilirubin produced within the hepatocytes from intracellular haemoproteins, conjugated to bilirubin diglucuronide. Conjugation of bilirubin aids aqueous solubilization and excretion via the biliary canaliculi.

After biliary excretion and gall bladder storage, bile is passed to the intestine via the common bile duct. Bile pigment is converted by intestinal bacteria to a number of faecal pigments, including stercobilin, which produce normal faecal colour. The pigment urobilinogen is also produced (see above).

Hyperbilirubinaemia can be caused by three basic mechanisms (Figure 12.14):

- Prehepatic causes – increased production of bilirubin exceeding the capacity for hepatic excretion
- Hepatic causes – abnormal uptake, conjugation or secretion by hepatocytes
- Posthepatic causes – obstruction of either intra- or extrahepatic biliary excretion or biliary tract rupture.

These three types of hyperbilirubinaemia can often be distinguished by a combination of other laboratory tests, such as haematocrit, cholesterol and hepatocellular and cholestatic marker enzymes. The van den Bergh test has been advocated for their differentiation by measuring the relative proportions of unconjugated and conjugated bilirubin. However, the results are unreliable and the test is *not* recommended. Its unreliablility is, in part, due to the variable presence of bilirubin bound irreversibly to serum albumin. This covalently-bound δ-bilirubin (biliprotein) cannot be taken up by hepatocytes and merely adds to the hyperbilirubinaemia. However, it is found in variable amounts between 2 and 96% of circulating bilirubin. The clearance of δ-bilirubin is as slow as the turnover of albumin (i.e. half-life up to 3 weeks), and jaundice can occasionally persist well beyond the time of resolution of the cause, both from a clinical and laboratory (except bilirubin) perspective. Persistent jaundice, after clinical recovery, occurs most frequently in dogs with obstructive jaundice associated with acute pancreatitis. Therefore, prolonged jaundice does not necessarily indicate persistent disease, and hyperbilirubinaemia should be interpreted in light of other clinical features.

Prehepatic jaundice: Increased production of bilirubin is almost invariably associated with haemolysis and typically a low haematocrit is present.

Mild hyperbilirubinaemia (often without clinically overt jaundice) may occur in some hyperthyroid cats, probably secondary to accelerated haemoprotein turnover in the cat's hypermetabolic state.

Increased bilirubin production may also occur during resorption of large haematomas, but rarely is sufficient to produce jaundice. Intracavitary haemorrhage (e.g. haemoperitoneum) does not produce jaundice, as many RBCs (approximately 40%) are resorbed intact. Similarly gastrointestinal haemorrhage does not cause jaundice because the haemoglobin is metabolized by bacteria to non-absorbable porphyrins.

Immune-mediated haemolytic anaemia is the most common cause of prehepatic jaundice, although other non-immune causes of haemolysis occur (see Chapter 4). The capacity of the liver for hepatic bilirubin processing is normally large, so development of jaundice depends not only on haemolysis of a large number of red blood cells, but also on the presence of concurrent hypoxic liver damage associated with the anaemia.

Initially during haemolytic jaundice the accumulated bilirubin is predominantly unconjugated, but gradually conjugated bilirubin accumulates as well. Spherocytosis and a positive Coombs' test support a diagnosis of immune-mediated haemolytic anaemia (see Chapter 4). Faeces may be orange coloured (due to excess bilirubin excretion), significant bilirubinuria will be present and urinary urobilinogen in the urine will be increased. Hypoxia may cause some increase in liver-specific enzymes (ALT, AST) that may be misleading, but, if the haematocrit is normal or there is only mild anaemia, any jaundice and liver enzyme elevations are not of haemolytic origin.

Hepatic jaundice: In primary liver disease hepatocyte abnormalities, affecting bilirubin uptake and conjugation, usually co-exist with intrahepatic cholestasis. Thus increased hepatocellular and cholestatic enzymes associated with jaundice are suggestive of primary hepatic disease, although it should be remembered that enzymes may be increased in haemolytic anaemia and may not be increased in terminal cirrhosis.

Hepatic jaundice is usually the result of a combination of hepatocyte dysfunction and intrahepatic cholestasis; both ALT and ALP are usually increased, whilst cholesterol is often decreased. Altered RBC integrity and consequent increased destruction may also contribute to the jaundice and thus both unconjugated and conjugated bilirubin may appear in the blood. Bilirubinuria and urobilinogen are expected on urinalysis.

Extrahepatobiliary disease can also cause cholestatic jaundice, but the exact mechanisms are poorly defined. Sepsis outside the hepatobiliary system can cause intrahepatic cholestasis and jaundice in dogs (Taboada and Meyer, 1989), probably through an effect of inflammatory cytokines and/or bacterial endotoxin.

Genetic defects of bilirubin uptake and secretion, as seen in Southdown and Corriedale sheep, respectively, have not been described in dogs and cats.

Posthepatic jaundice: Posthepatic jaundice occurs with bile duct obstruction, often associated with pancreaticoduodenal disease. Extrahepatic bile duct obstruction is characterized by hyperbilirubinaemia in association with hypercholesterolaemia, and increases in cholestatic enzymes greater than increases in hepatocellular enzymes.

Although an increase in conjugated bilirubin alone might be expected, as the defect in bilirubin excretion occurs after hepatic conjugation, this rarely occurs because, by the time clinical signs occur, there is significant dysfunction of hepatocyte conjugation mechanisms and bile salt induced damage. Increased cholestatic markers (ALP, GGT) and hypercholesterolaemia are found, and faeces are grey and acholic (Figure 12.15), whilst urine urobilinogen is absent if obstruction is complete. Ultrasound examination of the biliary tree can be helpful in confirming the obstruction and identifying its cause.

Passage of acholic faeces, where bile pigments are absent, is usually the result of persistent mechanical extrahepatic bile duct obstruction. In cats with severe cholangitis, obstruction is most commonly due to the accumulation of biliary sludge, but occasionally a clear viscous bile which lacks pigment is produced, resulting in acholic faeces even in the absence of obstruction.

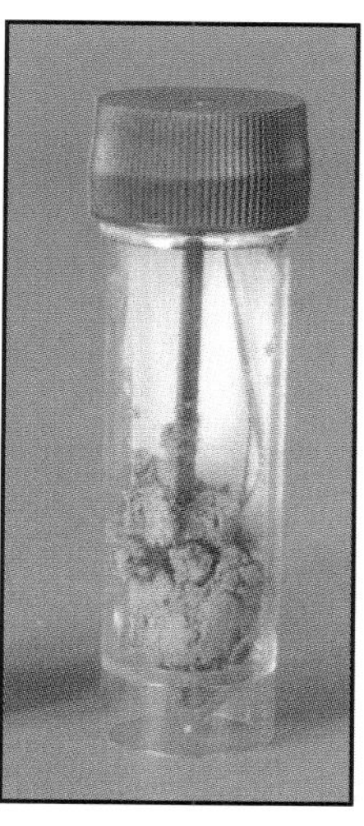

12.15 Acholic faeces. Pale faeces lacking bile pigments passed by a jaundiced dog with a complete bile duct obstruction caused by a pancreatic carcinoma.

Rupture of the biliary tract is either a result of trauma or spontaneous pathology (e.g. obstruction and perforation during passage of a gall stone), and leads to accumulation of bile in the peritoneal cavity (Figure 12.16). The severity of jaundice gradually increases as bile accumulates.

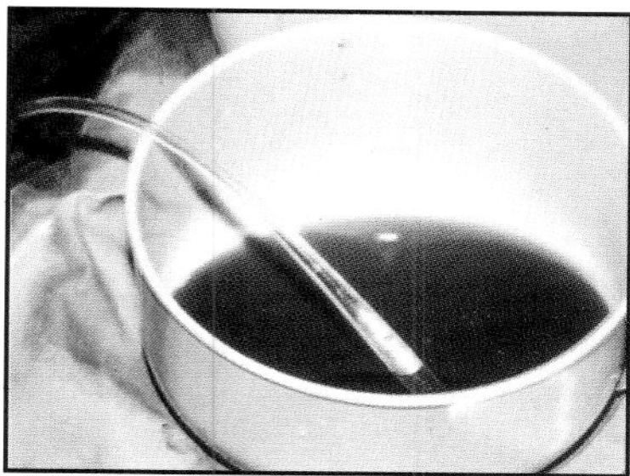

12.16 Bile peritonitis. Obvious bile-like fluid obtained by abdominocentesis in a dog 7 days after abdominal trauma in a road traffic accident.

Serum proteins

Total concentrations of albumin and globulin offer crude indices of liver function as discussed above. Serum protein electrophoresis offers prognostic information, and may demonstrate increased acute phase protein synthesis associated with inflammatory hepatopathies, or may identify production of abnormal proteins in certain liver diseases. The fetal liver-derived protein, α-fetoprotein, is not typically synthesized by normal adult liver, but is released into serum when hepatic regeneration takes place. It is present in serum in a number of liver diseases but the assay is not routinely available. Similarly, chronic hepatitis associated with α_1-antitrypsin accumulation can be characterized by demonstration of abnormal isoforms by isoelectric focusing (Sevelius and Jönsson, 1996). In contrast, copper hepatotoxicosis cannot be identified by assay of plasma ceruloplasmin but can only be confirmed on assay of copper in a liver biopsy or by genetic testing.

Liver autoantibodies (anti-nuclear antibody, anti-mitochondrial antibody, etc.) develop in human liver disease, and have been noted in canine chronic hepatitis. Their significance is not clear, and they are not routinely measured.

Coagulation times

The liver plays a central role in the coagulation and fibrinolytic systems, and subtle abnormalities may be detected by assay of individual factor activities. However, overall coagulation ability assessed by whole blood clotting time, one-stage prothrombin time (OSPT or PT) and activated partial thromboplastin time (aPTT) (see Chapter 6), is usually only significantly prolonged in severe disease. Whilst a bleeding diathesis will be expected if there is a history of gastrointestinal bleeding, an occult tendency should always be suspected, and a clotting profile is mandatory before a liver biopsy is performed. Coagulation factor proteins, synthesized in the liver, are activated through a vitamin K-dependent process. Measurement of inactive vitamin K-dependent coagulation factors, so-called 'proteins induced by vitamin K absence or antagonism' (PIVKAs), by their inhibition of the OSPT, detects subtle changes in production of active coagulation factors. However, the test for PIVKAs does not directly test for these inactive precursors; it is a modified PT performed on diluted plasma. Routine use of this test is not recommended due to limited availability and lack of clear superiority over PT and aPTT assays for disease diagnosis.

As well as deficiencies of clotting factors and failure of vitamin K-dependent activation, bleeding tendencies in liver disease may also reflect increased fibrinolysis, demonstrable as increased fibrin degradation products (FDPs) and D-dimers, and platelet dysfunction, which is most easily assessed by determining the buccal mucosal bleeding time (see Chapter 6). A buccal mucosal bleeding time should always be performed prior to hepatic biopsy, because some studies have suggested that complications arise more commonly due to platelet dysfunction resulting in primary haemostatic abnormalities, rather than secondary (coagulation factor) haemostatic abnormalities.

Occasionally bleeding occurs because of acquired vitamin K deficiency in complete bile duct obstruction; absence of bile salts precludes intestinal absorption of this fat-soluble vitamin, particularly following antibiotic therapy when bacterial synthesis of vitamin K is impaired. Both PT and aPTT are abnormal. This problem has occasionally been reported in feline biliary disease and in feline exocrine pancreatic insufficiency; it appears to be a rare feature of canine biliary disease.

Urea

Low serum concentrations of urea are sometimes seen in animals with PSS or severe liver dysfunction because of failure to convert ammonia to urea. However, this marker is unreliable because the normal lower limit for serum urea concentration is close to the limit of sensitivity of the assay, and prolonged anorexia can produce very low urea concentrations.

Uric acid

Uric acid is an excretory metabolite of hepatic purine degradation, and increased serum uric acid concentration can be used as a marker of hepatic dysfunction (Reyers *et al.*, 2001). Urate crystalluria is also a marker of hepatic dysfunction. However, uric acid also accumulates in dogs with inherited abnormalities of purine metabolism, such as Dalmatians.

Ascites

The accumulation of free fluid in the peritoneal cavity can be indicative of liver disease. Mechanisms of fluid accumulation can be identified by diagnostic abdominocentesis and measurement of the protein and cellular content. Classification of the fluid as transudate, modified transudate or exudate can be helpful (see Chapter 21). Assessment of the serum-ascites albumin gradient can help in classification of the effusion (Pembleton-Corbett *et al.*, 2000).

A pure, low-protein transudate will accumulate if there is hypoproteinaemia. However, liver disease in dogs and cats very rarely causes ascites by this mechanism alone, and hydrothorax or subcutaneous oedema are rarely seen in liver disease. Ascites in liver disease usually arises through a combination of hypoalbuminaemia and portal hypertension, resulting in accumulation of a modified transudate. The term 'modified transudate' is perhaps an unfortunate misnomer in liver disease, as it is usually not 'modified' after formation. Whilst modification by infection and inflammation can occur, in liver disease, ascitic fluid is more commonly just a transudate that results from increased hydrostatic pressure (i.e. portal hypertension). However, as hepatic sinusoids are highly permeable, the fluid entering the extracellular hepatic tissue spaces contains approximately 80% of serum proteins. Hepatic lymph is therefore protein-rich and, when the lymphatics are obstructed by intra- or posthepatic causes, it accumulates as protein-rich ascitic fluid. Only prehepatic portal hypertension (e.g. portal vein thrombosis, over-zealous PSS ligation), as well as simple hypoalbuminaemia, will cause a typical low-protein transudate. A modified transudate may indicate either primary hepatic disease or a 'posthepatic' problem, such as cardiac tamponade or right-sided heart failure causing hepatic venous congestion.

The presence of a protein-rich, cellular exudate, or the presence of significant amounts of blood, chyle or urine suggest extrahepatic diseases. The presence of a bile-like fluid is consistent with bile peritonitis associated with rupture of the extrahepatic biliary tree. Although the patient is jaundiced when suffering bile peritonitis, the bilirubin concentration is much greater in the peritoneal fluid. However, the gross appearance of the abdominal effusion is generally sufficient to make a diagnosis of bile peritonitis (Figure 12.16).

Dynamic liver function tests

These tests rely on analysis of paired blood samples to assess the capacity of the liver to clear endogenous (bile acids, ammonia) or exogenous (bromosulphthalein, indocyanine green) substances from the circulation. Impaired clearance is suggestive of hepatocellular dysfunction and/or portosystemic shunting, but does not differentiate the cause. Therefore, additional tests, including portovenography, ultrasonography and biopsy are required. Dynamic tests are not useful if the patient is icteric. Scintigraphy is also a dynamic test that can be used to assess both shunting and hepatic MPS function, but the need for radioisotopes and expensive equipment precludes its use in general practice.

Endogenous metabolism tests

These tests assess the metabolic capacity of the liver, and are feasible for veterinary surgeons in general practice.

Serum bile acids: Bile acids (bile salts) are major constituents of bile, but are *not* the same as bile pigments (i.e. bilirubin). Fasting serum total bile acid (FSBA) concentration is a reflection of the enterohepatic circulation of bile acids (Figure 12.17). Bile acids are

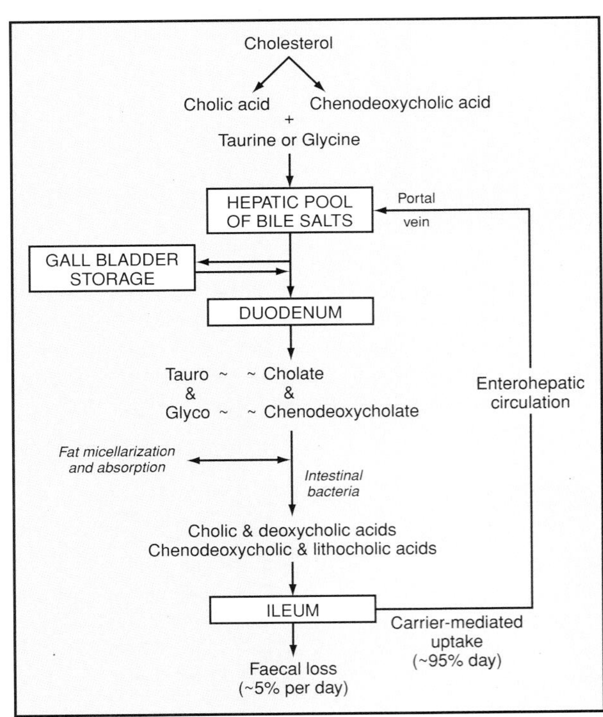

12.17 Schematic representation of normal enterohepatic circulation of bile salts.

synthesized in the liver at a rate to compensate for small faecal losses, whilst the enterohepatic circulation maintains a larger pool of bile acids that is recycled several times per meal. Hepatic dysfunction and/or portosystemic shunting permits bile acids to reach the systemic circulation where they can be measured. Measurement of urinary bile acids has also been proposed as a test of liver function (see below).

Bile acids (cholic and chenodeoxycholic acid) are synthesized in the liver from cholesterol, and are conjugated, predominantly with taurine, before biliary excretion as salts. Conjugated bile acids are ionized at the pH of the intestinal lumen and are lipid-insoluble, which prevents their absorption through the intestinal mucosa. Only when fat absorption, through micellarization, has been completed are bile acids reabsorbed on specific receptors in the ileum. Some of the primary bile acids (cholic and chenodeoxycholic acid) are metabolized by intestinal bacteria to secondary bile acids (deoxycholic and lithocholic acids) before reabsorption, and about 5% escape recycling and are lost in faeces. On return to the liver, bile acids are efficiently removed from the portal blood by hepatocytes and are re-excreted.

The rate of synthesis and the size and distribution of the bile acid pool can be abnormal in liver disease if there is one or a combination of the following:

- A reduction in hepatocellular mass
- Impaired hepatocyte function
- Disturbed enterohepatic circulation including:
  - Disruption of flow of portal blood to the liver
  - Obstruction of biliary flow from the liver.

Thus FSBA will be abnormal if hepatic function is suboptimal, or if there is portosystemic shunting, or if biliary obstruction occurs, and increases in serum bile acids (SBA) are *not* specific for certain disease types. They will be present in extrahepatic bile duct obstruction as well as primary liver disease and congenital PSS.

FSBA are most valuable for the detection of PSS and chronic hepatitis/cirrhosis before the development of jaundice. The test is simple and sensitive and is readily available to veterinary practitioners. However, given that FSBA can be increased by non-hepatic diseases (occasionally up to 100 μmol/l), the sensitivity and specificity for detecting primary hepatic diseases are not as good as initially hoped.

The sensitivity of the test is improved by measurement of 2-hour postprandial serum bile acid (PPSBA) concentration. Ingestion of food causes release of bile through stimulation of gall bladder contraction, and increases the amount of bile acids available for enterohepatic recycling. This provides a safe endogenous test of hepatic function.

The value of the PPSBA measurement is still controversial, although undoubtedly some patients with PSS do have normal FSBA and massively abnormal PPSBA concentrations. Yet, confusing decreases in the postprandial sample are sometimes found; possible explanations include inherent variability, failure to store all new bile in the gall bladder, incomplete gall bladder contraction on feeding and intestinal bacterial metabolism. The general recommendation is to interpret the higher of the two results. In posthepatic jaundice fasting levels can be very high, but often do not increase much postprandially.

Bile acids can be measured accurately by radioimmunoassay but, in most veterinary laboratories, enzymatic fluorimetric or spectrophotometric methods are used, and lipaemia, as well as haemolysis, can produce spurious results. Reference ranges for bile acids are somewhat controversial, not only because of methodological problems in some laboratories, but because of the effect of secondary hepatopathies. The initial criteria of <5 μmol FSBA and <10 μmol PPSBA are too strict, and clinically normal individuals can sometime have bile acid concentrations that are double these values. Specificity is improved by increasing the upper limit of the reference range, but at the expense of sensitivity. Concentrations >25 μmol/l, for both FSBA and PPSBA, correlate with the presence of histological lesions, although in some cases these may still be secondary hepatopathies.

An FSBA concentration of >40 μmol/l is usually taken as conclusive evidence of primary hepatic dysfunction and a need to perform further tests, such as a biopsy, unless an underlying disease can be identified. The magnitude of the FSBA over approximately 100 μmol/l apparently has little predictive value for the severity of any particular hepatopathy, and some cases of PSS have normal FSBA and massively raised (>800 μmol/l) PPSBA.

The interpretation of FSBA concentrations between 20 and 40 μmol/l is a grey area, and recommendations for these patients are:

- Look for extrahepatic disease
- Repeat FSBA with a PPSBA and look for at least a 2-fold increase
- Repeat FSBA in 2–4 weeks.

or

- If clinical signs and other results suggest primary liver disease, carry out further investigations.

Commercial bile acid assays measure total concentrations and do not distinguish between primary and secondary bile acids. In the future, fractionation of serum bile acids into specific acids, such as cholic and chenodeoxycholic, may have diagnostic utility in the identification of specific hepatopathies.

Urinary bile acids: Measurement of urinary bile acids has also been proposed as a test of liver function in dogs and cats as it theoretically provides an assessment of the cumulative production and excretion of bile acids (Balkman *et al.*, 2003; Trainor *et al.*, 2003). To correct for variations in urine specific gravity and dilution of bile acids, results are expressed as bile acid:creatinine ratio (similar to protein:creatinine ratio, see Chapter 10). Analysing the amounts of sulphated and non-sulphated bile acids was found to offer no advantage over measuring total urinary bile acids (TUBA), in contrast to the situation in humans. Some controversy exists as to the sensitivity and specificity of TUBA, and whether this offers any diagnostic advantages over dynamic SBA measurement (Steiner *et al.*, 2003).

Plasma ammonia and ammonia tolerance test: Ammonia, produced by intestinal bacteria, is normally cleared from the portal blood by the liver: normal portal blood contains up to 350 μmol/l ammonia, but <50 μmol/l enters the systemic circulation from the liver. Increased resting plasma ammonia concentration is evidence of hepatic dysfunction and/or portosystemic shunting (Figure 12.18). Very rarely, hyperammonaemia is caused by an abnormality in the urea cycle. This may be either due to a genetic defect, or secondary to cobalamin deficiency. In this circumstance, serum bile acids (see above) will be normal.

The degree of hyperammonaemia correlates crudely with the severity of hepatic encephalopathy, and so it is a reasonable marker for the condition, although the clinical signs of encephalopathy can develop secondary to the accumulation of other toxic metabolites. Further, fasting blood ammonia concentration only provides a relatively insensitive measure of hepatic function, because resting concentrations are frequently normal in patients with liver disease, including some with PSS. The sensitivity of the test can be improved by performing an ammonia tolerance test (ATT), administering exogenous ammonia either orally or *per rectum* to determine whether ammonia intolerance exists. Ammonium chloride is usually administered (100 mg/kg (maximum 3 g)) by either stomach tube or enema, and a blood sample is taken 30 minutes later. Plasma ammonia concentration does not increase significantly in normal patients; marked increases are seen in PSS. The peroral test is quite sensitive, but can cause vomiting and can be potentially dangerous in patients, especially cats, that are already encephalopathic. The rectal ammonia tolerance test has the advantage of not provoking immediate vomiting but the absorption of ammonia is more variable and samples must be taken at 20 and 40 minutes. The colon has to be prepared by enema, and, since the results are less sensitive, this method is rarely used. Measurement of postprandial ammonia has been advocated as a safer test of ammonia tolerance. It was sensitive for detecting congenital PSS but not for hepatocellular disease (Walker *et al.*, 2001).

The ATT test will detect PSS, but may not be able to detect subtler hepatic dysfunction. Further, methodological difficulties make the test difficult to perform in practice. Storage increases ammonia content of blood and so plasma must be harvested on ice and ammonia assayed within 30 minutes to produce meaningful results. Although dry chemistry ammonia tests are available in veterinary practice, results are frequently unreliable (Sterczer *et al.*, 1999). The test is, therefore, limited to institutions and practices with immediate access to a commercial laboratory.

Exogenous excretion tests

These tests are of historical interest, having been superseded by dynamic bile acid measurements.

- Bromosulphthalein (BSP) retention testing involved the intravenous administration of the organic dye, BSP, followed by blood sampling at 30 minutes and measurement of the percentage retention of the dye. Given that BSP is a potential carcinogen, it is no longer commercially available and the test is not now performed.

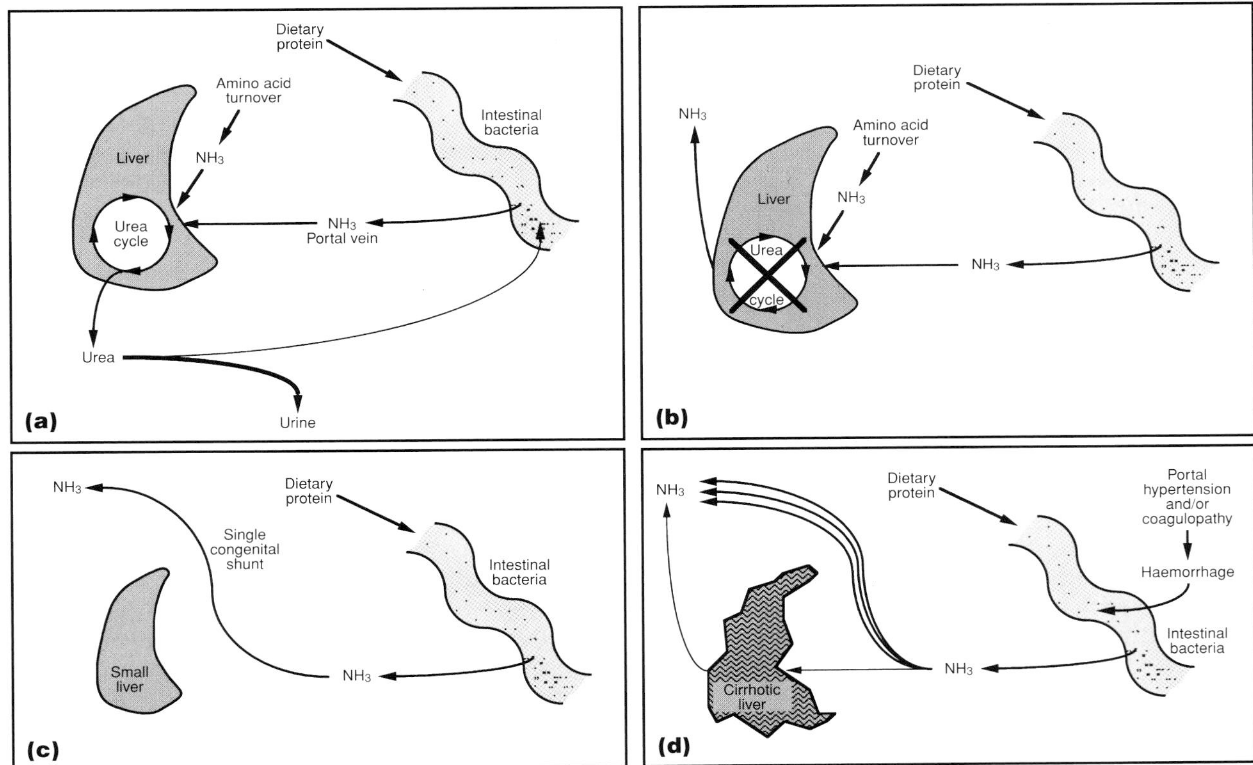

12.18 Metabolism of ammonia (NH_3) in (a) normal animals, and animals with (b) urea cycle enzyme defect (rare), (c) congenital portosystemic shunting and (d) cirrhosis with secondary acquired shunting.

- Indocyanine green (ICG) retention test. The ICG test was developed to replace BSP but offers no advantage over bile acid measurement (see above).

Exogenous metabolism tests

Aminopyrine test: Hepatic metabolism of intravenously administered ^{13}C-labelled aminopyrine results in formation of $^{13}CO_2$, which can be measured in breath. Preliminary tests suggest that it is a sensitive test of hepatic dysfunction (Moeller *et al.*, 2001; Chiaramonte *et al.*, 2003). The ^{13}C isotope is non-radioactive and therefore safe, but analysis requires mass spectroscopy.

P-450 cytochrome oxidase activity: Hepatic metabolic degradative capacity can be assessed by measuring clearance of antipyrine or caffeine by the hepatic P-450 cytochrome oxidase system or conversion of lidocaine to monoethylglyexylidide (MEGX). These tests have not yet been used in veterinary medicine.

Genetic testing

It is apparent that a number of chronic hepatopathies have a recognizable inheritance pattern and, in the future, specific genetic tests will be available. For copper hepatotoxicosis, an autosomal recessive condition of Bedlington Terriers, linkage analysis has been available for several years, allowing detection of affected dogs and selection of healthy breeding stock (Rothuizen *et al.*, 1999). Recently, a mutation in the *MURR* gene has been identified as the cause of this disease in affected dogs (Klomp *et al.*, 2003) and a genetic test for the condition has been patented.

Liver biopsy

Indications

Despite the plethora of clinicopathological tests of liver damage and dysfunction, identification of specific hepatopathies usually requires liver biopsy. Indications for liver biopsy include:

- Persistent elevations of liver enzymes with no apparent underlying disease
- Increased FSBA or PPSBA
- Altered liver size or ultrasonographic architecture
- Progressive signs of liver disease.

Cytology

It is possible to perform cytological examination of liver cells either by fine needle aspiration (FNA) or by a touch preparation of a liver biopsy specimen (see Chapter 20). However, the accuracy of FNA has been questioned. One recent study found only a 30% and 50% agreement between the cytological and histopathological diagnoses in canine and feline liver diseases respectively (Wang *et al.*, 2004).

The presence of intranuclear inclusion bodies is considered diagnostic of infectious canine hepatitis (Figure 12.19) but this is usually only found during a post-mortem examination.

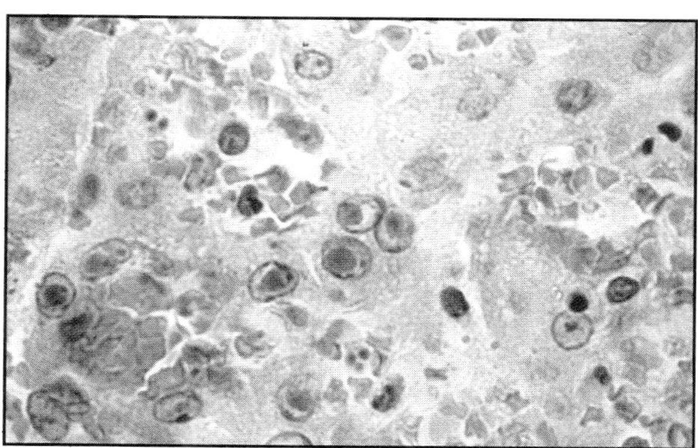

12.19 Impression smear of liver from a dog with infectious canine hepatitis showing characteristic intranuclear inclusions. (H&E; original magnification x400.)

Staining fine needle aspirates for copper granules with rubeanic acid can identify copper hepatotoxicosis (in Bedlington Terriers and other canine breeds), but histopathological staining and biochemical quantitation of copper content are necessary to avoid false negatives.

Many causes of vacuolar hepatopathies are listed in Figure 12.20; the cytological finding of enlarged cells with vacuolated cytoplasm may not be diagnostically helpful in dogs. Small foamy vacuoles may indicate glycogen accumulation, e.g. in steroid hepatopathy. Numerous larger discrete vacuoles in enlarged hepatocytes are highly suggestive of hepatic lipidosis in cats, although this may be secondary to underlying primary disease in the liver, such as inflammation and metabolic abnormalities (Wang *et al.*, 2004).

Chronic infections and inflammation:
Severe dental disease
Pyelonephritis
Diabetes mellitus
Hyperadrenocorticism
Hyperlipidaemia
Hypothyroidism
Inflammatory bowel disease
Neoplasia
Pancreatitis
Hepatic lipidosis
Treatment with glucocorticoids

12.20 Some causes of vacuolar hepatopathies.

Canine inflammatory liver disease cannot be diagnosed reliably by cytology: differentiation of chronic hepatitis and cirrhosis cannot be made as observation of the tissue architecture is needed. Similarly it is not usually possible to diagnose cholangiohepatitis in cats without solid biopsy.

Infiltration with malignant cells may be detected by FNA in primary and metastatic liver disease: malignant hepatic neoplasia, haemopoietic neoplasia (lymphoma, leukaemic infiltrates, mast cell tumours) and disseminated metastatic neoplasia may all be diagnosed cytologically. It is not possible to distinguish cytologically hepatoma from benign nodular hyperplasia.

Histopathology

Specimens for histopathological examination can be collected by a number of methods, but a coagulation profile must always be performed before biopsy because of the dangers of potential haemorrhage. Further, buccal mucosal bleeding time (BMBT) is recommended, since some studies have indicated that complications more closely correlate with problems of primary haemostasis. In practice liver biopsy is often limited to wedge biopsy at exploratory laparotomy. The techniques used are described in detail in the *BSAVA Manual of Canine and Feline Gastroenterology*.

Percutaneous biopsy techniques have been devised to provide a core of tissue, and are safest if performed under ultrasonographic visualization (Figure 12.21). However, percutaneous biopsy is now falling from favour because the size of a biopsy specimen is often inadequate for an accurate histopathological diagnosis. The diagnostic accuracy of two needle biopsies has been shown to be less than 50% compared with surgical biopsy (Cole *et al.*, 2002), and multiple biopsies are required. Laparoscopic biopsy is preferred as focal lesions can be visualized, larger biopsies obtained, and excessive bleeding identified.

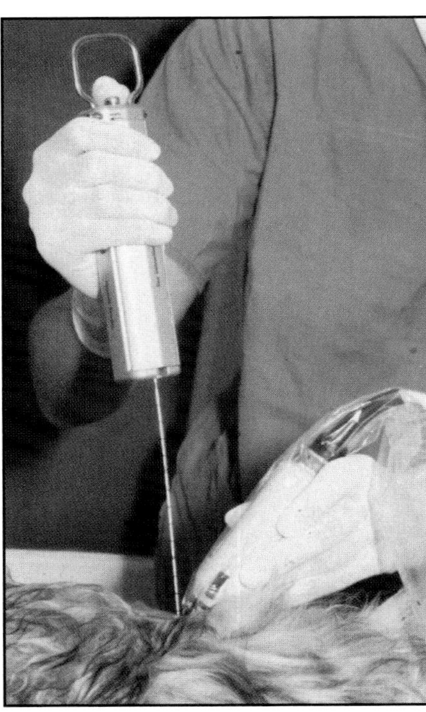

12.21 Ultrasound-guided percutaneous needle biopsy of the liver using an automated 'gun' to fire the biopsy needle. The ultrasound probe is covered in a sterile sleeve.

A number of stains, in addition to routine H&E, are available to facilitate characterization of hepatic pathology (Figure 12.22). However, the clinician needs to work with the pathologist, providing all the relevant historical, clinical and clinicopathological information, in order that appropriate stains are used and a relevant diagnosis is reached.

Pieces of hepatic tissue about the size of 1 cm cubes are required for accurate determination of hepatic copper content by atomic absorption spectrophotometry. Formalin-fixed tissue can be used.

Feature	Special stain
Amyloid	Congo red
Bacteria	Gram, Ziehl–Nielsen
Bile	Fouchet's, van Gieson
Collagen	Masson's trichrome, van Gieson
Copper	Rhodamine, rubeanic acid
Copper-associated protein	Orcein
Elastin	Elastic van Gieson, Weigert's
Fibrin, fibrinoid	Martius scarlet blue (MSB)
Glycogen	Periodic acid–Schiff (PAS) (diastase-positive), Best's carmine, Bauer–Feulgen (frozen)
α_1-Antitrypsin	PAS (unreliable), immunostaining
Iron (ferric)	Perl's Prussian blue
Lipid	Oil-red-O (frozen)
Lipofuscin	Schmorl, Ziehl–Nielsen
Reticulin	Reticulin stain

12.22 Some of the special stains available for characterization of hepatic pathological changes.

Prognostic indices

As well as identifying and helping to characterize hepatopathies, laboratory testing can provide some prognostic information.

Good prognostic signs

- Decreasing hyperbilirubinaemia
- Decreasing liver enzymes. With resolution of an acute hepatic insult, ALT should fall approximately 50% every 3–4 days in the dog. Initially increasing ALT may indicate regeneration rather than continued hepatocyte damage. ALP may continue to rise after the injury and take several weeks to normalize (see Figure 12.4)
- Normoglycaemia
- Normal coagulation times
- Increasing serum albumin, not due to dehydration. In inflammatory disease albumin is frequently subnormal as a negative acute phase response, but serum protein electrophoresis at that time will show normal to elevated haptoglobin and α_1-antitrypsin. This is a good prognostic sign (see Figure 12.9)
- Increasing cholesterol concentration (if previously low).

Bad prognostic signs

- Increases in AST and arginase as well as ALT, suggesting more severe hepatocellular damage
- Persistent elevation of ALT, AST, arginase etc., indicative of continuing damage

- Hypoglycaemia and prolonged PT in chronic hepatitis. In Dobermanns with copper-associated chronic hepatitis, these abnormalities were shown to be predictors of imminent death
- Hypoalbuminaemia due to failure of synthesis. A decrease in albumin and other acute phase proteins on serum protein electrophoresis is indicative of end-stage disease and carries a poor prognosis (see Figure 12.9).

Pattern recognition in liver disease

Apart from liver biopsy and visualization of PSS (i.e. by portovenography or ultrasonography), there is rarely any one test that provides a definitive diagnosis. Laboratory tests are only capable of identifying suspected liver disease, but particular patterns of clinicopathological abnormalities, when interpreted in light of the clinical findings, can often provide a high index of suspicion of certain diseases. The characteristic clinicopathological features of certain conditions are described below. However, whilst pattern recognition can assist the diagnostic approach, all results must be interpreted in light of the clinical picture. In this regard, laboratory artefacts may produce abnormal results, and laboratory errors may occur. The bile acid assay can be problematic, and some dry chemistry analysers are inaccurate, especially when measuring ammonia. Further, if poor quality or unsuitable samples are presented to the laboratory, the results may be inaccurate and misleading (see Chapter 2). Some of the common artefacts are summarized in Figure 12.23.

Analyte	False increase	False decrease
Bilirubin	Severe haemolysis Lipaemia	UV light Viscous serum (dry chemistry)
Bile acids	Hypertriglyceridaemia Increased serum dehydrogenases	Severe chylomicronaemia Haemolysis
Ammonia	Delayed assay Strenuous exercise Dry chemistry analyser	
ALT	Severe haemolysis Lipaemia	
AST	Severe haemolysis Lipaemia Ketoacidosis	
ALP	Jaundice Lipaemia Storage (haemolysis)	Fluoride Oxalate Citrate EDTA
GGT	Lipaemia Fluoride and oxalate	

12.23 Potential laboratory artefacts affecting liver test results.

Acute hepatitis and hepatic necrosis

Acute inflammatory conditions (whether due to toxic or infectious causes) usually cause rapid, moderate to marked increases in ALT (see Figure 12.4a). Other hepatocellular enzymes are likely to be increased, but rises in AST and arginase activity may be indicative of more severe damage. Intrahepatic cholestasis, caused by hepatocyte swelling, induces a slower rise in ALP and GGT. Depending on the severity of the hepatic damage there will be varying impairment of bile acid circulation, and, in severe cases, hyperbilirubinaemia will follow. Hypoalbuminaemia is not a feature because of the acuteness of the condition.

Chronic hepatitis

Histopathological assessment of liver tissue is usually required to differentiate specific types of chronic hepatitis; laboratory testing merely provides evidence of persistent damage and dysfunction, identifying the need for biopsy. In most disorders moderate to severe and persistent increases in ALT (or AST) and ALP (or GGT) are most characteristic (see Figure 12.4b). The absolute activities can fluctuate spontaneously and the clinician should not assume that a decrease in enzyme activity at one time point is necessarily indicative of remission.

Liver biopsy is indicated if there are persistent elevations in enzyme activity or increased FSBA. Jaundice suggests significant hepatic impairment and may herald the development of cirrhosis. Late in the disease, serum albumin is likely to be decreased and may be a poor prognostic indicator.

Cirrhosis

Hepatic fibrosis and nodular regeneration in cirrhosis, the end result of various forms of chronic hepatitis, are associated with significant hepatic dysfunction as demonstrated by increased SBA and, eventually, jaundice. Hypoalbuminaemia, low blood urea and, ultimately, coagulopathies and ascites may develop and animals often develop multiple secondary (acquired) PSS. Hypoglycaemia is a marker for end-stage cirrhosis, and is a poor prognostic indicator. Serum protein electrophoresis may demonstrate hypoalbuminaemia and decreases in acute phase proteins (see Figure 12.9). Serum enzyme activities may be elevated, but can be normal if there is no active inflammation or if minimal hepatocellular tissue remains.

Congenital portosystemic shunts

Given the absence of hepatic inflammation and cholestasis in most cases of congenital PSS, liver enzyme concentrations are often only mildly elevated or even normal. Shunting and hepatic bypass is characterized by increased FSBA and/or PPSBA; a typical 'shunt pattern', with normal FSBA and markedly elevated PPSBA, has also been described. Hyperammonaemia and/or ammonia intolerance may also be seen. Serum urea, albumin, cholesterol and, occasionally, glucose may all be decreased. Haematology quite frequently shows microcytic anaemia and poikilocytosis (see Figure 12.10), and urate crystalluria (see Figure 12.13) may be found.

Glucocorticoids

Both endogenous and exogenous glucocorticoids induce an increase in ALP/GGT with minimal increases in ALT/AST in dogs. Cats appear resistant to these changes. The response in dogs is quite variable and can persist for at least 6 weeks after the administration of even a single dose of steroid in some individuals. When severe steroid hepatopathy is present, moderate increases in ALT may develop but the increase is generally disproportionate to the magnitude of the increase in ALP. There may be mild hepatic impairment and mild to moderate increases in FSBA, very occasionally reaching as high as 100 μmol/l, but jaundice is exceptionally rare. There may also be hyperglycaemia and hypercholesterolaemia. If there is no history of exogenous steroid administration then dynamic hormone tests for hyperadrenocorticism (see Chapter 18) should be considered if clinical signs are compatible with the diagnosis.

Benign nodular hyperplasia

A common incidental finding in old dogs, nodular hyperplasia is usually considered to have no significant effect on overall liver function. However, there can be a marked rise in serum ALP with minimal changes in ALT (Meyer, 1996b). In this situation, the major differential diagnosis would be hyperadrenocorticism as there should be no signs consistent with liver disease. Nodular hyperplasia may thus explain occasional cases where hyperadrenocorticism is suspected because of increased ALP but the endocrine status is normal by dynamic hormone testing.

Primary hepatic neoplasia

Primary hepatocellular tumours may be associated with increases in ALT and/or ALP, dependent on the presence of associated inflammation or necrosis and/or intrahepatic cholestasis. Biliary carcinomas may cause increases in ALP and obstructive jaundice; other tumours cause jaundice infrequently. Hypoglycaemia may be noted with large hepatomas, but many are clinicopathologically 'silent'.

Metastatic liver disease

In primary hepatic or metastatic haemangiosarcoma there may be minimal increases in enzyme activity despite extensive tumour infiltration. Presentation with haemoperitoneum and haematological abnormalities, such as mild anaemia (which may be regenerative) and schistocytes (see Figure 12.11), are more commonly seen, although these findings are not specific for malignant disease. Focal metastatic disease is best detected ultrasonographically and confirmed by fine needle aspirate or biopsy; many, particularly older, animals will have areas of increased or decreased echogenicity due to pathology other than neoplasia.

Hepatic lymphoma

Enzyme elevation is an unreliable indicator of hepatic involvement in lymphoma but hepatomegaly, other clinical signs of lymphoma, increases in FSBA, and, sometimes, hypercalcaemia are usually enough to indicate the need for fine needle aspiration or, if required, biopsy.

Feline idiopathic hepatic lipidosis

Massive fatty infiltration of the liver in cats is associated with marked hepatic dysfunction with increased FSBA and often jaundice. Cholestatic markers would be expected to be increased, but there is often an increase in ALP but no significant rise in GGT. The reason for this unique discrepancy between ALP and GGT is not understood. The diagnosis can be confirmed by hepatic biopsy, although FNA cytology may be sufficient for a diagnosis.

Cholangiohepatitis

In dogs, cholangiohepatitis and associated cholecystitis appear to be most commonly associated with ascending infection, and an inflammatory leucogram may be seen. Increases in ALT as well as ALP suggest extension of the inflammation into the hepatic parenchyma in addition to intrahepatic cholestasis. Cholecystitis may be suspected by ultrasonographic changes in the gall bladder wall, but diagnosis is usually made on histological examination of liver biopsy tissue, supported by bacteriological culture of bile and/or liver tissue.

Lymphocytic cholangitis in cats is not uncommon and increases in liver enzymes and liver dysfunction are expected; occasionally lymphocytosis is seen. Sometimes protein-rich ascitic fluid is present, and the major differential diagnosis would be FIP.

Extrahepatic bile duct obstruction

Bile duct obstruction is classically associated with jaundice, hypercholesterolaemia and increased ALP; increases in hepatocellular marker enzymes are often smaller in magnitude. Initially, obstruction is associated with ALP and GGT increases but, if persistent, bilirubinuria and then hyperbilirubinaemia develop. The onset of obstruction is gradual if caused by biliary and pancreatic tumours or by chronic inflammatory lesions. Acute pancreatitis can also cause temporary bile duct obstruction, and onset of jaundice is often sudden and may be preceded by the more typical signs of pancreatitis. Abnormalities in hepatic parameters will not only reflect the bile duct obstruction, but also toxic hepatic changes secondary to pancreatic inflammation (see Chapter 14). In cases of biliary obstruction, ultrasonographic examination can be very helpful in determining a cause before exploratory surgery.

Drugs

Toxic hepatopathies may be associated with increases in hepatocellular enzyme markers, if hepatocellular damage is present. Drugs, such as glucocorticoids and anticonvulsants, induce production of ALP/GGT, and anticonvulsants, to a lesser extent, can induce synthesis of ALT. Figure 12.5 lists some of the more important known or suspected hepatotoxic drugs that can cause increases in ALT in dogs and cats. Epileptic dogs on chronic phenobarbital therapy sometimes develop chronic hepatitis and cirrhosis (Bunch, 1993). However, as barbiturates regularly induce liver enzymes, increased activities in the blood cannot be considered an indication of active liver damage. Such dogs should have liver function monitored by dynamic bile acid testing every 6 months.

Metabolic disease

Various hormonal and metabolic diseases cause secondary hepatopathies. Vacuolar hepatopathies with accumulation of lipid (e.g. diabetes mellitus, feline idiopathic hepatic lipidosis) or glycogen (e.g. hyperadrenocorticism) can cause increases in liver enzymes, but usually overall hepatic function is minimally impaired. Identification of the primary disorder usually precludes the need to investigate the liver beyond measuring SBAs.

Summary

There is a variety of markers of hepatic pathology with variable sensitivity and specificity. At a minimum, measurement of ALT, ALP and FSBA should be performed in suspected liver disease, and will identify most conditions. However, imaging and, ultimately, liver biopsy (after a coagulation profile) will be needed to reach a definitive diagnosis.

Case examples

Case 1

Signalment

13-year-old male Yorkshire Terrier.

History

Halitosis due to severe dental disease. Laboratory tests performed as a routine pre-anaesthetic screen.

Clinical pathology data

Haematology	Result	Reference interval
RBC (x 10^{12}/l)	6.9	5.50–8.50
Hb (g/dl)	14.8	12.0–18.0
HCT (l/l)	0.48	0.39–0.55
MCV (fl)	69.0	60.0–77.0
WBC (x 10^9/l)	8.3	6.0–15.0
Neutrophils (segmented) (x 10^9/l)	5.5	3.60–12.00
Lymphocytes (x 10^9/l)	1.3	0.70–4.80
Monocytes (x 10^9/l)	1.2	0.0–1.50
Eosinophils (x 10^9/l)	0.3	0.0–1.0
Basophils (x 10^9/l)	0	0.0–0.2
Platelets (x 10^9/l)	325	200–500

Biochemistry	Result	Reference interval
Sodium (mmol/l)	153	139–154
Potassium (mmol/l)	4.1	3.60–5.60
Glucose (mmol/l)	4.9	3.0–5.0
Urea (mmol/l)	6.5	1.7–7.4
Creatinine (μmol/l)	82	30–90
Calcium (mmol/l)	2.81	2.30–3.00
Inorganic phosphate (mmol/l)	1.1	0.90–1.20

▶

Biochemistry	Result	Reference interval
TP (g/l)	65.3	58.0–73.0
Albumin (g/l)	32.0	26.0–35.0
Globulin (g/l)	33.3	18.0–37.0
ALT (IU/l)	295	15–60
AST (IU/l)	12	7–50
ALP (IU/l)	95	20–60
GGT (IU/l)	2	0–8
Urine specific gravity	1.040	

What abnormalities are present?

- 5-fold increase in ALT, but normal AST
- Less than 2-fold increase in ALP and normal GGT.

How would you interpret these results and what are the likely differential diagnoses?

There is:

- A significant rise in ALT, and this is not an age-related finding
- Normal AST (the other hepatocellular marker)
- A less than a 2-fold rise in ALP is insignificant, and GGT is within the reference range.

This most likely a secondary (reactive) hepatopathy and there is unlikely to be any significant liver disease. Most likely, the rise in ALT is related to the periodontal disease.

What further tests would you recommend?

- If there was any doubt, liver function could be assessed by measuring pre- and postprandial serum bile acids before anaesthetizing the patient for dental treatment
- Alternatively, the ALT could be monitored after the dental treatment to ensure resolution. ALT should return to normal within 3–4 weeks
- If the raised ALT persists after dental treatment, then other underlying diseases should be searched for before considering liver biopsy.

Case 2 follows ▶

Case 2

Signalment

7-year-old, spayed female Labrador Retriever.

History

2-month history of poor appetite, increased thirst and weight loss. Sudden onset of jaundice.

Clinical pathology data

Haematology	Result	Reference interval
RBC (x 10^{12}/l)	4.8	5.50–8.00
Hb (g/dl)	10.6	12.0–18.0
HCT (l/l)	0.33	0.39–0.55
MCV (fl)	69.0	60.0–77.0
MCHC (g/dl)	32.1	32.0–36.0
Reticulocytes (x10^9/l)	50	<60
WBC (x 10^9/l)	15.5	6.00–15.00
Neutrophils (segmented) (x 10^9/l)	13.1	3.600–12.00
Lymphocytes (x 10^9/l)	0.9	0.70–4.80
Monocytes (x 10^9/l)	1.4	0.0–1.50
Eosinophils (x 10^9/l)	0.1	0.0–1.0
Basophils (x 10^9/l)	0.0	0.0–0.2
Platelets (x 10^9/l)	235	200–500

Biochemistry	Result	Reference interval
Sodium (mmol/l)	150	139–154
Potassium (mmol/l)	4.9	3.60–5.60
Glucose (mmol/l)	3.4	3.0–5.0
Urea (mmol/l)	1.1	1.7–7.4
Creatinine (µmol/l)	not measurable	30–90
Calcium (mmol/l)	2.2	2.30–3.00
Inorganic phosphate (mmol/l)	1.2	0.90–1.20
TP (g/l)	64.3	58.0–73.0
Albumin (g/l)	19.0	26.0–35.0
Globulin (g/l)	45.3	18.0–37.0
ALT (IU/l)	357	15–60
AST (IU/l)	95	7–50
ALP (IU/l)	220	20–60
GGT (IU/l)	23	0–8
Bilirubin (µmol/l)	157	0–10
Cholesterol (mmol/l)	2.1	3.5–9.0
Urine specific gravity	1.012	

What abnormalities are present?

There is:

- Mild normocytic, normochromic non-regenerative anaemia
- Slight leucocytosis and mature neutrophilia
- Marked hyperbilirubinaemia
- Moderate increase in both hepatocellular (ALT and AST) and cholestatic (ALP and GGT) marker enzymes
- Hypoalbuminaemia and hyperglobulinaemia
- Mild hypocalcaemia
- Low urea concentration
- Hypocholesterolaemia
- Isosthenuric urine specific gravity
- Creatinine could not be measured because severe hyperbilirubinaemia interferes with the colorimetric assay.

How would you interpret these results and what are the likely differential diagnoses?

- The anaemia is mild and likely to be an anaemia of chronic disease
- The WBC pattern probably indicates a stress response, though the neutrophilia may reflect an inflammatory response
- The jaundice is unlikely to be prehepatic in origin as the anaemia is not severe enough to explain the hyperbilirubinaemia
- Posthepatic jaundice is unlikely because of the similar magnitude in the increases in both ALT and ALP and the hypocholesterolaemia
- Changes in serum proteins are consistent with an inflammatory hepatopathy
- Mild hypocalcaemia is likely a reflection of mild hypoalbuminaemia
- Low urea concentration may reflect poor appetite, diuresis and hepatic dysfunction
- The isosthenuric urine is consistent with the history of increased thirst.

A chronic hepatopathy is likely:

- Prolonged history
- Evidence of hepatic damage
- Evidence of hepatic dysfunction (hypoalbuminaemia, hyperbilirubinaemia).

The most likely differentials are:

- Chronic hepatitis
  - Lobular dissecting hepatitis
  - Chronic active hepatitis
  - Copper hepatotoxicosis
- Cholangitis/cholangiohepatitis from ascending biliary infection
- Extensive primary hepatic tumour
  - Hepatocellular carcinoma
  - Biliary carcinoma
- Hepatic lymphoma.

What further tests would you recommend?

- Bile acid measurement is superfluous as hyperbilirubinaemia confirms hepatic dysfunction
- Radiographic and ultrasonographic imaging of the liver
- Assessment of coagulation profile (platelet count, PT, aPTT) and buccal mucosal bleeding time, to check for safety of liver biopsy
- Liver biopsy.

Case 3

Signalment

7-month-old, female entire West Highland White Terrier.

History

Depressed, thin with intermittent vomiting and diarrhoea.

Clinical pathology data

Haematology	Result	Reference interval
RBC (x 10^{12}/l)	4.9	5.50–8.00
Hb (g/dl)	9.1	12.0–18.0
HCT (l/l)	0.27	0.39–0.55
MCV (f/l)	55	60.0–77.0
MCHC (g/dl)	33.8	32.0–36.0
WBC (x 10^9/l)	23.3	6.00–15.00
Neutrophils (segmented) (x 10^9/l)	18.1	3.600–12.00
Lymphocytes (x 10^9/l)	2.9	0.70–4.80
Monocytes (x 10^9/l)	1.4	0.0–1.50
Eosinophils (x 10^9/l)	0.8	0.0–1.0
Basophils (x 10^9/l)	0.1	0.0–0.2
Platelets (x 10^9/l)	398	200–500

Biochemistry	Result	Reference interval
Sodium (mmol/l)	140	139–154
Potassium (mmol/l)	3.9	3.60–5.60
Glucose (mmol/l)	3.4	3.0–5.0
Urea (mmol/l)	0.9	1.7–7.4
Creatinine (µmol/l)	28	30–90
Calcium (mmol/l)	2.9	2.30–3.00
Inorganic phosphate (mmol/l)	1.6	0.90–1.20
TP (g/l)	44.0	58.0–73.0
Albumin (g/l)	21.0	26.0–35.0
Globulin (g/l)	23.0	18.0–37.0
ALT (IU/l)	298	15–60
ALP (IU/l)	301	20–60
Cholesterol (mmol/l)	3.7	3.5–9.0 ▶

Biochemistry *(continued)*	Result	Reference interval
Bilirubin (µmol/l)	2.1	0–10
Urine specific gravity	1.020	

What abnormalities are present?

There is:

- A moderate microcytic anaemia
- Leucocytosis due to a mature neutrophilia
- Hypoproteinaemia associated with hypoalbuminaemia
- Increases in ALT and ALP (five times upper limit of reference range)
- Low urea and creatinine concentrations.

How would you interpret these results and what are the likely differential diagnoses?

- Microcytic anaemia is associated with iron-deficiency anaemia and hepatic disease, especially portosystemic shunting. There is no gross evidence of blood loss. Hypochromasia of the red cells and thrombocytosis, characteristic of blood loss anaemia, are not present
- WBC response is suggestive of a stress response
- Raised ALT (x5) indicates some hepatocellular changes, but not severe hepatocellular damage
- Raised ALP may indicate cholestasis, undocumented steroid administration, or bone growth in a young animal
- Low urea and creatinine can indicate diuresis. Low urea could also indicate hepatic dysfunction, and low creatinine could reflect the dog's poor muscle mass.

The history and lab results are suggestive of:

- Congenital portosystemic shunt, although increases in liver enzymes are typically absent or mild
- Acquired juvenile hepatopathy
  - Lobular dissecting hepatitis
  - Idiopathic juvenile hepatic fibrosis.

What further tests would you recommend?

- Pre- and postprandial bile acids to assess hepatic function in a non-icteric dog. They are likely to be abnormal despite the normal bilirubin, although in congenital PSS a typical pattern of normal pre-prandial and elevated postprandial bile acids is often seen
- If bile acids are normal, assess faecal occult blood as possible cause of iron-deficiency anaemia
- Radiography to assess liver and kidney sizes. Microhepatica and renomegaly are typical of congenital PSS
- Ultrasonography to assess liver size and vasculature
- Portovenography
- Advanced imaging (scintigraphy).

References and further reading

Balkman CE, Center SA, Randolph JF, Trainor D, Warner KL, Crawford MA, Adachi K and Erb HN (2003) Evaluation of urine sulfated and nonsulfated bile acids as a diagnostic test for liver disease in dogs. *Journal of the American Veterinary Medical Association* **222,** 1368–1375

Bunch SE (1993) Hepatotoxicity associated with pharmacologic agents in dogs and cats. *Veterinary Clinics of North America: Small Animal Practice* **23,** 659–670

Center SA (1993) Serum bile acids in companion animal medicine. *Veterinary Clinics of North America: Small Animal Practice* **23,** 625–657

Center SA (1996) Chapters 30 and 32–35 In: *Strombeck's Small Animal Gastroenterology.* Eds: WG Guilford *et al.*, pp. 553–632 and pp. 654–846. WB Saunders, Philadelphia

Center SA, Erb HN and Joseph SA (1995) Measurement of serum bile acid concentrations for diagnosis of hepatobiliary disease in cats. *Journal of the American Veterinary Medical Association* **207,** 1048–1054

Center SA, Manwarren T, Slater MR and Wilentz E (1991) Evaluation of twelve-hour preprandial and two-hour postprandial serum bile acid concentration for diagnosis of hepatobiliary disease in dogs. *Journal of the American Veterinary Medical Association* **199,** 217–226

Chiaramonte D, Steiner JM, Broussard JD, Baer K, Gumminger S, Moeller EM, Williams DA, Shumway R (2003) Use of a C-13-aminopyrine blood test: first clinical impressions. *Canadian Journal of Veterinary Research* **67,** 183–189

Cole TL, Center SA, Flood SN, Rowland PH, Valentine BA, Warner KL and Erb HN. (2002) Diagnostic comparison of needle and wedge biopsy specimens of the liver in dogs and cats. *Journal of the American Veterinary Medical Association* **220,** 1483–1490

Dillon R (1985) The liver in systemic disease – an innocent bystander. *Veterinary Clinics of North America: Small Animal Practice* **15,** 97–117

Hall EJ, Simpson JW and Williams DA (2005) *BSAVA Manual of Canine and Feline Gastroenterology, 2nd edn.* BSAVA Publications, Gloucester

Klomp AEM, van de Sluis B, Klomp LWJ and Wijmenga C (2003) The ubiquitously expressed MURR1 protein is absent in canine copper toxicosis. *Journal of Hepatology* **39,** 703–709

Meyer DJ (1996a) Hepatic tests: reflections of hepatobiliary pathophysiology. WALTHAM Symposium, *Liver Disease. Practical Perspectives,* 8–11

Meyer DJ (1996b) Hepatic pathology. In: *Strombeck's Small Animal Gastroenterology,* ed. WG Guilford *et al.,* pp. 633–653. WB Saunders, Philadelphia

Moeller EM, Steiner JM, Williams DA and Klein PD (2001) Preliminary studies of a canine C-13-aminopyrine demethylation blood test. *Canadian Journal of Veterinary Research* **65,** 45–49

Pembleton-Corbett JR, Center SA, Schermerhorn T, Yeager AE and Erb HN (2000) Serum-effusion albumin gradient in dogs with transudative abdominal effusion. *Journal of Veterinary Internal Medicine* **14,** 613–618

Reyers F, Goddard A and Myburgh E (2001) Re-evaluation of serum uric acid as a liver function test. *Proceedings of the 44th Annual BSAVA Congress,* p. 562

Roth L and Meyer DJ (1995) Interpretation of liver biopsies. *Veterinary Clinics of North America: Small Animal Practice* **25,** 293–303

Rothuizen J, Ubbink GJ, van Zon P, Teske E, van den Ingh TSGAM and Yuzbasiyan-Gurkan V (1999) Diagnostic value of a microsatellite DNA marker for copper toxicosis in West-European Bedlington terriers and incidence of the disease. *Animal Genetics* **30,** 190–194

Sevelius E and Jönsson L (1996) Liver diseases. In: *Manual of Canine and Feline Gastroenterology,* ed. DA Thomas, JW Simpson and EJ Hall, pp. 191–220. BSAVA Publications, Cheltenham

Steiner JM, Willliams DA and Bunch SE (2003) Bile acids diagnostic test believed to contain limitations. *Journal of the American Veterinary Medical Association* **223,** 429

Sterczer A, Meyer HP, Boswijk HC and Rothuizen J (1999) Evaluation of ammonia measurements in dogs with two analysers for use in veterinary practice. *Veterinary Record* **144,** 523–526

Taboada J and Meyer DJ (1989) Cholestasis associated with extrahepatic bacterial infection in five dogs. *Journal of Veterinary Internal Medicine* **3,** 216–221

Trainor D, Center SA, Randolph JF, Balkman CE, Warner KL, Crawford MA, Adachi K and Erb HN (2003) Urine sulfated and nonsulfated bile acids as a diagnostic test for liver disease in cats. *Journal of Veterinary Internal Medicine* **17,** 145–153

Walker MC, Hill RC, Guilford WG, Scott KC, Jones GL and Buergelt CD (2001) Postprandial venous ammonia concentrations in the diagnosis of hepatobiliary disease in dogs. *Journal of Veterinary Internal Medicine* **15,** 463–466

Wang KW, Panciera DL, Al-Rukibat RK and Radi ZA (2004) Accuracy of ultrasound-guided fine-needle aspiration of the liver and cytological findings in dogs and cats: 97 cases (1990–2000). *Journal of the American Veterinary Medical Association* **224,** 75–78

13

Laboratory evaluation of gastrointestinal disease

Alexander J. German and Edward J. Hall

A diagnostic approach to gastrointestinal disease

Laboratory investigations are an important component of the diagnostic approach to gastrointestinal (GI) disease, although in most GI cases they do not provide a definitive diagnosis, and results of other investigations are equally important (Figure 13.1). Nevertheless, laboratory investigations narrow the list of differential diagnoses, and direct further investigation.

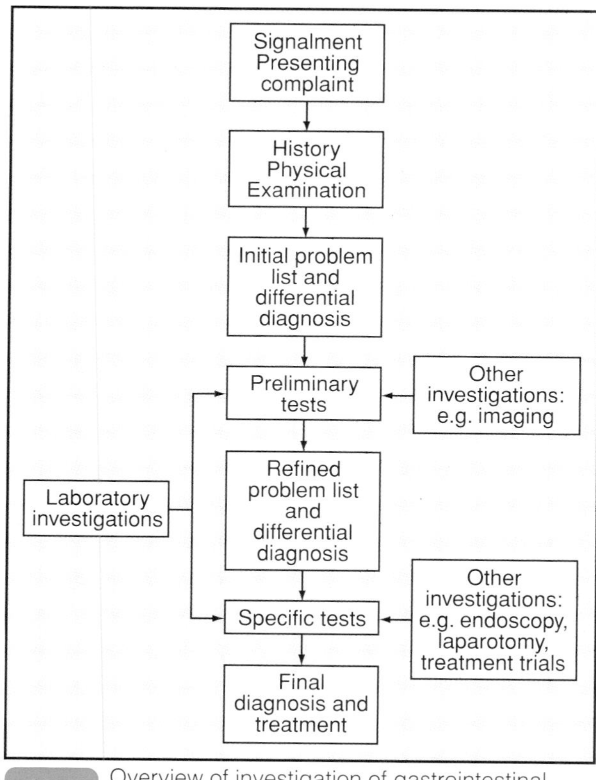

13.1 Overview of investigation of gastrointestinal disorders.

The usual diagnostic approach is first to eliminate diseases not involving the GI tract. It is important to take a full history (Figure 13.2) and to perform a complete physical examination (Figure 13.3). The main clinical signs associated with GI disease are vomiting, diarrhoea, weight loss, haematemesis and melaena.

Patient information
Age Gender Breed
Environmental history
Indoor vs. outdoor Free roaming Scavenging Exposure to parasites Contact with infected animals Recent change of environment Endemic disease area
Past medical history
Vaccination status Worming status Previous abdominal surgery Previous cutaneous mast cell tumour excision Drug history
Progression of clinical signs
Severity Duration Frequency Continuous or intermittent Length of sign-free intervals Moderating influences (improve or worsen signs) – e.g. treatments, diets Order of appearance of signs

13.2 History for cases of gastrointestinal disease.

General
Rule out other systems disease
Oropharynx
Mucous membranes: hydration status; cardiovascular status; anaemia; icterus Tongue: linear foreign body
Cervical region
Thyroid nodule (hyperthyroidism)

13.3 Physical examination for cases of gastrointestinal disease. (continues) ▶

Abdomen
Palpation: effusions; masses; bunching of intestinal loops; foreign bodies; associated pain; faeces; abnormal accumulations of ingesta; lymphadenopathy; diseases of other systems
Auscultation: ileus; borborygmi
Rectal examination
Digital examination: masses; foreign bodies; haemostatic disorders (blood); dehydration
Collection of stool sample: laboratory analysis; melaena
Rectal mucosal scrape: cytology
Cutaneous examination
Poor coat condition, scale: malnutrition
Pruritus: food hypersensitivity
Pedal pruritus: *Uncinaria stenocephala* infection (larval migration)

13.3 (continued) Physical examination for cases of gastrointestinal disease.

For emergency and critical care cases, analysis of samples for an emergency database should be performed at this stage (Figure 13.4), to enable selection of appropriate intravenous fluid therapy and initial treatment. In other cases, it is usually necessary to submit samples for haematological and serum biochemical analyses, full urinalysis and routine faecal analyses (bacteriological and parasitological examination). From this point, further investigations may be necessary, including diagnostic imaging (radiography and ultrasonography), exclusion of exocrine pancreatic insufficiency (EPI) and, ultimately, direct examination of the small intestine (SI) by endoscopy or surgery. This enables collection of tissue samples for histological examination. However, many cases with signs of GI disease are acute, non-fatal and self-limiting, and only require symptomatic support without a definitive diagnosis: detailed investigations are appropriate if systemic signs accompany vomiting and diarrhoea, or signs are unresponsive to symptomatic treatment.

Haematology
Packed cell volume (PCV)
Total protein (refractometer)
Blood smear examination
Biochemistry
Urea
Glucose
Electrolytes
Urinalysis
Dipstick tests
Specific gravity by refractometer
Additional (if available)
Blood gas analysis (acid–base): PCO_2, P_aO_2, HCO_3^-, etc.

13.4 Emergency database.

Vomiting

Vomiting can result from numerous causes (Figures 13.5, 13.6). The first aim is to differentiate vomiting from retching due to expectoration, and from regurgitation (Figure 13.7). Direct examination of the vomitus may assist in diagnosis. The presence of bile, digested blood or acidic contents (pH <5) confirms the material to be vomitus. A urine dipstick can be used to identify bilirubin and pH, for confirmation of bile and acidic contents, respectively. However, the absence of these findings does not exclude the presence of vomiting. If vomiting occurs shortly after eating, then contents will not be acidified, and if intestinal contents are present, the contents may have a pH >6. Bile will only be present if intestinal contents are vomited in addition to gastric contents, and will be absent if there is a pyloric obstruction. Once vomiting has been confirmed, non-GI diseases should be investigated next, and an integrated approach is required to achieve a diagnosis (Figure 13.8).

Gastroenteric causes
Acute gastritis–enteritis:
Infectious
Bacterial
Viral
Parasitic
Haemorrhagic gastroenteritis
Toxic
Gastrointestinal obstruction:
Foreign body
Complete obstruction
Linear
Intussusception
Gastric volvulus
Dietary indiscretion:
Ingestion of inappropriate or spoiled foods
Over-eating
Non-gastroenteric causes
Diseases of other systems:
Pancreatic disease
Hepatic disease
Renal disease
Endocrine disease
(Motion sickness)
CNS disease
Infection, bacteraemia, septicaemia
Drugs:
Chemotherapeutic drugs
Antibacterials (chloramphenicol)
Digitalis
Narcotics
Theophylline
Xylazine
Apomorphine
Toxins
Ethylene glycol
Herbicides
Plants
Organophosphates
Strychnine

13.5 Major causes of vomiting of acute onset.

Gastroenteric disease
Obstructive disease: Foreign objects Intussusception Neoplasia Pyloric stenosis Gastric antral mucosal hyperplasia Chronic partial gastric volvulus Congenital structural abnormalities Inflammatory disease: Inflammatory bowel disease Gastritis Enteritis Colitis Gastrointestinal ulceration, erosion Parasites (e.g. *Physaloptera*)
Non-gastroenteric diseases (systemic diseases stimulating chemoreceptor trigger zone ± vagal afferents)
Pancreatic disease: Pancreatitis Neoplasia Exocrine pancreatic insufficiency Hepatic disease: Chronic hepatitis Portovascular anomaly Neoplasia Hepatocellular dysfunction Toxic Infectious Renal disease Endocrinopathies/metabolic: Hypoadrenocorticism Diabetes mellitus Hyperthyroidism Hypercalcaemia Hypothyroidism CNS disease: Limbic epilepsy Neoplasia Encephalitis Raised intracranial pressure Vestibular disease Cardiac diseases: Heartworm Congestive heart failure

13.6 Major causes of chronic vomiting.

Clinical sign	Vomiting	Regurgitation
Abdominal effort	Marked	None
Signs of nausea	Yes	No
Timing of food ejection	Variable	Variable
Character of food	Undigested, partially digested or digested Bile stained Acid pH	Undigested, 'sausage-shape'
Associated signs	Retching	Dyspnoea Coughing Drooling

13.7 Differentiating vomiting from regurgitation.

Preliminary tests (all cases)
Haematology Serum biochemistry Urinalysis Faecal bacteriology Faecal parasitology Folate and cobalamin (for suspected small intestinal disease)
Additional tests to eliminate non-gastrointestinal diseases
Exocrine pancreatic insufficiency (all cases): Trypsin-like immunoreactivity Tests for pancreatitis (occasional indication): Canine pancreatic specific lipase (PLI) (Trypsin-like immunoreactivity) (Amylase) (Lipase) Endocrinopathies (occasional indication): Adrenocorticotropic hormone (ACTH) stimulation test Total T4/free T4 (cats) Gastrin measurement (for gastrinoma)
Tests specific for gastrointestinal disease
Histopathological assessment of stomach and small intestine (all cases) Cytological assessment (occasional cases)
Additional tests with limited indication
Tests for gastric spiral organisms Histopathological assessment Other
Suggested approach
• Preliminary tests should be performed in all cases • TLI should always be performed to eliminate the possibility of EPI • If abdominal pain is present and/or there is supportive evidence of pancreatitis on diagnostic imaging, tests for pancreatitis should be performed • Older cats should be tested for hyperthyroidism • An ACTH stimulation test should be considered (in both species), especially if supportive electrolyte changes are present • Gastrin measurement should be considered if a pancreatic mass is detected and/or hypertrophic gastropathy is detected on gastric biopsy specimens • Assuming non-gastrointestinal diseases have been eliminated, biopsy specimens should be procured for histopathological assessment • Exploratory laparotomy should be considered subsequent to endoscopic biopsy, if results do not fit or response to chosen therapy is poor • Additional tests listed have rare indications, and further advice should be sought prior to their consideration

13.8 Approach to laboratory testing for chronic vomiting.

Diarrhoea

There are numerous causes of diarrhoea in dogs and cats (Figure 13.9). Again, a thorough history is necessary to identify the origin of the diarrhoea, although SI diseases can provoke large intestine (LI) diarrhoea and some cases have signs consistent with both SI and LI disease (Figure 13.10). Physical findings may be helpful (see Figure 13.3). Given that signs of malabsorption are non-specific, a trypsin-like immunoreactivity (TLI) test should always be performed to eliminate the possibility of EPI. The general approach to chronic diarrhoea is summarized in Figure 13.11.

Gastrointestinal disease
Primary small intestinal disease
Primary large intestinal disease
Dietary-induced: Food poisoning Gluttony Sudden change of diet
Gastric disease: Achlorhydria (rare) Dumping syndromes (rare)
Pancreatic disease: Exocrine pancreatic insufficiency Pancreatitis Pancreatic neoplasia
Liver disease: Hepatocellular failure Intrahepatic and extrahepatic cholestasis
Non-gastrointestinal disease
Polysystemic infections: Dogs: distemper, leptospirosis, infectious canine hepatitis Cats: Feline infectious peritonitis (FIP), feline leukaemia virus (FeLV), feline immunodeficiency virus (FIV)
Endocrine disease: Hypoadrenocorticism Hyperthyroidism (rare in dogs only) Hypothyroidism APUDomas (gastrinoma/Zollinger–Ellison syndrome) (rare)
Renal disease: Uraemia Nephrotic syndrome
Miscellaneous: Toxaemia: pyometra; peritonitis Congestive heart failure Immune-mediated disease Metastatic neoplasia Various toxins and drugs

13.9 Causes of diarrhoea.

Clinical sign	Small intestine	Large intestine
Tenesmus	Rare	Common
Frequency	2–3 x normal/day	>3 x normal/day
Urgency	Uncommon	Common
Stool volume	Increased	Multiple small volumes
Mucus	Rare	Common
Fresh blood	Uncommon, melaena	Common
Vomiting	Occasionally	Uncommon
Weight loss	Common	Rare

13.10 Differentiation of small from large intestinal signs.

Preliminary tests (all cases)
Haematology Serum biochemistry Urinalysis Faecal bacteriology Faecal parasitology Folate and cobalamin
Additional tests to eliminate non-gastrointestinal diseases
Exocrine pancreatic insufficiency (all cases): Trypsin-like immunoreactivity Tests for pancreatitis (occasional indication): Canine pancreatic specific lipase (Trypsin-like immunoreactivity) (Amylase) (Lipase) Endocrinopathies (occasional indication): ACTH stimulation test Total T4/free T4 (cats)
Tests specific for gastrointestinal disease
Histopathological assessment of stomach and small intestine (all cases) Cytological assessment (occasional cases)
Additional tests with limited indication
Tests of intestinal function Protein loss: faecal α_1- proteinase inhibitor (α_1-PI) Malabsorption: sugar probe tests, breath hydrogen testing Permeability: sugar probe tests Immune function: serum IgA concentrations
Suggested approach
• Preliminary tests should be performed in all cases • TLI should always be performed to eliminate the possibility of EPI • If abdominal pain is present and/or there is supportive evidence of pancreatitis on diagnostic imaging, tests for pancreatitis should be performed • Older cats should be tested for hyperthyroidism • An ACTH stimulation test should be considered (in both species), especially if supportive electrolyte changes are present • Assuming non-gastrointestinal diseases are eliminated, biopsy specimens should be procured for histopathological assessment • Exploratory laparotomy should be considered subsequent to endoscopic biopsy, if results do not fit or response to chosen therapy is poor • Additional tests listed have rare indications, and further advice should be sought prior to their consideration

13.11 Approach to laboratory testing for chronic diarrhoea.

Weight loss

There are numerous differential diagnoses for weight loss in dogs and cats (Figure 13.12), but GI diseases are common causes. In some situations, intestinal disease can present with weight loss and no other localizing signs (e.g. vomiting or diarrhoea). A TLI test should be performed early in the investigation to rule out EPI before more involved investigations of the intestine are attempted. The general laboratory approach to the diagnosis of weight loss is similar to that described for chronic diarrhoea (see Figure 13.11).

Physiological
Excessive demand for energy with respect to intake:
Temperature
Exercise
Growth
Gestation/lactation
Inadequate intake/consumption:
Dietary factors
Intake problems
Poor quality food
Insufficient amount
No food
Pathological
Transfer of food:
Cranial/cervical injury
Dysphagia
Swallowing disorders
Regurgitation
Vomiting
Maldigestion:
Exocrine pancreatic insufficiency
Bile salt deficiency
Cholestasis
Hepatocellular dysfunction
Specific intestinal enzyme deficiency e.g. lactase
Malabsorption:
Inflammation (inflammatory bowel disease)
Infiltration
Neoplasia
Amyloidosis (rare)
Lymphangiectasia
Systemic diseases:
Hepatic disease
Cardiac disease
Diabetes mellitus
Renal disease
Cancer cachexia
Hypoadrenocorticism
Hyperthyroidism
Muscle wasting:
Myopathy
Neuropathy

13.12 Causes of weight loss in dogs and cats.

Ingestion of blood
Oral haemorrhage
Nasal haemorrhage
Pharyngeal haemorrhage
Haemoptysis
GI erosion/ulceration
Metabolic:
Uraemia
Hepatic disease
Inflammatory:
Gastritis
Enteritis
Haemorrhagic enteritis
Ulceration
Neoplastic:
Smooth muscle tumours
Lymphoma
Epithelial cell tumours
Paraneoplastic:
Mast cell tumours
Hypergastrinaemia
Vascular/ischaemic:
(Gastrinomas/APUDomas)
Arteriovenous fistula
Aneurysms
Hypovolaemia
Hypoadrenocorticism
Thrombosis
Infarction
Foreign bodies:
Reperfusion injury
Drug-induced:
NSAIDs
Haemostatic disorders
Primary:
Thrombocytopenia
Thrombocytopathy
von Willebrand's disease
Secondary:
Factor deficiencies
Coumarin toxicity
Mixed:
Disseminated intravascular coagulation

13.13 Causes of haematemesis and melaena.

Haematemesis and melaena

Possible causes of haematemesis and melaena are shown in Figure 13.13. Haematological parameters may confirm the presence of chronic blood loss and enable the severity of blood loss to be determined; they may be typical of chronic blood loss associated with iron deficiency (i.e. microcytosis, hypochromasia, thrombocytosis). Associated iron deficiency can be confirmed by a variety of laboratory tests (see Chapter 4). Serum biochemical parameters provide information on underlying causes of GI blood loss such as renal disease, hepatic disease and endocrinopathies. If GI haemorrhage is suspected but melaena has not been noted, faecal occult blood can be measured. However, whilst both faecal occult blood and assessment of iron status might confirm blood loss, they provide no information as to the underlying cause.

Routine diagnostic procedures

Preliminary investigations usually include routine haematological and serum biochemical analyses and urinalysis. Other general tests include routine faecal analyses (initially parasitology and bacteriology). Such investigations should be used in conjunction with other clinical interventions in an integrated diagnostic approach (see Figure 13.1).

Routine haematology

Red cell parameters

An increase in haematocrit, especially in conjunction with increased serum total protein, is often a marker of dehydration. This is typically associated with acute GI diseases and, depending on severity, may indicate the need for parenteral fluid therapy. The most marked haemoconcentration is typically seen in acute haemorrhagic gastroenteritis (HGE). The increase in haematocrit is marked, while total protein is usually normal or increased, but proportionately lower than would be expected from the corresponding increase in haematocrit.

Anaemia can be associated with GI disorders, and may indicate intestinal blood loss or chronic inflammation associated with intestinal disease. The anaemia associated with acute blood loss is usually markedly regenerative, assuming there has been sufficient time for a bone marrow response to occur. Characteristics that suggest chronic, iron-deficient, blood-loss anaemia include microcytosis, decreased red cell haemoglobin and thrombocytosis. Anaemia may also accompany other disorders causing secondary GI signs, such as chronic renal failure and endocrinopathies (e.g. hypoadrenocorticism, hypothyroidism), and microcytic anaemia can accompany some hepatic disorders.

See Chapter 4 for further details on red cell parameters.

White cell parameters

In GI disorders with an inflammatory aetiology, such as inflammatory bowel disease (IBD), neutrophilia with or without a left shift may be seen. Such changes are usually mild, and do not assist in differentiating GI inflammation from inflammation in other organs. Marked neutrophilia may be associated with severe inflammation, for example in diseases associated with bacteraemia/septicaemia, particularly when the mucosal barrier is severely compromised, i.e. mucosal ulceration is present. A degenerative left shift could also be seen in these circumstances. Neutrophilia is also a common finding in feline infectious peritonitis (FIP), and may be associated with anaemia and lymphopenia.

Eosinophilia may be associated with parasitism, dietary sensitivity and eosinophilic gastroenteritis (see Chapter 5). However, an eosinophil count slightly above the reference range established for healthy dogs of most breeds can be normal in German Shepherd Dogs. If eosinophilia is genuine, non-GI causes, such as ectoparasitism and hypoadrenocorticism, need to be excluded before considering food allergy or eosinophilic gastroenteritis.

If leucopenia is seen in cases of acute gastroenteritis, parvovirus infection should be suspected, as these enteric viruses also attack the rapidly dividing cells of the bone marrow. Cytotoxic drugs may also cause GI signs and leucopenia (see Chapter 5). Lymphopenia can be seen in lymphangiectasia, but other laboratory abnormalities would be expected, e.g. panhypoproteinaemia and hypocholesterolaemia. Circulating atypical lymphocytes are uncommon, but may be associated with lymphoproliferative disorders affecting the GI tract.

Routine serum biochemistry

A full panel of routine biochemical tests is recommended in all cases, primarily to identify dysfunction of other body systems, including renal, hepatic and endocrine disorders, which may present with GI signs.

Albumin and globulin

Decreases in protein concentrations may be noted in GI disease, particularly chronic intestinal diseases (protein-losing enteropathies (PLEs); Figure 13.14). Protein-losing gastropathies are rare. In most cases of PLE, panhypoproteinaemia is noted, in contrast to hepatic dysfunction or protein-losing nephropathy (PLN) where hypoalbuminaemia alone is typical. Historical and physical examination findings and the results of other laboratory analyses (e.g. haematological analysis, urinalysis) assist in differentiating causes of hypoalbuminaemia, so that PLN, liver dysfunction and other causes (e.g. blood loss, vasculitis, burns) can relatively easily be ruled out. Serum protein concentrations are insensitive indicators of GI protein loss, and tests that are more sensitive include measurement of α_1-proteinase inhibitor (α_1-PI) in faeces (see below).

Lymphangiectasia
Primary: Intestinal Generalized Secondary: Venous hypertension, e.g. right-sided cardiac failure, hepatic cirrhosis
Infectious
Parvovirus Salmonellosis
Structural
Intussusception
Neoplasia
Lymphoma
Inflammation
Inflammatory bowel disease: lymphoplasmacytic enteritis; eosinophilic enteritis; granulomatous enteritis
Endoparasitism
Giardia (*Ancylostoma*)
Gastrointestinal haemorrhage
Haemorrhagic enteritis Neoplasia Ulceration

13.14 Protein-losing enteropathies.

Increased protein concentrations usually indicate dehydration if the accompanying clinical picture fits. Hyperglobulinaemia can be seen in some GI disorders: those associated with intense inflammation (e.g. Basenji enteropathy), some infections (e.g. FIP) and lymphoproliferative diseases (lymphoma, myeloma).

See Chapter 7 for further details on serum proteins.

Sodium and potassium

Electrolyte abnormalities may be a feature of persistent vomiting, intestinal obstruction and secretory diarrhoea. Electrolyte measurements, ideally in association with blood-gas analysis, are important in determining the most appropriate type of fluid for initial replacement. Hypokalaemia is a common finding in GI disease as a result of anorexia and GI losses. Hyponatraemia and hyperkalaemia are suggestive of hypoadrenocorticism, which can cause GI signs. Other potential laboratory abnormalities in hypoadrenocorticism include azotaemia, hypercalcaemia, non-regenerative anaemia, lymphocytosis and eosinophilia. However, similar electrolyte changes (i.e. hyponatraemia and hyperkalaemia) can be associated with primary GI disease, especially with *Salmonella* and whipworm infections, and therefore an adrenocorticotropic hormone (ACTH) stimulation test should always be performed to confirm hypoadrenocorticism.

See Chapter 8 for further details on electrolyte abnormalities.

Liver enzymes

Liver enzymes routinely measured in small animals are broadly characterized as hepatocellular/leakage enzymes (most often alanine aminotransferase (ALT)) and biliary/cholestatic markers (most often alkaline phosphatase (ALP)) (see Chapter 12). Mild to moderate increases in the serum activities of these enzymes may be seen in primary GI disease. Such changes are likely to represent a reactive hepatopathy caused by delivery of luminally derived antigens, endotoxins and bacteria to the liver from the GI tract via the portal circulation. This is probably associated with permeability alterations of the mucosal barrier accompanying many GI diseases. It can, therefore, be difficult to differentiate primary GI disease with a secondary hepatopathy from primary hepatopathies associated with vomiting and diarrhoea. Measurement of serum bile acids can be helpful, although some GI diseases can be associated with mild increases in bile acid concentrations. In cats with IBD, moderate to marked increases in liver enzyme activities may suggest significant hepatic pathology as well as GI disease, since simultaneous inflammatory changes in related organs (SI, liver and pancreas) are recognized.

Cholesterol

Increased serum cholesterol concentrations are rarely associated with primary GI disease, but may be seen in diseases that cause secondary GI signs (e.g. endocrinopathies and renal, hepatic or pancreatic disease). Hypercholesterolaemia can be associated with PLN, which is also an important differential diagnosis for hypoalbuminaemia. As cholesterol is synthesized in the liver, low serum cholesterol concentrations are typically associated with diseases involving hepatocellular dysfunction, but hypocholesterolaemia may also be a feature of primary intestinal diseases, most notably in diseases that cause fat malabsorption. Marked hypocholesterolaemia is most consistently associated with lymphangiectasia.

Urea and creatinine

Low serum concentrations of urea, relative to serum creatinine, are sometimes seen in animals with GI signs caused by portosystemic shunts (PSSs) or severe liver dysfunction because of failure to convert ammonia to urea. Elevated urea and creatinine concentrations can be associated with prerenal (e.g. dehydration), intrinsic renal or postrenal azotaemia. Numerous diseases that cause vomiting and diarrhoea cause dehydration and, therefore, are associated with elevated urea and creatinine concentrations. Given that digestion and assimilation of protein leads to increased urea synthesis in the liver, elevated urea can also be associated with recent dietary protein intake. By a similar mechanism, gastric or upper intestinal haemorrhage can also increase urea concentrations.

Calcium and magnesium

Low total calcium and magnesium concentrations can be seen in cases with PLE. The reduction in total serum calcium can, in part, be explained by the concurrent hypoalbuminaemia, and a correction equation can be used to estimate its contribution in dogs (see Chapter 8). However, ionized hypocalcaemia and ionized hypomagnesaemia have been reported in some cases of PLE (Kimmel *et al.*, 2000), and other mechanisms are likely to be involved, such as vitamin D, calcium and magnesium malabsorption.

Serum bile acids

Serum total bile acid concentration is a reflection of the enterohepatic circulation of bile acids, and elevated concentrations are associated with hepatic dysfunction, biliary obstruction or portosystemic shunting (see Chapter 12). Hepatopathies secondary to a number of diseases, including those affecting the GI tract, can cause milder increases.

Folate and cobalamin

Serum folate and cobalamin assays are routinely available for dogs and cats and are widely used for the investigation of GI cases. However, many factors can affect concentrations of both folate and cobalamin (Figure 13.15). Therefore, clinicians should interpret

	Cobalamin	Folate
Factors increasing concentrations	High dietary intake Parenteral supplementation	High dietary intake Parenteral supplementation Intestinal bacterial metabolism Low intestinal pH Exocrine pancreatic insufficiency
Factors decreasing concentrations	Dietary deficiency Ileal disease Ileal resection Intestinal bacterial metabolism Exocrine pancreatic insufficiency	Dietary deficiency (rare) Proximal or diffuse small intestinal disease Drugs, e.g. sulfasalazine Low intestinal pH

13.15 Factors influencing serum folate and cobalamin concentrations.

the results with care. Currently, the main value of these tests is in documenting the presence of malabsorption rather than small intestinal bacterial overgrowth (SIBO).

Malabsorption: Folate is predominantly absorbed in the proximal SI, whilst cobalamin, bound to intrinsic factor, is absorbed by a specific carrier mechanism in the distal SI (Figure 13.16). Therefore, a subnormal concentration of folate suggests proximal small intestinal disease, a low cobalamin concentration can occur in diseases involving the distal intestine, and both low folate and cobalamin may be seen if diffuse disease is present. These tests are limited by their lack of specificity for particular primary diseases, but the presence of malabsorption can be confirmed and the need for vitamin supplementation assessed.

Cobalamin deficiency is documented more commonly as a sequel to small intestinal disease, particularly in cats, and systemic metabolic consequences have been recognized (Simpson *et al.*, 2001). Although any GI diseases (and some pancreatic diseases) can potentially cause a decreased serum cobalamin concentration in cats, most severe decreases have been documented in association with alimentary lymphoma. In Giant Schnauzers, a specific intrinsic factor–cobalamin receptor deficiency has been reported, which is associated with severe cobalamin deficiency (Fyfe *et al.*, 1991). If cobalamin deficiency is documented, parenteral supplementation with cobalamin is recommended or the response to treatment of the underlying GI disease may remain suboptimal. Decreased folate concentrations can also be seen secondary to malabsorption. If documented, supplementation (with oral folic acid) can be considered.

Small intestinal bacterial overgrowth: SIBO can occur secondary to many disorders. The aetiology of 'primary' or idiopathic SIBO has recently been re-evaluated, and the term idiopathic antibiotic-responsive diarrhoea (ARD) is preferred for these cases. The features of these two disorders are summarized in Figure 13.17. Folate and cobalamin are still used to diagnose SIBO in companion animals. Given that many bacterial species synthesize folate, whilst others can bind cobalamin, increased numbers of small intestinal bacteria may increase serum folate concentrations, decrease serum cobalamin concentrations, or do both.

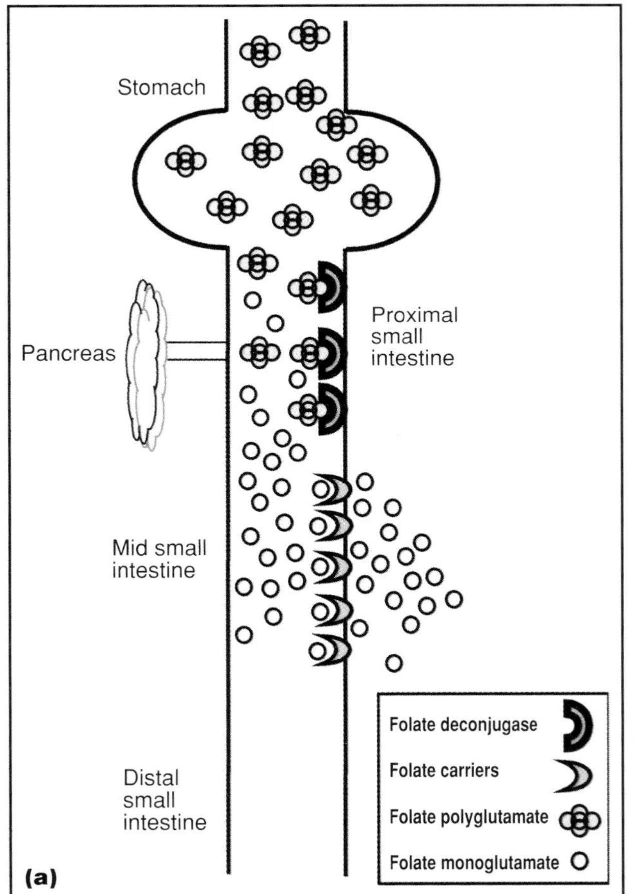

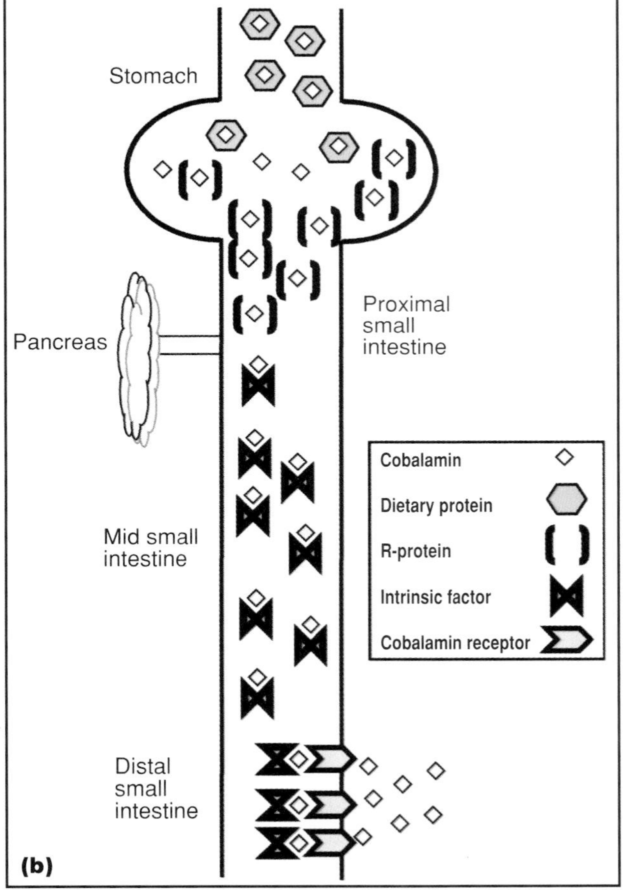

13.16 Assimilation of folate and cobalamin. (a) Dietary folate is present in food as a conjugated form, folate polyglutamate. This conjugate is digested by folate deconjugase, an enzyme on the microvillar membrane, which removes all but one residue. The resultant folate monoglutamate is taken up via specific carriers in the mid small intestine. (b) Following ingestion, cobalamin is released from dietary protein in the stomach. It then binds to non-specific binding proteins (e.g. 'R-proteins'). In the small intestine cobalamin transfers onto intrinsic factor (IF), which is synthesized by the stomach (dog) and pancreas (dog and cat). Cobalamin–IF complexes pass along the intestine until the distal small intestine, where cobalamin is transported across the mucosa and into the portal circulation.

	SIBO	ARD
Causes	Always occurs secondary to underlying disease: Exocrine pancreatic insufficiency Other causes of malabsorption? Partial obstruction Decreased gastric acid production (e.g. drug therapy, gastric surgery)	Idiopathic
Signalment	Cats and dogs Any age or gender Any breed	Dogs only Young dogs of either sex German Shepherd Dogs predisposed
History	Predominantly small intestinal diarrhoea, although other signs possible Signs of underlying disease? If partial obstruction, could be cyclical pattern	Predominantly small intestinal diarrhoea and weight loss/failure to gain weight
Physical examination	Signs of underlying disease If partial obstruction, may have abnormalities on abdominal palpation	Varies from no signs to poor body condition
Preliminary laboratory tests	Signs of underlying disease? No specific findings	No specific findings
Faecal analysis	Negative	Negative
Folate / cobalamin	Variable results	Variable results
Diagnostic imaging	Findings specific to underlying disease Evidence of partial obstruction	No specific findings
Intestinal biopsy	Not required	Normal or mild inflammatory change only
Recommended method of diagnosis	Diagnose underlying disease: e.g. TLI for EPI; ultrasonography for partial obstruction	Rule out all other GI diseases (see Figure 13.11) Response to antibacterial trial Remission often requiring antibacterials

13.17 Comparison of small intestinal bacterial overgrowth (SIBO) and antibiotic-responsive diarrhoea (ARD). (EPI: exocrine pancreatic insufficiency; TLI: trypsin-like immunoreactivity.)

However, measurement of serum folate and cobalamin concentrations has poor sensitivity and specificity for canine SIBO, and results do not correlate with quantitative duodenal juice culture (Walkely and Neiger, 2000). Some studies suggest that concurrently increased folate and decreased cobalamin concentrations are most specific for SIBO, but this has not been universally documented (German *et al.*, 2003). Moreover, neither changes in folate nor cobalamin (nor both) can reliably discriminate dogs with idiopathic ARD (idiopathic SIBO) from those with other aetiologies (German *et al.*, 2003). Thus, measurement of folate and cobalamin concentrations is of limited value in the diagnosis of SIBO/ARD.

Routine urinalysis

Routine urinalysis, involving biochemical assessment (dipstick analysis), assessment of specific gravity by refractometer and sediment analysis (see Chapter 10) is an important component of the preliminary diagnostic database and should be performed in all cases. Abnormalities can sometimes be identified on sediment analysis that assist in differentiating causes of vomiting and diarrhoea, e.g. ammonium biurate crystals would be suggestive of a PSS or hepatocellular dysfunction. Identification of proteinuria confirmed by a raised urine protein:creatinine ratio indicates the presence of PLN in cases of hypoalbuminaemia, although in Soft-Coated Wheaten Terriers, concurrent PLE and PLN can occur.

Serology

In cats, serological tests for feline leukaemia virus (FeLV) and feline immunodeficiency virus (FIV) should be considered, especially in cases presenting with chronic GI signs. Coronavirus serology may also be useful in some cases. Serology for infectious diseases, such as parvovirus, can sometimes be useful, although it is often complicated by titres derived from vaccination and the need to document rising titres to prove active infection.

Tests of endocrine disease

Routine haematological, serum biochemical and urinalysis findings can often increase the index of suspicion for endocrinopathies as the cause of GI signs. More specific diagnostic tests are then required (see Chapters 17 and 18).

Faecal analysis

Faecal examinations are an important part of the investigation of GI disease, and, in general practice, samples are regularly submitted for identification of parasites and bacteriological culture. Other investigations that are occasionally beneficial include description of faecal characteristics, direct faecal smear examination, assessment of parvovirus antigen and assessment of rectal cytology.

Character of faeces

Information on faecal character can be derived from the history or by direct examination of a stool sample (faecal material can be collected by digital rectal examination). The presence of diarrhoea can be confirmed, and the likely site of pathology can be deduced. If fresh blood or mucus is present, a large intestinal disorder is most likely, whilst changes in colour or volume more likely suggest small intestinal disease, with or without malabsorption.

Direct faecal smear

On occasion, a direct smear of fresh faeces can provide useful information. Unstained wet mounts can be used to identify protozoal trophozoites, such as *Giardia*. Identification of *Trichomonas*, *Tritrichomonas*, *Pentatrichomonas*, *Balantidium*, and *Entamoeba* species may be significant for LI diarrhoea. Further, given that enterotoxin production by *Clostridium perfringens* is a potential cause of diarrhoea, Diff-Quik-stained faecal smears can be examined for clostridial endospores. If large numbers of clostridial endospores (>5 per 100x oil immersion field) are detected, *C. perfringens* enterotoxicosis is possible; however, the correlation between sporulation and toxin elaboration is controversial since endospores can be found in stool samples from normal dogs (Marks *et al.*, 2002). Other diagnostic tests, such as detection of *C. perfringens* enterotoxin antigen by ELISA or reverse passive latex agglutination, are required to confirm diagnosis (see below).

A direct smear of faeces can also be used to detect fungal elements if fungal diseases are endemic in the area, although rectal cytology may be more appropriate (see below). *Cryptosporidium* spores can be detected if a direct smear is stained with an acid-fast stain. However, this organism is more commonly assessed using special faecal flotation techniques (see below). Faeces can also be stained for undigested starch granules (Lugol's iodine), fat globules (Sudan stain) and muscle fibres (Wright's or Diff-Quik stains) and their presence may indicate malabsorption, but these tests are unreliable.

Faecal concentration methods

Although direct examination of faecal samples can identify endoparasites, faecal concentration methods are usually more rewarding. Faeces can be 'concentrated' either with flotation (using sugar solution or zinc sulphate) or sedimentation techniques. The methods are described in Figure 13.18. Sugar solutions detect the majority of parasites (Figure 13.19), including coccidia and *Cryptosporidium*. Formalin–ether sedimentation techniques are suitable for metazoan ova (roundworms, hookworms and whipworms), or if a zoonotic infection (such as *Strongyloides*) is suspected. Zinc sulphate flotation is recommended to detect *Giardia* oocysts. A direct smear, sedimentation or the Baermann technique can identify larvae of *Strongyloides*, although the latter technique is more commonly used to detect lungworm (*Angiostrongylus vasorum* or *Oslerus osleri*) larvae.

As with any diagnostic test, interpretation is as important as methodology. Identification of a parasite does not necessarily prove causation, particularly in cases presenting with chronic GI signs. Most cestodes and nematodes do not cause clinical signs in adult dogs; ascarids can cause clinical signs in immature animals, but rarely cause significant clinical disease in adults. Further, coccidia and many other protozoans

Faecal flotation

1. Place 2–3 g faeces in 15 ml of solution: sugar solution (454 g sugar + 355 ml water) or 33 % zinc sulphate solution (33 g zinc sulphate in 100 ml distilled water, specific gravity 1.18).
2. Mix thoroughly.
3. Strain through tea strainer or cheesecloth. If there is excess fat after filtering, the sample can be mixed with 2–3 ml ethyl acetate or ether, centrifuged and the supernatant discarded.
4. Place in 15 ml polypropylene centrifuge tube.
5. Centrifuge at 1500 rpm for 5 minutes.
6. Place coverslip on top, touching the meniscus, for 3–4 minutes (alternatively use bacteriology loop).
7. Place coverslip on microscope slide and examine. Stain with Lugol's iodine for zinc sulphate flotation, if desired.

Faecal sedimentation

Water

1. Mix sample of fresh faeces with water and strain once to remove debris.
2. Allow sample to settle for between 30 minutes and 2 hours.
3. Place the sediment on a microscope slide, place a coverslip over the sediment and examine.

Formalin ether

1. Mix sample of fresh faeces with water and strain once to remove debris.
2. Centrifuge strained faeces and resuspend in 9 ml of 5% formalin solution.
3. Add 3 ml of ethyl acetate and shake vigorously.
4. Recentrifuge and discard the debris at the formalin–ethyl acetate interface.
5. Examine the sediment as above.

13.18 Methodologies for performing faecal examination for parasites.

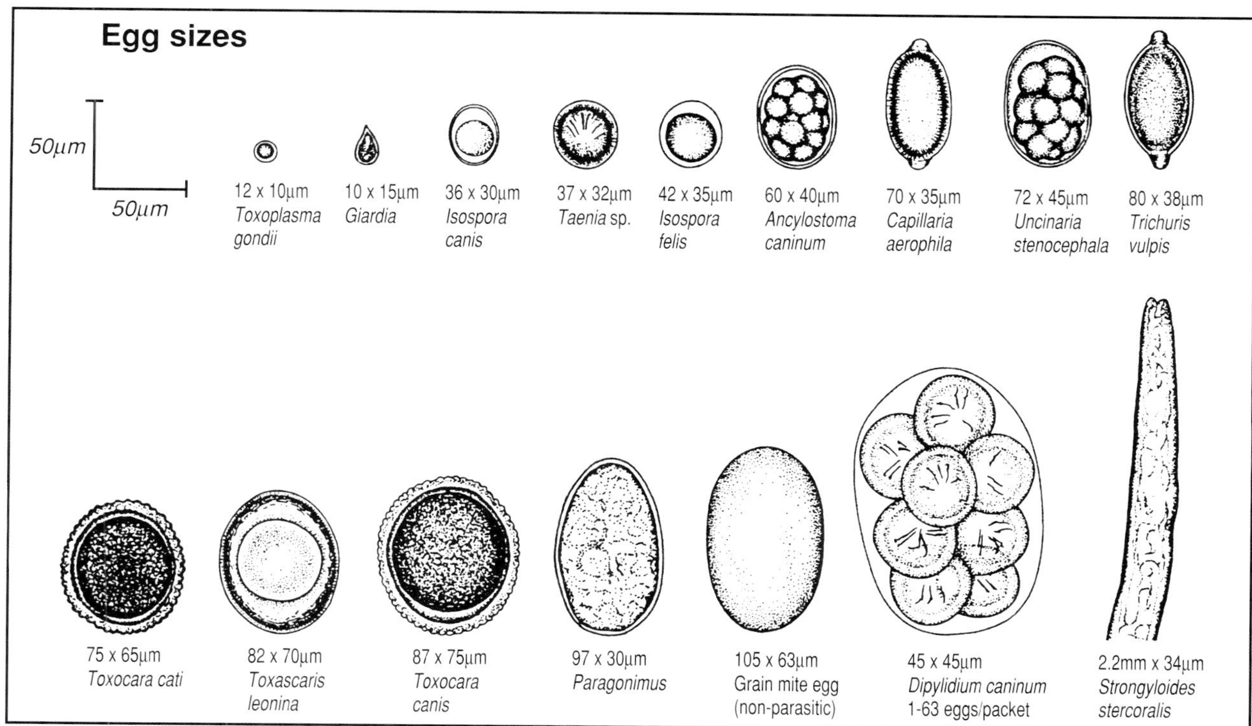

13.19 Faecal parasitology. (Courtesy of Hoechst–Roussel–Agri Vet Company, USA; permission requested)

are usually incidental findings on faecal examination. In contrast, parasites such as hookworms, whipworms, *Giardia* and *Cryptosporidium* are more often associated with clinical disease. Nevertheless, the presence of an underlying disease may allow such parasites to colonize the GI tract. Therefore, all positive findings should be interpreted in the light of the clinical presentation. If any doubt exists as to whether a particular agent is causal, a treatment trial is indicated.

Bacteria

Bacterial culture of faeces is most commonly indicated in animals with acute GI signs, particularly diarrhoea, and is especially important if cases present with haemorrhagic diarrhoea, pyrexia, an inflammatory leucogram, or if neutrophils are identified on rectal cytology (see below). Bacterial culture is also often performed in preliminary diagnostic screening of all cases with chronic GI signs. Use of inappropriate techniques is a common reason for false negatives, and samples of fresh faecal matter, rather than swabs, should be submitted promptly to laboratories that are equipped to culture the main pathogenic bacteria. However, given that many of the bacteria classed as pathogens can also be found in normal individuals, all results must be interpreted in light of the clinical presentation. Some laboratories recommend routine culture of faecal samples on the basis that changes in predominant populations of bacteria correlate with disease. However, there are currently no published studies to support such an approach, and the effect of postal delay on the relative growth rates of different organisms is often ignored. Further, whilst faecal flora might be representative of colonic bacterial populations, they correlate poorly with the small intestinal flora, and so are *not* suitable for the diagnosis of SIBO. Therefore, targetted evaluation for potential pathogens, e.g. *Salmonella*, *Campylobacter*, *Clostridium perfringens* and *Clostridium difficile*, by culture on selective media should be performed. *Escherichia coli* can also be cultured from most faecal samples but only certain strains are pathogenic, and it is more appropriate to use molecular probes to detect pathogenicity markers (enteropathogenic *E. coli* (EPEC)) (Turk *et al*., 1998). Molecular testing for EPEC is commercially available from the Royal Veterinary College, UK.

Given that all potential pathogens can be isolated both from healthy animals and those with clinical signs, determining the significance of positive results can be difficult. As it is a potential zoonosis, the isolation of *Salmonella* is invariably significant. However, the decision to treat a particular animal depends upon its individual circumstances because a carrier state may develop after therapy.

For *Campylobacter*, examination of a stained faecal smear for slender, seagull-shaped bacteria can yield a presumptive diagnosis. A positive diagnosis by culture is more likely from fresh faeces, because the bacteria are fragile. If shipment to a laboratory is required, Amies transport medium (containing charcoal) is recommended. *Campylobacter* are usually identified to genus rather than species level, and it is assumed that most isolates are potential pathogens such as *C. jejuni*. However, if identified to the species level, many are actually from a different species, including *C. upsaliensis*, for which pathogenicity is not established. Inappropriate treatment in these circumstances may allow the development of antimicrobial resistance.

Clostridia are common isolates from the faeces of healthy cats and dogs, and disease is thought to be more closely associated with periodic enterotoxin production. *Clostridium difficile* is responsible for antibiotic-associated pseudomembranous colitis in humans and has been incriminated as a cause of chronic diarrhoea in dogs. Enterotoxin-producing *C. perfringens* has also been associated with acute and chronic GI signs. As sporulation has been assumed to coincide with enterotoxin elaboration, examination of a Diff-Quik-stained faecal smear for 'safety-pin' shaped sporulating *C. perfringens* (>5 per 100x oil immersion field is supportive) has been suggested as a simple screening test. However, because endospores can be seen in the faeces of healthy dogs as well as those with clinical signs, their presence does not invariably confirm a diagnosis, and some studies have suggested that detection of the enterotoxin is more indicative of disease (Marks *et al.*, 2002). *C. perfringens* enterotoxin can be detected in faeces by reverse passive latex agglutination or by ELISA. The ELISA gives fewer false-positive and false-negative results, but the toxin may be found in healthy dogs. The test is available in the UK through some commercial laboratories.

Giardia

Trophozoites can sometimes be identified in very fresh stained or unstained faecal smears, but oocysts are best found by repeated zinc sulphate flotation. A commercially available ELISA and a rapid immunochromatographic method can be used to detect *Giardia* in faeces. However, whilst convenient to perform, they do not necessarily have greater accuracy than performing zinc sulphate flotation on three consecutive samples. Alternative approaches include examining duodenal fluid for *Giardia* trophozoites, although this has again not been shown to be superior to faecal methods. Molecular probes are available for detection of *Giardia* in humans, but these have yet to be adapted for small animals.

Parvovirus antigen

The diarrhoea caused by most viruses is usually acute and self-limiting with no need for a positive diagnosis. Electron microscopy has been used in the past to identify characteristic viral particles (e.g. rotavirus, coronavirus, parvovirus), but this is not used in clinical practice. The only virus that requires a specific diagnosis is parvovirus, and a faecal ELISA is commercially available. Indications for the test are listed in Figure 13.20. Fresh faeces samples should be submitted, ideally taken 24–36 hours after the onset of clinical signs. False-negative results can arise if samples are taken too early in the course of the disease, so the test should be repeated after 36–48 hours if clinical signs are still consistent with parvovirus. False-negative results can also occur if samples are taken too late in the disease process because shedding decreases after the first week, although the patient is still contagious. Theoretically, false-negative results can also occur due to interference from coproantibody, whilst weak false positives occur between 5 and 15 days after vaccination with a modified live vaccine.

Signalment and history
Young animal
Unvaccinated animal
Exposure or potential exposure to parvovirus (e.g. affected in-contact animal or contaminated environment)
Clinical signs
Acute/peracute gastrointestinal signs with or without:
Haematemesis, melaena or severe haematochezia
Pyrexia
Leucopenia or neutropenia

13.20 Indications for performing faecal parvovirus antigen ELISA.

Occult blood

The test is used to search for GI bleeding that is not apparent grossly as melaena or haematochezia. Haemorrhage can potentially occur at any level of the GI tract, and the test is sensitive enough to detect 2 ml blood per 30 kg body weight. Given that the test merely detects haemoglobin, false-positive results can arise from the ingestion of diets containing meat (and blood) and even, in some cases, fresh uncooked vegetables due to the presence of interfering peroxidases. Therefore, the patient must be fed a meat-free diet for at least 72 hours before samples are obtained.

Rectal cytology

Samples can be taken for cytological analysis by mildly abrading the rectal wall with a gloved finger after rectal examination. The material is then rolled onto a microscope slide and the smear stained. The test is easy to perform and non-invasive, but results are most often negative. Such examinations are of limited used for small intestinal disease, and are instead most appropriate for diseases involving the large intestine and, particularly, the rectum. Increased numbers of neutrophils may be suggestive of a bacterial problem and indicate the need for faecal culture. Clostridial endospores and fungal/oomycete elements (*Histoplasma*, *Aspergillus*, *Candida*, *Pythium*) may also be identified. However, perhaps the most specific results come from palpable masses within the rectum, from which samples can more readily be taken.

Analysis of cells and tissue specimens

Histopathology

Histopathology of gastric and intestinal biopsy specimens remains the gold standard for the diagnosis of GI disease (Figure 13.21), although it has many limitations. Biopsy specimens can be normal by light microscopy in almost half of cats and dogs with chronic GI disease, suggesting that either many diseases have a functional rather than morphological abnormality or that sampling problems have occurred. Another major problem with reliance on histopathological diagnoses is poor agreement between histopathologists (Willard *et al.*, 2002). Standardized criteria are currently being established as a means of improving agreement. However, the primary clinician should always interpret

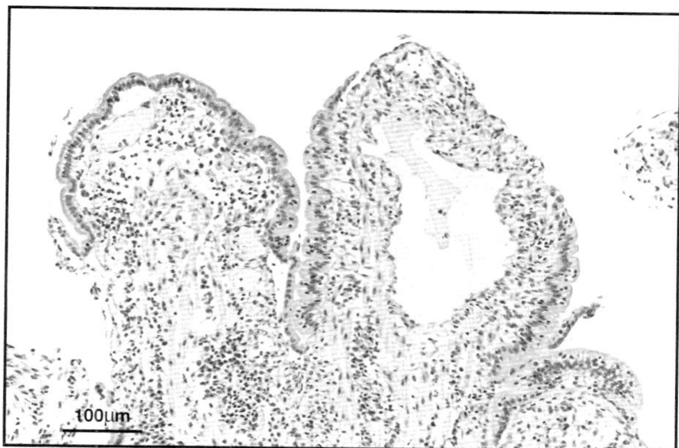

13.21 Photomicrograph of biopsy specimen from the duodenum of an 8-year-old neutered male crossbred dog with diarrhoea, ascites and severe panhypoproteinaemia (albumin 10 g/l, reference interval: 25–31 g/l; globulins 20 g/l, reference interval: 27–40 g/l). There is evidence of villous atrophy, epithelial erosions and mild lacteal dilatation. There is a variable, mixed inflammatory cell infiltrate within the mucosa. These findings would be consistent with a mixed inflammatory bowel disease. (HE stain; original magnification x10) (Courtesy of R. Fox, University of Liverpool.)

results cautiously in light of clinical presentation, and results should be questioned if the histopathological diagnosis does not fit the clinical picture. Tissue samples collected by endoscopy are superficial, small and often distorted. In some cases, therefore, full-thickness biopsy specimens may be required subsequent to endoscopy, if results are not representative.

Cytology

Cytology of endoscopic biopsy squash preparations or mucosal brushings (Figure 13.22) can be a useful adjunct to diagnosis of GI disease (Jergens *et al.*, 1998). Brush cytology provides superior information; it complements, rather than replaces, histopathology as it does not provide architectural information. Its greatest benefit is likely to be in the differentiation of severe lymphocytic–plasmacytic enteritis from alimentary lymphoma, as the cellular and nuclear characteristics of malignancy can be better assessed.

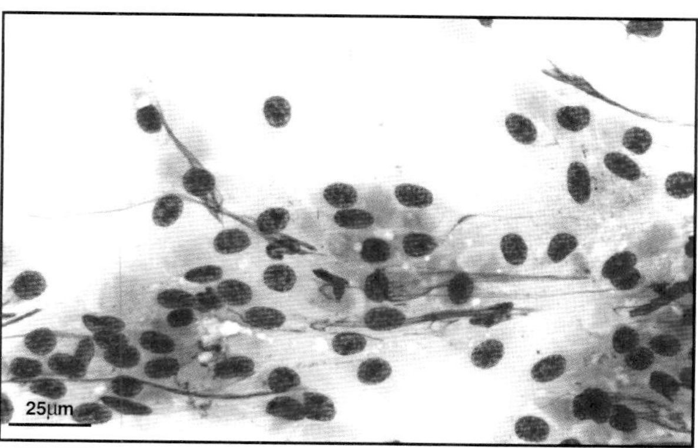

13.22 Cytological specimen (collected by cytology brush) from the duodenum of a 6-year-old neutered male Staffordshire Bull Terrier with chronic vomiting and diarrhoea. The preparation demonstrates clumps of normal epithelial cells. Streaks of nuclear material are due to rupture during smearing. The histopathological specimens from this case were unremarkable, and the dog responded to dietary management, suggesting an adverse reaction to food. (Rapid Romanowsky stain; original magnification x 40.)

Diagnostic procedures with occasional application

Numerous tests have been developed in an attempt to investigate GI diseases non-invasively. However, many of these tests are not commercially available, many have not properly been validated and many are more applicable to referral or research institutions rather than general practice. What follows is a summary of the main tests available, and their indications. However, these tests are not recommended for routine use at present.

Further tests for chronic vomiting

The main additional tests reported for cases that present with chronic vomiting are assessment of gastric lipase activity, assessment for gastric spiral organisms and measurement of serum gastrin.

Gastric lipase immunoreactivity

An assay for gastric lipase has been developed (Steiner *et al.*, 2002), but measurement of serum lipase activity did not aid in the diagnosis and differentiation of different gastric diseases. Further work would be required before such tests are adopted for companion animals. Gastric diseases can sometimes elevate serum pancreatic lipase activity, but rarely to the levels that are diagnostic for pancreatitis.

Tests for gastric spiral organisms

Tests used to assess the presence of gastric spiral organisms (GSO), include examination of biopsy specimens, light or electron microscopy, brush cytology, the rapid urease test, urea breath tests, PCR assay and serological assessment. Most of these methods have been modified from techniques used for detection of *Helicobacter pylori* in humans. However, the species of GSO seen in companion animals differ from that in humans, and they may be commensal organisms in the majority of healthy dogs and cats. These organisms could produce clinical disease through complex pathogenetic mechanisms, but their true significance as pathogens remains to be established.

Histopathology: The most routinely available test is histopathological examination of gastric biopsy material. Visualization is improved if special staining procedures are performed, e.g. Warthin–Starry silver stain. Some histopathologists comment on the presence of GSO within gastric glands, but there is no evidence to suggest that this correlates with pathogenicity. The presence of an inflammatory (lymphocytic–plasmacytic) infiltrate within the mucosa and lymphoid nodular hyperplasia may suggest an associated gastritis. Although similar findings have been documented in studies involving experimental infection of dogs and cats with *Helicobacter* organisms, the histopathological changes do not correlate with the presence of clinical signs. It is recommended that the documentation of GSO in biopsy material be interpreted with caution.

Other techniques for identifying GSO:

- In a research setting, electron microscopy and PCR are required to identify the exact species of GSO that is present
- The urease test is an indirect marker for the presence of 'pathogenic' GSO. Pathogenicity of GSO (at least in humans) correlates with their ability to produce urease, which neutralizes gastric acid by splitting urea into ammonia and bicarbonate. A mucosal biopsy specimen (usually endoscopic) is incubated in test medium; the production of ammonia by urease causes a pH-dependent colour change
- Urea breath test protocols are a method by which urease production can be assessed non-invasively, but such protocols are rarely used in practice.

Gastrin measurement

Gastrin is normally secreted by G-cells in the gastric and duodenal mucosa, and stimulates the secretion of gastric acid by parietal cells. On occasion, it is necessary to measure gastrin in clinical cases, and this can be performed either by radioimmunoassay or ELISA (using cross-reactive antibodies to human gastrin). Special handling is required to prevent gastrin degradation, and the test is currently limited to amenable hospital laboratories or research institutions.

Many gastric diseases can elevate serum gastrin concentrations, including chronic gastritis, gastric dilatation–volvulus and pyloric stenosis; increases also occur in chronic renal failure and secondary to drug administration (e.g. antacids, acid-blocking drugs and glucocorticoids). Therefore, routine use of the test is not helpful. The main indication for serum gastrin measurement is in cases of suspected gastrinoma, and marked increases (e.g. >500 pg/ml) are usually seen. Given that high gastrin concentrations could also arise if hyposecretion of gastric acid occurs (particularly where H_2 antagonists or proton pump inhibitors are in use), concurrent measurement of gastric luminal pH has been recommended. If gastrinoma is suspected, but only moderate increases in serum gastrin concentration are documented, a provocative test could be considered (Altschul *et al.*, 1997). Endoscopy and biopsy may provide further supportive evidence for a gastrinoma, by demonstrating gastric mucosal hypertrophy and ulceration.

Further tests for chronic diarrhoea

Alternative tests for small intestinal bacterial overgrowth

The only widely available tests for SIBO in dogs are folate and cobalamin concentrations (see above). However, given the problems associated with their use, attempts have been made at validating other methods. The current diagnostic gold standard for SIBO is quantitative bacterial culture of duodenal juice, whilst other 'indirect' methods include serum unconjugated bile acids and breath hydrogen analysis.

Quantitative bacterial culture of duodenal juice: Duodenal juice can be collected at duodenoscopy with sterile tubing, or at exploratory celiotomy by needle aspiration through the intestinal wall. However, collection of sufficient sample without blood, tissue and bile contamination can be difficult. Routine bacteriological methods are used to detect and quantify bacterial species. Isolates can be typed to the genus or species level, and values are obtained for total bacterial numbers and for numbers of aerobes and obligate anaerobes.

Unfortunately, there are limitations with the use of quantitative culture of duodenal juice (German *et al.*, 2003). The main concern is that large intra-individual variation exists in duodenal juice culture results; one report documented a seven log-unit difference between bacterial counts obtained on two separate occasions from the same animal (Delles *et al.*, 1994). Further, healthy dogs have been documented with small intestinal bacterial populations in excess of the suggested 'normal' upper limit (10^5 colony forming units/ml). A recent study suggested that the use of quantitative bacterial culture of duodenal juice does not aid in decision making for cases of GI disease (German *et al.*, 2003). The routine diagnostic use of duodenal juice bacterial culture is not recommended.

Serum unconjugated bile acids: Bile acids are synthesized and conjugated in the liver and subsequently excreted into the intestine via the biliary tract. Certain intestinal bacterial species deconjugate bile acids, which then are absorbed by the small intestine, and escape enterohepatic recycling by the liver. Therefore, in theory, increases in small intestinal bacterial numbers might result in increases in serum unconjugated bile acids (SUBA). Gas chromatography-mass spectrometry methods have been developed and validated for the major canine unconjugated bile acids (lithocholic acid, ursodeoxycholic acid, dexoycholic acid, chenodexoycholic acid and cholic acid) (Melgarejo *et al.*, 2000), and a value for total SUBA is most often used in diagnosis. Measurement of canine unconjugated bile acids (UBA) is commercially available in the USA and, since UBA are stable, no special handling requirements are required. Preliminary work suggested that increased SUBA concentrations were sensitive and specific for canine SIBO, although a recent study questioned their utility (German *et al.*, 2003). SUBA concentrations correlate poorly with quantitative bacteriology, and increased SUBA concentrations could not reliably discriminate dogs with idiopathic ARD from those with other GI diseases. Although test sensitivity can be increased if multiple (four to five) samples are taken, this makes the test too costly and impractical for routine use. Test sensitivity for human SIBO is improved by measuring postprandial increases in SUBA concentrations, and such an approach may prove useful in the future for dogs. More work is required to clarify the use of such markers for the investigation of GI diseases.

Breath hydrogen: Hydrogen breath tests have also been advocated for assessment of SIBO, either in a fasted state or after administration of a test meal. However, protocols have not been universally accepted and correlation with quantitative bacterial culture is poor (Walkley and Neiger, 2000). Therefore, breath hydrogen analysis remains a research technique.

Other tests for SIBO: A number of tests for intestinal bacterial metabolites have been devised for diagnosis of human SIBO; examples include the nitrosonaphthol test, urinary indican excretion, bacterial release of sulfapyridine from sulfasalazine and bacterial release of *p*-amino benzoic acid (PABA) from a bile salt conjugate (PABA-UDCA). However, none of these is currently used in companion animals.

Tests of gastrointestinal function

The main functions of the GI tract are assimilation of nutrients and immune integrity (immune responsiveness and immunological tolerance). Efficient assimilation of nutrients requires adequate digestive and absorptive function, and normal GI motility. Immune integrity requires appropriate functions of the immune system and adequate mucosal barrier function. Given that the clinical consequences of GI disease are usually the result of disruption to one or many of these mechanisms, methods have been developed to provide direct information on GI functionality. Numerous methods have been developed to assess absorptive function, protein absorption or loss, permeability and immune function. However, despite the promise that many research techniques show, few have been successfully adapted for clinical diagnosis. Further, since these tests rarely provide an aetiological diagnosis, they do not obviate the need for histopathological assessment. Therefore, none is currently recommended for routine use.

Malabsorption

The only widely available tests for detection of malabsorption are measurement of serum vitamins (folate and cobalamin – see above). Historically, tests that have been used to document malabsorption include the fat absorption test, the oral glucose absorption test, the starch digestion test and the D-xylose absorption test. However, all such methods require multiple blood samples or urine collection and are insensitive. More recently, protocols for breath hydrogen analysis have been described with potential use in the diagnosis of malabsorption. Breath hydrogen analysis has limited availability, and has not been widely adopted.

GI protein loss

GI protein loss is usually assessed by measuring serum protein concentrations (see above). However, these tests are insensitive and cannot detect early or mild disease because concentrations only decline once the capacity for hepatic production is overcome. Historically, intestinal protein loss has been detected by measuring the faecal loss of ^{51}chromium-labelled albumin. However, clinical application of this test is limited by the fact that the compound is radioactive. Therefore, this procedure is rarely used clinically, but remains the standard by which other tests are judged.

Faecal α_1-proteinase inhibitor (α_1-PI) concentration: In human gastroenterology, faecal α_1-PI is a reliable marker of GI protein loss. A canine-specific ELISA for this marker has recently been developed at Texas A&M University. α_1-PI is a serum protein with a molecular weight similar to albumin and intestinal protein loss will, therefore, lead to loss of both proteins at a similar rate. However, in contrast to albumin, α_1-PI is relatively resistant to proteolysis and thus can be measured in the faeces. Preliminary work has suggested that it is valuable for the diagnosis of PLE (Melgarejo *et al.*, 1998), and may prove to be a more sensitive marker than serum albumin concentrations for the detection of early disease (Murphy *et al.*, 2003). However, the assay is invalidated by the presence of blood in the faecal stool; digital rectal evacuation of faeces causes enough mucosal abrasion to increase faecal α_1-PI concentrations and invalidate the result. To improve diagnostic accuracy, three fresh faecal samples should be collected in a 48-hour period, and then shipped on ice to the laboratory. No UK laboratory currently offers the test, so its use is limited.

Intestinal permeability and absorptive function

Intestinal permeability: Intestinal permeability is an index of mucosal barrier function and is assessed by measuring unmediated uptake of non-digestible probe markers. Tests utilize a probe that is not metabolized after permeation; after absorption via the paracellular route (an index of permeability) the probe is measured in plasma or urine. ^{51}Cr-EDTA was used in original studies, but is not practical for routine clinical use. Non-absorbable sugars (e.g. lactulose or *o*-methyl-D-glucose) can be used as an alternative; when disrupted barrier function is present, increased amounts can be absorbed and detected either in plasma or urine. However, variability arises due to non-mucosal factors including gastric emptying rate, intestinal transit and completeness of urine collection (if the probe is measured in urine).

Absorptive function: If a sugar probe is chosen, that is normally completely absorbed via transcellular pathways (e.g. rhamnose or xylose), the efficiency of absorption can be assessed. Pathological processes that reduce the surface area for absorption (e.g. villus atrophy), will decrease the amount of test probe absorbed and hence that which appears in plasma or urine. Again, non-mucosal factors cause variability in results.

Combined tests: Variability caused by non-mucosal factors can be eliminated by concurrently measuring the absorption of two probes with different pathways of absorption (e.g. lactulose/rhamnose, xylose/*o*-methyl-D-glucose). Calculation of their excretion ratio eliminates variability from extramucosal factors, since both probes should be affected equally. Sensitivity is increased when decreased surface area and increased permeability are present concurrently. Again, either urine or plasma can be assayed.

GI immune function

There are three main indications for testing immune function: assessing immune competence; assessing for food allergy; and assessing for the presence of GI inflammation.

Immune integrity: IgA is the principle secretory immunoglobulin within the GI system and, theoretically, IgA deficiency could predispose to disease. There have been occasional reports of IgA deficiency in dogs, but it is unlikely that IgA deficiency plays an important part in predisposing to disease in the majority of dogs and cats, and routine assessment is not recommended. Further, there are currently no commercial laboratories in the UK that offer this service.

The main circumstances when assessment of IgA concentrations could be considered would be in young individuals suffering from repeated infections at body surfaces (mucosae and skin). Young animals have lower IgA concentrations than adults, so an appropriate age-matched control range should be used. Serum IgA concentrations provide a global assessment of IgA status, and are diagnostic if concentrations are absent, but correlation with mucosal concentrations within the GI tract is poor. Whole gut lavage is the only recommended method for assessment of GI immunoglobulins in humans, but is rarely performed in companion animals due to technical difficulties. Some studies have assessed faecal IgA concentrations but marked intra-individual variation and the fact that levels correlate poorly with total intestinal production mean this method is not recommended. More work is required before the routine measurement of IgA concentrations can be recommended.

Food hypersensitivity: Antigen-specific serum antibodies (IgE or IgG) to food components can be measured *in vitro* and a number of laboratories now offer this commercially. However, although tests are easy to perform, results do not correlate with actual clinical reactions in patients. Further, such food-specific antibodies can also be present in normal individuals. Therefore, such tests are not currently recommended.

Inflammation: Numerous methods have been described for assessing the role of the immune system in GI disease. These include immunohistochemistry and flow cytometry for mapping the distribution of mucosal immune cell populations (German *et al.*, 2001; Zentek *et al.*, 2002), and reverse transcriptase polymerase chain reaction (RT-PCR) for assessing cytokine mRNA (German *et al.*, 2000). However, none of the techniques described is yet appropriate to apply to clinical diagnosis.

Other recent studies have measured serum acute phase proteins (APPs), and increases in some markers (e.g. C-reactive protein) have been documented in samples from dogs with IBD (Jergens *et al.*, 2003). APPs are non-specific markers of inflammation, so these tests alone are not diagnostic for IBD. However, IBD indices (scoring systems for disease activity) are used widely in human IBD, and preliminary work in dogs has been encouraging (Jergens *et al.*, 2003). In combination, APPs and IBD indices may provide a non-invasive means of assessing disease severity and for monitoring response to treatment.

Case examples

Case 1

Signalment

8-year-old male, neutered crossbred dog.

History

4-week history of diarrhoea, weight loss and occasional vomiting. Abdominal distension detected on physical examination, otherwise unremarkable.

Clinical pathology data

Haematology	Result	Reference interval
RBC (x 10^{12}/l)	4.07	5.40–8.00
Hb (g/dl)	10.5	12–18
HCT (l/l)	0.28	0.35–0.55
MCV (fl)	69.0	65–75
MCHC (g/dl)	37.0	34–37
WBC (x 10^9/l)	17.8	6.0–18.0
Neutrophils (segmented) (x 10^9/l)	16.3	3.00–12.00
Lymphocytes (x 10^9/l)	0.49	0.80–3.80 ▶

Haematology *(continued)*	Result	Reference interval
Monocytes (x 10^9/l)	0.07	0.10–1.80
Eosinophils (x 10^9/l)	0.77	0.10–1.20
Basophils (x 10^9/l)	0.00	0.00–0.10
Platelets (x 10^9/l)	654	200–500

Biochemistry	Result	Reference interval
Sodium (mmol/l)	146.0	140–153
Potassium (mmol/l)	5.30	3.80–5.30
Chloride (mmol/l)	108.0	99–115
Glucose (mmol/l)	6.1	3.5–5.5
Urea (mmol/l)	6.8	3.5–6.0
Creatinine (μmol/l)	73.0	60–100
Calcium (mmol/l)	1.8	3.2–6.5 ▶

Case 1 continues ▶

Case 1 continued

Biochemistry *(continued)*	Result	Reference interval
Inorganic phosphate (mmol/l)	1.32	0.80–2.00
TP (g/l)	30.0	57.0–78.0
Albumin (g/l)	10.0	23.0–31.0
Globulin (g/l)	20.0	27.0–40.0
ALT (IU/l)	35	7–50
ALP (IU/l)	90	0–100
Cholesterol (mmol/l)	1.8	3.2–6.5

Faecal analysis	Results
Bacterial culture	Negative for *Campylobacter*, *Salmonella* or *Clostridium*
Parasitological examination	Negative for all parasites

What abnormalities are present?

Haematology

- Mild normocytic normochromic anaemia
- Mature neutrophilia
- Lymphopenia
- Thrombocytosis.

Biochemistry

- Severe panhypoproteinaemia
- Hypocalcaemia
- Hypocholesterolaemia.

How would you interpret these results and what are the likely differential diagnoses?

The mature neutrophilia most likely represents a 'stress' leucogram, since there were no signs to suggest hyperadrenocorticism, and exogenous glucocorticoids had not been administered. They may also reflect an inflammatory reponse. Lymphopenia could also be related to stress although chylothorax, chyloabdomen, lymphangiectasia or lymphoproliferative diseases would also be possible.

The mild anaemia (thrombocytosis is non-specific) could suggest blood-loss anaemia, which would normally be regenerative. Alternatively, the anaemia could represent anaemia of chronic disease. A reticulocyte count would help to clarify whether the anaemia was regenerative or not.

The major differentials for severely decreased serum protein concentrations would be decreased hepatic synthesis, protein-losing enteropathy (PLE) and protein-losing nephropathy (PLN). Blood loss cannot explain the hypoproteinaemia because, although anaemia is present, it is only mild and out of proportion to the hypoproteinaemia. PLE is most likely since this most often results in hypoalbuminaemia and hypoglobulinaemia, whilst PLN and decreased hepatic synthesis usually result in hypoalbuminaemia alone. However, neither renal nor hepatic disease can be completely discounted, and further tests (e.g. urinalysis and hepatic function testing) are required. The severe hypoalbuminaemia probably accounts for the ascites since, if albumin concentrations are below about 15 g/l, animals are at risk of developing abdominal effusions or subcutaneous oedema.

The hypocalcaemia is probably due to the hypoalbuminaemia, since the protein-bound fraction of calcium will be low. A formula can be used to correct for the degree of hypoalbuminaemia (see Chapter 8), to determine whether decreased albumin concentrations are to blame. Measurement of plasma ionized calcium concentrations would provide a more accurate assessment of the significance of this hypocalcaemia. Hypocholesterolaemia can result from either hepatic dysfunction or intestinal malabsorption.

What further tests would you recommend?

- Measurement of fasting and postprandial bile acid concentrations to assess liver function.
- Urinalysis and assessment of urine protein:creatinine ratio to look for evidence of PLN.
- Measurement of serum folate and cobalamin concentrations to assess for possible malabsorption.
- Abdominocentesis could also be performed to confirm the presence of ascites and determine the nature of the fluid. This might help to determine the pathophysiological mechanism, e.g. a transudate would probably be related to the hypoalbuminaemia.
- Plasma ionized calcium concentrations could also be measured, since this represents the active fraction.

Further clinical pathology data

Biochemistry	Result	Reference interval
Fasting bile acids (μmol/l)	1.8	0–15.0
Postprandial bile acids (μmol/l)	2.6	0–15.0
TLI (ng/ml)	18	<5
Folate (ng/ml)	2.4	3.5–8.5
Cobalamin (ng/l)	115	215–500
Ionized calcium (mmol/l)	0.96	1.12–1.40

Urine analysis	Result	Reference interval
pH	6.5	5.5–7.5
SG	1.038	1.001–1.070
Protein	-ve	
UP:C	0.18	<1
Blood	-ve	–
Glucose	-ve	–
Ketones	-ve	–
Deposit	Occasional RBC	

What abnormalities are present?

Biochemistry

- Low serum folate concentrations
- Hypocobalaminaemia
- Ionized hypocalcaemia.

Urinalysis

- No significant abnormalities detected.

How would you interpret these results and what are the likely differential diagnoses?

The normal bile acid stimulation test and absence of proteinuria make hepatic dysfunction and PLN unlikely. The normal TLI concentration excludes EPI. Therefore, the most likely cause of the clinical signs and laboratory analyses is intestinal disease with associated PLE. The most likely differential diagnoses for PLE are inflammatory bowel disease, lymphangiectasia and alimentary lymphoma. Further, there have been recent reports of PLE in association with crypt dilatation/abscessation but the underlying mechanism is not known. Intestinal histoplasmosis would be possible if in an endemic area.

The low folate and cobalamin concentrations suggest intestinal malabsorption in addition to PLE in this case.

Ionized hypocalcaemia is present but, at this level, is unlikely to cause clinical signs. Nevertheless, hypoalbuminaemia is not the

Case 1 continues ▶

Case 1 continued

only cause of the low total calcium concentration previously noted. The low ionized calcium is most likely related to malabsorption of calcium; this is dependent on vitamin D, which can also be low in cases of malabsorption.

What further tests would you recommend?

- Abdominocentesis could still be performed but, given that the site of pathology has now been determined, it is unlikely to contribute further useful information
- Diagnostic imaging may assist in establishing a diagnosis. Ultrasonography would confirm the presence of ascites and allow targeted aspiration of fluid (if necessary). The intestinal tract could be assessed subjectively and objectively (measurement of intestinal wall thickness). Other abdominal structures (e.g. liver, kidney, pancreas, spleen) could also be visualized to confirm that no other abnormalities were present elsewhere
- The most important step to establish a diagnosis would be intestinal biopsy, which could be performed either at endoscopy or exploratory celiotomy. The latter is more likely to give the definitive diagnosis since lymphoma and lymphangiectasia can sometimes be missed on endoscopic biopsy. However, it carries additional risk in this patient, given the severe hypoalbuminaemia.

Case 2

Signalment

15-week-old female crossbred dog (unvaccinated).

History

48-hour history of vomiting and severe haemorrhagic diarrhoea; a 24-hour history of generalized seizures. On physical examination: depressed, pale mucous membranes, mild pain on abdominal palpation, approximately 10% dehydrated.

Clinical pathology data

Haematology	Result	Reference interval
RBC (x 10^{12}/l)	3.84	5.40–8.00
Hb (g/dl)	9.5	12.0–18.0
HCT (l/l)	0.25	0.35–0.55
MCV (fl)	65.7	65–75
MCHC (g/dl)	37.7	34–37
WBC (x 10^9/l)	2.0	6.0–18.0
Neutrophils (segmented) (x 10^9/l)	0.12	3.00–12.00
Lymphocytes (x 10^9/l)	1.86	0.80–3.80
Monocytes (x 10^9/l)	0.02	0.10–1.80
Eosinophils (x 10^9/l)	<0.01	0.10–1.20
Basophils (x 10^9/l)	<0.01	0.00–0.10
Platelets (x 10^9/l)	246	200–500

Biochemistry	Result	Reference interval
Sodium (mmol/l)	119.0	140–153
Potassium (mmol/l)	3.48	3.80–5.30
Glucose (mmol/l)	5.0	3.5–5.5
Urea (mmol/l)	5.6	3.5–6.0
Creatinine (μmol/l)	68.0	60–100
Calcium (mmol/l)	1.88	3.2–6.5
Inorganic phosphate (mmol/l)	1.49	0.80–2.00
TP (g/l)	31.0	57.0–78.0
Albumin (g/l)	15.0	23.0–31.0
Globulin (g/l)	16.0	27.0–40.0
ALT (IU/l)	44	7–50
ALP (IU/l)	346	0–100
Cholesterol (mmol/l)	3.8	3.2–6.5

What abnormalities are present?

Haematology

- Normocytic normochromic anaemia
- Severe leucopenia, largely due to severe neutropenia.

Biochemistry

- Panhypoproteinaemia
- Hypocalcaemia
- Hyponatraemia
- Hypokalaemia
- Increase ALP concentrations.

How would you interpret these results and what are the likely differential diagnoses?

Care should be exercised in interpreting all of these values, because adult rather an age-matched reference range is quoted. Healthy dogs of equivalent age to the patient are likely to have mild reductions in red cell mass and proteins, and increases in calcium, inorganic phosphate and ALP compared to the reference range. This probably explains the increased ALP and contributes to the apparent anaemia and hypoproteinaemia.

The severe neutropenia could be caused by consumption of neutrophils (e.g. overwhelming sepsis, immune-mediated destruction) or decreased production (secondary to: infections, e.g. parvovirus, ehrlichiosis; bone marrow toxicity, e.g. oestrogen, drug toxicity; bone marrow neoplasia; myelopthisis; immune-mediated destruction of precursors). Increased destruction is unlikely, given the lack of left shift; there is no history of drug use, and bone marrow neoplasia is unlikely given the age. The types of *Ehrlichia* that cause bone marrow suppression are not endemic to the UK. Given that the dog is unvaccinated and has compatible clinical signs, parvovirus infection is most likely, although overwhelming sepsis and immune-mediated destruction cannot be excluded completely.

In light of the haemorrhagic nature of the diarrhoea, the mild anaemia most likely represents blood loss. The full extent of the anaemia may not yet be evident, because the history is short, and insufficient time has elapsed to allow complete redistribution of fluids between body compartments. Further, there has been insufficient time to determine whether or not the anaemia is regenerative (usually takes 3–5 days). Sequential blood samples, which included a reticulocyte count, would be the best way to determine the kinetics of anaemia in this case.

The possible decreased serum protein concentrations can result from decreased synthesis (hepatic insufficiency, inadequate intake, malabsorption), sequestration (body cavity effusion, vasculopathy), increased loss (protein-losing enteropathy or nephropathy, cutaneous loss (e.g. burns), blood loss) or dilution. With respect to the severe haemorrhagic diarrhoea, the most probable causes are either blood loss or gastrointestinal protein loss, or a combination.

The hypocalcaemia is most likely due to the hypoproteinaemia since 40% of calcium is protein-bound. Measurement of plasma ionized calcium concentrations would be required to provide a more accurate assessment of the significance of this hypocalcaemia.

Case 2 continues ▶

Case 2 continued

Changes in sodium are primarily due to changes in free water distribution (e.g. loss or gain). Given the presence of hypovolaemia in this case (based on history and physical examination), the most likely explanation is increased loss of sodium (with water) from gastrointestinal tract. In light of the acute onset, the hyponatraemia may well explain the seizures.

Other possible causes of hyponatraemia include increased loss via the kidneys, hypoadrenocorticism, or third-space loss (e.g. pancreatitis, peritonitis, etc). A pseudohyponatraemia has also been reported with hyperlipidaemia (not present here).

The hypokalaemia is mild in comparison with the hyponatraemia. Hypokalaemia can result from decreased intake, translocation (extracellular to intracellular), or increased loss (gastrointestinal tract, urinary tract etc). In this case, hypokalaemia has probably occurred secondary to the severe gastrointestinal signs.

What further tests would you recommend?

- The presence of parvovirus antigen could be confirmed by performing a faecal ELISA
- Measurement of fasting and postprandial bile acid concentrations to assess liver function
- Urinalysis to exclude renal protein
- Plasma ionized calcium concentrations could also be measured, since this represents the active fraction.

References and further reading

Altschul M, Simpson KW, Dykes NJ, Mauldin EA, Reubi JC and Cummings JF (1997) Evaluation of somatostatin analogues for the detection and treatment of gastrinoma in a dog. *Journal of Small Animal Practice* **38,** 286–291

Delles EK, Willard MD, Simpson RB, Fossum TW, Slater M, Kolp D, Lees GE, Helman R and Reinhart G (1994) Comparison of species and numbers of bacteria in concurrently cultured samples of proximal small intestinal fluid and endoscopically obtained duodenal mucosa in dogs with intestinal bacterial overgrowth. *American Journal of Veterinary Research* **55,** 957–964

Fyfe JC, Giger U, Hall CA, Jezyk PF, Klumpp SA, Levine JS and Patterson DF (1991) Inherited selective intestinal cobalamin malabsorption and cobalamin deficiency in dogs. *Pediatric Research* **29,** 24–31

German AJ, Helps CR, Hall EJ and Day MJ (2000) Cytokine mRNA expression in mucosal biopsies from German Shepherd Dogs with small intestinal enteropathies. *Digestive Diseases and Sciences* **45,** 7–17

German AJ, Day MJ, Ruaux CG, Steiner JM, Williams DA and Hall EJ (2003) Comparison of direct and indirect tests for small intestinal bacterial overgrowth and antibiotic-responsive diarrhea in dogs. *Journal of Veterinary Internal Medicine* **17,** 33–43

German AJ, Hall EJ and Day MJ (2001) Immune cell populations within the duodenal mucosa of dogs with enteropathies. *Journal of Veterinary Internal Medicine* **15,** 14–25

Jergens AE, Andreassen CB, Hagemoser WA, Ridgway J and Cambell KL (1998) Cytologic examination of exfoliative specimens obtained during endoscopy for diagnosis of gastrointestinal tract disease in dogs and cats. *Journal of the American Veterinary Medical Association* **213,** 1755–1759

Jergens AE, Schreiner CA, Frank DE, Niyo Y, Ahrens FE, Eckersall PD, Benson TJ, Evans R (2003) A scoring index for disease activity in canine inflammatory bowel disease. *Journal of Veterinary Internal Medicine* **17,** 291

Kimmel SE, Waddell LS and Michel KE (2000) Hypomagnesemia and hypocalcemia associated with protein-losing enteropathy in Yorkshire terriers: five cases (1992–1998). *Journal of the American Veterinary Medical Association* **217,** 703–706

Marks SL, Kather EJ, Kass PH and Melli AC (2002) Genotypic and phenotypic characterisation of *Clostridium perfringens* and *Clostridium difficile* in diarrheic and healthy dogs. *Journal of Veterinary Internal Medicine* **16,** 533–540

Melgarejo T, Williams DA and Asem EK (1998) Enzyme-linked immunosorbent assay for canine alpha 1-protease inhibitor. *American Journal of Veterinary Research* **59,** 127–130

Melgarejo T, Williams DA, O'Connell NC and Setchell KDR (2000) Serum unconjugated bile acids as a test for intestinal bacterial overgrowth in dogs. *Digestive Diseases and Sciences* **45,** 407–414

Murphy KF, German AJ, Ruaux CG, Steiner JM, Williams DA and Hall EJ (2003) Faecal alpha-1 protease inhibitor concentrations in dogs with chronic gastrointestinal disease. *Veterinary Clinical Pathology* **32,** 67–72

Simpson KW, Fyfe J, Cornetta A, Sachs A, Strauss-Ayali D, Lamb SV and Reimers TJ (2001) Subnormal concentrations of serum cobalamin (vitamin B_{12}) in cats with gastrointestinal disease. *Journal of Veterinary Internal Medicine* **15,** 26–32

Steiner JM, Berridge BR, Wolcieszyn J, Williams DA (2002) Cellular immunolocalization of gastric and pancreatic lipase in various tissues obtained from dogs. *American Journal of Veterinary Research* **63,** 722–727

Turk J, Maddox C, Fales W, Ostlund E, Miller M, Johnson G, Pace L, Turnquist S and Kreeger J (1998) Examination for heat-labile, heat-stable, and Shiga-like toxins and for the eaeA gene in *Escherichia coli* isolates obtained from dogs dying with diarrhea: 122 cases (1992–1996). *Journal of the American Veterinary Medical Association* **212,** 1735–1736

Walkley HM and Neiger R (2000) Accuracy of three non-invasive tests to diagnose small intestinal bacterial overgrowth in dogs. *Journal of Small Animal Practice* **41,** 478

Willard MD, Jergens AE, Duncan RB, Leib MS, McCracken MD, DeNovo R, Herlman RG, Harbison JL (2002) Interobserver variation among histopathologic evaluations of intestinal tissues from dogs and cats. *Journal of the American Veterinary Medical Association* **220,** 1177–1182

Zentek J, Hall EJ, German A, Haverson K, Bailey M, Rolfe V, Butterwick R and Day MJ (2002) Morphology and immunopathology of the small and large intestine in dogs with non-specific dietary sensitivity. *Journal of Nutrition* **132,** 1652S–1654

14

Laboratory evaluation of exocrine pancreatic disease

Penny Watson

Introduction

Exocrine acinar cells comprise about 98% of the normal pancreas, and insulin-secreting endocrine islets about 2%. The acinar cells secrete enzymes involved in the initial digestion of food, including lipase (for which the pancreas is the main source), alpha-amylase, phospholipase and the proteolytic enzymes trypsin, chymotrypsin and elastase. Proteases are stored and released as inactive zymogens, which are cleaved in the small intestine to active enzymes. Trypsinogen is split by intestinal enterokinase, and activated trypsin then cleaves the other proteases.

Diseases of the exocrine pancreas are relatively common but often misdiagnosed in dogs and cats, because of non-specific clinical signs and a lack of sensitive and specific clinicopathological tests. Pancreatitis, acute and chronic and varying from severe to subclinical, is the most common disease of the exocrine pancreas in both species. Exocrine pancreatic insufficiency, although less common, is also recognized frequently. Pancreatic abscesses, pseudocysts and pancreatic neoplasia are less common.

There are important differences between cats and dogs in pancreatic structure, disease associations and clinical pathology (Figure 14.1).

Pancreatitis

Pathophysiology

The aetiopathogenesis of pancreatitis is incompletely understood, but the 'final common pathway' of pancreatitis appears to be the inappropriate early activation of trypsinogen within the pancreas, as a result of increased autoactivation and/or reduced autolysis (Naruse *et al.*, 1999). Activated trypsin then activates other enzymes and the result is pancreatic autodigestion, inflammation and peripancreatic fat necrosis. There is an associated systemic inflammatory response (SIR) in even the mildest pancreatitis. Many other organs may be involved and, in the most severe cases, there is multi-organ failure and disseminated intravascular coagulation (DIC). The circulating protease inhibitors α_1-antitrypsin (α_1-protease inhibitor) and α-macroglobulin remove trypsin and other proteases from the circulation, and saturation of these inhibitors by excessive circulating proteases contributes to systemic inflammation. However, generalized neutrophil activation and cytokine release is probably the primary cause of SIR (Norman, 1998).

Potential trigger factors for pancreatitis in dogs and cats are outlined in Figure 14.2. Unlike human cases, 90% of canine and feline cases remain idiopathic and some of these are likely to represent hereditary disease.

Feature	Dogs	Cats
Anatomy	Usually two pancreatic ducts: • Large accessory duct from right limb to minor papilla in duodenum • Small pancreatic duct from left limb to major duodenal papilla in duodenum next to (but not joining) bile duct	Usually single major pancreatic duct joins the common bile duct before entering duodenum at duodenal papilla 3 cm distal to pylorus. 20% of cats have second, accessory duct. Occasionally bile duct and major pancreatic duct remain separate
Disease associations	Pancreatitis commonly associated with endocrine disease (see text). Association with liver and small intestinal disease not studied/recognized	Pancreatitis commonly associated with cholangiohepatitis and/or inflammatory bowel disease. Often concurrent hepatic lipidosis. May also be associated with nephritis
Pancreatitis: spectrum of disease	Most cases acute. Low-grade chronic disease increasingly recognized	Most cases low-grade, chronic interstitial and a challenge to diagnose. Acute severe cases occur less frequently
Pancreatitis: diagnosis	Histology gold standard. Variety of catalytic and immunoassays available. Ultrasonography quite sensitive. Obvious/suggestive clinical signs in acute cases	Histology gold standard. Catalytic assays no help. Immunoassays less sensitive and specific than in dogs. Ultrasonography less sensitive than in dogs. More low-grade, non-specific clinical signs
Causes of exocrine pancreatic insufficiency	Often pancreatic acinar atrophy, increased incidence in certain breeds (especially German Shepherd Dogs). End-stage chronic pancreatitis does occur	Most cases end-stage chronic pancreatitis. Pancreatic acinar atrophy not reported

14.1 Comparison of pancreatic structure and disease in dogs and cats.

Risk factors	Causes
Idiopathic (90%)	Unknown (some may be hereditary)
Duct obstruction ± hypersecretion ± bile reflux into pancreatic duct	Experimental Neoplasia Surgery ± cholangitis + role in chronic pancreatitis
Hypertriglyceridaemia	Inherent abnormal lipid metabolism (breed-related, e.g. Miniature Schnauzers) Endocrine: diabetes mellitus, hyperadrenocortism, hypothyroidism
Breed/sex?	Increased risk terriers ± spayed females, may reflect risk of hypertriglyceridaemia (also Miniature Schnauzers – see above)
Diet	Dietary indiscretion, high fat diet Malnutrition Obesity?
Trauma	Road traffic accident Surgery 'High rise syndrome'
Ischaemia/reperfusion	Surgery (not just pancreas) Gastric dilatation–volvulus Shock Severe anaemia (common association)
Hypercalcaemia	Experimental Hypercalcaemia of malignancy (uncommon association clinically) Primary hyperparathyroidism
Drugs/toxins	Organophosphates, azathioprine, asparaginase, thiazides, furosemide, oestrogens, sulpha drugs, tetracycline, procainamide, potassium bromide. Possibly steroids, propofol
Infections	*Toxoplasma* Others (uncommon)

14.2 Risk factors and potential clinical causes of pancreatitis in dogs and cats.

Diagnosis

Overview

Pancreatitis may be defined as acute or chronic (Figures 14.3, 14.4) but these terms are histopathological rather than clinical: disease severity does not differentiate acute from chronic pancreatitis. In dogs, chronic pancreatitis is often recurrent, and a long subclinical phase can culminate in a dramatic acute-on-chronic episode, which is clinically and clinicopathologically identical to a single, acute bout of pancreatitis. However, acute-on-chronic disease may lead to more significant long-term sequelae, such as the development of exocrine pancreatic insufficiency (EPI) and/or diabetes mellitus. In general, chronic disease is more challenging to diagnose, as the clinical signs, diagnostic imaging findings and clinicopathological changes are less dramatic than in acute disease. Cats show a high incidence of low-grade, chronic disease with particularly low-grade, non-specific clinical signs. They also have a high incidence of concurrent disease (particularly cholangiohepatitis and/or inflammatory bowel disease) and a lack of specific diagnostic tests, making the diagnosis of pancreatitis difficult. In dogs, acute disease is believed to be commonest, but chronic disease may also be frequent and under-recognized (Watson, 2003).

The gold standard for diagnosis of pancreatitis is biopsy and histopathological examination, but this is often neither practical nor indicated. No single clinicopathological test currently available has 100% sensitivity and specificity for the diagnosis of pancreatitis in dogs and cats, and non-invasive diagnosis remains presumptive, based on supportive results from clinical and diagnostic imaging findings as well as the results of blood tests.

	Acute	Chronic	Chronic active
Histology	Pancreatic inflammation with neutrophils. Varying degrees of pancreatic necrosis, oedema and peripancreatic fat necrosis	Inflammatory infiltrate, mainly mononuclear cells. Fibrosis, nodular hyperplasia, architectural disruption	As chronic but with neutrophilic inflammation
Reversibility of histological features	Histological changes potentially completely reversible	Architectural disruption irreversible	Architectural disruption irreversible
Clinical features	Varies from severe and fatal (usually necrotizing) to mild and subclinical (usually interstitial inflammation)	Generally mild	May be severe. Can present as a single bout of acute disease

14.3 Features of acute and chronic pancreatitis.

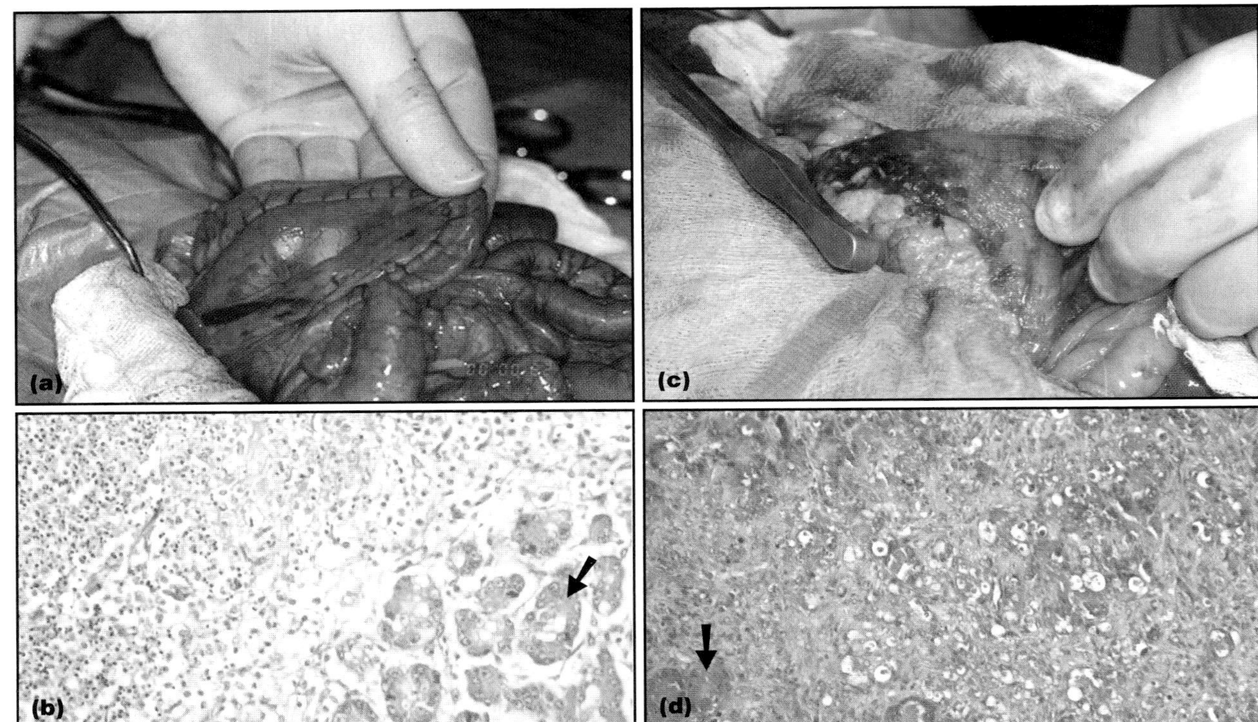

14.4 Pancreatitis. (a) Gross appearance of acute pancreatitis in a cat at laparotomy, demonstrating generalized hyperaemia. (b) Histopathological appearance of acute (fatal) pancreatitis in a dog. Note extensive neutrophilic infiltrate and inflammatory exudate but absence of fibrosis. A normal acinus is arrowed. (H&E stain; original magnification X100.) (Courtesy of *In Practice* and Aude Roulois.) (c) Gross appearance of chronic pancreatitis at laparotomy (right, duodenal limb). Note nodular appearance of pancreas and extensive adhesions to duodenum obscuring the mesentery. (Courtesy of *In Practice* and Dr Stephen Baines.) (d) Histopathological appearance of chronic pancreatitis in a dog (the same dog as Figure 14.4c). Extensive fibrous tissue between the acini completely disrupts the normal architecture. A normal acinus is arrowed. (H&E stain; original magnification X200.) (Courtesy of *In Practice* and Aude Roulois.)

Haematology and biochemistry

Haematology and biochemical screens are important in animals with pancreatitis.

- Significant changes often occur due to the SIR associated with pancreatitis. A modified organ-scoring system based on clinical and clinicopathological changes on admission is very useful in assessing prognosis and treatment in dogs (Figures 14.5 and 14.6).
- Pancreatitis may be secondary to another disease, which may be suggested by biochemical changes, and which requires treatment or prevention to control the pancreatitis. Concurrent disease is common, particularly in severe pancreatitis. The most important concurrent diseases in dogs are diabetes mellitus (especially ketoacidotic diabetes), hyperadrenocorticism and hypothyroidism; up to 50% of dogs with severe pancreatitis have one or more of these endocrinopathies. There are also associations with gastrointestinal (GI) disease and with epilepsy (which may represent the effects of treatment). The most important associated diseases in cats are diabetes mellitus, hepatic lipidosis, inflammatory bowel disease and cholangiohepatitis. Cats with pancreatitis may also have an increased incidence of interstitial nephritis.
- Pancreatitis may lead to secondary complications and sequelae that require recognition and treatment (see Figure 14.7).

Severity	Disease score	Prognosis	Expected mortality (%)
Mild	0	Excellent	0
Moderate	1	Good to fair	11
	2	Fair to poor	20
Severe	3	Poor	66
	4	Grave	100

14.5 A modified organ scoring system for canine acute pancreatitis. The severity scoring system is based on the number of organ systems apart from the pancreas that show evidence of failure or compromise at initial presentation. The organ system involvement is assessed clinicopathologically as shown in Figure 14.6. This scoring system was developed for acute pancreatitis in dogs. It is unclear whether this system can be applied to cats or to acute-on-chronic pancreatitis (Ruaux and Atwell, 1998; Ruaux, 2000).

Organ system	Criteria for scoring	Laboratory reference interval
Hepatic	One or more of alkaline phosphatase (ALP), aspartate aminotransferase (AST) or alanine aminotransferase (ALT) >3x upper reference range	Varies between laboratories
Renal	Urea >14 mmol/l Creatinine >265 µmol/l	Urea 2.5–9.5 mmol/l Creatinine 53–159 µmol/l
Leucocytic	>10% band neutrophils or total white cell count >24 x 10^9/l	Band neutrophils 0.0–0.2 x 10^9/l WBC 4.5–17 x 10^9/l
Endocrine pancreas	Blood glucose >13 mmol/l and/or β-hydroxybutyrate >1 mmol/l	Blood glucose 3.3–6.8 mmol/l β-Hydroxybutyrate 0.0–0.6 mmol/l
Acid–base	Bicarbonate <13 or >26 mmol/l and/or anion gap <15 or >38 mmol/l	Bicarbonate 15–24 mmol/l Anion gap 17–35 mmol/l

14.6 Criteria to assess organ system compromise for severity scoring system in canine acute pancreatitis. An abnormality in each system adds one point to the score, with the exception that if increased glucose, butyrate and acidosis co-exist (e.g. in diabetic ketoacidosis), endocrine pancreas and acid–base are counted as one system (Ruaux and Atwell, 1998).

Acute sequelae
Dehydration Metabolic acidosis Pre-renal azotaemia Electrolyte disturbances • Hypokalaemia (most important) • Hyponatraemia • Hypochloraemia • Mild hypocalcaemia and hypomagnesaemia (not usually clinically significant) Hepatic involvement Systemic inflammatory response syndrome Systemic hypotension Acute respiratory distress syndrome Cardiac arrhythmias Coagulopathies Diffuse intravascular coagulation Pancreatic abscesses Pancreatic pseudocysts
Chronic sequelae
Exocrine pancreatic insufficiency (90% enzyme loss) Diabetes mellitus (80% beta cell loss) Fibrosis around bile duct/chronic biliary obstruction Potentially neoplastic transformation Pancreatic abscesses Pancreatic pseudocysts

14.7 Potential sequelae of acute and chronic pancreatitis.

Haematological and biochemical abnormalities seen in pancreatitis are summarized in Figures 14.8 and 14.9.

Electrolyte changes seen with acute pancreatitis often include significant hypokalaemia due to loss through vomiting, reduced intake and fluid therapy increasing renal loss. Hypokalaemia must be recognized and treated, as it can cause ongoing GI atony and become life-threatening if marked.

Parameter	Change	Frequency of change in dogs	Frequency of change in cats	Reason/comments
Neutrophils	Increased ± left shift	Common (55–60%)	Less common than dogs (about 30%)	Systemic inflammatory response
	Decreased ± degenerative left shift	Very uncommon	Uncommon (up to 15%)	'Degenerative' response due to overwhelming inflammation – poor prognostic indicator in cats?
Haematocrit	Increased	Moderately common (up to 20%)	Moderately common (up to 13–20%)	Dehydration (may become low in some once rehydrated)
	Decreased (both regenerative and non-regenerative anaemia seen)	Moderately common (24%)	26–55%	Anaemia of chronic disease ± Bleeding gastrointestinal ulcers ± Shortened red cell lifespan (azotaemia and sepsis) ± Reduced production (above + anorexia)
Fibrinogen	Increased	Common	?	Inflammatory response
	Decreased	Uncommon	?	Consumption in DIC
Fibrin degradation products (and also probably D-dimers)	Increased	Uncommon (16% of severe cases)	?	Coagulation abnormalities associated with circulating proteases ± DIC
Platelets	Decreased	Common in severe cases (59%)	Uncommon, usually normal or only slightly decreased	Coagulation abnormalities associated with circulating proteases ± DIC

14.8 Potential non-specific findings on haematology screens in pancreatitis in dogs and cats. These figures are from dogs and cats with severe, acute pancreatitis; there is very little information on chronic, low grade disease but changes are likely to be less dramatic (Schaer, 1979; Hill and Van Winkle, 1993; Hess *et al.*, 1998; Mansfield and Jones, 2001). (continues) ▶

Parameter	Change	Frequency of change in dogs	Frequency of change in cats	Reason/comments
Coagulation times	Increased	Prolonged prothrombin time in 43% cases, prolonged partial thromboplastin time in 61% cases	Only measured in small numbers of cases but often prolonged in those. N.B. Up to 20% of cats have thromboembolic disease	Coagulation abnormalities associated with circulating proteases ± DIC

14.8 (continued) Potential non-specific findings on haematology screens in pancreatitis in dogs and cats. These figures are from dogs and cats with severe, acute pancreatitis; there is very little information on chronic, low grade disease but changes are likely to be less dramatic (Schaer, 1979; Hill and Van Winkle, 1993; Hess *et al.*, 1998; Mansfield and Jones, 2001).

Parameter	Change	Frequency of change in dogs	Frequency of change in cats	Reason/comments
Urea ± creatinine	Increased	Common Urea: 53–65% Creatinine: 50–59%	Common Urea: 57% Creatinine: 33%	Prerenal failure due to dehydration ± Hypotension (classically urea elevated most) ± Intrinsic renal failure (sepsis, immune complexes, underlying or pre-existing disease)
Potassium	Decreased	Relatively common (20%)	Very common (56%)	Increased loss in vomiting Fluid therapy Reduced intake + aldosterone release secondary to hypovolaemia
Sodium	Increased	Uncommon (12%)	Uncommon (4%)	Dehydration
	Decreased	Relatively common (33%)	Relatively common (23%)	Loss in GI secretions with vomiting
Chloride	Decreased	Very common (81%)	Unknown but likely to be common	Loss in GI secretions with vomiting
Calcium	Increased	Uncommon (9%)	Uncommon (5%)	May be cause rather than effect?
	Decreased	Uncommon (3%) Not a prognostic indicator	Very common and poor prognostic indicator (up to 40–45% reduced total calcium, up to 60% reduced ionized calcium)	Saponification in peripancreatic fat (unproven) Increased glucagon release increasing calcitonin (shown in some)
Phosphate	Increased	Common (55%)	Quite common (27%)	Usually due to reduced renal excretion, and animal also azotaemic
	Decreased	Uncommon (0% in one study)	Quite common (14%)	Usually secondary to treatment of diabetes mellitus or increased insulin increasing cellular uptake. Can become clinically important in cats
Magnesium	Decreased	Reported but unknown frequency	Reported but unknown frequency	Saponification in peripancreatic fat
Glucose	Increased	Common (30–88%)	Common (64%)	Increased glucagon, cortisol and catecholamines and reduced insulin. 40% became normal, 30% permanently diabetic (Hess *et al.*, 1998)
	Decreased	Common (up to 40%)	Uncommon (4%)	Sepsis/systemic inflammatory response Anorexia and malnutrition (especially small breeds) Concurrent liver disease
Albumin	Increased	Common (39–50%)	Quite common (8–30%)	Dehydration
	Decreased	Quite common (17%)	Quite common (24%)	Gut loss Anorexia or malnutrition Concurrent liver disease ± Renal loss
Total protein	Increased	Common (27%)	Common (24%)	Dehydration with inflammation increasing globulins
	Decreased	Common (45%)	Uncommon (14%)	As albumin

14.9 Potential non-specific changes on biochemistry screen in pancreatitis in dogs and cats. These figures are from dogs and cats with severe, acute pancreatitis; there is very little information on chronic, low grade disease but changes are likely to be less dramatic (Schaer, 1979; Hill and Van Winkle, 1993; Hess *et al.*, 1998; Mansfield and Jones, 2001). (continues) ▶

Parameter	Change	Frequency of change in dogs	Frequency of change in cats	Reason/comments
Hepatocellular enzymes (ALT and AST)	Increased	Common (61%)	Common (68%)	Hepatic necrosis and lipidosis due to sepsis, local effects of pancreatic enzymes ± Concurrent disease (most important in cats)
Cholestatic enzymes (ALP and gamma-glutamyl transferase (GGT))	Increased	Very common (79%)	Common (50%) In lipidosis ALP high but GGT often normal	Biliary obstruction caused by inflamed pancreas (common cats and dogs) ± Primary or concurrent disease (cholangitis or lipidosis in cats) ± Steroid-induced ALP isoenzyme (in dogs only)
Bilirubin	Increased	Common (53%)	Very common (64%)	As ALP
Cholesterol	Increased	Common (48–80%)	Common (64%)	Commonly elevated: see text. May also increase with secondary cholestasis
Triglycerides	Increased	Common leads to lipaemic serum	Uncommon (10%?) but rarely measured	Commonly elevated: see text

14.9 (continued) Potential non-specific changes on biochemistry screen in pancreatitis in dogs and cats. These figures are from dogs and cats with severe, acute pancreatitis; there is very little information on chronic, low grade disease but changes are likely to be less dramatic (Schaer, 1979; Hill and Van Winkle, 1993; Hess *et al.*, 1998; Mansfield and Jones, 2001).

Azotaemia is commonly prerenal, and assessment of a concurrent urine sample before commencing fluid therapy is important to determine whether there is also intrinsic renal compromise.

Pancreatic oedema, fibrosis or neoplasia can cause partial or complete biliary obstruction, and consequent increases in liver enzymes. Dogs with pancreatitis may present with jaundice. In cats, pancreatitis and cholangiohepatitis often occur concurrently. There is also a high incidence of hepatic lipidosis in cats with severe acute pancreatitis.

Increased cholesterol and triglycerides are common and may represent either a cause or an effect of the disease. However, experimental pancreatitis does not cause elevations in cholesterol and triglycerides in dogs, even though it alters the patterns of lipoproteins (Whitney *et al.*, 1987). Many of the risk factors for pancreatitis in dogs (particularly the endocrinopathies) are associated with lipaemia, so it has been concluded that the increase in lipids is more likely to be a cause than an effect.

Other clinicopathological tests

Urinalysis: A high urine specific gravity with azotaemia suggests acute prerenal failure due to dehydration and shock. However, dogs with severe pancreatitis often have isosthenuric urine, suggesting concurrent intrinsic renal damage. Proteinuria is seen in up to 78% of dogs (Hess *et al.*, 1998), probably due to a combination of SIR and tubular damage. Glucosuria may be seen in both dogs and cats and may be temporary due to increased insulin resistance and a 'pre-diabetic' response. Blood and urine glucose should be monitored after the pancreatitis has resolved to assess whether the animal is truly an insulin-dependent diabetic. The presence of ketones in the urine in both dogs and cats with pancreatitis indicates diabetic ketoacidosis which requires immediate and urgent treatment. Concurrent pancreatitis in a diabetic animal increases the risk of ketoacidosis and mortality.

Coagulation screens: Coagulation abnormalities are common, particularly in severe acute disease in both dogs and cats due to DIC. In addition, proteolytic enzymes (proteases) released from the pancreas catabolize complement and von Willebrand factor, contributing to the haemostatic abnormalities.

Analysis of effusions: Body cavity effusions are common in pancreatitis and may be pleural as well as peritoneal. They are usually serosanguineous exudates, although transudates and chylous effusions have been reported in cats. Effusions form due to focal peritonitis and fat necrosis in the abdomen, and more generalized vasculitis, inflammation and fat necrosis in the pleural space. Amylase and lipase levels in the fluid may be elevated, although the diagnostic or prognostic usefulness of these measurements has not been assessed in small animals.

Blood gas analysis: Blood gas analysis in animals with pancreatitis shows metabolic acidosis in most cases. There may also be concurrent respiratory acidosis and hypoxia if there is acute respiratory distress syndrome associated with the pancreatitis.

Specific enzyme assays

Non-invasive diagnosis of pancreatitis in dogs and cats requires the use of specific pancreatic enzyme assays, but these assays vary greatly in sensitivity and specificity between species and individuals, and no single assay is totally sensitive and specific.

In dogs and cats, the time of onset of the episode of pancreatitis is rarely known. Pancreatic enzymes have distinct half-lives: in dogs the half-life of amylase is approximately 5 hours and that of lipase is approximately 2 hours. Many animals are examined an unknown period, often days, after the onset of the disease, by which time the enzymes may have returned to normal. In addition, the pancreas can respond to inflammation by shutting off production of enzymes and, in ongoing, chronic disease, there is progressive loss of pancreatic mass with an associated overall reduction in enzyme production. All these factors contribute to the variable, often poor sensitivity of enzyme assays. Finally, assays are often affected by renal clearance and drug therapy, particularly steroids. Each assay has advantages and disadvantages (Figure 14.10).

Pancreatic enzyme assays currently available for use in dogs and cats are divided into catalytic assays and immunoassays.

Catalytic assays: These measure plasma levels of the pancreatic acinar enzymes, amylase and lipase, by measuring the enzyme's ability to catalyse a specific reaction. Catalytic assays do not measure inactive precursors, such as zymogens, so are not used for proteases (e.g. trypsin). They are neither species- nor organ-specific: a catalytic lipase assay will potentially detect any lipase reaching the circulation, including gastric lipase, intestinal acidic lipase, lipoprotein lipase and other extrapancreatic lipases. There is a high background non-pancreatic activity for both amylase and lipase: plasma levels of amylase and lipase are normal in dogs after total pancreatectomy. Plasma lipase is also often normal in dogs with EPI, which equates to loss of 90% of exocrine enzyme output (Steiner *et al.*, 2001). Thus these assays are neither sensitive nor specific. Hess *et al.* (1998) found a sensitivity of only 69% for amylase and 39% for lipase in dogs with fatal acute pancreatitis.

Small elevations in amylase or lipase are unlikely to be significant, because of the high background level; generally only elevations of 3–5 times normal (or above) are considered suggestive of pancreatitis (provided none of the secondary causes of elevations outlined in Figure 14.10 are present). In the cat, plasma amylase and lipase, although measurable, are of no use at all in the diagnosis of pancreatitis as they may be elevated in normal cats and normal in pancreatitis cases.

Immunoassays: These are organ-specific, and may be species-specific and can measure precursors in addition to active enzymes. They use an antibody directed against part of the enzyme molecule (usually distinct from the active site) which is detected by either radioimmunoassay (RIA) or an enzyme-linked immunosorbent assay (ELISA).

Trypsin-like immunoreactivity (TLI): This measures trypsin and trypsinogen. It is species-specific. Canine and feline (and human) TLI are available. The canine TLI (cTLI) test used in the UK was developed at the GI Laboratory at Texas A and M University, and is an RIA. The feline TLI (fTLI) test is currently only available in Texas (UK laboratories will forward samples) and is an ELISA. The TLI test was originally developed in cats and dogs for the diagnosis of exocrine pancreatic insufficiency, but can be used as an additional test in pancreatitis, although it may be no more useful than lipase in the diagnosis of pancreatitis in dogs. Specificity has been reported as about 65% but sensitivity only 33% (Steiner, 2003). Some dogs may have elevated TLI and normal lipase and vice versa, so it may be worth measuring both.

Assay	Advantages	Disadvantages
Catalytic assays (N.B. Dogs only; no use in cats)		
Amylase	Widely used. Available on in-house analysers. Not affected (or possibly reduced) by steroids	Low sensitivity and specificity. High background level because released from other sources including small intestine. Less often elevated than other pancreatic enzymes. Renally excreted: elevated 2–3-fold in azotaemia. May be normal in severe/chronic pancreatitis due to enzyme depletion ± loss of tissue. No prognostic value
Lipase	As sensitive as canine TLI if other causes ruled out. Degree of elevation may have prognostic significance. Steroids elevate up to 5-fold	High background level because released from other sources. Renally excreted: elevated 2–3-fold in azotaemia. May be normal in severe/chronic pancreatitis due to enzyme depletion and inhibition
Immunoassays		
Canine TLI	Elevations highly specific for pancreatitis. May be no more sensitive than lipase	Said to rise and fall more quickly than lipase/amylase but elevations often persist in clinical cases. Renally excreted: elevated 2–3-fold in azotaemia. May be inappropriately low in severe/chronic pancreatitis due to pancreatic depletion ± loss of tissue mass. No clear prognostic significance
Feline TLI	One of only two assays available for cats	Lower sensitivity and specificity than canine TLI. Renally excreted so elevated in azotaemia
Canine PLI	Early indications more sensitive and specific than TLI. Organ-specific so no interference from extrapancreatic sources	Currently only available in USA (time delay before receiving results). Unclear yet if affected by steroids. Increased in renal disease but may not be significant
Feline PLI	Very new test. Appears more sensitive and specific than fTLI	Only available in USA. Very little published data on its use

14.10 Advantages and disadvantages of enzyme assays in the diagnosis of pancreatitis in dogs and cats (TLI, trypsin-like immunoreactivity; PLI, pancreatic lipase immunoreactivity).

In cats, TLI is the only established blood test available for the diagnosis of pancreatitis. Unfortunately, fTLI has a lower sensitivity and specificity for diagnosis of pancreatitis in cats than cTLI in dogs. Most concerningly, false positives have been reported in cats with hepatic or GI disease, which are the conditions most likely to be confused clinically with pancreatitis in cats. Swift *et al.* (2000) found a sensitivity of 55% and specificity of 56% for diagnosis of pancreatitis with fTLI. However, they used a lower cut-off than currently recommended (>82 ng/l) and used the RIA rather than the ELISA. Gerhardt *et al.* (2001) used the ELISA and found a sensitivity of 62% if the cut-off were 82 ng/l, a sensitivity of 33% with a cut-off of 100 ng/l (currently accepted cut-off for diagnosis of canine pancreatitis) and a sensitivity of 86% if the cut off were 49 ng/l (top of normal range).

Pancreatic lipase immunoreactivity (PLI): This measures lipase of pancreatic origin only. Therefore, it is pancreas-specific and, unlike lipase, PLI is not only high in pancreatitis but also very low in EPI. It is species-specific and both canine and feline PLI are available. Both are new tests and currently only available in Texas (UK laboratories will forward samples). The canine PLI is an ELISA and the feline PLI an RIA. Published work on canine PLI is currently limited, but early work suggests it has a higher sensitivity than TLI or lipase for the diagnosis of pancreatitis in dogs. Early work on the clinical use of PLI suggests it may be more sensitive and specific than fTLI and may remain elevated for longer than fTLI in experimental feline pancreatitis (Williams *et al.*, 2003).

Trypsin activation peptide (TAP): An assay for TAP has been recently developed. TAP is the peptide cleaved from trypsinogen by enterokinase in the small intestine, resulting in active trypsin. It is highly conserved between species, so the human ELISA can be used in both dogs and cats.

Theoretically, there should be no TAP in the plasma in healthy animals if all the trypsinogen is activated within the small intestine. However, the finding of low but significant levels of TAP in the plasma of healthy dogs (Mansfield and Jones, 2000) suggests that a small amount of normal trypsinogen autoactivation occurs in the pancreas. Elevations in plasma TAP levels should be diagnostic of pancreatitis, but elevated plasma TAP has a specificity of only 76% and sensitivity of 53% for pancreatitis in dogs. Urinary TAP:creatinine ratio has a higher specificity but lower sensitivity than plasma TAP. There is a much wider range of urinary TAP concentration in healthy dogs than in humans, and urinary TAP is also increased in renal disease (Mansfield and Jones, 2000).

Summary

The non-invasive diagnosis of pancreatitis is problematical. In both dogs and cats, a combination of history, clinical findings, diagnostic imaging findings (radiography to rule out intestinal obstruction as a cause of acute vomiting and other pathology, and ultrasonography of the pancreas) and the results of appropriately chosen pancreatic enzyme assays should be used to reach a presumptive diagnosis of pancreatitis. Definitive diagnosis is only gained by histological examination of the pancreas which is not appropriate in many acute cases.

Prognostic indicators

In dogs, the best prognostic indicator currently available is the calculated organ score (Figures 14.5 and 14.6). Of the individual clinicopathological tests, urinary TAP:creatinine ratio is the most useful (Mansfield *et al.*, 2003), although elevations in serum lipase, creatinine and phosphate and low urine SG have shown some value as negative prognostic indicators. The degree of elevation of TLI does not appear to be prognostically useful. The prognostic relevance of the degree of elevation in cPLI is unknown.

Recognized negative prognostic indicators in cats include low ionized calcium and leucopenia (Kimmel *et al.*, 2001). Urinary or plasma TAP do not seem to be prognostically helpful in cats.

Other tests which have been assessed as prognostic indicators but are not clinically useful include α-macroglobulin (circulating protease inhibitor) (Ruaux and Atwell, 1999) and circulating α_1-protease inhibitor–trypsin complexes, which have too short a half-life to be clinically useful (Suchodolski *et al.*, 2001).

Exocrine pancreatic insufficiency

Exocrine pancreatic insufficiency (EPI) is a functional lack of pancreatic enzymes resulting in clinical signs of steatorrhoea and weight loss. Unlike pancreatitis, it is diagnosed by clinical signs and pancreatic function tests and not on the results of pancreatic histopathology.

Causes

Pancreatic acinar atrophy (PAA) is believed to be the predominant cause of EPI in dogs but end-stage chronic pancreatitis is also important (Keller, 1990; Watson, 2003). PAA is particularly recognized in German Shepherd Dogs, in which an autosomal mode of inheritance has been demonstrated; it has also been described in Rough Collies, in English Setters and sporadically in other breeds. Histological studies in German Shepherd Dogs suggest an immune-mediated disease directed against the acini. The islet cells are spared and dogs with PAA are not typically diabetic. Most dogs develop the disease in young adulthood, but a proportion of German Shepherd Dogs remain subclinical for a prolonged period, in spite of clinicopathological evidence of pancreatic enzyme insufficiency, and only develop clinical signs late in life. PAA has not been recognized in cats and end-stage pancreatitis is the commonest cause of feline EPI.

EPI can also develop as a consequence of chronic pancreatitis in which there is extensive loss of pancreatic acini. As chronic disease may be largely subclinical or only present as occasional clinical acute-on-chronic episodes, the degree of underlying pancreatic damage may be under-estimated. Many dogs with end-stage chronic pancreatitis also develop diabetes mellitus either before or after EPI as a result of concurrent islet cell destruction (Keller, 1990; Watson, 2003) and the situation is likely to be similar in cats.

EPI may develop secondary to pancreatic tumours in dogs and cats, usually due to blockage of pancreatic ducts by the tumours, although destruction of acinar tissue by the mass and associated pancreatitis also play a role.

Finally, clinical EPI may develop in the presence of adequate pancreatic output as a result of hyperacidity of the duodenum inactivating lipase in the intestinal lumen. This is rare in small animals.

Diagnosis

The diagnosis of EPI relies on demonstrating reduced pancreatic enzyme output. The most sensitive and specific way of doing this is by measuring reduced circulating enzyme activity. However, there are problems interpreting these results in the presence of concurrent pancreatitis. In these cases, measurement of reduced enzyme activity in the gut, by measuring reduced faecal enzyme activity, may be useful.

Blood tests: immunoassays

Measurement of reduced TLI in the blood has a high sensitivity and specificity for the diagnosis of EPI in dogs and cats, and is currently the single test of choice in small animals. A fasting serum sample is required because the release of pancreatic enzymes associated with feeding can raise the levels. It is **not** necessary to stop exogenous pancreatic enzyme supplementation before measuring TLI because the test is an immunoassay which does not cross-react with the TLI of other species (and very little exogenous pancreatic enzyme is absorbed). There are some problems in interpreting the results, particularly in dogs, as outlined below:

- A low serum TLI (<2.5 ng/l in dogs) alone does not diagnose clinical EPI if there are no compatible clinical signs. Serum TLI should be measured several times, over several weeks to months, and be persistently low to demonstrate EPI. Occasionally, a single TLI may be low in a dog with pancreatitis as a result of a temporary reduction in enzyme production. A dog with persistently low TLI but no steatorrhoea or weight loss would be considered to have 'subclinical' EPI and should not be treated but be monitored for any evidence of clinical disease. Subclinical EPI is uncommon but has been reported in a small number of German Shepherd Dogs with PAA (Wiberg *et al.*, 1999); it has not yet been reported in cats. A TLI stimulation test may give more information about the status of the animal but is rarely performed (Wiberg *et al.*, 1999; Wiberg, 2004)
- A TLI in the 'grey area' (2.5–5.0 ng/l in dogs) is not diagnostic of EPI and the test needs to be repeated a few weeks to months later. In a proportion of dogs (45% in one study: Wiberg *et al.*, 1999), the TLI will return to the normal range. In about 10% of dogs, the TLI will drop down to the level diagnostic of EPI, while in the rest it remains in the grey area
- A single normal or high TLI in a breed of dog other than a German Shepherd, with suspicious clinical signs, does not rule out EPI. TLI can increase to or above the normal range in dogs with EPI secondary to chronic end-stage pancreatitis, if it is measured during a bout of disease (Keller, 1990; Watson, 2003). This is because EPI reduces TLI, but pancreatitis elevates it. A similar situation may arise in cats, but this has not been well documented. Therefore, in any animal with suspected EPI secondary to chronic pancreatitis, TLI measurements should be repeated, preferably when the animal is showing no clinical signs of pancreatitis. Alternatively, a test for enzyme activity in the gut, such as a faecal elastase test, could be used in these animals, since pancreatitis leads to enzyme release into the abdomen and blood stream but not into the pancreatic ducts which drain into the gut.

A low cPLI also has good sensitivity and specificity for the diagnosis of EPI in dogs (Steiner *et al.*, 2001), but is not superior to TLI and the latter is more readily available. PLI is also likely to be low in cats with EPI.

Unlike in humans, amylase and lipase are **not** consistently low in dogs and cats with EPI. This is because of the high background levels of enzyme from other organs.

Faecal tests

Faecal trypsin activity: Measurement of faecal trypsin activity has such a low sensitivity and specificity for the diagnosis of EPI that it is not worth doing! Likewise, microscopic examination or faeces for undigested fat, starch and muscle fibres is not helpful: as with plasma turbidity, other conditions apart from EPI can cause maldigestion/malabsorption. Observation of a subjectively 'marked' increase in faecal fat is usually associated with EPI, but this has a very low sensitivity; most dogs with EPI have only mild to moderate increases in faecal fat, overlapping with normal dogs and dogs with other diseases. In addition, animals with EPI often have intermittently normal faeces. Faecal proteolytic activity can be assessed in a number of ways, but again these tests generally have poor sensitivity and specificity. Bacteria in the gut can also produce proteolytic enzymes, and these certainly produce false negative results in tests such as the gelatine (radiographic film) digestion tests. Normal dogs, unlike humans, show intermittent excretion of pancreatic proteases, so levels may be low on single faecal samples from normal animals. The tests can be improved by stimulation with a test food (e.g. soybean) but the tests remain difficult to perform and interpret (Westermarck and Sandholm, 1980).

Faecal elastase: This appears to have higher sensitivity and specificity than the other faecal tests for the diagnosis of EPI in dogs. Elastase is a pancreatic enzyme and a species-specific ELISA for canine elastase has been developed and is available for commercial use in dogs (Spillman *et al.*, 2001). As with canine TLI, there is no cross-reaction with elastase from other species, so dogs can remain on enzyme supplementation while the test is performed. There is marked variation in elastase levels in normal canine faeces compared with humans. The sensitivity and specificity of the test are improved by taking three separate faecal samples on 3 days or using a cut-off value for diagnosis of EPI which is below this variation in most dogs. Measurement may be particularly useful in animals with end-stage pancreatitis and/or pancreatic duct blockage where TLI results might be misleading (Spillman *et al.*, 2000).

Faecal culture and sensitivity, and parasite examination: At least one faecal culture and sensitivity and parasite examination (see Chapter 13) should be carried out on all animals with EPI. Concurrent GI infections are not uncommon in these dogs, secondary to disruption of the GI environment and immunity. Treatment of the EPI will not be successful unless concurrent infections are also recognized and treated.

Additional tests

It is advisable to measure serum cobalamin (B12) concentration in animals with EPI because cobalamin is often reduced due to a deficiency of pancreatic intrinsic factor (Hall *et al.*, 1991). In cats with end-stage pancreatitis, the low cobalamin is compounded by the high incidence of concurrent inflammatory bowel disease, which often further reduces cobalamin by reducing ileal absorption. Cobalamin deficiency has been reported to cause villous atrophy and reduced GI function, weight loss and diarrhoea in cats. If low cobalamin is documented in dogs and cats with EPI it is important to supplement with parenteral B12 injections.

Serum folate concentrations may also be measured in these animals, and are elevated in about a third of dogs. This may indicate small intestinal bacterial overgrowth (SIBO), although the sensitivity and specificity of a high serum folate for the diagnosis of SIBO is poor (see Chapter 13). Up to 75% of dogs with EPI also have SIBO, secondary to increased undigested nutrients in the gut, reduction in the antibacterial effects of pancreatic secretions and chronic maldigestion leading to malnutrition and reduced gut immunity. The definition and diagnosis of SIBO is problematical and it is better to assume SIBO in newly diagnosed dogs with EPI and treat appropriately, rather than rely on the results of diagnostic tests. The importance of SIBO in cats with EPI is unknown.

A small number of dogs with EPI have low serum folate levels (4% in the study by Hall *et al.*, 1991). In some cases, this may be due to concurrent inflammatory bowel disease reducing jejunal absorption of folate.

Haematology and biochemistry screens in dogs and cats with EPI are often normal. In very cachexic animals, they may show subtle changes associated with malnutrition, negative nitrogen balance and breakdown of body muscle, such as low albumin and globulin, mildly elevated liver enzymes, low cholesterol and triglycerides and lymphopenia. Animals with EPI, particularly German Shepherd Dogs, often present with dermatological problems due to poor coat quality and may have a neutrophilia resulting from chronic pyoderma.

Finding a marked hypoproteinuria or more severe changes on haematology and biochemistry screens in an animal with EPI should trigger a search for another disease. Cats and dogs with end-stage pancreatitis may present with more severe secondary changes on blood screens as outlined in the pancreatitis section. A high percentage of these end-stage pancreatitis animals (up to 50%) will also have concurrent diabetes mellitus and will show typical clinicopathological changes.

Pancreatic neoplasia

Neoplasia of the exocrine pancreas is uncommon in cats and dogs.

Pancreatic adenocarcinomas are generally very malignant and have usually disseminated widely by the time of diagnosis. They are often subclinical but can result in single or repeat bouts of pancreatitis and/or the development of EPI. Although the development of EPI secondary to neoplasia is rare (<10% of cases in man), it has been reported in both dogs (Bright, 1985) and cats. It occurs due to a combination of duct blockage and pancreatic parenchymal destruction. Occasionally, pancreatic carcinomas can cause paraneoplastic hypercalcaemia, although this is rare.

Pancreatic adenomas are rare in small animals but have been reported in cats (Bjorneby and Kari, 2002). Nodular hyperplasia of the exocrine pancreas is common in older dogs and cats. This usually presents as multiple small masses, whereas pancreatic tumours are usually single; histology is necessary definitively to differentiate hyperplasia from neoplasia.

Pancreatic tumours are not associated with any specific clinicopathological changes and they may cause no changes in enzyme activities at all. However, some cases have been associated with very marked elevations in serum lipase concentration (Quigley *et al.*, 2001). Alternatively, they can result in recurrent bouts of pancreatitis, with typical associated blood changes, and EPI can develop. In the latter cases, TLI may be low or normal, or even elevated if the EPI is due to duct blockage and there is plenty of remaining acinar tissue to produce trypsin. In cases with suspected EPI due to pancreatic tumours, tests of enzyme function, such as the faecal elastase test, are likely to be a more sensitive means to diagnose the insufficiency. Marked elevations in liver enzymes and jaundice may be seen in some cases as a result of extrahepatic obstruction of the bile duct by the mass (Mayhew *et al.*, 2002).

Ultrasound-guided fine needle aspiration cytology may help to differentiate between inflammatory and neoplastic lesions of the pancreas (Bennet *et al.*, 2001; Bjorneby and Kari, 2002). Care must be taken, as dysplastic changes in epithelial cells in the presence of inflammation may appear very similar to neoplasia.

Pancreatic abscesses, cysts and pseudocysts

Pancreatic abscesses, cysts and pseudocysts are uncommonly reported in dogs and cats and are usually a complication of pancreatitis.

- Pancreatic cysts may be congenital (e.g. as part of the polycystic renal disease in Persian cats) or secondary to cystic neoplasia, but most commonly are secondary to pancreatitis.
- Pseudocysts have been recognized in association with pancreatitis in both cats and dogs. A pseudocyst is a collection of fluid containing pancreatic enzymes and debris in a non-epithelialized sac. Fluid analysis generally shows a modified transudate, and the levels of amylase and lipase can be measured. In humans, the enzymes are more elevated in pseudocysts associated with pancreatitis than in those associated with cystic carcinomas, but the value of this measurement in small animals is unknown. Cytologically, a pseudocyst contains amorphous debris, some neutrophils and macrophages and, rarely, small numbers of reactive fibroblasts.
- A true pancreatic abscess is a collection of septic exudate which results from secondary infection of necrotic pancreatic tissue or a pancreatic pseudocysts. Cytologically, there are many degenerative neutrophils and variable numbers of pancreatic acinar cells which may appear atypical or dysplastic as a result of inflammation. They are fortunately rare in dogs and cats as they are associated with a poor prognosis.

Case examples

Case 1

Signalment

3-year-old entire female Miniature Dachshund.

History and clinical findings

10-day history of severe vomiting (food and then bile) and anorexia. On clinical examination the dog was thin, depressed and about 5% dehydrated. There was no palpable intestinal foreign body.

Clinical pathology data

Haematology	Result	Reference interval
RBC (x 10^{12}/l)	7.8	5.5–8.5
Hb (g/dl)	17.1	12–18
HCT (l/l)	0.47	0.37–0.55
MCV (fl)	60.3	60–77
MCHC (g/dl)	60.3	32–37
WBC (x 10^9/l)	37.2	6.0–17.0
Neutrophils (x 10^9/l)	36.5	3.0–11.5
Neutrophils (band) (x 10^9/l)	0	0–0.3
Lymphocytes (x 10^9/l)	0.4	1.0–4.8
Monocytes (x 10^9/l)	0.3	0.2–1.5
Eosinophils (x 10^9/l)	0	0.1–1.3
Platelets (x 10^9/l)	406	175–500
Fibrinogen (g/l)	3.0	2.0–4.0

Biochemistry	Result	Reference interval
Sodium (mmol/l)	155.4	135.0–155.0
Potassium (mmol/l)	2.28	3.7–5.8
Glucose (mmol/l)	1.7	3.4–5.3
Urea (mmol/l)	11.5	3.3–6.7
Creatinine (μmol/l)	66	70–170
Calcium (mmol/l)	2.33	2.2–2.7
Inorganic phosphate (mmol/l)	2.17	0.6–1.3
TP (g/l)	43.1	55.0–80.0
Albumin (g/l)	22.8	25–45
Globulin (g/l)	20.3	25–45
ALT (IU/l)	21	21–59 ▶

Biochemistry *(continued)*	Result	Reference interval
AST (IU/l)	29	20–32
ALP (IU/l)	1129	3–142
Amylase (IU/l)	3585	167–1126
Lipase (IU/l)	3471	0–200

Urine analysis

SG 1.050, nothing remarkable on dipstick.

What abnormalities are present?

Haematology

- Mature neutrophilia
- Lymphopenia.

Biochemistry

- Hypoglycaemia
- Marked elevation in ALP
- Mildly elevated urea
- Marked elevations in both amylase and lipase
- Hypokalaemia
- Hypoproteinaemia and hypoalbuminaemia.

The SG of the urine confirms adequate renal concentrating ability.

How would you interpret these results?

The neutrophilia probably reflects inflammation, although it may also reflect stress. Lymphopenia is most likely to be a stress response.

Marked elevations in both amylase and lipase are strongly suggestive of pancreatitis. There is prerenal azotaemia, with mild elevation urea but high urine SG. However, the degree of elevations of amylase and lipase in this case could not be explained by reduced renal excretion alone. Hypokalaemia is probably secondary to vomiting and low glucose secondary to malnutrition and hypermetabolism (particularly in a small dog). Low protein and albumin may reflect malnutrition and probable gut loss (there is no renal loss as there is no protein in the urine). Both the low potassium and the low glucose could become life-threatening so need immediate treatment. Marked elevation in ALP is most likely to be due to a combination of cholestasis, associated with pancreatitis, and stress, increasing steroid-induced isoenzyme.

Results of further tests

Abdominal radiographs showed poor abdominal contrast but no other abnormalities. Abdominal ultrasonography showed mixed, hyperechoic echogenicity of pancreas and hyperechoic adjacent mesentery. TLI and cPLI were not measured during this visit.

Case 1 continues ▶

Case 1 continued

Diagnosis

Acute pancreatitis was diagnosed (organ score 2 therefore moderately severe). The dog recovered after 2 weeks of intensive management with fluid therapy, anti-emetics, analgesics and nutritional support.

Follow-up

The dog was followed up at regular intervals with repeat measurements of TLI and cPLI as outlined below (neither immunoassay was performed at the first presentation).

	TLI (ng/ml) Normal >5.0 EPI <2.5 Pancreatitis >35	**cPLI** (ng/ml) Normal 2.2–102 Pancreatitis >200
T + 1 month	2.5	–
T + 5.5 months	3.7	–
T + 18 months	1.8	–
T + 77 months	11.6	134
T + 78 months	1.7	5.6

T = time at initial presentation with acute pancreatitis

At T + 77 months, the dog was showing signs of gastrointestinal disease. The dog was treated long term with a low fat diet and pancreatic enzyme supplementation.

How would you interpret these results?

These results showed that the dog had developed EPI by 1 month after the apparent single episode of 'acute pancreatitis' confirming that this was probably, in fact, an acute-on-chronic episode which had resulted in extensive loss of pancreatic acinar tissue. The cPLI is also low (T + 78 months). The dog's clinical signs supported this. There are elevations in TLI and cPLI associated with a recurrent bout of pancreatitis (T + 77 months) elevating both assays into the normal range. This would complicate diagnosis of EPI if these had been the only samples taken.

Case outcome

The dog is doing well nearly 7 years from original presentation on a low-fat diet and pancreatic enzyme supplementation. The dog has not yet become overtly diabetic, but dynamic testing shows she has markedly reduced insulin release consistent with markedly reduced pancreatic beta cell function.

Case 2

Signalment

7-year-old neutered male Domestic Shorthair cat.

History and clinical findings

Re-presented 1 week after stifle surgery for investigation of inappetence. Clinically, the cat was depressed and weak with a thready peripheral pulse and pale, jaundiced mucous membranes. There was a palpable cranial abdominal mass, which was painful.

Clinical pathology data

Haematology	Result	Reference interval
RBC (x 10^{12}/l)	8.3	5.0–10.0
Hb (g/dl)	12.6	8.0–15.0
HCT (l/l)	0.38	0.26–0.45
MCV (fl)	45.9	39–55
MCHC (g/dl)	33.3	30–36
WBC (x 10^9/l)	26.2	5.5–19.5
Neutrophils (x 10^9/l)	24.6	2.5–12.5
Neutrophils (band) (x 10^9/l)	0	0–0.3
Lymphocytes (x 10^9/l)	1.15	1.5–7.0
Monocytes (x 10^9/l)	0.2	0.0–1.5
Eosinophils (x 10^9/l)	0.20	0.0–1.5
Platelets (x 10^9/l)	156	200–800
Fibrinogen (g/l)	2.0	1.0–3.0

Film comment

Red cells appear normocytic and normochromic. WBC morphology appears normal. Platelets consistent with count given.

Coagulation tests

PT 31 s (normal <7–12 s)
aPTT >2 minutes (normal <15 s)

Biochemistry	Result	Reference interval
Sodium (mmol/l)	150.9	135.0–155.0
Potassium (mmol/l)	3.66	3.6–4.5
Glucose (mmol/l)	6.5	4.0–5.3
Urea (mmol/l)	5.7	6.7–10.0
Creatinine (μmol/l)	118	45–150
Calcium (mmol/l)	2.38	1.9–2.4
Inorganic phosphate (mmol/l)	1.35	0.7–1.2
TP (g/l)	82	55.0–80.0
Albumin (g/l)	27	25–45
Globulin (g/l)	55	25–45
ALT (IU/l)	698	16–44
AST (IU/l)	275	0–32
ALP (IU/l)	564	16–68
Total bilirubin (μmol/l)	85	0–15

Urine analysis	
SG	>1.050
Protein	2+
Blood	>3+
pH	6
Microscopy	Packed fields of red blood cells, white cells 40 per hpf. Many bilirubin crystals

Case 2 continues ▶

Case 2 continued

What abnormalities are present?

Haematology

- Marked neutrophilia
- (Mild thrombocytopenia)
- Coagulation screen shows marked prolongations of PT and aPTT.

Biochemistry

- Mildly elevated glucose
- Markedly elevated ALP, ALT and AST
- Markedly elevated bilirubin
- Slight hyperphosphataemia
- Elevated globulin (and total protein).

How would you interpret the results?

The neutrophilia is consistent with inflammation. The slightly reduced platelets, accompanied by the prolonged coagulation times, may reflect DIC.

The increased urine SG probably reflects dehydration, but may also be contributed to by the proteinuria. Sediment examination suggests urinary tract inflammation.

The mild elevation in glucose most likely reflects stress. The marked elevation of liver enzymes, including ALP (latter very significant in cats), is suggestive of cholangitis and/or hepatic lipidosis. The elevated bilirubin may be either hepatic or posthepatic. The presence of the cranial abdominal mass could be consistent with an obstructive lesion and posthepatic jaundice.

Slight hyperphosphataemia may be the first sign of prerenal azotaemia developing. Similarly, the elevated total protein and globulin probably reflect hypovolaemia. This may be masking hypoalbuminaemia.

What further tests would be useful?

- Diagnostic imaging (radiology, ultrasonography)
- fTLI
- B12 and folate
- Fibrin degradation products or D-dimers
- GGT to help differentiate cholangitis and hepatic lipidosis (see Chapter 12)
- Urine culture and sensitivity.

Results of further tests

Abdominal radiographs showed mild hepatomegaly, displacement of the transverse colon caudally by a visible soft tissue mass and a gravel sign in the pylorus, suggestive of delayed gastric emptying. Abdominal ultrasonography showed a markedly enlarged pancreas, which was assumed to be the mass visible on radiographs, with normal echogenicity but markedly dilated pancreatic ducts. There was no peristalsis in the stomach. The gall bladder was dilated and the cystic duct was tortuous but the hepatic parenchyma was of normal echogenicity.

Feline TLI was measured and the result (which came back after the cat had died) was 272 ng/ml (reference interval 12–82) suggestive of pancreatitis. Folate and B12 were also measured and were normal.

Diagnosis

Acute pancreatitis was tentatively diagnosed. The cat died 8 hours after admission in spite of intensive management with intravenous fluids, antibiotics and analgesics. Post-mortem examination confirmed acute necrotizing pancreatitis.

Case 3

Signalment

12-month-old neutered female German Shepherd.

History and clinical findings

Weight loss, polyphagia, vomiting bile and intermittent diarrhoea with mucus passed 3–4 times a day for several months. Clinical examination revealed poor body condition with a dry coat but was otherwise unremarkable.

Clinical pathology data

Haematology	Result	Reference interval
RBC (x 10^{12}/l)	8.76	5.5–8.5
Hb (g/dl)	19.1	12–18
HCT (l/l)	0.60	0.37–0.55
MCV (fl)	68.7	60–77
MCHC (g/dl)	31.7	32–37
WBC (x 10^9/l)	13.1	6.0–17.0
Neutrophils (x 10^9/l)	11.4	3.0–11.5
Lymphocytes (x 10^9/l)	0.4	1.0–4.8
Monocytes (x 10^9/l)	1.0	0.2–1.5
Eosinophils (x 10^9/l)	0.2	0.1–1.3
Platelets (x 10^9/l)	180	175–500
Fibrinogen (g/l)	1.0	2.0–4.0

Biochemistry	Result	Reference interval
Sodium (mmol/l)	149.3	135.0–155.0
Potassium (mmol/l)	5.13	3.7–5.8
Glucose (mmol/l)	2.9	3.4–5.3
Urea (mmol/l)	5.7	3.3–6.7
Creatinine (μmol/l)	112	70–170
Calcium (mmol/l)	2.64	2.2–2.7
Inorganic phosphate (mmol/l)	0.87	0.6–1.3
TP (g/l)	62.5	55.0–80.0
ALT (IU/l)	52	21–59
AST (IU/l)	57	20–32
ALP (IU/l)	42	3–142

Gastrointestinal panel	Result	Reference interval
TLI (ng/ml)	<1.5	EPI <2.5 Normal >5.0
Folate (ng/ml)	2.6	3–13
Cobalamin (pg/ml)	534	>200

Case 3 continues ▶

Case 3 continued

Faecal culture

Campylobacter cultured. Negative parasitology and *Giardia*.

What abnormalities are present?

Haematology

- Lymphopenia
- Mild eythrocytosis.

Biochemistry

- Hypoglycaemia.

Gastrointestinal panel

- Subnormal TLI
- Low folate
- Normal cobalamin.

Faecal culture

- *Campylobacter*.

How would you interpret these results?

Haematology is normal except for a lymphopenia (most likely to be stress related), and a mild erythrocytosis, possibly secondary to mild hypovolaemia. The mild reduction in glucose may be due to malnutrition, or inappropriate sample handling (wrong anticoagulant).

The low TLI in a German Shepherd Dog with this history is highly suggestive of clinical EPI due to PAA, but at least one repeat test is advisable. The low folate is unusual (it should be increased due to small intestinal bacterial overgrowth). Cobalamin is normal, although it is often reduced in EPI. The *Campylobacter* infection is probably secondary but should be treated as it may worsen the clinical signs.

Diagnosis and treatment

EPI was diagnosed, probably due to PAA, and concurrent *Campylobacter* infection. The dog was treated with a low-fat diet, pancreatic enzyme supplementation and a course of erythromycin for the *Campylobacter* followed by metronidazole for possible secondary small intestinal bacterial overgrowth. The faecal quality improved and she gained a little weight but the vomiting continued.

	TLI (ng/ml) (EPI <2.5, normal >5)	**Folate** (ng/ml) (normal 3–13)	**Cobalamin** (pg/ml) (normal >200)
2 months later	1.8	1.1	294
5 months later	1.5	4.1	<100

Follow-up

Final diagnosis and outcome

The persistently low TLI confirmed EPI. The persistently low folate and progressive reduction in cobalamin in spite of enzyme supplementation suggested infiltrative disease in the small intestine reducing absorption. The owner declined any further work-up or biopsies, so a novel protein diet and steroid therapy were commenced with a presumptive diagnosis of concurrent inflammatory bowel disease. The improvement was dramatic: the vomiting stopped and the dog gained weight.

References and further reading

Bennett PF, Hahn KA, Toal RL and Legendre AM (2001) Ultrasonographic and cytopathological diagnosis of exocrine pancreatic carcinoma in the dog and cat. *Journal of the American Animal Hospital Association* **37,** 466–473

Bjorneby JM and Kari S (2002) Cytology of the pancreas. *Veterinary Clinics of North America: Small Animal Practice* **32,** 1293–1312

Bright JM (1985) Pancreatic adenocarcinoma in a dog with a maldigestion syndrome. *Journal of the American Veterinary Medical Association* **187,** 420–421

Cook AK, Breitschwerdt EB, Levine JF, Bunch SE and Linn LO (1993) Risk factors associated with acute pancreatitis in dogs: 101 cases (1985–1990). *Journal of the American Veterinary Medical Association* **203,** 673–679

Gerhardt A, Steiner J M, Williams DA, Kramer S, Fuchs C, Janthur M, Hewicker-Trautwein M and Nolte I (2001) Comparison of the sensitivity of different diagnostic tests for pancreatitis in cats. *Journal of Veterinary Internal Medicine* **15,** 329–333

Hall EJ, Bond PM, McLean C, Batt RM and McLean L (1991) A survey of the diagnosis and treatment of canine exocrine pancreatic insufficiency. *Journal of Small Animal Practice* **32,** 613–619

Hess RS, Saunders M, Van Winkle TJ, Shofer FS and Washabau RJ (1998) Clinicopathological, radiographic and ultrasonographic abnormalities in dogs with fatal acute pancreatitis: 70 cases (1986–1995). *Journal of the American Veterinary Medical Association* **213,** 665–670

Hill RC and Van Winkle TJ (1993) Acute necrotizing pancreatitis and acute suppurative pancreatitis in the cat: a retrospective study of 40 cases (1976–1989). *Journal of Veterinary Internal Medicine* **7,** 25–33

Keller ET (1990) High serum trypsin-like immunoreactivity secondary to pancreatitis in a dog with exocrine pancreatic insufficiency. *Journal of the American Veterinary Medical Association* **196,** 623–626

Kimmel SE, Washabau RJ and Drobatz KJ (2001) Incidence and prognostic value of low plasma ionised calcium concentration in cats with acute pancreatitis: 46 cases (1996–1998). *Journal of the American Veterinary Medical Association* **219,** 1105–1109

Mansfield CS and Jones BR (2000) Plasma and urinary trypsinogen activation peptide in healthy dogs, dogs with pancreatitis and dogs with other systemic diseases. *Australian Veterinary Journal* **78,** 416–422

Mansfield CS and Jones BR (2001) Review of feline pancreatitis part two: clinical signs, diagnosis and treatment. *Journal of Feline Medicine and Surgery* **3,** 125–132

Mansfield CS, Jones BR and Spillman T (2003) Assessing the severity of canine pancreatitis. *Research in Veterinary Science* **74,** 137–144

Mayhew PD, Holt DE, McLear RC and Washabau RJ (2002) Pathogenesis and outcome of extrahepatic biliary obstruction in cats. *Journal of Small Animal Practice* **43,** 247–253

Naruse S, Kitagawa M and Ishiguro H (1999) Molecular understanding of chronic pancreatitis: a perspective on the future. *Molecular Medicine Today* **5,** 493–499

Norman J (1998) The role of cytokines in the pathogenesis of acute pancreatitis. *American Journal of Surgery* **175,** 76–83

Quigley KA, Jackson ML and Haines DM (2001) Hyperlipasemia in 6 dogs with pancreatic or hepatic neoplasia: evidence for tumour lipase production. *Veterinary Clinical Pathology* **30,** 114–120

Ruaux CG (2000) Pathophysiology of organ failure in severe acute pancreatitis in dogs. *Compendium on Continuing Education for the Practicing Veterinarian* **22,** 531–542

Ruaux CG and Atwell RB (1998) A severity score for spontaneous canine acute pancreatitis. *Australian Veterinary Journal* **76,** 804–808

Ruaux CG and Atwell RB (1999) Levels of total α-macroglobulin and trypsin-like immunoreactivity are poor indicators of clinical severity in spontaneous canine acute pancreatitis. *Research in Veterinary Science* **67,** 83–87

Schaer M (1979) A clinicopathological survey of acute pancreatitis in 30 dogs and 5 cats. *Journal of the American Animal Hospital Association* **15,** 681–687

Spillmann T, Wiberg ME, Teigelkamp S, Failing K, Chaudhry YS, Kirsch A, Eifler R, Westermarck E, Eigenbrodt E and Sziegoleit A (2000) Canine pancreatic elastase in dogs with clinical exocrine pancreatic insufficiency, normal dogs and dogs with chronic enteropathies. *The European Journal of Comparative Gastroenterology* **5,** 1–6

Spillmann T, Wittker S, Teigelkamp S, Eim C., Burkhardt E, Eigenbrodt E and Sziegoleit A (2001) An immunoassay for canine pancreatic elastase 1 as an indicator of exocrine pancreatic insufficiency in dogs. *Journal of Veterinary Diagnostic Investigation* **13,** 468–474

Steiner JM (2003) Diagnosis of pancreatitis. *Veterinary Clinics of North America: Small Animal Practice* **33,** 1181–1195

Steiner JM, Gumminger SR, Rutz GM and Williams DA (2001) Serum canine pancreatic lipase immunoreactivity in dogs with exocrine pancreatic insufficiency. *Journal of Veterinary Internal Medicine* **15,** 274

Steiner JM and Williams DA (2000) Serum feline trypsin-like immunoractivity in cats with exocrine pancreatic insufficiency. *Journal of Veterinary Internal Medicine* **14,** 627–629

Strombeck DR, Wheeldon E and Harrold D (1984) Model of chronic pancreatitis in the dog. *American Journal of Veterinary Research* **45,** 131–136

Suchodolski JS, Ruaux CG, Steiner JM, Collard JC, Simpson KW and Williams DA (2001) Serum α_1-proteinase-inhibitor/trypsin complex as a marker for canine pancreatitis. *Journal of Veterinary Internal Medicine* **15,** 273

Swift NC, Marks SL, MacLachlan NJ and Norris CR (2000) Evaluation of serum feline trypsin-like immunoreactivity for diagnosis of pancreatitis in cats. *Journal of the American Veterinary Medical Association* **217,** 37–42

Watson PJ (2003) Exocrine pancreatic insufficiency as an end stage of pancreatitis in four dogs. *Journal of Small Animal Practice* **44,** 306–312

Weiss DJ, Gagne JM and Armstrong PJ (1996) Relationship between inflammatory hepatic disease and inflammatory bowel disease, pancreatitis and nephritis in cats. *Journal of the American Veterinary Medical Association* **206,** 1114–1116

Westermarck E and Sandholm M (1980) Faecal hydrolase activity as determined by radial enzyme diffusion: a new method for detecting pancreatic dysfunction in the dog. *Research in Veterinary Science* **28,** 341–346

Whitney MS, Boon GD, Rebar AH and Ford RB (1987) Effects of acute pancreatitis on circulating lipids in dogs. *American Journal of Veterinary Research* **48,** 1492–1497

Wiberg ME (2004) Pancreatic acinar atrophy in German Shepherd Dogs and Rough-coated Collies. Aetiopathogenesis, diagnosis and treatment: a review. *Veterinary Quarterly* **26,** 62–75

Wiberg ME, Nurmi AK and Westermarck E (1999) Serum trypsin-like immunoreactivity measurement for the diagnosis of subclinical exocrine pancreatic insufficiency. *Journal of Veterinary Internal Medicine* **13,** 426–432

Williams DA and Batt RM (1988) Sensitivity and specificity of radioimmunoassay of serum trypsin-like immunoreactivity for the diagnosis of canine exocrine pancreatic insufficiency. *Journal of the American Veterinary Medical Association* **192,** 195–201

Williams DA, Steiner JM, Ruaux CG and Zavros N (2003) Increases in serum pancreatic lipase immunoreactivity (PLI) are greater and of longer duration than those of trypsin-like immunoreactivity (TLI) in cats with experimental pancreatitis. *Journal of Veterinary Internal Medicine* **17,** 445–446

15

Laboratory evaluation of lipid disorders

Joan Duncan

Introduction

The lipids, including triglycerides and cholesterol (Figure 15.1), are essential for normal physiological function. Triglycerides are a source of chemical energy, while cholesterol is a structural component of cell membranes and an essential precursor in steroid hormone synthesis. Decreased or increased plasma lipid concentrations are identified relatively frequently in veterinary patients. Hyperlipidaemia, an increase in plasma cholesterol and/or triglyceride, is most common. It may arise as the result of a primary defect in lipoprotein metabolism or as a consequence of an underlying systemic disease. This chapter outlines the major events in lipid metabolism and the investigation of hyperlipidaemia.

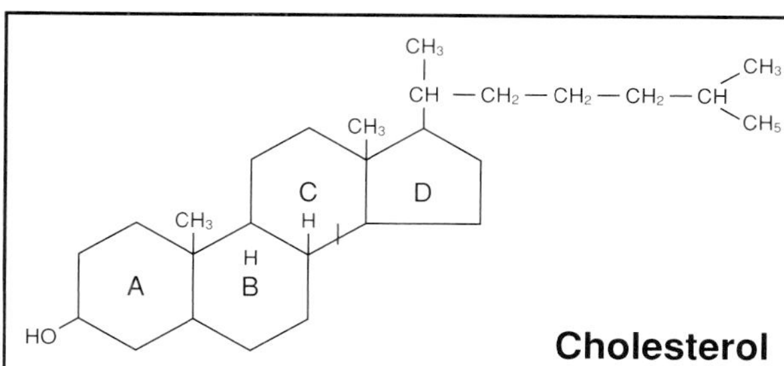

15.1 Chemical structures of cholesterol and a triglyceride. Triglycerides are the result of esterification of three fatty acids and glycerol.

Lipid metabolism in the dog and cat

Lipids and lipoproteins

Lipids are insoluble and are transported through the plasma to their sites of utilization in lipid–protein complexes called lipoproteins. The interactions between lipoproteins and tissues ensure the efficient transport of lipid in response to physiological demand. Lipoproteins are composed of a surface coat, containing phospholipid, free cholesterol and apolipoproteins, surrounding a hydrophobic lipid centre containing triglyceride and cholesterol esters (Figure 15.2). The apolipoproteins (designated apoA, apoB, etc.) are specific proteins that direct the lipoproteins to their sites of metabolism and act as cofactors in the enzymatic reactions of lipid metabolism.

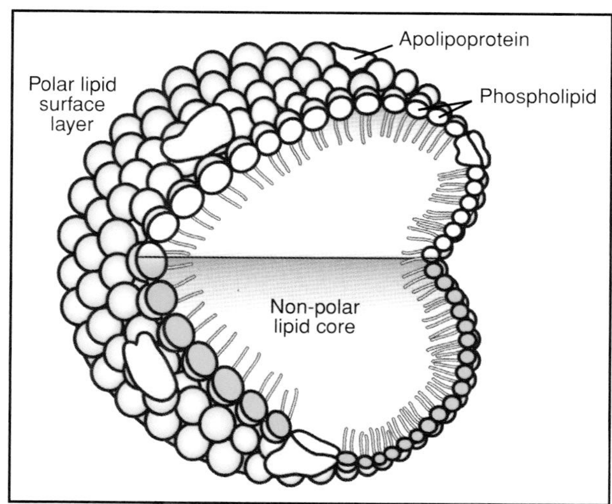

15.2 Schematic representation of a lipoprotein. The polar surface layer is composed of phospholipids, cholesterol and apolipoproteins. The non-polar core contains triglyceride and cholesterol esters.

There are four discrete populations of lipoproteins recognized in the dog and cat, classified on the basis of their size, density, lipid and apolipoprotein content, and electrophoretic mobility. Each lipoprotein species has a specific function (Figure 15.3). The classes recognized in the dog are:

- Chylomicrons
- Very low density lipoproteins (VLDLs), which transport primarily triglyceride (TG), with a small amount of cholesterol
- Low density lipoproteins (LDLs), which transport primarily cholesterol
- High density lipoproteins (HDLs), which also transport primarily cholesterol.

Figure 15.4 shows an outline of lipid metabolism which is based on observations in dogs, cats and humans.

Lipoprotein	Function
Predominantly triglyceride transport	
Chylomicrons	Transport of dietary lipid (predominantly triglyceride) from the intestines to the peripheral tissues and liver.
Very low density lipoproteins (VLDL)	Export of hepatic triglyceride and cholesterol to peripheral tissues. Modified by the action of lipases to form LDL (see below).
Predominantly cholesterol transport	
Low density lipoproteins (LDL)	Delivery of cholesterol to peripheral tissues.
High density lipoproteins (HDL)	Transport of excess cholesterol from peripheral tissues to the liver (for excretion or export elsewhere). Donates apoC and apoE to chylomicrons and VLDL, facilitating delivery of the contents of these lipoproteins to the tissue, and their remnants to the liver.

15.3 Functions of the lipoproteins involved in lipid metabolism.

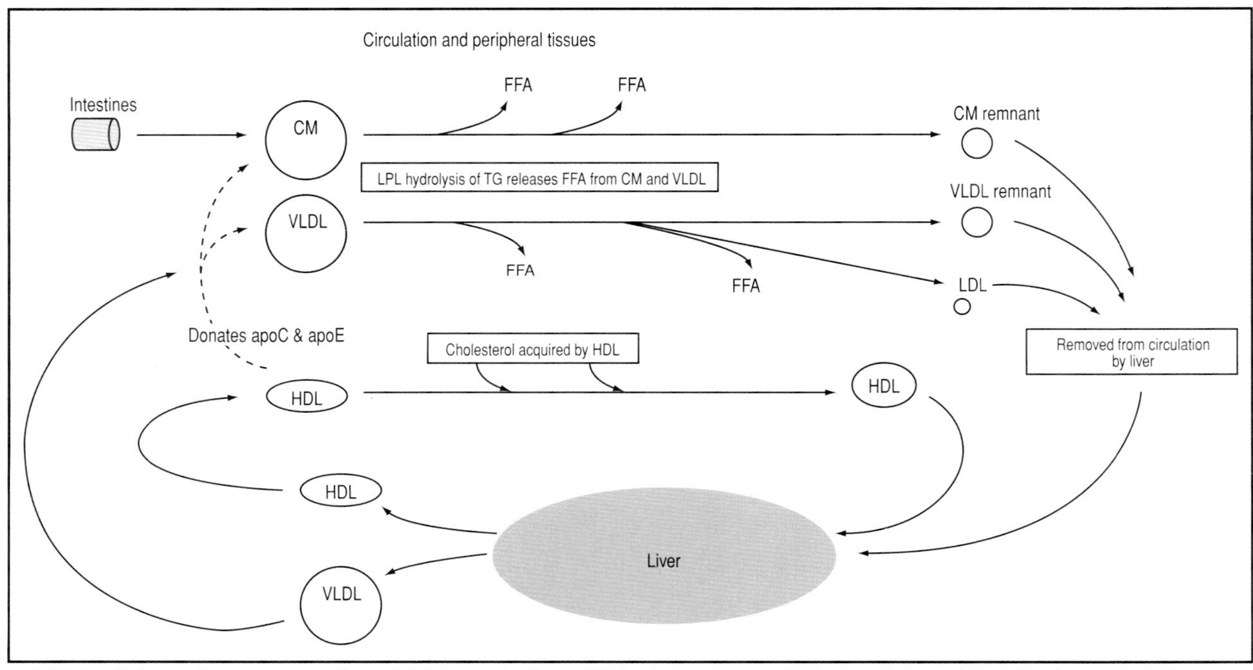

15.4 Schematic representation of lipid metabolism. (CM, chylomicrons; FFA, free fatty acids; LPL, lipoprotein lipase; TG, triglyceride)

Dietary lipid metabolism

Ingested TG is broken down in the intestine into fatty acids and monoglyceride, which are then taken up by intestinal luminal cells and reassembled into TG. This TG is assembled with cholesterol, phospholipids and the apolipoprotein, apoB_{48}, to form chylomicrons. Following secretion from the luminal cells, the chylomicrons enter the intestinal lacteals and lymphatics, where they transfer to the thoracic duct and, finally, the circulation. Chylomicron synthesis, therefore, accompanies fat absorption and this lipoprotein class is detected in postprandial plasma. After entering the circulation, the chylomicrons acquire apoC and apoE from HDL. ApoC-II activates the enzyme lipoprotein lipase (LPL), which hydrolyses the chylomicron core TG, liberating fatty acids for uptake by the peripheral tissues. LPL is bound to the endothelium of a number of tissues, particularly skeletal muscle and adipose tissue. The activity of adipose tissue LPL correlates positively with plasma insulin concentrations, ensuring delivery of fatty acids to the adipose tissue during the postprandial period. The remaining chylomicron remnant is removed from the circulation by hepatocytes, via a receptor which recognizes apoE.

Endogenous lipid metabolism

Lipoproteins are synthesized continuously in the liver in the form of VLDLs and HDLs, although secretion is influenced by nutritional and metabolic changes which alter demand for the lipids carried in the lipoprotein core.

VLDL and LDL

VLDLs are large macromolecules that contain predominantly TG, with a small amount of cholesterol and apoB_{100} (also apoB_{48} in the dog). Upon entering the circulation, the core lipid of VLDL is subjected to the lipolytic action of LPL, in a similar fashion to chylomicrons, liberating fatty acids from hydrolysed

TG. The resulting remnant may be removed from the circulation by a hepatic receptor, or further modified to intermediate-density lipoproteins (IDL), and then LDLs. LDLs are removed from the circulation by a cell surface receptor (apoB,E receptor) found in the liver and peripheral tissues, ensuring delivery of cholesterol to a wide variety of tissues.

HDL

In the dog and cat, HDLs are the major carrier of plasma cholesterol. They accept cholesterol from the peripheral tissues and transport it to the liver where it may be stored, used in the synthesis of bile acids, excreted or redistributed. In addition, HDLs donate apoC and apoE to chylomicrons and VLDLs, facilitating the metabolism of these lipoproteins.

HDLs are synthesized primarily in the liver in the form of a disc-shaped phospholipid bilayer containing cholesterol and apoA-I (a crucial structural protein of this lipoprotein class). The immature lipoprotein circulates through the peripheral tissues where it collects tissue cholesterol, thus forming a mature HDL. During HDL maturation, free cholesterol at the surface of the HDL is esterified by the action of lecithin:cholesterol acyltransferase (LCAT) and the cholesteryl ester enters the lipid core of the lipoprotein. In this way, cholesterol is drawn from the peripheral tissues into the immature lipoprotein. Progressive accumulation of cholesterol results in expansion of the macromolecule, which is ultimately returned to the liver and removed from the circulation by hepatic receptors. The cholesteryl esters in the core of HDL are not transferred to other lipoprotein species, but are directed to the liver for excretion. The containment of cholesteryl esters within the HDL class and their efficient uptake by hepatic receptors may play a major role in the protection of the dog from atherosclerosis. In contrast, LDL is the main cholesterol carrier species in humans, and is considered to be the major participating lipoprotein in the development of atherosclerosis.

Measurement of lipids and lipoproteins

The measurement of plasma cholesterol and TG can easily be performed using enzymatic, colorimetric methods designed for patient-side biochemistry analysers and large-scale commercial analysers. Serum or heparinized plasma are usually acceptable, and a fasted sample (ideally 12 hours) is preferred. Where immediate analysis is not possible, the serum or plasma should be separated from the cells and the sample may be stored for 4 days at 2–8°C without significant effect on either analyte.

Cholesterol is often included in routine screening profiles, especially where endocrine disease is suspected, and hypercholesterolaemia is relatively commonly identified. Estimation of the TG concentration is less commonly included in routine profiles, but measurement should be performed when lipaemia is detected on visual appraisal of the plasma. Lipaemia is the milky turbidity of plasma caused by the accumulation of triglyceride-rich lipoproteins (chylomicrons, VLDL) (Figure 15.5), and is not secondary to hypercholesterolaemia. This turbidity of the sample is important, since it may interfere with the production of accurate laboratory results. The magnitude and direction of error depends upon the degree of lipaemia and the methodology of the test; potential effects are listed in Figure 15.6. Diagnostic laboratories and the manufacturers of patient-side analysers are able to provide information regarding the effect of lipaemia on their specific methodologies. The visual appraisal of a spun serum or plasma sample for the presence of lipaemia is therefore an essential component of any biochemical analysis, and allows the operator to predict potential interference with laboratory analyses. The effect of lipaemia on laboratory tests may be compounded by *in vitro* haemolysis. The degree of haemolysis may be related to the length of contact time

Hyperlipidaemia
Increased concentrations of plasma cholesterol and/or triglyceride. Hypertriglyceridaemia may be accompanied by lipaemia.
Lipaemia
The turbidity of whole blood, serum or plasma caused by an increased concentration of triglycerides, carried in triglyceride-rich lipoproteins.

15.5 Definition of terms.

Parameter	Potential effect
Haemoglobin	Increased
Mean corpuscular haemoglobin concentration (MCHC)	Increased
Electrolytes by ion-specific electrode	Not affected
Glucose	Increased
Blood urea nitrogen	Variable
Creatinine	Increased
Calcium	Increased
Phosphate	Increased
Total protein (refractometer)	Increased
Albumin	Decreased
Alanine aminotransferase (ALT)	Increased
Aspartate aminotransferase (AST)	Increased
Alkaline phosphatase (ALP)	Increased
Gamma-glutamyl transferase (GGT)	Variable
Amylase	Decreased
Lipase	Decreased
Cholesterol	Variable
Bile acids	Increased
Bilirubin	Increased

15.6 The potential effects of lipaemia on the results of biochemical tests. Diagnostic laboratories and manufacturers of patient-side analysers will provide details for their specific test methods.

with erythrocytes. Therefore, rapid analysis or immediate separation of the cells from the plasma can reduce this phenomenon. For biochemical tests, preparation of plasma (which can be separated immediately), rather than serum, can be helpful.

When lipaemia is present, the possibility of physiological hyperlipidaemia secondary to a recent meal should be considered initially. If the lipaemia is present to a degree which will interfere with routine analysis then it would be prudent to collect a fasting sample (12–16 hours) for repeat analysis. Measurement of the TG concentration in the fasting sample allows confirmation or exclusion of pathological hyperlipidaemia. In some patients, there may still be considerable lipaemia present, even after fasting. The TG concentration must be measured in an aliquot of the lipaemic sample, but manipulation is then required to clear the turbidity for further analysis. Refrigeration of the sample helps to clear the sample of chylomicrons, which float to the top, forming a cream layer. Plasma collected from below the cream layer may be suitable for analysis. Clearing agents can be used to remove the offending lipoproteins, however the manufacturer recommends that the effects of the agent on biochemical results should be established for each laboratory system.

Investigation of hyperlipidaemia

Where lipaemia is present in a fasted sample it is possible to characterize further the abnormalities of lipid metabolism, i.e. is the lipaemia associated with an increased concentration of chylomicrons, VLDL or both? The serum or plasma is stored overnight at 4°C. Chylomicrons float to the top of the sample forming a 'cream layer', while an increase in the VLDL concentration is characterized by a generalized opalescence of the plasma (Figure 15.7). Laboratory confirmation of the presence of these and the other classes of lipoproteins can be achieved by lipoprotein electrophoresis and combined ultracentrifugation/precipitation methods. These techniques are not routinely available for veterinary patients but are available through some university clinical pathology laboratories in the UK and elsewhere.

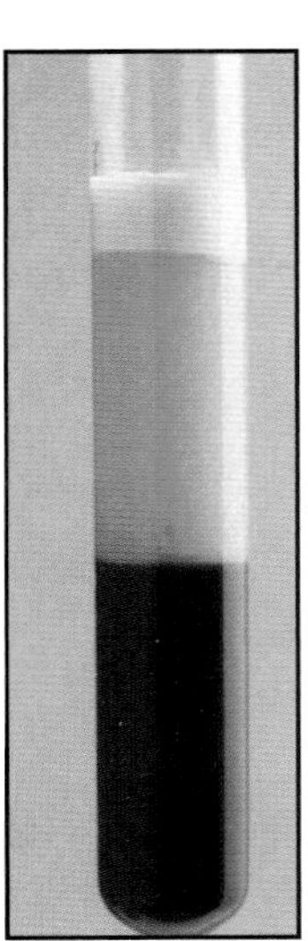

15.7 A cream layer of chylomicrons above an opalescent plasma containing VLDL in a sample from a dog with concurrent diabetes mellitus and hypothyroidism.

The demonstration of fasting hyperlipidaemia should initiate routine screening (clinical and laboratory) for underlying endocrine or systemic disease (Figures 15.8 and 15.9). A full haematology and biochemistry screen, urinalysis and specific endocrine testing may be required. If underlying disease is recognized then further lipid investigation is usually unnecessary. Where no underlying disease or inherited basis is proven, the hyperlipidaemia is classified as idiopathic. In these cases it may be necessary to categorize the lipoprotein disturbances further in order to select a management strategy.

Physiological hyperlipidaemia
Postprandial hypertriglyceridaemia
Secondary hyperlipidaemia
Diabetes mellitus Hypothyroidism Hyperadrenocorticism Cholestatic liver disease Glomerulonephritis Non-nephrotic renal disease Glucocorticoid therapy Megoestrol acetate (cats)
Inherited hyperlipidaemia (proven or suspected)
Inherited hyperchylomicronaemia in the cat Idiopathic hyperlipidaemia in the Miniature Schnauzer Hypercholesterolaemia in the Briard
Idiopathic hyperlipidaemia

15.8 The potential causes of hyperlipidaemia (increased cholesterol and/or triglyceride).

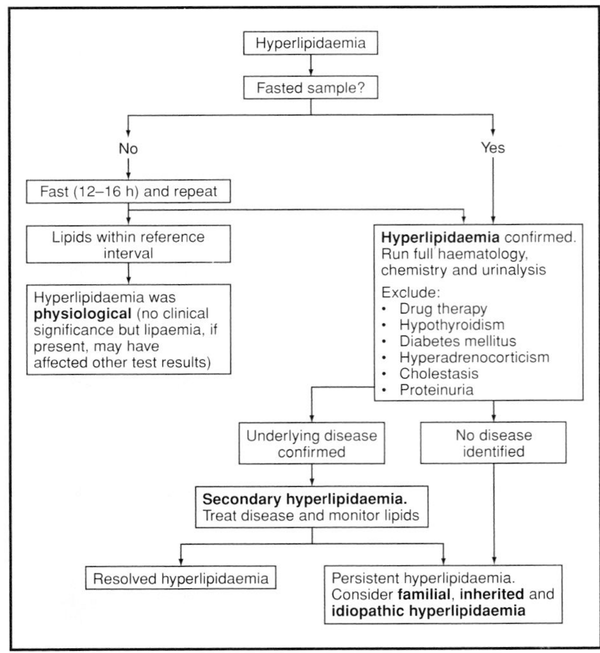

15.9 The investigation of hyperlipidaemia.

Abnormalities of lipid metabolism: potential causes

Physiological

The absorption of dietary fat from the intestines is accompanied by the formation of chylomicrons. The accumulation of these TG-rich lipoproteins lends a turbidity (lipaemia) to the serum or plasma of normal individuals, which clears by 4–6 hours after eating.

Diabetes mellitus

Hyperlipidaemia is commonly associated with endocrine disease. Canine diabetes mellitus (DM) is often accompanied by mild to moderate hypercholesterolaemia (<15 mmol/l) and hypertriglyceridaemia. Mechanisms for hyperlipidaemia in DM include impaired LPL activity (this enzyme requires insulin for its activation) and increased mobilization of body fat. Hyperlipidaemia has also been noted with feline diabetes mellitus.

Hypothyroidism

Two thirds of dogs with hypothyroidism are reported to have an increased serum cholesterol concentration. Hypertriglyceridaemia may or may not be present. The lipid abnormalities are probably secondary to reduced hepatic clearance of LDLs and reduced LPL activity (Barrie *et al.*, 1993). Hypercholesterolaemia secondary to hypothyroidism may be mild to marked and, in the author's experience, marked hypercholesterolaemia (>15 mmol/l) is most commonly associated with hypothyroidism alone, or a combination of endocrine disorders.

There are occasional reports of an unusual lipoprotein (β-VLDL) in the plasma of dogs with marked hypercholesterolaemia and hypothyroidism. The factors which determine the appearance of this lipoprotein are not clear, but in man it has been proposed that this lipoprotein has a marked atherogenic potential.

The clinical consequences of mild or moderate hypercholesterolaemia are not usually serious. However, spontaneous atherosclerosis is a potential complication of marked hypercholesterolaemia. Hess *et al.* (2003) demonstrated that dogs with atherosclerosis are more likely to have concurrent DM or hypothyroidism than dogs without vascular changes. The clinical signs of vascular disease depend upon the organ or tissue affected but neurological signs have been described, including stupor, seizures and paresis secondary to iliac thrombosis (Zeiss and Waddle, 1995).

Hyperadrenocorticism

Hyperadrenocorticism is often accompanied by mild to moderate hypercholesterolaemia (usually <15 mmol/l) and hypertriglyceridaemia, secondary to increased concentrations of LDLs and VLDLs.

Liver, intestinal and pancreatic disease

Cholestatic disease is commonly associated with moderate to marked hypercholesterolaemia, largely due to reduced biliary excretion of cholesterol. The lipid abnormalities resolve with correction of the underlying biliary stasis. Hypocholesterolaemia has been observed in patients with severe hepatic dysfunction, especially cirrhosis, and as a consequence of protein-losing enteropathies.

Historically, it was proposed that canine pancreatitis caused hypertriglyceridaemia, but more recently it has become accepted that marked hypertriglyceridaemia (> 5 mmol/l) may predispose an individual to pancreatitis. Although not all patients with hypertriglyceridaemia develop pancreatitis, dietary intervention is warranted in an attempt to reduce the TG concentration. Moderate hypercholesterolaemia is also noted in some cases of pancreatitis (Bauer, 2000), possibly secondary to biliary obstruction.

Renal disease

Glomerulonephritis and non-nephrotic renal disease have been associated with a variety of lipid abnormalities (Down and Krawiec, 1996) including mild to moderate hypertriglyceridaemia and hypercholesterolaemia. The relationship between renal function and lipid metabolism has not been extensively studied in dogs and cats but exclusion of proteinuria is an important step in the investigation of hyperlipidaemia.

Neoplasia

Cancer cachexia in man and animals has been associated with abnormalities of lipid metabolism. In one study of canine lymphoma (Ogilvie *et al.*, 1994), dogs with disease had significantly higher TG concentrations. In man, it is proposed that the metabolic alterations may be related to the tumour type, but extensive research on the effect of tumour type on lipid metabolism in veterinary patients has not been performed.

Drug therapy and diet

Drugs which may cause hypercholesterolaemia include corticosteroids, phenytoin and methimazole (Burkhard and Meyer, 1995). An increase in TG concentration may be noted with corticosteroids, oestrogens and cholestyramine (Burkhard and Meyer, 1995). Megestrol acetate is reported to cause hyperlipidaemia in cats (Bauer, 1992).

The effect of diet should also be considered when evaluating lipid abnormalities. Diets which provide many of the calories as fat may be associated with mildly increased cholesterol concentrations (Bauer, 2000).

Familial hyperchylomicronaemia in cats

An inherited defect of LPL activity is recognized as the cause of familial hyperchylomicronaemia in cats (Peritz *et al.*, 1990). The defect, which has been recognized in kittens and young adults, results in the accumulation of chylomicrons and VLDL in the plasma of fasted cats. Peritz *et al.* (1990) identified a point mutation which prevents LPL binding with the endothelial surface. However, more recently reported cases of feline hyperchylomicronaemia in the United Kingdom have not demonstrated this mutation (Gunn-Moore *et al.*, 1997).

Some of the kittens with hypertriglyceridaemia have presented with concurrent, profound anaemia (Gunn-Moore *et al.*, 1997) and, in many cases, the owners have sought veterinary advice because of a high kitten mortality rate within individual litters. The cause of the anaemia and the nature of its relationship to the hypertriglyceridaemia have not been determined. In other cats and kittens, additional signs have been described, including the development of xanthomas (lipid granulomas) over bony prominences and at sites of trauma, Horner's syndrome, other peripheral neuropathies (Jones, 1993), lipaemia retinalis (pale pink appearance of the retinal vessels) and lipid-laden aqueous humour.

Hyperlipidaemia of the Miniature Schnauzer

Idiopathic hyperlipidaemia in the Miniature Schnauzer is thought to be the result of an inherited defect, the exact nature of which has not been elucidated. The clinical entity is characterized by hypertriglyceridaemia associated with increased VLDLs, with or without accompanying hyperchylomicronaemia (Whitney *et al.*, 1993). Proposed mechanisms include increased production of VLDL, reduced clearance of this lipoprotein secondary to decreased LPL activity and the presence of a hepatic membrane receptor defect with impaired lipoprotein remnant clearance (Bauer, 2000). Clinical signs may be noted with moderate to marked hypertriglyceridaemia and include abdominal pain, anorexia, intestinal signs, seizures, lipaemia retinalis and lipid-laden aqueous humour.

Idiopathic hypercholesterolaemia of the Briard

Mild hypercholesterolaemia (<9 mmol/l) has been reported in Briards in the United Kingdom (Watson *et al.*, 1993).

Therapy for hyperlipidaemia

With the possible exception of the lipid changes associated with neoplasia, the plasma lipid alterations of dogs and cats with secondary hyperlipidaemia resolve after successful stabilization or treatment of the underlying disease process. Where the abnormalities do not resolve, or inherited/idiopathic hyperlipidaemia is suspected, then dietary, and possibly therapeutic, intervention, is indicated (Duncan, 2004).

Case examples

Case 1

Signalment

10-year-old male Boxer.

History

Gradual onset of polyuria, polydipsia and abdominal enlargement. Signs present for several months.

Clinical pathology data

Biochemistry	Result	Reference interval
Glucose (mmol/l)	8.22	4.3–6.9
Urea (mmol/l)	2.6	2.5–9.6
Creatinine (μmol/l)	74	44–159
Calcium (mmol/l)	2.47	1.98–3.0
Albumin (g/l)	31	27–38
ALT (IU/l)	220	10–100
ALP (IU/l)	444	23–212
Cholesterol (mmol/l)	10.82	2.8–8.3
Bilirubin (μmol/l)	10	0–15

Sample quality

No lipidaemia noted.

What abnormalities are present?

Increased liver enzyme activities (both ALP and ALT twice upper limit of the normal range), hyperglycaemia and hypercholesterolaemia.

How would you interpret these results?

The results, taken with the clinical presentation, could support a diagnosis of hyperadrenocorticism. Hypothyroidism is also a possibility, though less likely due to the polydipsia and polyuria, and the elevated ALT.

What further tests would you recommend?

An ACTH stimulation test or low dose dexamethasome suppression test (see Chapter 18) should be performed to confirm the diagnosis of hyperadrenocorticism: the ACTH stimulation test is the usual first test performed as it is less likely to produce false positive results in other disease states. This would not differentiate between pituitary and adrenal dependent disease, however. Total T4 and TSH could be measured (see Chapter 17).

Case outcome

The dog was confirmed to have hyperadrenocorticism using the ACTH stimulation test.

Case 2

Signalment

6-year-old Cocker Spaniel.

History

2–3 week history of polyuria, polydipsia and anorexia, mild weight loss.

Clinical pathology data

Biochemistry	Result	Reference interval
Sodium (mmol/l)	141.0	135–155
Potassium (mmol/l)	5.45	3.6–5.6
Sodium/potassium ratio	25.87	28–40
Chloride (mmol/l)	108.0	100–116
Glucose (mmol/l)	5.6	3.3–5.8
Urea (mmol/l)	32.3	2.5–6.7
Creatinine (μmol/l)	322.5	20.0–150.0
Calcium (mmol/l)	2.73	2.40–2.90
Inorganic phosphate (mmol/l)	4.16	0.8–1.6

Case 2 continues ▶

Case 2 continued

Biochemistry *(continued)*	Result	Reference interval
TP (g/l)	49.9	55.0–75.0
Albumin (g/l)	20.6	25.0–41.0
Globulin (g/l)	29.3	20.0–45.0
ALT (IU/l)	19.0	5.0–60.0
ALP (IU/l)	43.1	<130
Cholesterol (mmol/l)	17.00	3.2–6.2
Bile acids (fasting) (μmol/l)	6.5	0.1–5.0
Total bilirubin (μmol/l)	1.6	0.1–5.1

Sample quality

No lipidaemia noted.

Urine analysis	
Specific gravity	1.022
Protein	++++
RBC	<5
WBC	<5
Protein:creatinine ratio	14.96 (reference interval <1)

What abnormalities are present?

Biochemistry

- Hypoalbuminaemia
- Hypercholesterolaemia
- Azotaemia, hyperphosphataemia
- Na:K ratio is slightly decreased

Urinalysis

- Marked proteinuria
- Submaximal concentration of the urine
- Markedly increased protein:creatinine ratio

How would you interpret these results?

The azotaemia, hyperphosphataemia and submaximal concentration of the urine support renal insufficiency and renal azotaemia. The marked proteinuria is likely to have affected (increased) the urine specific gravity. The urinary protein loss is further quantified by a protein:creatinine ratio, which in this case is markedly increased. In the absence of significant haematuria and inflammation, such marked proteinuria is consistent with glomerular protein loss, such as might be noted with glomerulonephritis.

Both the hypoalbuminaemia and hypercholesterolaemia noted in the biochemistry screen could be a consequence of renal protein loss. Other causes of hypoalbuminaemia include hepatic and intestinal disease, while endocrine disease (especially hypothyroidism) could be a potential cause of the hypercholesterolaemia. In the absence of current signs supportive of thyroid disease, the lipid abnormalities are attributable to the renal disease. Further testing for hypothyroidism may be warranted but the presence of non-thyroidal disease would be expected to have an impact on thyroid hormone concentrations (see Chapter 17).

The Na^+:K^+ ratio is slightly decreased, which could be noted in association with hypoadrenocorticism; other disease processes, including primary renal disease, should also be considered.

References and further reading

Barrie J, Watson TDG, Stear MJ and Nash AS (1993) Plasma cholesterol and lipoprotein concentrations in the dog: The effects of age, gender and endocrine disease. *Journal of Small Animal Practice* **34**, 507–512

Bauer JE (1992) Diet-induced alterations of lipoprotein metabolism. *Journal of the American Veterinary Medical Association* **201**, 1691–1694

Bauer JE (2000) Hyperlipidemias. In: *Textbook of Veterinary Internal Medicine, 5th edn,* ed. SJ Ettinger and EC Feldman, pp. 283–292. WB Saunders, Philadelphia

Burkhard MJ and Meyer DJ (1995) Causes and effects of interference with clinical laboratory measurements and examinations. In: *Kirk's Current Veterinary Therapy XII*, ed. JD Bonagura, pp. 14–20. WB Saunders, Philadelphia

Down LK and Krawiec DR (1996) Dyslipoproteinemia of chronic renal failure: its relevance to canine progressive kidney disease. *Compendium on Continuing Education for the Practicing Veterinarian* **18**, 65–74

Duncan J (2004) Hyperlipidaemia. In: *BSAVA Manual of Endocrinology, 3rd edn,* ed. CT Mooney and M Peterson. pp. 49–56. BSAVA, Gloucester

Gunn-Moore DA, Watson TDG, Dodkin SJ, Blaxter AC, Crispin SM and Gruffydd-Jones T (1997) Transient hyperlipidaemia and anaemia in kittens. *Veterinary Record* **140**, 355–359

Hess RS, Kass PH and Van Winkle TJ (2003) Association between diabetes mellitus, hypothyroidism or hyperadrenocorticism and atherosclerosis in dogs. *Journal of Veterinary Internal Medicine* **17**, 489–494

Jones BR (1993) Inherited hyperchylomicronaemia in the cat. *Journal of Small Animal Practice* **34**, 493–499

Ogilvie GK, Ford RB, Vail DM, Walters LM, Salman MD, Babineau C and Fettman MJ (1994) Alterations in lipoprotein profiles in dogs with lymphoma. *Journal of Veterinary Internal Medicine* **8**, 62–66

Peritz LN, Brunzell JD, Harvey-Clarke C, Pritchard PH, Jones BR and Hayden MR (1990) Characterization of a lipoprotein lipase class III type defect in hypertriglyceridemic cats. *Clinical and Investigative Medicine* **13**, 259–263

Watson P, Simpson KW Odedra RM and Bedford PGC (1993) Hypercholesterolaemia in Briards in the United Kingdom. *Research in Veterinary Science* **54**, 80–85

Whitney MS, Boon GD, Rebar AH, Story JA and Bottoms GD (1993) Ultracentrifugal and electrophoretic characteristics of the plasma lipoproteins of Miniature Schnauzer dogs with idiopathic hyperlipoproteinemia. *Journal of Veterinary Internal Medicine* **7**, 253–260

Zeiss CJ and Waddle G (1995) Hypothyroidism and atherosclerosis in dogs. *Compendium on Continuing Education for the Practicing Veterinarian* **17**, 1117–1128

16

Laboratory evaluation of hyperglycaemia and hypoglycaemia

Clare Knottenbelt

Glucose homeostasis

Glucose homeostasis is maintained by an interaction between dietary intake, liver storage and release, and the effects of the major hormones controlling blood glucose concentrations (insulin and glucagon) (Figure 16.1). The liver acts as storage organ where glucose is stored as glycogen. Glucose can be released from the liver by the breakdown of these glycogen stores (glycogenolysis) or by breakdown of fatty acids or amino acids (gluconeogenesis) (Figure 16.2). Other hormones (growth hormone, glucocorticoids, progesterone and oestrogen) alter glucose concentrations by affecting the cellular response to insulin or enhancing hepatic glucose release.

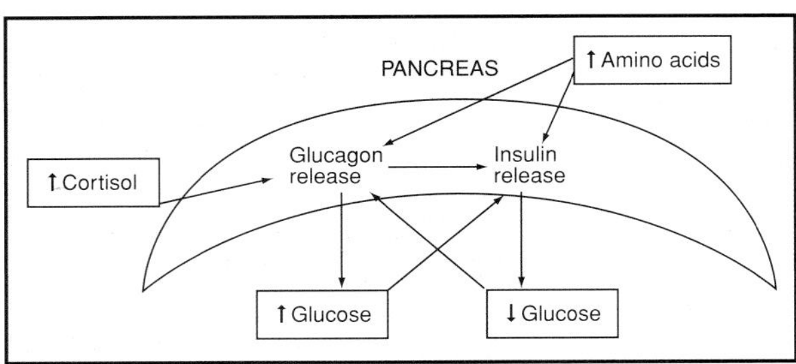

16.1 Glucose homeostasis: effects of insulin and glucagon on blood glucose concentrations in normal animals.

Insulin

Insulin is produced by the beta islet cells of the pancreas and is the major controller of plasma glucose concentrations. When blood glucose increases, insulin is released by the islet cells, resulting in increased cellular uptake of glucose and a reduction in the blood glucose concentration (Figure 16.3). When blood glucose concentrations are low, insulin release is suppressed and the blood insulin concentration falls. Insulin release is also stimulated by fatty acids, some amino acids, ketones and glucagons.

The peripheral effects of insulin include:

- Inhibition of gluconeogenesis
- Increased glucose utilization by cells
- Prevention of fat breakdown.

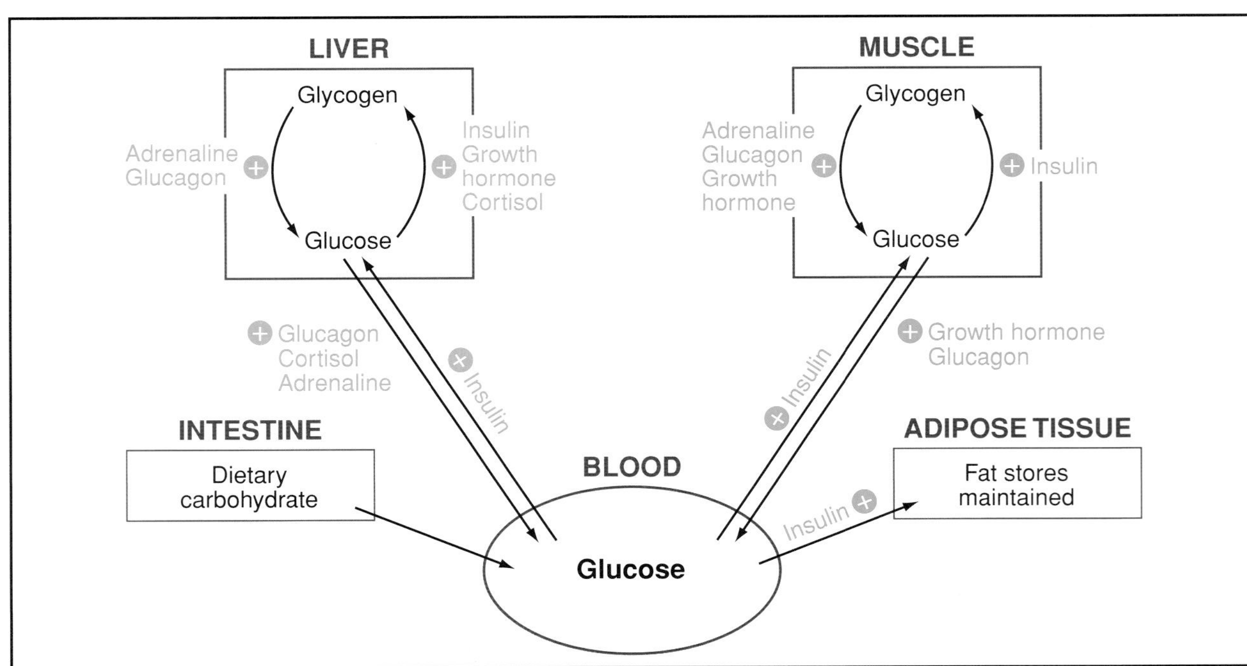

16.2 Glucose homeostasis: effects of counter-regulatory hormones.

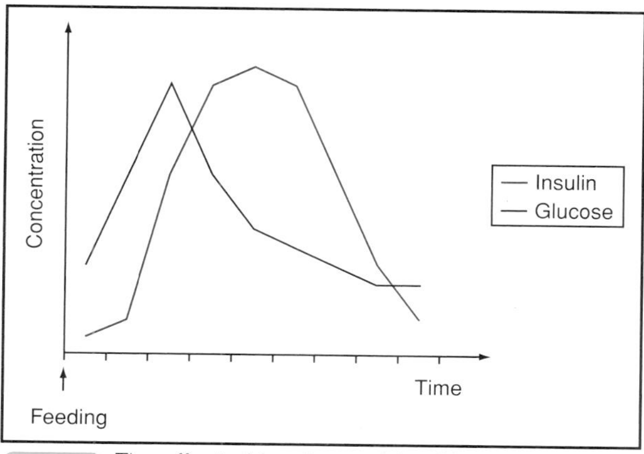

16.3 The effect of feeding on blood levels of glucose and insulin in normal patients.

The effects of insulin are inhibited by growth hormone, glucocorticoids, oestrogen and progesterone: these hormones cause a resistance to the peripheral effects of insulin so that greater concentrations of insulin are required to achieve the same reduction in blood glucose concentrations (see Figure 16.2).

Glucagon

Glucagon is produced by the endocrine pancreas. Its main role is to increase glucose concentration by increasing gluconeogenesis and glycogenolysis in the liver. Increased glucagon secretion occurs when blood glucose concentrations fall, while increases in blood glucose suppress secretion of glucagon.

Other hormones

Growth hormone

Growth hormone is produced in the pituitary gland, and in the mammary gland of entire bitches, under the stimulation of progesterone. Growth hormone stimulates hepatic glucose production and adipocyte lipolysis. It antagonizes insulin activity by causing a decrease in the number of peripheral insulin receptors and by inhibiting glucose transport into cells. This may be mediated by a reduction in the expression of glucose transporter genes.

Progesterone

Progesterone is produced by the corpus luteum during dioestrus, whether or not the bitch or queen is pregnant. Progesterone reduces insulin binding and glucose transport in peripheral tissues, and also stimulates secretion of growth hormone in dogs. Progesterone levels will decline 7 days after spaying or spontaneous regression of the corpus luteum.

Cortisol

Glucocorticoids antagonize both the peripheral and hepatic effects of insulin by reducing the number and efficacy of glucose transporters and increasing circulating concentrations of glucagon and fatty acids. The precise mechanism is unclear, however, as glucocorticoids stimulate receptor gene transcription suggesting that they influence the receptors after the transcription process. Glucocorticoids also promote gluconeogenesis, lipolysis and muscle breakdown, thereby increasing circulating blood glucose concentrations.

Catecholamines

Catecholamines stimulate gluconeogenesis, glycogenolysis and lipolysis by inhibiting peripheral glucose use through a β-adrenergic mechanism, which may involve a decrease in cellular glucose transport.

C-peptide

C-peptide is part of the pro-insulin molecule in dogs and is secreted at the same time as insulin. Its presence in the circulation means that there is still some residual beta cell insulin production. However this does not influence the management of diabetes mellitus.

Assessment of blood glucose

Plasma glucose

Plasma glucose can be assessed using a glucometer, in-house dry chemistry analyser or submitted to an external laboratory (Figure 16.4). As glucose is only contained within the plasma component of blood, glucose concentration is influenced by the packed cell volume (PCV) when whole blood is used for glucose assessment . This means that glucose concentrations will be overestimated in anaemic patients and underestimated in patients with increased PCVs. Measurements of glucose concentration made using whole blood will also be lower than those made using plasma.

If blood for glucose estimation is to be stored, plasma should be separated as soon as possible after collection. Glucose concentrations will fall by 5–10% per hour due to continued utilization of glucose by red and white blood cells. This decline in glucose concentration will be more marked if there is significant erythrocytosis or leucocytosis. Fluoride oxalate anticoagulant is an enzyme inhibitor, which prevents cellular glucose utilization.

It is vital that a number of factors are considered prior to collection of blood for glucose measurement:

- Glucose concentrations will increase after feeding
- Stress or excitement before and during sampling can cause increased blood glucose concentrations.

When measuring blood glucose the following should be observed:

- Fast the patient for 12 hours (unless the patient is immature)
- Avoid stress and excitement throughout sampling
- Avoid the use of certain sedatives (especially medetomidine and ketamine) (see Figure 16.5)
- Separate serum from cellular components within 30 minutes of collection
- Use fluoride oxalate anticoagulant if plasma separation is not possible.

Method of assessment	Advantages	Disadvantages
Glucometer	Small volumes of blood required Rapid results Cheap Useful for assessing trends	Underestimates blood glucose as designed to prevent hypoglycaemia in humans Affected by PCV (see text) Reliability of results can vary between glucometers Fluoride oxalate anticoagulant interferes with the enzyme reaction on some glucometer strips
In-house dry chemistry	Rapid results	Fluoride oxalate anticoagulant cannot be used because glucose oxidase enzyme in most assays is blocked by fluoride. Must assay heparinized samples within 1 hour of collection (see text)
External laboratory	Most accurate assessment of glucose concentrations	Fluoride oxalate must be used as glucose concentration will fall if other anticoagulants are used and cells are left in contact with serum (see text) Relatively expensive

16.4 Methods of assessing glucose.

Glycated proteins

Proteins bind irreversibly to glucose and measurement of glycated proteins can therefore provide an indication of mean blood glucose concentrations over a period of time. The half-life of the protein determines the period over which the glycated proteins reflect blood glucose concentration. When blood glucose concentrations increase there is an increase in glucose binding and therefore an increase in glycated protein concentrations. This increase is also affected by the duration of the increase in blood glucose. If the increase in glucose is transient, there will be no significant increase in glycated protein concentrations (Marca *et al.*, 2000). In addition to the glucose concentrations, any disease that significantly affects the half-life of the protein concerned will influence the result. The most commonly measured glycated proteins are fructosamine and glycated haemoglobin.

Serum fructosamine

Fructosamine is irreversibly glycated albumin and is useful for assessing mean blood glucose concentrations in both dogs and cats. Albumin has a shorter half-life than haemoglobin (see below) and fructosamine reflects glycaemic control over the 2–3 weeks prior to sampling. Fructosamine concentrations are not affected by transient stress hyperglycaemia and are therefore useful in distinguishing between diabetes mellitus and stress- or excitement-associated hyperglycaemia. Fructosamine concentration may be low in patients with recurrent hypoglycaemia, and assessment of fructosamine can therefore be helpful in the diagnosis of insulinoma (Thoresen *et al.*, 1995) especially when hypoglycaemia cannot be documented (Mellanby and Herrtage, 2002). Fructosamine can only be measured in serum samples.

Factors affecting serum fructosamine concentrations:

- **Albumin/protein concentration:** reductions in serum protein concentrations can reduce the fructosamine concentration; fructosamine will, however, remain elevated in patients with concurrent hypoproteinaemia and poorly controlled diabetes mellitus, unless severe hypoproteinaemia is present (Jensen, 1993)
- **Hyperthyroidism and hypothyroidism:** the increased protein turnover associated with hyperthyroidism results in a reduction in fructosamine concentrations (due to a shortened half-life). This may be an important confounding factor in the diagnosis of diabetes mellitus in cats with hyperthyroidism. Conversely, dogs with hypothyroidism (and some cats after thyroidectomy) may have elevated fructosamine concentrations because of decelerated protein turnover (Reusch *et al.*, 2002)
- **Azotaemia in dogs:** azotaemia has been associated with fructosamine concentrations below the reference range in some normoglycaemic dogs, due to denaturation of albumin (Reusch and Harberer, 2001). The significance in dogs with diabetes mellitus has not been investigated.

Glycated haemoglobin

Glycated haemoglobin reflects the glycaemic control over the previous 4–8 weeks as it is dependent on red blood cell half-life. EDTA or heparinized whole blood must be submitted for analysis. Glycated haemoglobin can be useful for monitoring glycaemic control in dogs, but it can be normal in recently diagnosed diabetics and fructosamine is usually preferred. Cats have lower reference concentrations, which may be due to a shorter red blood cell life-span, or the presence of fewer glucose binding sites on feline haemoglobin (Hasegawa *et al.*, 1992), so fructosamine is generally preferred for both diagnosis and monitoring in cats. Glycated haemoglobin is not currently available at commercial laboratories in the United Kingdom.

Glycated haemoglobin must always be interpreted in light of the haemoglobin concentration:

- **Anaemia.** Anaemia is, by definition, a reduction in haemoglobin concentration. Therefore, in patients with anaemia there will be less haemoglobin and fewer binding sites for glucose. The glycated haemoglobin concentration will be lower
- **Erythrocytosis/polycythaemia.** Increased haemoglobin concentrations (as occurs in polycythaemia) will result in increased availability of glucose binding sites and false elevations in glycated haemoglobin.

Hyperglycaemia

The common causes of hyperglycaemia are summarized in Figure 16.5.

Cause	Mechanism
Postprandial	Normal due to absorption of dietary derived glucose. Should return to normal within 4 hours
Stress or excitement (may be significant in cats)	'Stress' hormone associated: predominantly catecholamines
Diabetes mellitus	Insulin deficiency (failure of production) or insulin resistance
Glucose-containing fluids	Ongoing glucose administration
Hyperadrenocorticism (rare in cats, common in dogs)	Insulin antagonism and peripheral resistance
Acromegaly (rare)	Insulin resistance and gluconeogenesis
Acute pancreatitis	Inadequate insulin production due to beta cell damage, peripheral resistance
Peracute liver damage	Inhibition of hepatic insulin action
Sedatives	Reduced insulin production (medetomidine) Stress hormone associated (ketamine)
Drugs	Insulin resistance (glucocorticoids, progestogens) Possible pancreatic toxicity in humans (furosemide, thiazide diuretics)

16.5 Causes and mechanisms of hyperglycaemia.

Diabetes mellitus

Pathophysiology

Diabetes mellitus is caused by inadequate insulin activity. This may result from a failure of beta cell insulin production and/or release, or may be associated with peripheral insulin resistance. The absence of appropriate insulin activity causes persistent hyperglycaemia. In human medicine, diabetes has been classified into three types:

- Type 1 diabetes mellitus (insulin-dependent diabetes mellitus, IDDM) is thought to be associated with immune-mediated destruction of the pancreatic beta cells. Almost all diabetic dogs and many diabetic cats have IDDM. Dogs are thought to have immune-mediated islet destruction, and 50% of newly diagnosed diabetics have increased anti-beta cell antibodies. There appears to be a genetic susceptibility, but a trigger is required to precipitate beta cell autoimmunity. Anti-beta cell antibodies have not been found in untreated diabetic cats (Hoenig *et al.*, 2003) and chronic pancreatitis may be responsible for islet destruction and amyloid deposition in this species. Chronic pancreatitis may also cause diabetes mellitus in dogs (Figure 16.6)

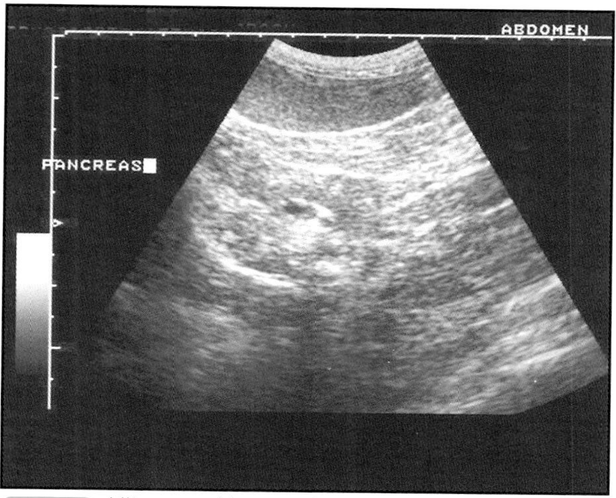

16.6 Ultrasound image showing an enlarged heterogenous pancreas in a dog with chronic pancreatitis. Chronic pancreatitis and pancreatic neoplasia can cause diabetes mellitus, due to destruction of the islet cells of the pancreas.

- Type 2 diabetes (non-insulin dependent diabetes mellitus, NIDDM) is thought to be related to obesity and islet amyloidosis in humans. These mechanisms are potential causative factors in feline diabetes mellitus. Obesity results in reversible insulin resistance by causing down-regulation of insulin receptors, impaired receptor binding and post-receptor defects. This results in an increase in insulin production and concurrent amylin production, which may result in amyloid deposition in the pancreas. Initially insulin production increases to compensate for the effects of obesity, but eventually the islet cells become exhausted (glucose toxicity) and fail to produce sufficient insulin. Obesity-associated diabetes has been reported in dogs but is relatively rare
- Type 3 diabetes mellitus results from insulin resistance due to antagonizing hormones, such as growth hormone, progesterone, glucocorticoids and catecholamines.

When blood glucose concentrations exceed the renal threshold (11–18 mmol/l in cats and 10–12 mmol/l in dogs), glucose is excreted in the urine. This glucosuria prevents normal water resorption and causes an osmotic diuresis, resulting in polyuria. There is a compensatory polydipsia in order to maintain body water. Patients with diabetes mellitus, therefore, frequently present with polyuria and polydipsia.

Patients with untreated diabetes mellitus can develop ketoacidosis due to the ongoing failure of insulin inhibition of lipolysis and gluconeogenesis, which results in production of ketones (see below).

Clinicopathological features

- Persistent marked hyperglycaemia. Note: In cats, stress hyperglycaemia can be marked and may be confused with diabetes mellitus; measurement of glycated proteins may therefore be more useful in cats in which diabetes mellitus is suspected.

- Concurrent glucosuria. Note: in cats, stress-associated hyperglycaemia can be so marked that it exceeds the renal threshold and is, therefore, associated with glucosuria. In cats that have been chronically or repeatedly stressed, glucosuria may be detected on routine urine sampling.
- Increased glycated proteins (fructosamine or glycated haemoglobin).
- Elevations in liver enzymes (alkaline phosphatase and alanine aminotransferase) due to diabetic vacuolar hepatopathy (hepatic lipidosis) or concurrent pancreatitis.
- Elevated triglyceride concentration due to insulin deficiency resulting in impaired lipoprotein lipase (LPL) activity. Without LPL, triglycerides are not hydrolysed and taken up by cells and so accumulate in the bloodstream. Obesity, high calorific intake and excess hepatic production of triglyceride also contribute to the increase in triglycerides commonly seen in diabetic patients.
- Elevated cholesterol concentration occurs to a lesser degree than elevated triglycerides. In humans it is associated with increased hepatic production, impaired clearance due to reduced receptor activity and increased intake of saturated fatty acids.
- Electrolyte changes (hyper/hyponatraemia, hypokalaemia). (See Chapter 8.)
- High incidence of urinary tract infections, which may be detected on routine analysis and culture (see Chapters 10 and 25) or may be occult (clinically silent). It is important to culture urine in any diabetic patient with evidence of urinary tract infection or if diabetes is difficult to stabilize.
- Urine specific gravity will be increased by the presence of glucose and is therefore usually higher than expected in a patient with polyuria.
- The presence of ketonuria is associated with diabetic ketoacidosis (see below).

Diagnosis of diabetes mellitus

Diabetes mellitus is diagnosed on the basis of appropriate clinical signs (Figure 16.7), persistent hyperglycaemia and concurrent glucosuria. In cats stress hyperglycaemia can exceed the renal threshold and result in glucosuria, particularly if the stress has been prolonged. Elevations in glycated proteins must, therefore, be used to confirm the diagnosis in cats and provide a useful baseline for monitoring in dogs.

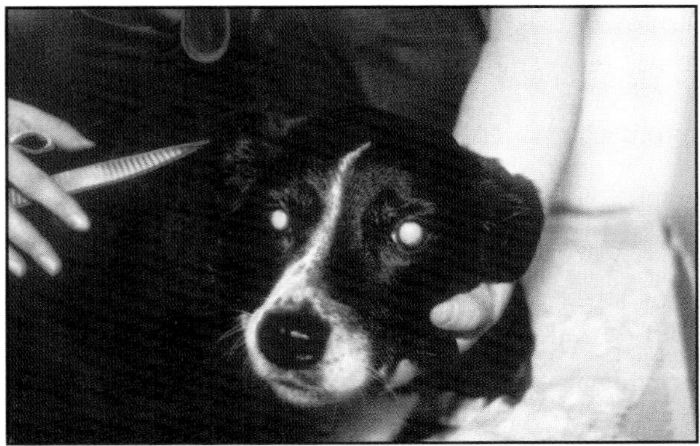

16.7 Cataracts develop in dogs with uncontrolled diabetes mellitus due to trapping of sorbitol within the lens. They are not seen in cats with diabetes mellitus.

Monitoring the diabetic patient

Stability of diabetes mellitus is most readily assessed by resolution of clinical signs (normal thirst, appetite and urination) and maintenance of body weight in both cats and dogs.

Monitoring urine glucose and ketones provides useful information regarding stability of diabetic animals. In dogs this is relatively simple and has been the mainstay of many traditional diabetic regimes. Alteration of insulin dose on the basis of morning urine glucose measurement is no longer recommended, however twice daily urine monitoring can provide useful information for dose adjustment, particularly in the early stages of diabetic stabilization, and can be performed at home.

The glycated proteins (see above) provide a useful method of documenting improved glycaemic control. In a well controlled diabetic, glycated protein concentration should be just above the reference range. In a patient that has been recently diagnosed as a diabetic, glycated proteins should only be measured once an appropriate period of time has elapsed (at least one half-life) so that significant changes are evident. Changes in the glycated protein concentration can only be used to determine that a change in insulin dose is required, and should not be used as the sole basis for increasing dose. In patients that have been on insulin for prolonged periods or have been receiving steadily increasing insulin doses, glycated proteins do not provide information on whether the insulin dose should be increased or decreased. For example, a patient receiving too much insulin will develop a rebound hyperglycaemia (Somogyi effect) (see Figure 16.10) and the glycated proteins will be elevated despite too high a dose of insulin being given. In this situation a glucose curve is required to determine what dose modification is required. Generally fructosamine is more useful in monitoring diabetics since it has a shorter half-life than glycated haemoglobin.

Serial blood glucose curves are used to establish the duration of insulin effect and determine if the dose is providing adequate glycaemic control (Figures 16.8 to 16.10). Glucose curves have traditionally been performed with the patient hospitalized. In cats it may be helpful to place an intravenous catheter for blood sampling in order to minimize the stress associated with 2-hourly blood sampling. In some dogs, owners may be able to sample blood glucose using ear-prick glucometers. This system will minimize the effect of stress associated with hospitalization, allows for more frequent glucose assessment and provides a more realistic curve based on the patient's home lifestyle.

Continuous glucose monitoring systems are being investigated in both cats and dogs. These devices assess interstitial fluid glucose concentrations using a subcutaneous sensor. Early studies suggest that interstitial fluid glucose concentrations may not reflect blood glucose concentrations postprandially and glucose results are not available in real time (Davison *et al.*, 2003b). Further studies are required to calibrate these devices.

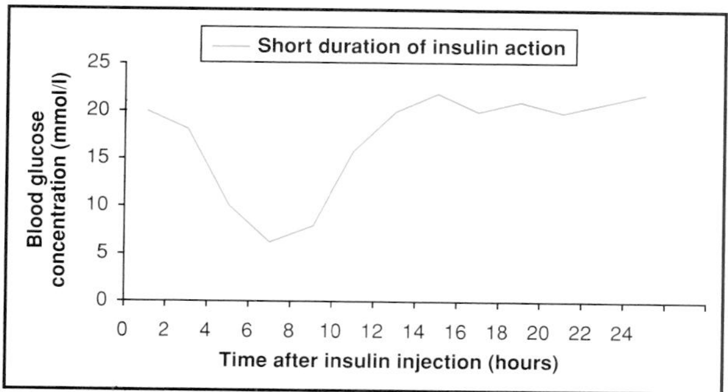

16.8 24-hour glucose curve consistent with short duration of insulin action. There is an initial good response to insulin injection at 0 hours. By 12 hours post-insulin, blood glucose concentrations are markedly elevated.

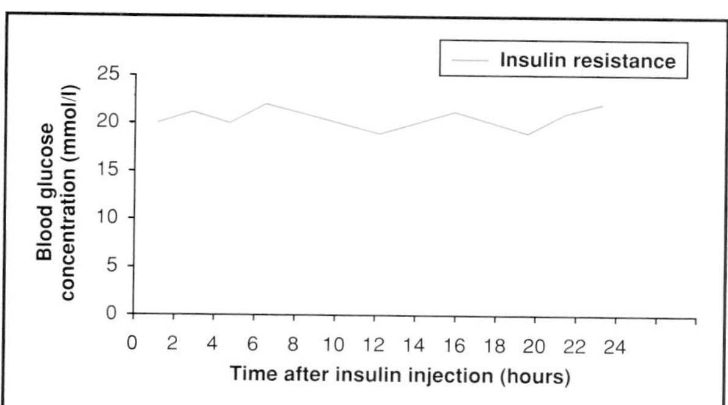

16.9 24-hour glucose curve consistent with insulin resistance. There is no response to insulin given at 0 hours.

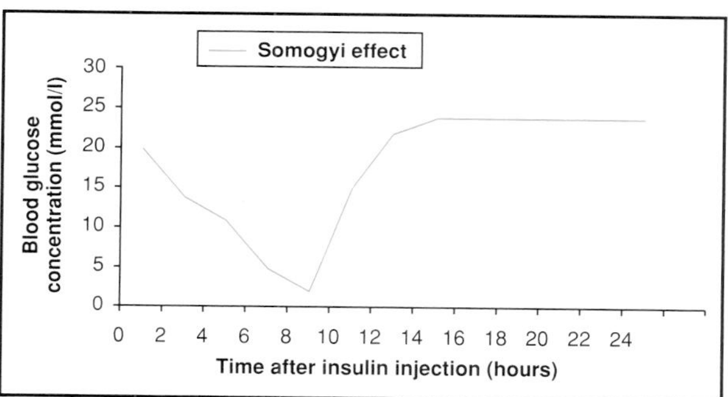

16.10 24-hour glucose curve consistent with the Somogyi effect. Insulin injection at 0 hours results in hypoglycaemia. There is then an immediate marked increase in blood glucose concentrations, which can be maintained for up to 72 hours.

Insulin resistance

Failure to respond to insulin is often termed insulin resistance, however this term should only be used in patients receiving more than 2 IU/kg of insulin at each injection. In this situation the serial glucose curve would reveal no response to insulin administration (Figure 16.9). Where true resistance is documented investigations should be undertaken to rule out diseases associated with increased concentrations of the counter-regulatory hormones, such as urinary tract infections (catecholamines), hyperadrenocorticism (cortisol) or acromegaly (growth hormone or IGF-1). In a few patients antibodies against the exogenous insulin can develop, which may warrant changing the type of insulin from bovine (most similar to feline) to porcine (most similar to canine) or *vice versa*. However, there appears to be cross reactivity of anti-insulin antibodies and variable reactivity to the different insulin subunits (Davison *et al.*, 2003a). Antibodies against exogenous insulin have also been reported in four diabetic cats (Hoenig *et al.*, 2003).

Diabetic ketoacidosis

Pathophysiology

In ketotic diabetic animals, increased fat breakdown (lipolysis) results in formation of the ketones, acetone, acetoacetate and betahydroxybutyrate, and hyperketonaemia. These ketones exceed the renal threshold and ketonuria results. Ketones are also known as ketone acids, as accumulation of ketones overwhelms the buffering mechanisms resulting in increased hydrogen ions and decreased bicarbonate (i.e. a metabolic acidosis). Ketosis is confirmed by ketonuria, and ketoacidosis by documentation of metabolic acidosis. The pathophysiology of diabetic ketoacidosis (DKA) is not fully understood but is thought to be multifactorial (Figure 16.11). It results from a low insulin:glucose ratio due to an absolute or relative insulin deficiency and the effects of counter-regulatory diabetogenic hormones (see above). It has been suggested that DKA is more common in patients with low levels of endogenous insulin, but it has recently been shown that dogs with DKA do have detectable concentrations of insulin (Parsons *et al.*, 2002). Ketogenesis is also increased during fasting and dehydration, both of which may exacerbate DKA. Ketosis itself results in dehydration, anorexia and increased amounts of diabetogenic hormones, thereby exacerbating the lipolysis and ketone formation resulting in ketoacidosis (see Figures 16.2 and 16.11). Patients receiving even low doses of insulin rarely develop ketosis, unless there is a concurrent predisposing cause. Dogs and cats diagnosed with DKA should be investigated to determine any potential cause of insulin resistance. DKA is commonly associated with infections (especially those of the urinary tract), pancreatitis, heart disease, gastrointestinal problems or any disease that can result in an increase in 'stress' hormones.

Clinicopathological features

The diagnosis of diabetic ketoacidosis is based on the presence of persistent hyperglycaemia (or elevated glycated proteins) glucosuria and ketonuria with a history of signs consistent with diabetes mellitus.

Dipstick tests for ketonuria detect acetoacetate but do not detect β-hydroxybutyrate (BHB). However, BHB rarely exists alone in the urine of patients with DKA. It is worth remembering that, at the start of insulin therapy, BHB is converted to acetoacetate, so the ketonuria will initially appear to worsen as the concentrations of measured ketones increases.

If the animal is clinically unwell, then the DKA is assumed to be severe. Patients with diabetes mellitus and ketonuria but no overt clinical signs have mild DKA, which is not an emergency.

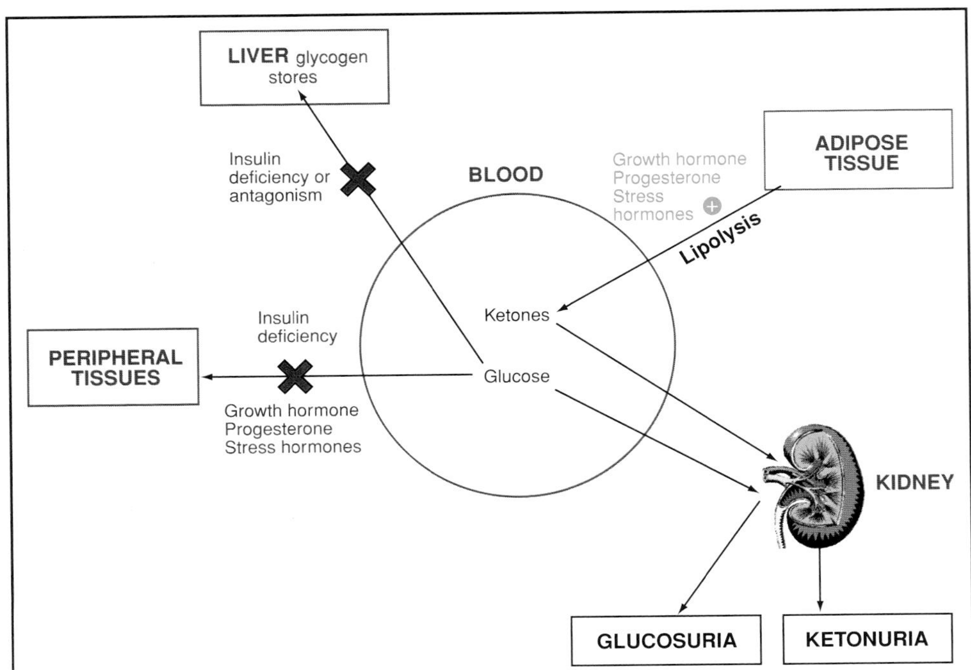

16.11 The pathophysiology of diabetic ketoacidosis. Insulin deficiency or antagonism, and counter-regulatory diabetogenic hormones (shown in red), result in failure of glucose uptake in the periphery and liver (red crosses). In the absence of insulin, the hormones (in green) stimulate lipolysis and the formation of ketones. Both glucose and ketones are excreted in the urine.

During the development of DKA, ketone anions are excreted into urine and, since electrical neutrality is always maintained, this is accompanied by an obligatory loss of sodium and potassium. Hyponatraemia may therefore be present. The total body potassium is depleted with developing acidosis, as cells increase uptake of hydrogen ions in exchange for potassium ions. This results in a normal blood potassium concentration despite total body depletion. As treatment with insulin is started, glucose and potassium move back into the cells and blood potassium falls dramatically. Phosphate is also lost during DKA, but cellular mechanisms similar to those described for potassium result in a normal blood phosphate concentration at presentation. Blood phosphate concentrations will fall dramatically after approximately 24 hours of insulin therapy in patients with DKA. The ensuing severe hypophosphataemia may result in red cell haemolysis and associated anaemia. Intravenous fluids should be supplemented with potassium phosphate and potassium chloride in all patients with DKA.

Blood osmolality can increase in some patients with DKA, however, many will have concurrent hyponatraemia, which protects them from this dangerous complication. The presence of a metabolic acidosis will result in respiratory compensation (seen clinically as hyperventilation), but a marked anion gap will develop in some patients (see Chapter 9).

Blood osmolality is calculated by the following equation:

$$\text{Osmolality (mOsm/kg)} = 2(\text{Na} + \text{K})(\text{mmol/l}) + \text{Urea (mmol/l)} + \text{Glucose (mmol/l)}$$

(Normal osmolality is 290–313 mOsm/kg in dogs. Cats may have a slightly higher reference range.)

Osmolality is rarely calculated in animals with DKA, but is important in the diagnosis of hyperosmolar non-ketotic diabetes mellitus as these patients often need emergency treatment.

Hyperosmolar non-ketotic diabetes mellitus

Patients may rarely develop hyperosmolar non-ketotic diabetes mellitus (HNDM), which is characterized by severe hyperglycaemia (>35 mmol/l), hyperosmolality (>350 mOsm/kg) and dehydration without ketosis or acidosis (unless there is lactic acidosis) (Peterson, 1998). This condition is thought to reflect the presence of remaining functional beta cells. These cells produce enough insulin to prevent fat breakdown (lipolysis) thereby preventing development of ketosis. The clinical signs usually associated with early DKA do not occur, and dehydration due to concurrent diseases, inadequate intake and excess fluid loss can, therefore, be severe. This dehydration results in a failure of renal glucose excretion due to reduced glomerular filtration rate and further increases blood glucose. The total body electrolyte abnormalities in HNDM are usually similar to those in DKA, however hyponatraemia is rare (as it would protect against hyperosmolality). Azotaemia is usually severe.

Hypoglycaemia

The common causes of hypoglycaemia are summarized in Figure 16.12.

Insulinoma

An insulinoma is a neoplasm of the pancreatic beta cells, which remain functional and produce insulin. The neoplastic cells remain sensitive to positive feedback

Cause	Mechanism
Laboratory error	Inappropriate anticoagulant Delayed serum or plasma separation, especially if there is leucocytosis or erythrocytosis
Insulinoma	Insulin production and release by neoplastic beta cells despite normo- or hypoglycaemia
Iatrogenic	Overdose of insulin or other hypoglycaemic agents, e.g. glipizide
Hypoadrenocorticism	Absence of cortisol
Hypopituitarism	Absence of growth hormone or ACTH (and therefore cortisol)
Endotoxaemia	Decreased hepatic glucose production and increased tissue utilization
Congenital portosystemic shunts	Insufficient glycogen stores and poor gluconeogenesis
Severe liver disease (failure)	Absence of glycogenolysis and gluconeogenesis
Juvenile hypoglycaemia (puppies, especially miniature and toy breeds)	Inadequate glycogen stores, limited fat and muscle mass
Hunting dogs	Excessive glucose demand and inadequate glycogen stores
Glycogen storage diseases	Deficiency of enzymes required for glycogen conversion
Starvation	Loss of glycogen stores and inadequate intake
Paraneoplastic (leiomyoma, leiomyosarcoma, lymphoma, haemangiosarcoma, large hepatic tumours, others)	Excessive glucose utilization or production of insulin-like growth factor-2 or other insulin-like factors (with similar effects to insulin)
Polycythaemia/leukaemia	Increased glucose utilization post sampling (artefactual)
Chronic renal failure	Impaired hepatic glucose production

16.12 Causes and mechanisms of hypoglycaemia.

and therefore increase insulin production and release when there is hyperglycaemia (for example after a meal) but fail to stop insulin release when the patient is normoglycaemic or hypoglycaemic. These patients can therefore become severely hypoglycaemic when food is withheld, and may also show signs after eating or exercise. Compensatory sympathoadrenal stimulation results in muscular tremors, nervousness, restlessness and hunger and often precedes the onset of neuroglycopenic signs, such as lethargy, weakness, ataxia, abnormal behaviour and convulsions or coma. These compensatory mechanisms mean that clinical signs are usually short-lived due to prompt recovery after each episode of hypoglycaemia.

Diagnosis

Diagnosis is dependent on demonstration of an elevated serum insulin concentration in the face of hypoglycaemia (i.e. an inappropriate hyperinsulinaemia). High insulin concentrations in the presence of hyperglycaemia are appropriate and therefore are not necessarily consistent with insulinoma. Elevated insulin concentrations in the presence of normoglycaemia may be consistent with insulinoma, provided the hyperinsulinaemia is severe enough. The use of the glucose:insulin ratio may improve the diagnosis of insulinomas in these circumstances. However, the best method of diagnosis remains hyperinsulinaemia in the presence of hypoglycaemia.

Patients with insulinoma usually develop hypoglycaemia within 12 hours of fasting, so it vital to ensure that blood glucose is monitored regularly whilst withholding food from a suspected insulinoma patient. Fructosamine concentrations may be subnormal in patients with insulinoma and may be useful when hypoglycaemia cannot be documented.

In the past Whipple's triad (symptoms after fasting or exercise; symptoms associated with hypoglycaemia; and response to administration of glucose) was used to diagnose an insulin-secreting tumour; however, most causes of hypoglycaemia will meet the three criteria of Whipple's triad and it is of no diagnostic value.

Insulin concentrations: Insulin concentrations can be measured in serum. Some laboratories prefer the serum to be frozen immediately after collection. Interpretation of insulin concentrations is easier if the sample is collected when there is concurrent hypoglycaemia. In patients where hypoglycaemia cannot be documented the insulin:glucose ratio can be used (see below). The amended insulin:glucose ratio is not thought to offer any diagnostic advantage in small animals, as it is based on work in humans.

Interpretation of insulin concentrations should consider the following:

- Reference range = <20 μIU/l
- >20 μIU/l = absolute hyperinsulinaemia consistent with an insulinoma
- 10–20 μIU/l = relative hyperinsulinaemia consistent with an insulinoma
- 5–10 μIU/l = possible insulinoma
- <5 μIU/l = inconsistent with insulinoma.

For the insulin:glucose ratio, insulin concentration (μIU/l) is divided by glucose concentration (mmol/l). An insulin:glucose ratio >4.2 IU/mol is consistent with insulinoma.

Case examples

Case 1

Signalment

2-year-old male Malemoise dog.

History

1-month history of large volume diarrhoea with occasional haematochezia and increased mucus, decreased appetite and weight loss. The dog collapsed yesterday and has remained very weak since then.

Clinical pathology data

Haematology	Result	Reference interval
RBC (x 10^{12}/l)	8.64	5.5–8.5
Hb (g/dl)	19	12.0–18.0
HCT (l/l)	0.52	0.37–0.55
MCV (fl)	60.5	60.0–77.0
MCH (pg)	21.9	19.5–24.5
MCHC (g/dl)	36.3	32.0–36.0
WBC (x 10^9/l)	21.7	6.0–12.0
Neutrophils (x 10^9/l)	14.5	3.0–11.8
Neutrophils (band) (x 10^9/l)	0.217	0.0
Lymphocytes (x 10^9/l)	3.3	1.0–4.8
Monocytes (x 10^9/l)	0.2	0.15–1.35
Eosinophils (x 10^9/l)	3.3	0.1–1.25

Biochemistry	Result	Reference interval
Sodium (mmol/l)	131.7	136–159
Potassium (mmol/l)	8.99	3.4–5.8
Glucose (mmol/l)	3.1	3.3–5.5
Urea (mmol/l)	64.2	2.7–9.2
Creatinine (μmol/l)	533	91–180
Calcium (mmol/l)	3.32	2.34–3.0
Inorganic phosphate (mmol/l)	5.1	1.29–2.9
Albumin (g/l)	22	28–42
Globulin (g/l)	40	27–45
Biochemistry (continued)		
ALT (IU/l)	69	<90
AST (IU/l)	106	<40
ALP (IU/l)	86	<230
Na:K ratio	14.6	>27

What abnormalities are present?

Haematology

Leucocytosis, eosinophilia, neutrophilia and normal lymphocyte count. Eosinopenia and lymphopenia would be expected due to the stress of chronic illness.

Biochemistry

Subnormal Na:K ratio, hyperkalaemia, hyponatraemia, hypoglycaemia, hypercalcaemia, hyperphosphataemia, marked azotaemia, hypoalbuminaemia, elevated AST.

How would you interpret these results and what are the likely differential diagnoses?

Hypoadrenocorticism with secondary, severe azotaemia, associated with marked dehydration is most likely, based on the electrolyte disturbance, renal abnormalities, hypercalcaemia, hypoglycaemia and eosinophilia and lymphocytosis.

Hypoadrenocorticism causes hypoglycaemia due to a deficiency in cortisol, which normally increases blood glucose concentrations and antagonizes insulin. Glucose concentrations normalized following treatment for hypoadrenocorticism with mineralocorticoid and glucocorticoid supplementation.

What further tests would you recommend?

- **Adrenocorticotropic hormone (ACTH) stimulation test.** The results in this case were:
  - Pre-ACTH cortisol = <6.0 nmol/l
  - Post-ACTH cortisol = <6.0 nmol/l

  This result is consistent with hypoadrenocorticism.
- **Urinalysis** will not differentiate pre-renal azotaemia (reversible) from renal azotaemia (potentially irreversible) in patients with hypoadrenocorticism as sodium depletion causes isosthenuria in these animals (see Chapter 11).

Case 2

Signalment

13-week-old female Pomeranian puppy.

History

Episode of weakness at 5 weeks of age, subsequently has remained quieter than littermates. Over last 24 hours not eating, soft faeces and lifeless. Seizure prior to presentation, collapsed for the previous 1 hour.

Clinical pathology data

Results limited by volume of blood and emergency facilities.

Haematology	Result	Adult reference interval
HCT (l/l)	0.36	0.37–0.55

Biochemistry	Result	Adult reference interval
Sodium (mmol/l)	149	136–159
Potassium (mmol/l)	2.4	3.4–5.8
Glucose (mmol/l)	1.7	3.3–5.5

What abnormalities are present?

Hypoglycaemia and hypokalaemia.

How would you interpret these results and what are the likely differential diagnoses?

Puppies are prone to hypoglycaemia and when severe this can cause seizures. Hypokalaemia probably reflects inadequate intake. A tentative diagnosis of juvenile hypoglycaemia can therefore be made.

What further tests would you recommend?

Response to intravenous glucose bolus.

Case 3

Signalment

6-year-old female, neutered Cairn Terrier.

History

Marked increase in thirst and urination over previous 2 weeks. Now drinking about 240 ml/kg/day. Some weight loss and development of cloudy eyes over a similar period.

Clinical pathology data

Haematology	Result	Reference interval
RBC (x 10^{12}/l)	7.88	5.5–8.5
Hb (g/dl)	17.3	12.0–18.0
HCT (l/l)	0.53	0.37–0.55
MCV (fl)	67.2	60.0–77.0
MCH (pg)	22	19.5–24.5
MCHC (g/dl)	32.5	32.0–36.0
WBC (x 10^9/l)	15.8	6.0–12.0
Neutrophils (x 10^9/l)	13.59	3.0–11.8
Neutrophils (band) (x 10^9/l)	0.32	0
Lymphocytes (x 10^9/l)	1.11	1.0–4.8
Monocytes (x 10^9/l)	0.47	0.15–1.35
Eosinophils (x 10^9/l)	0.16	0.1–1.25
Basophils (x 10^9/l)	0	0.0–0.6
Normoblasts (x 10^9/l)	0.16	0
Platelets (x 10^9/l)	201	200–500

Biochemistry	Result	Reference interval
Sodium (mmol/l)	144.4	136–159
Potassium (mmol/l)	4.54	3.4–5.8
Glucose (mmol/l)	17.8	3.3–5.5
Urea (mmol/l)	4.5	2.7–9.2
Creatinine (μmol/l)	78	91–180
Calcium (mmol/l)	2.63	2.34–3.0
Inorganic phosphate (mmol/l)	1.29	1.29–2.9
Albumin (g/l)	34.0	28–42
Globulin (g/l)	36.0	27–45
ALT (IU/l)	88	<90
AST (IU/l)	41	<40 ▶

Biochemistry *(continued)*	Result	Reference interval
ALP (IU/l)	428	<230
Cholesterol (mmol/l)	4.47	2.0–7.0
Na:K ratio	31.8	>27
Triglycerides (mmol/l)	1.45	<0.6

Urine analysis	
Protein	+
Glucose	++
Ketones	+++
Blood	-ve
pH	6.5
Specific gravity	1.048
Protein:creatinine ratio	1.32
Sediment	Few WBC, few small epithelial cells

What abnormalities are present?

Haematology

Leucocytosis due to mature neutrophilia.
Increased ALP (just under twice normal), insignficantly small increase in AST, hypertriglyceridaemia, hyperglycaemia, increased fructosamine.

Biochemistry

Proteinuria, glucosuria, ketonuria. White blood cells on urine sediment.

How would you interpret these results and what are the likely differential diagnoses?

Biochemistry and urinalysis abnormalities are all consistent with diabetes mellitus. The specific gravity is not consistent with polyuria; this is because of the presence of glucose in the urine, which has a higher density than water. The presence of ketones is consistent with ketosis and this patient therefore requires prompt treatment. The proteinuria and white blood cells in the urine may be due to a urinary tract infection, which is common in patients with diabetes mellitus.

What further tests would you recommend?

- **Fructosamine** is useful to provide a baseline for monitoring glucose control and also helps to confirm diabetes mellitus in equivocal cases. In this case fructosamine was 546 μmol/l (reference range 162–310 μmol/l).
- **Urine culture** may be warranted to confirm urinary tract infection and provide antimicrobial sensitivity.

Case 4 follows ▶

Case 4

Signalment

10-year-old male entire Staffordshire Bull Terrier.

History

3-week history of intermittent hindlimb weakness approximately three times weekly. Usually associated with exercise in the afternoon (prior to feeding).

Clinical pathology data

Haematology	Result	Reference interval
RBC (x 10^{12}/l)	7.49	5.5–8.5
Hb (g/dl)	17.0	12.0–18.0
HCT (l/l)	0.46	0.37–0.55
MCV (fl)	61.0	60.0–77.0
MCH (pg)	22.6	19.5–24.5
MCHC (g/dl)	37.1	32.0–36.0
WBC (x 10^{9}/l)	8.0	6.0–12.0
Neutrophils (x 10^{9}/l)	5.49	3.0–11.8
Neutrophils (band) (x 10^{9}/l)	0	0
Lymphocytes (x 10^{9}/l)	1.96	1.0–4.8
Monocytes (x 10^{9}/l)	0.24	0.15–1.35
Eosinophils (x 10^{9}/l)	0.24	0.1–1.25
Basophils (x 10^{9}/l)	0	0.0–0.6
Normoblasts (x 10^{9}/l)	0.08	0

Biochemistry	Result	Reference interval
Sodium (mmol/l)	148	136–159
Potassium (mmol/l)	3.7	3.4–5.8
Glucose (mmol/l)	2.6	3.3–5.5
Urea (mmol/l)	3.4	2.7–9.2
Creatinine (µmol/l)	97	91–180
Calcium (mmol/l)	2.74	2.34–3.0
Inorganic phosphate (mmol/l)	1.6	1.29–2.9
Albumin (g/l)	41.0	28–42
Globulin (g/l)	33.0	27–45
ALT (IU/l)	61	<90
AST (IU/l)	27	<40
ALP (IU/l)	157	<230
Na:K ratio	40	>27

What abnormalities are present?

Haematology

Mild increase in MCHC (artefactual; see Chapter 4).

Biochemistry

Hypoglycaemia.

How would you interpret these results and what are the likely differential diagnoses?

First, confirm that glucose result is not a laboratory error. If result is correct, the most likely differential given the history and signalment is insulinoma.

What further tests would you recommend?

- **Fructosamine** may confirm persistent hypoglycaemia.
- **Insulin concentration** with concurrent hypoglycaemia will confirm hyperinsulinaemia. Insulin concentration in this case was 22 µIU/l .
- **Ultrasonography, exploratory laparotomy and histopathology** will be required to confirm that hyperinsulinaemia is related to an insulinoma in the pancreas.

Case 5

Signalment

12-year-old, female neutered Domestic Shorthair cat.

History

Increased urination and thirst for the previous 2 months. Increased appetite for the previous 4 years and long-term obesity.

Clinical pathology data

Haematology	Result	Reference interval
RBC (x 10^{12}/l)	9.40	5.50–10.0
Hb (g/dl)	13.1	8.0–14.0
HCT (l/l)	0.44	0.24–0.45
MCV (fl)	47.0	39.0–55.0
MCHC (g/dl)	29.6	30.0–36.0
WBC (x 10^{9}/l)	11.7	7.0–20.0
Neutrophils (segmented) (x 10^{9}/l)	8.307	2.5–12.8
Neutrophils (band) (x 10^{9}/l)	0.0	0.0
Lymphocytes (x 10^{9}/l)	2.340	1.500–7.000
Monocytes (x 10^{9}/l)	0.585	0.07–0.85
Eosinophils (x 10^{9}/l)	0.468	0.0–1.0
Basophils (x 10^{9}/l)	0.0	0.0–0.2

Biochemistry	Result	Reference interval
Sodium (mmol/l)	152	145–156
Potassium (mmol/l)	4.26	4.00–5.00
Glucose (mmol/l)	21.8	3.3–5.0
Urea (mmol/l)	15.4	2.8–9.8
Creatinine (µmol/l)	120	26–118
Calcium (mmol/l)	2.43	2.10–2.90
TP (g/l)	72.2	69.0–79.0
Albumin (g/l)	29.5	28.0–35.0
Globulin (g/l)	42.7	23.0–50.0
ALT (IU/l)	34	15–60
ALP (IU/l)	116	20–100
Total T4 (nmol/l)	60	13–48

Case 5 continues ▶

Case 5 continued

What abnormalities are present?

Haematology

Very mild increase in MCHC.

Biochemistry

Hyperglycaemia, increased total T4, azotaemia, increased ALP.

How would you interpret these results and what are the likely differential diagnoses?

Hyperglycaemia is significant but could be stress-associated or due to diabetes mellitus. Increased T4 is consistent with hyperthyroidism. Mild azotaemia (urea increased more than creatinine), which may reflect dehydration secondary to hyperthyroidism, due to polyuria with inadequate water intake, or may reflect renal failure (especially if cat has reduced muscle mass). Increased ALP is consistent with hyperthyroidism or diabetes mellitus. The very mild increase seen in MCHC is not significant (see Chapter 4). This cat has hyperthyroidism; however, the T4 concentration does not reflect the severity of clinical signs. It is possible that a second disease is suppressing the T4 concentration.

What further tests would you recommend?

- **Urinalysis** for presence of glucose, ketones and specific gravity. In this case marked glucosuria was present.
- **Fructosamine** is useful to confirm if there has been persistent hyperglycaemia but is affected by hyperthyroidism. In this case fructosamine = 3.90 mmol/l (laboratory reference range 2.19–3.47 mmol/l). As hyperthyroidism tends to reduce fructosamine concentrations, this increase is significant. Combined with the urine results it suggests that this cat has both hyperthyroidism and diabetes mellitus. The increased T4 may promote ketogenesis so both diseases require management.

References and further reading

Bennett N (2002) Monitoring techniques for diabetes mellitus in the dog and the cat. *Clinical Techniques in Small Animal Practice* **17**, 65–69

Briggs CE, Nelson RW, Feldman EC, Elliott DA and Neal LA (2000) Reliability of history and physical examination findings for assessing control of glycemia in dogs with diabetes mellitus: 53 cases (1995–1998). *Journal of the American Veterinary Medical Association* **217**, 48–53

Bruskiewicz KA, Nelson RW, Feldman EC and Griffey SM (1997) Diabetic ketosis and ketoacidosis in cats: 42 cases (1980–1995). *Journal of the American Veterinary Medical Association* **211**, 188–192

Cohn LA, McCaw DL, Tate DJ and Johnson JC (2000) Assessment of five portable blood glucose meters, a point-of-care analyzer, and color test strips for measuring blood glucose concentration in dogs. *Journal of the American Veterinary Medical Association* **216**, 198–202

Davison LJ, Podd SL, Ristic JM, Herrtage ME, Parnham A and Catchpole B (2002) Evaluation of two point-of-care analysers for measurement of fructosamine or haemoglobin A1c in dogs. *Journal of Small Animal Practice* **43**, 526–532

Davison LJ, Ristic JME, Herrtage ME, Ramsey IK and Catchpole B (2003a) Anti-insulin antibodies in dogs with naturally occurring diabetes mellitus. *Veterinary Immunology and Immunopathology* **91**, 53–60

Davison LJ, Slater LA, Herrtage ME, Church DB, Judge S, Ristic JME and Catchpole B (2003b) Evaluation of a continuous glucose monitoring system in diabetic dogs. *Journal of Small Animal Practice* **44**, 435–442

Greco DS (2004) Diabetic ketoacidosis. In: *BSAVA Manual of Canine and Feline Endocrinology, 3rd edn,* ed. CT Mooney and ME Peterson, pp. 142–149. BSAVA Publications, Gloucester

Feldman EC and Nelson RW (1996) The endocrine pancreas. In: *Canine and Feline Endocrinology and Reproduction, 2nd edn,* ed EC Feldman and RW Nelson, pp 338–453. WB Saunders, Philadelphia

Hasegawa S, Sako T, Takemura N, Koyama H, Motoyoshi S (1992a) Glycated haemoglobin fractions in normal and diabetic dogs measured by high performance liquid chromatography. *Journal of Veterinary Medical Science* **53**, 65–68

Hasegawa S, Sako T, Takemura N, Koyama H, Motoyoshi S (1992b) Glycated haemoglobin fractions in normal and diabetic cats measured by high performance liquid chromatography. *Journal of Veterinary Medical Science* **54**, 789

Hoenig M, Reusch C and Peterson ME (2000) Beta cell and insulin antibodies in treated and untreated diabetic cats. *Veterinary Immunology & Immunopathology* **77,** 93–102

Jensen AL (1993) Various protein and albumin corrections of the serum fructosamine concentration in the diagnosis of canine diabetes mellitus. *Veterinary Research Communications* **17**, 13–23

Loste A and Marca MC (2001) Fructosamine and glycated hemoglobin in the assessment of glycaemic control. *Veterinary Research* **32**, 55–62

Marca MC, Loste A and Ramos J. (2000) Effect of acute hyperglycaemia on the serum fructosamine and blood glycated haemoglobin concentrations in canine samples. *Veterinary Research Communications* **24,** 11–16

Mellanby RJ and Herrtage ME (2002) Insulinoma in a normoglycaemic dog with low serum fructosamine. *Journal of Small Animal Practice* **43**, 506–508

Miller E (1995) Long-term monitoring of the diabetic dog and cat. Clinical signs, serial blood glucose determinations, urine glucose, and glycated blood proteins. *Veterinary Clinics of North America: Small Animal Practice* **25**, 571–584

Nichols R and Crenshaw KL (1995) Complications and concurrent disease associated with diabetic ketoacidosis and other severe forms of diabetes mellitus. *Veterinary Clinics of North America: Small Animal Practice* **25**, 617–624

Parsons SE, Drobatz KJ, Lamb SV, Ward CR and Hess RS. (2002) Endogenous serum concentration in dogs with diabetic ketoacidosis. *Journal of Veterinary Emergency and Critical Care* **12**, 147–152

Peterson M (1998) Endocrine emergencies. In: *BSAVA Manual of Canine and Feline Endocrinology 2nd edn,* ed. AG Torrance and CT Mooney, pp. 163–172. BSAVA Publications, Cheltenham

Reusch CE, Gerber B, Boretti FS (2002) Serum fructosamine concentrations in dogs with hyperthyroidism. *Veterinary Research Communications* **26,** 531–536

Reusch CE and Tomsa K (1999) Serum fructosamine concentration in cats with overt hyperthyroidism. *Journal of the American Veterinary Medical Association* **215**, 1297–1300

Reusch CE and Haberer B (2001) Evaluation of fructosamine in dogs and cats with hypo- or hyperproteinaemia, azotaemia, hyperlipidaemia and hyperbilirubinaemia. *Veterinary Record* **148**, 370–376

Siliart B and Stambouli F (1996) Laboratory diagnosis of insulinoma in the dog: a retrospective study and a new diagnostic procedure. *Journal of Small Animal Practice* **37**, 367–370

Thoresen SI, Aleksandersen M, Lonaas L, Bredal WP, Grondalen J and Berthelsen K (1995) Pancreatic insulin-secreting carcinoma in a dog: fructosamine for determining persistent hypoglycaemia. *Journal of Small Animal Practice* **36**, 282–286

17

Laboratory evaluation of hypothyroidism and hyperthyroidism

Peter A. Graham and Carmel T. Mooney

Introduction

Hypothyroidism and hyperthyroidism are the most common endocrine disorders of dogs and cats, respectively, and testing for these diseases is frequently carried out in practice. Interpretation relies on a good understanding of thyroid physiology and the myriad factors, other than thyroid disease, that can affect tests of thyroid function.

Physiology of the thyroid gland

The thyroid gland of dogs and cats exists as two separate lobes located on either side of the trachea extending downwards over the first five or six tracheal rings. Each thyroid lobe is composed of microscopic spherical follicles lined by a single layer of thyroid epithelium; the lumen of which contains colloid, a gelatinous storage substance for thyroglobulin secreted by the follicular cells (Figure 17.1). Thyroglobulin is a large glycoprotein containing iodotyrosines that serve as precursors for thyroid hormone synthesis. Most of the steps involved in thyroid hormone synthesis are catalysed by the enzyme thyroid peroxidase (TPO).

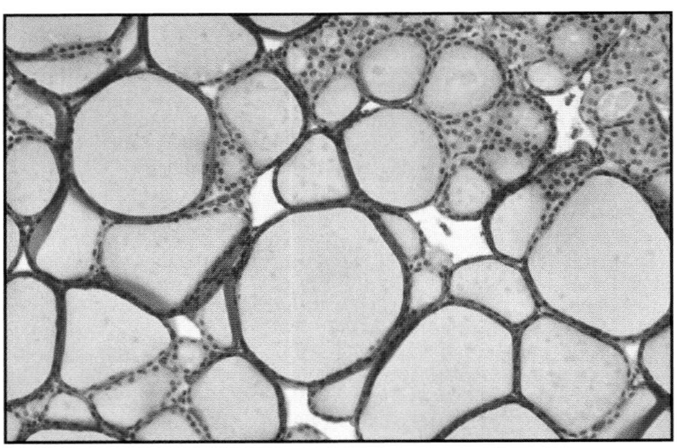

17.1 Histological appearance of healthy canine thyroid tissue. Note the follicular architecture.

The metabolically active thyroid hormones are the iodothyronines: 3,5,3',5'-L-tetraiodothyronine (thyroxine (T4)) and 3,5,3'-L-triiodothyronine (triiodothyronine (T3)). T4 is the main secretory product of the thyroid gland. Only small amounts of T3, the more metabolically active hormone, and 3,3',5'-L-triodothyronine (reverse T3 (rT3)), an inactive product, are produced by the thyroid gland. The majority of circulating T3 and rT3 is produced by peripheral monodeiodination of T4, which occurs mainly in the liver and kidney (Figure 17.2); so T4 is often considered to be a prohormone. Activation to T3 is potentially autoregulated in the periphery.

The thyroid hormones circulate bound to plasma proteins. The exact proteins and their binding affinities vary between species. In dogs, circulating T4 is bound to thyroxine-binding globulin (TBG) and to a lesser extent thyroxine-binding prealbumin (TBPA), albumin, a high density lipoprotein (HDL_2) and a very low density lipoprotein. Cats depend primarily on albumin and TBPA. Approximately 99.9% of T4 is protein-bound in both species, and the remaining fraction is free and metabolically active. T3 is slightly less protein-bound with a free fraction of approximately 1%. For both hormones, the bound fraction acts as a reservoir to buffer hormone delivery to target tissues.

17.2 The structure of thyroxine (T4), triiodothyronine (T3) and reverse T3 (rT3) and the effects of 5– and 5'–deiodinases.

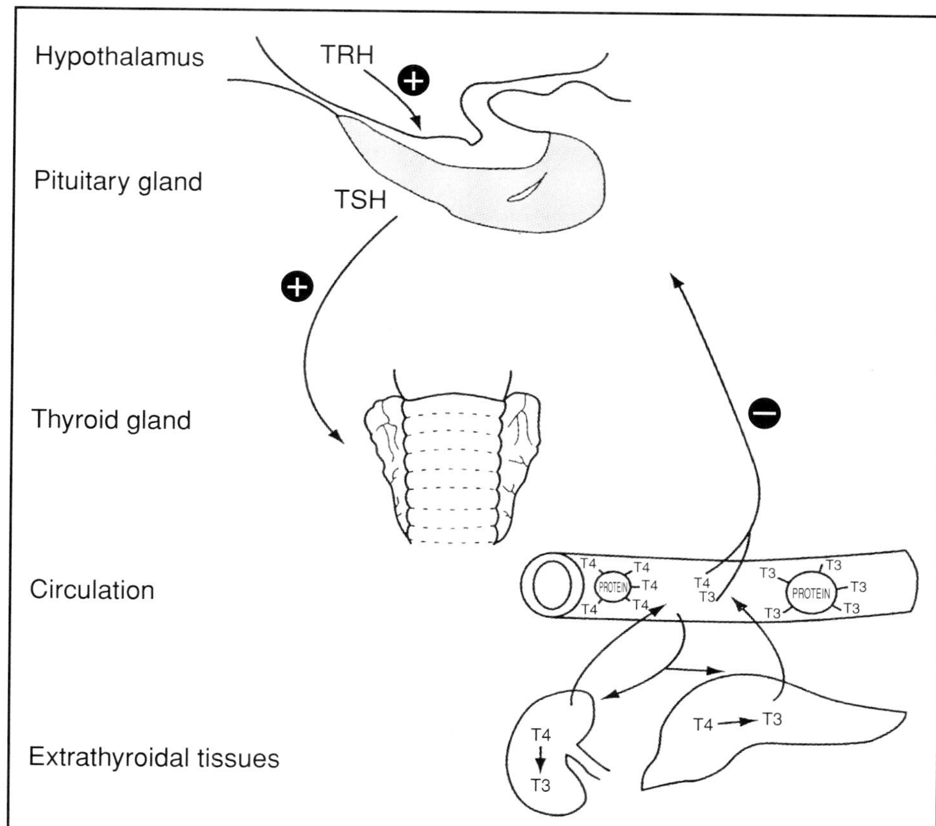

17.3 The hypothalamic–pituitary–thyroid–extrathyroid axis, demonstrating the interaction between the various factors controlling thyroid function (TRH, thyrotropin releasing hormone; TSH, thyroid stimulating hormone (thyrotropin); T4, thyroxine; T3, triiodothyronine; +, stimulation; –, inhibition).

Control of thyroid hormone production is mediated via negative feedback (Figure 17.3). The hypothalamus secretes thyrotropin releasing hormone (TRH) into the hypophyseal portal system and this acts on the anterior pituitary promoting the synthesis and secretion of thyrotropin (thyroid stimulating hormone (TSH)). TSH acts on the thyroid cells, promoting trapping of iodide and synthesis and release of the thyroid hormones. The presence of excess circulating free T4 and T3 produces a negative feedback effect on the anterior pituitary, which serves to decrease TSH synthesis and release and, subsequently, thyroid hormone production. Peripherally, protein binding, cytosolic buffers and the activities of the deiodinase enzymes offer additional areas for control of thyroid hormone action.

Thyroid hormones have numerous functions but their major influence is on metabolic rate, growth and tissue turnover. They also interact with the nervous system by increasing overall sympathetic drive. The clinical presentations in animals with a deficiency of thyroid hormone, therefore, can include stunting, skin and hair abnormalities, lethargy and increased body weight. Conversely, in hyperthyroid individuals, there is weight loss, hyperactivity, intermittent vomiting/diarrhoea and signs of hypertrophic cardiomyopathy. The effect of thyroid hormone on tissues is relatively slow and, consequently, clinical signs can take some time (weeks to months) to develop after loss of thyroid function or as hyperfunction commences. Similarly it takes time for clinical signs to disappear after appropriate treatment has been initiated.

Laboratory methods for assessment of thyroid function

A variety of tests and methodologies is available for measurement of total and free thyroid hormone concentrations, thyroid autoantibodies and pituitary hormones that may play a role in assessment of thyroid function. In addition, the hypothalamic-thyroid-pituitary axis can be manipulated through the administration of various stimulatory and suppressive agents. A description of the methodology of the most commonly used tests is provided elsewhere (*BSAVA Manual of Canine and Feline Endocrinology*).

In general, thyroid hormones are pretty robust and stable with some notable exceptions (Figure 17.4). There is no effect of time of day for diagnostic sampling, but time post-medication is important for therapeutic monitoring. Haemolysis and lipaemia rarely affect the results of radioimmunoassays (RIAs) but this may not be the case for non-isotopic methods.

Total thyroid hormone measurement

Both total T4 and total T3 can be readily measured in serum (or plasma) samples from dogs and cats. RIA is the preferred laboratory method but, because of the necessary use of radioisotopes, is generally confined to commercial laboratories. Assays that avoid the use of radioisotopes offer several advantages including longer shelf-life, no exposure to radioactive material, easier disposal and potential application in the practice laboratory. They include enzyme-linked immunosorbent assay (ELISA), enzyme immunoassay (EI) and several

Analyte	Sample type	Handling considerations	Indications
Total T4	Serum/plasma	None	Diagnosing hyperthyroidism Diagnosing hypothyroidism (with TSH) Therapeutic monitoring TRH/TSH response tests T3 suppression test
Total T3	Serum/plasma	None	No advantage over total T4 for diagnostic purposes Assessment of absorption for T3 suppression test
Free T4	Serum/plasma	Avoid delayed transport Severe hyperlipaemia	Diagnosing hypo- and hyperthyroidism
cTSH	Serum/plasma	None	Diagnosing canine hypothyroidism (with T4) Therapeutic monitoring TRH response test
Thyroglobulin autoantibody	Serum or blood spot	None	Assessment of thyroid pathology
T4 and T3 autoantibodies	Serum/plasma	None	Assessment of thyroid autoimmunity Assessment of immunoassay interference

17.4 Sample requirements, special handling considerations and uses of the analytes for assessment of thyroid disease.

automated systems that use advanced signal generation and detection systems (e.g. chemiluminescence). Although early reports were critical, there have been improvements in these methods over recent years and, in some circumstances, they correlate well with RIA (Lurye *et al.*, 2002; Peterson *et al.*, 2003). However, it is usually recommended that one test method is used exclusively with its own test-specific reference range.

Many of the kits available for total thyroid hormone concentrations are designed primarily for use with human serum. In dogs and cats the binding affinities and overall concentrations of the major binding proteins are lower than in humans. Consequently kits designed for human use must be modified to allow for the measurement of the lower circulating total thyroid hormone concentrations in dogs and cats, and validated to account for differences in plasma protein binding.

Free thyroxine measurement

Despite the differences in circulating concentrations of total T4 between dogs, cats and man, absolute free T4 concentrations are similar. Free T4 measurement is difficult, not least because of its circulation in minute quantities (pmol/l rather than nmol/l). Several methods of measurement are available and include direct and analogue radio- and chemiluminescent immunoassay methods. These assays have been primarily developed for use in humans and remain controversial as accurate assessments of true free hormone concentrations. In dogs and cats, this controversy is exacerbated. Although not all methods have been evaluated in dogs and cats, it is clear that results from analogue methods offer no further information than total T4 measurement alone.

Assessment of free T4 concentrations by equilibrium dialysis or ultrafiltration is preferred. Most commercial laboratories use the equilibrium dialysis technique as it is available in kit form. In this method, the patient sample undergoes a dialysis step and the dialysate is subsequently subjected to an ultrasensitive RIA. The dialysis step ensures that free T4 measurement is not affected by altered protein binding and crossreacting substances. Care should be taken to avoid prolonged transport (>5 days) as measured free T4 concentrations can increase with time. In regions with very high environmental temperatures this effect can be seen in as little as 2 days. This presumably results from degradation or loss of affinity of the binding proteins, allowing the free fraction to become greater. High serum concentrations of free fatty acids have a similar effect.

Thyrotropin measurement

A species-specific assay (chemiluminescent or immunoradiometric (IRMA)) for measurement of canine TSH (cTSH) is available. A species-specific feline assay is not yet available.

Thyroid autoantibody measurement

A variety of antibodies can be produced during immune-mediated thyroid disease. A species-specific method for measurement of canine thyroglobulin autoantibodies (TgAA) is readily available commercially. In a proportion of TgAA positive cases, T3 and T4 autoantibodies (T3AA and T4AA) are produced because the TgAA is formed against an epitope containing an iodothyronine site. These antibodies have limited impact on the availability of thyroid hormones *in vivo*. However, they can have a dramatic impact on laboratory test procedures and can result in spuriously high or low total thyroid hormone concentrations, depending on the particular assay and separation system used.

Dynamic thyroid function tests

Dynamic thyroid function tests are often recommended to confirm or refute a diagnosis of thyroid dysfunction, particularly when baseline test results are equivocal. They can also be used to determine the site of the lesion.

	T3 suppression	TSH stimulation		TRH stimulation
Drug	Liothyronine	Bovine TSH	Human TSH	TRH
Dose	20 µg 8-hourly for 7 doses (cats only)	0.1 IU/kg (dogs) 0.5 IU/kg (cats)	50–75 µg/dog 0.025–0.20 mg/cat	100–600 µg (dogs) 0.1 mg/kg (cats)
Route	Oral	Intravenous	Intravenous	Intravenous
Sampling times	0 and 2–4 hours after last dose	0 and 6 hours	0 and 6 hours (dogs) 0 and 6–8 hours (cats)	0 and 4 hours
Assay	Total T4	Total T4	Total T4	Total T4
Reference range	<20 nmol/l with >50% suppression	50% increase exceeding approximately 23 nmol/l (dogs) >100% increase (cats)	As for bovine TSH	At least >20% increase or >6 nmol/l (dogs) >60% increase (cats)

17.5 Commonly used protocols for dynamic thyroid function tests in dogs and cats. Values quoted for interpretation are guidelines only. Each individual laboratory should furnish its own reference interval.

In most cases, the total T4 response to either exogenous TRH, TSH or synthetic T3 is assessed, although cTSH can be measured after administration of TRH. Both exogenous TRH and T3 are readily available. Bovine TSH, previously used for the TSH response test, is no longer available as a pharmaceutical preparation. A recombinant human β-subunit TSH is now available and, although expensive, appears to work well in healthy dogs and cats (Sauve and Paradis, 2000; Stegeman *et al.*, 2003). The most commonly used protocols for these tests are outlined in Figure 17.5.

Hypothyroidism

Hypothyroidism is primarily a concern in dogs although occasionally investigation is required in cats.

Canine hypothyroidism

A range of possible causes of canine hypothyroidism exists. Primary hypothyroidism refers to disease arising as a consequence of pathology within the thyroid gland itself. Hypothyroidism may also arise because of a deficiency of TSH or TRH, so-called secondary and tertiary hypothyroidism. Although the former has been recognized in dogs and cats, the latter has never been reported. The distinction is not always clear, however, and many refer to this type of hypothyroidism as central. The overwhelming majority of hypothyroid cases arise from irreversible acquired thyroid gland disease. Only a small percentage of hypothyroidism results from nutritional, congenital, pituitary or other conditions.

Adult-onset hypothyroidism

Primary, irreversible destruction of the thyroid gland accounts for almost all of the naturally occurring cases of hypothyroidism in adult dogs. The histopathological description is either lymphocytic thyroiditis or idiopathic thyroid degeneration (atrophy), each of which occurs with approximately equal frequency.

Lymphocytic thyroiditis, also referred to as autoimmune thyroiditis, is characterized by lymphocytic infiltration of the thyroid glands with progressive destruction of thyroid follicles. There is a variation in the rate of progression of this process but extensive pathological changes must have occurred prior to the appearance of clinical signs of hypothyroidism (Graham *et al.*, 2001). This condition is recognized as a heritable trait.

Idiopathic thyroid degeneration is characterized by a loss of thyroid parenchyma with replacement by adipose or fibrous tissue. The cause is not yet defined, but there is evidence that these lesions may be an end stage of lymphocytic thyroiditis (Graham *et al.*, 2001).

Congenital hypothyroidism (cretinism)

Dogs that are hypothyroid at birth fail to grow and develop normally; they are usually described as having disproportionate dwarfism. If goitre is present a defect in one of the steps of hormonogenesis or, less commonly, iodine deficiency is the likely cause. Defects in TPO have been described in Toy Fox Terriers with congenital hypothyroidism and goitre (Fyfe *et al.*, 2003). However, goitre is absent in most reports of congenital hypothyroidism. A lack of production of TSH is the suspected cause of juvenile hypothyroidism in Giant Schnauzers (Greco *et al.*, 1991), Boxers (Mooney and Anderson, 1993) and Scottish Deerhounds (Robinson *et al.*, 1988). However, most reports were published prior to the availability of the cTSH assay, so this is unproven.

Laboratory diagnosis of canine hypothyroidism

Canine hypothyroidism is difficult to diagnose because of the long preclinical phase, the variety of presenting complaints and the poor specificity of several of the diagnostic tests. It is probably one of the most overdiagnosed conditions in veterinary medicine, but certain circumstances can lead to underdiagnosis.

A common physiological response to any illness is a lowering of circulating thyroid hormone concentrations. It is, therefore, often difficult to distinguish between pathological and physiological thyroid-deficient states, and the diagnostic specificity of thyroid hormone measurements is consequently poor. In addition, early in the disease, animals may be overtly hypothyroid on laboratory testing but may not display classic or well defined clinical features for many months thereafter. Finally, hypothyroid dogs may have reference range serum thyroid hormone concentrations because of analytical interference by crossreacting anti-thyroid hormone antibodies.

A variety of clinical pathology abnormalities can be seen in hypothyroid dogs although none is truly specific (Figure 17.6) (Panciera, 1994a; Dixon *et al.*, 1999). Historically, hypothyroidism was suggested to have an adverse effect on von Willebrand factor antigen and clotting times but this has been disproved (Avgeris *et al.*, 1990; Panciera and Johnson, 1994).

Clinical pathological abnormality	% of hypothyroid dogs
Haematology	
Mild normocytic anaemia	18–40
Serum biochemistry	
Elevated cholesterol	73–78
Elevated triglyceride	88
Elevated creatine kinase	18–35
Elevated alkaline phosphatase	30

17.6 Clinical pathological abnormalities in hypothyroid dogs (Panciera, 1994a; Dixon *et al.*, 1999).

Laboratory tests for directly investigating thyroid disease can be divided into those that assess thyroid function and those that provide evidence of pathology (thyroiditis).

Thyroid hormones: Low concentrations of thyroid hormones are poorly specific for hypothyroidism. Concentrations can be decreased in response to general non-thyroidal illness or administration of many drugs. Exogenous thyroid hormone supplementation therapy can also interfere with diagnostic testing and a greater than 4-week withdrawal period is required before retesting (Panciera *et al.*, 1990).

Total thyroxine: Total T4 is a reasonably sensitive test (up to 100%) but it is poorly specific (as low as 70%) (Figure 17.7). (For discussions of sensitivity and specificity, see Chapters 2 and 26.) Unfortunately, total T4 concentrations can be low in a variety of situations other than hypothyroidism. If used as the sole diagnostic test for hypothyroidism, many false positive results would ensue.

Total T4 is lowered in non-thyroidal illness as a normal physiological response to that illness. Although several mechanisms are responsible, not all are clearly defined in the dog. Possible explanations include:

- Glucocorticoid-mediated TSH suppression
- Reduced serum protein binding
- Altered peripheral hormone metabolism.

The suppressive effect of non-thyroidal illness can be profound and has been demonstrated in both acute and chronic illnesses (Panciera, 1994b; Elliot *et al.*, 1995; Calvert *et al.*, 1998; Panciera *et al.*, 2003; Torres *et al.*, 2003). In general, the more severe the illness, the greater the effect on thyroid hormone concentrations (Kantrowitz *et al.*, 2001). In some chronic conditions, such as osteoarthritis, there appears to be little effect (Paradis *et al.*, 2003). The preferred terminology for this effect is the 'low-T4 state of medical illness' although the phrase 'euthyroid sick syndrome' has also been used.

A similar phenomenon occurs with a variety of drugs, including glucocorticoids, long-term phenobarbital, acetylsalicylic acid, amiodarone, clomipramine and sulphonamide-containing antibiotics (Bicer *et al.*, 2002; Gulikers and Panciera, 2003; Williamson *et al.*, 2002; Daminet and Ferguson, 2003; Daminet *et al.*, 2003).

Sulphonamide therapy warrants specific mention as it potentially causes a true but reversible hypothyroidism, presumably mediated through inhibition of TPO, an enzyme essential for thyroid hormone production. As a result, circulating total T4 concentrations can be severely depressed. The effects of sulphonamide therapy is relatively long-lived after withdrawal, with full recovery in a few weeks. A withdrawal period of 3 weeks is recommended prior to assessing thyroid function.

Whilst total T4 concentrations should be interpreted cautiously in dogs being treated with the drugs listed above, more recent studies have shown that some drugs have no or minimal effects on thyroid function including bromide, propanolol, etodolac, ketoprofen, meloxicam, carprofen and chondroitin sulfate/glucosamine (Panciera and Johnston, 2002; Daminet and Ferguson, 2003; Daminet *et al.*, 2003; Sauve *et al.*, 2003). Thyroid function can be reasonably reliably assessed in animals receiving these medications.

Study	TT4		FT4d		TSH		TT4/TSH		FT4d/TSH		TgAA	
	Sen	Spec	Sen	Spec	Sen	Spec	Sen	Spec	Sen	Spec	Sen	Spec
Iversen *et al.*, 1998											91	97
Nachreiner *et al.*, 1998											100	100
Beale and Torres, 1991											86	94
Nelson *et al.*, 1991	98	73	97	78								
Peterson *et al.*, 1997	89	82	98	93	76	93	67	98	74	98		
Scott-Moncrieff *et al.*, 1998	100	78			63	88	63	100				
Dixon and Mooney, 1999b	100	75	80	94	87	82	87	92	80	97		

17.7 Published diagnostic performance of tests used in the diagnosis of canine hypothyroidism and thyroid pathology. All values expressed as percentage (TT4, total thyroxine; FT4d, free thyroxine by equilibrium dialysis; TSH, thyroid stimulating hormone (thyrotropin); TgAA, thyroglobulin autoantibodies; Sen, sensitivity; Spec, specificity).

Several physiological mechanisms are also responsible for low circulating total T4 concentrations in dogs. Of the potential factors, time of year, age, dioestrus, exercise and nutritional status, do not effect total T4 concentrations enough to misdiagnose eu- or hypothyroidism, although extreme diet alteration may (Castillo *et al.*, 2001). Breed, on the other hand, can be very important. Greyhounds, other 'sighthounds' and sled dogs usually have values at the low end or below the general reference range (Gaughan and Bruyette, 2001; Lee *et al.*, 2004). Values may even be undetectable in healthy individuals of these breeds.

Relying on a reference range total T4 concentration alone to rule out a diagnosis of hypothyroidism also has its drawbacks particularly if T4AAs are present (see below). Thus, neither a reference range or low total T4 concentration result can be relied upon accurately to confirm or refute hypothyroidism. The use of a serial testing protocol, only progressing to additional thyroid test if an initial 'screening' total T4 is abnormal, is a flawed approach.

Assessment of total T4 concentrations has several advantages including its relative inexpense and ready availability.

Free thyroxine by equilibrium dialysis: Measurement of free T4 concentrations is a more specific diagnostic test for hypothyroidism than measurement of total T4 alone (see Figure 17.7). It is most helpful when:

- There is significant non-thyroidal illness present suppressing total T4 concentrations
- The animal is receiving medication that can influence protein binding and ultimately total T4 concentrations
- When T4AAs are present resulting in falsely elevated total T4 concentrations.

In these cases serum free T4 concentrations are expected to remain within reference range. However, although it is less affected by non-thyroidal illness and drug therapies, free T4 concentrations may be suppressed by severe illness and glucocorticoids, long-term phenobarbital therapy and clomipramine.

In addition, free T4 is a less sensitive diagnostic test than total T4, particularly in the early stages of the illness (Dixon and Mooney, 1999b). It is also susceptible to endogenous and exogenous sample effects (see above).

Total triiodothyronine: The measurement of serum total T3 offers no real advantage over the measurement of total or free T4 concentrations (see Figure 17.7). It is a relatively poor predictor of thyroid function for the following reasons:

- A high prevalence of interfering T3AAs in hypothyroid dogs
- Possible up-regulation of deiodinase activity in animals with failing thyroid function resulting in maintenance of circulating total T3 concentrations
- Suppressive effect of non-thyroidal illness which presumably is metabolically protective and a beneficial response to illness
- Suppressive effect of various drug therapies, including sulphonamides, acetylsalicylic acid, glucocorticoids, amiodarone and clomipramine.

In animals which are known to be TgAA negative, measurement of serum total T3 may be helpful in specific circumstances, e.g. the 'sighthound' reference range for total T3 may be more similar to that of the general population than that for total or free T4.

Thyrotropin: Dogs with primary hypothyroidism are expected to have an elevated serum cTSH concentration because of the loss of the negative feedback effect of the thyroid hormones. Unfortunately, not all cases of primary hypothyroidism exhibit elevated values and some euthyroid (sick and healthy) dogs have been shown to have elevated values. Clinical studies of cTSH measurement for the diagnosis of hypothyroidism report sensitivity between 63% and 87% and specificity between 82% and 100% (see Figure 17.7).

The poor diagnostic sensitivity of cTSH measurement could arise for several reasons, not all of which are well understood:

- The presence of concurrent non-thyroidal illness could potentially suppress a previously high cTSH into the reference range in a dog with primary hypothyroidism
- Concurrent drug therapy, particularly with glucocorticoids, potentially suppresses cTSH concentrations into the reference range in hypothyroid dogs
- Random fluctuation of cTSH into the reference range in hypothyroid animals, particularly if only minimally elevated initially
- Existence of central rather than primary hypothyroidism
- The possible existence of various isomers of cTSH not all of which are measured using current assay techniques.

Elevated cTSH values in euthyroid dogs are less common but also not well understood. Possible explanations include:

- Recovery of thyroid function from the effects of previous non-thyroidal illness or drug use
- Treatment with sulphonamide-containing or phenobarbital drugs
- During the prolonged progression of thyroid pathology from normal to thyroid failure, an intermediate step is a compensated phase in which much higher concentrations of TSH are generated to stimulate the decreasing thyroid mass and maintain normal thyroid hormone concentrations.

The use of cTSH measurements alone is not recommended: it should be interpreted in conjunction with other thyroid hormone results.

Thyroglobulin autoantibodies: The majority of canine hypothyroidism is caused by lymphocytic thyroiditis. As part of this inflammatory process, antibodies to thyroid antigens may be expressed and released into the circulation. Thyroglobulin is the principal antigen for which measurable serum antibodies are present. Measurement of TgAA therefore provides evidence for an active inflammatory process in the thyroid glands. A positive TgAA status cannot provide any information on thyroid function *per se* because thyroid dysfunction does not occur until at least 60–70% of the gland is destroyed. Consequently, both lymphocytic thyroiditis and TgAAs can be present in dogs which are not yet functionally hypothyroid. It may take several months to years for hypothyroidism to develop and, in some cases, a functional problem never arises.

Limited studies have been published comparing TgAA results and histological examination of thyroid biopsy material. However, of those published, there is excellent diagnostic sensitivity and specificity (>90% in each case) (see Figure 17.7). Lymphocytic thyroiditis, as determined by serum TgAA measurement, does occur in the general healthy canine population with prevalence estimates of between 2% and 3% (Nachreiner *et al.*, 1998; Dixon and Mooney, 1999a).

Measurement of TgAA provides advantages in detecting thyroid pathology long before a change in thyroid function is apparent. This may have implications for breeding selection. In addition, it may allow timely institution of therapy without waiting for dramatic clinical signs to develop. Although widespread studies are limited, approximately 20% of dogs with positive TgAA status and no other thyroid hormone abnormality progress to thyroid dysfunction within 1 year (Graham *et al.*, 2001). Assuming a similar proportion would progress in each subsequent year, the majority could be hypothyroid within 4 years or so. However, longer term studies are currently lacking.

Despite the excellent diagnostic performance reported for this test in the assessment of thyroid pathology, there are some reports that false weak positive results occasionally occur in recently vaccinated dogs as a result of non-specific binding of immunoglobulin G (IgG).

Thyroid hormone autoantibodies: Autoantibodies to T4 and T3 only develop in a proportion of TgAA positive dogs. However, the high prevalence of T3AAs in the dog is one of the main reasons that measurement of T3 has limited value in the diagnosis of hypothyroidism. In most commonly used assay systems, autoantibodies cause falsely elevated values that can be extreme, and they may result in elevation of a low value into the reference range. Similarly, the presence of T4AAs potentially results in an underdiagnosis of hypothyroidism in approximately 10% of cases if the diagnosis is solely reliant on demonstration of low total T4 values, as T4AAs increase measured values into the reference range. T3AAs have an estimated prevalence of 34% in hypothyroid dogs compared with 15% for T4AAs (Graham *et al.*, 2001).

Putting it all together – thyroid profiles: The introduction of methods for free T4, cTSH and TgAA measurement have significantly improved the diagnostic capability for hypothyroidism compared with total T4 measurement alone. When used together the diagnostic short-comings of each test are minimized. In most situations, a combined thyroid 'profile' is better for investigating hypothyroidism than serial individual tests. In combination, the gain from the high sensitivity of T4 and high specificity cTSH measurements is maximized.

The minimum recommended thyroid profile is total T4 and cTSH.

Free T4 should be added or used instead of total T4 when the patient is known to have non-thyroidal illness or to be receiving potentially interfering therapies (e.g. glucocorticoids and barbiturates) or when T4-crossreacting TgAA are suspected. The addition of TgAA to the initial profile serves as a screen to determine whether the total T4 result can be believed to be free from interference by T4AA and helps define the pathogenesis of thyroid dysfunction. In addition, it may help with some equivocal cases and identify subclinical thyroid disease.

The most common diagnostic dilemma is finding low T4 and reference range cTSH results in a dog. This could indicate:

- The animal is responding appropriately to a physiological stress (such as non-thyroidal illness)
- The animal is on medication that suppresses T4 concentrations
- It is one of the proportion of hypothyroid dogs (approximately 15% or more) in which an elevated TSH result is not detected.

In such cases, free T4 and TgAA assessment may be warranted. Free T4 serves to differentiate the low T4 state of medical illness or the effect of drug therapies from true hypothyroidism in many cases. If a diagnosis remains unclear, retesting at a later date, instituting a therapeutic trial or embarking on a TSH stimulation test is recommended.

In interpreting the results of tests which have less than perfect diagnostic sensitivity and specificity, the effect of prevalence on the predictive value of positive and negative test results must be considered (see Chapter 26). In large thyroid diagnostic laboratories, a rough estimate can be made of the prevalence of hypothyroidism in the population being tested. Clear-cut diagnoses of hypothyroidism were made in approximately 8% of samples submitted to one laboratory (Diagnostic Center for Population and Animal Health, Michigan State University) and unclassified cases (low total or free T4 but reference range cTSH) accounted for a further 17%. Figure 17.8 compares the predictive values of positive and negative test results for total T4 measured alone and for total T4 measured in combination with cTSH and illustrates the enhanced diagnostic confidence for combined results.

Test			Pre-test probability					
			10%		25%		50%	
	Sensitivity	Specificity	PPV	NPV	PPV	NPV	PPV	NPV
TT4 alone	89	75	28	98	54	95	78	87
T4/TSH	87	98	83	99	94	96	98	88

17.8 Positive and negative predictive values for the measurement of TT4 and the combination of TT4 and TSH at three different levels of pre-test probability (or prevalence of hypothyroidism in tested group) at example levels of diagnostic sensitivity and specificity. The table shows that a pre-test probability of 10% (similar to that experienced by diagnostic laboratories) means that less than 30% of dogs with a low total T4 result alone have hypothyroidism. Even at the relatively high pre-test probability of 25%, a low total T4 still only has a positive predictive value of approximately 50%, similar to the clinician guessing whether or not hypothyroidism is present. The combination of TT4 and TSH measurement gives more useful PPV and NPV over a range of pre-test probabilities consistent with clinical practice (10–25%). All values presented as percentages. See Chapter 2 for methods of calculation (PPV, positive predictive value; NPV, negative predictive value; TT4, total thyroxine; TSH, thyroid stimulating hormone (thyrotropin)).

Dynamic thyroid function tests: The ideal tools for investigating endocrine disorders are the dynamic function (stimulation and suppression) tests. Certainly the TSH stimulation test is considered by many to be the closest to a 'gold standard' test of thyroid function. Unfortunately, pharmaceutical grade TSH now has limited availability. More recently, a recombinant human β-subunit TSH has become available (Sauve and Paradis, 2000). Given its expense and the improved diagnostic performance of multiple concurrent basal thyroid hormone assessments, it is unlikely to gain widespread use except in diagnostically equivocal cases.

The TRH response test gained some support following the reduced availability of TSH but the results of this test are difficult to interpret and many euthyroid dogs are classified erroneously as hypothyroid (Frank, 1996). It may have some use in assessing the pituitary production of TSH in rare cases of suspected pituitary hypothyroidism.

Monitoring thyroid hormone replacement therapy

The exogenous T4 used for treating hypothyroidism is immunologically identical to endogenous T4, so the same assays can be used to measure its circulating concentration. In addition, the negative feedback effect of exogenous T4 decreases production of cTSH. Thus, the measurement of both T4 and cTSH concentrations can provide useful indications of the adequacy of thyroid hormone supplementation.

The measurement of serum total T4 concentrations provides an indication of the adequacy of therapy on the day of the test; peak concentrations are usually achieved around 3 hours post pill. Common recommendations for therapeutic monitoring are to measure T4 4–6 hours after medication. With few evidence based studies available, an assumption has often been made that good therapy implies serum T4 concentrations at least a little above the lower limit of the reference range throughout the day. Given the half-life of T4 of between 6 and 10 hours, it is clear that to achieve such a goal with once daily medication usually requires peak concentrations to be a little above the reference range. With twice daily therapy peak concentrations would only need to be in the top part of the reference range to achieve the same goal. The sampling time can be flexible if the clinician can apply knowledge of the half-life of T4 in extrapolating between these targets (high-normal or slightly above at peak, low-normal at the trough). The serum concentration of cTSH takes several days to change and therefore the measurement of this hormone provides information on the adequacy of therapy in the preceding few days rather than just on the day of the test. Compared to the measurement of total T4 alone, combined total T4 and cTSH helps identify long-term compliance failures and avoids unnecessary dose adjustment. Reasonable clinical response can be expected when peak thyroid hormone concentrations are in the top end or above the reference range and cTSH concentrations are within reference range (Dixon *et al.*, 2002).

Feline hypothyroidism

Hypothyroidism occurs rarely in cats. Usually this is iatrogenic following treatment for hyperthyroidism but there have also been some spontaneous cases (Sjollema *et al.*, 1991; Tanase *et al.*, 1991; Rand *et al.*, 1993). The measurement of TSH using the widely available canine assay may be of some help in making a diagnosis of primary or iatrogenic hypothyroidism with similar test performance characteristics to its use in dogs (i.e. imperfect sensitivity).

Hyperthyroidism

Hyperthyroidism is primarily a concern in cats and only rarely is investigation required in dogs.

Feline hyperthyroidism

Feline hyperthyroidism (thyrotoxicosis) was first definitively diagnosed in 1979 and its incidence has increased dramatically since then. It is now the most common endocrine disorder of the cat and a disease frequently encountered in practice. It is unclear if this is because it is truly a new disease or because it is being diagnosed more frequently as a result of improved practitioner and client awareness, a growing cat population, increased longevity or a combination of these factors.

Hyperthyroidism is a multisystemic disorder arising from increased thyroid hormone production by an abnormally functioning thyroid gland. Histopathologically, the normal thyroid follicular architecture is replaced by multiple, well defined, hyperplastic nodules ranging from <1 mm to >2 cm in diameter and usually described as adenomatous hyperplasia (adenoma). This results in enlargement of either one (<30 % of cases) or more commonly both (>70% of cases) thyroid lobes (goitre). Thyroid carcinoma is a rare cause of hyperthyroidism in the cat, accounting for less than 2% of cases.

Hyperthyroidism typically affects older cats (usually >10 years of age) of either sex and any breed. There has been a recent report of hyperthyroidism in a kitten but, given that the histopathological appearance was different to that seen in older cats, it probably represents a distinct and rare clinical entity (Gordon *et al.*, 2003).

The aetiology of the disorder remains unclear and prevention is therefore not possible. However, because of the benign nature of the lesions in the majority of cases, the disease carries an excellent prognosis with effective therapy.

Laboratory diagnosis of feline hyperthyroidism

Classically hyperthyroidism is associated with weight loss, despite an increased or normal appetite, hyperactivity, tachycardia, intermittent gastrointestinal signs of vomiting and diarrhoea, cardiac murmur and goitre. However, cats are less highly symptomatic now compared to 15 years ago, presumably because of increased awareness. This, coupled with its high prevalence, means that many older cats undergo testing for hyperthyroidism that may actually have the disease, or that may be suffering from a variety of non-thyroidal illnesses or that may indeed be healthy. This impacts the performance of the diagnostic tests used in confirming, but probably more importantly in refuting a diagnosis of hyperthyroidism.

Routine clinicopathological features: Routine haematological and biochemical investigations are useful in providing supportive evidence of hyperthyroidism (Figure 17.9). However, they prove more useful in eliminating or diagnosing non-thyroidal illnesses in animals presenting with similar clinical signs or in depicting concurrent disorders that may ultimately affect the prognosis.

Clinical pathological abnormality	% of cases
Haematology	
Erythrocytosis	50
Macrocytosis	50
Serum biochemistry	
Elevated liver enzymes	90
Azotaemia	20
Hyperphosphataemia	36–43

17.9 Common haematological and biochemical abnormalities associated with hyperthyroidism (Peterson *et al.*, 1983; Thoday and Mooney, 1992; Broussard and Peterson, 1995).

Haematology: In early reports of hyperthyroidism, mild to moderate erythrocytosis and macrocytosis were considered to be relatively common (Peterson *et al.*, 1983). These changes may reflect increased erythropoietin production, resulting from increased oxygen consumption, or direct thyroid hormone-mediated β-adrenergic stimulation of erythroid marrow. However, these findings have not been confirmed in all studies (Thoday and Mooney, 1992) and when they do occur they are clinically insignificant.

Anaemia, on the other hand, appears to be rare and is usually associated with severe hyperthyroidism. It may result from bone marrow exhaustion or iron or other micronutrient deficiency. A significantly higher incidence of Heinz body formation and increased platelet size have been reported in cats with hyperthyroidism compared with healthy cats (Mooney, 2001). However, these abnormalities appear to have minimal clinical significance.

Changes in white blood cell parameters are not unusual in hyperthyroidism but are relatively non-specific. The most frequent changes include leucocytosis, mature neutrophilia, lymphopenia and eosinopenia, presumably reflecting a stress response. However, eosinophilia and lymphocytosis may occur in a small number of cats potentially resulting from a relative decrease in available cortisol because of enhanced metabolism induced by thyroid hormone excess.

Serum biochemistry: The most striking biochemical abnormalities are elevations in the liver enzymes, alanine aminotransferase (ALT), alkaline phosphatase (ALP), lactate dehydrogenase (LDH) and aspartate aminotransferase (AST). At least one of these enzymes is elevated in over 90% of hyperthyroid cats (Peterson *et al.*, 1983; Thoday and Mooney, 1992; Broussard and Peterson, 1995). The elevations in these enzymes can be dramatic (>500 IU/l) but are usually significantly correlated to total T4 concentrations (Foster and Thoday, 2000). Liver enzyme elevation may be minimal, if present at all, in early or mild cases of hyperthyroidism and concurrent hepatic disease should be suspected if there are marked elevations in these enzymes but only mildly elevated serum thyroid hormone concentrations. When elevated as a result of hyperthyroidism, liver enzyme concentrations decrease to within the reference range with successful management of the thyrotoxicosis (Mooney *et al.*, 1992).

Despite the marked elevations in hepatic enzymes, histological examination of hyperthyroid cat livers has revealed only modest and non-specific changes, possibly caused by malnutrition, congestive cardiac failure, infections, hepatic anoxia and direct toxic effects of thyroid hormones on the liver. Several recent reports have shown that both liver and bone contribute to increased ALP activity in hyperthyroid cats (Mooney, 2001).

Hyperphosphataemia, in the absence of azotaemia, was originally reported in approximately 20% of cases but has more recently been reported in a higher percentage (36–43%) of hyperthyroid cats (Peterson *et al.*, 1983; Archer and Taylor, 1996; Barber and Elliott, 1996). Serum total calcium is largely unaffected by hyperthyroidism but ionized calcium is decreased and circulating parathormone (PTH) increased. Circulating osteocalcin concentration, a measure of osteoblastic activity and bone remodelling, is elevated in some hyperthyroid cats (Archer and Taylor, 1996). The aetiology of these changes is unknown but, given the increased concentrations of the bone isoenzyme of ALP, it may reflect alterations in bone turnover. The clinical consequences are unclear.

Mild to moderate azotaemia occurs in just over 20% of hyperthyroid cats (Broussard and Peterson, 1995). While this is not unexpected in a group of aged cats, the increase could be exacerbated by the increased protein catabolism and prerenal uraemia of thyrotoxicosis. In hyperthyroid cats without azotaemia, serum creatinine concentration is significantly lower compared with that in age-matched, healthy animals (Barber and Elliott, 1996). This may be related to reduced muscle mass. Whatever its cause, it has implications when assessing renal function in hyperthyroid cats prior to deciding on the best option for treatment, particularly because renal function may deteriorate after commencing therapy (see below). A number of other clinicopathological abnormalities have been described in hyperthyroid cats, although these remain rare. Clinically significant hypokalaemia has been reported in four hyperthyroid cats but the aetiology remains unclear (Nemzek *et al*., 1994). Two separate studies (Graham *et al*., 1999; Reusch and Tomsa, 1999) have shown that serum fructosamine concentration is significantly lower in hyperthyroid compared with healthy cats, presumably as a result of increased protein turnover. Importantly, 17–50% of cases had values below the respective reference range and caution is therefore advised in interpreting serum fructosamine concentration in hyperthyroid cats, particularly if they are concurrently diabetic, since the hyperglycaemia associated with diabetes may not be reflected by high fructosamine in hyperthyroid cats.

Other analytes (e.g. cholesterol, sodium, chloride, bilirubin, albumin and globulin) are largely unaffected by hyperthyroidism. Circulating glucose may be elevated, presumably reflecting a stress response.

Urinalysis: Examination of urine in thyrotoxic cats is non-contributory. Urine specific gravity is variable and in one study ranged from 1.009–1.050 (mean 1.031) in 57 hyperthyroid cats with only two values (4%) below 1.015 (Peterson *et al*., 1983).

Assessment of thyroid function: Unlike the situation in canine hypothyroidism, there are no laboratory tests that depict the underlying thyroid pathology in hyperthyroid cats. Elevated circulating concentrations of the thyroid hormones serve as the biochemical hallmark of hyperthyroidism, irrespective of underlying pathology.

Thyroid hormones: For the diagnosis of hyperthyroidism, total T3, total T4 and free T4 can be measured, although the diagnostic performance of each varies. Measurement of TSH concentration, frequently used in humans, is not recommended in cats. A species-specific assay does not exist and, although preliminary reports suggest that the canine assay can be used for feline TSH, the relatively high lower limit of detection curtails its usefulness in hyperthyroidism.

- Total thyroxine concentration: most hyperthyroid cats exhibit an elevated circulating total T4 concentration with values up to approximately 20 times the upper limit of the reference range reported. Total T4 is a highly specific diagnostic test for hyperthyroidism, as elevated values do not occur in euthyroid cats. It is relatively inexpensive and readily accessible. However, approximately 10% of hyperthyroid cats have serum total T4 concentrations within the reference range (Peterson *et al*., 2001). This increases to 40% of cases if only those with mild clinical disease are selected. In most of these cats total T4 values are within the mid to high reference range. Thus hyperthyroidism cannot be excluded in cats by demonstration of a single reference range total T4 concentration alone. There are several explanations for reference range total T4 values in hyperthyroid cats:
  - Non-specific thyroid hormone fluctuation may result in reference range total T4 values in cats with marginal elevations. A circadian rhythm does not exist in cats but circulating hormone concentrations vary both within and, more pronouncedly, between days (Peterson *et al*., 1987). Increased thyroidal production and fluctuations in binding proteins or other undefined haemodynamic changes possibly account for these changes. Serum total T4 concentrations will often increase into the thyrotoxic range on retesting 3–6 weeks later. However, in some cats, a longer interval is required and testing when more overt clinical signs develop may be more appropriate. (In cats with markedly elevated circulating total T4 concentration, the degree of fluctuation is of little diagnostic significance)
  - Non-thyroidal illness has a suppressive effect on circulating total T4 concentration in cats resulting in mid to high reference range values in mild hyperthyroidism. The mechanisms remain unclear but are more likely to involve changes in peripheral thyroid hormone metabolism or protein binding rather than any effect on the hypothalamic-pituitary axis. Similar to the phenomenon of fluctuation, the degree of suppression has little diagnostic significance in hyperthyroid cats with markedly elevated circulating total T4 concentration. In euthyroid cats, non-thyroidal illness tends to suppress total T4 concentrations into the low end or below the reference range, depending on the severity of the illness. Total T4 measurement can be used as a prognostic indicator (Mooney *et al*., 1996; Peterson *et al*., 2001) (Figure 17.10). Consequently, concurrent hyperthyroidism should always be suspected in cats with severe non-thyroidal illness and serum total T4 concentrations within the mid to high reference range. It is likely that serum total T4 concentrations would increase into the thyrotoxic range upon treatment or recovery

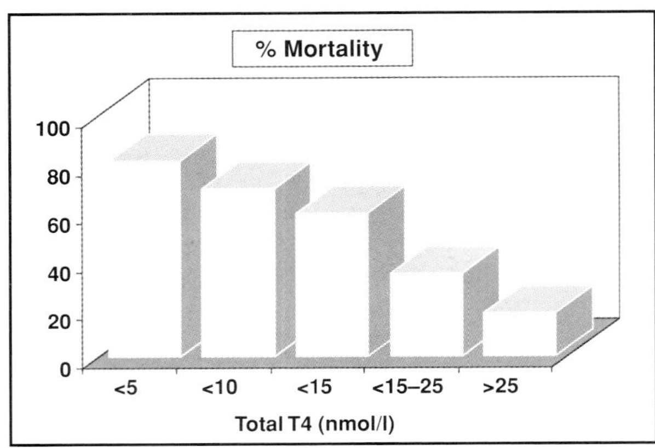

17.10 The relationship of mortality to serum total T4 concentrations in 107 cats with a variety of non-thyroidal illnesses.

from the non-thyroidal illness. Occasionally serum total T4 concentrations are suppressed to the lower half of the reference range in hyperthyroid cats that have extreme non-thyroidal illnesses. However, in these cases, the non-thyroidal illness dictates the prognosis and pursuing hyperthyroidism is of less clinical importance. In large studies of hyperthyroid cats, approximately 20% of cats with reference range total T4 values have an identifiable concurrent illness. The overwhelming majority are classified as mild or early cases (Peterson *et al.*, 2001)

- Free thyroxine by equilibrium dialysis: in human thyrotoxicosis, assessment of free T4 is considered a better diagnostic test for hyperthyroidism because it is less affected by non-thyroidal factors than total T4 and provides a more accurate reflection of thyroid status. In addition, when serum total T4 concentration is increased, the concentration of free T4 is disproportionately increased. In hyperthyroid cats, serum free and total T4 concentrations are highly significantly correlated. In all cats with markedly elevated total T4 concentrations, free T4 concentration is concurrently elevated, adding little diagnostic information to that already obtained. However, as in humans, it is a more sensitive indicator of hyperthyroidism than total T4 measurement alone. Estimates suggest that up to 98% of hyperthyroid cats have an elevated circulating free T4 concentration. More significantly, approximately 95% of hyperthyroid cats with reference range total T4 values, because of mild disease or the suppressive effects of concurrent non-thyroidal illness, have concurrent elevated free T4 concentrations (Peterson *et al.*, 2001). Measurement of free T4 concentrations is difficult. It is more expensive and less readily available than total T4 and is more subject to sample handling errors. More significantly, it is a less specific diagnostic test for hyperthyroidism, as elevated values have been demonstrated in up to 12% of sick euthyroid cats (Mooney *et al.*, 1996; Peterson *et al.*, 2001). Most of these cats had serum total T4 concentrations in the lower end of or below the reference range. As a consequence, caution is advised in interpreting an elevated free T4 value alone. A stepwise approach is recommended: serum total T4 concentrations should be assessed first in cats suspected of hyperthyroidism. If values are found within the mid to high reference range, consideration should be given to measurement of the corresponding free T4 concentration. If elevated, hyperthyroidism is confirmed
- Total triiodothyronine concentration: serum total T4 and T3 concentrations are highly correlated in hyperthyroid cats. However, over 30% of hyperthyroid cats have reference range serum total T3 concentrations (Peterson *et al.*, 2001). The majority of cats with such values has serum total T4 concentrations either within the reference range or only marginally elevated (e.g. usually <65 nmol/l, always <100 nmol/l). These cases are usually classified as early or mildly affected and it is likely that total T3 concentrations would increase into the diagnostic thyrotoxic range if the disorder were allowed to progress untreated. It is possible that this phenomenon reflects a compensatory decrease in peripheral conversion of T4 to the more active T3 as hyperthyroidism is developing, although in a small number of cases the suppressive effect of severe concurrent non-thyroidal illness may play a role. Due to the poor diagnostic sensitivity of total T3 measurement, it is no longer recommended for the evaluation of hyperthyroidism.

Dynamic thyroid function tests: In the majority of hyperthyroid cats with reference range total T4 concentrations the diagnosis can be confirmed by consideration of the presence of concurrent non-thyroidal illness, retesting at a later date or by simultaneous assessment of free T4 concentrations. Dynamic thyroid function tests, previously recommended for confirming hyperthyroidism in equivocal cases, are therefore almost obsolete. They should only be considered in cats with clinical signs of hyperthyroidism when repeated serum total T4 concentrations remain within the reference range, or free T4 analysis is unavailable or diagnostically unhelpful. A brief description of these tests is given here and in Figure 17.5. Further details can be found elsewhere (Mooney, 2001).

- T3 suppression test: in healthy individuals, T3 has a suppressive effect on pituitary TSH secretion and subsequently on T4 production by the thyroid gland. In hyperthyroidism, because of autonomous production of thyroid hormones and chronic suppression of TSH, this suppressive effect is lost. Thus, serum total T4 concentrations show minimal or no decrease in hyperthyroid cats following exogenous T3 administration and values remain higher than approximately 20 nmol/l with less than 35% suppression over the duration of the test. Simultaneous measurement of serum total T3 concentrations is required to ensure compliant administration and adequate absorption of the drug and thus avoid false positive results. Generally, the test is most useful in ruling out, rather than confirming, hyperthyroidism

- TSH stimulation test: due to its poor diagnostic performance this test has largely been superseded, although the availability of recombinant human TSH may renew interest in its application in cats. Exogenous TSH is a potent stimulator of thyroid hormone secretion but serum total T4 concentrations show little or no increase following exogenous TSH administration in hyperthyroid cats. This is presumably because the thyroid gland of affected cats secretes thyroid hormones independently of TSH control or because T4 is already being produced at a near maximal rate with limited reserve capacity. Cats with equivocally elevated serum total T4 concentrations tend to exhibit results indistinguishable from those in healthy animals and thus the test has limited diagnostic value
- TRH stimulation test: TRH is less expensive and easier to obtain than TSH. Serum total T4 concentrations increase minimally (<50%) after TRH administration in mildly hyperthyroid cats. Compared to the T3 suppression test, this test is quicker and avoids tablet administration. However, TRH is associated with transient adverse reactions, such as salivation, vomiting, tachypnoea and defecation. In addition, results of the test are largely indistinguishable between sick euthyroid and hyperthyroid cats with concurrent disease and total T4 concentrations within or below the reference range (Tomsa *et al.*, 2001).

Monitoring response to therapy

Irrespective of the therapeutic modality chosen, measurement of serum total T4 concentrations is of most value in monitoring efficacy.

In cats treated with the antithyroid drugs, methimazole and carbimazole, assessment of total T4 concentration is recommended 3 weeks after commencing therapy or after each dose adjustment. Once cats are stable, serum total T4 concentrations should be checked every 3–6 months, or more frequently if indicated clinically. Regular assessment is necessary as antithyroid drugs have no effect on the underlying lesions and the thyroid nodules continue to grow and enlarge, necessitating an increased dosage in the long term.

The aim of therapy is to suppress serum total T4 concentrations to within the lower half or slightly below the reference range. Even if T4 is suppressed, clinical signs of hypothyroidism do not develop, presumably because corresponding total T3 (the more metabolically active hormone) concentrations tend to remain within the reference range. This is thought to be because of preferential thyroidal secretion of T3, although increased peripheral production may play a role (Mooney *et al.*, 1992). In addition, serum free T4 concentrations appear to remain relatively higher than total T4 during antithyroid medication.

Laboratory analysis may be required to assess adverse reactions specifically associated with antithyroid drug administration. Early in the course of therapy, mild and transient haematological abnormalities, including lymphocytosis, eosinophilia or leucopenia, occur in up to 15% of cases but without any apparent clinical effect (Peterson *et al.*, 1988; Mooney *et al.*, 1992). More serious haematological complications occur in <5% of cases, usually within the first 3 months of therapy, and include agranulocytosis and thrombocytopenia, either alone or concurrently; more rarely, immune-mediated haemolytic anaemia is seen. Fortnightly complete blood and platelet counts have been recommended, in order to detect such reactions. However, because of their rarity and unpredictability, assessment of a complete blood count if clinical signs indicate is more cost-effective. A hepatopathy characterized by marked increases in liver enzymes and bilirubin concentration occurs in <2% of treated cats. Serum antinuclear antibodies develop in approximately 50% of hyperthyroid cats treated with methimazole for longer than 6 months, usually in cats on high dose therapy (>15 mg/day) (Peterson *et al.*, 1988).

Serum total T4 concentrations are usually low for weeks to months after surgical thyroidectomy or radioactive iodine therapy but will eventually increase into the reference range. Treatment for hypothyroidism is only indicated if cats exhibit definite clinical signs and is rarely required.

Effect of therapy on renal function

Hyperthyroidism is known to increase glomerular filtration rate (GFR), decrease circulating creatinine concentration and mask underlying renal disease. All treatments for hyperthyroidism have been associated with a decrease in GFR capable of unmasking latent renal disease (Mooney, 2001). Therefore, renal dysfunction should always be considered a potential adverse reaction of treatment and assessed if clinical signs develop. Several studies have attempted to predict those cats in which renal failure is likely to develop. However, the only successful methods have involved estimating GFR and are not readily applicable in practice. Serum urea and creatinine concentrations and urine specific gravity should be carefully evaluated in all cats. If both serum parameters are within reference range and the urine is concentrated, the risk of developing renal failure after treatment is minimal. However, creatinine concentration should be evaluated in light of the animal's muscle mass, with lower values expected in emaciated cats. If the serum parameters are higher than expected and the urine is dilute, there is a risk of developing renal failure upon treatment of the hyperthyroidism.

Canine hyperthyroidism

Hyperthyroidism is exceptionally rare in dogs and almost always the result of thyroid carcinoma with only sporadic reports associated with thyroid adenoma (Lawrence *et al.*, 1991; Bezzola, 2002). However, hyperthyroidism only occurs in approximately 10–20% of thyroid carcinomas. Measurement of serum total T4 is adequate for diagnosis but elevations are usually modest compared to the marked increases often seen in hyperthyroid cats.

Case examples

Case 1

Signalment

6-year old neutered female Labrador cross.

History

Generalized weakness. On clinical examination there was obesity, bradycardia (60 bpm) and mild thinning of the coat.

Clinical pathology data

Haematology	Result	Reference interval
RBC (x 10^{12}/l)	5.75	5.4–8.5
Hb (g/dl)	14.2	12–18
HCT (l/l)	0.39	0.37–0.56
MCV (fl)	68.0	65–75
MCHC (g/dl)	36	31–35
WBC (x 10^9/l)	7.9	5–18
Neutrophils (x 10^9/l)	5.37	3.7–13.32
Neutrophils (band) (x 10^9/l)	0.00	0–0.54
Lymphocytes (x 10^9/l)	1.42	1.00–3.60
Monocytes (x 10^9/l)	0.32	0.20–0.72
Eosinophils (x 10^9/l)	0.79	0.10–1.25
Basophils (x 10^9/l)	0.00	0.05–0.18
Platelets (x 10^9/l)	591	200–900

Film comment

Platelet comment – appear consistent with count
No morphological abnormalities observed

Biochemistry	Result	Reference interval
Sodium (mmol/l)	150	135–150
Potassium (mmol/l)	5.6	3.5–5.6
Chloride (mmol/l)	107	95–124
Glucose (mmol/l)	4.6	3.0–5.5
Urea (mmol/l)	8.5	3.5–7.0
Creatinine (μmol/l)	95	0–130
Calcium (mmol/l)	2.52	2.3–3.0
Inorganic phosphate (mmol/l)	1.7	0.9–1.6

Biochemistry *(continued)*	Result	Reference interval
TP (g/l)	67	55–75
Albumin (g/l)	34	29–35
Globulin (g/l)	33	18–38
Albumin:globulin ratio	1.03	0.50–1.20
ALT (IU/l)	59	0–40
AST (IU/l)	38	0–45
ALP (IU/l)	187	0–135
GGT (IU/l)	3	0–14
GDH (IU/l)	8	0–9
CK (IU/l)	108	0–400
Amylase (IU/l)	256	400–2750
Lipase (IU/l)	230	0–500
Cholesterol (mmol/l)	12.9	3.8–7.9
Total bilirubin (μmol/l)	1.3	0–5.0
Total T4 (nmol/l)	<6	13–52
TSH (ng/ml)	3.85	<0.68

What abnormalities are present?

- Slight elevations in ALP and ALT
- Moderate elevation in cholesterol
- Subnormal total T4
- Moderately elevated TSH

How would you interpret these results?

- The elevations in ALP and ALT are slight, and GGT and GDH are within reference ranges. Such a finding is non-specific and observed in many medically ill dogs and in some hypothyroid dogs.
- The combination of low total T4 and moderately elevated TSH provides very strong support for primary hypothyroidism, provided the animal has not recently been receiving 'sulpha' type medications or other reversible thyroid inhibitors.

Even in cases where a confident diagnosis of hypothyroidism can be made, some of the classically reported clinical pathology features (e.g. normocytic normochromic anaemia, elevated creatine kinase) are absent. A positive clinical response to adequate thyroid replacement therapy would confirm the diagnosis further. If the elevations in ALP and ALT continued, further investigation for hepatic disease may be warranted.

Case 2

Signalment

4-year old entire male German Shorthaired Pointer.

History

The owners had noticed circular crusting erythematous patches on the ventral abdomen over the previous few weeks and the dog had lost some of his energy. Clinical examination was unremarkable except for the skin lesions, consistent with superficial pyoderma.

Clinical pathology data

Haematology	Result	Reference interval
RBC (x 10^{12}/l)	4.89	5.4–8.5
Hb (g/dl)	10.9	12–18

Case 2 continues ▶

Case 2 continued

Haematology *(continued)*	Result	Reference interval
HCT (l/l)	0.32	0.37–0.56
MCV (fl)	65.1	65–75
MCHC (g/dl)	34	31–35
WBC (x 10^9/l)	13.1	5–18
Neutrophils (x 10^9/l)	9.17	3.7–13.32
Neutrophils (band) (x 10^9/l)	0.00	0–0.54
Lymphocytes (x 10^9/l)	3.54	1.00–3.60
Monocytes (x 10^9/l)	0.13	0.20–0.72
Eosinophils (x 10^9/l)	0.26	0.10–1.25
Basophils (x 10^9/l)	0.00	0.05–0.18
Platelets (x 10^9/l)	198	200–900

Film comment

Platelets – numbers appear adequate on the smear
Red cells – normochromic, normocytic
White cells – no morphologic abnormalities

Biochemistry	Result	Reference interval
Sodium (mmol/l)	141	135–150
Potassium (mmol/l)	4.7	3.5–5.6
Chloride (mmol/l)	103	95–124
Glucose (mmol/l)	4.7	3.0–5.5
Urea (mmol/l)	4.9	3.5–7.0
Creatinine (μmol/l)	61	0–130
Calcium (mmol/l)	2.36	2.3–3.0
Inorganic phosphate (mmol/l)	1.5	0.9–1.6
TP (g/l)	64	55–75
Albumin (g/l)	30	29–35
Globulin (g/l)	34	18–38
Albumin:globulin ratio	0.88	0.50–1.20
ALT (IU/l)	38	0–40
AST (IU/l)	37	0–45
ALP (IU/l)	189	0–135
GGT (IU/l)	5	0–14
GDH (IU/l)	3	0–9
CK (IU/l)	340	0–400
Amylase (IU/l)	598	400–2750
Lipase (IU/l)	319	0–500
Cholesterol (mmol/l)	4.6	3.8–7.9
Total bilirubin (μmol/l)	1.6	0–5.0
Total T4 (nmol/l)	52	13–52

What abnormalities are present?

- Mild normocytic, normochromic anaemia. No evidence of regeneration given absence of polychromasia
- Mild elevation in ALP
- Borderline total T4

How would you interpret these results?

- Mild non-regenerative anaemia can result from many chronic illnesses, bone marrow disease or may reflect pre-regeneration in cases of very recent haemorrhage or haemolysis.
- Mild elevation in ALP with no other evidence of hepatopathy is a common non-specific finding in cases of medical illness.

Has hypothyroidism been ruled out?

Hypothyroidism has not been ruled out by this single normal total T4 result. In particular, in this case, there is cause to be suspicious. In dogs with significant non-thyroidal illness a low or low normal T4 concentration would normally be expected. In this patient, there is some evidence in both haematology and clinical chemistry that a medical illness may be present. The presence of T4 cross-reacting anti-thyroglobulin antibodies (T4AA) causes false increases in reported total T4 concentrations. Such antibodies are observed in around 10% of hypothyroid dogs.

If not, what further tests would you recommend?

Measuring TSH would help identify primary hypothyroidism, and free T4 by equilibrium dialysis is free from interference by T4AA. Measuring thyroglobulin autoantibody (TgAA) (or direct measurement of T4AA) will help identify any potentially cross-reacting antibodies.

Further clinical pathology results

Endocrinology	Result	Reference interval
TSH (ng/ml)	2.79	<0.68
Free T4 by equilibrium dialysis (pmol/l)	<2.0	7–40
TgAA (%)	1026	<200
T4AA	3.5	<2.0

Note: TgAA is expressed as a percentage of the reading for negative control sera which are assigned a value of 100%. Greater than 200 is deemed abnormal. Similarly, T4AA is expressed relative to the measured activity of negative control sera which are assigned a value of 1, and >2 is deemed abnormal.

How would you interpret this further set of results?

- The combination of elevated TSH and low free T4 confirms primary hypothyroidism.
- The positive TgAA result confirms lymphocytic thyroiditis as the underlying pathology, and suggests T4AA was an interfering substance in the total T4 result: this is confirmed by the positive T4AA.

In this case, and in cases where the effect of T4AA is so great as to cause an above-reference-range-result, there is reason to be suspicious and continue with further thyroid testing but in many cases which have T4AA, the total T4 result is not clearly high. A minimum canine thyroid investigation, therefore, should include at least TSH (if not also TgAA) in addition to total T4.

Case 3 continues ▶

Case 3

Signalment

6-year old spayed female Dobermann Pinscher.

History

1–2 weeks of polydipsia and polyuria. Obesity over the last few years. A urine sample presented a few days prior to this visit was strongly positive for glucose.

Clinical pathology data

Haematology	Result	Reference interval
RBC (x 10^{12}/l)	5.08	5.4–8.5
Hb (g/dl)	11.9	12–18
HCT (l/l)	0.35	0.37–0.56
MCV (fl)	68.2	65–75
MCHC (g/dl)	34	31–35
WBC (x 10^9/l)	7.3	5–18
Neutrophils (x 10^9/l)	5.4	3.7–13.32
Neutrophils (band) (x 10^9/l)	0.00	0–0.54
Lymphocytes (x 10^9/l)	1.10	1.00–3.60
Monocytes (x 10^9/l)	0.15	0.20–0.72
Eosinophils (x 10^9/l)	0.66	0.10–1.25
Basophils (x 10^9/l)	0.00	0.05–0.18
Platelets (x 10^9/l)	279	200–900

Film comment

Platelets – numbers appear appropriate on the smear
Red cells – normocytic normochromic
White cells – no morphological abnormalities

Biochemistry	Result	Reference interval
Glucose (mmol/l)	22.3	3.0–5.5
Urea (mmol/l)	3.5	3.5–7.0
Creatinine (μmol/l)	106	0–130
Calcium (mmol/l)	2.53	2.3–3.0
Inorganic phosphate (mmol/l)	1.1	0.9–1.6
TP (g/l)	68	55–75
Albumin (g/l)	34	29–35
Globulin (g/l)	34	18–38
Albumin:globulin ratio	1.00	0.50–1.20
ALT (IU/l)	65	0–40
AST (IU/l)	26	0–45
ALP (IU/l)	215	0–135
GGT (IU/l)	18	0–14
GDH (IU/l)	20	0–9
CK (IU/l)	136	0–400
Amylase (IU/l)	428	400–2750
Lipase (IU/l)	489	0–500
Cholesterol (mmol/l)	10.4	3.8–7.9
Total bilirubin (μmol/l)	1.2	0–5.0

Endocrinology	Result	Reference interval
Total T4 (nmol/l)	<6	13–52
TSH (ng/ml)	0.09	<0.68
TgAA (%)	108	<200

What abnormalities are present?

- Mild normocytic normochromic anaemia. No evidence of regeneration given absence of polychromasia.
- Mild elevation in alkaline phosphatase, alanine aminotransferase, gammaglutamyl transferase and glutamate dehydrogenase.
- Moderately elevated cholesterol.
- Markedly elevated glucose.
- Subnormal thyroxine.

How would you interpret these results?

- The dominating result is the glucose concentration. As suspected from the urine result, a diagnosis of diabetes mellitus is confirmed. The haematology and clinical chemistry findings are all consistent with such a diagnosis.
- There is a subnormal total T4 but the TSH is normal. The negative TgAA rules out the presence of active immune-mediated thyroid pathology. It could be that this dog is one of the proportion of hypothyroid dogs in which an elevated TSH is not detected. This proportion is variably reported but may be as low as 13%. TgAA-negative cases account for only around half of this proportion, so this dog could be one of as few as 7% of hypothyroid dogs that could give this pattern of test results. A more likely explanation is that this dog has a low total T4 as a physiologic consequence of medical illness. In this case, where diabetes mellitus has been confirmed the chances of a low T4 state of medical illness is high.
- The hypercholesterolaemia in this case cannot be used to provide support for a diagnosis of hypothyroidism since it would also be expected because of the confirmed diabetes mellitus.

Is hypothyroidism confirmed? If not what further tests would you recommend?

No. To further elucidate whether hypothyroidism could be a contributing factor in this dog's obesity, it would be wise to wait until the non-thyroidal illness was controlled before repeating total T4 and TSH measurements. An alternative would be to measure free T4 by equilibrium dialysis as it is less commonly affected by the presence of non-thyroidal illness than is total T4.

Further clinical pathology results

After 4 weeks of insulin therapy a repeat sample was taken.

Endocrinology	Result	Reference interval
Total T4 (nmol/l)	28	13–52
TSH (ng/ml)	0.12	<0.68

How would you interpret these additional results?

Taken along with the previous negative TgAA result, hypothyroidism has been conclusively ruled out.

Case 4

Signalment

5-year old intact male Golden Retriever weighing 35 kg.

History

Hypothyroidism was confirmed 2 months ago. TgAA was negative at the time of diagnosis. Since that time the dog has been receiving 0.8 mg L-thyroxine once daily. The two owners disagree about whether there has been a clinical response to the medication.

Clinical pathology data

Endocrinology	Result	Reference interval
Total T4 (nmol/l)	32	13–52
TSH (ng/ml)	1.05	<0.68

How would you interpret the total T4 result?

- The total T4 result can be believed because this patient was recently shown to be TgAA-negative. It is very unlikely that TgAA (including T4 cross reacting subsets) would start to appear after diagnosis and the initiation of therapy.
- The total T4 value seems reasonable; it is well inside the reference range for normal dogs.

Would you interpret the total T4 result any differently with the information that the sample was obtained 4 hours post-pill?

At 4 hours post-pill, the peak T4 concentration has passed and values will continue to decline until the time of the next pill. The rate of decline will be equivalent to a half-life of 6–10 hours. The next pill is due in 20 hours. At a half-life of 6 hours, we can expect more than three half-lives to pass and can predict a trough concentration < 4 nmol/l (32, 16, 8, 4). Even with a half-life of 10 hours, the predicted trough concentration would be subnormal (8 nmol/l). Given the interval post-pill, this total T4 concentration may reflect inadequate therapy.

What is your overall interpretation of the results?

The TSH value is elevated, confirming continued physiological hypothyroidism. The TSH concentration takes days to change and therefore additionally confirms that therapy has been suboptimal for some time and not just on the day of the test. What initially appear to be conflicting therapeutic monitoring results are in fact supporting one another when combined with knowledge of the interval post-pill.

Case 5

Signalment

7 year-old female, neutered Domestic Shorthair cat.

History

Prolonged history of polyuria/polysipsia, more recent (3 days) history of anorexia and profound depression after returning from being missing for several days. On physical examination the cat was dehydrated, pale and had small bilateral palpable nodules in the cervical area.

Clinical pathology data

Haematology	Result	Reference interval
RBC (x 10^{12}/l)	9.00	5.5–10.0
HCT (l/l)	0.36	0.27–0.45
Hb (g/dl)	12.6	8.00–14.00
MCV (f/l)	40.2	39–55
MCHC (g/dl)	34.6	30.0–36.0
WBC (x 10^9/l)	11.8	8–20
Neutrophils (segmented) (x 10^9/l)	11.7	2.8–15.0
Lymphocytes (x 10^9/l)	0.10	1.8–11
Monocytes (x 10^9/l)	0.0	0.0–1.5
Eosinophils (x 10^9/l)	0.0	0.0–1.0
Basophils (x 10^9/l)	0.0	0.0–0.1
Platelets (x 10^9/l)	673	300–800

Biochemistry	Result	Reference interval
Sodium (mmol/l)	154	147–156
Potassium (mmol/l)	4.50	4.00–5.50
Glucose (mmol/l)	11.7	3.3–5.0
Urea (mmol/l)	119.8	6.6–10
Creatinine (μmol/l)	1704	40–170
Calcium (mmol/l)	2.38	2.00–3.00
Inorganic phosphate (mmol/l)	6.64	1.6–2.5
TP (g/l)	90.9	59.0–78.0
Albumin (g/l)	36.2	23.0–35.0
Globulin (g/l)	54.7	24.0–48.0
ALT (IU/l)	24	5–25
ALP (IU/l)	22	5–40
Amylase (μmol/l)	1554	< 730
Lipase (IU/L)	90	< 200

Urine specific gravity 1.012

Free T4 by equilibrium dialysis 75.54 pmol/l (reference interval 8.14–41.45)

What abnormalities are present?

- Eosinopenia and lymphopenia
- Hyperproteinaemia: elevated globulin and albumin
- Markedly elevated urea and creatinine
- Mildly elevated glucose
- Elevated phosphate
- Elevated amylase
- Isosthenuria
- Elevated free T4 concentration

Case 5 continues ▶

Case 5 continued

How would you interpret these results and what are the likely differential diagnoses?

- The haematology results of lymphopenia and eosinopenia are consistent with stress. Given the clinical dehydration, the relatively normal red cell parameters may be masking mild anaemia.
- The biochemical changes are dominated by marked azotaemia with hyposthenuria in the face of clinical dehydration, suggestive of severe renal failure. The elevated protein and amylase concentrations result from this.
- Mildly elevated plasma glucose is most likely due to stress, a common phenomenon in cats.
- The free T4 concentration is suggestive of hyperthyroidism, as is the finding of palpable nodules in the cervical area. However, free T4 analysis lacks specificity for diagnosing hyperthyroidism and can be inappropriately elevated in cats with non-thyroidal illness. Parathyroid enlargement can occur in renal failure and can result in palpable lesions in cats.

What further tests would you recommend?

Total T4 analysis is preferred for assessing thyroid function in cats as it is 100% specific and therefore unlikely to be elevated in cats with non-thyroidal illness. However, it can be decreased into the reference range in hyperthyroid cats by concurrent non-thyroidal disorders. The severity of the illness dictates the degree of suppression. In this cat, assessment of thyroid function is less of a concern because of the severity of renal failure. However, total T4 analysis would have been a better choice. A suppressed value is supportive of euthyroidism while a value of within the mid to high end of the reference range suggests concurrent hyperthyroidism. Without concurrent total T4 analysis, interpretation of a mildly elevated free T4 concentration cannot be made.

References

Archer FJ and Taylor SM (1996) Alkaline phosphatase bone isoenzyme and osteocalcin in the serum of hyperthyroid cats. *Canadian Veterinary Journal* **37,** 735–739

Avgeris S, Lothrop CD Jr and McDonald TP (1990) Plasma von Willebrand factor concentration and thyroid function in dogs. *Journal of the American Veterinary Medical Association* **196,** 921–924

Barber PJ and Elliott J (1996) Study of calcium homeostasis in feline hyperthyroidism. *Journal of Small Animal Practice* **37,** 575–582

Beale K and Torres S (1991) Thyroid pathology and serum antithyroglobulin antibodies in hypothyroid and healthy dogs. *Journal of Veterinary Internal Medicine* **5,** 128

Bezzola P (2002) Thyroid carcinoma and hyperthyroidism in a dog. *Canadian Veterinary Journal* **43,** 125–126

Bicer S, Nakayama T and Hamlin RL (2002) Effects of chronic oral amiodarone on left ventricular function, ECGs, serum chemistries, and exercise tolerance in healthy dogs. *Journal of Veterinary Internal Medicine* **16,** 247–254

Broussard JD and Peterson ME (1995) Changes in clinical and laboratory findings in cats with hyperthyroidism from 1983 to 1993. *Journal of the American Veterinary Medical Association* **206,** 302–305

Calvert CA, Jacobs GJ, Medleau L, Pickus CW, Brown J and McDermott M (1998) Thyroid-stimulating hormone stimulation tests in cardiomyopathic Doberman pinschers: a retrospective study. *Journal of Veterinary Internal Medicine* **12,** 343–348

Castillo VA, Lalia JC, Junco M, Sartorio G, Marquez A, Rodriguez MS and Pisarev MA (2001) Changes in thyroid function in puppies fed a high iodine commercial diet. *Veterinary Journal* **161,** 80–84

Daminet S, Croubels S, Duchateau L, Debunne A, van Geffen C, Hoybergs Y, van Bree H and de Rick A (2003) Influence of acetylsalicylic acid and ketoprofen on canine thyroid function tests. *The Veterinary Journal* **166,** 224–232

Daminet S and Ferguson DC (2003) Influence of drugs on thyroid function in dogs. *Journal of Veterinary Internal Medicine* **17,** 463–472

Dixon RM and Mooney CT (1999a) Canine serum thyroglobulin autoantibodies in health, hypothyroidism and non-thyroidal illness. *Research in Veterinary Science* **66,** 243

Dixon RM and Mooney CT (1999b) Evaluation of serum free thyroxine and thyrotropin concentrations in the diagnosis of canine hypothyroidism. *Journal Small Animal Practice* **40,** 72–78

Dixon RM, Reid SW and Mooney CT (1999) Epidemiological, clinical, haematological and biochemical characteristics of canine hypothyroidism. *Veterinary Record* **145,** 481–487

Dixon RM, Reid SW and Mooney CT (2002) Treatment and therapeutic monitoring of canine hypothyroidism. *Journal of Small Animal Practice* **43,** 334–340

Elliot DA, King LG, and Zerbe CA (1995) Thyroid hormone concentrations in critically ill intensive care patients. *The Journal of Veterinary Emergency and Critical Care* **5,** 17–23

Foster DJ and Thoday KL (2000) Tissue sources of serum alkaline phosphatase in 34 hyperthyroid cats: a qualitative and quantitative study. *Research in Veterinary Science* **68,** 89–94

Frank LA (1996) Comparison of thyrotropin-releasing hormone (TRH) to thyrotropin (TSH) stimulation for evaluating thyroid function in dogs. *Journal of the American Animal Hospital Association* **32,** 481–487

Fyfe JC, Kampschmidt K, Dang V, Poteet B, He Q, Lowrie C, Graham PA and Fetro VM (2003) Congenital hypothyroidism with goiter in toy fox terriers. *Journal of Veterinary Internal Medicine* **17,** 50–57

Gaughan KR and Bruyette DS (2001) Thyroid function testing in Greyhounds. *American Journal of Veterinary Research* **62,** 1130–1133

Gordon JM, Ehrhart EJ, Sisson DD and Jones MA (2003) Juvenile hyperthyroidism in a cat. *Journal of the American Animal Hospital Association* **39,** 67–71

Graham PA, Mooney CT and Murray M (1999) Serum fructosamine concentrations in hyperthyroid cats. *American Journal of Veterinary Research* **67,** 171–175

Graham PA, Nachreiner R, Refsal KR and Provencher-Bolliger AL (2001) Lymphocytic thyroiditis. *Veterinary Clinics of North America: Small Animal Practice* **31,** 915–933

Greco DS, Feldman EC, Peterson ME, Turner JL, Hodges CM and Shipman LW (1991) Congenital hypothyroid dwarfism in a family of giant schnauzers. *Journal of Veterinary Internal Medicine* **5,** 57–65

Gulikers KP and Panciera DL (2003) Evaluation of the effects of clomipramine on canine thyroid function tests. *Journal of Veterinary Internal Medicine* **17,** 44–49

Iversen L, Jensen AL, Hoier R *et al.* (1998) Development and validation of an improved enzyme-linked immunosorbent assay for the detection of thyroglobulin autoantibodies in canine serum samples. *Domestic Animal Endocrinology* **15,** 525

Kantrowitz LB, Peterson ME, Melian C and Nichols R (2001) Serum total thyroxine, total triiodothyronine, free thyroxine, and thyrotropin concentrations in dogs with nonthyroidal disease. *Journal of the American Veterinary Medical Association* **219,** 765–769

Lawrence D, Thompson J, Layton AW, Calderwood-Mays M, Ellison G and Mannella C (1991) Hyperthyroidism associated with a thyroid adenoma in a dog. *Journal of the American Veterinary Medical Association* **199,** 81–83

Lee JA, Hinchcliff KW, Piercy RJ, Schmidt KE and Nelson S (2004) Effects of racing and nontraining on plasma thyroid hormone concentrations in sled dogs. *Journal of the American Veterinary Medical Association* **224,** 226–231

Lurye JC, Behrend EN and Kemppainen RJ (2002) Evaluation of an in-house enzyme-linked immunosorbent assay for quantitative measurement of serum total thyroxine concentration in dogs and cats. *Journal of the American Veterinary Medical Association* **221,** 243–249

Mooney CT (2001) Feline hyperthyroidism: diagnostics and therapeutics. *Veterinary Clinics of North America: Small Animal Practice* **31,** 963–983

Mooney CT and Anderson TJ (1993) Congenital hypothyroidism in a boxer dog. *Journal of Small Animal Practice* **34,** 31–35

Mooney CT, Little CJ and Macrae AW (1996) Effect of illness not associated with the thyroid gland on serum total and free thyroxine concentrations in cats. *Journal of the American Veterinary Medical Association* **208,** 2004–2008

Mooney CT, Thoday KL and Doxey DL (1992) Carbimazole therapy of feline hyperthyroidism. *Journal of Small Animal Practice* **33,** 228–235

Nachreiner RF, Refsal KR, Graham PA, Hauptman J and Watson GL (1998) Prevalence of autoantibodies to thyroglobulin in dogs with nonthyroidal illness. *American Journal of Veterinary Research* **59,** 951–955

Nelson RW, Ihle SL, Feldman EC and Bottoms GD (1991) Serum free thyroxine concentration in healthy dogs, dogs with hypothyroidism, and euthyroid dogs with concurrent illness. *Journal of the American Veterinary Medical Association* **198,** 1401–1407

Nemzek JA, Kruger JM, Walshaw R and Hauptman JG (1994) Acute onset of hypokalaemia and muscular weakness in four hyperthyroid cats. *Journal of the American Veterinary Medical Association* **205,** 65–68

Panciera DL (1994a) Hypothyroidism in dogs: 66 cases (1987–1992). *Journal of the American Veterinary Medical Association* **204,** 761–767

Panciera DL (1994b) Thyroid function in dogs with spontaneous and induced congestive heart failure. *Canadian Journal of Veterinary Research* **58,** 157–162

Panciera DL and Johnson GS (1994) Plasma von Willebrand factor antigen concentration in dogs with hypothyroidism. *Journal of the American Veterinary Medical Association* **205,** 1550–1553

Panciera DL and Johnston SA (2002) Results of thyroid function tests and concentrations of plasma proteins in dogs administered etodolac. *American Journal of Veterinary Research* **63,** 1492–1495

Panciera DL, MacEwen EG, Atkins CE, Bosu WT, Refsal KR and Nachreiner RF (1990) Thyroid function tests in euthyroid dogs treated with L-thyroxine. *American Journal of Veterinary Research* **51,** 22–26

Panciera DL, Ritchey JW and Ward DL (2003) Endotoxin-induced nonthyroidal illness in dogs. *American Journal of Veterinary Research* **64,** 229–234

Paradis M, Sauve F, Charest J, Refsal KR, Moreau M and Dupuis J (2003) Effects of moderate to severe osteoarthritis on canine thyroid function. *Canadian Veterinary Journal* **44,** 407–412

Peterson ME, DeMarco CL and Sheldon KM (2003) Total thyroxine testing: comparison of an in-house test kit with radioimmuno- and chemiluminescent assays. *Journal of Veterinary Internal Medicine* **17,** 396

Peterson ME, Graves TK and Cavanagh I (1987) Serum thyroid hormone concentrations fluctuate in cats with hyperthyroidism. *Journal of Veterinary Internal Medicine* **1,** 142–146

Peterson ME, Kintzer PP, Cavanagh PG, Fox PR, Ferguson DC, Johnson GF and Becker DV (1983) Feline hyperthyroidism: pretreatment clinical and laboratory evaluation of 131 cases. *Journal of the American Veterinary Medical Association* **183,** 103–110

Peterson ME, Kintzer PP and Hurvitz AI (1988) Methimazole treatment of 262 cats with hyperthyroidism. *Journal of Veterinary Internal Medicine* **2,** 150–157

Peterson ME, Melian C and Nichols R (1997) Measurement of serum total thyroxine, triiodothyronine, free thyroxine, and thyrotropin concentrations for diagnosis of hypothyroidism in dogs. *Journal of the American Veterinary Medical Association* **211,** 1396–1402

Peterson ME, Melian C and Nichols R (2001) Measurement of serum concentrations of free thyroxine, total thyroxine, and total triiodothyronine in cats with hyperthyroidism and cats with nonthyroidal disease. *Journal of the American Veterinary Medical Association* **218,** 529–536

Rand JS, Levine J, Best SJ and Parker W (1993) Spontaneous adult-onset hypothyroidism in a cat. *Journal of Veterinary Internal Medicine* **7,** 272–276

Reusch CE and Tomsa K (1999) Serum fructosamine concentration in cats with overt hyperthyroidism. *Journal of the American Veterinary Medical Association* **215,** 1297–1300

Robinson WF, Shaw SE, Stanley B and Wyburn RS (1988) Congenital hypothyroidism in Scottish Deerhound puppies. *Australian Veterinary Journal* **65,** 386–389

Sauve F and Paradis M (2000) Use of recombinant human thyroid-stimulating hormone for thyrotropin stimulation test in euthyroid dogs. *Canadian Veterinary Journal* **41,** 215–219

Sauve F, Paradis M, Refsal KR, Moreau M, Beauchamp G and Dupuis J (2003) Effects of oral administration of meloxicam, carprofen, and a nutraceutical on thyroid function in dogs with osteoarthritis. *Canadian Veterinary Journal* **44,** 474–479

Scott-Moncrieff JC, Nelson RW, Bruner JM and Williams DA (1998) Comparison of serum concentrations of thyroid-stimulating hormone in healthy dogs, hypothyroid dogs, and euthyroid dogs with concurrent disease. *Journal of the American Veterinary Medical Association* **212,** 387–391

Sjollema BE, den Hartog MT, de Vijlder JJ, van Dijk JE and Rijnberk A (1991) Congenital hypothyroidism in two cats due to defective organification: data suggesting loosely anchored thyroperoxidase. *Acta Endocrinology (Copenhagen)* **125,** 435–440

Stegeman JR, Graham PA and Hauptman JG (2003) Use of recombinant human thyroid-stimulating hormone for thyrotropin-stimulation testing of euthyroid cats. *American Journal of Veterinary Research* **64,** 149–152

Tanase H, Kudo K, Horikoshi H, Mizushima H, Okazaki T and Ogata E (1991) Inherited primary hypothyroidism with thyrotrophin resistance in Japanese cats. *Journal of Endocrinology* **129,** 245–251

Thoday KL and Mooney CT (1992) Historical, clinical and laboratory features of 126 hyperthyroid cats. *Veterinary Record* **131,** 257–264

Tomsa K, Glaus TM, Kacl GM, Pospischil A and Reusch CE (2001) Thyrotropin-releasing hormone stimulation test to assess thyroid function in severely sick cats. *Journal of Veterinary Internal Medicine* **15,** 89–93

Torres SMF, Feeney DA, Lekcharoensuk C, Fletcher TF, Clarkson CE, Nash NL and Hayden DW (2003) Comparison of colloid, thyroid follicular epithelium, and thyroid hormone concentrations in healthy and severely sick dogs. *Journal of the American Veterinary Medical Association* **222,** 1079–1085

Williamson NL, Frank LA and Hnilica KA (2002) Effects of short-term trimethoprim-sulfamethoxazole administration on thyroid function in dogs. *Journal of the American Veterinary Medical Association* **221,** 802–806

18

Laboratory diagnosis of adrenal diseases

Ian Ramsey and Michael Herrtage

Introduction

Each adrenal gland is composed of a cortex and a medulla, which are embryologically and functionally separate endocrine glands. The cortex is essential for life, but the medulla is not. The most common disorders affect the adrenal cortex and cause either hyperadrenocorticism (HAC) or hypoadrenocorticism. Conditions affecting the adrenal medulla are rare, the most common being neoplasia (phaeochromocytoma).

The adrenal cortex produces about 30 different hormones, many of which have little or no clinical significance. The hormones can be divided into three groups based on their predominant actions:

- Mineralocorticoids are responsible for electrolyte and water homeostasis. Aldosterone, the most important, is produced by the zona glomerulosa
- Glucocorticoids promote gluconeogenesis, lipolysis and protein catabolism. They also antagonize the effect of insulin and are anti-inflammatory and immunosuppressive. Cortisol, the most important, is produced in the zonas fasciculata and reticularis
- Sex hormones, particularly male hormones that have weak androgenic activity, are produced in small quantities in the zonas fasciculata and reticularis.

Adrenal steroid synthesis and release

Glucocorticoid release is controlled almost entirely by adrenocorticotropic hormone (ACTH) secreted by the anterior pituitary, which, in turn, is regulated by corticotropin releasing hormone (CRH) from the hypothalamus (Figure 18.1). ACTH causes cortisol release from the adrenal cortex, with serum concentrations rising almost immediately. Cortisol has direct negative feedback effects on:

- The hypothalamus to decrease formation of CRH
- The anterior pituitary gland to decrease formation of ACTH.

There is probably an internal or 'short loop' negative feedback control by ACTH on CRH. These feedback mechanisms help to regulate the plasma concentration of cortisol.

The principal mineralocorticoid released by the adrenal cortex is aldosterone. The secretion of aldosterone is mainly regulated by the renin–angiotensin system and the serum potassium concentration. ACTH only has a permissive effect on its secretion at physiological doses (Figure 18.2). Pharmacological doses of ACTH will, however, induce the secretion of aldosterone, e.g. in performing an ACTH stimulation test. Aldosterone primarily acts on the proximal convoluted tubule to increase sodium reabsorption and on the distal convoluted tubule to increase sodium

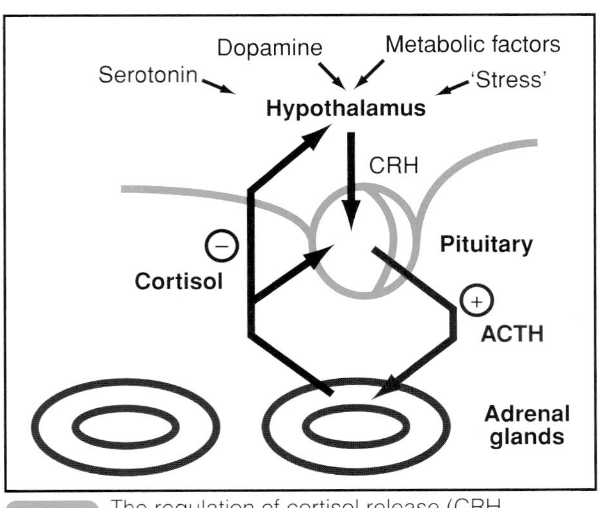

18.1 The regulation of cortisol release (CRH, corticotropin releasing hormone).

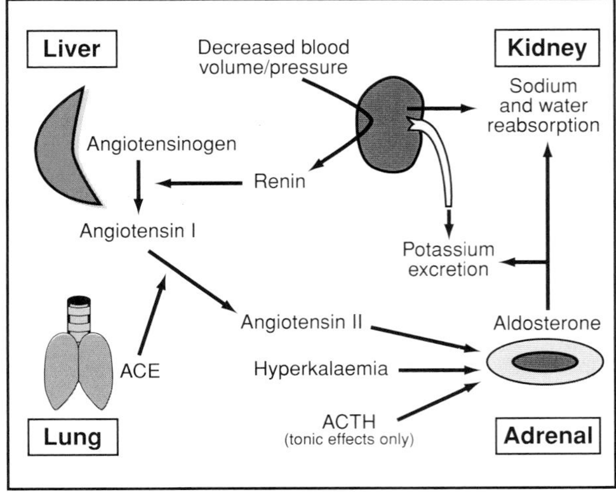

18.2 The regulation of aldosterone release (ACE, angiotensin converting enzyme).

reabsorption in exchange for potassium ions. Osmotic forces ensure that this results in an increase in water retention.

Further details on adrenal steroid synthesis and regulation of their release can be found in the *BSAVA Manual of Endocrinology*.

Canine hyperadrenocorticism

Hyperadrenocorticism (HAC), results from a chronic excess of glucocorticoid secretion. The disease has two spontaneous forms and may also be produced iatrogenically by the administration of steroids. The most common cause of spontaneous HAC is the overproduction of ACTH by a small benign pituitary microadenoma (pituitary-dependent HAC (PD-HAC) or Cushing's disease). Excessive secretion of ACTH results in bilateral adrenocortical hyperplasia and overproduction of cortisol and its precursors. Other causes of PD-HAC include larger tumours (macroadenomas) and diffuse hyperplasia of the ACTH-secreting cells (corticotrophs). PD-HAC accounts for about 85% of all spontaneous canine HAC. Macroadenomas are seen in about 10% of these cases. Rarely, pituitary adenocarcinoma has been documented. The incidence of pituitary corticotroph hyperplasia is debated in the literature.

Adrenal-dependent HAC (AD-HAC) results from the overproduction of cortisol by an adrenal tumour. Adrenal tumours may show a range of biological (including metastatic) behaviour and the neoplastic cells release variable amounts of cortisol (and other precursor steroids). Approximately half these tumours are malignant. The release of cortisol from the tumour may, or may not, be influenced by ACTH. Moreover, the extent of the effect of ACTH is variable. Therefore adrenal tumours do not behave predictably in any endocrine test. The contralateral adrenal gland is usually atrophic.

The clinical signs of HAC are summarized in Figure 18.3. Signs of AD-HAC are indistinguishable from those of PD-HAC (Reusch and Feldman, 1991). AD-HAC is more common in larger breeds than PD-HAC, and is more common in bitches (about 70% of cases are in females).

HAC is much less common in the cat than in the dog. Although fewer studies have been published in the cat, it appears that PD-HAC accounts for a similar proportion of HAC cases to those seen in dogs (Nelson *et al.*, 1988; Watson and Herrtage, 1998). The clinical and clinicopathological findings of feline HAC are described later in this chapter.

Iatrogenic HAC may be produced by the administration of glucocorticoids. It is fairly common in the dog but relatively rare in the cat. Clinical and clinicopathological presentations are similar to spontaneous HAC but the results of specific endocrine tests are different. The differences observed depend on the dose and type of glucocorticoid administered. Obtaining a reliable history can prevent expensive and unnecessary testing.

Common signs of hyperadrenocorticism
Polydipsia, polyuria, polyphagia
Lethargy
Dermatological changes: • Symmetrical alopecia, poor hair regrowth, comedones, skin thinning • Hyperfragile skin (in cats)
Abdominal distension ('pot belly')
Excessive panting
Muscle weakness
Anoestrus and genital atrophy
Uncommon signs of hyperadrenocorticism
Dermatological changes: • Coat colour changes, hyperpigmentation, calcinosis cutis • Excessive bruising and poor wound healing
Stiff hindlimb gait (due to pseudomyotonia)
Dyspnoea (due to pulmonary thromboembolism)
Neurological signs (due to rapid tumour growth): • Ataxia, depression, apparent blindness, inappetance, aimless walking, seizures, alteration in normal behaviour patterns

18.3 Clinical signs of canine hyperadrenocorticism. It is important to employ specific endocrine tests only in animals that have appropriate clinical signs.

Investigation of hyperadrenocorticism

The process of investigating and confirming canine HAC is summarized in Figure 18.4. Before performing any laboratory tests for HAC it is important to obtain an accurate history and perform a thorough clinical examination. Hyperadrenocorticism is a chronic disease and many of the changes develop slowly and so are missed by the owners. Clinical signs (Figure 18.3) vary considerably between individual animals and a few cases may only show one or two signs.

Full blood and urine profiles are carried out to:

- Identify any non-specific indicators of the disease
- Exclude other causes of polyuria/polydipsia, polyphagia, etc.
- Identify intercurrent disease that might affect subsequent therapy.

The more common laboratory changes that are seen in canine HAC are summarized in Figure 18.5 and below.

Blood profiles

Alkaline phosphatase (ALP): Serum ALP concentrations are increased in over 90% of cases of canine HAC. The increase is commonly 5–40 times the upper end of the reference range, and this is perhaps the most sensitive biochemical indicator of HAC. Glucocorticoids, both endogenous and exogenous, induce a specific isoenzyme of ALP that is unique to the dog. However, increases in serum ALP occur in many other conditions and a normal serum ALP concentration does not exclude a diagnosis of HAC.

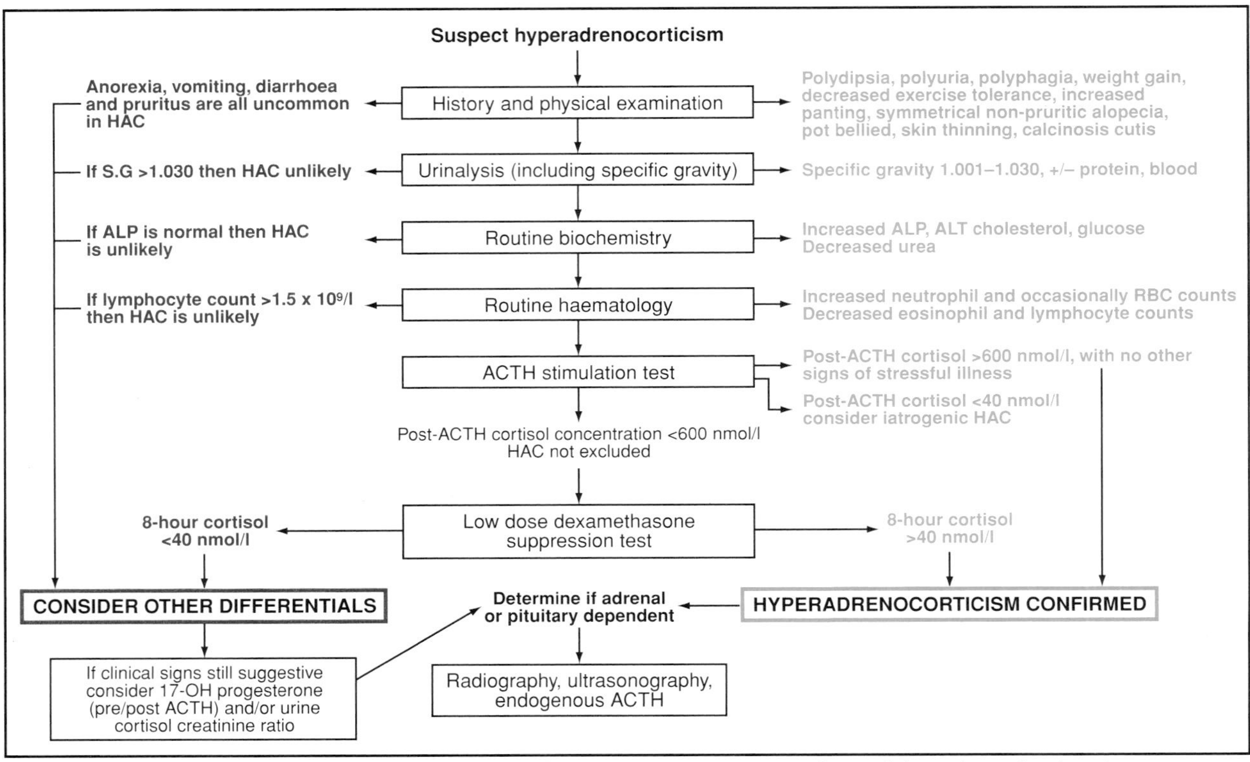
Suspect hyperadrenocorticism
History and physical examination
Anorexia, vomiting, diarrhoea and pruritus are all uncommon in HAC
Polydipsia, polyuria, polyphagia, weight gain, decreased exercise tolerance, increased panting, symmetrical non-pruritic alopecia, pot bellied, skin thinning, calcinosis cutis
Urinalysis (including specific gravity)
If S.G >1.030 then HAC unlikely
Specific gravity 1.001–1.030, +/– protein, blood
Routine biochemistry
If ALP is normal then HAC is unlikely
Increased ALP, ALT cholesterol, glucose
Decreased urea
Routine haematology
If lymphocyte count >1.5 x 10⁹/l then HAC is unlikely
Increased neutrophil and occasionally RBC counts
Decreased eosinophil and lymphocyte counts
ACTH stimulation test
Post-ACTH cortisol >600 nmol/l, with no other signs of stressful illness
Post-ACTH cortisol <40 nmol/l consider iatrogenic HAC
Post-ACTH cortisol concentration <600 nmol/l HAC not excluded
Low dose dexamethasone suppression test
8-hour cortisol <40 nmol/l
8-hour cortisol >40 nmol/l
CONSIDER OTHER DIFFERENTIALS
HYPERADRENOCORTICISM CONFIRMED
Determine if adrenal or pituitary dependent
If clinical signs still suggestive consider 17-OH progesterone (pre/post ACTH) and/or urine cortisol creatinine ratio
Radiography, ultrasonography, endogenous ACTH

18.4 Summary of the investigation of canine HAC. It is not necessary to perform all these investigations in every case. Text in green refers to typical features of HAC; text in red refers to uncommon findings.

Haematology
Increased total WBC Neutrophilia Eosinopenia Lymphopenia Monocytosis
Biochemistry
Increased ALP – high proportion of dogs but only 30% of cats Increased ALT Hypercholesterolaemia Hyperglycaemia – more pronounced in cats (overt diabetes mellitus is common) Decreased circulating total T4
Urinalysis
Specific gravity is generally low (<1.015), sometimes isosthenuric or hyposthenuric Proteinuria Glucosuria common in cats, less so in dogs Urinary tract infections (blood, protein, pH changes, active sediment, occult UTI)

18.5 Summary of changes seen on routine haematology, biochemistry and urinalysis in HAC in approximate order of frequency.

The steroid-induced alkaline phosphatase (SIALP) can be quantified (see Chapter 12) and initial studies suggested that SIALP measurement provided an accurate differentiation of the causes of increased ALP. However subsequent studies have concluded that, while measurement of SIALP is quite sensitive, it is not specific for spontaneous canine HAC: SIALP can be increased in primary hepatopathies, diabetes mellitus and with anticonvulsant and exogenous glucocorticoid therapy (Teske *et al.*, 1989).

Alanine aminotransferase (ALT): ALT is commonly mildly elevated in HAC, as a result of hepatocyte damage due to glycogen accumulation. Increases of more than five times the upper limit of the reference range warrant further investigation as they may affect subsequent therapy.

Bile acid concentrations: Resting and postprandial serum bile acid concentrations may show a mild to moderate elevation (up to 60 μmol/l pre- and postprandially) in some cases of HAC, due to steroid hepatopathy. When abnormal results are obtained, HAC is best differentiated from primary liver disorders by the clinical history, physical examination and diagnostic imaging.

Glucose: Glucose concentration is usually in the high normal range. About 10% of cases develop overt diabetes mellitus, which is caused by antagonism to the action of insulin by the gluconeogenic effects of excess glucocorticoids. Initially serum insulin concentrations increase to maintain normoglycaemia, but eventually the pancreatic islet cells become exhausted giving rise to overt diabetes mellitus.

Urea and creatinine: Creatinine concentration usually tends to be in the low to normal range. This may reflect loss of muscle mass as well as the effects of glucocorticoid-induced polyuria. Urea is variable: increased protein catabolism and glucocorticoid-induced diuresis are conflicting factors and blood urea may be normal, increased or decreased.

Cholesterol and lipaemia: Cholesterol and triglyceride concentrations are usually increased due to glucocorticoid stimulation of lipolysis. Cholesterol is usually >8 mmol/l but is also raised in hypothyroidism, diabetes mellitus, chronic pancreatitis, cholestatic liver disease and protein-losing nephropathy, all of which may be differential diagnoses. Elevated triglyceride and consequent lipaemia can also occur, although less frequently than elevated cholesterol.

Electrolytes: Sodium, potassium and calcium concentrations are usually in the reference range. Phosphate is often increased when compared with age-matched controls (Tebb *et al.*, 2003a). This probably reflects the increased bone metabolism in dogs with HAC.

Urinalysis

Urine specific gravity: Urine specific gravity (SG) is usually <1.015, and is often hyposthenuric (<1.008) provided water has not been withheld. This is due to antagonism of antidiuretic hormone (ADH) leading to a secondary nephrogenic diabetes insipidus. Dogs with HAC can usually concentrate their urine if deprived of water, but their concentrating ability is frequently reduced. However, in some cases of PD-HAC due to a macroadenoma, compression of the posterior lobe of the pituitary and extension into the hypothalamus may cause disruption of ADH production and release. This will result in signs of central diabetes insipidus (see Chapter 10). Confirmation of this diagnosis using a water deprivation test can only be made after the HAC has been controlled.

Urinary tract infection: Urine (collected by cystocentesis) should be cultured, because urinary tract infections occur in about 50% of cases of HAC. Urinary tract infection occurs because voiding is never complete due to muscle weakness. Immunosuppression may also play a role. There is often little evidence of inflammatory cells in the sediment of the urine and, indeed, there are often few clinical signs of urinary tract infection, due to the immunosuppressive action of excess glucocorticoids. Lower urinary tract infections can ascend to the kidneys to cause pyelonephritis.

Urine protein: Up to 45% of dogs with untreated HAC may have proteinuria, defined as a urine protein: creatinine ratio (UPCR) >1.0, in the absence of urinary tract infection (Hurley and Vaden, 1998). Proteinuria is usually mild (UPCR <5.0), but can be severe (>10.0), and may be associated with systemic hypertension. Despite the severity of proteinuria in some cases, HAC has not been shown to produce nephrotic syndrome or hypoalbuminaemia.

Urine glucose: Glucosuria occurs in 10% of dogs with HAC: these represent cases with overt diabetes mellitus.

Standard endocrine tests

Specific endocrine tests should only be undertaken in animals with clinical evidence of HAC. Indiscriminate testing alters diagnostic efficiency and makes accurate interpretation difficult (Kaplan *et al.*, 1995).

Basal cortisol measurements are of no value in the diagnosis of hyperadrenocorticism, as normal dogs, those with HAC and those stressed by another illness have cortisol concentrations that fluctuate widely and overlap to a considerable extent.

There are two long-established tests used for the diagnosis of canine HAC; the ACTH stimulation test and the low dose dexamethasone suppression test (LDDST). The test chosen depends on individual owner, dog and veterinary factors, including time constraints, cost, personal preference and the particular form of HAC that is suspected.

About 80% of all dogs with hyperadrenocorticism are positive on the ACTH stimulation test, and 90–95% are positive on the LDDST. The sensitivity of ACTH stimulation testing in the diagnosis of adrenal dependent disease is much lower (as low as 60%). Some dogs with functional adrenal tumours can give normal results on both tests (Norman *et al.*, 1999). It should be noted that the reported sensitivity and specificity, and positive and negative predictive values for these two tests vary with the population sampled. For example, if dogs with clinical presentations not suggestive of hyperadrenocorticism and final diagnoses of non-adrenal illnesses are examined then 14% are (falsely) positive on ACTH stimulation and 56% are (falsely) positive on low dose dexamethasone suppression testing (Kaplan *et al.*, 1995). False positive results may be seen, for example with diabetes mellitus, renal failure or pyometra. However, this group of dogs is not normally tested for hyperadrenocorticism. (See Chapters 2 and 26 for discussions of sensitivity, specificity and positive and negative predictive values.)

Some cases of HAC are presented with highly suggestive clinical signs but diagnostic tests prove equivocal or negative. In these circumstances it is sensible to check for other endocrine diseases (particularly hypothyroidism) and then to repeat the tests. If this approach is unsuccessful at determining the cause of the dog's presenting signs then two other tests for HAC, the 17-hydroxyprogesterone (17-OHP) test and the urine corticoid:creatinine ratio, are sometimes useful. Neither test is a replacement for the ACTH stimulation test or LDDST.

ACTH stimulation test: The test method is described in Figure 18.6.

Cortisol is stable for many weeks at 4°C. Cortisol is measured using radioimmunoassays, and immunoradiometric assays are considered the most reliable. Interpretation is summarized in Figure 18.7. In normal dogs, pre-ACTH cortisol concentrations are usually

1. 2 ml blood sample obtained in a heparin or plain tube.
2. Synthetic ACTH administered intravenously (preferably) or intramuscularly (painful). Dose is 250 µg in dogs >5 kg or 125µg in dogs < 5 kg.
3. Obtain another 2 ml blood sample 30–90 minutes (if ACTH given intravenously) or 1–2 hours (if ACTH given intramuscularly) later.

Serum or plasma should be separated before transport to laboratory.

18.6 The ACTH stimulation test.

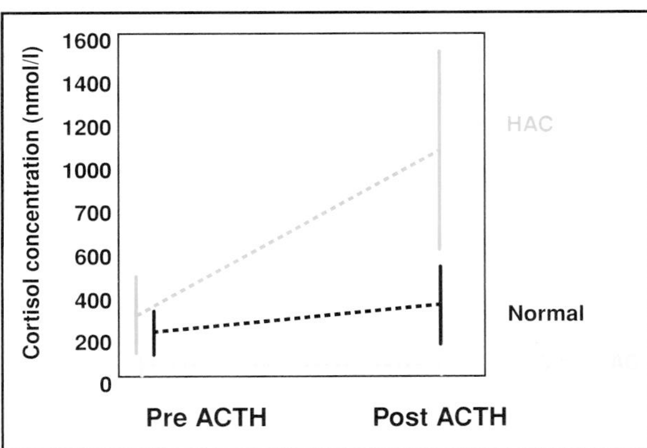

18.7 Interpretation of the ACTH stimulation test. Normal dogs show a 2–3-fold increase in cortisol concentrations but these remain <450 nmol/l. Most dogs with HAC have post-ACTH cortisol concentrations >600 nmol/l. False positive results occur with 'stressful' illnesses, such as unstable diabetes mellitus. The expected results in cases of iatrogenic HAC (iHAC) and hypoadrenocorticism (hAC) are also shown.

between 20 and 250 nmol/l and post-ACTH cortisol concentrations are between 200 to 450 nmol/l. Regardless of the pre-ACTH cortisol value, a diagnosis of HAC is confirmed by a post-ACTH cortisol concentration >600 nmol/l in dogs with compatible clinical signs and no evidence of acute stressful illnesses. Values between 450 and 600 nmol/l should be regarded as indicative of an abnormal adrenal cortex but the cause (HAC or stress) cannot be determined. Post-ACTH cortisol concentrations <40 nmol/l in dogs with obvious clinical signs of hyperadrenocorticism are consistent with the diagnosis of iatrogenic hyperadrenocorticism.

When interpreting ACTH stimulation tests it is important to remember that other steroids will be detected in the cortisol assay. The degree of cross reactivity between cortisol and pharmaceutical steroids varies: for example, prednisolone cross reacts about 30% whereas dexamethasone does not cross react. Prednisolone can be detected by a cortisol assay for up to 24 hours after administration.

Advantages of the ACTH stimulation test include:

- Simple, quick and specific
- Best screening test for distinguishing spontaneous from iatrogenic HAC
- Provides baseline information for monitoring mitotane and trilostane therapy (see below).

Disadvantages of the ACTH stimulation test include:

- Minimal value in differentiating pituitary from adrenal HAC
- False negative results (i.e. a normal response) may occur, especially in AD-HAC
- False positive results (i.e. an exaggerated response) may occur with chronic stress due to non-adrenal illness. The highest post-ACTH cortisol concentration recorded in one series of 59 dogs with non-adrenal illnesses was about 850 nmol/l (although 95% of the dogs had values <600 nmol/l) (Kaplan *et al.*, 1995).

Low dose dexamethasone suppression test: The method for the LDDST is described in Figure 18.8.

The expected results of LDDSTs are shown in Figure 18.9. Interpretation must be based on the laboratory's reference range. As a guide, normal dogs show >50% suppression of cortisol concentrations at 3 hours and suppress to <30 nmol/l at 8 hours. If the dose of dexamethasone fails to suppress circulating cortisol concentrations adequately (i.e. the 8-hour cortisol is >40 nmol/l) in a dog with compatible clinical signs, a diagnosis of HAC is confirmed.

1. Obtain a 2 ml blood sample in a plain or heparin tube early in the morning.
2. Inject 0.015 mg/kg dexamethasone i.v.
3. Collect blood samples 3–4 hours and 8 hours after administration of dexamethasone.
4. Serum or plasma should be separated before transport to laboratory.

The basal and 8-hour post-dexamethasone samples are the most important for interpretation of the test. The intermediate sample is not essential but may be useful in some cases.

18.8 The low dose dexamethasone suppression test.

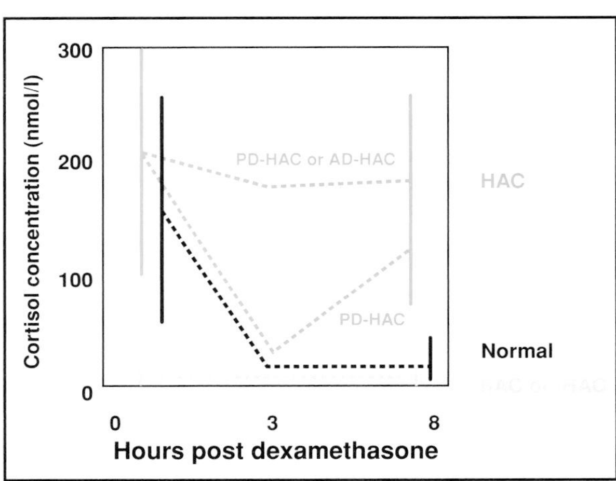

18.9 Interpretation of the low dose dexamethasone suppression test. Normal dogs show >50% suppression of cortisol concentrations at 3 hours with values <30 nmol/l at 8 hours. Dogs with HAC show little or no suppression at 8 hours. Cases with PD-HAC may show an initial suppression at 3 hours. The effects of iatrogenic HAC (iHAC) and hypoadrenocorticism (hAC) are also shown.

If the 3–4 hour sample is suppressed normally or near-normally (to <40 mmol/l), while the 8-hour sample shows escape from suppression (i.e. is >40 nmol/l), then a diagnosis of PD-HAC can be made (Peterson, 1984). A failure to suppress plasma cortisol at both 3–4 hours and 8 hours is not helpful in determining the cause of the HAC (i.e. it could be pituitary or adrenal dependent).

Some cases show a pattern of low cortisol production that is not suppressed throughout the test. This abnormal pattern should prompt further investigation for an adrenal tumour, as some adrenal tumours may principally release cortisol precursors.

Advantages of the LDDST include:

- More sensitive than the ACTH stimulation test in confirming HAC
- May confirm the diagnosis of PD-HAC.

Disadvantages of the LDDST include:

- Not as specific as the ACTH stimulation test, i.e. it is more likely to produce false positives, especially if it is performed in a stressful environment. In chronically ill animals that do not have hyperadrenocorticism it can be (falsely) positive in up to 56% of cases
- Takes longer to perform than ACTH stimulation
- Does not provide pre-treatment information that may be used in monitoring the effects of therapy.

Additional tests for atypical HAC

Some cases of HAC have classical clinical signs and changes on routine haematology and biochemistry but equivocal results on the specific endocrine tests described above; these are termed atypical HAC. If, on repetition of the standard tests outlined above, the results remain inconclusive and the clinical signs persist, then further tests for atypical forms of HAC can be undertaken. It is often best to perform both of the tests outlined below to obtain as much evidence as possible.

Urinary corticoid:creatinine ratio: Cortisol and its metabolites (corticoids) are excreted in urine. By measuring urine corticoids in the morning sample, the concentration will reflect cortisol release over several hours, thereby adjusting for fluctuations in plasma cortisol concentrations. Urine corticoid concentration increases with increased plasma cortisol concentration. Relating the urine corticoid concentration to urine creatinine concentration provides a correction for any differences in urine concentration. Evaluation of urinary corticoid:creatinine ratio (UCCR), rather than the more laborious 24-hour urinary corticoid excretion, has been shown to be a simple and valuable screening test (Rijnberk *et al.*, 1988). However, urine corticoids may not always reflect plasma cortisol concentrations. Rate of cortisol breakdown can be influenced by other factors (e.g. hepatic disease, drug administration).

The owner should obtain a urine sample at home every morning for 3 days and then these samples can either analysed separately (preferred) or 1 ml aliquots can be mixed together before analysis (cheaper). Urine samples obtained in a clinical environment are unsuitable as the stress of being taken to the clinic is sufficient to increase the urine cortisol to levels that are suggestive of HAC (Vonderen *et al.*, 1998). A single sample obtained at home is also unsuitable.

The UCCR is calculated as:

$$\frac{\text{urine cortisol concentration } (\mu\text{mol/l})}{\text{urine creatinine concentration } (\mu\text{mol/l})}.$$

It may be necessary to convert values in other units:

- Cortisol μg/dl x 27.59 = Cortisol nmol/l
- Cortisol nmol/l / 1000 = Cortisol μmol/l
- Creatinine mmol/l x 1000 = Creatinine μmol/l.

As a guide, the reference ratio for normal dogs is $<10 \times 10^{-6}$ (Stolp *et al.*, 1983). The ratio is increased in dogs with HAC but also in many dogs with non-adrenal illness (Smiley and Peterson, 1993). Therefore this test is not very specific, but is useful for screening for HAC since it is highly sensitive. Values in the reference range make a diagnosis of HAC highly unlikely and the test is best used to exclude the diagnosis of HAC. The test cannot reliably differentiate PD- from AD-HAC unless the ratio exceeds 100×10^{-6}, when it becomes very likely that the dog is suffering from PD-HAC (Galac *et al.*, 1997). It is of little value in monitoring the response to mitotane therapy in dogs with HAC.

ACTH stimulation of 17-hydroxyprogesterone: Recently, the measurement of 17-OHP before and after ACTH stimulation has been shown to be useful in helping to confirm the diagnosis of atypical HAC (Ristic *et al.*, 2002). In atypical HAC there may be a derangement of the steroid production pathway and some of the precursors of cortisol, such as 17-OHP, may be abnormally increased. Both pituitary-dependent and adrenal-dependent atypical HAC cases have been reported (Norman *et al.*, 1999; Ristic *et al.*, 2002).

The method is identical to that described above for the standard ACTH stimulation test and thus measurements of 17-OHP can be made on the same samples after cortisol concentrations have been measured. 17-OHP concentrations are stable in plasma at 4°C for several weeks.

Figure 18.10 summarizes the interpretation. In normal dogs, post-ACTH 17-OHP concentrations are mostly between 1.0 and 8.0 nmol/l. In dogs with classical and atypical hyperadrenocorticism plasma 17-OHP concentrations show an exaggerated response to ACTH stimulation with concentrations increasing to between 6.5 and 38 nmol/l after stimulation (Ristic *et al.*, 2002). There is a degree of overlap between normal and affected animals and there is some controversy over the cut off value for the diagnosis of HAC. A recent study suggested a post-ACTH stimulation 17-OHP concentration of

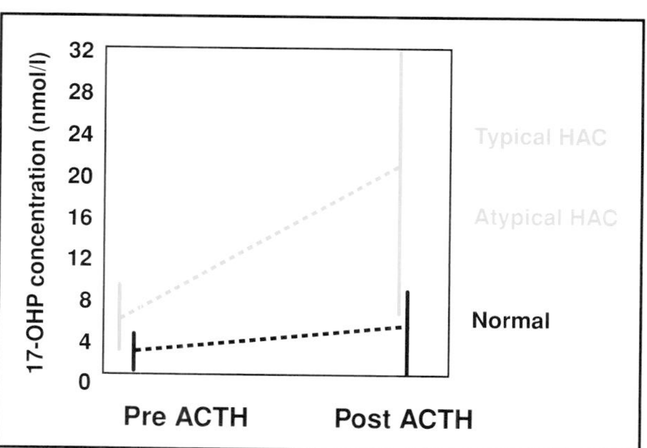

18.10 Interpretation of 17-hydroxyprogesterone assay. Normal dogs show a 2–3-fold increase in 17-OHP concentrations but these remain <10 nmol/l. Most dogs with typical or atypical HAC have post-ACTH 17-OHP concentrations >8 nmol/l. False positive results may occur with 'stressful' illnesses, such as unstable diabetes mellitus, neoplasia and liver disease. False negatives can also occur but are uncommon.

>8.5 nmol/l could be used as a cut off with a sensitivity and specificity of about 70%; but a few normal dogs may have post-ACTH 17-OHP concentrations as high as 17 nmol/l and dogs with 'stressful' diseases may be as high as 38 nmol/l (Chapman *et al.*, 2003).

The test is best used to identify confirmatory evidence of abnormalities of steroid metabolism in animals with considerable clinical evidence of such abnormalities. The test should not be used to distinguish between diseased and healthy animals.

Distinguishing pituitary- and adrenal-dependent HAC

Distinguishing the two major forms of HAC is useful in the management and essential for prognosis of the condition, though it is not necessary to make the distinction in all cases. Both endocrine tests and adrenal ultrasonography are used. The best endocrinological test is the endogenous ACTH assay, although the low dose dexamethasone and high dose dexamethasone tests may contribute. It is usually assumed that if an adrenal tumour is not detected the disease is pituitary in origin. It is only necessary to confirm the presence and size of a suspected pituitary tumour in dogs with HAC and neurological signs. Magnetic resonance imaging is the best method for examining the pituitary gland. In its absence, high resolution computed tomography (HRCT) is an acceptable alternative.

Sometimes conflicting results are obtained, such as low ACTH concentrations with evidence of mild bilateral adrenomegaly. In these cases the only solution is repeating some or all of the tests. In rare cases pituitary and adrenal tumours have been found in the same animal. This situation is identified after in-depth investigations of animals that have conflicting results from the investigations outlined in this section or after failure of conventional therapy.

Endogenous ACTH: Endogenous ACTH concentration is usually high or normal in PD-HAC (>25 pg/ml), but low in AD-HAC (<5 pg/ml). Equivocal results (5–25 pg/ml) are sometimes seen. The assay should be repeated in these circumstances, as some of these results are due to poor sample handling (see below). On rare occasions low ACTH values (<5 pg/ml) have been recorded in PDH cases but high ACTH values have never been recorded in adrenal tumours. The assay is therefore less specific for the diagnosis of adrenal-dependent disease than for pituitary-dependent disease. The test is easy to perform but is less accurate than ultrasonography when performed by an experienced operator in the exclusion of adrenal tumours (Gould *et* al., 2001).

Endogenous ACTH is measured (by radio-immunoassay) after collecting a single blood sample into EDTA and rapidly separating and freezing the plasma (within 15 minutes). The sample must be sent by a guaranteed express delivery service in a special freezer pack that can be borrowed from a specialist laboratory.

Low dose dexamethasone suppression test: As discussed above the LDDST may help in distinguishing between causes of HAC because some cases of PD-HAC show suppression of cortisol at 3 hours but not at 8 hours. However, if this does not occur, then PD-HAC cannot be excluded. Some cases of AD-HAC may show low concentrations of cortisol throughout the test without any suppression (Norman *et al.*, 1999).

High dose dexamethasone suppression test: The high dose dexamethasone suppression test is probably now unnecessary in most situations, due to the availability of other, more convenient, tests. The procedure is as outlined in Figure 18.8 for the LDDST except that the dose of dexamethasone used is increased to 0.1 mg/kg. Suppression of cortisol at 3 hours or at 3 and 8 hours is consistent with PD-HAC. However, if this does not occur, then PD-HAC cannot be excluded. Lack of adequate suppression (i.e. cortisol concentrations >40 nmol/l at 3–4 hours and at 8 hours) is seen in all AD-HAC cases and in 20–30 % of PD-HAC cases. The high dose dexamethasone suppression test cannot be used to distinguish between normal dogs and those with HAC (unlike the LDDST).

Effects on other endocrine tests

Thyroxine (T4) concentrations: Basal thyroxine concentrations are decreased in about 70% of dogs with HAC (Peterson *et al.*, 1984). This is thought to be due to inhibition of pituitary secretion of thyroid stimulating hormone (TSH) and so TSH levels are usually low (Ramsey and Herrtage, 1998). The response of thyroxine to TRH or TSH stimulation usually parallels a normal response, but thyroxine concentrations both pre- and post-TRH or TSH are subnormal (Peterson *et al.*, 1984). However, in some cases of spontaneous HAC, canine TSH concentrations are normal or even increased; in these cases, the low T4 may be due to cortisol altering thyroid hormone binding to plasma proteins or enhancing the metabolism of thyroid hormone.

Parathyroid hormone concentrations: Glucocorticoids are known to increase urinary calcium excretion in canine HAC. In order to maintain normal circulating concentrations of calcium, parathyroid hormone (PTH) concentrations are increased in over 80% of cases of HAC (Ramsey and Herrtage, 2001). PTH concentrations decrease with treatment, but not usually to normal concentrations (Tebb *et al.*, 2003b).

Growth hormone and insulin-like growth factor 1 concentrations: HAC reduces spontaneous and stimulated growth hormone (GH) secretion by enhanced release of somatostatin from the hypothalamus. Reduced GH secretion from the pituitary may result in reduced serum insulin-like growth factor 1 (IGF-1) concentrations.

Insulin and C-peptide concentrations: Both insulin and C-peptide (which is released in equimolar concentrations to insulin) concentrations are increased in dogs with hyperadrenocorticism (Montgomery *et al.*, 2003).

Tests for monitoring therapy

Trilostane

Trilostane is a steroid synthesis inhibitor that is licensed for the treatment of HAC in the UK and is used in other countries as an alternative to mitotane. It is recommended that ACTH stimulation tests are performed at 10–14 days, 30 days and 90 days after starting therapy (Neiger *et al.*, 2002). As trilostane has a short plasma half-life, it is important that this test is performed 4–6 hours after the drug has been administered.

- If the post-ACTH cortisol concentration is <20 nmol/l, trilostane is stopped for 48 hours and then re-introduced at a lower dose.
- If the post-ACTH cortisol concentration is between 20 nmol/l and 120 nmol/l and the patient appears to be clinically well controlled then the dose is unaltered.
- If the post-ACTH cortisol concentration is >120 nmol/l and the clinical signs appear poorly controlled then the dose of trilostane may need to be increased to twice daily administration. An ACTH stimulation test can be performed 24 hours after trilostane administration (i.e. just before the next trilostane administration) to investigate this. If the post-ACTH cortisol concentration is >250 nmol/l at 24 hours after trilostane, but the post-ACTH cortisol concentration 4 hours after trilostane is <120 nmol/l then an increase to twice daily dosing is justified.
- If an ACTH stimulation test is performed inadvertently at times other than 4–6 hours after dosing with trilostane, the post-ACTH cortisol concentration should be >20 nmol/l and <250 nmol/l.

Once the clinical condition of the animal and the dose rate have been stabilized, the dog should be examined and an ACTH stimulation test performed every 3–6 months. Serum biochemistry should be performed periodically to check for hyperkalaemia (which may reflect low aldosterone concentrations in some, but not all, cases).

In atypical HAC treated with trilostane, measurement of 17-OHP is not helpful in monitoring since the concentrations are massively increased. This is presumably due to cross reactivity in the assay with 17-hydroxypregnenolone, which would be expected to increase because of inhibition of 3ß-hydroxysteroid dehydrogenase by trilostane.

It is important to note that many aspects of trilostane's use in canine HAC are still under investigation and, therefore, the above recommendations are likely to change.

Mitotane

Mitotane is the mainstay of medical management of PD-HAC in most countries. It is a cytotoxic agent that principally causes necrosis of the zona fasciculata and zona reticularis of the adrenal glands.

Mitotane is initially given as an induction course which results in the suppression of the ACTH stimulation test. Generally a post-ACTH cortisol of between 20 and 120 nmol/l indicates satisfactory control (Kintzer and Peterson, 1991; Dunn *et al.*, 1995). Maintenance therapy is then given and monitored by ACTH stimulation tests, initially monthly and then every 3–6 months. Further details on mitotane therapy are available in the *BSAVA Manual of Endocrinology*.

Dogs treated with mitotane, particularly when they have been treated for several months, may develop acute signs of hypoadrenocorticism (see below). Occasionally, there may be evidence of hyperkalaemia and hyponatraemia. Should this occur, treatment should be stopped and an ACTH stimulation test should be performed: post-ACTH cortisol would be expected to be <20 nmol/l.

Plasma 17-OHP concentrations can be used to monitor treatment of atypical HAC cases when mitotane is used.

Other medical therapy

In some countries, ketoconazole is used for the treatment of PD-HAC, particularly in those dogs that cannot tolerate mitotane. Ketoconazole therapy is monitored in a similar fashion to that described for trilostane. Ketoconazole can cause hepatotoxicity: increases in liver enzymes in dogs treated with this drug are a cause for concern and require withdrawal of the drug in most cases.

In the USA and some other countries, selegiline (L-deprenyl) is licensed for the treatment of PD-HAC. The current evidence indicates that there is minimal endocrinological improvement but some clinical improvement; no laboratory monitoring is recommended (Reusch *et al.*, 1999).

Feline hyperadrenocorticism

Adrenal diseases in the cat are uncommon compared with those in the dog: HAC is the most common of these, but has been reported in less than 100 cats. Primary hyperaldosteronism (or Conn's Syndrome) is also reported in cats (see later). Most (80%) cats with confirmed HAC have concurrent diabetes mellitus. As well as showing most of the same signs of HAC as dogs, many also have hyperfragile skin. Hyperglycaemia (about 80%) and hypercholesterolaemia (about 50%) are the most common serum biochemistry abnormalities. High serum ALP activity is uncommon, developing in only a third of cats. Urine SG is generally <1.020.

The ACTH stimulation test is the most useful test for the diagnosis of feline HAC. However, as the peak response in cats is variable, samples must be obtained at 30, 60 and 120 minutes after the intravenous injection of 0.125 mg ACTH (0.25 mg if >5kg) (Schoeman *et al.*, 2000). The sensitivity of the test is variably reported from 50–80%. It can also give a positive result in cats with non-adrenal diseases. As in the dog, values >600 nmol/l are very suggestive of HAC.

The low dose (0.015 mg/kg) dexamethasone suppression test is not considered to be useful in the diagnosis of feline HAC as false positive test results are seen in many cats with non-adrenal illness. Dexamethasone suppression testing using a higher dexamethasone dosage (0.1 mg/kg) has been advocated as a screening test with a reported sensitivity of 78%. Serum cortisol values in all normal cats and most cats with non-adrenal illness are said to be suppressed with this dose, whilst all cats with AD-HAC and most cats with PD-HAC fail to suppress cortisol at either 3–4 or 8 hours. However, too few cases have been evaluated to assess accurately the sensitivity and specificity. The higher dose dexamethasone suppression test is used in cats as a screening test, not for distinguishing between adrenal and pituitary forms of the disease.

A combined dexamethasone suppression/ACTH stimulation test protocol was suggested for use in cats: however, it has not been sufficiently investigated to recommend its routine use.

The value of any test for distinguishing reliably between pituitary- and adrenal-dependent forms of feline HAC has not been assessed. A very high dose (1.0 mg/kg) dexamethasone suppression test or measurement of basal endogenous ACTH concentration have been used to differentiate cats with PD-HAC from those with AD-HAC. Normal to high plasma ACTH levels support a diagnosis of PD-HAC, whereas low concentrations are consistent with AD-HAC.

The urinary corticoid:creatinine ratio is not widely used in cats but is likely to be sensitive if non-specific. Urine should always be collected at home (not in the hospital environment) as all stressful situations will elevate the urinary corticoid:creatinine ratio. A value of less than 10×10^{-6} probably rules out hypercortisolaemia (Rochlitz, 1999). Almost all cats with HAC will be positive, but false positive test results may be seen frequently in cats with non-adrenal illness. Importantly, hyperthyroid cats have increased ratios. Recent results suggest that laboratory extraction of corticoids may improve the diagnostic efficiency but larger scale studies are needed before this can be recommended.

There are no reliable reports of using ACTH stimulation tests to monitor the treatment of large numbers of cats with HAC and so target values have to be extrapolated from dogs (see above). Cats have been successfully treated with trilostane using these extrapolated values (Neiger *et al.*, 2004).

Canine hypoadrenocorticism

Hypoadrenocorticism is defined as the absolute lack of adrenocortical steroids. This includes a lack of mineralocorticoids and glucocorticoids. Isolated deficiencies in glucocorticoids have been reported but not isolated deficiencies in mineralocorticoids (Dunn and Herrtage, 1998). Canine hypoadrenocorticism can be classified according to the underlying cause, of which four are of importance:

- Spontaneous hypoadrenocorticism (= idiopathic hypoadrenocorticism)
- Mitotane-induced hypoadrenocorticism
- Trilostane-induced hypoadrenocorticism
- Iatrogenic hypoadrenocorticism (due to sudden withdrawal of glucocorticoid therapy).

Different causes of hypoadrenocorticism are associated with varying degrees of mineralocorticoid and glucocorticoid deficiency.

Investigation of hypoadrenocorticism

Many cases are presented with signs that could be suggestive of hypoadrenocorticism, such as lethargy, weight loss, poor appetite, vomiting, diarrhoea or episodic collapse (Figure 18.11). Figure 18.12 summarizes the approach to a suspected case of canine hypoadrenocorticism.

Routine biochemistry, haematology and urinalysis

A routine blood profile often provides the first indication that hypoadrenocorticism may be present. The common biochemical, haematological and urinalysis findings in cases of hypoadrenocorticism are shown in Figure 18.13.

Body system/organ	Examples	Similarities in presenting signs
Kidney	Decompensated renal failure	Dehydration Polyuria/polydipsia Vomiting Anorexia
Exocrine pancreas	Acute pancreatitis	Abdominal pain, dehydration Anorexia Vomiting Diarrhoea
Gastrointestinal tract	Infectious enteritis (various)	Anorexia Vomiting Haemorrhagic diarrhoea
Hepatobiliary tract	Hepatitis (toxic, inflammatory)	Vomiting Diarrhoea
Neuromuscular system	Myaesthenia gravis	Episodic weakness Regurgitation/vomiting
Endocrine system	Hypothyroidism	Bradycardia Dullness
Cardiovascular system	Third degree heart block	Bradycardia Episodic collapse
Haemopoietic system	Anaemia	Pale mucous membranes Collapse
Systemic disease	Neoplasia (e.g. lymphoma)	Many!

18.11 Conditions that may resemble canine hypoadrenocorticism in at least two major presenting signs.

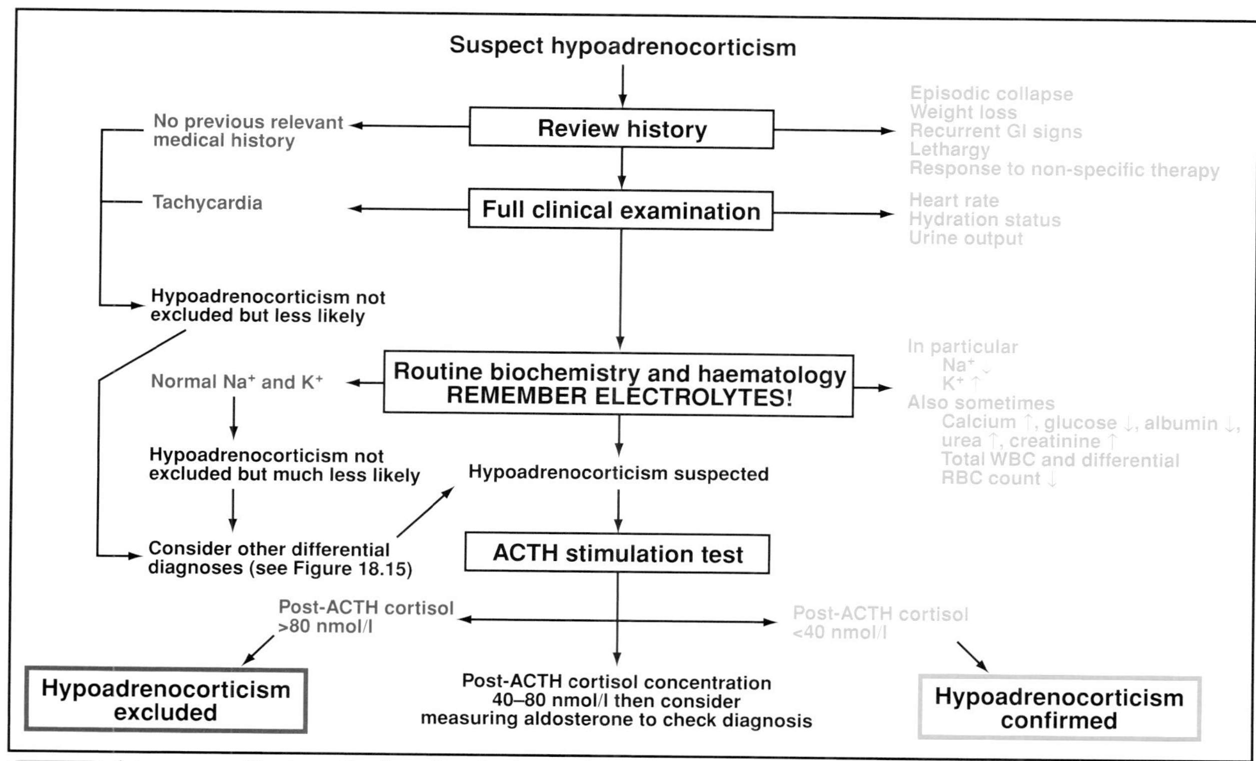

18.12 A summary of the investigation of canine hypoadrenocorticism. It is not necessary to perform all these investigations in every case. Text in green refers to typical features of HAC; text in red refers to uncommon findings.

Test	Abnormality
Biochemistry	
Azotaemia	Increased urea and creatinine (can be very high)
Electrolytes	Increased potassium Decreased sodium Decreased chloride Decreased sodium:potassium ratio (<27:1)
Calcium	May be increased (however usually <4.0 mmol/l)
Glucose	May be decreased (only rarely clinically significant)
Albumin	May be decreased
Haematology	
Red blood cells	Normally mild non-regenerative anaemia May be masked by haemoconcentration May be severe due to haemorrhage Occasionally severe due to concurrent immune-mediated haemolytic anaemia
White blood cells	Total count is normal to low Lymphocytes may be increased Neutrophil:lymphocyte ratio decreased Eosinophilia
Urinalysis	
Specific gravity	Usually low normal (1.015–1.030) SG may not increase in dehydrated dogs with hypoadrenocorticism and it can be difficult to distinguish prerenal azotaemia from intrinsic renal failure

18.13 Common abnormalities in routine laboratory profiles of dogs with hypoadrenocorticism.

Biochemistry: In cases of canine hypoadrenocorticism biochemistry will nearly always (>90%) demonstrate hyperkalaemia and hyponatraemia, with hypochloraemia being seen in about 80% of cases (Peterson *et al.*, 1996). Whilst hypoadrenocorticism is the commonest cause of a combination of reduced sodium and increased potassium, individual changes are associated with a wider range of conditions (Figure 18.14; see also Chapter 8).

Many laboratories quote the sodium:potassium ratio. Whilst a reduced sodium:potassium ratio (<27:1) is suggestive of hypoadrenocorticism, it is not diagnostic of the condition. This is particularly true when one of the electrolytes is within its reference range. A ratio of <20:1 is very suggestive of hypoadrenocorticism but is

Metabolic
Hypoadrenocorticism Severe gastrointestinal disease with haemorrhage into intestines Renal disease Chylothorax/pleural effusions Pregnancy (+ vomiting)
Drugs/poisons
Trilostane Mitotane Combination therapy for cardiac disease, especially if combined with sodium-restricted diet

18.14 Differential diagnosis of combined hyponatraemia and hyperkalaemia. Conditions that may cause isolated hyponatraemia or hyperkalaemia are listed in Appendix 1.

not very sensitive. Absolute electrolyte concentrations are more reliable indicators of hypoadrenocorticism. Cases of hypoadrenocorticism with normal sodium and potassium concentrations are very rare. In such cases, further testing (ACTH stimulation test) should always be performed before starting therapy.

Biochemistry may also demonstrate azotaemia (90% of dogs), hypercalcaemia (30%), hypoglycaemia (16%) and hypoalbuminaemia (6%) (Peterson *et al.*, 1996). Metabolic acidosis is often evident on blood gas analysis. None of these changes is as specific or as sensitive as the changes in electrolyte concentrations. Azotaemia may be very severe and is caused by prerenal factors (predominantly hypovolaemia, but gastrointestinal haemorrhage may contribute to the increased urea concentration). Dehydration may also mask some of the changes noted above. See below and Chapter 11 for further discussion of how to make the important distinction between renal failure and hypoadrenocorticism.

Haematology: Haematology profiles of dogs with hypoadrenocorticism are characterized more by the absence of abnormalities than their presence. In many ill (and therefore stressed) dogs neutrophil numbers are high normal to increased, whereas eosinophils and lymphocytes are low normal to decreased. In hypoadrenocorticism white blood cell counts are lower than would be expected for a sick dog and sometimes there may be a reverse stress leucogram (low normal numbers of neutrophils with increased numbers of lymphocytes and eosinophils).

Anaemia is present in about one quarter of dogs at presentation but the actual incidence may be much higher as it will often be masked by concurrent dehydration. Usually this anaemia is mild, normocytic and normochromic. However, in some cases, gastrointestinal haemorrhage or concurrent immune-mediated haemolytic anaemia may produce a more severe anaemia with evidence of regeneration.

Urinalysis: Urinalysis may often demonstrate a normal to low normal SG. This can make the distinction between hypoadrenocorticism and renal failure difficult in the azotaemic patient. Clinical history and laboratory findings must be combined to make this distinction (Figure 18.15). Decompensated chronic renal failure will only rarely be associated with hyperkalaemia and/or hyponatraemia. Acute renal failure, whilst associated with electrolyte changes, can usually be distinguished from acute hypoadrenocorticism by the reduction in urinary output and the short clinical history. Moreover, with adequate fluid therapy, the increased urea and creatinine concentrations of a dog with hypoadrenocorticism will return to normal within 24 hours, whereas in renal failure the urea and creatinine concentrations will take longer to recover (if at all).

The most practical implication of this discussion is that any dog, but particularly younger dogs, should have their electrolytes measured when presented with signs that are suggestive of renal failure to avoid missing the alternative diagnosis of hypoadrenocorticism.

	Acute (oliguric) renal failure	Chronic renal failure	Hypoadrenocorticism
History			
Weight loss	No	Yes	Yes
PU/PD	Can develop later	Yes – often severe	Uncommon and usually mild
Others: vomiting, diarrhoea, collapse, depression, recent 'stressful' incident	Yes	Yes	Yes
Clinical examination			
Urine output	Poor or none	Excessive	Normal or mildly increased
Uraemic glossitis	Uncommon	Rare	Never reported
Normal heart rate	Tachycardia more likely	Tachycardia more likely	Bradycardia possible
Pale mucous membranes	No	Likely	Likely
Clinical pathology			
Urine specific gravity	>1.030	Between 1.008 and 1.020	Variable but can be as low as 1.008
Hyperkalaemia	Possible	Normo- or hypokalaemic	Very common
Hyponatraemia	Possible	No	Very common
Increased urea	Yes	Yes	Yes
Urea >40 mmol/l	Rare	Common	Occasional
Increased creatinine	Yes	Yes	Yes
Increased calcium	Rare	Rare	About 30%
Increased phosphate	After 4 days	Very common	About 30%
'Stress' leucogram	Yes	Yes	No
Anaemia	No	Yes	Yes

18.15 Summary of the differences between hypoadrenocorticism and renal failure, one of its commonest differential diagnoses. This table presents only a general overview. In some clinical cases the distinction may be less clear than suggested. Some forms of each category have subtle differences, e.g. hypercalcaemia is relatively common in chronic renal failure due to juvenile nephropathies. Categories are also not mutually exclusive, for example, acute decompensation may occur with chronic renal failure.

Specific endocrine tests

It is not acceptable to diagnose hypoadrenocorticism on the basis of a therapeutic trial of steroids. There are several conditions that may present with clinical signs similar to those seen in hypoadrenocorticism (and/or electrolyte changes), which will also improve significantly with glucocorticoid administration.

ACTH stimulation test: The ACTH stimulation test is a highly sensitive and specific test for hypoadrenocorticism (>95% in both cases) (Peterson *et al*., 1996) and should be performed in all suspected cases. It is not suggested that an ACTH stimulation test is performed on every case that is presented with recurrent vomiting and diarrhoea, but a routine haematology and biochemistry profile (including electrolyte analysis) should be obtained, looking for evidence of hypoadrenocorticism. For cases with a greater range of the clinical signs of hypoadrenocorticism (e.g. vomiting, diarrhoea, weight loss and episodic collapse) the clinician may elect to perform an ACTH stimulation test at the same time as the routine laboratory profiles. The test is performed as described in Figure 18.6.

Note that hypoadrenocorticism cannot be diagnosed using the LDDST.

The diagnosis is confirmed if the post-ACTH cortisol concentration is <40 nmol/l. However a small percentage of cases of hypoadrenocorticism with classical laboratory abnormalities and consistent clinical signs may have post-ACTH cortisol concentrations as high as 80 nmol/l (see Figure 18.7). Note that if a supranormal result (500–800 nmol/l) is obtained this is unlikely to indicate *hyper*adrencorticism but rather the metabolic stress of another illness that more closely resembles hypoadrenocorticism in its presentation.

As discussed above, the test can be influenced by the administration of exogenous glucocorticoids. Hydrocortisone and prednisolone cross react in the assay and therefore give false increases. Other glucocorticoids, such as dexamethasone, do not cross react but may suppress the response. The duration and dose of such therapy will determine the degree of suppression of the response. Sometimes clinicians are presented with suspected cases of hypoadrenocorticism that have been given a single dose of dexamethasone the previous evening. In such circumstances, it is prudent to support the animal with fluid therapy for 24 hours before performing an ACTH stimulation test. It is highly unlikely that the ACTH stimulation test will be sufficiently suppressed to give a false positive result for hypoadrenocorticism 36 hours after a single dose of dexamethasone. Prednisolone should not be given during the 24 hours before an ACTH stimulation test as it may cross react with cortisol in the assay.

Measurement of aldosterone: In some cases of hypoadrenocorticism it is valuable to measure the response of aldosterone to ACTH stimulation. In dogs with normal electrolytes, measurement of aldosterone will distinguish between true hypocortisolism and dogs with a mineralocorticoid deficiency that has not produced electrolyte abnormalities at the time of examination. Aldosterone should also be measured in cases with post-ACTH cortisol concentrations between 40 and 80 nmol/l. The normal aldosterone values post-ACTH stimulation lie between 100 and 600 pmol/l (Willard *et al*., 1987; Dunn and Herrtage, 1998).

Tests for monitoring therapy

Urea and creatinine should be monitored initially to ensure adequate hydration status. Serum electrolytes should initially be checked weekly for the first month, then monthly. Once the regimen has been adapted to the individual patient then the frequency of rechecks can be reduced to every 3 months. Many dogs require increased doses of fludrocortisone during their lives and so some form of electrolyte monitoring is advisable. Relying on clinical signs is a relatively poor indicator of the quality of control achieved.

Feline hypoadrenocorticism

Hypoadrenocorticism has been reported in fewer than 20 cats. The largest series (of 10) suggested that the clinicopathological changes seen in cats with hypoadrenocorticism are similar to those seen in dogs (Peterson *et al*., 1989). The sodium:potassium ratio is particularly unreliable in cats, and is decreased by several other conditions such as gastrointestinal diseases and body cavity effusions.

Other adrenal diseases

Hyperaldosteronism (Conn's syndrome)

Several examples of functional adrenal tumours that release aldosterone have been reported in cats (Flood *et al*., 1999), and similar tumours have been reported in dogs.

The major laboratory finding is hypokalaemia, and associated cervical ventroflexion is seen in most affected cats. Metabolic alkalosis and hypertension may also be seen in these cases. Alkalosis rarely requires specific treatment, but hypertension, if found, should be treated. Electrolytes should continue to be monitored during treatment

Basal aldosterone is often increased >600 pmol/l. However, in equivocal cases, ACTH stimulation tests should be used to demonstrate an inappropriate aldosterone response. Normal values have not been published for post-ACTH aldosterone concentrations in cats. However, from extrapolation from dogs a value of >600 pmol/l would be regarded as suggestive of hyperaldosteronism.

Phaeochromocytomas

The laboratory diagnosis of a phaeochromocytoma is complicated by the rapid breakdown of the vasoactive amines by plasma enzymes. Tests for adrenaline metabolites in urine collected over 24 hours have been described; however, reference ranges have not been established for veterinary patients.

Case examples

Case 1

Signalment

Pyrennean Mountain Dog, male, weighing 57 kg.

History and clinical findings

Non-pruritic alopecia of 18 months' duration. More recently progressive polyuria/polydipsia (approximately 100 ml/kg/day), polyphagia and mild loss of muscle mass. No weight loss or gain, and good exercise tolerance. Clinical examination demonstrated abnormal skin thinning, comedones, loss of skin elasticity and a pot-bellied appearance with a pendulous prepuce.

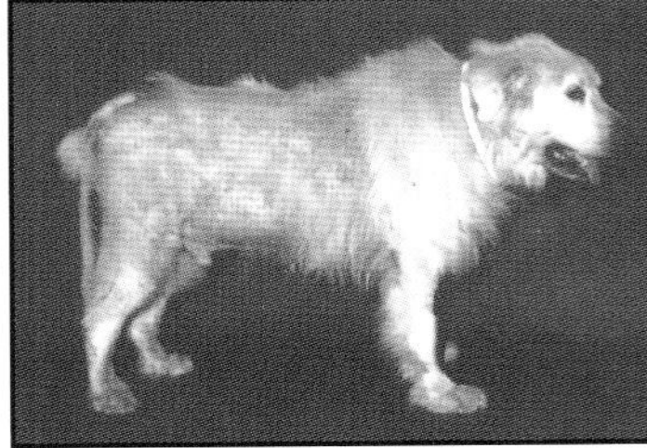

Clinical pathology data

Haematology	Result	Reference interval
RBC (x 10^{12}/l)	7.99	5.5–8.5
Hb (g/dl)	17.9	12–18
HCT (l/l)	0.47	0.37–0.55
MCV (fl)	60	60–77
MCH (pg)	22.4	19.5–24.5
MCHC (g/dl)	37.6	32–37
WBC (x 10^9/l)	11.2	6–17
Neutrophils (segmented) (x 10^9/l)	7.2	3–11.5
Neutrophils (band) (x 10^9/l)	0	0–0.3
Lymphocytes (x 10^9/l)	0.45	1–4.8
Monocytes (x 10^9/l)	3.5	0.2–1.5
Eosinophils (x 10^9/l)	0.05	0.1–1.3
Basophils (x 10^9/l)	0	0
Platelets (x 10^9/l)	381	175–500

Biochemistry	Result	Reference interval
Sodium (mmol/l)	144	135–155
Potassium (mmol/l)	4.0	3.5–5.8
Chloride (mmol/l)	109	95–115
Glucose (mmol/l)	6.1	3.3–5.5
Urea (mmol/l)	3.3	2.5–8.5
Creatinine (μmol/l)	91	45–155
Calcium (mmol/l)	2.6	2.3–3.0
Inorganic phosphate (mmol/l)	1.45	1.3–1.9
TP (g/l)	57	50–78
Albumin (g/l)	30	25–35
Globulin (g/l)	27	25–40
ALT (IU/l)	128	0–90
ALP (IU/l)	278	0–230
GGT (IU/l)	10	0–20
Cholesterol (mmol/l)	11.7	2.0–7.0

What abnormalities are present?

Haematology

- Eosinopenia
- Lymphopenia
- Monocytosis.

Biochemistry

- Mildly increased ALP and ALT
- Mildly increased glucose
- Increased cholesterol.

How would you interpret these results and what are the likely differential diagnoses?

The history and appearance of the dog are suggestive of an endocrinopathy, specifically hyperadrenocorticism. Lymphopenia, monocytosis and eosinopenia may all be caused by exogenous or endogenous corticosteroids, although neutrophilia is not present.

The most specific change on the routine biochemistry is the increased cholesterol which is consistent with a number of endocrinopathies (diabetes mellitus, hypothyroidism and hyperadrenocorticism) as well as some liver diseases. Postprandial effects might also cause increased cholesterol.

The very slightly increased glucose concentration is consistent with stress, and effectively excludes diabetes mellitus.

The mild increases in ALT and ALP are very non-specific and could be due to almost any systemic metabolic, inflammatory, toxic or neoplastic condition as well as any hepatopathy.

Hyperadrenocorticism is the most likely differential diagnosis.

What further tests would you recommend?

- ACTH stimulation test
- Low dose dexamethasone test (if ACTH stimulation test negative)
- Combined T4 and TSH measurement.

Endocrinology	Result	Reference interval
Total T4 (nmol/l)	12	15–45
TSH (ng/ml)	0.44	0–0.69
Cortisol pre ACTH (nmol/l)	45	50–250
Cortisol post ACTH (nmol/l)	254	<400
Cortisol basal (nmol/l)	31	50–250
Cortisol 3 hour post dex (nmol/l)	34	<40
Cortisol 8 hour post dex (nmol/l)	34	<40

How would you interpret these results and what are the likely differential diagnoses?

The ACTH stimulation test is within reference limits. The low dose dexamethasone suppression test is difficult to interpret. The absolute values are below the normal reference range for cortisol throughout the assay. However, there is no suppression of the cortisol following dexamethasone administration. This pattern may be consistent with an adrenal tumour but persistent adrenal suppression or failure to inject the dexamethasone properly are also possible interpretations.

Case 1 continues ▶

Case 1 continued

The low total thyroxine concentration and normal TSH concentration are consistent with the so-called sick euthyroid syndrome (or low T4 state of medical illness, see Chapter 17)

What further tests would you recommend?

As this dog is still likely to have hyperadrenocorticism, a test that is less specific but more sensitive than the standard ACTH stimulation test is probably the best option. Measurement of 17-hydroxyprogesterone was undertaken on pre- and post-ACTH samples. The results were 1.0 ng/ml pre-ACTH and 4.6 ng/ml post-ACTH. These results are within reference ranges and hyperadrenocorticism is not confirmed. Cortisol measured on the same samples was 117 and 459 nmol/l, respectively. Note the post-ACTH cortisol concentration is now greater than 400 nmol/l (which is the upper limit of the reference range) but is still less than 600 nmol/l which is the level at which hyperadrenocorticism could be confirmed in this case.

What advice would you give the owner?

There several possible courses of action:

- Wait for 1–2 months and then repeat the ACTH stimulation test and/or low dose dexamethasone test
- Diagnostic imaging (looking for an adrenal tumour with ultrasonography and then looking for a pituitary tumour with MRI or CT)
- Trial therapy with trilostane or mitotane (but may be inappropriate and potentially hazardous for the dog).

2 months later an ACTH stimulation test and a low dose dexamethasone suppression test were performed and the results of both were diagnostic of hyperadrenocorticism:

Endocrinology	Result	Reference interval
Cortisol pre ACTH (nmol/l)	146	50–250
Cortisol post ACTH (nmol/l)	610	<400
Endogenous ACTH (pg/ml)	<5	20–80
Cortisol basal (nmol/l)	147	50–250
Cortisol 3 hour post dex (nmol/l)	135	<40
Cortisol 8 hour post dex (nmol/l)	117	<40

Endogenous ACTH levels are consistent with an adrenal tumour. Medical therapy was successful in controlling the clinical signs for 2 years. The dog died of unrelated causes and at post-mortem examination a unilateral adrenal mass was found with no evidence of metastasis.

Case 2

Signalment

4-year-old female Standard Poodle.

History and clinical findings

2-month history of lethargy, exercise intolerance and decreased appetite. Clinical examination revealed that the dog was a little thin and was generally weak. Mucous membranes were dry but pink. No other abnormalities were detected (heart rate was 90 per minute).

Clinical pathology data

Haematology	Result	Reference interval
RBC (x 10^{12}/l)	6.26	5.5–8.5
Hb (g/dl)	14.4	12–18
HCT (l/l)	0.39	0.37–0.55
MCV (fl)	63	60–77
MCH (pg)	22.9	19.5–24.5
MCHC (g/dl)	36.3	32–37
WBC (x 10^9/l)	15.8	6–17
Neutrophils (segmented) (x 10^9/l)	5.85	3–11.5
Neutrophils (band) (x 10^9/l)	0	0–0.3
Lymphocytes (x 10^9/l)	7.43	1.0–4.8
Monocytes (x 10^9/l)	0.63	0.2–1.5
Eosinophils (x 10^9/l)	1.9	0.1–1.3
Basophils (x 10^9/l)	0	0
Platelets (x 10^9/l)	364	175–500

Film comment

Some of the lymphocytes appear to be reactive

Biochemistry	Result	Reference interval
Sodium (mmol/l)	143	135–155
Potassium (mmol/l)	6.5	3.5–5.8 ▶
Chloride (mmol/l)	117	95–115
Glucose (mmol/l)	4.2	3.3–5.5
Urea (mmol/l)	20.7	2.5–8.5
Creatinine (μmol/l)	184	45–155
Calcium (mmol/l)	2.7	2.3–3.0
Inorganic phosphate (mmol/l)	2.11	1.3–1.9
TP (g/l)	62	50–78
Albumin (g/l)	23	25–35
Globulin (g/l)	39	25–40
ALT (IU/l)	67	0–90
ALP (IU/l)	45	0–230
GGT (IU/l)	5	0–20
Cholesterol (mmol/l)	2.8	2.0–7.0

Urinalysis

Specific gravity	1.024
Dipstick analysis	No protein, blood, glucose or ketones pH = 6.5

What abnormalities are present?

Haematology

- Eosinophilia
- Lymphocytosis.

Biochemistry

- Mild hypoalbuminaemia
- Azotaemia
- Hyperkalaemia
- Mild hyperchloraemia
- Hyperphosphataemia.

Urinalysis

- SG suggests concentrating ability compromised.

Case 2 continues ▶

Case 2 continued

How would you interpret these results and what are the likely differential diagnoses?

The most striking haematological abnormality is lymphocytosis. Infectious diseases (particularly viral infections), lymphoproliferative diseases and hypoadrenocorticism may all produce this change. The increased eosinophil count and the neutrophil count within the lower part of the reference range are also consistent with hypoadrenocorticism. There is no anaemia (which may occur in about 30% of cases of hypoadrenocorticism), although anaemia may be masked by dehydration.

There is a hyperkalaemia without hyponatraemia, with a sodium:potassium ratio of 22 (reference >27). The hyperkalaemia is consistent with hyperadrenocorticism, some forms of renal failure, liquorice poisoning and poor sample handling.

The azotaemia is significant, with relatively higher urea then creatinine concentrations, which is common in prerenal azotaemia or where there is gastrointestinal haemorrhage. In prerenal azotaemia, increased urine SG is expected, while in azotaemia of renal origin isosthenuria is expected. In this case the urine SG is intermediate, a common feature of hypoadrenocorticism. Response to fluid therapy will be needed to further assess the renal function.

Mild hypoalbuminaemia is consistent with hypoadrenocorticism, liver diseases and mild cases of protein-losing enteropathy and nephropathy.

What further tests would you recommend?

An ACTH stimulation test, and possibly measurement of endogenous ACTH.

Endocrinology	Result	Reference interval
Cortisol pre ACTH (nmol/l)	<5	50–250
Cortisol post ACTH (nmol/l)	<5	<400
Endogenous ACTH (pg/ml)	259	20–80

The results of the ACTH stimulation test confirm this as a case of hypoadrenocorticism. The increased endogenous ACTH concentration indicates that this is a case of primary (i.e. adrenal-dependent) hypoadrenocorticism.

References

Chapman PS, MooneyCT, Ede J, Evans H, O'Connor J, Pfeiffer DU and Neiger R (2003) Evaluation of the basal and post-adrenocorticotrophic hormone serum concentrations of 17-hydroxyprogesterone for the diagnosis of hyperadrenocorticism in dogs. *Veterinary Record* **153,** 771–775

Dunn KJ and Herrtage ME (1998) Hypocortisolaemia in a Labrador retriever. *Journal of Small Animal Practice* **39,** 90–93

Dunn KJ, Herrtage ME and Dunn JK (1995) Use of ACTH stimulation tests to monitor the treatment of canine hyperadrenocorticism. *Veterinary Record* **137,** 161–165

Flood SM, Randolph JF, Gelzer ARM and Refsal K (1999) Primary hyperaldosteronism in two cats. *Journal of the American Animal Hospital Association* **35,** 411–416

Galac S, Kooistra HS, Teske E and Rijnberk A (1997) Urinary corticoid/creatinine ratios in the differentiation between pituitary-dependent hyperadrenocorticism and hyperadrenocorticism due to adrenocortical tumour in the dog. *Veterinary Quarterly* **19,** 17–20

Gould SM, Baines EA, Mannion PA, Evans H and Herrtage ME (2001) Use of endogenous ACTH concentration and adrenal ultrasonography to distinguish the cause of canine hyperadrenocorticism. *Journal of Small Animal Practice* **42,** 113–121

Herrtage ME (2004) Canine hyperadrenocorticism. In: *BSAVA Manual of Canine and Feline Endocrinology, 3rd edn*, ed. CT Mooney and ME Peterson, pp.150–171. BSAVA Publications, Gloucester.

Hurley KJ and Vaden SL (1998) Evaluation of urine protein content in dogs with pituitary-dependent hyperadrenocorticism. *Journal of the American Veterinary Medical Association* **212,** 369–373

Kaplan AJ, Peterson ME and Kemppainen RJ (1995) Effects of disease on the results of diagnostic tests for use in detecting hyperadrenocorticism in dogs. *Journal of the American Veterinary Medical Association* **207,** 445–451

Kemppainen RJ and Sartin JL (1984) Evidence for episodic but not circadian activity in plasma concentrations of adrenocorticotrophin, cortisol and thyroxine in dogs. *Journal of Endocrinology* **103,** 219–226

Kintzer PP and Peterson ME (1991) Mitotane (o,p'-DDD) treatment of 200 dogs with pituitary-dependent hyperadrenocorticism. *Journal of Veterinary Internal Medicine* **5,** 182–190

Montgomery TM, Nelson RW, Feldman EC, Robertson K and Polonsky KS (2003) Basal and glucagon-stimulated plasma C-peptide concentrations in healthy dogs, dogs with diabetes mellitus, and dogs with hyperadrenocorticism. *Journal of Veterinary Internal Medicine* **10,** 116–122

Neiger R, Ramsey I, O'Connor J, Hurley KJ and Mooney CT (2002) Trilostane treatment of 78 dogs with pituitary dependent hyperadrenocorticism. *Veterinary Record* **150,** 799–804

Neiger R, Witt AL, Noble A and German AJ (2004) Trilostane therapy for treatment of pituitary-dependent hyperadrenocorticism in 5 cats. *Journal of Veterinary Internal Medicine* **18,** 160–164

Nelson RW, Feldman EC and Smith MC (1988) Hyperadrenocorticism in cats: seven cases (1978–1987). *Journal of the American Veterinary Medical Association* **193,** 245–250

Norman EJ, Thompson H and Mooney CT (1999) Dynamic adrenal function testing in eight dogs with hyperadrenocorticism associated with adrenocortical neoplasia. *Veterinary Record* **144,** 551–554

Peterson ME, Ferguson DC, Kintzer PP and Drucker WD (1984) Effects of spontaneous hyperadrenocorticism on serum thyroid hormone concentrations in the dog. *American Journal of Veterinary Research* **45,** 2034–2038

Peterson ME, Greco DS and Orth DN (1989) Primary hypoadrenocorticism in ten cats. *Journal of Veterinary Internal Medicine* **3,** 55–58

Peterson ME, Kemppainen RJ and Graves TK (1988) Episodic but not circadian activity in plasma concentrations of ACTH, cortisol and thyroxine in the normal cat. (Abstract) *American College of Veterinary Internal Medicine Scientific Proceedings*, 721

Peterson ME, Kintzer PP and Kass PH (1996) Pretreatment clinical and laboratory findings in dogs with hypoadrenocorticism: 225 cases (1979–1993). *Journal of the American Veterinary Medical Association* **208,** 85–91

Ramsey IK and Herrtage ME (1998) The effect of thyrotropin releasing hormone on thyrotropin concentrations in euthyroid, hypothyroid and hyperadrenocorticoid dogs. (Abstract) *Journal of Veterinary Internal Medicine* **12,** 235

Reusch CE and Feldman EC (1991) Canine hyperadrenocorticism due to adrenocortical neoplasia. Pretreatment evaluation of 41 dogs. *Journal of Veterinary Internal Medicine* **5,** 3–10

Reusch CE, Steffen T and Hoerauf A (1999) The efficacy of L-Deprenyl in dogs with pituitary-dependent hyperadrenocorticism. *Journal of Veterinary Internal Medicine* **13,** 291–301

Rijnberk A, Wees Av and Mol JA (1988) Assessment of two tests for the diagnosis of canine hyperadrenocorticism. *Veterinary Record* **122,** 178–180

Ristic JME, Ramsey IK, Heath FM, Evans HJ and Herrtage ME (2002) The use of 17-hydroxyprogesterone in the diagnosis of canine hyperadrencorticism. *Journal of Veterinary Internal Medicine* **16,** 433–439

Rochlitz I (1999) Use of urinary cortisol to creatinine ratios and behavioural measures to monitor the adaption of cats to new environments. (Abstract) *BSAVA Congress Proceedings*, 306

Schoeman JP, Evans HJ, Childs D and Herrtage ME (2000) Cortisol response to two different doses of intravenous synthetic ACTH (tetracosactrin) in overweight cats. *Journal of Small Animal Practice* **41,** 552–557

Tebb AJ, Herrtage ME and Ramsey IK (2003a) Calcium and phosphate measurements in dogs with hyperadrenocorticism (Abstract). *Journal of Veterinary Internal Medicine* **17,** 737

Tebb AJ, Herrtage ME and Ramsey IK (2003b) The effects of therapy on parathyroid hormone concentrations in dogs with hyperadrenocorticism (Abstract). *Journal of Veterinary Internal Medicine* **17,** 737

Teske E, Rothuizen J, Bruijne JJ and Rijnberk A (1989) Corticosteroid-induced alkaline phosphatase isoenzyme in the diagnosis of canine hypercorticism. *Veterinary Record* **125,** 12-14.

Vonderen IK, Kooistra HS and Rijnberk A (1998) Influence of veterinary care on the urinary corticoid:creatinine ratio in dogs. *Journal of Veterinary Internal Medicine* **12,** 431–435

Watson PJ and Herrtage ME (1998) Hyperadrenocorticism in six cats. *Journal of Small Animal Practice* **39,** 175–184

Willard MD, Refsal K and Thacker E (1987) Evaluation of plasma aldosterone concentrations before and after ACTH administration in clinically normal dogs and in dogs with various diseases. *American Journal of Veterinary Research* **48,** 1713–1718

19

Laboratory evaluation of the reproductive system

Gary England and Marco Russo

Introduction

Investigation of diseases of the reproductive tract requires a detailed breeding history and a thorough clinical examination, followed by careful application of a number of laboratory tests. The purpose of this chapter is to describe the logical application of laboratory testing to common clinical presentations met by veterinary surgeons in first opinion practice.

Female

The bitch

The bitch differs from many of the domestic species in that she is monoestrous, with a long period of anoestrus between successive periods of oestrus, whether she is pregnant or not. There does not seem to be a seasonal cyclicity in most breeds and the average interval between oestrus periods is 7 months. Understanding the normal physiology is essential so that these normal, but unusual, features of reproductive function are not confused with pathology.

Reproductive physiology

Puberty generally commences between 6 and 24 months of age, often within 1 to 6 months of the bitch attaining adult height and weight. Before puberty, and during each period of anoestrus, the ovaries appear to be in a quiescent state.The onset of oestrus (or puberty) is initiated by increased secretion of gonadotrophin releasing hormone (GnRH) from the hypothalamus and a subsequent release of follicle stimulating hormone (FSH) and luteinizing hormone (LH) from the pituitary gland; these, in turn, stimulate follicular growth and the production of oestrogen. A raised plasma oestrogen concentration initiates the onset of pro-oestrus, when vulval oedema and a sanguineous discharge occur. The bitch is attractive to the male at this time, but will not accept mating. A subsequent decline in oestrogen and slight increase in plasma progesterone initiates oestrus, at which time the bitch will allow mating. During oestrus, the vulva becomes less oedematous and the discharge clearer and less sanguineous. The rise in plasma progesterone concentration is the result of pre-ovulatory luteinization and the low oestrogen:progesterone ratio causes a surge in LH from the pituitary gland. Most ovulations begin 48 hours after peak LH concentrations are reached. Formation of the corpus luteum occurs quickly after ovulation. High concentrations of progesterone occur approximately 7 days after ovulation and in many bitches this signifies the end of standing oestrus.

There is a similar duration of progesterone secretion in the non-pregnant and pregnant bitch (Figure 19.1). The non-pregnant luteal phase is termed metoestrus or dioestrus (these terms are used synonymously). In both pregnancy and non-pregnancy, progesterone is associated with mammary enlargement. Progesterone production during the luteal phase is maintained principally by the luteotrophic effects of the pituitary hormone prolactin.

During the non-pregnant luteal phase progesterone causes mammary gland enlargement and, when combined with an increase in plasma prolactin (caused by a decline in plasma progesterone), results in the

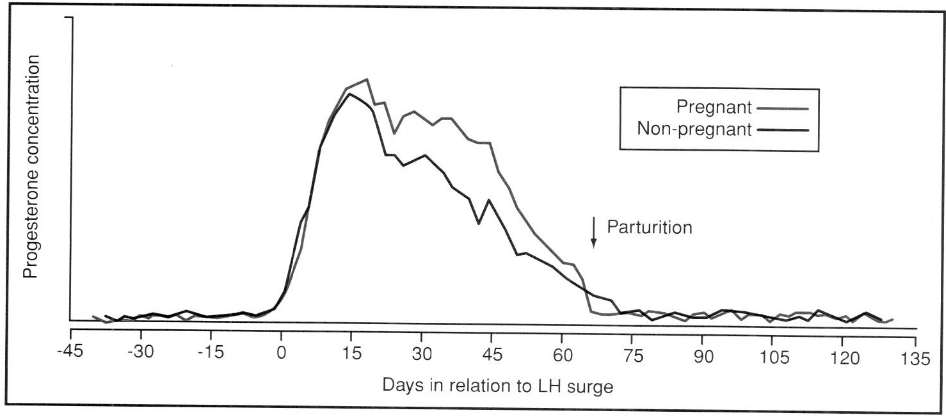

19.1 Schematic representation of progesterone concentrations during pregnant and non-pregnant luteal phases of the bitch.

secretion of milk and in behavioural changes that are typical of pregnancy. This latter condition, termed pseudopregnancy, is a normal event that is observed in all non-pregnant bitches. In some cases the changes are severe and produced marked clinical signs, whilst in others the signs may be unnoticed by the owner.

Following pregnancy or the non-pregnant luteal phase, the quiescent anoestrus state resumes, and plasma progesterone concentrations return to baseline values. The factors which result in cessation of progesterone secretion are unknown.

The queen

The queen is a polyoestrous breeder in which ovulation is induced by coitus. Cyclicity in the queen is influenced by photoperiod.

Reproductive physiology

In most queens ovulation must be induced by coitus (or artificial stimulation), although it may occur in a small number of queens without an obvious stimulus. In the majority, copulation produces a rapid pituitary-mediated release of LH. Ovulation occurs once LH concentration exceeds a threshold value.

Usually multiple copulations within a short time are required to produce an LH surge of sufficient magnitude to induce ovulation. Progesterone concentration remains basal until after the mating-induced LH surge, and increases after ovulation; peak values are reached 1 month after mating. In pregnant queens progesterone concentration declines slowly until day 60 and remains relatively low for the last week, before declining abruptly at parturition; the duration of pregnancy is usually 64–68 days from mating. In a queen that has been mated but does not become pregnant, progesterone concentration is initially identical to that of early pregnancy but then rapidly returns to basal values, with the luteal phase lasting between 30 and 45 days before the queen returns to oestrus (Figure 19.2). These queens are said to be pseudopregnant, although the only clinical sign is an absence of oestrus. Non-ovulating (non-mated or inadequately mated) queens do not have a luteal phase and return to oestrus after an interval of approximately 21 days. Throughout pregnancy the primary source of progesterone is the ovary, and there does not appear to be a significant contribution from the placenta.

Oestradiol concentration is elevated during the last week of pregnancy and prolactin concentration is elevated in the last third of pregnancy and throughout lactation. Prolactin has a luteotrophic action similar to that in the bitch. There are no significant changes in prolactin concentration during pseudopregnancy.

Relaxin is present in the plasma from approximately day 25, and, similarly to relaxin in the bitch, it increases to peak values at approximately day 50, and declines after parturition.

Laboratory techniques

Techniques available for the investigation of reproductive tract disease include measurement of concentrations of the reproductive sex steroids (progesterone, oestrogen and testosterone) and luteinizing hormone (LH), and cytological investigation of collected fluids or aspirates. Endocrinological evaluation frequently requires radioimmunoassays performed in specialist laboratories, but enzyme-linked immunosorbent assays (ELISAs) are available for the measurement of both progesterone and LH. All hormone determinations can be made in either plasma or serum.

Failure to cycle

A common clinical presentation of bitches is a failure to cycle. In many cases this may be an apparent absence of oestrus or an apparent delay in puberty because the owner has not observed the signs of oestrus. Elevated plasma progesterone concentrations (>2.0 ng/ml (6.5 nmol/l)) demonstrate that ovulation has occurred within the last 60 days (i.e. the oestrus or puberty has been missed).

In the queen there is a normal period of anoestrus during winter. This influences the timing of the onset of puberty since most queens reach puberty in the spring. Cyclicity may therefore commence at 6 months of age (or slightly less) for queens born in the autumn, but queens born in spring often do not reach puberty until the next spring when they are 12 months old. Vaginal cytology will enable the documentation of normal cyclical activity.

In those cases where it is clear that lack of oestrus is not the result of failure of observation by the owner, failure to cycle may be primary (no oestrus before 24 months, i.e. delayed puberty) or secondary (no oestrous activity within 12 months of a previous cycle, i.e.

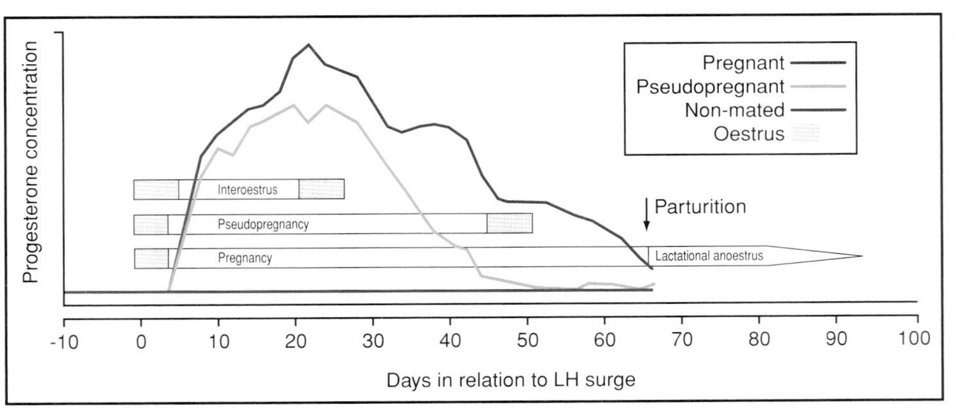

19.2 Schematic representation of progesterone concentrations in pregnant, pseudopregnant and non-mated queens.

prolonged anoestrus). In most cases a specific disease process may be responsible, and careful investigation of the underlying cause is important for appropriate treatment and prognosis.

Delayed puberty

In general, bitches that do not reach puberty by 2½ years of age are considered to have delayed puberty. Investigation involves evaluating housing and diet (since poor environmental conditions and nutrition may be associated with failure to cycle), and clinical examination to rule out chronic disease. Chromosomal abnormalities may cause delayed puberty and establishing the karyotype is key to diagnosis. EDTA blood samples need to be transported rapidly to the laboratory. Normally there are 78 chromosomes (77XX); common abnormalities include either absence (77XO) or additional chromosomes (79XXX, 79XXY) or, in some cases, mixed chromosome aberrations (78XX/78XY). Many of these bitches are phenotypically abnormal (having a small cranially positioned vulva and developing clitoral enlargement at puberty). A smaller proportion of bitches are phenotypically normal but the abnormal complement of sex chromosomes results in ovarian hypoplasia or ovarian dysgenesis.

There is little information available for queens, although it is clear that chromosomal abnormalities can influence the onset of puberty in the same manner as in the bitch.

Prolonged anoestrus

Prolonged anoestrus in the bitch represents an interoestrous interval greater than anticipated for that particular animal (usually more than 12 months from the previous cycle). In the queen it represents an animal that does not resume cyclical activity after winter.

There are several causes of failure of normal cyclicity, including chronic systemic disease, drug-induced anoestrus (glucocorticoids, anabolic steroids, androgens and progestogens) and hypothyroidism (see Chapter 17). Although hypothyroidism has been associated with prolonged anoestrus, the mechanism of this abnormality has not been fully established. Following replacement therapy most bitches return to oestrus within 6 months, although a consistent relationship between thyroid disease and reproductive function has yet to be established.

Progesterone-producing ovarian cysts have also been described in the bitch and queen, producing prolonged interoestrous intervals and cystic endometrial hyperplasia. The ovarian cysts may be identified ultrasonographically and the diagnosis confirmed by persistently elevated plasma progesterone concentrations. Hormone concentrations that remain on a plateau over a period of 6 weeks would be suspicious, as in the normal luteal phase progesterone concentrations decline during this time; plateau values for >8 weeks would be diagnostic.

In some cases, ovarian neoplasms that produce either progesterone or androgens result in a failure to return to cyclical activity. They may be diagnosed by serial estimation of plasma progesterone and testosterone concentrations.

Optimal time to breed

The most common cause of infertility in the bitch is mating at an inappropriate time. In the queen, on the other hand, coitus is the trigger for ovulation, and the optimal mating time is generally thought to be the first few days of oestrus.

Bitches ovulate approximately 12 days after the onset of pro-oestrus; however, some normal bitches may ovulate as early as 5 days whilst others ovulate as late as 30 days after the onset of pro-oestrus. Many breeders try to impose standard mating regimes on days 10 and 12, but for many bitches this is not appropriate. Careful monitoring of oestrus is important to establish the time of ovulation and therefore the most appropriate time for mating (Figure 19.3). Observation of the behaviour of the bitch has limited value, and although there may be clear changes affecting the external genitalia (the onset of vulval softening, for example, occurs 1 to 2 days prior to ovulation), laboratory investigation can be extremely useful.

Hormone measurement

Measurement of peripheral plasma concentrations of LH is a potentially useful method of determining the optimum time to mate, although assay kits are not always readily available. Plasma progesterone concentrations begin to increase towards the end of pro-oestrus at the time of the LH surge, so serial monitoring of plasma progesterone concentration allows the anticipation of ovulation (Figure 19.4). Progesterone may be

Period	Days from LH surge	Days from ovulation
Period of potential fertility: the 'fertile period'	-3 to +7 (or later)	-5 to +5 (or later)
Period of potential fertilization of mature oocytes: the 'fertilization period'	+4 to + 6 (or later)	+2 to +4 (or later)
Time of oocyte maturation (estimated)	+4 to +5	+2 to +3
Period of peak fertility in bitches of high fertility at natural mating	0 to +6	-2 to +4
Preferred time for managed breeding of natural service or fresh semen insemination	+2 to +6	0 to +4
Time for critical managed breeding or frozen semen artificial insemination	+4 to +6	+2 to +4
Period of reduced fertility with matings or inseminations late in oestrus	+7 to +9	+5 to +7

19.3 The timing of peak fertility in relationship to the day of the LH surge and day of ovulation. Note that day 0 is not the same for both: ovulation occurs 2 days after the LH surge.

	Day 7 (before LH surge)	Day of LH surge	Days 4–5 after LH surge (when oocytes mature)	Days 8–11 after LH surge
Plasma progesterone (ng/ml)	<0.5	0.9–3.0	3.5–12	8.0–25

19.4 Plasma progesterone concentrations in relationship to the fertile period of the bitch.

measured using ELISA test kits designed for in-practice use or in commercial laboratories using radioimmunoassay. Both methods have been shown to be useful for predicting the optimum mating time in the bitch.

Breeding or insemination should be planned between 4 and 6 days after progesterone concentrations exceed 2.0 ng/ml (6.5 nmol/l) (the concentration typically observed at the time of the LH surge). Some reports suggest that breeding should commence one day after progesterone concentrations exceed 8.0–10.0 ng/ml (25.0–32.0 nmol/l), which is commonly seen 2 days after ovulation when oocytes become fertilizable.

Vaginal cytology

Examination of exfoliative vaginal epithelial cells is frequently used to monitor the oestrous cycle. During pro-oestrus, increased plasma oestrogen concentrations cause thickening of the vaginal mucosa, which becomes a keratinized squamous epithelium. Surface vaginal epithelial cells may be collected using a saline-moistened swab or by aspiration. The relative proportions of different types of epithelial cells can be used as a marker of the endocrine environment. The fertile period can be predicted by calculating the percentage of cornified or anuclear epithelial cells using a modified Wright–Giemsa stain. Breeding should be attempted throughout the period when >80% of epithelial cells are anuclear (Figures 19.5 and 19.6). Whilst this is a useful guide, some bitches reach peak values of only 60% cornification, whilst in others there may be two peaks of cornification.

Neutrophils are generally absent from the vaginal smear during oestrus because the keratinized epithelium is impervious to these cells. Their reappearance during late oestrus reflects the breakdown of this epithelium. The return of neutrophils to the vaginal smear has been used by some workers as an indicator of the time of optimum fertility. Typical changes in vaginal cytology are shown in Figure 19.7.

At the Guide Dogs for the Blind Association in the UK, mating on the basis of vaginal cytology was found to increase the pregnancy rate and litter size of bitches compared with a similar group mated only on the basis of the onset of pro-oestrus (England, 1992). Whelping rates have been consistently maintained above 90% over a 10-year period since the introduction of this regime.

Feature	Anoestrus	Early pro-oestrus	Pro-oestrus	Early oestrus	Oestrus	Early metoestrus
Anuclear cells (%)	0	10	30	50	80	5
Erythrocytes	–	+++	++	+	–	–
Neutrophils	++	+	–	–	+	++++
Debris and mucus	++	+++	++	–	–	+++

19.5 Periovulatory changes in the vaginal smear of bitches.

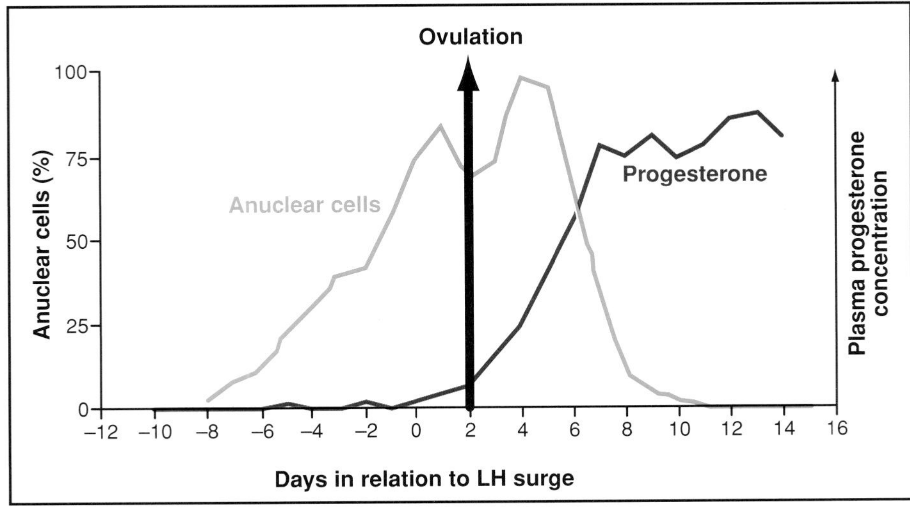

19.6 Changes in the percentage of anuclear vaginal epithelial cells in relation to ovulation and the peri-ovulatory changes in progesterone concentration in the bitch.

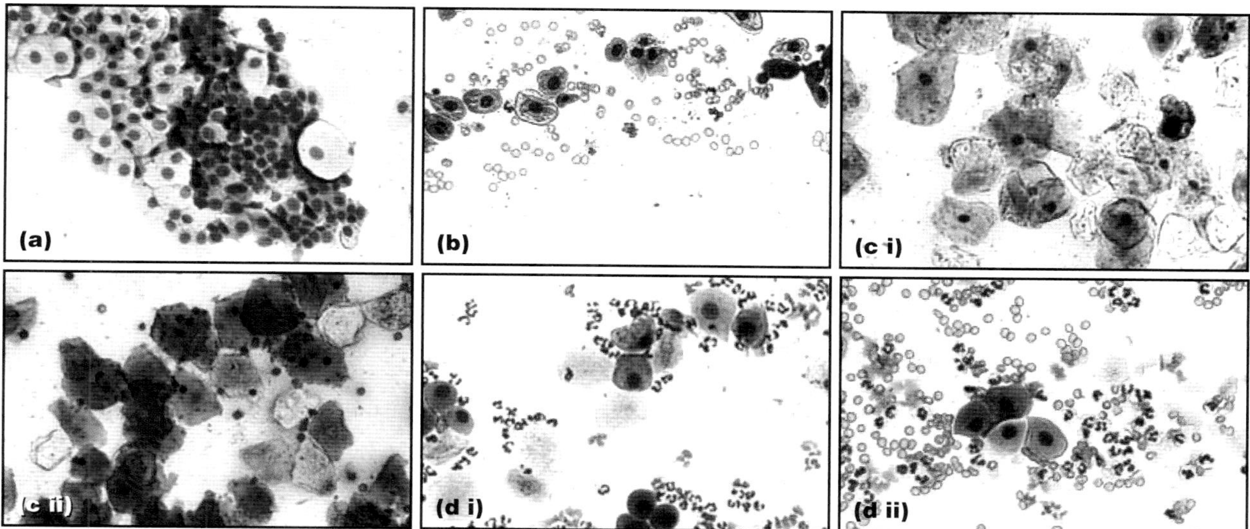

19.7 Exfoliative vaginal cytology from bitches. **(a)** Anoestrus. The predominant cell types are small parabasal epithelial cells, which have a small volume of cytoplasm compared to the size of the nucleus. The majority of cells are roughly circular in shape. Neutrophils may be present in small numbers but are not evident in this example.
(b) Pro-oestrus. The predominant cell types are small intermediate epithelial cells, which have an increased volume of cytoplasm compared to the size of the nucleus. The cells are irregular in shape and appear somewhat flattened with sharp edges. Erythrocytes are present in large numbers. Neutrophils may be present in small numbers as in this sample.
(c) Oestrus. The predominant cell types are large intermediate epithelial cells and anuclear epithelial cells, which have a large volume of cytoplasm compared to the size of the nucleus, and an absent nucleus, respectively. The cells are two dimensionally flattened and are very irregular in shape (often referred to as 'cornflake' cells). Erythrocytes are present in small numbers. Neutrophils are absent from the smear. **(d)** Metoestrus. The predominant cell types are large and small intermediate epithelial cells. Large numbers of neutrophils are again present. Erythrocytes may be present in small numbers. (Diff-Quik stain; original magnification X400)

Abnormal oestrus

There are many presentations of abnormal oestrous cycles, including those that appear shorter or longer than normal, or where there is a short period between one cycle and the next. Investigations involve careful monitoring of each cycle, and vaginal cytology and progesterone measurements are often useful.

Split oestrus

In bitches, a short interval between clinical signs of oestrus is often described as a split oestrus. This occurs most frequently at puberty, but can occur at any age. After an initial phase of follicular growth and oestrogen secretion, the follicles regress and signs of oestrus disappear. Vaginal cytology shows an initial (normal) progressive increase of anuclear cells, followed by a decline, usually before maximum cornification is reached. Often there is only a maximum of 50% anuclear cells. There is no increase in plasma progesterone. Usually a second follicular phase appears 2–12 weeks later. In some cases this may be repeated several times until finally the bitch ovulates normally. This syndrome is confusing since it may be thought that the bitch has failed to ovulate or that fertilization with subsequent resorption/abortion has occurred.

Ovulation failure

Ovulation failure is probably one of the most common causes of infertility in the queen. Several matings in a short period of time are necessary to ensure that the LH surge occurring after coitus is of sufficient magnitude to exceed the threshold value necessary to stimulate ovulation. Frequent matings are likely to produce a larger LH surge if they occur on the first or second day of oestrus. Inappropriate mating regimes imposed by the breeder may result in a failure of ovulation. This can readily be detected by an absence of elevated plasma progesterone after the end of oestrus; queens that do not ovulate generally return to oestrus with a short interval whilst ovulating queens either enter pseudopregnancy or become pregnant.

In cases of ovulation failure in the bitch, vaginal cytological changes are similar to those observed in a normal cycle, although there is a less rapid decline in anuclear cells and a smaller influx of neutrophils just prior to the end of the signs of oestrus compared with a normal oestrus. The accurate diagnosis is made by detecting an absence of an increase in plasma progesterone concentration on serial samples.

Prolonged pro-oestrus or oestrus

Although unusual, some normal bitches may show pro-oestrous or oestrous behaviour lasting up to 30 days or more (for bitches ovulating 30 days after the onset of pro-oestrus). These animals do not require treatment but careful assessment of the optimum mating time, usually by evaluation of vaginal cytology or measurement of plasma progesterone.

In some cases, however, there is an underlying pathology. Oestrogen-secreting follicular cysts may produce persistent oestrus. This is often inconvenient for the owner and may ultimately lead to bone marrow suppression with anaemia, leucopenia and thrombocytopenia. In these bitches there is persistence of a large proportion of anuclear vaginal epithelial cells and no increase in plasma progesterone. In addition, large (8–12 mm diameter) fluid-filled follicles may be identified using ultrasonography.

This syndrome is not recognized in the queen.

Ovarian neoplasia

Epithelial tumours are the most frequently identified ovarian neoplasms seen in bitches and queens but are not common and account for approximately 1% of all neoplasms. Tumours that release oestrogen may produce signs of persistent oestrus and bone marrow suppression, although clinical signs are also often related to a mass effect or ascites (the latter is usually due to widespread metastasis throughout the abdominal cavity, often termed carcinomatosis). Signs of persistent oestrus relate to persistently elevated plasma oestrogen (>50 pg/ml). There is thickening of the vaginal wall and subsequent increase in the percentage of anuclear cells found on vaginal cytology. In some cases the principal hormone produced is either progesterone or testosterone; in these cases serial estimation of these hormones may confirm the diagnosis.

Neoplasia may be suspected on the basis of an ultrasound examination, although confirmation requires cytological or histological investigation.

Presence of ovarian tissue

Alleged oestrous activity following routine 'spay' (ovariohysterectomy) is not an uncommon presentation in clinical practice. In some cases, owners observe mounting and/or thrusting behaviour and assume that this is a sign of oestrus (although it is commonly observed in both neutered and entire bitches). In other cases, males are attracted to the bitch because of a non-oestrous vulval discharge (e.g. vaginitis), or because of other odours (e.g. in skin disease). Determination of true remnant ovarian tissue is most simply done by examination of the female during periods of apparent attractiveness (see later). Examination at other times usually requires measurement of plasma hormones.

Bitch or queen during periods of attractiveness

In these cases the simplest diagnostic tool is collection of a vaginal smear and evaluation for changes typical of pro-oestrus or oestrus, as described above. Plasma hormone testing may be useful but requires consideration of the time at which the sample has been taken. Plasma oestrogen concentrations are elevated (25–50 pg/ml) during late anoestrus, pro-oestrus and early oestrus; they decline to basal during mid and late oestrus. In the bitch plasma progesterone measurement in late oestrus is very useful, as progressive luteinization of pre-ovulatory follicles results in increased in plasma progesterone to values >2.0 ng/ml (6.5 nmol/l) around the time of ovulation.

In the queen there will be no increase in progesterone unless ovulation has been stimulated. Ovulation can be induced by the administration of either human chorionic gonadotrophin (hCG) or gonadotrophin releasing hormone (GnRH); detection of elevated plasma progesterone between 7 and 30 days later is diagnostic of an ovarian remnant.

Bitch up to 60 days after a period of attractiveness

Bitches with ovarian remnants usually have normal ovulation and a resultant increase in plasma progesterone, which remains elevated for approximately 60 days after the end of oestrus. A single sample demonstrating elevated progesterone is diagnostic of remnant ovarian tissue (remember in the queen there will be no elevated progesterone unless ovulation has been stimulated).

Bitch or queen remote from a period of attractiveness

In bitches that do not currently have signs of oestrus, or are not within 60 days of the last oestrus, it is necessary to consider stimulation tests for the confirmation of remnant ovarian tissue. Gonadotrophins stimulate the release of 17β-oestradiol from theca internal cells within the ovarian remnant and can be given directly in the form of hCG (which is LH-like in activity), or GnRH can be used to stimulate the release of endogenous gonadotrophin. A blood sample is taken for assay of basal oestrogen, either hCG (25 IU/kg s.c.) or GnRH analogue (2.2 μg/kg i.m. or 0.01 μg/kg i.v.) is injected, and a second blood sample is taken 2 hours later. With both tests oestrogen concentrations increase by a factor of 2–3 when there is ovarian tissue. These tests are also applicable in the queen.

Pregnancy diagnosis

Measurement of plasma relaxin, acute phase proteins, progesterone and prolactin may all be used for pregnancy diagnosis, although plasma relaxin concentration is considered the most reliable method.

Plasma relaxin

Relaxin is a pregnancy-specific protein that is produced by the placenta. Relaxin concentrations increase in pregnant bitches and queens from approximately 24 days after ovulation, and continue to increase progressively until the last 2 weeks prior to parturition, when there is a slight decrease. Relaxin may be measured using ELISA test kits designed for in-practice use. This assay has high accuracy and precision. Some studies suggest that higher concentrations of relaxin are present with a larger litter (presumably due to a greater total placental tissue), but other studies have disputed this relationship.

Acute phase proteins

Acute phase proteins (fibrinogen, C-reactive protein, haptoglobin) are elevated in pregnant bitches compared with concentrations in non-pregnant bitches. Pregnancy can be diagnosed as early as 20 days after ovulation by measuring fibrinogen or C-reactive protein, although false positive diagnoses may occur with other conditions that stimulate release of these proteins (e.g. some inflammatory conditions such as pyometra). Unlike the situation with plasma relaxin, there is no relationship between absolute concentrations and the number of fetuses.

Plasma progesterone

In the bitch there are great similarities between the endocrinology of pregnancy and non-pregnancy. Importantly, there is a long non-pregnant luteal phase. Similarly in the queen there is a significant elevation of progesterone when ovulation occurs but pregnancy does not ensue. Thus, for both species, the measurement of plasma progesterone alone has no value for the diagnosis of pregnancy. However, in bitches the combination of plasma progesterone and acute phase protein concentrations is a more useful indicator and some commercial diagnostic laboratories 'weight' the measure of acute phase proteins in blood (see above) according to the concentration of progesterone. In this method the laboratory would pay greater attention to a 'medium' concentration of acute phase protein in the face of a 'high' concentration of progesterone, than in the face of a 'medium' or 'low' concentration of progesterone. It is suggested that this algorithm improves the reliability of the acute phase protein assay. The combined assay can be used to diagnose pregnancy from 3 weeks after mating onwards, but is most accurate from 28 days after mating onwards.

Prolactin

Prolactin is produced in the pregnant and non-pregnant bitch, although prolactin concentrations are greater during pregnancy.

Other changes that occur during pregnancy

Pregnant bitches normally develop a significant decrease in haematocrit, reaching minimum values by day 60 of pregnancy. This finding is attributed to a pregnancy-related increase in blood volume.

Vulval discharge

Vulval discharge is a relatively common problem in the bitch and queen. It is most frequently seen in prepubertal animals with prepubertal vaginitis. There are many causes of vulval discharge that may result in discharge from the urinary or reproductive tract (Figure 19.8).

Investigation of vulval discharge involves collection of the breeding history and a full breeding soundness examination, including endoscopy of the caudal genitourinary tract and ultrasonography of the uterus, ovaries, bladder and kidneys. Laboratory investigation of any discharge should include routine cytology. In some specific cases, bacteriological and virological investigation may also be useful.

Nature of the discharge	Condition	History	Condition of the vulva	Cytological findings	Comments
Clear or straw coloured	Oestrus	Expected in 'heat'	Swollen or slightly soft	LIEC, AEC, RBC, no WBC	Attractive to male
Mucoid	Metoestrus	Recent oestrus	Large but soft	PBC, SIEC, VSIEC, WBC	No malaise
Mucoid	Normal pregnancy	Pregnant / recent oestrus	Large but soft	PBC, SIEC, WBC	No malaise; does not threaten pregnancy
Purulent	Juvenile vaginitis	Before first 'heat'	Normal	PBC, SIEC, WBC	May respond to antibiotics but recurs. Recovery after puberty
Purulent	Vaginitis	Variable but often excessive licking, attractive to male	Depends on the stage of the cycle	Depends on the stage of the cycle	Specific causes include chemical irritation (urine), mechanical irritation (FB), neoplasia, anatomical abnormalities and certain bacterial or viral infections
Purulent/haemorrhagic	Pyometra	Oestrus 2–8 weeks previously	Slightly swollen	WBC, SIEC, LIEC, RBC, bacteria, cell debris	Diagnosis using ultrasonography or radiography. Often malaise
Purulent/haemorrhagic	Metritis	Recent parturition	Large	Multinucleated cells, LIEC, LIEC, uterine cells	Severe malaise
Haemorrhagic	Pro-oestrus	Expected in 'heat'	Swollen	SIEC, LIEC, RBC, WBC	Attractive to male
Haemorrhagic	Oestrus	Expected in 'heat'	Swollen or slightly soft	LIEC, AEC, RBC, no WBC	Attractive to male
Haemorrhagic	Follicular cysts	Persistent discharge	Swollen	LIEC, RBC, ± WBC	No malaise; attractive to male; may develop bone marrow suppression
Haemorrhagic	Vaginal ulceration	Recent trauma or mating	Depends on the stage of the cycle	RBC, depends on the stage of the cycle	Rare; may start up to 2 weeks after mating

19.8 Differential diagnosis of vulval discharge in the bitch. (AEC: anuclear epithelial cells; FB: foreign body; LIEC: large intermediate epithelial cells; PBC: parabasal cells; RBC: erythrocytes; SIEC: small intermediate epithelial cells; VSIEC: vacuolated small intermediate epithelial cells ('metoestrus cells'); WBC: polymorphonuclear leucocytes) (continues)

▶

Nature of the discharge	Condition	History	Condition of the vulva	Cytological findings	Comments
Haemorrhagic	Placental separation	Pregnant	Normal or slightly swollen	RBC, mucus	Ultrasonography, radiography etc. will confirm pregnancy
Haemorrhagic	Sub-involution of placental sites	Persistent discharge after whelping	Normal or slightly swollen	RBC, large polynucleated vacuolated cells	No malaise; refractory to treatment
Haemorrhagic	Transmissible venereal tumour	Not all countries of the world	Depends on the stage of the cycle	RBC, tumour cells (round cells)	If tumour identified on vulva or in vagina, cytological/histological confirmation is required
Haemorrhagic	Cystitis	Frequent urination	Depends on the stage of the cycle	RBC, mucus	Small volumes of urine, dysuria
Haemorrhagic	Urinary tract neoplasia	Dysuria	Depends on the stage of the cycle	RBC, tumour cells (most often transitional cells)	Endoscopy may show origin of haemorrhage, and positive contrast cysto- or urethrography may reveal a mass. Cytological or histological confirmation is required
Haemorrhagic/brown	Abortion	Pregnant	Slightly enlarged	RBC, mucus	Ultrasonography shows uterus with similar appearance to post-partum
Green/brown	Parturition	Pregnant	Slightly swollen	RBC, SIEC, uterine cells	Panting, nest making, milk production
Green/brown	Dystocia, placental separation	Non-productive straining	Slightly swollen	RBC, SIEC, uterine cells	Ultrasonography will confirm pregnancy and fetal viability

19.8 (continued) Differential diagnosis of vulval discharge in the bitch. (AEC: anuclear epithelial cells; FB: foreign body; LIEC: large intermediate epithelial cells; PBC: parabasal cells; RBC: erythrocytes; SIEC: small intermediate epithelial cells; VSIEC: vacuolated small intermediate epithelial cells ('metoestrus cells'); WBC: polymorphonuclear leucocytes)

Cytology

Cytological examination of vulval discharge may be useful (Figure 19.8) to determine its aetiology, although cytology is only part of the investigation and clinical examination, radiography and ultrasonography also need to be employed.

Microbiology

Bacteriology: In the UK there are no bacterial venereal pathogens, although *Brucella canis* is widely present in much of continental Europe. In both the bitch and queen, routine bacteriological screening of a vulval discharge normally results in the isolation of mixed bacterial commensal organisms, including *Escherichia coli*, staphylococci, streptococci (including beta haemolytic streptococci) and others, such as *Pseudomonas* and *Proteus*. Rarely, a pure growth of bacteria is isolated, but even in these cases it is very unusual for the organism to be the primary pathogen; rather, it is an opportunistic invasion secondary to an underlying disease. Currently in the UK there is no rationale for the routine bacteriological screening of bitches or stud dogs prior to breeding.

In countries where *Brucella canis* is present, it may be a recognized cause of infertility in bitches and be associated with a vulval discharge. There is possibility of this organism entering the UK with the increased transportation of dogs to other countries for the purpose of breeding.

Virology: Canine herpesvirus is found with a low prevalence in the UK, and may be associated with a vulval discharge if it causes resorption or abortion. In some cases small vesicles are identified within the vestibule and vagina and virus may be isolated from these. In other cases paired serology samples are useful for documenting acute infection.

In the queen serological screening (see Chapter 27) is used to test for organisms that may result in pregnancy failure and result in a vulval discharge (feline herpesvirus 1, feline panleucopenia virus, feline leukaemia virus, feline coronavirus).

Male

The dog and tom cat

Reproductive dysfunction appears to be common in the male dog, with the authors observing increased referrals for male factor infertility over the last 3–5 years.

Reproductive physiology

The control of testicular function is via the gonadotrophin system previously described in the female. Luteinizing hormone (LH) (also called interstitial cell stimulating hormone) stimulates the Leydig cells to produce testosterone, dihydrotestosterone and small quantities of oestradiol. LH secretion is regulated by a feedback mechanism involving testosterone and oestradiol. Androgens mediate the development and maintenance of primary and secondary sexual characteristics and normal sexual behaviour and potency, as well as playing an important role in the initiation and maintenance of spermatogenesis. Follicle stimulating hormone (FSH) stimulates spermatogenesis indirectly by an action upon the Sertoli cells. These cells also secrete inhibin, which acts upon the pituitary to regulate the secretion of FSH. Concentrations of testosterone, LH and FSH fluctuate throughout the day. Spermatozoa are produced in the seminiferous tubules and then transported into the epididymides for maturation and storage. Sperm acquire the ability to fertilize during the phase of epididymal maturation and there is good evidence that dihydrotestosterone is pivotal in this event.

Breeding soundness

A breeding soundness examination involves collection of a breeding history, detailed clinical examination (including ultrasonography of the testes) and laboratory investigation of a semen sample. Methods of semen collection are described in standard texts.

The ejaculate of the dog has three distinct fractions, of which the first and third originate from the prostate gland. In the tom cat the ejaculate is relatively homogenous. Normally only the second fraction of the dog's ejaculate, but the entire ejaculate of the tom, is evaluated for the purpose of investigating fertility. Cytological and bacteriological examination of the third fraction of the dog's ejaculate may be useful for demonstrating the cause of prostatic disease.

Assessment of semen quality

Evaluation of a semen sample can be useful for confirmation of normal fertility in an animal prior to breeding, or when there is concern over infertility. Furthermore, detailed semen evaluation should be undertaken in potential stud dogs prior to purchase, before importation and before embarking upon semen preservation.

Spermatozoal number: Measurement of the total number of sperm within the ejaculate is the most accurate assessment of sperm production. The total sperm output is calculated by multiplying the volume of the sperm-containing (second) fraction by the sperm concentration. Sperm concentration is conventionally measured using a haemocytometer counting chamber after dilution of the sample, usually with distilled water at a ratio of 1 in 200. A traditional Neubauer counting chamber (see Figure 23.3) is usually used; the number of sperm in five of the large squares (each comprising 16 small squares) are counted and that total multiplied by a factor of 10×10^6 (e.g. if after a 1:200 dilution, 36 sperm are counted in this area, the sperm concentration will be 360 million sperm per ml (360×10^6/ml)).

A relationship has been demonstrated between breed and the number of sperm ejaculated. Larger breeds produce more sperm. There is, however, a wide normal range of total sperm output for fertile dogs (Figure 19.9) and tom cats (Figure 19.10).

Spermatozoal morphology: Sperm morphology can be examined using a background stain such as Indian ink, or by staining with Giemsa. Spermac® is a stain that facilitates evaluation of acrosomal morphology and nigrosin–eosin allows assessment of live/dead ratios.

For nigrosin and eosin staining a drop of semen is mixed with 5 drops of stain and a smear is made immediately and allowed to dry. Examination with oil immersion microscopy allows determination of both vital staining (dead or membrane-damaged sperm are stained pink by the eosin, live sperm remain unstained) and individual sperm morphology. One hundred sperm are examined and noted as being either dead (pink) or live (white) and their individual morphology are recorded. An example of a table for recording sperm morphology and vital staining is given in Figure 19.11.

	Progressive motility (%)	Sperm-rich volume (ml)	Sperm concentration ($\times 10^6$/ml)	Total sperm output ($\times 10^6$)	Live normal sperm (%)
Mean	82.1	1.2	328.6	410.8	73.5
SEM	0.9	0.05	15.3	21.3	2.1
Range	40–95	0.3–3.2	50–610	36–1550	50–92

19.9 Seminal characteristics from 121 dogs that were fertile in the 6 months prior to semen collection and the 6 months after semen collection (unpublished observations). SEM = standard error of the mean.

	Progressive motility (%)	Sperm-rich volume (ml)	Sperm concentration ($\times 10^6$/ml)	Total sperm output ($\times 10^6$)	Live normal sperm (%)
Mean	62.5	0.65	95.2	145.0	56.4
SEM	2.8	0.02	25.3	34.3	4.2
Range	40–65	0.25–1.10	52–120	32–178	39–69

19.10 Seminal characteristics from 5 fertile tom cats (collected by artificial vagina) (unpublished observations). SEM = standard error of the mean.

Morphology	Number of live sperm	Number of dead sperm
Normal		
Proximal droplets		
Distal droplets		
Coiled tail		
Detached head		
Other morphological abnormalities		

19.11 Example of a table used for recording the morphological and vital status of sperm stained with nigrosin–eosin.

For normal fertility there are usually >60% live normal spermatozoa; values <60% are associated with reduced fertilty, although some fertile dogs have values below this (see Figure 19.9). Normal and abnormal sperm morphology are demonstrated in Figure 19.12.

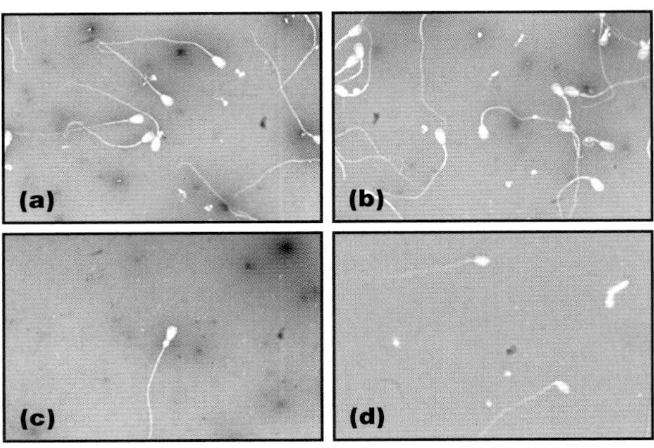

19.12 Dog semen stained with nigrosin/eosin. **(a)** Normal sperm morphology (one centrally positioned sperm has a coiled tail). Nigrosin provides the background colour and eosin stains dead sperm (none is present in this field). **(b)** A large number of sperm have significant bending of the tails and midpieces. These morphological changes are either secondary or tertiary sperm abnormalities. The sperm positioned in the top right corner has a distal cytoplasmic droplet. **(c)** Individual dog sperm with a spherical swelling at the region of the neck. This is a typical proximal cytoplasmic droplet. **(d)** Two sperm with broken/abnormal necks and a significant tail abnormality.

Spermatozoal motility: Dog sperm motility is conventionally evaluated by placing a drop of semen on a microscope slide under a coverslip and observing sperm movement at X200 and X400 magnification. Importantly, sperm motility is influenced by temperature and samples should be examined at a standard temperature, commonly 38°C. Not all sperm that are motile have normal motility, and it is important to record the type of motility and the percentage of sperm with that motility. Sperm that have normal motility swim very quickly in straight lines across the field of view (they have good progression). An example of a table used for recording sperm motility is given in Figure 19.13.

Category	Description	Percentage of sperm
0	Immotile sperm	
I	Sperm that are motile but not progressive	
II	Sperm that have sluggish motility and poor progression	
III	Sperm with reasonable motility and moderate progression	
IV	Sperm with rapid forward progressive motility	

19.13 Example of a table used for recording estimated sperm motility in unstained sperm examined at body temperature.

For normal fertility there are usually > 60% of sperm with normal motility defined as rapid forward progression (category IV in Figure 9.13). Note that motile sperm in categories I–III do not have normal motility. The cut-off point for a reduction in fertility is when the percentage of sperm with rapid forward progression reduces below 60%, although some fertile dogs have values slightly below this (see Figure 19.9).

Microbiological screening: In some countries, routine screening of dogs for *Brucella canis* is recommended. This organism is not currently present in the UK and so screening here is unnecessary. Dogs may harbour herpes virus in small vesicle lesions present on the penis and mucosa of the sheath, but clinical inspection usually reveals the lesions, and virological screening of the prepuce is unlikely to detect virus in the absence of lesions.

Absence of testicular tissue

Males with an absence of scrotal testes are either previously castrated or are bilateral cryptorchids. Anorchia is very rare in both the dog and tom cat.

In normal entire dogs there is significant variation in testosterone production throughout the day with testosterone concentrations of 0.5–1.5 ng/ml (1.7–5.2 mmol/l) at the trough of production, and 3.5–6.0 ng/ml (12.1–20.8 mmol/l) at the peak of production. In dogs with no testes, testosterone concentrations are <0.5 ng/ml (<1.7 mmol/l). Single samples could potentially be taken at the trough of production, resulting in a false diagnosis of absent testicular tissue. For this reason stimulation tests are normally performed using either hCG or a GnRH analogue. A basal plasma/serum sample is obtained, hCG (44 IU/kg i.m.) or GnRH analogue (2.0 μg/kg i.m.) is injected and a second blood sample is taken 60–120 minutes later. In both cases a significant increase in testosterone concentration (to >5.0 ng/ml (17 mmol/l)) in the post-stimulation sample is diagnostic of testicular tissue. There should be no false positive diagnoses.

The infertile male

Males with presumed infertility should have semen collected and evaluated as described above. Such examination may reveal the cause of the infertility. In addition it may also be prudent to undertake a more detailed examination of the seminal plasma.

Semen quality

Laboratory investigation of a semen sample in an alleged infertile male may reveal a number of different abnormalities, including abnormalities of sperm number, sperm morphology or sperm motility. These abnormalities may be identified concurrently.

Azoospermia: Azoospermia is an apparently normal ejaculation producing an ejaculate that contains no sperm. There is a number of causes, including incomplete ejaculation, obstructive azoospermia and gonadal dysfunction (which may be congenital or acquired). In the dog, measurement of alkaline phosphatase concentration in seminal plasma may be helpful in differentiating these conditions (see seminal plasma below).

Oligozoospermia: Oligozoospermia is an ejaculate containing low numbers of morphologically normal sperm. This is rare in dogs but may occur for one of several reasons:

- Incomplete ejaculation
- Retrograde ejaculation
- Frequent ejaculation
- Recent testicular insult.

Confirmation of retrograde ejaculation can be made by preventing the dog from urinating prior to semen collection, and then after attempted semen collection, catheterizing the bladder, collection of urine and lavage of the bladder with 10–20 ml of saline. The collected urine and flushings should be centrifuged to look for the presence of sperm. Large numbers of sperm (>10 per low power field) in a wet preparation of the centrifuged pellet is diagnostic.

Teratozoospermia: Teratozoospermia is abnormal sperm morphology, which, in many cases, results in impaired sperm motility. When present in large numbers, abnormal midpiece droplets, other midpiece defects, and abnormalities of the base/midpiece region are associated with infertility. Sperm with midpiece defects and deformed acrosomes have been found following experimental *Brucella canis* infection.

Primary spermatozoal abnormalities (abnormalities that occur during spermatogenesis, for example malformations of the sperm head) may result from orchitis, congenital defects of spermatogenesis, toxin exposure, administration of hormonal or chemotherapeutic agents or elevated scrotal temperature. Secondary spermatozoal abnormalities (abnormalities that occur after sperm formation but during sperm maturation, e.g. bending of the midpiece or tail) may occur with epididymal disorders or following the administration of agents that influence epididymal function. Tertiary abnormalities, such as broken tails, occur as a result of poor semen collection or handling.

Asthenozoospermia: Asthenozoospermia is normal sperm morphology but a reduction in motility. The condition is rare in the dog without concurrent oligozoospermia. Recognized causes include:

- Contamination of the ejaculate with toxic compounds (latex artificial vagina liners, lubricants, certain plastic syringes, urine, water, sterilizing agents)
- Agglutination of sperm in dogs that produce antisperm antibodies (seen in some dogs with *Brucella canis* infection).

Seminal plasma

Measurement of alkaline phosphatase concentration in the seminal plasma may be useful for the diagnosis of dogs with obstruction of the tubular genitalia. This enzyme originates from the epididymides, and therefore a low concentration may indicate either incomplete ejaculation or tubular obstruction. Normal concentrations (5000–40,000 IU/l) combined with an absence of sperm indicate azoospermia.

The ejaculate of the tom cat contains significant concentrations of alkaline phosphatase.

Cytology

Common haematology stains can be used for cytological examination of ejaculate. It is not uncommon for low numbers of inflammatory cells to be identified within the semen sample; most originate from the prepuce during semen collection. High numbers of inflammatory cells are seen in cases of epididymitis, orchitis and prostatitis. Red blood cells and prostatic cells are commonly identified in the prostatic fluid of dogs with benign prostatic hyperplasia, and multinucleate cells may be identified in dogs with prostatic neoplasia. Many dogs with significant prostatic disease will not ejaculate and therefore prostatic fluid needs to be collected via lavage of the prostatic urethra after massage of the gland per rectum, or via ultrasound-guided fine needle aspiration.

Microbiology

There is little information available for the tom cat.

Bacteriology: There has been considerable debate concerning the role of bacteria within the prostatic fluid and seminal plasma of dogs. However many aerobic and anaerobic organisms are frequently isolated from the prepuce of the dog and the bacterial flora is usually mixed. These bacteria are similar to those identified in the bitch, including beta haemolytic *Streptococcus* and are now considered normal commensal organisms. *Brucella canis* may cause epididymitis, orchitis and infertility and is a known venereal pathogen, but is not currently present in the UK. Recent data suggests that mycoplasmas and ureaplasmas are also commensal organisms, although some authors have suggested that they are implicated in cases of infertility.

Virology: Herpesvirus may cause vesicular lesions on the penis and prepuce. These lesions are usually asymptomatic, although in some cases there is secondary infection and pain at coitus. The main concern is potential of transmission to the bitch at coitus. Virus may be isolated from the vesicles or exposure may be detected serologically.

Hormone measurement

There is little published information concerning measurement of plasma hormones and their relationship to infertility in dogs and tom cats. In some infertile males there may be normal plasma concentrations of testosterone and LH, and elevated concentrations of FSH (presumably due to reduced production of inhibin by the Sertoli cells). Serial measurement of FSH may therefore be useful in these cases; normal FSH values are 70–85 ng/ml.

Low serum testosterone and LH concentrations indicate a possible hypothalamic, pituitary or testicular dysfunction. Pituitary or hypothalamic disease can be further demonstrated by persistently low LH concentrations following GnRH challenge (2.0 μg/kg i.m.), whereas increased LH following such administration confirms the problem to be testicular in origin.

Testicular disease

In males with known testicular disease (small testes or testes of abnormal texture), the primary diagnostic tool is testicular ultrasonography. In addition it may be helpful to collect a semen sample (see above), or to perform fine needle aspiration for cytological evaluation.

Ultrasonography is useful in evaluation of suspected testicular tumours. Oestrogen-secreting tumours (usually Sertoli cell tumours) can be diagnosed by documenting increased concentration of oestradiol after stimulation with GnRH or hCG (see Presence of ovarian tissue, above).

Testicular biopsy is widely recommended in standard texts for the investigation of a wide range of disease processes. It is now clear however that testicular biopsy may itself result in severe testicular pathology. Whilst the sample collected may be diagnostic, the diagnostic benefit of the procedure rarely justifies the risk to future fertility in the authors' opinion.

Cytological investigation of prostatic disease is discussed in Chapter 20.

Case examples

Case 1

Signalment

11-year-old female Springer Spaniel, spayed at 1 year of age.

History

Episodes of male attractiveness that have waxed and waned over the last 5 months. Small volume vulval discharge and increased licking of the vulva. No signs of pseudopregnancy following the episodes of male attractiveness.

Clinical pathology data

Vaginal cytology collected at the time of attractiveness revealed approximately 20 neutrophils per hpf, moderate amounts of mucus, and 95% parabasal cells with 5% small intermediate cells. Large numbers of bacteria were evident with many being engulfed by neutrophils. Bacterial culture was not performed

A blood sample collected 2 weeks after the end of the period of attractiveness showed that plasma progesterone was <0.5 ng/ml.

How would you interpret these results and what are the possible differential diagnoses?

Vaginal cytological results confirm the absence of oestrus in the bitch. A failure of progesterone to increase after the period of attractiveness confirms that the bitch does not have an ovarian remnant. The most likely diagnosis is male attraction to the vulval discharge, the cause of which has not yet been elucidated. An atrophic vaginitis would be consistent with the history of neutering 10 years previously and the presence of neutrophils and mucus identified on the vaginal smear.

Case 2

Signalment

6-year-old male Labrador Retriever.

History

Experienced stud dog that had produced 12 litters. Last four bitches, mated over a period of 7 months, had failed to become pregnant. Normal libido. Testes of normal size but somewhat soft in texture.

Clinical pathology data

There was no clear separation of the semen sample into three fractions. No sperm were present. What was thought to be the third fraction was heavily contaminated with erythrocytes

ALP concentration in the combined first and second fractions was 35,000 IU/l (reference interval 5000–40,000 IU/l).

How would you interpret these results and what are the possible differential diagnoses?

The presence of high (normal) concentrations of ALP in the absence of sperm indicate azoospermia. The clinical findings fit with this as a diagnosis (based on the soft testes). Ultrasonography of the testes is warranted. Autoimmune degenerative orchitis is recognized as a cause of azoospermia in the Labrador.

References and further reading

England GCW (1992) Vaginal cytology and cervico vaginal mucus arborisation in the breeding management of bitches. *Journal of Small Animal Practice* **33,** 577–582

England GCW (2000) Semen evaluation, artificial insemination and infertility in the male dog. In: *Textbook of Veterinary Internal Medicine, 5th edn*, ed. SJ Ettinger and EC Feldman, pp. 1571–1580. WB Saunders, Philadelphia

Mooney CT and Peterson ME (2004) *BSAVA Manual of Canine and Feline Endocrinology, 3rd edn.* BSAVA Publications, Gloucester

Simpson G, England GCW and Harvey M (1998) *BSAVA Manual of Small Animal Reproduction and Neonatal Care.* BSAVA Publications, Cheltenham

20

Diagnostic cytology

John K. Dunn and Karen Gerber

Introduction

Diagnostic cytology (cytopathology) is most frequently used to investigate superficial cutaneous or subcutaneous masses, lymphadenopathy and body cavity effusions. The examination of body cavity effusions is reviewed in Chapter 21; indications for cytological examination are listed in Figure 20.1.

- Soft tissue masses:
  - cutaneous/subcutaneous lesions
  - enlarged lymph nodes
  - intrathoracic or intra-abdominal masses
- Suspected splenic or hepatic pathology
- Body cavity effusions (pleura, peritoneal, pericardial)
- Upper and lower respiratory tract disease:
  - nasal flush
  - tracheal wash
  - bronchoalveolar lavage
  - pulmonary aspirates
- Synovial fluid analysis
- Cerebrospinal fluid analysis
- Urogenital disease:
  - prostatic aspirates/washes
  - kidney aspirates
  - urine sediment examination
- Staging of the oestrous cycle (vaginal cytology)
- Bone marrow evaluation

20.1 Indications for cytological examination.

Cytology is a useful diagnostic tool in a practice setting, since samples can be collected quickly, easily and inexpensively. There is usually no requirement for a general anaesthetic (although light sedation may be required), the processing time is short, and results are available in minutes. The collection techniques are less invasive than surgical biopsy and therefore give rise to fewer complications. Potential complications include haemorrhage, pneumothorax (intrathoracic lesions), sepsis, bacteraemia and tumour seeding, either along the needle tract or via the haematogenous route. In reality, such complications are extremely rare. The risk of haemorrhage is greater if the animal has an underlying coagulopathy (more so with aspirates from liver and kidneys than the spleen since the spleen has a fibroelastic capsule). Tumour seeding has occasionally been reported with aspirates from transitional cell carcinomas of the bladder wall.

Diagnostic accuracy

The diagnostic accuracy of cytology is influenced by many factors, including:

- the quality of the sample submitted
- the organ and disease process being investigated
- the experience and training of the cytopathologist.

Sample quality is affected by operator experience, in both sample harvesting and handling prior to submission. For example, excessive downward pressure when preparing a crush smear can render a good-quality aspirate non-diagnostic by causing cell rupture. Some organs exfoliate cells easily (e.g. lymph nodes), whereas it may be more difficult to harvest diagnostic samples from other organs (e.g. kidney, bone). In suspected neoplasia, tumour type will also influence cell yield. Discrete round cell and epithelial tumours tend to exfoliate cells in sheets or large clusters whereas aspirates from tumours of mesenchymal origin are more frequently non-diagnostic because the cells within the tumours are bound together in a matrix material such as collagen or osteoid.

A study by Kristensen *et al.* (1990) showed a positive correlation between cytological and histological diagnoses in 86% of cases of canine and feline liver disease. The specimens that did not correlate well originated from livers affected by diseases in which the cells did not readily exfoliate or where lesions were discrete (focal or multifocal). Correlation is improved where there is diffuse change: Roth (2001) showed good correlation, especially in cases of fatty change and lymphoma. Discordance between the cytological and histological findings occurred most frequently with fibrosis and hepatitis (where evidence of inflammation was not seen on the cytology specimens). Where mass lesions are visualized by ultrasonography, or other imaging techniques, it might be expected that accuracy may be improved, but this is not borne out by recent work (Wang *et al.*, 2004.) This study, comparing the results of cytology of ultrasound-guided fine needle aspirates of the liver with histological diagnoses in dogs and cats, reported a much lower rate of agreement (30% for dogs; 51% for cats). The highest percentage of agreement occurred in vacuolar hepatopathy. Inflammation was correctly identified in <40% of cases (Wang *et al.*, 2004). In contrast to the poor agreement for hepatic diseases, Villiers *et al.,* (1995) showed good correlation (82%) between cytological and histological diagnoses for canine intrathoracic lesions. More recently, Bonfanti *et al.* (2004) reported 89.4% agreement between cytology and histology of deep thoracic and abdominal masses, and 100% specificity for neoplasia. Similarly, Chalita *et al.* (2001) reported 89% accuracy using fine needle aspirate cytology in canine skin and soft tissue tumours.

Limitations of diagnostic cytology

Cytology can be performed either independently or in conjunction with histological examination of a surgical biopsy. Biopsy specimens have the advantage of preserving tissue architecture, and therefore provide more information regarding the tissue of origin and biological behaviour of a tumour (e.g. grading, degree of tissue infiltration, presence or absence of necrosis).

The requirement for histological examination depends to a large extent on the type of lesion under investigation. Small mobile or very firm lesions, for example, are unlikely to yield sufficient material for cytological evaluation. Virtually all mast cell tumours and histiocytomas can be diagnosed definitively on the basis of cytological examination alone (although histology is usually required to grade mast cell tumours); in contrast, poorly differentiated tumours, especially those of mesenchymal origin, nearly always require concurrent histological examination of a biopsy specimen in order to define tissue type accurately.

It is important also to realize that a cytological specimen may not always be representative of the lesion under investigation; e.g. perilesional fat may be aspirated in animals that are particularly obese. Large lymphomatous lymph nodes may become necrotic and yield non-diagnostic aspirates. Impression smears or scrapings of ulcerated lesions may contain only superficial cells and secondary inflammation/infection may result in dysplastic changes which can mimic those associated with neoplasia (see below).

Artefacts

Failure to recognize artefacts or non-diagnostic samples can lead to serious and often dangerous errors in interpretation. The worst scenario is when a poor-quality or hypocellular smear is over-interpreted. Many artefacts arise because of poor sample collection, smear preparation or staining techniques (Figure 20.2a–d). Some problems are unavoidable; splenic aspirates, for example, invariably contain a lot of blood, reflecting the vascularity of the organ. Smears that are too thick or heavily contaminated with blood are difficult to interpret. Poor smear preparation may result in large numbers of smudged cells, 'bare' nuclei or cytoplasmic strands, and other degenerative changes such as nuclear and cytoplasmic vacuolation. Other common artefacts include excessive stain precipitate, dirty slides, water artefact, starch granules (from surgical gloves; Figure 20.2e) and ultrasound gel aspirated when fine needle aspiration is performed under ultrasound guidance (Figure 20.2f).

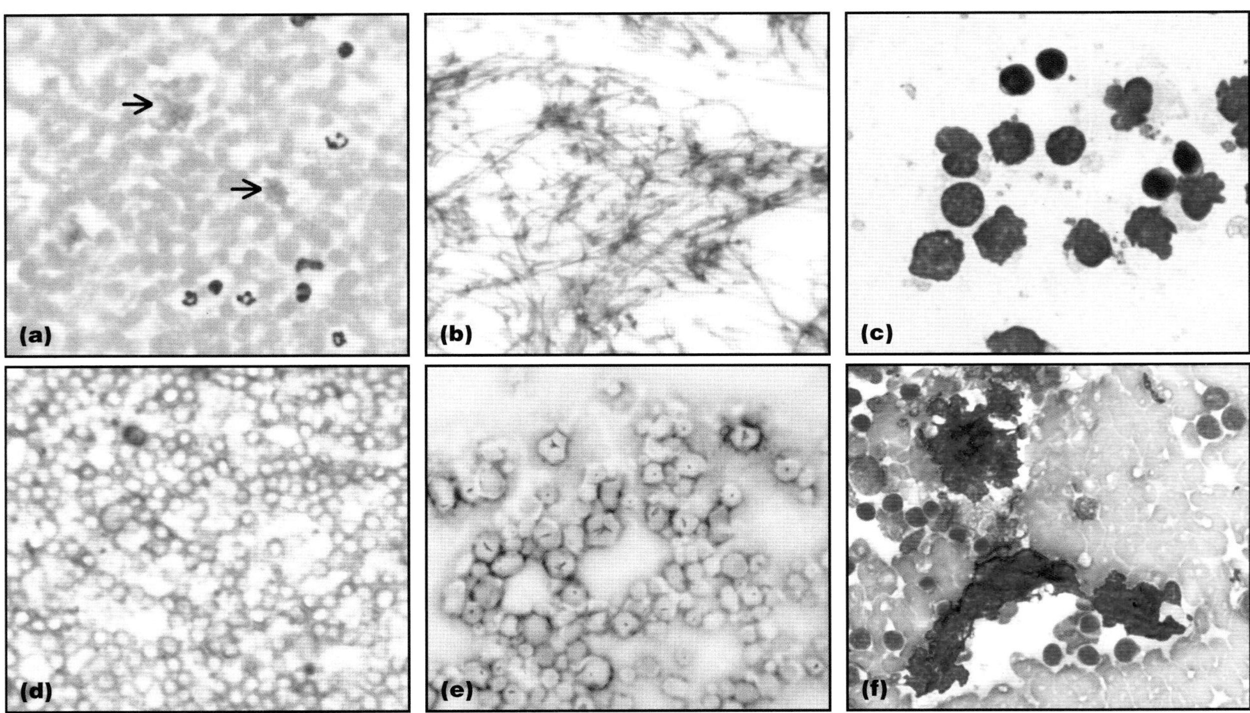

20.2 Fine needle aspirates: artefacts. (a) This aspirate from a small cutaneous mass consists only of blood; there are numerous small platelet clusters (arrowed). (b) In this lymph node aspirate there are ruptured nuclei and strands of nuclear protein, resulting from damage during the smearing process. (c) The lymphoid cells have been stripped of their cytoplasm, leaving numerous 'bare' nuclei. (d) This aspirate appears to consist of a population of small round cells, but the thickness of the smear is such that more precise cytological interpretation is not possible. (e) This aspirate contains a large number of glove powder (starch) granules. (f) Aspirate from the spleen of a dog with lymphoma; the pink granular material is ultrasound gel. (f, Courtesy of L Blackwood.) (Wright's stain (a–e, Rapi-Diff II (f); original magnification X400 (f), X500 (a,b,d,e), X1000 (c))

Collection techniques

The choice of collection technique depends on the anatomical location and characteristics of the lesion, and also the temperament of the patient.

Fine needle aspiration

Indications for fine needle aspiration (FNA) for cytology are as listed in Figure 20.1.

FNA technique

The area in which the lesion is located is clipped and cleaned with alcohol (if a body cavity or joint space is to be penetrated, or the sample is required for microbiology, the site should be surgically prepared). The mass is immobilized with one hand and a 21 or 23 gauge needle with 5 ml syringe attached inserted into the lesion (Figure 20.3a,b). Suction is applied, either continuously or intermittently.

- **Continuous suction** is used for firm masses, e.g. suspected sarcomas, which are less likely to exfoliate large numbers of cells. Withdraw the plunger to one half to three quarters of the volume of the syringe (to apply 2–3 ml suction) (Figure 20.3c). Maintain suction and move the needle to and fro, redirecting the needle several times within the lesion. Release the suction and remove the needle from the mass. Disconnect the needle from the syringe.
- **Intermittent suction** is a variation of this technique and is more suitable for smaller lesions, where it is not possible to advance or redirect the needle without exiting the mass. Withdraw and release the plunger several times with the needle inserted in the mass. Release the suction and withdraw the needle from the lesion.
- Fine needle aspirates can also be obtained using a **non-suction** (needle-only) technique (Figure 20.3d). This method causes less damage to fragile cells, e.g. lymphoid cells, and minimizes blood contamination. It is therefore useful for aspirating highly vascular masses and lymph nodes, and for obtaining ultrasound-guided samples of lesions within body cavities (see below). The needle is moved to and fro several times within the lesion and then withdrawn.

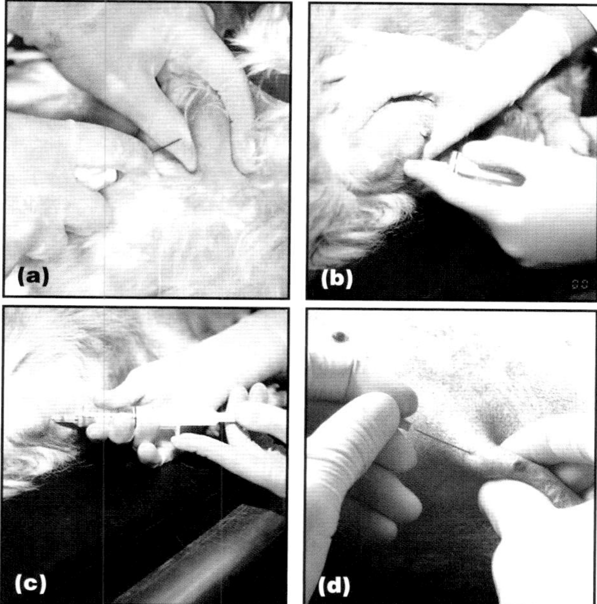

20.3 Fine needle aspiration technique. A needle, with a 5 ml syringe attached, is inserted into: (a) an enlarged prescapular lymph node; (b) a mammary gland mass. (c) Suction is applied to the syringe by withdrawing the plunger. (d) Non-suction (needle-only) method. (d, Courtesy of L Blackwood)

No matter which technique is used, an air-filled syringe is attached to the needle (if a syringe is already attached, it is disconnected from the needle and filled with air). The contents of the needle containing the sample are then expelled on to one or more clean glass sides (see Figure 20.5), and smears prepared using one of the techniques described below. Aspirates from fluid-filled lesions should be transferred into an EDTA tube (and a plain tube if microbiology is required). A fresh smear should be prepared immediately using a blood film or line concentration technique (see below).

Special considerations:

- Fine needle aspirates from internal organs (liver, spleen, kidney) and intrathoracic or intra-abdominal masses are best performed under ultrasound guidance (Figure 20.4). This ensures that large vessels are avoided and the aspirate is collected from a representative part of the lesion. The procedure is generally well tolerated; light sedation may be necessary in some cases. The overlying chest or abdominal wall should be surgically prepared. Continuous or intermittent suction or non-suction techniques can be used to obtain the sample, keeping the needle in a single plane and advancing it to and fro
- For splenic aspirates, which are excessively contaminated with blood, aspirated samples can be applied to slides prepositioned at 45 degrees or more to the horizontal, e.g. against a sandbag (as for a bone marrow aspirate), or the slides can be held vertically to allow excess blood to run down the slide before making the smear
- Long spinal needles can be used for very deep lesions (the stylet being removed and needle attached once the needle is positioned within the lesion).

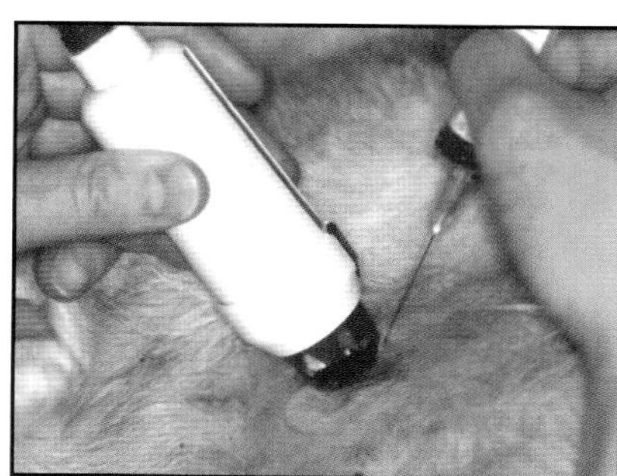

20.4 FNA of intrathoracic or intrabdominal masses is best performed under ultrasound guidance. (Reproduced with permission from *In Practice*.)

- A coagulation profile and platelet count should be performed if a haemostatic defect is considered likely, such as in liver disease, although significant haemorrhage is rarely encountered following FNA.

Smear preparation

A smear can be prepared using one of the following methods.

Squash preparation: The aspirate is expelled on to the centre of a glass slide (Figure 20.5a). A second spreader slide is placed horizontally and at right angles to spread the sample, taking care not to exert too much downward pressure to avoid rupturing the cells. The spreader slide is then drawn quickly and smoothly across the bottom slide (Figure 20.5b). In most cases the weight of the spreader slide is sufficient to spread the cells. Note that it is the smear produced on the *underside of the spreader slide* that is examined under the microscope.

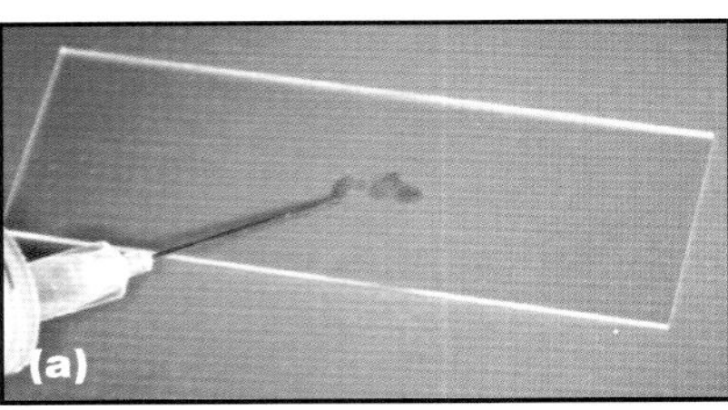

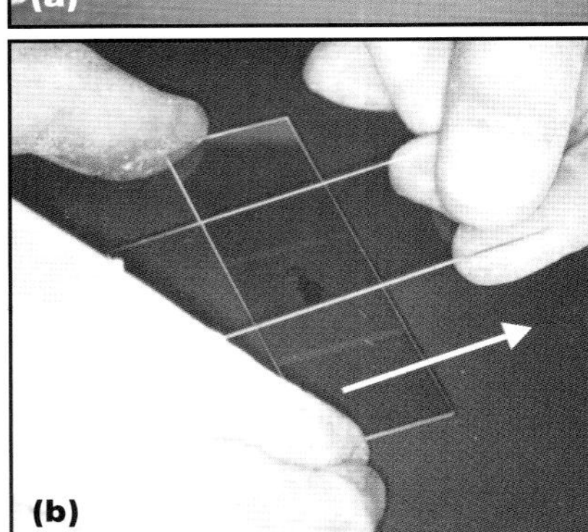

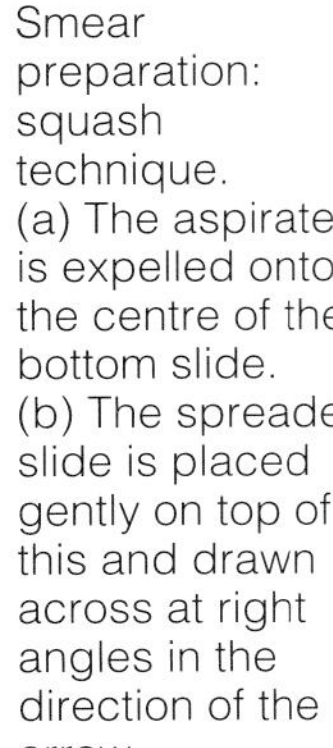

20.5 Smear preparation: squash technique. (a) The aspirate is expelled onto the centre of the bottom slide. (b) The spreader slide is placed gently on top of this and drawn across at right angles in the direction of the arrow.

Blood film technique: A 'spreader' slide with one corner missing is used to prepare the smear in order to avoid spreading the cells over the edges of the slide. The aspirate is expelled from the syringe towards one end of the slide. The spreader slide should be angled at 20–45 degrees in front of the sample and then drawn back until it comes into contact with the sample drop (see Figure 3.12). After the sample has spread along the interface of the two slides, the spreader slide is advanced gently forwards to create a smear with a feathered edge. This technique is useful for fluid aspirates (but not those with low cellularity).

A modification of this technique is the 'line concentration' technique. The sample is smeared as for a blood film but after the spreader has been advanced about two-thirds of the way along the bottom slide it is lifted abruptly upwards (Figure 20.6). This has the effect of concentrating cells along a line at the end of the smear. This technique is useful for hypocellular fluid aspirates, e.g. aspirates from cystic masses, or for samples heavily contaminated with blood.

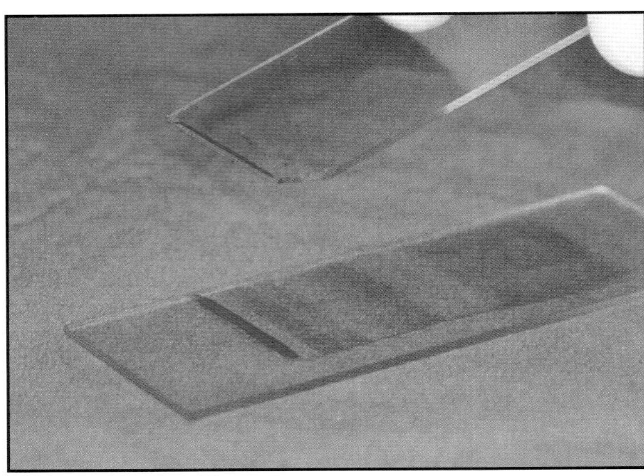

20.6 Smear preparation: line concentration technique. After the spreader has been advanced two thirds of the way along the bottom slide it is lifted abruptly upwards in order to concentrate cells at the end of the smear.

Processing fluid samples

Fluid aspirates should be collected into EDTA and also into a plain tube if microbiology will be required. The sample is then processed using the methods described for effusions in Chapter 21.

Fluids of low cellularity, such as transudates, peritoneal fluid and CSF samples, should be centrifuged at slow speed (1000–1500 RPM) for 5 minutes to concentrate the cells. The sediment is then resuspended in a few drops of supernatant, and a smear made. It should be noted, however, that centrifugation and resuspension may create additional cellular artefacts. Most commercial laboratories use a cytospin centrifuge, which deposits cells directly on a predefined area of the slide.

Impression smears and scrapings

Impression smears

Impression smears can be prepared from the surface of ulcerated cutaneous lesions (Figure 20.7a,b). Imprints should be taken before and after cleaning the lesion with a saline-moistened gauze swab. Several imprints can be prepared on one slide simply by making contact with the surface of the lesion (the slide should not be smeared across the lesion). Impression smears can also be prepared from the cut surface of surgically excised or post-mortem specimens (Figure 20.7c–e). Excess blood or tissue fluid is removed before making the smear, by blotting the surface dry with a clean paper towel (Figure 20.7d).

The disadvantages of this technique are:

- It collects relatively few cells
- The cells collected may not necessarily be representative of the lesion under investigation. For example, ulcerated lesions are often secondarily inflamed or infected, which may result in only inflammatory cells being harvested or may induce in the cells of interest dysplastic changes that mimic those associated with neoplasia.

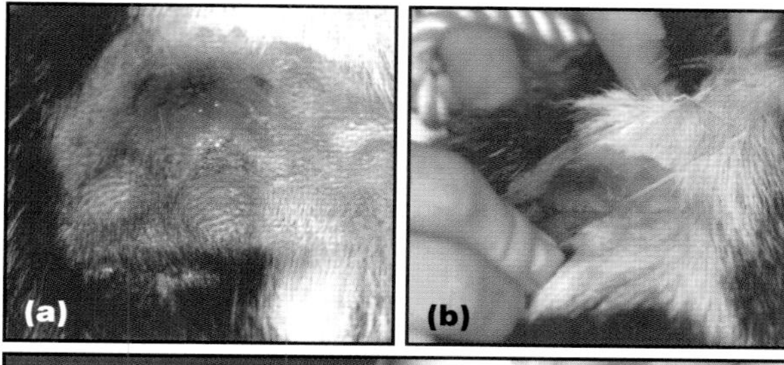

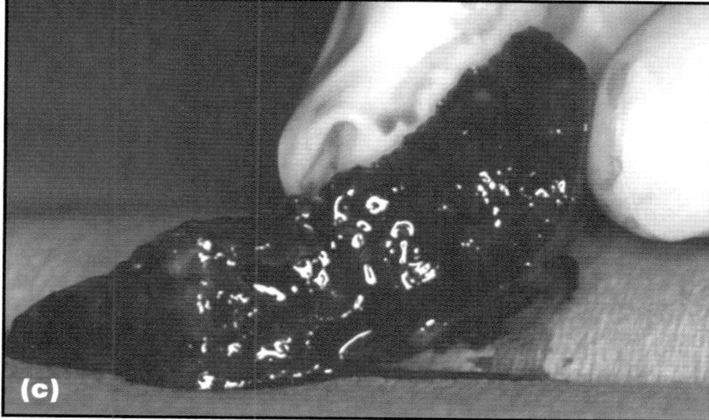

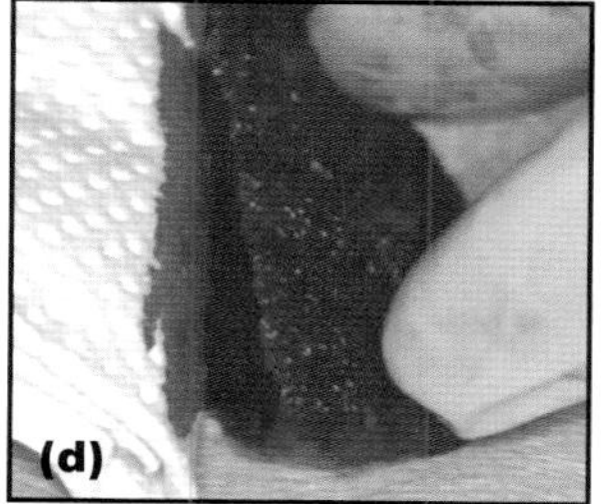

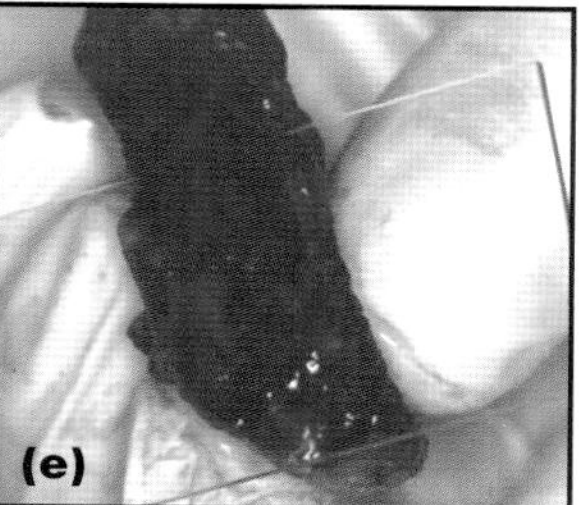

20.7 Impression smears can be prepared from the surface of an ulcerated cutaneous lesion, e.g. cutaneous lymphoma (a,b). The technique is also useful for collecting cells from the cut surface of a surgically excised or postmortem specimen, e.g. spleen (c). Excess blood is first removed by blotting the cut surface with a clean paper towel (d). Several imprints can be prepared on the same slide (e). (Reproduced with permission from *In Practice*.)

Impression smears are therefore of limited use in the diagnosis of superficial neoplastic lesions, but can be useful for intraoperative confirmation of neoplasia when impression smears from biopsy samples or excised tissue are examined.

Scrapings

Scrapings collect more cells than impression smears but are otherwise subject to the same disadvantages. Scraping is a useful technique for harvesting cells from lesions that are unlikely to yield large numbers of cells on fine needle aspiration, e.g. mesenchymal tumours that are ulcerated. The technique is similar to that used to collect skin scrapings for dermatological investigations (see Chapter 24). The material collected on the scalpel blade is teased on to a glass slide with a needle and the smear prepared using the squash preparation technique (see above).

Swab smears

A swab or cotton bud can be used to collect cells from fistulous tracts and from the vagina. The swab should be first moistened with normal saline to minimise cell damage. It should be rubbed against the surface of the lesion or vaginal wall, and then gently rolled on to a clean glass slide (not dragged across it).

Brushings

Brushings are useful for obtaining cells from very soft friable specimens, e.g. splenic haemangiosarcomas. Cells are transferred from the cut surface of the excised tissue to a glass slide with a fine camel hair paintbrush. This technique can also be used to evaluate the gastrointestinal tract by passing a brush through the biopsy channel of an endoscope.

Stains

Romanowsky stains

Romanowsky stains, such as Wright's, Giemsa, Wright's–Giemsa and May–Grünwald–Giemsa, generally provide excellent cytoplasmic and nuclear detail, and have the advantage of staining bacterial organisms. Several alcohol-based 'fast' staining kits such as Diff-Quik are also commercially available.

Smears should be air-dried or, if staining is to be delayed for more than a few days, cell preservation can be enhanced by fixing in methyl alcohol for 2–3 minutes. A good smear consists of a monolayer of cells that 'fix' to the slide within 30–60 seconds. Smears that are too thick dry slowly, resulting in poor morphological detail and condensation and shrinking of nuclei. Thicker smears, such as those prepared from lymph node or bone marrow aspirates, may have to be stained for twice the recommended time or even longer.

It is important to realize that the tinctorial properties of the different Romanowsky stains vary considerably (some stain more blue or more pink than others) and also that some of the rapid staining kits may not stain mast cell granules.

New methylene blue

New methylene blue (NMB) is rarely used as a cytological stain. It is an aqueous stain that allows immediate examination of a smear after application to air-dried cells. It provides excellent nuclear and nucleolar detail and is useful for staining thick, haemodiluted smears that contain large clumps of cells.

Trichrome stains

Trichrome stains, such as Papanicolaou or Sano's modified stain, are applied to cells that have been immediately wet-fixed in alcohol or by using a spray fixative. Air-dried cells can be rehydrated for 30 seconds in saline and then wet-fixed in the same way. Like NMB, these stains provide superior nuclear and nucleolar detail but cytoplasm stains weakly. Wet fixation also causes red cell lysis, which may improve visual examination of any clumps of cells that are present. These stains are useful for very thick smears or those heavily contaminated with blood. However, the staining techniques are time-consuming and not generally practical for a veterinary practice laboratory.

Other stains

Other special stains are sometimes used on cytological specimens; for example, toluidine blue (mast cell granules in poorly differentiated mast cell tumours), Fontana stain (malignant melanomas with very few melanin pigment granules), and periodic acid–Schiff (fungal hyphae and fungal spores).

Microscopic evaluation of a cytological specimen

1. The smear should be scanned at low magnification (4X or 10X objective) to identify areas of increased cellularity or areas with different staining characteristics. Crystals, foreign bodies and parasites are usually visible at low magnification.
2. The 20X objective lens can be used to assess cellularity and cellular composition, i.e. the relative numbers of different cell types (e.g. inflammatory cells, epithelial cells).
3. Changing to the 40X objective (or 50X or 60X 'dry' lens) and then to the 100X oil immersion lens allows evaluation of cell morphology in greater detail.

The basic aim of cytological evaluation is to establish an aetiological and/or morphological diagnosis in order to obtain a more accurate prognosis. An attempt should be made to answer the following questions:

- Is the quality of the specimen good enough to evaluate?
- Are the cells present normal for this anatomical site?
- Is the lesion inflammatory/reactive or non-inflammatory?
- If inflammatory, what is the predominant inflammatory cell type(s) and is an aetiological agent present; i.e. is there evidence of bacterial or fungal infection?
- If non-inflammatory, is the lesion neoplastic, hyperplastic or dysplastic?
- If neoplastic, what is the origin of the cells present and is the lesion benign or malignant?

Some cytological terminology is explained in Figure 20.8.

Cytology of inflammatory disease

Classification

An inflammatory response can be classified as acute, subacute, chronic active or chronic. These terms refer more to different types of inflammation than to the duration of the inflammatory response (see below) since, in reality, the relative percentages of inflammatory cell types do not reliably predict duration.

Inflammation can also be categorized, according to the predominant inflammatory cell type(s) present, as: purulent/suppurative (neutrophils); eosinophilic (eosinophils); mixed (mixed cell types including neutrophils, lymphocytes, plasma cells and macrophages); or granulomatous (mixed cell types but predominantly mononuclear cells and macrophages).

The authors prefer to use these two classification systems in combination. Henceforth, throughout this chapter:

- **Acute** equates to a purulent, suppurative or neutrophilic inflammatory response
- **Chronic active** equates to a mixed inflammatory response
- **Chronic** equates to a granulomatous inflammatory response (although some authors use the term granulomatous only when inflammatory giant cells and a significant number of epithelioid macrophages are present).

Term	Definition
Anisocytosis	Variation in cell size
Anisokaryosis	Variation in nuclear size
Emperipolesis	The presence of one cell type within the cytoplasm of another; sometimes seen in neoplastic epithelial cells in squamous cell carcinoma
Hyperplasia	A reversible increase in cell numbers, brought about by increased mitotic activity in response to a stimulus
Neoplasia	Cell multiplication is uncontrolled, progressive and irreversible. The neoplastic proliferation of cells is driven by somatic mutations and/or alterations in cell cycle control, and cell differentiation is often impaired (see Anaplasia)
Metaplasia	A reversible process where one mature cell type is replaced by another mature cell type. This represents the adaptive replacement of a normal cell population by cells less sensitive to a stimulus. For example, in response to chronic upper airway irritation, ciliated columnar epithelial cells of the trachea and bronchi are replaced by stratified squamous epithelial cells
Dysplasia	Reversible proliferative cellular changes that occur in response to irritation or inflammation. Dysplastic change is characterized by abnormal size, shape and organization of mature cells. Some of the morphological abnormalities, particularly those resulting in alterations in nuclear morphology, are cytologically similar to those commonly associated with neoplasia
Anaplasia	Describes a lack of cellular differentiation. Poorly differentiated tumours are generally more malignant
Chromatin pattern	The microscopic appearance of the nuclear chromatin. The chromatin pattern can be described as smooth (fine), finely or coarsely stippled, lacey (reticular), coarse (ropey), clumped or smudged. It becomes more coarse as malignant potential increases

20.8 Definitions of some common terms used in the interpretation of cytology samples.

This terminology emphasizes the fact that different categories of inflammation are not mutually exclusive. For example, some mixed inflammatory responses characterized by a mixed population of neutrophils and macrophages are often referred to as pyogranulomatous.

The severity of the inflammatory response can be assessed subjectively as mild, moderate or severe.

Acute inflammation

If >70% of the total number of nucleated cells are neutrophils, the inflammatory response is classified as acute, suppurative or purulent (although some authors only use the terms suppurative or purulent when the number of neutrophils exceeds 85% of the total number of nucleated cells present) (Figure 20.9). The remaining cells are a mixture of mononuclear cells (monocytes, macrophages, lymphocytes and plasma cells). Cell morphology may provide a clue to the aetiology.

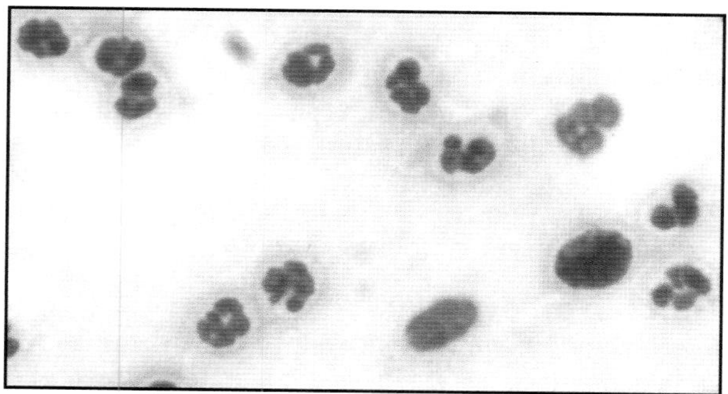

20.9 Synovial fluid from a dog with immune-mediated polyarthritis. The neutrophils appear well preserved and many are hypersegmented. (Wright's stain; original magnification X1000)

Neutrophils

Neutrophils can show a variety of degenerative changes:

- Swelling and hyalinization of nucleus (the nucleus assumes a 'glass-like' appearance, i.e. it is shiny but not refractile)
- Loss of nuclear lobulation and rupture of nuclear membrane (karyolysis; Figure 20.10a)
- Nuclear fragmentation and formation of 'nuclear dust' (karyorrhexis)
- Shrinkage of nuclear material into dark staining hyperchromatic masses (pyknosis; Figure 20.10b).

Well preserved (non-degenerate) neutrophils tend to be associated with non-septic conditions such as immune-mediated polyarthritis, although it is important to realize that the absence of degenerative change does not exclude a bacterial aetiology. For example, bacteria are rarely seen in joint fluid aspirates, even from cases of confirmed septic arthritis, and the neutrophils can often appear surprisingly well preserved. Neutrophil morphology may also be expected to improve rapidly if an animal has already received antibiotics. Conversely, neutrophils in body cavity effusions, particularly in effusions with a high protein content or that contain a lot of blood, start to degenerate if there is a significant delay in processing the sample (this ageing process occurs *in vitro* and does not necessarily indicate an infectious aetiology).

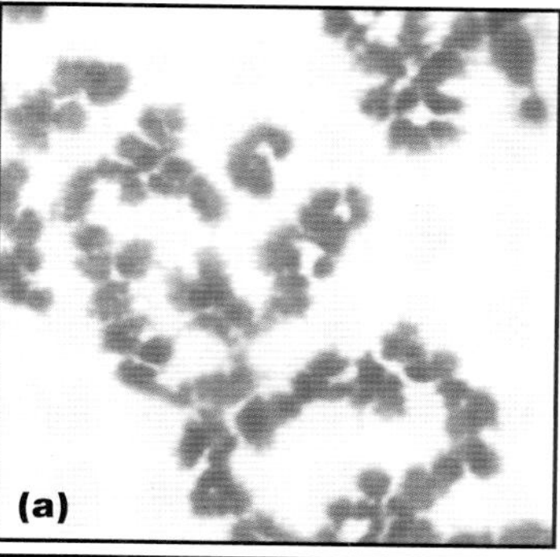

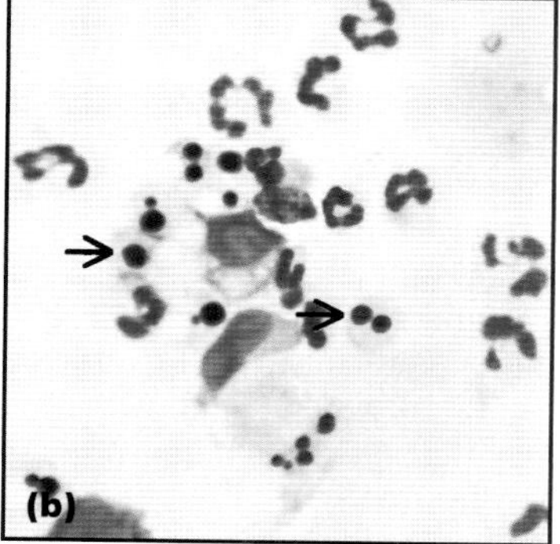

20.10 Degenerative neutrophils. (a) Peritoneal fluid from a 6-year-old Domestic Shorthair cat with peritonitis. The neutrophils show severe degenerative changes (karyolysis). (b) Peritoneal fluid from a dog with right-sided congestive heart failure. There are numerous pyknotic neutrophils. Note the round dark-staining 'balls' of nuclear chromatin (arrowed). (Wright's stain; original magnification X1000) (Reproduced with permission from *In Practice*.)

Karyolysis and karyorrhexis indicate sudden cell death. Degenerate neutrophils, particulary those showing karyolytic changes, are usually associated with septic lesions especially those caused by endotoxin-producing or pyogenic bacteria, e.g. in pyothorax.

Pyknosis implies slower cell death, associated with ageing of neutrophils in the inflammatory process, and is less indicative of sepsis. Some bacterial infections, e.g. *Nocardia,* do not produce marked degenerative changes.

Neutrophils should always be examined for the presence of ingested bacteria (Figure 20.11), since the presence of intracellular bacteria makes contamination after sampling less likely and supports a diagnosis of bacterial infection.

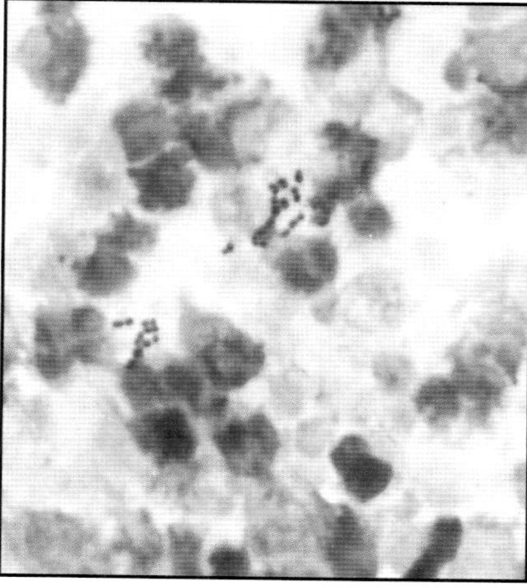

20.11 Degenerate neutrophils containing ingested bacteria in peritoneal fluid from a Springer Spaniel with septic peritonitis. (Wright's stain; original magnification X1000)

Special considerations

It is important to realize that in some lesions the inflammatory response may either mask, or be secondary to, another pathological process.

- Ulcerated cutaneous lesions are invariably covered with inflammatory cells and bacteria. Impression smears taken from such lesions may therefore not be representative of the underlying pathological process. Prior removal of superficial exudate and cellular debris with a saline-soaked gauze swab may provide a more representative impression smear.
- Certain tumours, e.g. squamous cell carcinomas, frequently elicit an intense inflammatory response. Thorough examination of a smear may be required to detect neoplastic cells.
- Inflammation may be expected to induce dysplastic changes in normal cells adjacent to the lesion (Figure 20.12). These morphological changes often resemble those associated with neoplasia: variation in cell size and shape; variation in nuclear/nucleolar size, shape and number; increased nuclear:cytoplasmic (N:C) ratio; and coarser nuclear chromatin. Since the morphological changes associated with dysplasia can resemble some of those associated with neoplasia/malignancy it is very difficult, if not often impossible, to determine with the aid of cytology alone whether an inflammatory response is secondary to neoplasia or whether it is the inflammatory response that is initiating the dysplastic changes.

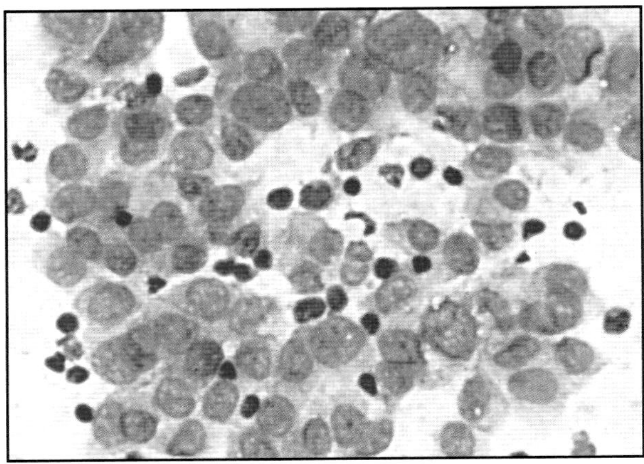

20.12 Nasal flush from a dog with nasal aspergillosis. This cluster of cuboidal epithelial cells shows dysplastic changes: they are larger than normal and a moderate degree of anisocytosis, anisokaryosis and variation in N:C ratio is evident. Some nuclei contain a visible nucleolus. Neutrophils and lymphocytes are also present. No tumour was identified on post-mortem examination (Wright's stain; original magnification X500) (Reproduced with permission from *In Practice*.)

Eosinophilic inflammatory response

An eosinophilic inflammatory response is a subcategory of acute inflammation characterized by an increased number (usually >10%) of eosinophils in the sample (Figure 20.13). The presence of a large number of eosinophils suggests either a hypersensitivity component to the inflammatory response or the presence of a parasitic agent (e.g. *Oslerus osleri* or *Angiostrongylus vasorum* larvae in bronchoalveolar lavage fluid). Large numbers of eosinophils and neutrophils are frequently

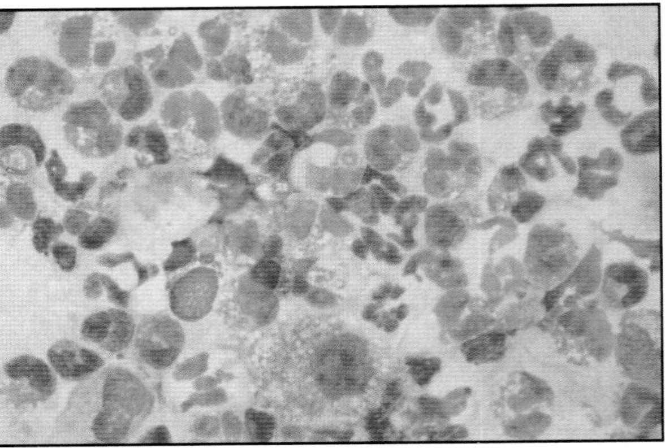

20.13 Fine needle aspirate from a cutaneous mass in a young German Shepherd Dog. There is a mixed population of eosinophils and neutrophils, consistent with an eosinophilic granuloma. A macrophage is also seen in the field. (Wright's stain; original magnification x1000)

observed on impression smears of feline eosinophilic granuloma complex lesions. Increased numbers of eosinophils are often present in aspirates from mast cell tumours and, less frequently, lymphomas and histiocytic tumours, presumably in response to the release of cytokines from the neoplastic cells.

Chronic inflammation

The chronic inflammatory response is characterized by a predominance of mononuclear inflammatory cells, i.e. monocytes, macrophages, lymphocytes and plasma cells. At least 50% of the inflammatory cells present are macrophages and the remaining nucleated cell population may consist of a mixture of fairly well preserved neutrophils, lymphocytes and plasma cells. Possible aetiologies for this type of response include: low-grade irritants (inert foreign material); fungi (e.g. *Histoplasma capsulatum*); and certain bacteria (e.g. *Mycobacterium, Actinomyces, Nocardia*). Resolving acute inflammatory reactions may also show this type of mixed population.

Macrophages

Macrophages are readily identified by: size (diameter 20–100 μm; 3–12 times the diameter of a red blood cell); an oval or bean-shaped nucleus; and abundant pale blue cytoplasm (with Romanowsky stains), which may contain numerous vacuoles and/or phagocytosed cellular material (Figure 20.14). The nucleus is often eccentrically placed and has a lacey or reticulated chromatin pattern.

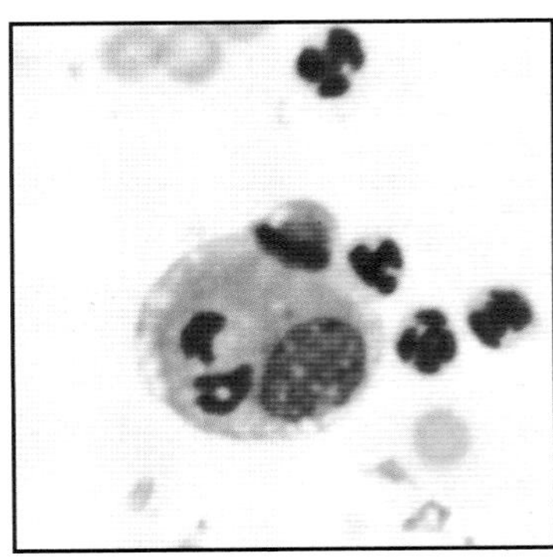

20.14 This large reactive macrophage contains two phagocytosed neutrophils. (Wright's stain; original magnification X1000).

Granulomatous inflammation

This is a subcategory of chronic inflammation, characterized by significant numbers of large reactive and smaller epithelioid macrophages and, in some cases, inflammatory giant cells as well as smaller numbers of neutrophils, lymphocytes and plasma cells.

Epithelioid macrophages

These are smaller macrophages (Figure 20.15) that are not actively phagocytic; they resemble epithelial cells in appearance and are often seen in small clusters.

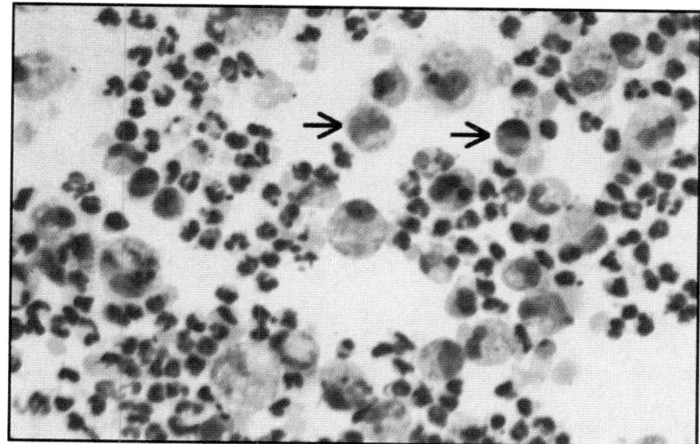

20.15 Pyogranulomatous inflammatory response. The smaller mononuclear cells (arrowed) are epithelioid macrophages. (Wright's stain; original magnification X500).

Inflammatory giant cells

These are large multinucleated cells (Figure 20.16), which must be differentiated from multinucleated neoplastic cells. The nuclei of inflammatory giant cells are usually uniform in size and shape (in contrast to the more pleomorphic nuclei seen in multinucleated neoplastic cells) and are usually arranged around the periphery of the cell. Increased numbers of inflammatory giant cells are a feature of many foreign body reactions.

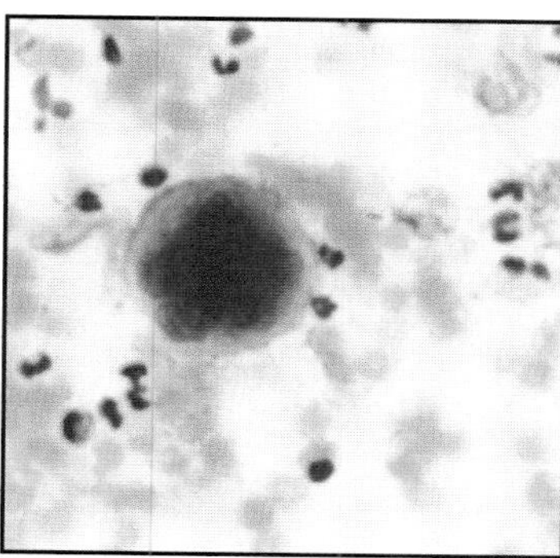

20.16 A multinucleate giant cell in exudate from a fistulous tract associated with a penetrating foreign body on the flank of a German Shepherd Dog. (Wright's stain; original magnification X500) (Reproduced with permission from *In Practice*.)

Chronic active inflammation

The term chronic active inflammation describes a mixed inflammatory response with both chronic and active components. By definition, 50–70% of the inflammatory cells are neutrophils and 30–50% are mononuclear cells (lymphocytes and macrophages). When macrophages and neutrophils are the major cell types present, this is sometimes referred to as a pyogranulomatous inflammatory response (see Figure 20.15). The causes of this type of inflammatory response are fairly similar to those that can initiate chronic or granulomatous inflammation: migrating grass awns; release of keratin from a ruptured epidermal inclusion or sebaceous cyst; fungal infections; and certain bacterial infections, e.g. *Mycobacterium, Actinomyces, Nocardia.*

Cytology of neoplasia

Cytology is a useful diagnostic tool for determining whether a lesion is neoplastic and, secondly, if it is neoplastic, for establishing whether it is benign or malignant. It should be emphasized, however, that some tumours, cytologically at least, can appear 'benign' when they are actually highly malignant, e.g. thyroid carcinomas. Cytological examination should not be regarded as a substitute for histological examination, since it provides no information regarding the architecture of the tumour and its relationship to adjacent structures, nor can it determine whether a tumour is well demarcated or locally invasive. Cytological examination, certainly in the case of most spindle cell tumours, rarely provides a histiogenic diagnosis. Nevertheless, it often provides vital diagnostic and prognostic information regarding tumour type and may also help to determine whether surgical intervention, either to excise or biopsy, is required.

Criteria for malignancy

The cytological criteria for differentiating reactive or dysplastic cells from neoplastic cells, and for assessing the degree of malignancy, rely heavily on changes in nuclear and nucleolar morphology. Cytoplasmic changes associated with malignancy are less specific; similar changes may be seen with hyperplasia and in response to inflammation (dysplasia).

Non-specific cellular criteria

- Aspirates from malignant tumours tend to contain more cells.
- Cellular pleomorphism, i.e. variation in cell size (anisocytosis) and shape, is greater in malignancy. There is an increased number of larger cells, showing variation in the N:C ratio.
- A population of cells in an abnormal location is a good indicator of neoplasia (even if the cell population is monomorphic and nuclear criteria for malignancy are absent). For example, a population of small well differentiated lymphocytes aspirated from a cutaneous mass is consistent with a diagnosis of cutaneous lymphoma.

Cytoplasmic criteria (less definitive than nuclear criteria)

- Increased cytoplasmic basophilia (due to increased RNA content) may be seen in any metabolically active population of cells (e.g. hyperplastic cells, secretory glandular epithelial cells) and is therefore not necessarily indicative of neoplasia.

- Cytoplasmic margins may be less well defined and the cytoplasm may appear vacuolated or excessively granulated in malignant cells.
- The presence of large coalescing vacuoles or 'signet ring' cells, where the nucleus is 'pushed' to the periphery of the cell by a single large cytoplasmic vacuole (Figure 20.17a), and evidence of acinus formation (Figure 20.17b) are highly suggestive of malignancy (carcinoma).

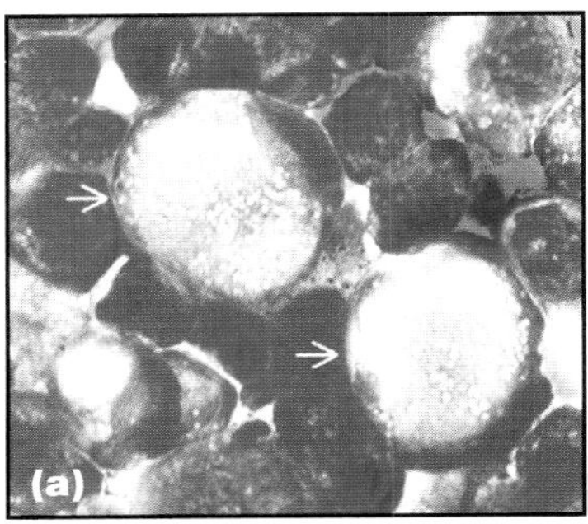

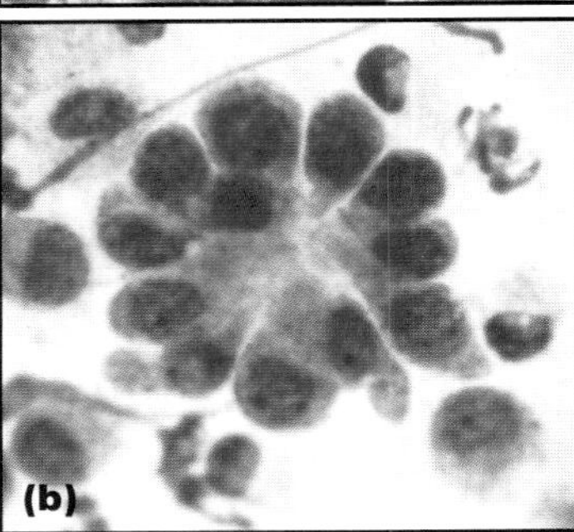

20.17 Cytoplasmic features suggesting malignancy. (a) Pleural fluid from a bitch with pulmonary metastases from a mammary adenocarcinoma. The large 'signet ring' cells (arrowed) each have one large cytoplasmic vacuole and a nucleus that has been 'pushed' to the periphery of the cell. (b) An acinus in a fine needle aspirate from a dog with pulmonary adenocarcinoma. (Wright's stain; original magnification X1000)

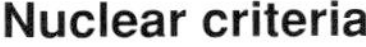

Nuclear criteria

The following are suggestive of malignancy:

- Variation in nuclear size (anisokaryosis) and shape (Figure 20.18a)
- Increased N:C ratio or variation in N:C ratio within the same population of cells
- Multiple (>4) nucleoli in one nucleus or a single very large nucleolus (approaching the size of a red cell)
- Variation in nucleolar size, shape and number, especially within the same nucleus. The presence of extremely large, angular or irregularly shaped nucleoli is highly suggestive of malignancy (Figure 20.18b)
- Coarse, ropey or reticulated nuclear chromatin pattern
- The nucleus may become distorted (nuclear moulding) as it is compressed by adjacent neoplastic cells or by a second nucleus within the same neoplastic cell
- Multinucleation (more significant if the nuclei within the same cell vary in size; Figure 20.18c)
- Increased numbers of mitotic figures. This may also be seen with benign hyperplasia; the presence of abnormal mitotic figures where nuclei divide in more than two directions or nuclear division is uneven is more significant and is highly suggestive of malignancy (Figure 20.18c).

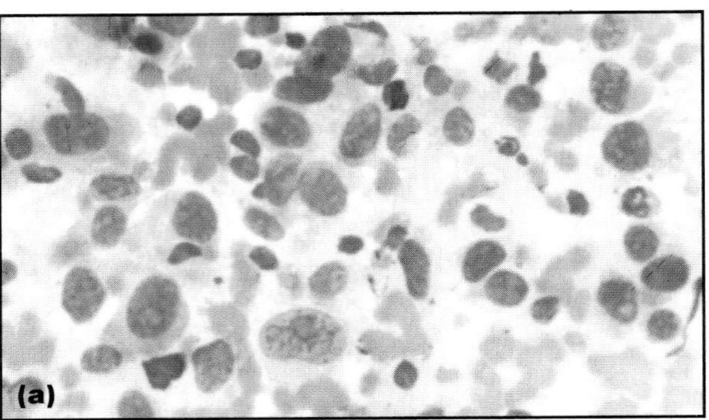

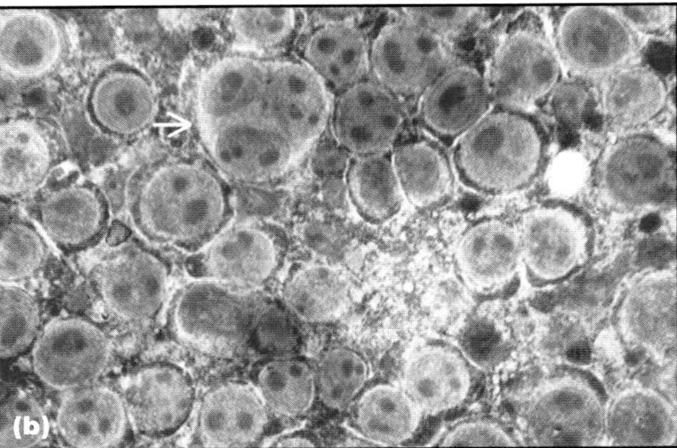

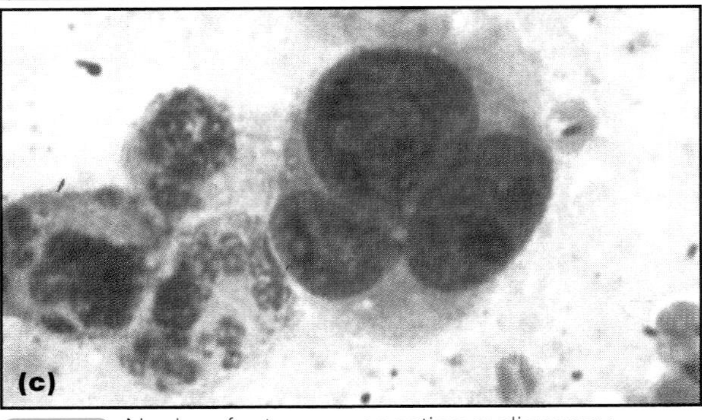

20.18 Nuclear features suggesting malignancy. (a) Marked anisocytosis, anisokaryosis and variation in N:C ratio in an aspirate from a dog with haemangiopericytoma. Some cells also show a coarse reticulated chromatin pattern and unusually large nucleoli. (b) Considerable variation in the size, shape and number of nucleoli within the nuclei of cells from a mammary adenocarcinoma. One large multinucleated cell is present (arrowed). (c) Three abnormal mitotic figures are seen to the left of a cell with three nuclei of variable size in this aspirate from a soft tissue (giant cell) sarcoma in a Flat-coated Retriever. (Wright's stain; original magnification X500 (a), X1000 (b,c)) (b,c © Axiom Veterinary Laboratories)

A single population of cells containing young immature blastic nuclei is highly suggestive of malignancy, especially if there is evidence of nuclear and nucleolar pleomorphism. Recognition of more than three of the above nuclear criteria is regarded as strong evidence for malignancy.

Classification of tumour cell type

Tumours may be broadly classified as epithelial, mesenchymal (spindle cell) or discrete round cell tumours. The morphological features of each of these categories are described below. Classification into one of these three tumour types is primarily based on the size and shape of cells aspirated and on their tendency to exfoliate singly or in clusters. While this system is useful for classifying the majority of tumours it is not flawless. For example, a poorly differentiated tumour may be clearly malignant but demonstrate insufficient morphological characteristics to allow further classification as either a carcinoma or sarcoma. Conversely, some tumours, for example thyroid carcinomas, may show few cytological criteria of malignancy and may be diagnosed erroneously as benign.

Epithelial tumours

Epithelial cells line the oral and nasal cavities, and the gastrointestinal, urogenital and respiratory tracts. Secretory and non-secretory epithelial cells are also present in the skin and glandular tissue. Adenomas or carcinomas/adenocarcinomas may therefore arise at all these sites.

Epithelial cells may be round, cuboidal or columnar, and have common adjoining borders.

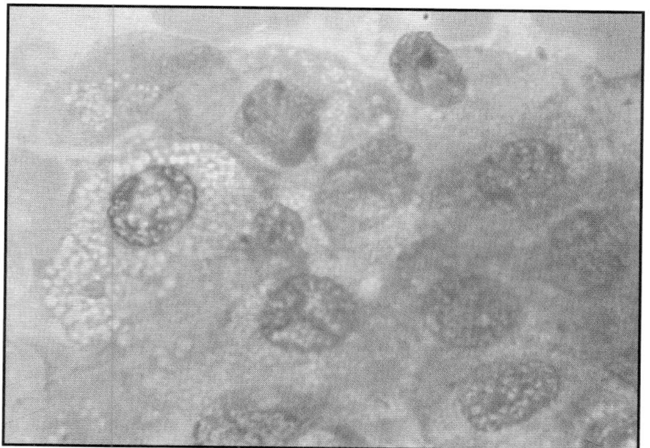

20.19 Cluster of epithelial cells from a sebaceous gland adenoma on the back of a 7-year-old Toy Poodle. The cells and their nuclei are of uniform size and shape. The cytoplasm appears finely vacuolated, suggesting the cells have a secretory capacity. (Wright's stain; original magnification X1000)

Tumours of epithelial origin tend to exfoliate cells in sheets or cohesive clusters. The cells vary in shape, depending on the tissue of origin. They are usually round or polyhedral, with abundant cytoplasm and well defined cytoplasmic margins (Figure 20.19). Columnar or cuboidal epithelial cells are present in the respiratory and gastrointestinal tracts.

The character of the cytoplasm varies greatly with respect to colour, granularity and degree of vacuolation, depending on the location, and function of the cells. The presence of intracellular secretory product or acinus formation (see Figure 20.17b) suggests the cells are of glandular epithelial origin.

The nucleus is usually round, with a smooth or finely stippled chromatin pattern (which becomes coarser as the malignant potential increases). One or more nucleoli are usually present (nucleoli can also be seen in hyperplastic and dysplastic epithelial cells, especially those with a secretory capacity). These become larger and more irregular in shape as the cells undergo malignant transformation (Figure 20.20).

Epithelial cells become dysplastic in response to localized inflammation or irritation. Dysplastic changes (see Figure 20.12) include: variations in size and shape of cell, nucleus and nucleoli; increased N:C ratio; and coarser nuclear chromatin. These changes can resemble those associated with neoplasia.

Commonly encountered tumours of epithelial origin include sebaceous gland adenomas/adenocarcinomas (see Figure 20.19), perianal adenomas/adenocarcinomas, squamous cell carcinoma (see Figure 20.31), transitional carcinomas of the bladder, basal cell tumours (see Figures 20.26 and 20.30), mammary gland tumours (see Figure 20.18b) and tumours of other glandular epithelial tissue, e.g. prostatic adenocarcinomas (see Figure 22.63).

Mesenchymal tumours

Mesenchymal cells (spindle cells) are present in adipose tissue, muscle, bone, cartilage, fibrous tissue and in blood and lymphatic vessels. They typically have elongated cytoplasmic tails and a round or oval nucleus.

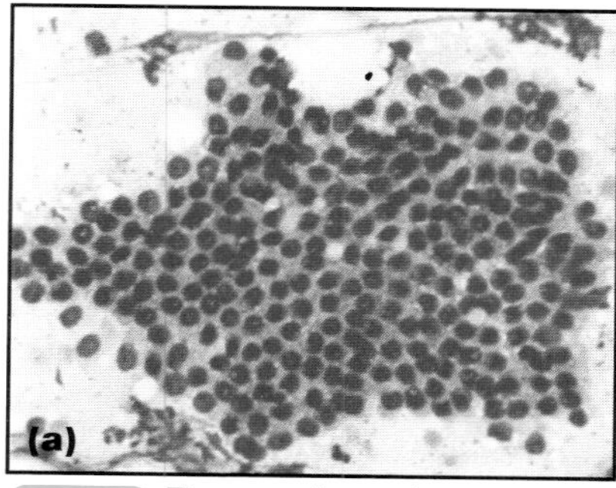

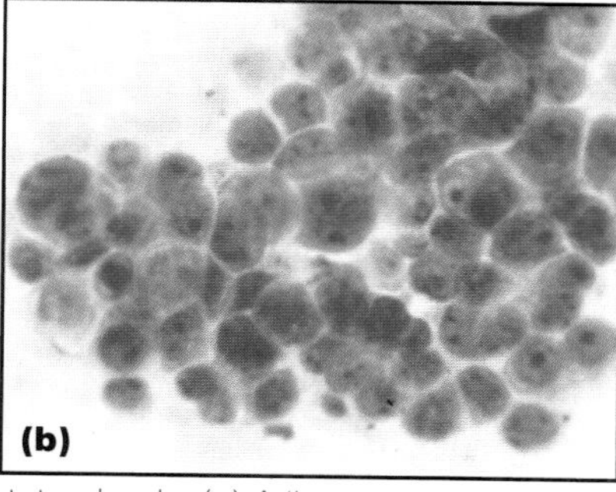

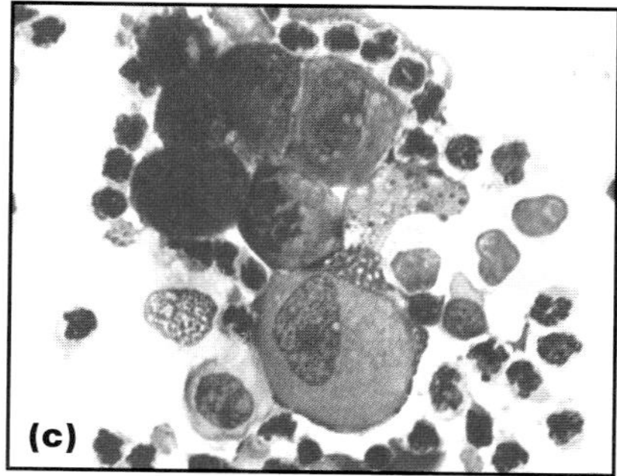

20.20 Fine needle aspirates from prostate glands. (a) A 'honeycomb' cluster of hyperplastic prostatic epithelial cells from a dog with benign prostatic hyperplasia. (b) An irregularly arranged cluster of neoplastic cells from a prostatic carcinoma. The cells show marked anisocytosis, anisokaryosis and variation in N:C ratio. Considerable variation in the size, shape and number of nucleoli is also evident. (c) These prostatic epithelial cells showing similar changes to those in (b). Some of the nuclei appear to contain more than one nucleolus. However, there is also evidence of an associated inflammatory response, with numerous neutrophils. On a cytological basis, and without histological back-up, it would be difficult to determine whether this was a prostatic carcinoma (in which case the inflammatory response may be secondary) or whether the inflammation was the primary problem and had induced dysplastic or reactive changes in the prostatic epithelial cells. (Wright's stain; original magnification X500 (a), X1000 (b,c,)) (a,b, Reproduced with permission from *In Practice*. c, © Axiom Veterinary Laboratories)

Mesenchymal tumours (commonly referred to as spindle cell tumours) are derived from connective tissue. Fine needle aspirates from these tumours are often hypocellular because the cells are embedded in an extracellular matrix (e.g. osteoid (bone), chondroid (cartilage), collagen (fibrous tissue)). The aspirated cells, therefore, are often discrete, although a few small clusters may be present.

Well differentiated mesenchymal cells are usually of small to medium size and are classically spindle-shaped, with cytoplasmic tails trailing away from the nucleus (Figure 20.21). Cytoplasmic borders are often poorly defined, and the nuclei are oval or elliptical with a smooth or fine lacey chromatin pattern. As malignant potential increases, the nucleus enlarges and the cells may become rounder and/or assume a stellate (star-like) appearance with short, blunt cytoplasmic projections rather than long cytoplasmic tails. Nuclear chromatin becomes coarser and the nucleoli become more prominent.

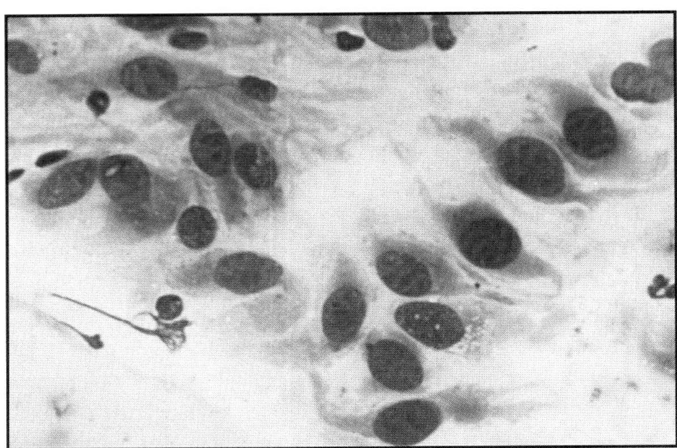

20.21 Spindle-shaped cells with cytoplasmic tails trailing away from the nucleus in an aspirate from an oral fibrosarcoma. The nuclei contain several nucleoli. A moderate degree of anisocytosis is evident. There is eosinophilic matrix material towards the top left hand corner, which is probably collagen. (Wright's stain; original magnification X1000) (Reproduced with permission from *In Practice*)

Accurate identification of tissue type in many instances is not possible on a cytological basis alone. This is especially true of poorly differentiated mesenchymal tumours, although the type of extracellular matrix, location of the lesion, and its clinical and/or radiographic appearance often provide important clues.

Mesenchymal cells become dysplastic in response to local inflammation or irritation and these cells may be very difficult to differentiate from neoplastic cells. If granulation tissue is present in the lesion, young fibroblasts may similarly be mistaken for neoplastic cells.

Common mesenchymal tumours include lipoma/liposarcoma (see Figure 20.34), chondroma/chondrosarcoma, osteoma/osteosarcoma, fibroma/fibrosarcoma (see Figure 20.21), haemangioma/haemangiosarcoma (see Figure 20.36), haemangiopericytoma (see Figure 20.35), neurofibroma/neurofibrosarcoma, and myxoma/myxosarcoma.

Round cell tumours

Round cell tumours exfoliate discrete round cells with well defined cytoplasmic margins and a round or indented nucleus. They are often haemopoietic in origin. Aspirates from round cell tumours are usually extremely cellular. The cells exfoliate individually or in small clusters.

Tumours classified as discrete round cell tumours include lymphoma (Figure 20.22), plasmacytoma (see Figure 20.39), histiocytoma (Figure 20.23), mast cell tumour (Figure 20.24) and transmissible venereal tumour (see Figure 20.41). Most round cell tumours can be accurately identified cytologically because of their specific cytoplasmic, nuclear and tinctorial properties. The cytological features of different round cell tumours are described in the section on Cytology of cutaneous and subcutaneous lesions.

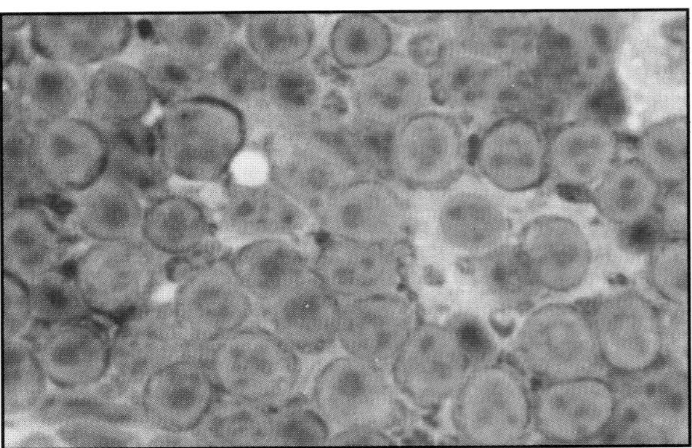

20.22 Multicentric lymphoma. This lymph node aspirate consists of a population of large lymphoblasts with multiple nucleoli; the nuclei are approximately three times the diameter of a red blood cell. (Wright's stain; original magnification X1000) (© Axiom Veterinary Laboratories)

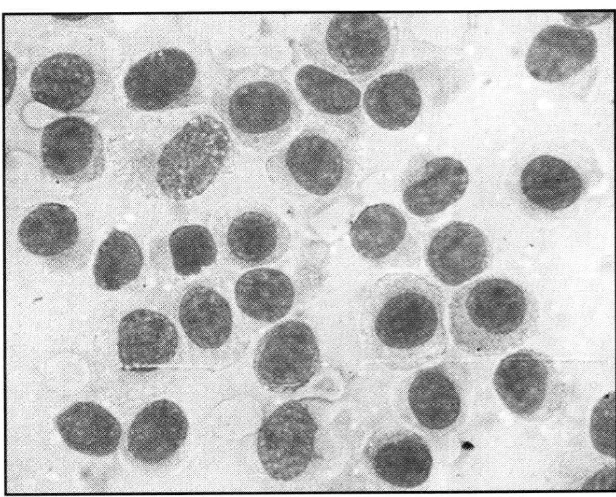

20.23 Fine needle aspirate from a canine histiocytoma on the pinna of a 1-year-old terrier cross. The cells are round, with discrete cytoplasmic margins. Although the cells in aspirates from histiocytomas almost always show a mild to moderate degree of anisocytosis and anisokaryosis, these tumours are benign and usually regress spontaneously. (Wright's stain; original magnification X1000) (Courtesy of E Villiers)

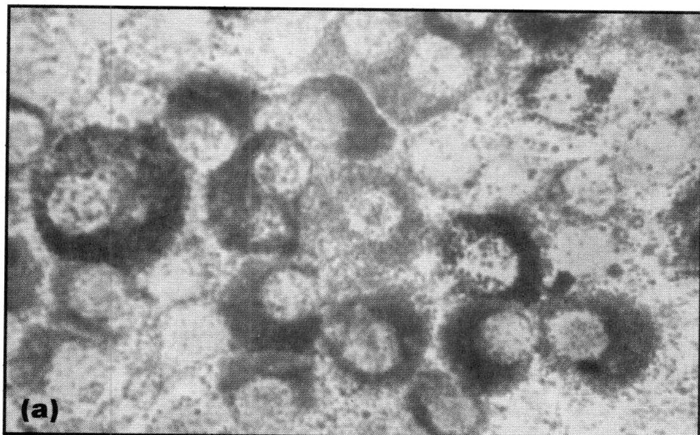

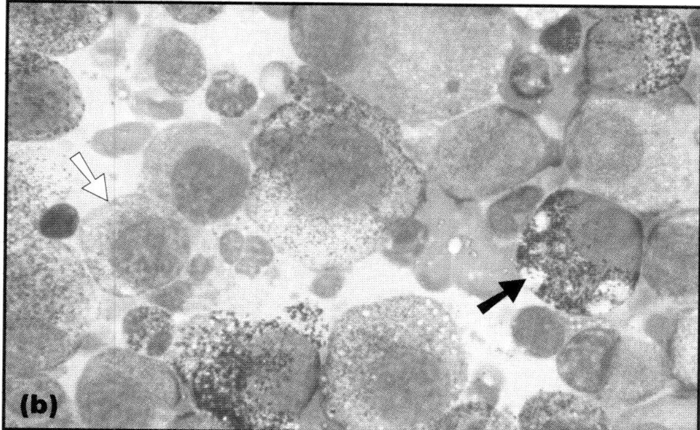

20.24 Mast cell tumours. (a) Aspirate from an MCT on the lower limb of a crossbred dog. The mast cells contain densely packed azurophilic cytoplasmic granules. The nuclei are relatively unstained because the stain is 'soaked up' by the granules. (b) Aspirate from an MCT on the prepuce of a Boxer. Compared with (a), the mast cells are much larger, with marked variation in cell and nuclear size. The cytoplasmic granules are variable: some cells have abundant granules (black arrow) but in other cells the granules are scant and fine (white arrow). A binucleated cell is seen in the top right corner. (Wright's stain; original magnification X1000)

Although malignant melanomas (Figure 20.25) and basal cell tumours (Figure 20.26) may yield discrete round cells on cytological smears, they are not included in this category (they are usually classified as mesenchymal and epithelial tumours, respectively).

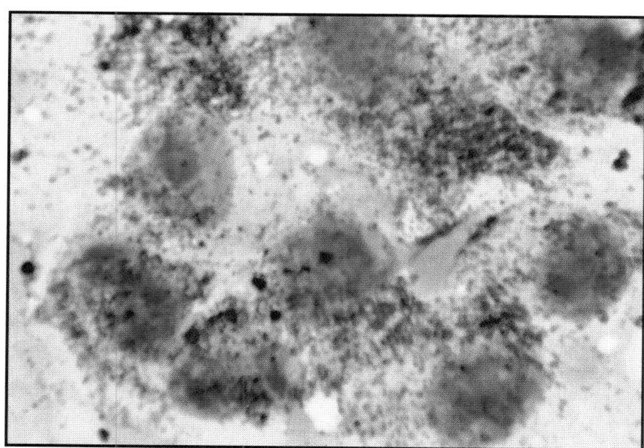

20.25 Fine needle aspirate from a malignant melanoma. Although the cells are round, malignant melanomas are classified as mesenchymal tumours. Note the melanin pigment granules. The nuclei contain at least one large nucleolus. (Wright's stain; original magnification X1000) (Reproduced with permission from *In Practice*.)

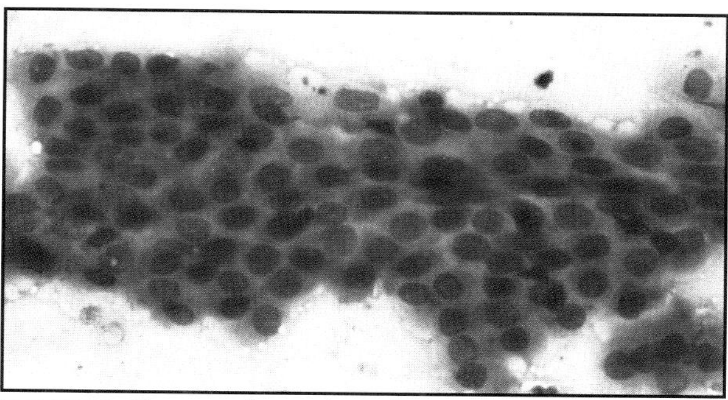

20.26 Fine needle aspirate from a basal cell tumour (trichoblastoma) on the distal limb of a dog. There is a monomorphic population of basal epithelial cells. Basal cells usually exfoliate in cohesive clusters or sheets. (Wright's stain; original magnification X500) (© Axiom Veterinary Laboratories.)

Cytology of cutaneous and subcutaneous lesions

Most cutaneous and subcutaneous lesions can be categorized sufficiently to provide useful clinical guidance. Specimens for cytological examination are usually obtained by FNA or, if the lesion is ulcerated, by impression smears. The disadvantages and limitations of the latter technique have been discussed earlier.

Normal skin is composed of several layers of squamous epithelial cells. Basal epithelial cells are round and deeply basophilic with a high N:C ratio. The cells in the most superficial layer become cornified (keratinized) and their nuclei become pyknotic or disappear completely. Hence, aspirates from cutaneous or subcutaneous lesions may contain variable numbers of cornified squamous epithelial cells or anucleated keratinized squames (also referred to as keratin scrolls or bars). As the cells become keratinized, the cytoplasm becomes light blue (Romanowsky) and the cell outline becomes angular.

The adnexal structures of the epidermis include hair follicles, sweat glands and sebaceous glands. Immediately below the epidermis is the dermis and below this is the subcutis. Aspirates of the dermis and subcutis may contain adipose tissue, collagen and glandular elements.

Subcutaneous non-neoplastic lesions

Abscess

Skin or subcutaneous abscesses are especially common in cats, and are often the result of a bite wound. A creamy white purulent exudate is usually aspirated. Cytological examination reveals a large number of extremely degenerate neutrophils, many of which may contain intracellular bacteria (see Figure 20.11). Staphylococci usually appear in small clusters, whereas streptococci tend to form chains. Gram's stain may be helpful to identify organisms in aspirates containing a lot of cell debris.

Actinomyces, Nocardia, Mycobacterium and certain fungal infections tend to elicit a mixed (pyogranulomatous) or granulomatous inflammatory response.

Penetrating foreign bodies are more likely to be associated with either *Nocardia* or *Actinomyces* infection. The subcutaneous swellings that result may rupture, leaving either a raw ulcerated lesion or fistulous tracts that discharge reddish brown fluid. *Actinomyces* and *Nocardia* are slender filamentous branching rods, which often have a beaded appearance with Romanowsky staining. *Actinomyces* is Gram-positive but acid-fast-negative; *Nocardia* is also Gram-positive and may stain slightly acid-fast-positive with Ziehl–Neelsen (ZN) stain. Myobacteria can cause deep-seated abscesses, especially in cats. Large numbers of negatively staining rods can be seen within the cytoplasm of macrophages on a Romanowsky-stained smear (these stain positive with ZN stain).

Haematoma

Haematomas are large blood-filled masses, usually resulting from trauma. An aspirate from a recently formed haematoma has the appearance of blood, except that platelets are usually absent. This is followed by an increase in the number of macrophages, many of which may contain phagocytosed red cells (Figure 20.27). Macrophages in longer standing haematomas may contain haemoglobin breakdown products in the form of bluish black haemosiderin granules or haematoidin crystals (see Figure 20.28b). As the haematoma continues to organize, plump fibroblasts may be seen in aspirated fluid.

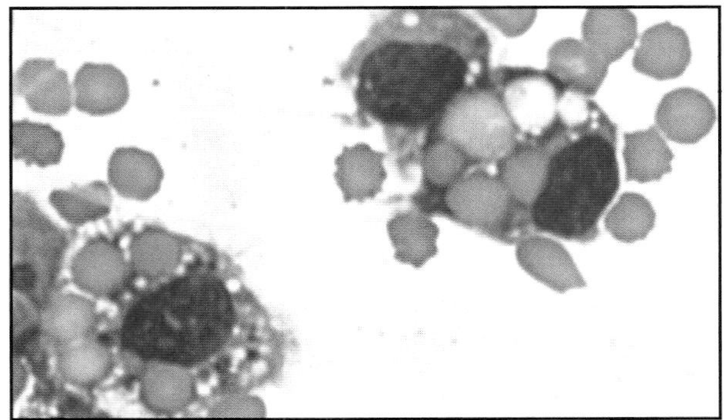

20.27 Fine needle aspirate from a large haematoma on the shoulder of a Labrador Retriever. This consists of red blood cells and large reactive macrophages, many of which contain phagocytosed red cells (erythrophagocytosis). (Wright's stain; original magnification X1000) (© Axiom Veterinary Laboratories.)

Sialocele

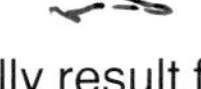

Sialoceles (or salivary gland cysts) usually result from trauma or infection. They often form in the submandibular region and contain clear or blood-tinged fluid that may appear quite viscous and stringy. Aspirates are usually contaminated with blood and contain a variable number of large, finely vacuolated mononuclear cells (Figure 20.28a). These are probably macrophages but it has also been suggested that some of the non-phagocytic cells may be reactive glandular epithelial cells. Some of the macrophages may contain phagocytosed red cells or haemoglobin breakdown products in the form of haematoidin crystals, indicating previous intracavitatory haemorrhage (Figure 20.28b).

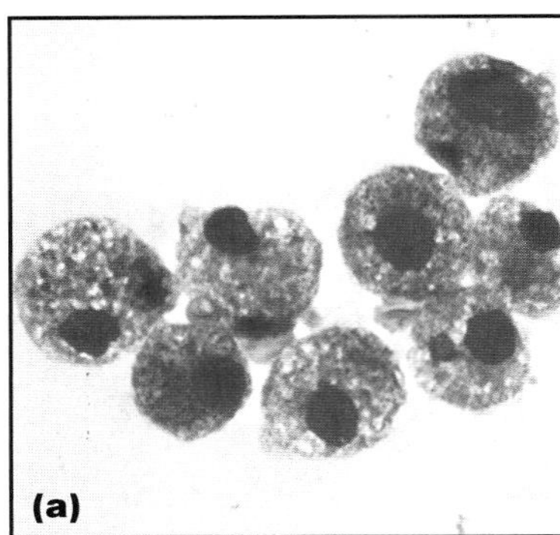

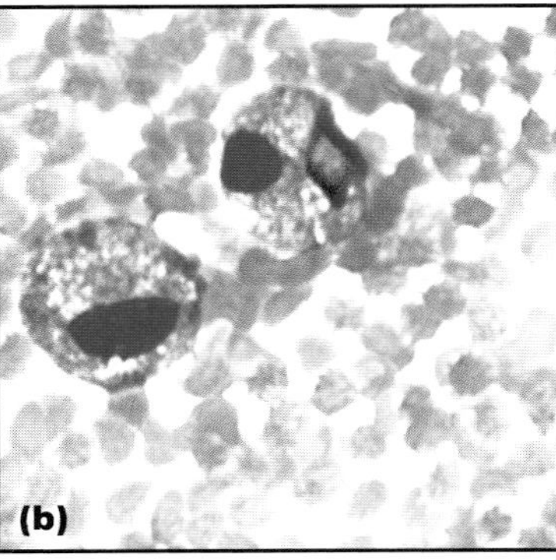

20.28 Fine needle aspirate from a submandibular salivary gland cyst (sialocele) in a Springer Spaniel. (a) A cluster of cells with abundant finely vacuolated cytoplasm. Some of these cells contain phagocytosed red cells, suggesting they are probably macrophages. (b) The cell on the right contains a rhomboid crystal of haematoidin, indicating previous intracavitatory haemorrhage. (Wright's stain; original magnification X1000) (© Axiom Veterinary Laboratories.)

Nodular panniculitis (steatitis)

Nodular panniculitis is characterized by the appearance of discrete solitary or multiple fluctuant lesions on the dorsal trunk and neck. The lesions usually rupture releasing a whitish or yellow brown oily fluid. Aspirates from such lesions contain a mixed population of non-degenerate neutrophils and macrophages located in a 'fatty' background deposit. A similar type of lesion (lipogranuloma) can be seen with injection site reactions. Variable numbers of small lymphocytes, plasma cells and mesenchymal-type cells may also be seen. Culture and histological examination are recommended to rule out infectious causes of panniculitis.

Cutaneous non-neoplastic lesions

Eosinophilic plaque/granuloma

Feline eosinophilic plaques tend to occur on the face, neck, abdomen and medial thighs. The lesions ulcerate and become secondarily infected with bacteria. Aspirates or impression smears from such lesions consist of large numbers of eosinophils and neutrophils (see Figure 20.13). Mast cells may also be present.

Epidermal inclusion cyst or epidermoid cyst

Epidermal inclusion cysts occur in middle-aged or older dogs. They are usually firm or fluctuant and well circumscribed. They are often located on the dorsum or on the tail head. Aspirates consist almost entirely of keratinized squames and cellular debris; cholesterol crystals and a few small clusters of normal or dysplastic epithelial cells may also be seen (Figure 20.29). Rupture of the cyst can induce an intense localized pyogranulomatous response, necessitating surgical excision.

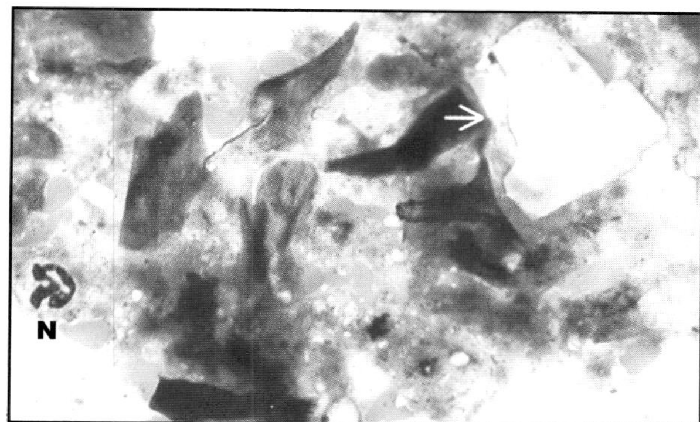

20.29 Fine needle aspirate from an epidermal inclusion cyst from a dog's back. This consists of a large number of keratinized squames. A cholesterol crystal can be seen (arrowed) and a neutrophil is present (N). (Wright's stain; original magnification X1000) (© Axiom Veterinary Laboratories.)

Tumours of epithelial origin

Basal cell tumours

Basal cell tumours are typically single, well circumscribed, intradermal lesions. Occasionally they may ulcerate or become cystic but they are almost always benign. They are most frequently located on the neck and limbs. Basal cells exfoliate in compact clusters. They have scant basophilic cytoplasm, which may contain melanin or keratohyaline granules. Basal cell tumours in which basal cells predominate are also called trichoblastomas (see Figure 20.26). Some basal cell tumours show evidence of adnexal differentiation. Those with sebaceous differentiation contain sebaceous epithelial cells with more abundant vacuolated cytoplasm and a round centrally located nucleus (Figure 20.30). Basal cell tumours that become cystic or have follicular differentiation may contain keratinized epithelial cells or keratinized debris.

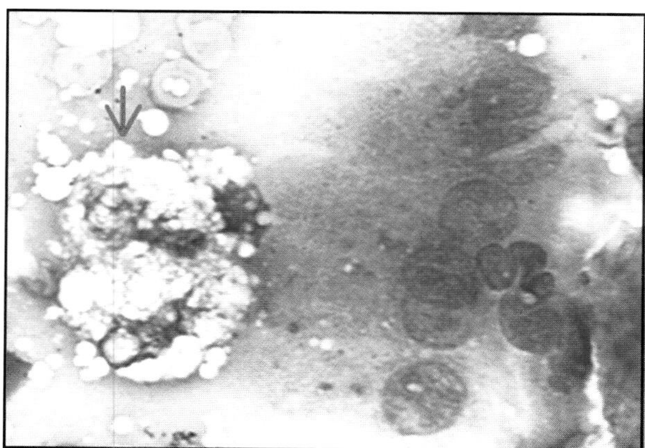

20.30 Fine needle aspirate from a basal cell tumour with sebaceous differentiation. The epithelial cells have a round, basally located nucleus and an extended 'sock' of cytoplasm; if these cells were seen end on, they would resemble those in Figure 20.27. The arrow points to sebaceous epithelial cells. (Wright's stain; original magnification X1000) (© Axiom Veterinary Laboratories.)

Sebaceous adenoma

These tumours are often mistakenly referred to as 'warts'. They are often small multilobulated lesions and tend to occur most frequently on the head, neck and trunk of older dogs. Sebaceous epithelial cells contain a moderate amount of pale, finely vacuolated cytoplasm and a small centrally located nucleus (see Figure 20.19). Sebaceous adenocarcinomas are relatively rare. They are often ulcerated and poorly circumscribed, and the sebaceous epithelial cells show obvious criteria of malignancy.

Squamous cell carcinoma

Squamous cell carcinoma (SCC) is a common tumour in dogs and, especially, cats. In cats, the tumours most commonly occur on the tips of the pinnae or face, whereas in dogs they are more common on the limbs, especially the digits, nailbeds and footpads. The tumours tend to ulcerate. They are locally invasive and may metastasize to the regional lymph node.

SCCs often elicit an intense inflammatory response. The cells may exfoliate singly or in clusters and may show varying degrees of differentiation. A mixture of intermediate, superficial and anucleated squamous epithelial cells with angular cell borders may be seen in well differentiated tumours. Some epithelial cells may contain other cell types, e.g. neutrophils (this is termed emperipolesis), and there may be evidence of perinuclear vacuolation. Poorly differentiated SCCs, in contrast, show a more marked degree of anisocytosis and anisokaryosis and the cells have a higher N:C ratio. Nuclear chromatin often has a coarse ropey or 'moth-eaten' appearance (Figure 20.31).

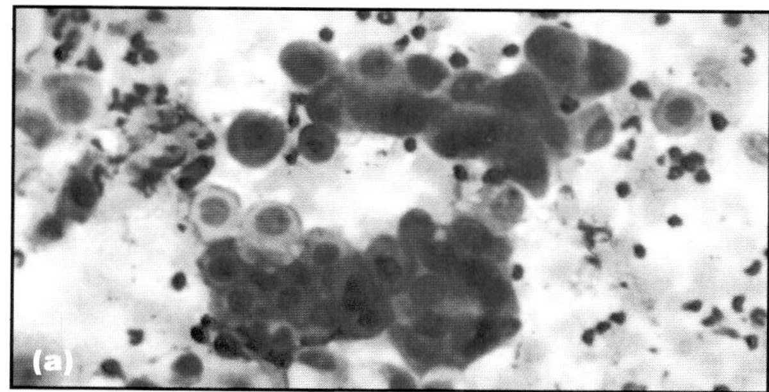

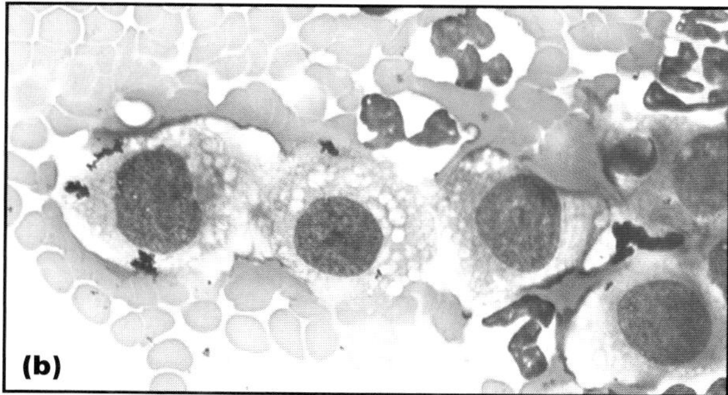

20.31 Squamous cell carcinoma. (a) Fine needle aspirate from an SCC on the nose of a 15-year-old cat. The cells have round nuclei, containing several prominent nucleoli, and moderate to abundant, intensely basophilic, cytoplasm. A mixed population of small lymphocytes and neutrophils, with dark condensed nuclear chromatin, is also present. (b) Fine needle aspirate from an SCC below the mandible of a cat. Note the perinuclear vacuolation of the cytoplasm, coarse nuclear chromatin and large irregularly shaped nucleoli. Several non-degenerate neutrophils can also be seen. (Wright's stain; original magnification X500 (a), X1000 (b))

Perianal adenoma

These are usually seen in intact male dogs (very occasionally in females) and most are located on the perineum adjacent to the anus. They can also be found occasionally on the tail and prepuce. The lesions tend to lobulate or ulcerate as they increase in size. On FNA the cells exfoliate in clusters and are hepatoid in appearance (i.e. they resemble hepatocytes; Figure 20.32). The cells have abundant granular pinkish/blue cytoplasm (Romanowsky) and a round nucleus containing a single centrally located nucleolus. Perianal adenomas are benign; perianal adenocarcinomas are rarely encountered. They tend to show more obvious criteria of malignancy but some may appear well differentiated and cannot reliably be differentiated from adenomas on a cytological basis.

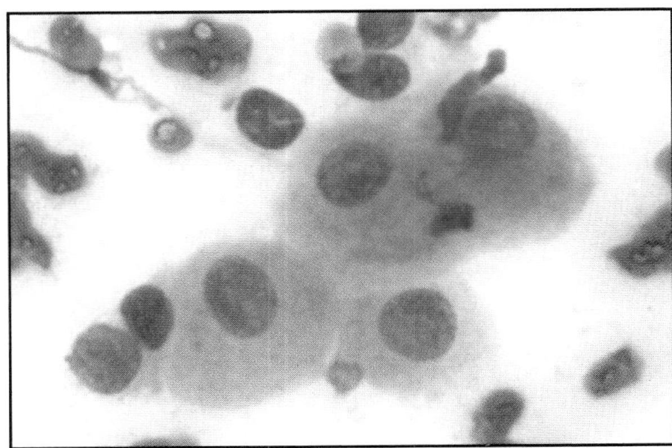

20.32 Fine needle aspirate from a small perianal mass on an entire male Cocker Spaniel. There is a small cluster of epithelial cells with round uniform nuclei and abundant basophilic, grainy cytoplasm resembling hepatocyte cytoplasm (hence the term hepatoid tumour). (Wright's stain; original magnification X1000) (Courtesy of E Villiers)

Apocrine gland adenocarcinoma of the anal sac

These tumours arise from the glands in the walls of the anal sacs. They have a greater tendency to occur in older female dogs. Adenocarcinomas of the anal sac are malignant and have often spread to the sublumbar lymph nodes by the time they are diagnosed. For this reason it is important they are differentiated from perianal adenomas. Up to 50% of cases have a paraneoplastic hypercalcaemia (see Chapter 8). Cells from these tumours usually exfoliate in large sheets or clusters and have a moderate amount of pale basophilic cytoplasm and a round or oval nucleus; cytoplasmic margins are poorly defined (Figure 20.33). Malignant characteristics are usually present but may not be as pronounced as with carcinomas involving other tissues.

Tumours of mesenchymal origin

Lipoma

Lipomas are common benign mesenchymal tumours. They usually affect older obese dogs and occur most commonly on the trunk and proximal limbs. Most lipomas are soft discrete masses that arise in the subcutis. Although they may be quite large, they usually grow slowly. Some lipomas may infiltrate between muscles.

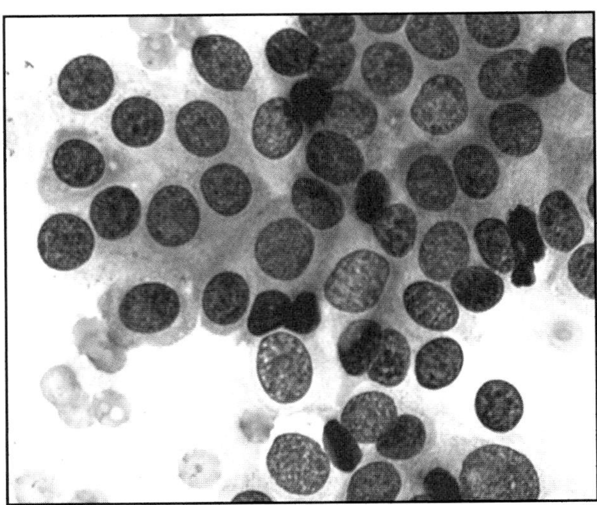

20.33 Fine needle aspirate from an apocrine gland tumour of the anal sac in a 7-year-old German Shepherd bitch. Cells from these tumours often exfoliate in large sheets, have a moderate amount of pale basophilic cytoplasm and a round nucleus. Only a mild degree of anisocytosis and anisokaryosis is evident. (Wright's stain; original magnification X1000) (© Axiom Veterinary Laboratories.)

Grossly, aspirates from lipomas have a greasy appearance and consist of numerous fat droplets that can be stained with Sudan red. Intact adipocytes may be aspirated either singly or in large aggregates. Adipocytes have abundant clear cytoplasm and a small dark nucleus, which is compressed on the periphery of the cell (Figure 20.34a). Small blood vessels may also be seen. Since normal adipose tissue appears similar cytologically, diagnosis of a lipoma is based on an assumption that the aspirate is representative of the lesion under investigation and that the aspirate has not been taken from perilesional fat.

Liposarcomas are rare tumours. They have been reported most frequently on the ventral abdomen. They are firm, poorly demarcated and adhere to underlying tissue. Some may ulcerate. Aspirates consist of dense aggregates of plump spindle-shaped mesenchymal cells containing numerous variably sized lipid vacuoles. The cells show obvious malignant features such as large vesicular nuclei with prominent nucleoli, variation in N:C ratio and multinucleation (Figure 20.34b).

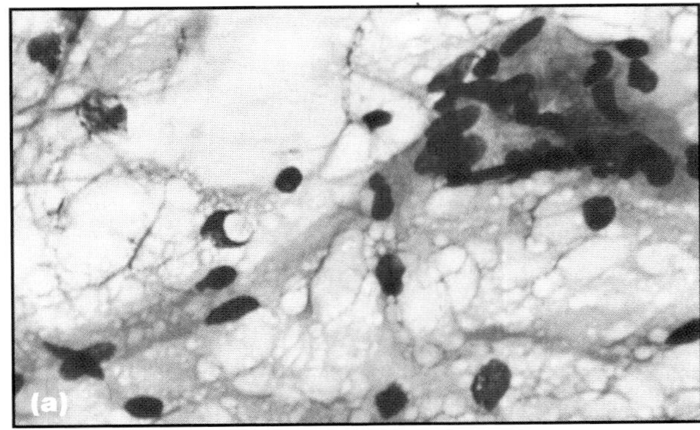

20.34 (a) Lipoma: the aspirate resembles normal adipose tissue. (Wright's stain; original magnification X1000) (© Axiom Veterinary Laboratories.) ▶

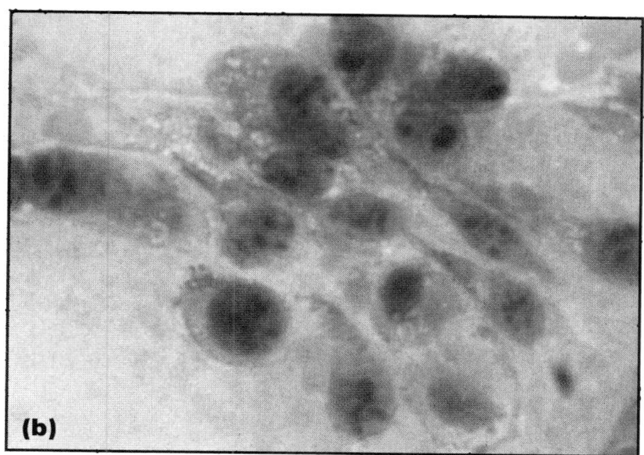

20.34 (b) Liposarcoma: the aspirate contains a population of mesenchymal cells showing several criteria of malignancy. (Wright's stain; original magnification X1000) (© Axiom Veterinary Laboratories.)

Haemangiopericytoma

Haemangiopericytomas are relatively common tumours, which are thought to arise from the cells that line blood vessels. They occur in dogs and are most frequently located on the limbs. Although they usually do not metastasize, haemangiopericytomas are locally invasive and with conservative excision the rate of recurrence is high. Fine needle aspirates are often quite cellular and consist of plump spindle cells (Figure 20.35) with an oval-shaped nucleus and basophilic cytoplasm, which may be vacuolated. Nuclear chromatin has a coarse stippled or reticulated appearance (see Figure 20.20a). Some cells may be seen adhering to the surface of capillaries.

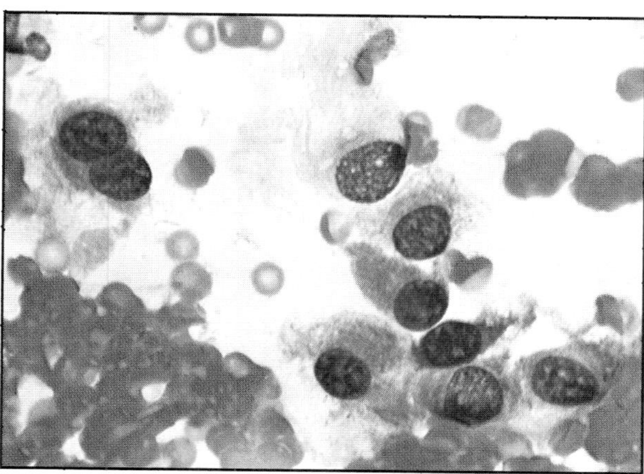

20.35 Fine needle aspirate from a haemangiopericytoma on the thigh of a Bull Mastiff bitch. The plump spindle-shaped cells have wispy cytoplasmic tails and round or oval nuclei. The nuclear chromatin is quite coarse and some nuclei contain one or more small bluish nucleoli. (Wright's stain; original magnification X1000) (© Axiom Veterinary Laboratories.)

Haemangioma and haemangiosarcoma

Haemangiomas are benign tumours arising from vascular endothelial cells and are more common in dogs than cats. They may be solitary or multiple, are dark red in colour, and aspirates usually contain a lot of blood. Small elongated endothelial cells are often present in very low numbers and may be difficult to identify if the aspirate is severely contaminated with blood.

Cutaneous or subcutaneous haemangiosarcomas are relatively rare tumours of older dogs and cats. Some haemangiosarcomas appear well differentiated and cannot be differentiated from haemangiomas. In contrast, the cells aspirated from anaplastic haemangiosarcomas have a high N:C ratio, oval nuclei with a coarse nuclear chromatin pattern and prominent nucleoli, and basophilic cytoplasm that may be vacuolated (Figures 20.36 and 20.56). There may be evidence of erythrophagocytosis and/or chronic haemorrhage (haemosiderin-laden macrophages may be present).

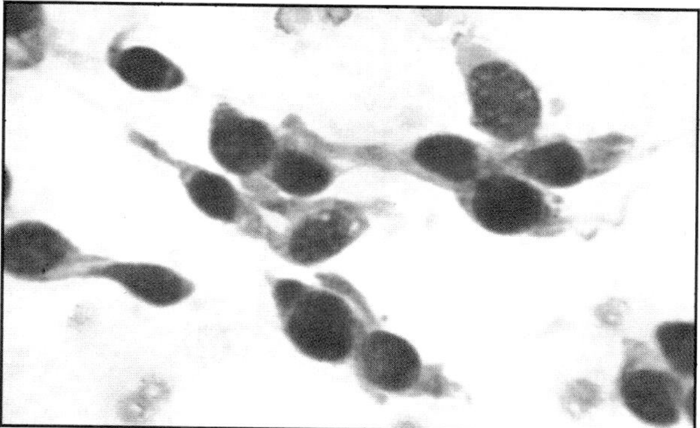

20.36 Fine needle aspirate from a cutaneous haemangiosarcoma located over the elbow joint of a Boxer, showing a population of spindle-shaped cells with elongated cytoplasmic tails. A mild to moderate degree of anisocytosis and anisokaryosis is evident. Cytologically, it would be difficult to differentiate this tumour from the haemangiopericytoma shown in Figure 20.35 (although from a clinical perspective the mass would appear quite different). Histological examination would almost certainly be required to provide a definitive diagnosis. (Wright's stain; original magnification X1000) (© Axiom Veterinary Laboratories.)

Fibroma and fibrosarcoma

Fibromas are relatively rare tumours and are composed of well differentiated spindle cells with an oval nucleus and elongated cytoplasmic tails extending away from the nucleus. Fibrosarcomas are more common, particularly in the cat, and have a predilection for the oral cavity, head and limbs. These tumours are poorly circumscribed and may ulcerate. Vaccine-induced fibrosarcomas are locally invasive and slow to metastasize. Aspirates taken from reactive granulation tissue, fibromas and well differentiated fibrosarcomas may appear remarkably similar, making cytological differentiation difficult (if not impossible). Cells from less well differentiated fibrosarcomas are plumper and have a higher N:C ratio (see Figures 20.21 and 20.37). Nuclear pleomorphism is more pronounced and the occasional multinucleated giant cell may be present. The cells may be located in an eosinophilic matrix material (collagen). Histology is often required to differentiate fibrosarcomas from other spindle cell tumours.

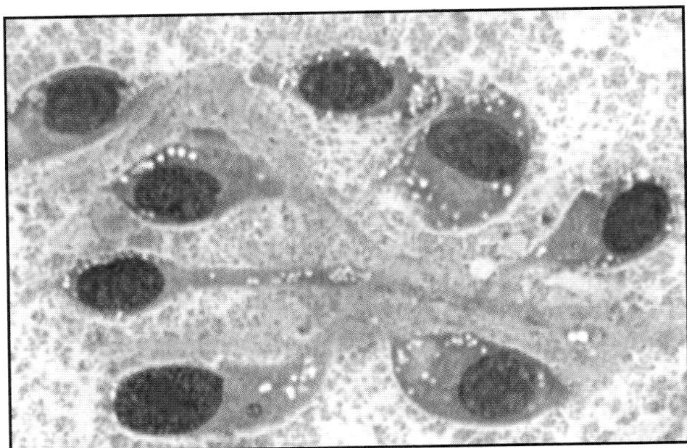

20.37 Fine needle aspirate from a suspected vaccine-induced sarcoma on the neck of a cat. The cytoplasm of these spindle cells is vacuolated and there is marked anisocytosis, anisokaryosis and variation in N:C ratio. Nuclear chromatin appears coarse and each nucleus contains a large irregular nucleolus. The cells are located in a granular eosinophilic background deposit. (Wright's stain; original magnification X1000) (© Axiom Veterinary Laboratories.)

Melanoma

Benign and malignant melanomas occur more frequently in dogs than in cats. The capacity of a melanoma to metastasize depends on its location. Tumours arising in the digits, oral cavity or mucocutaneous junctions, e.g. on the lip, generally carry a much poorer prognosis than cutaneous melanomas. The cytological appearance of cells in aspirates from melanomas varies from epithelioid to mesenchymal; in some cases the cells can even resemble those seen in discrete round cell tumours. Melanin pigment granules can usually be seen within the cells, although the degree of pigmentation is often quite variable. Cells from well differentiated melanomas contain numerous fine black–green granules, which may obscure nuclear morphology. Cells from poorly differentiated tumours, in contrast, may contain scant melanin pigment granules and the cells usually have large nuclei containing several large irregular nucleoli. Anisocytosis and anisokaryosis are usually evident (see Figure 20.25). Amelanotic melanomas are quite rare; with careful examination, a few melanin granules can usually be seen in at least a few of the cells.

Discrete round cell tumours

Canine histiocytoma

Histiocytomas are very common tumours that originate from epidermal Langerhans' cells. Most occur in young dogs less than 5 years of age. They are small, well circumscribed tumours and can occur on the head (especially the pinnae), paws, limbs and trunk. Some may ulcerate; most regress spontaneously. Despite the fact that these tumours are benign, the cells can show a mild to moderate degree of anisocytosis and anisokaryosis. The nuclei are round, oval or indented and the cells have a moderate amount of pale basophilic cytoplasm (see Figure 20.23). Some nuclei may contain one or more poorly defined nucleoli. An increased number of lymphocytes may be seen as the tumour starts to regress.

Other histiocytic neoplasms

Other histiocytic neoplasms that can involve the skin include cutaneous histiocytosis, systemic histiocytosis and malignant histiocytosis.

Canine cutaneous histiocytosis is characterized by the development of multifocal lesions similar to those described for cutaneous histiocytoma. The lesions may wax and wane over a period of months to years.

Systemic histiocytosis occurs in young adult male Bernese Mountain Dogs but has also been reported in other breeds. The skin is consistently affected but regional lymph nodes and ocular sites (e.g. conjunctiva) may also be involved. Like cutaneous histiocytosis, this disorder follows a chronic waxing and waning course. The histiocytes in systemic histiocytosis do not show the degree of malignant atypia seen in malignant histiocytosis. Aspirates may also contain moderate numbers of lymphocytes and neutrophils.

Malignant histiocytosis is a rapidly progressive disease that occurs in older Bernese Mountain Dogs and, less frequently, in other breeds. It has also been reported in cats. Malignant histiocytes may infiltrate the spleen, lymph nodes, lung and bone marrow; the skin is only occasionally involved. Aspirates contain large mononuclear cells with abundant vacuolated cytoplasm showing marked anisocytosis and anisokaryosis (see Figure 20.58). There may be evidence of cytophagia. Nuclear chromatin appears coarse and the nuclei often contain large prominent nucleoli. In addition, there may be evidence of multinucleation, and numerous abnormal mitotic figures may be present.

Mast cell tumour

This is an extremely common tumour in dogs, occurring most frequently on the trunk and limbs. The prevalence is highest in the Boxer, Pug and Boston Terrier.

Mast cell tumours occur less frequently in cats. They tend to occur on the head, neck and limbs. Most solitary lesions are benign. Multiple 'histiocytic type' mast cell tumours have been reported in young Siamese cats. The lesions often regress spontaneously.

Mast cells contain azurophilic cytoplasmic granules that can obscure the nuclei. It should be noted that some water-soluble rapid Romanowsky stains may not stain mast cell granules. The degree of cytoplasmic granularity is quite variable. Mast cells with densely packed cytoplasmic granules and nuclei of uniform size are generally regarded as being well differentiated (see Figure 20.24a). As the malignant potential of the tumour increases, the cytoplasm contains fewer granules, the nuclei contain large prominent nucleoli, and a more marked degree of anisocytosis, anisokaryosis and variation in N:C ratio becomes evident (see Figure 20.24b). Toluidine blue can be used to stain the granules in these poorly differentiated cells. Determining the frequency of agyrophilic nucleolar organizer regions (AGNORs) has been shown to correlate well with the histological grade of the tumour in dogs (Kravis *et al.*, 1996). Aspirates from most canine mast cell tumours also contain a moderate number of eosinophils. Mesenchymal cells are also frequently observed (Figure 20.38).

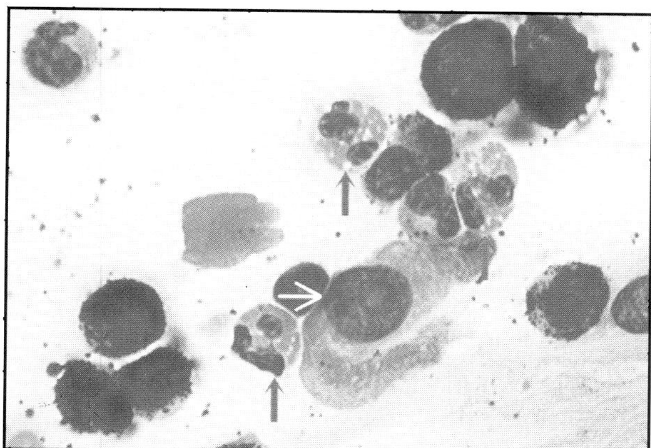

20.38 Fine needle aspirate from a mast cell tumour on the flank of a Boxer. There are numerous mast cells with dense azurophilic cytoplasmic granules. Three eosinophils are present (red arrows) and one large mesenchymal cell, probably a reactive fibrocyte, can also be seen (white arrow). (Wright's stain; original magnification X1000) (© Axiom Veterinary Laboratories.)

Extramedullary plasmacytoma

Plasmacytomas are neoplastic proliferations of plasma cells. They have been reported on the skin (especially the digits and ears), oral cavity, gingiva and tongue of older dogs, but are rare in cats. Although the cells can appear extremely pleomorphic, most plasmacytomas are benign and surgical excision is usually curative. Aspirates are usually quite cellular. The cells have a variable amount of dark basophilic cytoplasm and a round eccentrically placed nucleus with a coarse chromatin pattern. A moderate degree of anisocytosis, anisokaryosis and variation in N:C ratio is usually evident. Binucleated and/or multinucleated cells are often present (Figure 20.39). Pink amorphous material (amyloid) may be intimately associated with the plasmacytoid cells.

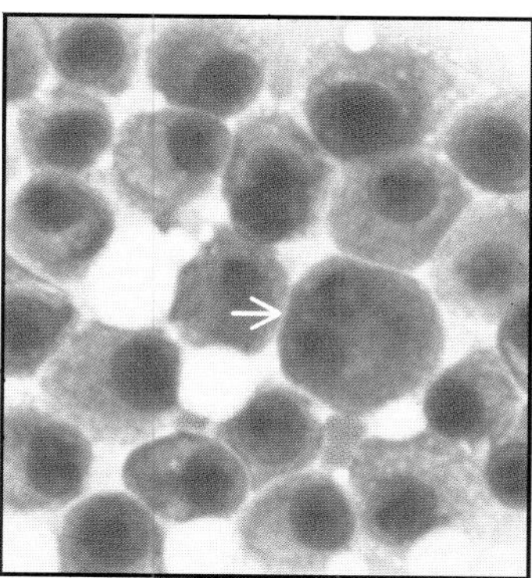

20.39 Fine needle aspirate from a plasmacytoma on the muzzle of a terrier cross. The cells have dark basophilic cytoplasm and a round eccentrically placed nucleus. One large binucleated cell is present (arrowed). (Wright's stain; original magnification X1000) (© Axiom Veterinary Laboratories.)

Cutaneous lymphoma

Lymphoma may arise primarily in the skin or, occasionally, as a manifestation of generalized lymphoma. Cutaneous lymphoma usually presents as solitary or multiple nodules or plaques. It can be classified as epitheliotrophic (also known as mycosis fungoides) or non-epitheliotrophic. Epitheliotrophic lymphoma is the more common form and is usually of T cell origin. The neoplastic T cells infiltrate the epidermis and adnexa. They vary in size from small to large, with round, indented or convoluted nuclei that may contain visible nucleoli. The cells possess a variable amount of pale basophilic cytoplasm (Figure 20.40). Occasionally, in addition to generalized skin involvement, circulating T cells are present in the blood, i.e. the animal is leukaemic (this is known as Sézary syndrome). The non-epitheliotrophic form of cutaneous lymphoma involves the infiltration of the dermis and subcutis by neoplastic lymphoid cells.

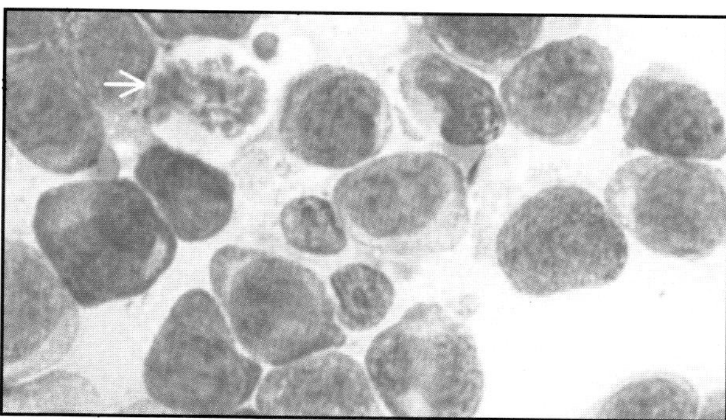

20.40 Fine needle aspirate from an 11-year-old German Pointer with epitheliotrophic lymphoma (mycosis fungoides). The cells are quite large (the nuclei are approximately three times the diameter of a red blood cell) and have a variable amount of basophilic cytoplasm. The nuclei are round, indented or convoluted. One mitotic figure is present (arrowed). (Wright's stain; original magnification X1000) (© Axiom Veterinary Laboratories.)

Canine transmissible venereal tumour

Transmissible venereal tumours (TVTs) are most frequently seen in young, roaming, sexually active dogs. They arise as a result of sexual contact and transplantation of intact cells. In the UK they are usually only seen in dogs imported from temperate climates. The lesions are usually located on the external genitalia or oronasal area, and are poorly circumscribed, ulcerated and haemorrhagic. Superficial secondary bacterial infection is common. The cells from TVTs are large and round with a moderate amount of pale basophilic cytoplasm that may contain small punctate vacuoles (Figure 20.41). The nuclei are round, with coarse nuclear chromatin and one or two prominent nucleoli. Mitotic figures and a mixed inflammatory cell population may be present. The lesions may regress spontaneously. Metastasis is rare but the rate of recurrence is high.

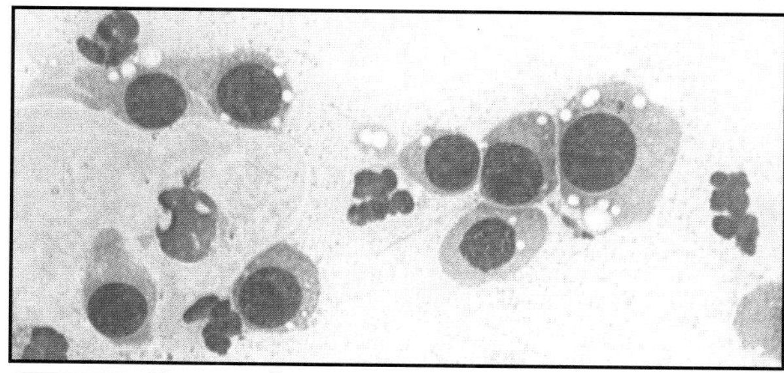

20.41 Fine needle aspirate from a transmissible venereal tumour in the vagina of a crossbred bitch that had been living in Spain, showing a population of round cells with some variation in N:C ratio. Note the punctate cytoplasmic vacuoles. Neutrophils are also present. Secondary superficial inflammation and/or infection is common with these tumours. (Wright's stain; original magnification X1000) (© Axiom Veterinary Laboratories.)

Cytology of lymph nodes

Direct FNA cytology is a useful diagnostic tool to identify the cause of lymphadenopathy in a patient without the need for anaesthesia. Cytology may help in the diagnosis of benign lymph node hyperplasia, lymphoma, lymphadenitis (where infectious agents (e.g. *Leishmania*) may be identified) and metastatic neoplasia.

Sampling

FNA is performed using the needle-only or continuous suction method as described earlier. Impression smears of biopsied lymph nodes can also be examined. If multicentric lymphadenopathy is present, more then one lymph node should always be aspirated. The best samples are often harvested from the popliteal node: the submandibular lymph node is often very reactive, reflecting oral/dental disease; and prescapular lymph node aspirates frequently contain variable amounts of cell-free fat that often increases the fragility of the lymphocytes, resulting in rupture of cells or poor preservation.

Normal findings

In a smear from a 'normal' non-enlarged lymph node, small well differentiated lymphocytes predominate (≥90%), with lower numbers of medium-sized and large lymphocytes (lymphoblasts).

- Small lymphocytes have a diameter approximately 1.5 times that of a red blood cell, a single round nucleus, densely clumped chromatin, no nucleoli and scant basophilic cytoplasm.
- Lymphoblasts (Figure 20.42) are 2–4 times the size of a red blood cell. They have abundant pale basophilic cytoplasm and a lower N:C ratio than small lymphocytes, diffuse finely stippled chromatin, and a variable number of nucleoli.

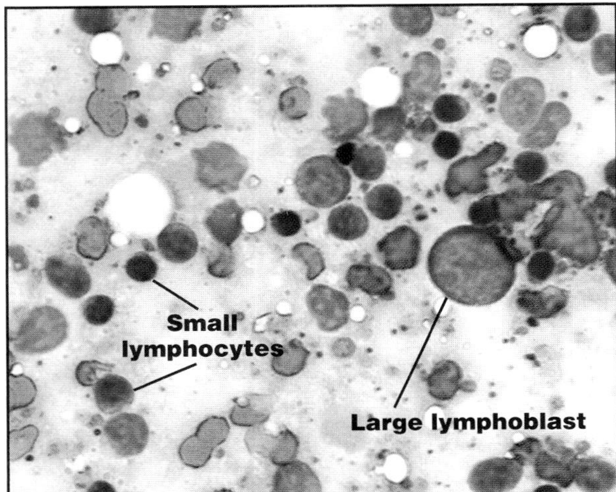

20.42 Fine needle aspirate from the submandibular lymph node. Observe the difference in size between a 'normal' small lymphocyte and a large lymphocyte/lymphoblast. (Wright's stain; original magnification X500) (© Axiom Veterinary Laboratories.)

A few tingible body macrophages, lymphoglandular bodies, and very low numbers of plasma cells may be seen.

- Tingible body macrophages are large mononuclear cells with abundant basophilic vacuolated cytoplasm. In areas of high cell turnover the macrophages contain phagocytosed basophilic cellular debris, hence the name tingible body macrophages.
- Lymphoglandular bodies are basophilic fragments of lymphoid cytoplasm, which are approximately a quarter the size of a red blood cell. Their presence reflects the increased fragility of neoplastic lymphocytes.
- Bare nuclei that lack intact cytoplasm can have prominent nucleoli. These nuclei must not be confused with lymphoblasts as they are of no diagnostic significance.
- Plasma cells (see Figure 20.43) have a moderate N:C ratio, an eccentric nucleus with clumped chromatin (often arranged like the spokes of a wheel) and deeply basophilic cytoplasm; many have a pale perinuclear area compatible with a Golgi zone.

In addition, smears from normal nodes may contain the occasional mast cell. Feline lymph nodes may contain a higher proportion of mast cells compared to canine lymph nodes. It can be difficult to distinguish relatively well differentiated metastatic mast cells from reactive mast cells that are part of the 'normal' cell population within lymph nodes. Some authors quote up to 3% mast cells or 6 mast cells per slide as acceptable.

Abnormal findings

Lymph node hyperplasia

Lymph node hyperplasia occurs in response to any antigenic stimulus. Cytologically, small lymphocytes still predominate but medium-sized lymphocytes and lymphoblasts may constitute up to 20% of the lymphoid population. Increased numbers of plasma cells and macrophages may also be seen. Mott cells may be present; these are plasma cells containing numerous large, lightly basophilic spherical structures (Russell bodies) that contain immunoglobulin (Figure 20.43).

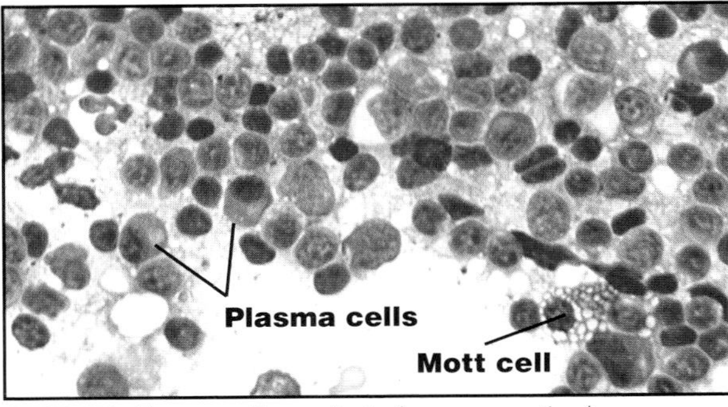

20.43 Fine needle aspirate from a reactive/hyperplastic lymph node in a dog. The presence of increased numbers of plasma cells and Mott cells indicates a response to a strong immunological stimulus. (Wright's stain; original magnification X500) (© Axiom Veterinary Laboratories.)

Lymphoma

Lymphoma is characterized by the proliferation of neoplastic lymphocytes formed as a result of proliferation of a malignant clone of lymphoid cells. Most lymphomas in dogs are of high grade and thus the proliferating cells are lymphoblasts (Figure 20.44). A cytological diagnosis of lymphoma is established when a single population of lymphoblasts forms >50% of the total lymphoid population. In early cases of lymphoma, where the population of malignant lymphoblasts is increased but does not exceed 50% of the total population, the cytological interpretation will be equivocal and histological evaluation is required. Histological investigation entails assessment of architecture of the node and features of malignancy not appreciable on cytology.

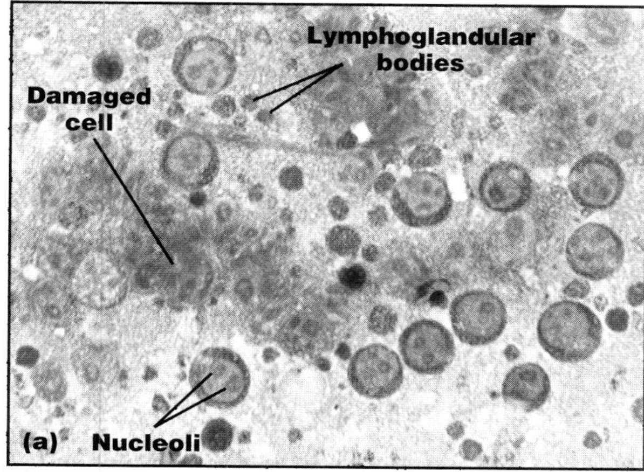

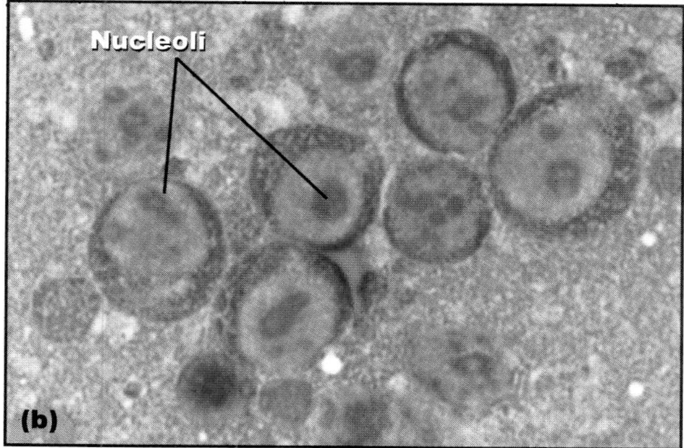

20.44 Centroblastic subtype of B cell lymphoma: fine needle aspirate from the popliteal lymph node of an adult dog with generalized lymphadenopathy. The cells have a round nucleus, fine chromatin pattern, two to four prominent small basophilic marginally placed nucleoli and scant basophilic cytoplasm. Centroblastic lymphoma is the most common subtype in dogs, representing about half of all canine lymphoma cases. (Wright's stain; original magnification X500 (a), X1000 (b)) (© Axiom Veterinary Laboratories.)

Tingible body macrophages, which phagocytose lymphocyte remnants, may increase in number with lymphoma due to increased rates of cell death (apoptosis). Lymphoglandular bodies may be present in low numbers in normal or hyperplastic lymph nodes but are usually present in high numbers in lymphoma. This may be due to the increased fragility of the neoplastic lymphocytes, which are more susceptible to rupture.

In dogs, low-grade lymphomas occur less commonly and are difficult to diagnose cytologically because the proliferating neoplastic cells are small, well differentiated lymphocytes that are morphologically indistinguishable from normal small lymphocytes. If a fine needle aspirate of a markedly enlarged lymph node consists of a monomorphic population of small lymphocytes without reactive change, small cell lymphoma should be considered (Figure 20.45). However, definitive diagnosis often requires excision and histological evaluation of the lymph node. Mixed (small and large lymphocytes) lymphomas are similarly difficult to diagnose on cytology and require histological confirmation.

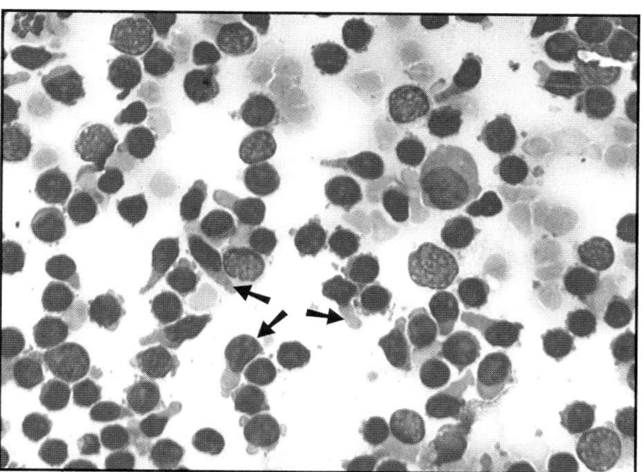

20.45 Fine needle aspirate from a lymph node of a patient with prominent multicentric lymphadenopathy. The majority of cells are small lymphocytes. Some have comet tails of cytoplasm extending from the nucleus (so-called 'hand-mirror' morphology); these tails extend in different directions, distinguishing them from artefacts caused during smear preparation. The monomorphic population of small lymphocytes is suggestive of small cell (lymphocytic) lymphoma; this was confirmed by histopathology. (Wright's stain; original magnification X500) (© Axiom Veterinary Laboratories.)

In cats, lymphoma may be more difficult to diagnose with cytology because mixed- or low-grade lymphomas are more common. In addition, certain forms of reactive hyperplasia may be very marked and can be confused with lymphoma.

Morphological features of neoplastic cells may be used to classify lymphomas. In veterinary medicine the updated Kiel Classification, which considers morphology and immunophenotype, is most frequently used (Fournel-Fleury *et al.,* 1997; Raskin, 2001). Immunophenotyping can be carried out on cytological as well as histological specimens to identify B, T or null cell lymphomas (Figure 20.46). In general, lymphomas of B cell phenotype have a better prognosis then T cell lymphomas. However, a recent study demonstrated Burkitt-like B cell lymphoma was associated with a very poor prognosis, whilst one subtype of T cell lymphoma (classified as clear cell lymphoma) was associated with a relatively favourable prognosis (Ponce *et al.,* 2004). Thus, simply classifying lymphoma as B cell or T cell appears to be an oversimplification; morphological classification is also important.

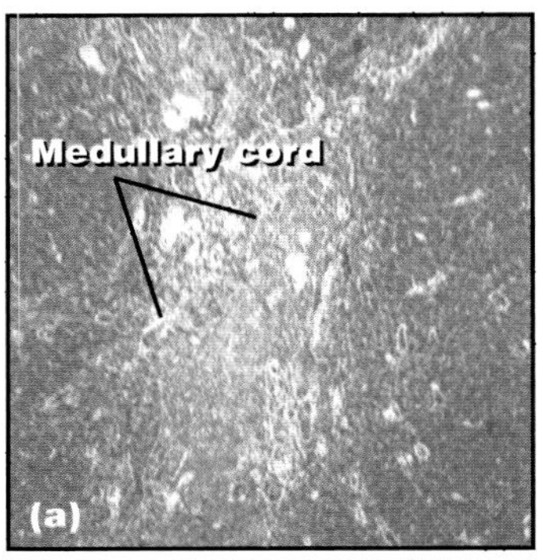

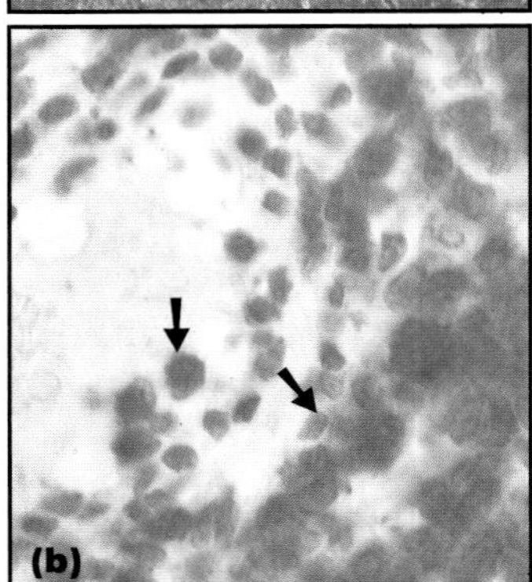

20.46 Immunophenotyping. Immunohistochemical staining with CD79a of a section of canine lymph node. Strong positive (brown) staining of the lymphoid population, which has effaced most of the lymph node, indicates that this is a B cell lymphoma. Residual T lymphocytes in the medullary cords are negative for CD79a but stained positively for CD3. Arrows in (b) indicate CD79a+ lymphoid cells. (Original magnification X40 (a), X100 (b)) (Courtesy of KC Smith and M A Silkstone)

Lymphadenitis

Lymphadenitis is characterized by an increased number of inflammatory cells in the lymph node, usually accompanied by reactive lymphoid hyperplasia. Three types of lymphadenitis may be seen:

- **Suppurative lymphadenitis:** Increased numbers of neutrophils (Figure 20.47a) may be associated with metastatic rapidly expanding tumours (especially squamous cell carcinoma), bacterial infections and fungal or protozoal (e.g. *Toxoplasma*) infections
- **Granulomatous/pyogranulomatous lymphadenitis:** Increased numbers of macrophages, with or without increased numbers of neutrophils, may be associated with leishmaniasis or mycobacterial infections
- **Eosinophilic lymphadenitis:** Increased numbers of eosinophils (Figure 20.47b), mast cells and sometimes melanophages may be observed with chronic skin conditions ('dermatopathic lymphadenopathy'), allergic conditions involving the respiratory or gastrointestinal tract (where tracheobronchial or mesenteric lymphadenopathy may be observed) or in association with metastatic mast cell tumours. Eosinophilic lymphadenitis is also seen occasionally in feline lymphoma.

Metastatic neoplasia

Malignant tumours often metastasize to regional lymph nodes via haematogenous or lymphatic routes. Metastasis to a lymph node occurs more commonly with epithelial (Figure 20.48a) or glandular tumours, round cell tumours (e.g. mast cell tumours; Figure 20.48b) and melanomas than with sarcomas.

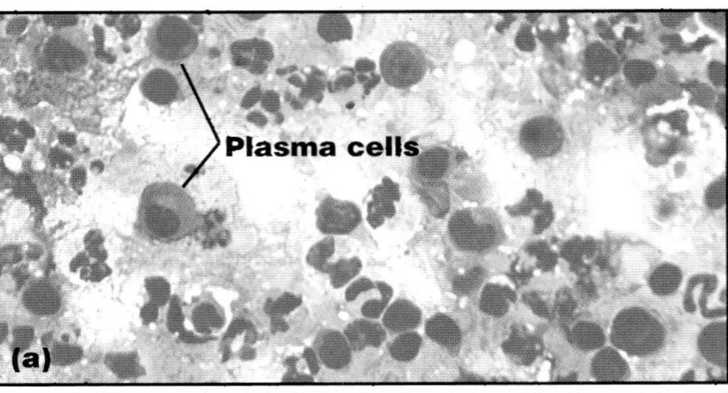

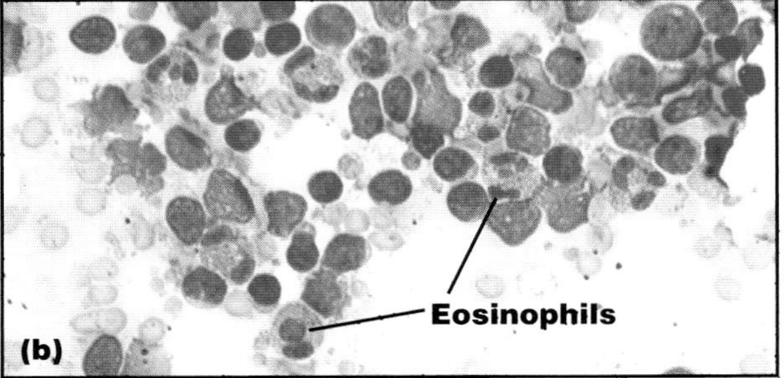

20.47 (a) Suppurative lymphadenitis. Lymph node aspirate showing increased numbers of neutrophils and plasma cells, in addition to the resident lymphoid population. (b) Eosinophilic lymphadenitis. Lymph node aspirate from a West Highland White Terrier with a history of chronic skin disease. There are increased numbers of eosinophils, plasma cells and macrophages, and also increased numbers of medium-sized and large lymphoid cells. (Wright's stain; original magnification X500 (a), X400 (b)) (© Axiom Veterinary Laboratories.)

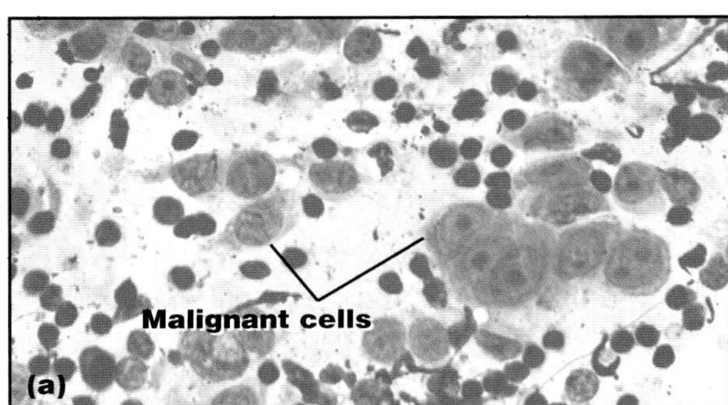

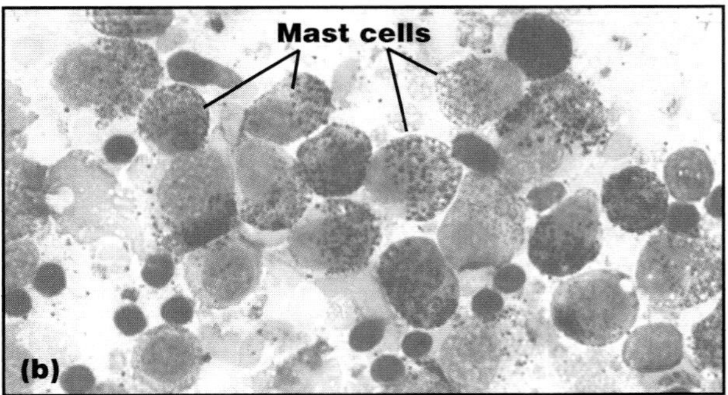

20.48 Metastatic lymph node tumours. (a) Carcinoma. There are clusters and individual epithelial cells that are not normally resident in this regional lymph node. These cells exhibit several criteria of malignancy: large nuclei, variable N:C ratio and prominent nucleoli. (b) Mast cell tumour. There are high numbers of mast cells in this aspirate from a lymph node draining an area from which a histologically diagnosed poorly differentiated mast cell tumour was removed. (Wright's stain; original magnification X100 (a), X500 (b)) (© Axiom Veterinary Laboratories.)

Cytological examination reveals a background population of lymphoid cells compatible with a reactive/ hyperplastic node. Metastatic tumour cells are seen either as scattered individual cells, or as groups of cells concentrated in one area of the smear. The cells are non-haemopoietic in origin and are morphologically distinct from the lymphoid and inflammatory cell populations seen in benign disease. The cell type may be apparent (e.g. epithelial, mesenchymal) or the cells may appear anaplastic (poorly differentiated). As noted earlier, it can be difficult to distinguish a metastatic well differentiated mast cell tumour from mast cells that are part of the 'normal' cell population within the lymph node. Higher percentages of mast cells or poorly granulated mast cells suggest potential metastasis. Concurrent lymphadenitis may be present if the tumour is rapidly expansile.

A recent study in dogs and cats found that FNA cytology showed 100% sensitivity and 96% specificity in detecting tumour metastases in lymph nodes, where histological examination of the entire node was the gold standard (Langenbach *et al.,* 2001). However, while a positive identification of metastasis is always significant, a negative result on cytology does not rule out the presence of metastatic disease.

Haemopoietic neoplasia

Lymphoma is discussed above. Other haemopoietic tumours, including lymphoid leukaemia (Figure 20.49), myeloid leukaemia and malignant histiocytosis, may also infiltrate lymph nodes. Diagnosis is made in the context of peripheral blood and bone marrow evaluation.

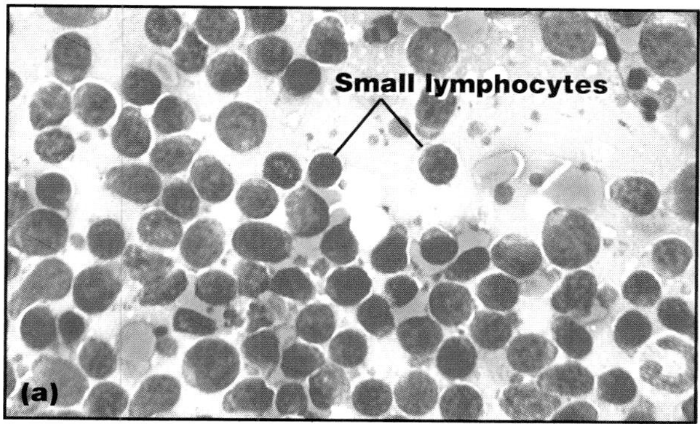

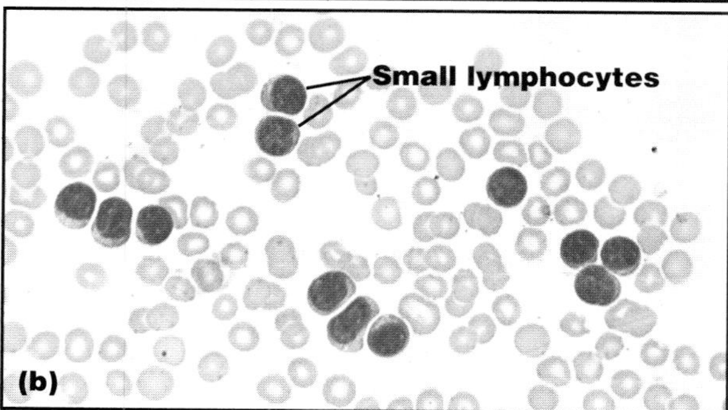

20.49 Chronic lymphocytic leukaemia. (a) Infiltration of a lymph node. Interpretation was made based on other haematological findings, as it is not possible to distinguish the neoplastic small lymphocytes from the 'normal' resident small lymphocytes using light microscopy. (b) Peripheral blood from the patient, which had presented with marked lymphocytosis and hepato/splenomegaly. (Wright's stain; original magnification X500 (a), X400 (b))

Cytology of the liver, spleen and kidney

Sampling

Specimens of liver, spleen and kidney for cytological examination can be collected by percutaneous FNA. Smears are prepared using the methods described above (the squash technique is preferred). Aspirates are best collected under ultrasound guidance to ensure that a representative sample is obtained. This is especially important when sampling nodular or focal lesions. Impression smears can be prepared from biopsy samples.

FNA is usually performed with the animal in dorsal or right lateral recumbency. The technique is similar to that described earlier, except that a slightly longer 22 gauge 1–1.5 inch needle is usually required. Spinal needles are also suitable. Aspirates from these organs are invariably contaminated with blood, and this must be taken into consideration when examining and interpreting smears. The degree of blood contamination can be minimized by using the non-suction (needle-only) technique.

Liver

Clotting times (one-stage prothrombin and activated partial thromboplastin times) and buccal mucosal bleeding time should be checked in animals with severe diffuse hepatic dysfunction as these patients may have clinically significant coagulation defects that contraindicate sampling. Samples can be collected easily from livers that are palpably enlarged and which project beyond the costal arch. If the liver cannot be palpated, the needle should be inserted craniomedially into the liver through the left 12th or 13th intercostal space. Focal lesions should be visualized using ultrasonography. Complications are rare.

Normal findings

Liver aspirates are usually quite cellular. Hepatocytes exfoliate readily, either as single cells or in clusters. Normal hepatocytes have a moderate amount of pale basophilic cytoplasm and a round nucleus with a single prominent nucleolus (Figure 20.50). The cytoplasm often appears granular and has a pinkish tinge (Romanowsky). Some cells may appear vacuolated or contain scant greenish–black bile pigment granules. Cytoplasmic margins are well defined. Compact clusters of smaller cuboidal or low columnar epithelial cells, with a round nucleus and relatively little cytoplasm, may also be present; these are biliary epithelial cells.

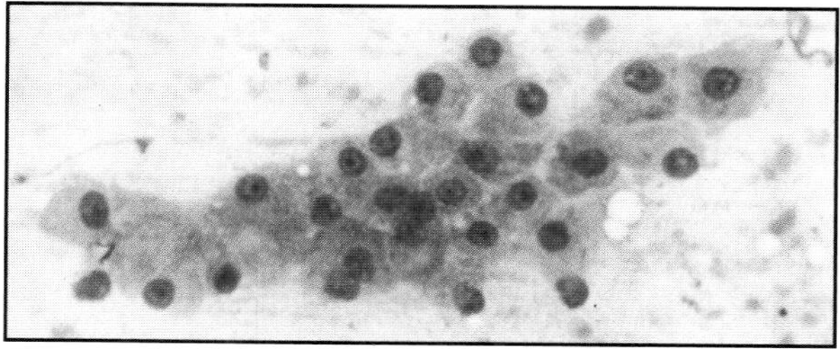

20.50 Normal feline hepatocytes. The cells have a round nucleus and a moderate amount of rather granular pale basophilic cytoplasm. Each nucleus contains a single, centrally located nucleolus. The cells and their nuclei are of uniform size and shape. (Wright's stain; original magnification X500) (© Axiom Veterinary Laboratories.)

Common non-neoplastic disorders

Cholestasis: This results in the accumulation of intracytoplasmic bile pigment and formation of canalicular bile casts (Figure 20.51). Cholestasis is often accompanied by other cytological abnormalities such as evidence of inflammation.

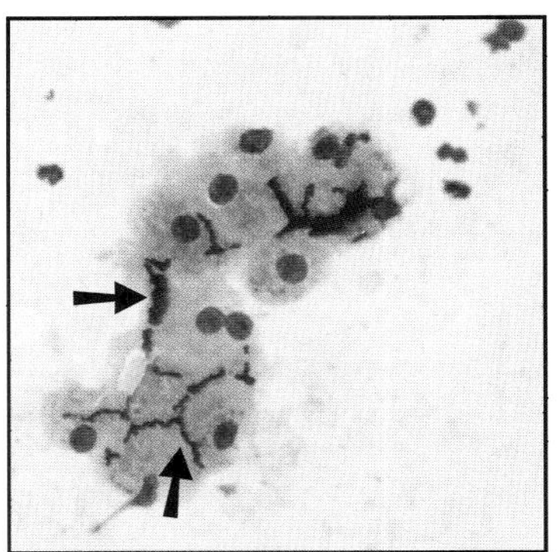

20.51 Cholestasis results in the accumulation of intracytoplasmic bile pigment and the formation of bile casts (arrowed). (Wright's stain; original magnification X500) (© Axiom Veterinary Laboratories.)

Inflammation (cholangitis or cholangiohepatitis): Cholangiohepatitis occurs more frequently in cats than in dogs and can be classified as suppurative or lymphocytic. Diagnosis of inflammation is often difficult, especially in animals with a marked neutrophilia, because fine needle aspirates from liver are always contaminated with blood.

Suppurative cholangiohepatitis can arise as a result of an ascending biliary tract infection. Aspirates contain a large number of neutrophils that are intimately associated with clusters of hepatocytes. Bacteria may be seen in some cases. In contrast, lymphocytic cholangiohepatitis is characterized by the presence of increased numbers of lymphocytes and plasma cells. Differentiation of lymphocytic cholangioheptitis from chronic lymphocytic leukaemia or small cell lymphoma infiltrating the liver may require biopsy. Cytological evidence of cholestasis may be seen in both the suppurative and lymphocytic forms of the disease.

Cytological examination of liver aspirates from a cat with feline infectious peritonitis may show evidence of a pyogranulomatous inflammatory response characterized by the presence of significant numbers of non-degenerate neutrophils and reactive macrophages. Other causes of chronic pyogranulomatous inflammation of the liver include mycobacterial infection, mycotic infections such as aspergillosis and histoplasmosis, and certain protozoal infections, e.g. leishmaniasis.

Feline hepatic lipidosis: Hepatic lipidosis tends to occur in obese cats. Clinical signs include anorexia, jaundice and hepatomegaly. Affected animals usually have a marked increase in alkaline phosphatase (ALP) concentration with little or no increase in gamma-glutamyl transferase (GGT) (see Chapter 12). The condition is easy to diagnose on a cytological basis. Hepatocytes become distended with multiple discrete lipid vacuoles of varying size (Figure 20.52) and the nuclei may be pushed to the periphery of the cell. A milder degree of lipid accumulation in hepatocytes can occur secondary to diabetes mellitus in dogs.

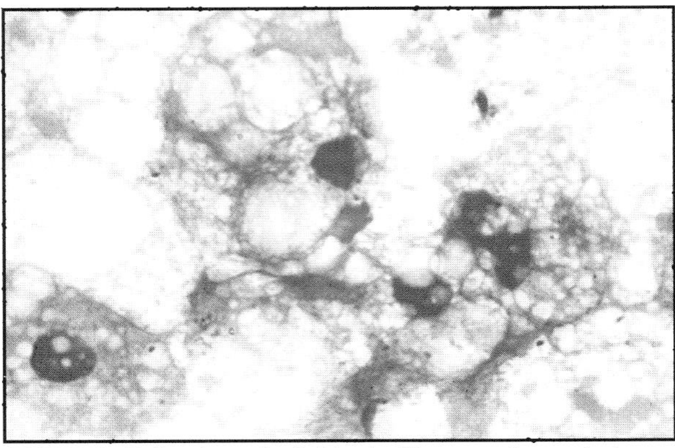

20.52 Feline hepatic lipidosis. Fine needle aspirate from the liver of an adult British Shorthair cat with hepatomegaly and jaundice. The hepatocytes' cytoplasm is distended with numerous large clear vacuoles, consistent with accumulation of fat. (Wright's stain; original magnification X1000) (Courtesy of E Villiers)

Glucocorticoid hepatopathy: Glucocorticoid administration to dogs results in a moderate to marked increase in serum ALP activity with less pronounced increases in other liver enzymes such as GGT and alanine aminotransferase (ALT). The hepatocytes become swollen with glycogen and water (hydropic degeneration). Cytologically, this manifests as diffuse cytoplasmic vacuolation (Figure 20.53) (the vacuoles are less discrete than those seen in cases of hepatic lipidosis). Similar abnormalities in hepatocyte morphology can be seen in response to toxic insult and ischaemia.

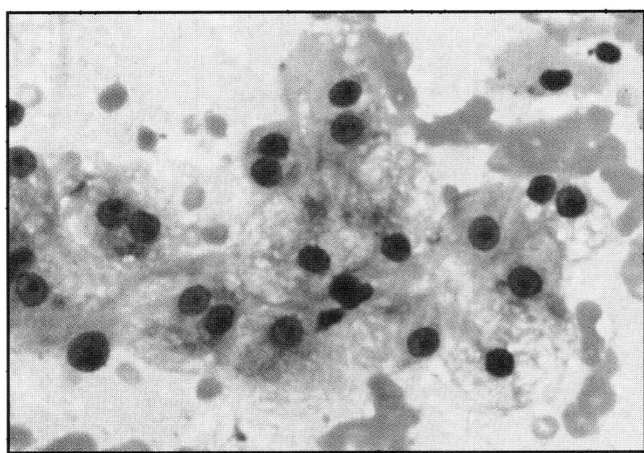

20.53 Glucocorticoid hepatopathy. Fine needle aspirate from the liver of a dog with hyperadrenocorticism. Hypercortisolaemia results in glycogen accumulation and hydropic degeneration of hepatocytes, characterized by diffuse cytoplasmic vacuolation. (Wright's stain; original magnification X500) (© Axiom Veterinary Laboratories.)

Extramedullary haemopoiesis: This occurs most frequently in response to chronic anaemia and is characterized by the presence of late erythroid precursors in the liver (and spleen; see Figure 20.55); myeloid precursors and megakaryocytes may also be present in low numbers. Extramedullary haemopoiesis can also be observed in dogs with chronic hepatitis and nodular regenerative hyperplasia. A few haemopoietic precursors may be present in aspirates from normal livers.

Nodular hyperplasia: Hyperplastic nodules of hepatic parenchyma and fibrous tissue can be seen in the livers of older dogs. On ultrasound examination these nodules may resemble primary or metastatic neoplasia. Fine needle aspirates of these regenerative nodules yield hepatocytes that often appear morphologically normal. The hepatocytes may be slightly larger than normal, and a mild degree of anisocytosis and anisokaryosis may be evident. An increased number of binucleated hepatocytes may also be present. On a cytological basis such lesions are difficult, if not impossible, to differentiate from hepatocellular adenomas and, in some cases, well differentiated carcinomas.

Miscellaneous disorders resulting in pigment accumulation within hepatocytes:

- Copper toxicity occurs primarily in Bedlington and West Highland White Terriers. Fine needle aspirates from affected animals contain a mixed inflammatory cell population. Rubeanic acid can be used to demonstrate copper within hepatocytes as pale green granules
- Increased stores of haemosiderin within hepatocytes may be associated with immune-mediated haemolytic disease. Haemosiderin stains bluish black with Prussian blue
- Lipofuscin pigment granules stain blue with Luxol blue. Lipofuscin accumulation does not represent a pathological process. It is most frequently observed in the hepatocytes of older cats and may be confused with bile pigment.

Primary liver tumours

Primary epithelial tumours of the liver include hepatocellular adenomas/adenocarcinomas and cholangiocellular (bile duct) adenomas/carcinomas. Fine needle aspirates from liver tumours are typically hypercellular and contain large cell clusters.

Hepatomas are relatively rare tumours, which tend to involve one liver lobe. Cytological differentiation of hepatomas from nodular hyperplasia is difficult, if not impossible. Hepatocellular carcinomas also tend to involve a single liver lobe. Diagnosis of hepatocellular carcinoma is based on the presence of hepatocytes that are showing obvious signs of malignancy (e.g. dark basophilic cytoplasm, high N:C ratio, large nuclei with large prominent nucleoli and evidence of multinucleation) (Figure 20.54a). Poorly differentiated hepatocellular carcinomas may be impossible to differentiate from metastatic carcinoma, e.g. of the pancreas. Conversely, some hepatocellular carcinomas contain hepatocytes that do not appear overtly malignant, and these lesions cannot be differentiated from nodular hyperplasia and hepatomas.

Cholangiocellular carcinomas (bile duct carcinomas) are composed of cells that are approximately the same size as, or slightly bigger than, normal biliary epithelial cells and show few of the normal criteria associated with malignancy (Figure 20.54b). They are often arranged in sheets or clusters, and there may be evidence of tubule or acinus formation. The lesions are multiple and diffuse, involving all liver lobes.

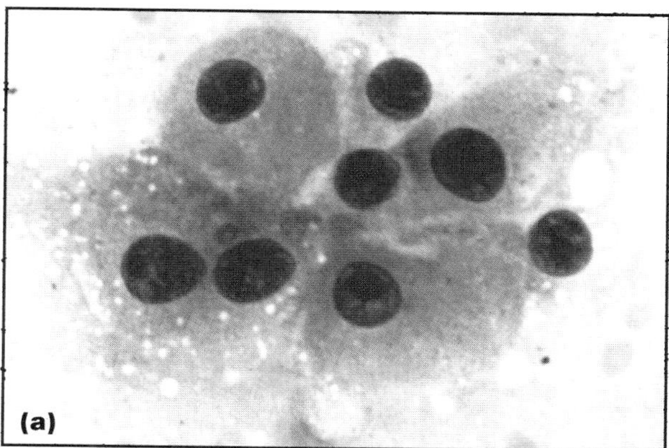

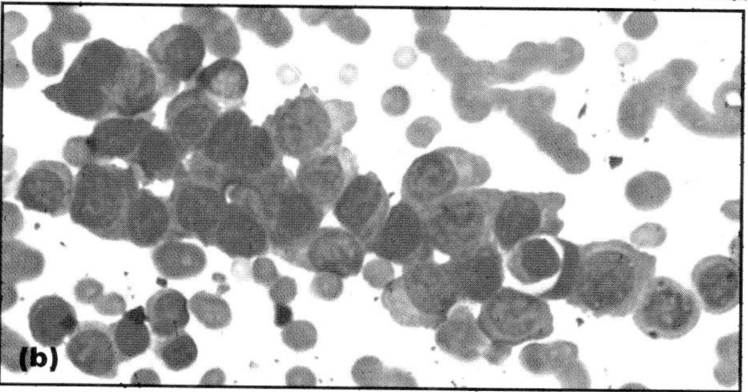

20.54 Primary liver tumours. (a) Hepatocellular carcinoma in a dog. The hepatocytes have darker and more basophilic cytoplasm; the nuclei contain multiple prominent nucleoli. Some of the nucleoli are exceptionally large. (b) Bile duct carcinoma in a cat. The cells in this aspirate are approximately the same size as normal biliary epithelial cells. They are smaller and contain less cytoplasm than hepatocytes and show few of the normal criteria associated with malignancy. A diagnosis of bile duct carcinoma was confirmed histologically. (Wright's stain; original magnification X1000(a), X500(b)) (© Axiom Veterinary Laboratories.)

Tumour metastases and liver involvement in haemopoietic neoplasia

Tumour metastases in the liver can often be detected cytologically. Metastasis to the liver may be expected with neuroendocrine tumours (e.g. pancreatic islet cell tumours), disseminated mastocytosis, carcinoma (e.g. pancreas, intestinal tract) or sarcoma (e.g. haemangiosarcoma). Similarly, malignant histiocytosis (see Figure 20.58) and haemolymphatic neoplasia (particularly lymphoma, acute lymphoblastic leukaemia and acute myeloid leukaemia; see Spleen, below) commonly involve the liver. Although in most cases the neoplastic cells can be classified into one of the previously mentioned categories, special immunocytochemical staining techniques may be required to define cell type accurately.

Spleen

The main indications for FNA of the spleen are splenomegaly or the presence of a splenic mass. The most common causes of splenomegaly in dogs and cats include lymphoproliferative and myeloproliferative disease, haemangiosarcoma, immune-mediated haemolytic anaemia, extramedullary haemopoiesis, and certain infectious conditions, e.g. histoplasmosis. Unless a diffuse lesion (e.g. lymphoma) is expected, the technique is best performed under ultrasound guidance. The risk of intra-abdominal haemorrhage and seeding of tumour metastases within the peritoneal cavity should be considered if attempting to aspirate a suspected haemangiosarcoma.

Normal findings

The spleen is part of the haemolymphatic system and its cytological appearance generally resembles that of a normal lymph node, with small lymphocytes predominating in most fields (see Figure 20.42); lymphoblasts, plasma cells and macrophages are also present but in lower numbers. Some of the macrophages may contain haemosiderin. Small endothelial-lined capillaries and a few mast cells may also be seen. Aspirates from the capsular surface may contain sheets of mesothelial cells. Splenic aspirates are always severely contaminated with blood and therefore contain variable numbers of white blood cells and platelets. Small numbers of haemopoietic precursors, including the occasional megakaryocyte, may be seen in aspirates from normal spleens.

Common non-neoplastic disorders

Splenic hyperplasia: This occurs in response to systemic infection (e.g. babesiosis, leishmaniasis, ehrlichiosis, histoplasmosis) and immune-mediated disease (e.g. immune-mediated haemolytic anaemia (IMHA), thrombocytopenia). Small and medium-sized lymphocytes remain the predominant cell types but there are relative increases in the numbers of lymphoblasts, plasma cells and macrophages. Increased numbers of macrophages, containing either haemosiderin and/or phagocytosed red cells, may be seen in some cases of IMHA.

Splenitis or splenic abscessation: A marked increase in the number of neutrophils occurs with splenitis and splenic abscessation, both relatively rare conditions.

***Extramedullary haemopoiesis*:** This occurs in any condition where the bone marrow cannot sustain an increased demand for red blood cells. Precursors from all three cell lines may be present but members of the erythroid series usually predominate (Figure 20.55).

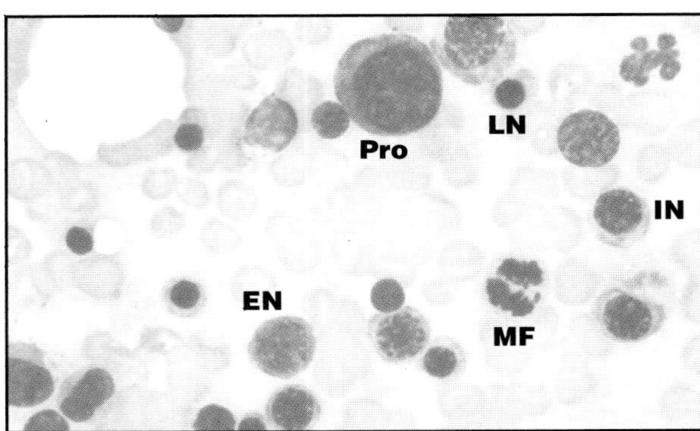

20.55 Extramedullary haemopoiesis seen in fine needle aspirates from spleen. All stages of red cell development are present: Pro = proerythroblast (rubriblast); EN = early normoblast (prorubricyte); IN = intermediate normoblast (rubricyte); LN = late normoblast (metarubricyte). A mitotic figure is present (MF). (Wright's stain; original magnification X1000) (Courtesy of E Villiers)

Primary splenic neoplasia

The most common primary splenic tumour in dogs is haemangiosarcoma. Fibrosarcomas, leiomyosarcomas and other undifferentiated sarcomas are less frequently encountered.

Haemangiosarcoma is characterized by the presence of mesenchymal-type cells with poorly defined cytoplasmic margins (Figure 20.56). The neoplastic cells have dark basophilic cytoplasm that may be vacuolated. Marked anisocytosis, anisokaryosis and variation in N:C ratio is usually evident. Some cells are quite clearly spindle-shaped; others are rounder and plumper. Nuclear chromatin tends to be coarsely clumped or has a coarse stippled appearance. Scrapings or impression smears of splenic tissue tend to be more reliable than smears prepared from fine needle aspirates, which are relatively insensitive for the diagnosis of splenic haemangiosarcoma.

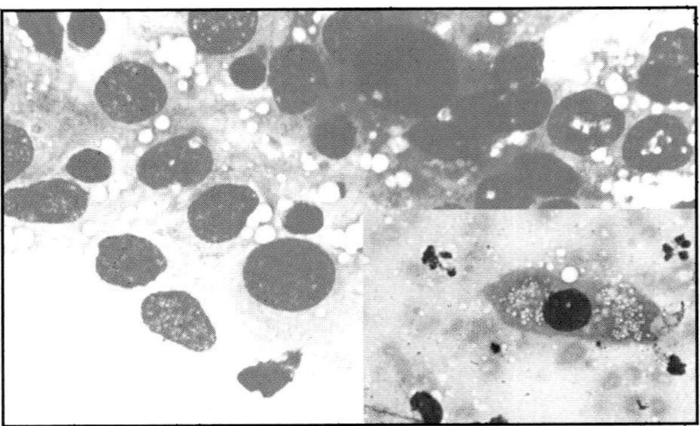

20.56 Haemangiosarcoma: fine needle aspirate from the spleen of a 7-year-old German Shepherd Dog. There is a cluster of mesenchymal cells with dark basophilic cytoplasm. The cytoplasm of the neoplastic cells may be vacuolated (inset). (Wright's stain; original magnification X1000) (© Axiom Veterinary Laboratories.)

Haemolymphatic neoplasia

Haemolymphatic tumours similar to those which can infiltrate the liver can also involve the spleen. These include lymphoma, acute myeloid or lymphoblastic leukaemia, chronic lymphocytic or myeloid leukaemia, multiple myeloma (Figure 20.57), malignant histiocytosis (Figure 20.58), and disseminated mastocytosis (more common in cats).

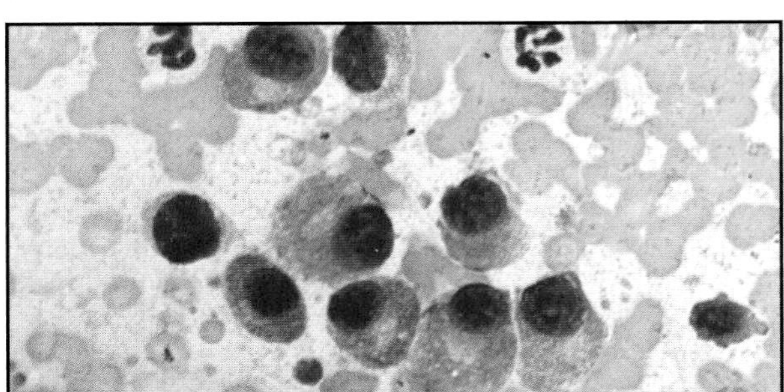

20.57 Multiple myeloma: fine needle aspirate from the spleen of a dog. The plasma cells have a moderate amount of dark basophilic cytoplasm and an eccentrically placed nucleus. Note the prominent perinuclear 'halo' which represents the Golgi apparatus. (Wright's stain; original magnification X1000) (© Axiom Veterinary Laboratories.)

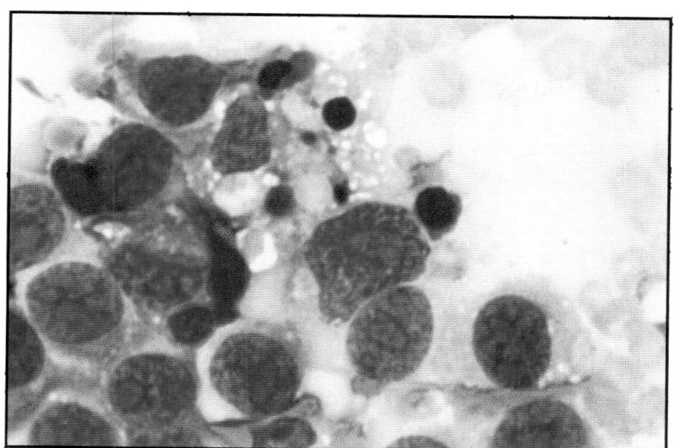

20.58 Malignant histiocytosis: splenic aspirate from a dog. There are several large round histiocytes with large nuclei and prominent nucleoli. One cell is phagocytosing red blood cells. (Wright's stain; original magnification X500)

Kidney

FNA of the kidney is a useful procedure for the investigation of suspected neoplasia, especially renal lymphoma in dogs and cats. FNA also lends itself to cystic and inflammatory lesions, e.g. in feline infectious peritonitis. If possible FNA is best performed under ultrasound guidance, using a non-aspiration technique without redirection, in order to ensure the needle is not directed into the renal hilus.

Normal findings

Renal tubular epithelial cells are round to polygonal cells with abundant basophilic granular cytoplasm and a round nucleus containing a small single nucleolus (Figure 20.59). The cells exfoliate singly or in clusters and are of uniform size and shape. Tubular fragments or casts may sometimes be seen. The renal tubular epithelial cells of cats may be vacuolated due to the presence of lipid droplets. Similar cells may be seen in dogs with diabetes mellitus or which have received long-term corticosteroids.

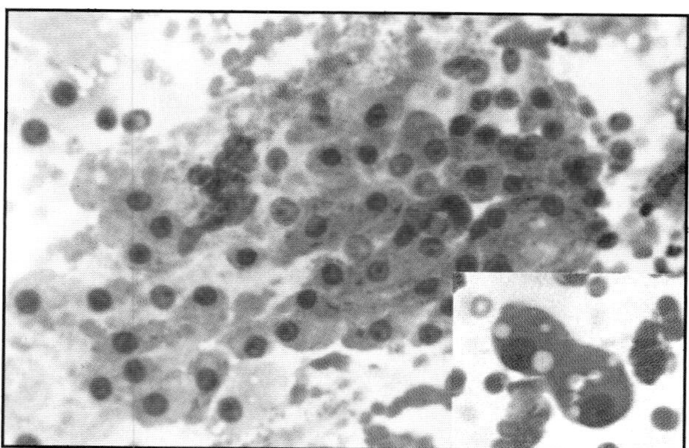

20.59 Fine needle aspirate from a feline kidney, showing a cluster of normal renal tubular epithelial cells with granular basophilic cytoplasm and a round nucleus containing a single nucleolus. The cytoplasm may be vacuolated, especially in cats, due to the presence of lipid droplets (inset). (Wright's stain; original magnification X500) (© Axiom Veterinary Laboratories.)

Non-neoplastic disorders

Inflammation: A large number (>90%) of degenerate neutrophils (with or without bacteria) in a renal aspirate is consistent with acute pyelonephritis. A pyogranulomatous inflammatory response may be seen in feline infectious peritonitis.

Renal cysts and abscesses: Renal cysts may be single or multiple, congenital or acquired. Aspirated fluid is usually clear or slightly straw-coloured and contains very few cells (the occasional epithelial cell, neutrophil or macrophage may be seen). Renal carcinomas can sometimes become cystic; these tumours rarely exfoliate malignant cells into the cystic fluid.

Renal abscesses are uncommon in dogs and cats. They occasionally occur secondary to pyelonephritis. The aspirated material is typical of an acute septic inflammatory exudate.

Neoplasia

Primary renal carcinomas are uncommon in dogs and cats, but may be cystic (see above). Diagnosis is based on the presence of a population of epithelial cells demonstrating adequate criteria of malignancy (although the degree of cytological atypia may not be as pronounced as in carcinomas involving other organs, such as the lung).

Lymphoma is the most common renal tumour, especially in the cat, and usually involves both kidneys. Cytological diagnosis is relatively straightforward. Aspirates are usually hypercellular and consist almost entirely of large lymphoblasts with a high N:C ratio (see Figures 20.22 and 20.44).

Cytology of the prostate gland

The prostate may be sampled by performing a prostatic wash or by direct FNA. Common indications for sampling are prostatomegaly, other abnormalities in shape, symmetry or consistency, and prostatic pain.

Sampling

Prostatic wash

1. The bladder is emptied by inserting a sterile urethral catheter. The bladder may be flushed with saline and emptied again at this point to ensure that all urine has been removed. A sample of the saline flush can be collected for comparison with the prostatic wash to help clarify the site of pathology (bladder *versus* prostate).
2. The catheter is partially withdrawn to the level of the prostate, guiding the catheter per rectum.
3. The prostate is massaged per rectum and transabdominally and then 5 ml of sterile saline is injected into the urinary catheter.
4. After further massage, material is aspirated into the catheter using a 10 or 20 ml syringe. It is important to ensure that the contents of the catheter as well as those of the syringe are harvested.

For turbid samples a direct smear of the wash is prepared. It is usually necessary to concentrate the sample by centrifugation (see Chapter 21); however, if this cannot be done on site, placing some of the wash into an EDTA tube in addition to the direct smear is advisable. A sample should also be placed in a sterile plain pot for culture if infection is suspected.

Prostatic FNA

This is performed percutaneously via the caudal abdomen using ultrasound guidance. The prostate may be pushed cranially with a gloved finger in the rectum. Squash smears are prepared as described earlier. FNA may be more helpful then a prostatic wash, especially for the diagnosis of neoplasia, since cells may not exfoliate into the prostatic urethra. In addition, FNA avoids the possibility of contamination by material from the urinary bladder: distinction between squamous metaplasia and squamous cell contamination from the distal urethra can be made with greater certainty. Preservation and morphological detail of prostatic cells obtained by FNA are superior to cells obtained by a prostatic wash, since the cells are not in direct contact with urine. FNA should not be performed if a prostatic abscess is suspected because of the risk of rupture of the abscess and subsequent peritonitis.

Normal findings

A prostatic wash from a 'normal' patient consists of prostatic epithelial cells; it may also contain cells from the proximal and distal urinary tract, as well as spermatozoa. Prostatic epithelial cells are small uniform cuboidal cells, usually found in small cohesive clusters. They have a moderate N:C ratio, a single round centrally located nucleus, finely stippled chromatin and moderate amounts of basophilic cytoplasm. Some may have a small inconspicuous nucleolus.

Cells from the distal urethra are usually large superficial squamous epithelial cells with abundant blue cytoplasm (Romanowsky) and a round pyknotic nucleus. Transitional epithelial cells, collected from the proximal urethra and bladder, are larger than prostatic epithelial cells, have a lower N:C ratio and lighter cytoplasm.

Non-neoplastic disorders

Inflammation: Neutrophilic inflammation characterizes prostatitis and is usually due to bacterial infection. The neutrophils are usually degenerate due to the effects of bacterial toxins. Intracellular bacteria are often identified (Figure 20.60). Prostatic epithelial cells are seen in clusters and may be dysplastic or undergo squamous metaplasia secondary to the inflammatory reaction.

Squamous metaplasia: Prostatic epithelial cells develop morphological and staining characteristics of squamous epithelium (Figure 20.61), due to the influence of increased circulating concentrations of oestrogen, e.g. a functional Sertoli cell tumour, chronic irritation, or inflammation. It may be difficult to distinguish squamous metaplasia from 'normal' squamous epithelium that originates from the distal urethra and is obtained by contamination during the prostatic wash procedure.

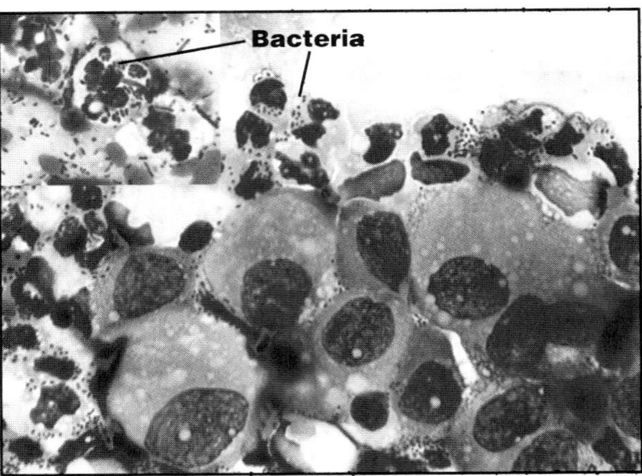

20.60 Septic suppurative prostatitis/prostatic abscess. Neutrophils have phagocytosed bacteria, indicating active infection. Prostatic epithelial cells show typical cytological features of dysplasia, which include marked anisocytosis and increased cytoplasmic basophilia. (Wright's stain; original magnification X500) (© Axiom Veterinary Laboratories.)

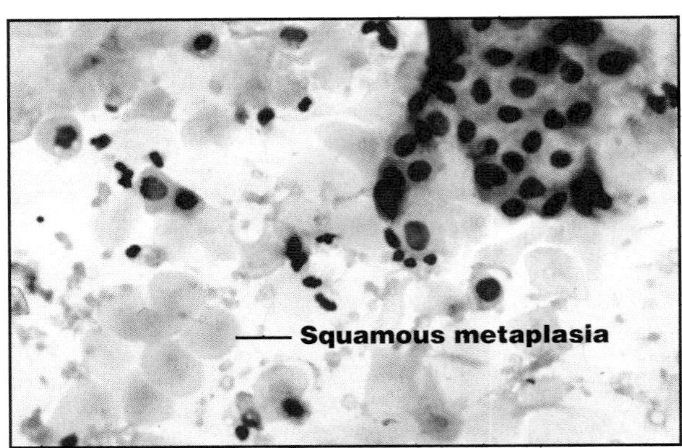

20.61 Ultrasound-guided direct fine needle aspirate from a bilaterally enlarged prostate. Prostatic epithelial cells that have undergone squamous metaplasia have abundant hyalinized basophilic cytoplasm and occasionally contain a small pyknotic nucleus. Compare the normal prostatic epithelial cells in the top right hand corner with the squamous epithelial cells in the rest of the field. (Wright's stain; original magnification X100) (© Axiom Veterinary Laboratories.)

Benign prostatic hyperplasia: This is characterized by symmetrical enlargement of the prostate, and occurs under hormonal influence in intact older male dogs (mediated mainly by dihydrotestosterone in the presence of an altered androgen:oestrogen ratio).

Cytologically, there may be an increased cell yield of prostatic epithelial cells, which are of uniform size and shape, and similar in appearance to 'normal' prostatic epithelium. They may have a mild increase in N:C ratio, and small indistinct nucleoli may be seen (Figure 20.62). Prostatic hyperplasia can occur in association with inflammation and squamous metaplasia.

Prostatic cyst: Prostatic cysts may be single or multiple, intraprostatic or paraprostatic (arising from a remnant of the uterus masculinus). They can occur in association with BPH or squamous metaplasia. Serosanguineous to brown fluid is usually aspirated. This

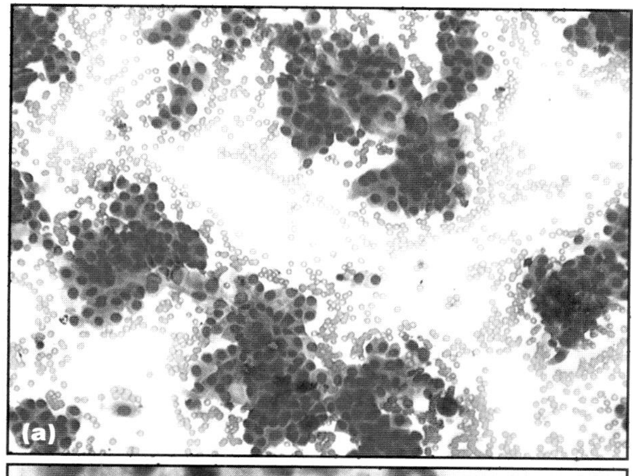

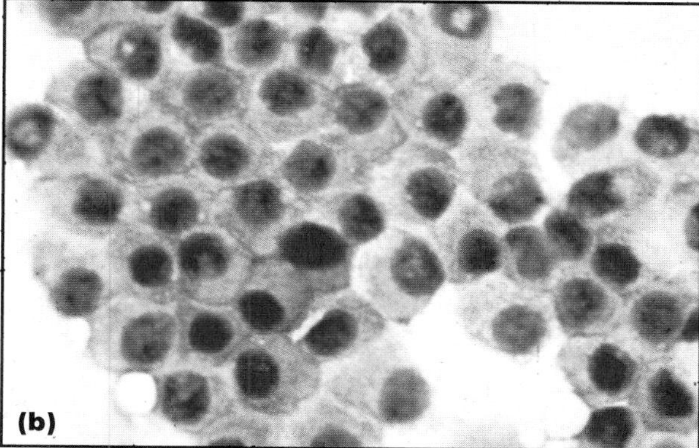

20.62 Fine needle aspirate from a bilaterally enlarged prostate in an entire middle-aged dog. The prostatic epithelial cells are of uniform size and shape and are arranged in large 'honeycomb' clusters. The appearance is consistent with benign prostatic hyperplasia. The higher power view shows a sheet of cells resembling a honeycomb mosaic. Cytoplasm is finely vacuolated and nucleoli are not visible. (Wright's stain; original magnification X100(a), X400(b)) (a, © Axiom Veterinary Laboratories; b, courtesy of E Villiers.)

may be acellular or may contain variable amounts of cellular debris and/or low numbers of red blood cells or neutrophils and macrophages plus a few benign prostatic or squamous epithelial cells. The cysts may become secondarily infected, in which case higher numbers of neutrophils will be present.

Neoplasia

Prostatic neoplasia, in contrast to other prostatic diseases, can be seen in both intact and neutered dogs (Obradovich *et al.*, 1987; Teske *et al.*, 2002). Adenocarcinomas of prostatic origin are the most common tumours, followed by transitional cell carcinoma from the prostatic urethra. Prostatomegaly is usually asymmetrical but can be symmetrical. On microscopic examination, cell clusters are often very disorganized and show typical cytological features of malignancy, including prominent anisokaryosis, anisocytosis, pleomorphic nuclei and nucleoli that are often multiple, prominent or large (Figure 20.63). FNA may be more sensitive than prostatic wash for detecting adenocarcinoma if the tumour has not invaded the urethra. The prognosis for prostatic neoplasia is poor.

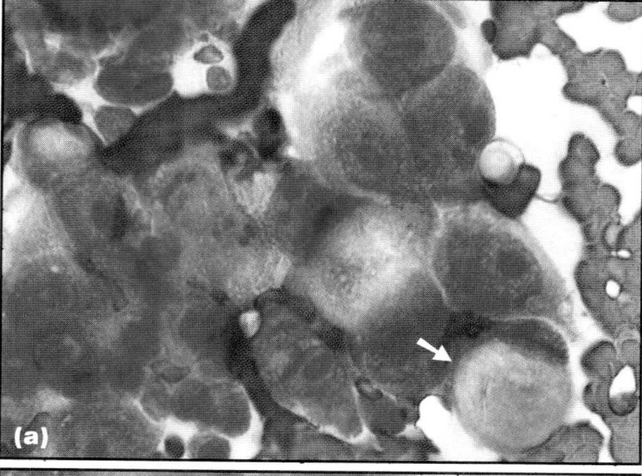

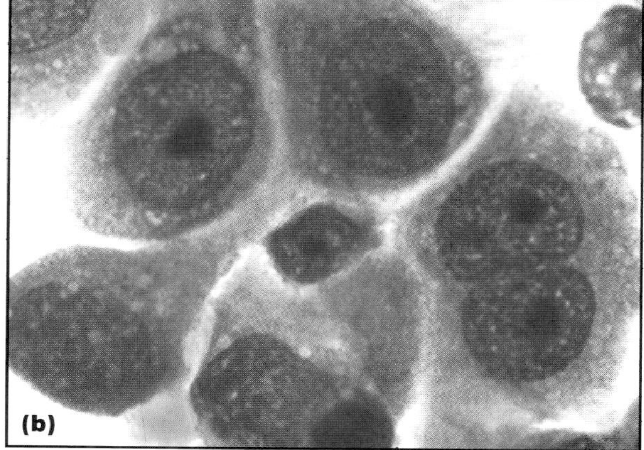

20.63 Prostatic carcinoma: direct fine needle aspirate from an asymmetrically enlarged prostate in a dog that presented with a clinical history of tenesmus and haematuria. There are multiple atypical features, including anisocytosis, anisokaryosis, nuclear moulding and prominent pleomorphic nucleoli. The eosinophilic intracytoplasmic material is a secretary product that may be seen in prostatic glandular tissue. The higher power view demonstrates a coarse nuclear chromatin pattern and increased cytoplasmic basophilia, both indicators of malignancy. (Wright's stain; original magnification X500(a), X1000 (b))

Cytology of the respiratory tract

Samples for cytology can be obtained directly from the respiratory tract using an endoscope or, blindly, through an endotracheal tube or by transtracheal aspiration. These are useful techniques for investigating animals with tracheal, bronchial or lower respiratory tract disease, especially airway or diffuse alveolar disease. They are inexpensive and minimally invasive tools. However, they have limited application with parenchymal (interstitial or focal) disease that does not cross the bronchial walls. Thus, where there is generalized interstitial disease or where a focal lesion can be visualized (e.g. with ultrasonography) FNA may be more appropriate. There is a significant risk of pneumothorax when aerated lung is penetrated whilst taking a fine needle aspirate from the lungs. This risk can be minimized by using a fine needle, by performing the procedure under general anaesthesia, and by controlling respiration during the sampling procedure.

Sampling equipment

The basic equipment required for obtaining cytology specimens from the respiratory tract is:

- Catheter: jugular catheter; male urinary catheter plus intravenous cannula; or biopsy channel catheter
- Syringes containing warm saline (0.9% sodium chloride)
- 20 ml syringe for suction or mucus extractor attached to suction machine (Figure 20.64)
- Transport containers – EDTA for cytology, plain sterile tube for culture
- Glass slides for direct smears of mucus flecks.

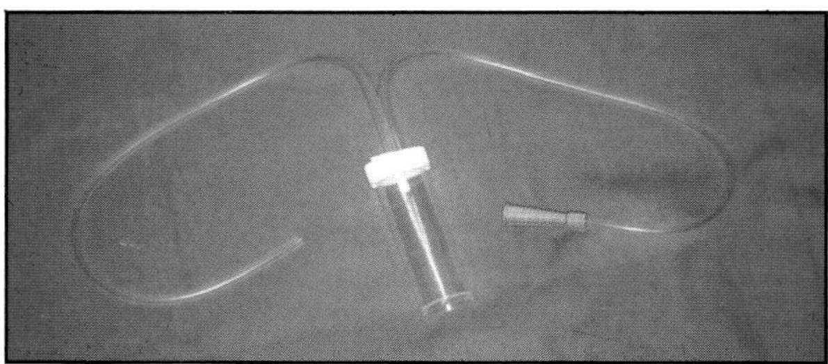

20.64 A mucus extractor can be used to harvest material from tracheal washing or bronchoalveolar lavage. The green-ended tube is attached to a suction machine (low setting) and the other tube is attached to the tracheal catheter. (Courtesy of E Villiers)

Sampling techniques

There are three techniques for obtaining a sample: via a bronchoscope; through an endotracheal tube; or by transtracheal collection. The latter two techniques generally yield samples representative of the trachea and primary or (at best) secondary bronchi (referred to as a tracheal wash (TW)), although some material from the lower bronchioles and alveoli may be collected. For patients with deep parenchymal disease the endoscopic technique is preferred, since this is most likely to yield material from the lower bronchioles or alveoli (i.e. bronchoalveolar lavage). In practice, the choice of procedure is determined by the site of respiratory pathology, the suitability of the patient for general anaesthesia and the equipment available.

Bronchoalveolar lavage

Bronchoalveolar lavage (BAL) can be performed using a flexible endoscope:

1. Under general anaesthesia the endoscope is inserted into a bronchus, until it fits snugly.
2. A catheter is inserted into the biopsy channel of the endoscope.
3. A large volume of saline (10 ml for dogs up to 8 kg and for cats; 25 ml for larger dogs) is injected, flooding the alveoli associated with that bronchus.
4. The exfoliated material is aspirated using a mucus extractor attached to a suction machine (see Figure 20.64) or a large syringe attached via a 3-way tap (multiple suctions).

Only a small proportion of the injected saline is usually aspirated. The yield may be improved by coupage during the collection procedure. If more than one site is of interest the procedure can be repeated but samples must be labelled appropriately.

Sampling through an endotracheal tube

Blind sampling by passing a catheter through a sterile endotracheal (ET) tube while the patient is anaesthetized is commonly used in cats and small dogs. Care should be taken to minimize contact between the tip of the ET tube and the oropharynx during intubation to avoid oropharyngeal contamination. Coupage and turning the patient may improve cell yield.

1. A jugular catheter or sterile polypropylene male dog urinary catheter (2.0 mm, 2.7 mm or 3.3 mm depending on patient size) is passed through the ET tube. The tip of the catheter can be cut off to remove the side holes, but care must be taken to ensure that the tip is not sharp.
2. The distance the catheter is inserted varies depending on the anatomical location from which a sample is required.
3. 0.3–0.5 ml/kg of warmed saline is injected into the catheter and aspirated back as described for BAL.

Transtracheal collection

This technique can be used where general anaesthesia is a risk to the patient. Mild sedation may be necessary, depending on the patient's temperament.

Suitable catheters are:

- Through-the-needle long jugular catheter (19–22 gauge, 8 inches long for cats and small (< 10 kg) dogs; 19 gauge, 12 or 24 inches long for larger dogs)
- 3.5 French polyethylene male urinary catheter, together with a 16 gauge through-the-needle intravenous cannula
- Transtracheal lavage set (Figure 20.65).

The technique is as follows:

1. The patient is restrained in a sternal position with the head elevated.
2. The area over the larynx or proximal trachea is clipped and surgically prepared. The usual site is the cricothyroid ligament but an alternative site is between two tracheal rings (measure against radiograph or the patient).
3. Local anaesthetic is injected into the skin and subcutis over the cricothyroid ligament, which can be palpated. A small skin incision is made over the ligament.
4. If a through-the-needle catheter is used, the needle is inserted through the ligament into the trachea. The catheter is then passed through the needle and down the trachea. The needle can then be retracted. Alternatively, an intravenous cannula is passed through the cricothyroid ligament, the stylet removed, and the urinary

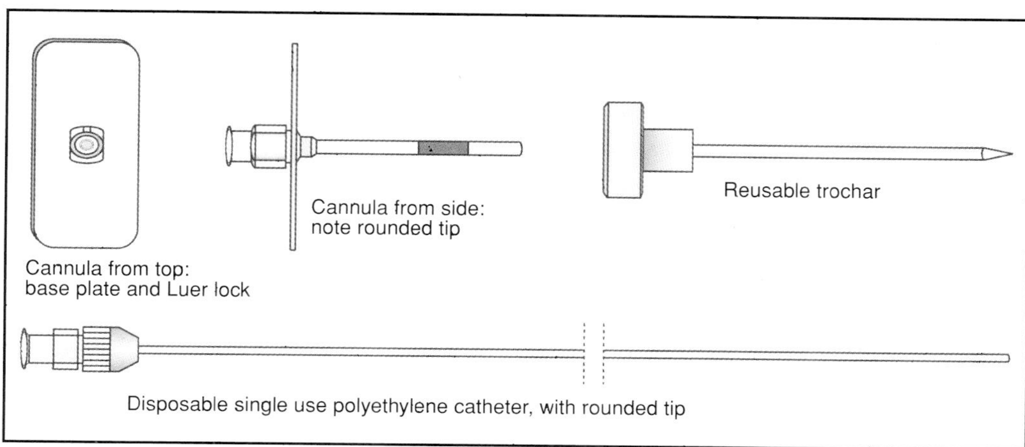

20.65 Transtracheal lavage set: re-useable stainless steel trocar and cannula plus catheter. The catheter has a rounded tip to prevent tracheal trauma and is only intended for one-time use.

catheter threaded through the cannula and down the trachea. The catheter should be long enough to reach the tracheal bifurcation or carina, approximately at the level of the 4th intercostal space.

5. An aliquot of warmed saline (2–4 ml for cats and small (< 10 kg) dogs; 10–20 ml for larger dogs) is injected into the catheter and aspirated back, as described for BAL.

Up to 40–50% of the aliquot is retrieved. Patients may cough during the procedure, which may help sample collection, but coughing can also result in the catheter tip being coughed into the pharynx, and this should be avoided as it may result in oropharyngeal contamination.

Repeating a TW or BAL

This may be necessary if the initial procedure is unsuccessful or if there is marked oropharyngeal contamination. Repeating the wash or lavage within 24 hours is inadvisable, as it is not possible to distinguish between pathological neutrophilic inflammation and an increase in neutrophils secondary to the sampling procedure. Thus, sampling should only be repeated after an interval of at least 48 hours.

Sample handling

In a successful wash sample there are usually at least a few small flecks of flocculent material and/or mucus in the aspirated fluid. Larger flecks or strands of mucus should be harvested using a pipette, placed directly on a slide, and a squash smear prepared (see earlier).

The remaining material should be divided between an EDTA tube for cytology and a plain sterile tube or swab for bacterial culture if necessary. If the sample is to be posted out, some laboratories recommend placing a third aliquot into another EDTA tube to which a drop of 10% formalin has been added, although these samples require specialized staining. It is important to label this tube as formalin-fixed and to package it separately, since formalin fumes frequently result in poor uptake of Romanovsky-type stains, used by the majority of laboratories.

If the sample is to be examined in-house a sediment smear should be prepared from the EDTA sample (see Chapter 21).

Limitations

- Cytology may be unsuccessful if an inappropriate medium is used for the wash. For example, sterile water will lyse any cells harvested, due to the effects of osmosis.
- Cytology samples may be non-diagnostic if there are large amounts of mucus (e.g. in chronic bronchitis) and direct smears are not submitted in addition to the sample in EDTA. Cells of diagnostic significance may be difficult to identify if trapped in dry mucus, as they dry more slowly and shrivel up (round up).
- As a general rule, if there is no macroscopic evidence of floccules, foamy fluid or mucus, the sample may be acellular or is unlikely to contain an adequate number of cells on which to base a diagnosis.
- Cytology results compatible with findings in a 'healthy' patient do not exclude the possibility of pulmonary disease, since the sample might not be representative.

Normal findings

In normal animals the appearance of samples from TW and BAL differs.

A normal TW sample consists of:

- A small amount of mucus, seen as wispy basophilic or pink material (Romanowsky)
- Columnar or cuboidal epithelial cells. These should be the predominant cell type. Cells generally have a single round nucleus in a basal location. One end of the cell can terminate in a tail and the other may be ciliated (Figure 20.66a). Many free cilia, originating from these cells, can be seen in the background as a result of trauma during sampling
- Small numbers of goblet cells (Figure 20.66b). These have a similar appearance to columnar cells, but also contain variable amounts of round dark-staining mucus granules in their cytoplasm
- Small numbers of alveolar macrophages and neutrophils
- Occasional lymphocytes.

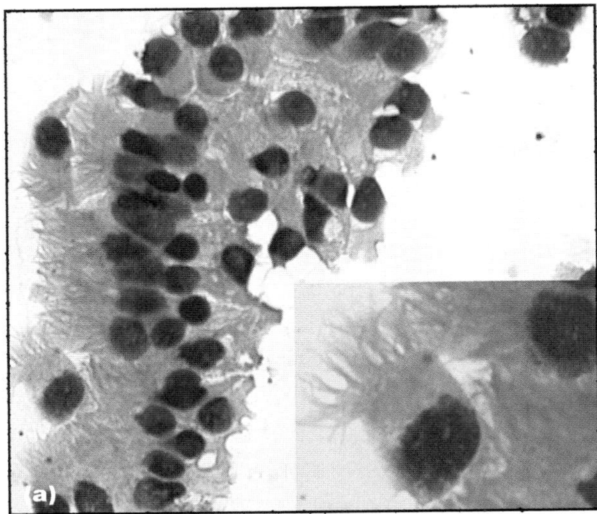

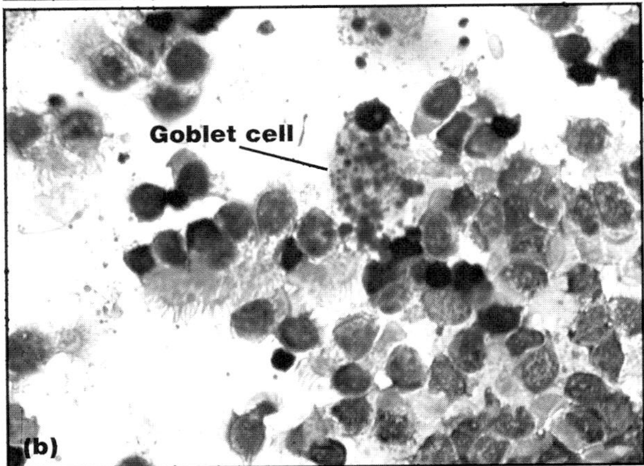

20.66 Normal tracheal wash: centrifuged smears from a dog. (a) There are 'normal' columnar ciliated epithelial cells with basal nuclei, pale cytoplasm and cilia at one pole. The insert highlights the cilia that identify these cells. (b) A goblet cell with dark basophilic mucus granules surrounded by columnar epithelial cells is also seen. (Wright's stain; original magnification X100) (© Axiom Veterinary Laboratories.)

For BAL samples:

- The proportion of epithelial cells is much lower (1–15%)
- Macrophages are generally the predominant cell type
- Neutrophils and lymphocytes generally each form <5% of the total cell population
- In dogs, eosinophils usually constitute <5% of the population; in cats 5–25% of cells may be eosinophils (Padrid *et al.,* 1991).

Contamination

Oropharyngeal contamination may occur with BAL or ET sampling but is very rare with tracheal washing, unless the catheter was inserted craniodorsally instead of caudoventrally during placement or changed direction when the patient coughed. The presence of superficial squamous epithelial cells, with or without a mixed population of adherent bacteria (in particular *Simonsiella* spp., which have a railroad-track appearance) are markers of oral contamination (Figure 20.67).

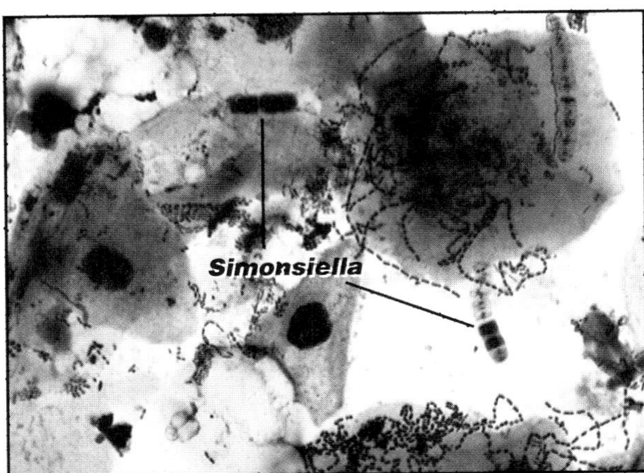

20.67 Oropharyngeal contamination. Squash smear of a large fleck of material, harvested with a pipette, from an endotracheal wash. There are superficial squamous epithelial cells (large angular cells) and a mixed bacterial population, including *Simonsiella* sp. (Wright's stain; original magnification X400) (© Axiom Veterinary Laboratories.)

Abnormal findings

Neutrophilic or suppurative inflammation

Non-infectious: Neutrophils are generally non-degenerate and no bacteria are present. Neutrophils entrapped in mucus may appear degenerate due to poor cell preservation rather than the lytic effect of bacterial toxins. Neutrophils may also appear degenerate if there is a delay between sampling and making smears. Neutrophils are present in both acute and chronic inflammation.

In chronic bronchitis the most prominent features are neutrophilic (or mixed) inflammation and goblet cell hyperplasia, resulting in increased mucus production. The cytological pattern of chronic bronchitis may also include activated macrophages, identified as large round cells (often bi- or multinucleate) and epithelial hyperplasia (characterized by variation in size, and deeply basophilic cytoplasm). The respiratory tract is very sensitive to tissue irritation, and even sterile saline can result in suppurative inflammation, which is important to bear in mind when a TW or BAL has to be repeated.

Other causes of tissue irritation are diverse and include early foreign body reaction, chemicals, noxious substances (including smoke) and underlying neoplasia.

Neutrophilic inflammation may predominate in allergic disease. For example, the inflammatory response seen in feline asthma may be primarily neutrophilic or mixed (neutrophils, macrophages and eosinophils) or primarily eosinophilic. Eosinophils are not seen consistently. Neutrophils are generally non-degenerate unless secondary bacterial infection is present. Thus a TW sample consisting predominantly of neutrophils (± bacteria) without eosinophils could be due to allergic disease or to primary bacterial infection. In such cases, persistence of neutrophilic inflammation but disappearance of bacteria after antibiotic therapy, with appropriate clinical changes, would be more supportive of allergic disease.

Infectious:

- **Bacterial** infection usually results in a marked increase in cellularity, with a predominance of neutrophils, which often appear degenerate. Bacteria may be seen intra- or extracellularly (Figure 20.68). They must be distinguished from bacteria due to oropharyngeal contamination, which are extracellular or on the surface of squamous cells and are not associated with an inflammatory response.
- **Parasitic worms,** particularly *Oslerus* (*Filaroides*), can cause an eosinophilic inflammation or neutrophilic inflammatory response, due to dying adult worms or larvae, respectively (Figure 20.69).
- **Fungal and protozoal** infections generally cause granulomatous inflammation, but may also be associated with a neutrophilic response (Figure 20.70).

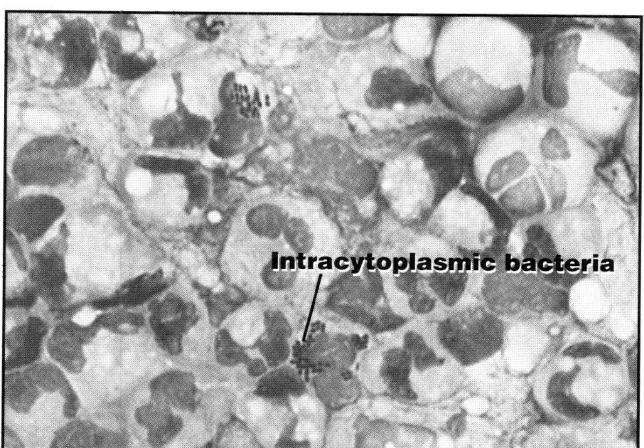

20.68 Septic suppurative respiratory tract inflammation: BAL from an adult male dog with a history of regurgitation and pyrexia. Numerous degenerate bacteria are seen in a proteinaceous background. Bacteria have been phagocytosed by the neutrophils, indicating active infection. (Wright's stain; original magnification X1000) (© Axiom Veterinary Laboratories.)

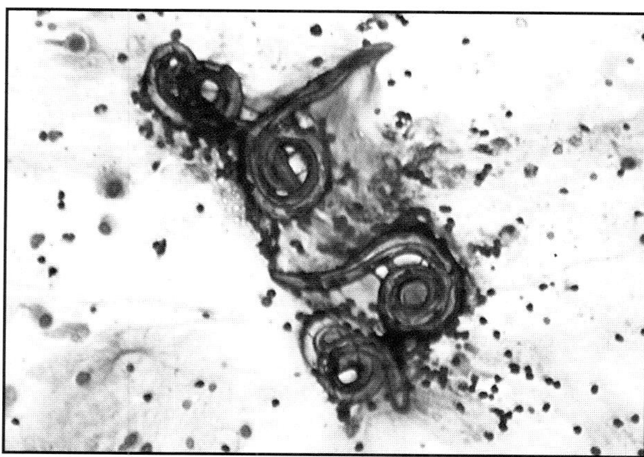

20.69 Parasitic helminth larvae (*Oslerus* spp.) in a tracheal wash from a dog. Higher power views revealed a mixed eosinophilic and neutrophilic inflammatory reaction. (Wright's stain; original magnification X40) (© Axiom Veterinary Laboratories.)

Fungi
Blastomyces dermatitidis *Cryptococcus neoformans* *Coccidioides immitis* *Histoplasma capsulatum* *Sporothrix schenckii* *Aspergillus* spp.
Protozoa
Toxoplasma gondii *Neospora caninum* *Cytauxzoon felis* *Pneumocystis carinii*

20.70 Fungal and protozoal infections that can cause a neutrophilic inflammation in the respiratory tract.

Eosinophilic inflammation

Eosinophils can be present in healthy (asymptomatic) patients, and the precise percentage present is contentious. Normal values vary widely: from <5% in dogs (although some publications mention <24%) to <25% in cats. The significance of cytological findings must be interpreted in the context of history, clinical signs and results obtained from other diagnostic tests. Bearing this in mind, if there is increased cellularity (often marked) and the number of eosinophils exceeds 10% of the total nucleated cell count, then there may be a significant hypersensitivity component to the inflammatory response. Conversely, if the total cell count is low, or only slightly increased, care should be taken not to overinterpret the significance of the eosinophils, especially in cats. Eosinophilic or mixed inflammation, composed of variable numbers of eosinophils, neutrophils, macrophages, small lymphocytes and plasma cells, characterizes some allergic and parasitic conditions.

Eosinophilic inflammation may be seen with:

- Allergy (Figure 20.71): allergic bronchitis; feline asthma; eosinophilic bronchopneumonopathy (EBP), also known as pulmonary infiltrate with eosinophils (PIE)
- Paraneoplastic syndromes, e.g. in association with T cell lymphoma
- Parasitic larvae or ova (Figure 20.72)

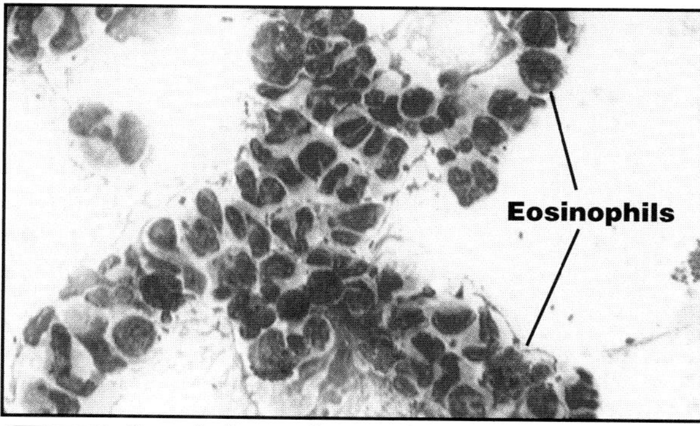

20.71 Sample from a 6-year-old dog with a history of chronic coughing, recent deterioration and pyrexia, showing an eosinophilic respiratory tract inflammation with a secondary septic suppurative component. The eosinophils seen here have prominent pink granules, but these may sometimes be less obvious. (Wright's stain; original magnification X400)

Species	Host	Morphology	Diagnostic tests
Larvae			
Oslerus (Filaroides) osleri	Dog	232–266 µm long; S-shaped tail (Figure 20.74)	Bronchoscopy; Baermann technique
Filaroides hirthi	Dog	240–290 µm long	Zinc sulphate flotation (not always reliable)
Aelurostrongylus abstrusus	Cat	360 µm long; notched tail (1st-stage larvae have dorsal and ventral cuticular spines on tails)	Baermann technique
Angiostrongylus	Dog	2.5 cm; resemble *Aelurostrongylus*; small cephalic button and wavy tail	Baermann technique
Crenosoma vulpis	Dog	<16 mm long; straight tail, well developed bursae and large dorsal ray	Baermann technique
Ova			
Capillaria aerophila	Cat, Dog	60–35 µm; oval; bipolar (double-operculated)	Zinc sulphate flotation; BAL
Paragonimus spp.	Cat, Dog	80–115 µm; oval; unipolar (single operculum)	Zinc sulphate flotation

20.72 Parasitic larvae and ova that may cause eosinophilic inflammation in the respiratory tract of dogs and cats.

Differentiation of the various parasitic lung infections is based on morphological criteria of the parasites (see Figure 20.72). Faecal examination by Baermann or zinc sulphate flotation is often necessary to confirm the presence of an underlying parasite and is also useful when the pathogenesis of the parasite only involves deep lung parenchyma, not alveoli or bronchioles normally harvested via BAL or TW. For example, *Paragonimus* is only present in a focal location in the caudal right lung lobe. Faecal examination to diagnose *Capillaria* is not always necessary since they live in the trachea and bronchi, so are readily identified on wash samples, unlike *Paragonimus*.

Mixed inflammation

A combination of macrophages and/or neutrophils with eosinophils and lymphocytes can be seen in acute or chronic inflammation. Macrophages become activated and appear larger, with bi- or multinucleation in chronic inflammation. The inflammatory response may be accompanied by epithelial and/or goblet cell hyperplasia and/or increased mucus production. Curschmann's spirals (Figure 20.73) are tight spiral coils of inspissated mucus formed in small bronchioles, which can also form with chronic small airway disease.

The underlying causes of mixed inflammation are numerous and include: foreign bodies; chronic allergy (including feline asthma); canine chronic bronchitis; inhalation pneumonia; and necrosis secondary to neoplasia.

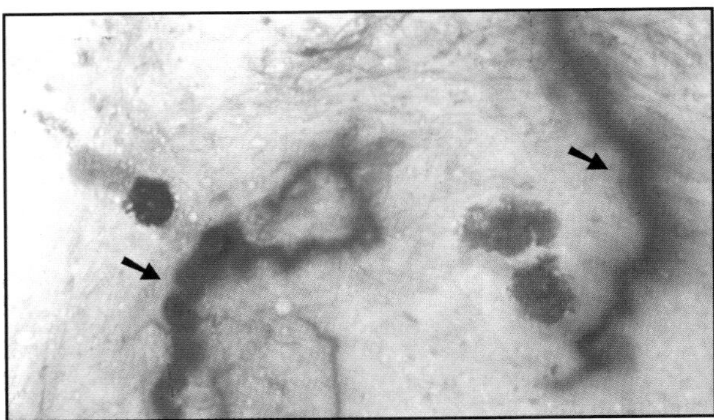

20.73 Curschmann's spirals, deeply basophilic tight spiral coils composed of inspissated mucus, in a tracheal wash from an elderly Poodle with chronic coughing exacerbated by exercise but improved somewhat with steroid administration. The spirals form when there is increased mucus production due to goblet cell hyperplasia. (Wright's stain; original magnification X40) (© Axiom Veterinary Laboratories.)

Haemorrhage

Red blood cells in a TW or BAL sample may indicate true haemorrhage but can also be iatrogenic in origin. Erythrophagocytosis (macrophages engulfing red cells), haemosiderin-laden macrophages (Figure 20.74a) and

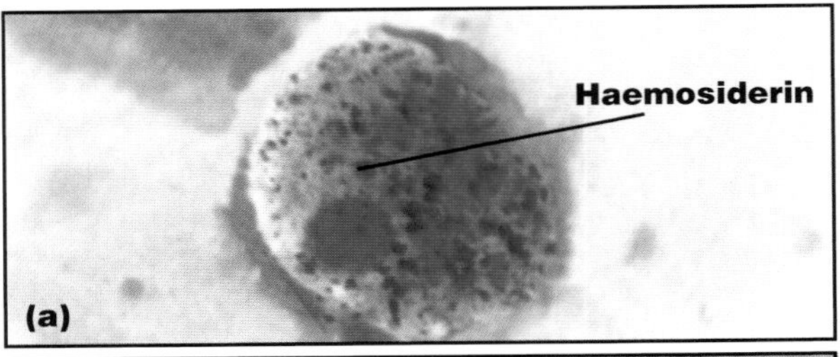

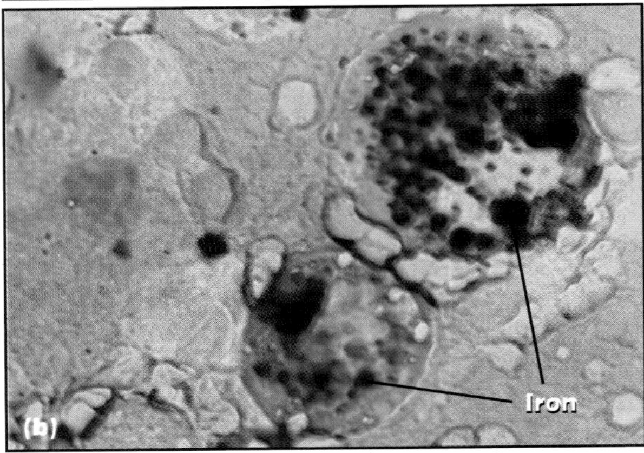

20.74 Respiratory tract samples suggesting haemorrhage. (a) Macrophage filled with black granules. (Wright's stain; original magnification X500) (b) Perls-positive staining confirms that the black globular material in the macrophages is haemosiderin rather than mucin or carbon. (Perl's stain; original magnification X500) (© Axiom Veterinary Laboratories.)

haematoidin crystals all indicate pre-existing airway haemorrhage and are useful in distinguishing true from iatrogenic haemorrhage. Granular material in macrophages may be haemosiderin, mucin or carbon. Haemosiderin, a blood breakdown pigment, contains iron which stains positively with Prussian blue (Perl's stain) (Figure 20.74b).

Haemorrhage into the airways may be due to:

- Vascular damage due to neoplasia, infectious diseases, or trauma (including coughing in cats with chronic asthma)
- Increased diapedesis (movement of blood cells through intact vessel walls) associated with congestive heart failure or coagulopathies.

Neoplasia

Cytological evidence of either primary and metastatic neoplasia is rare in TW or BAL samples.

Neoplastic cells are only seen if the pathological process breaks through into the alveoli or bronchi; neoplasia involving the respiratory tract is usually confined to the interstitium of the pulmonary parenchyma. Exceptions include canine lymphoma, where cytological evaluation of an endoscopic BAL sample is more sensitive than radiography for identifying pulmonary involvement (Hawkins *et al.*,1993).

Metastatic neoplasia (Figure 20.75) is more common than primary respiratory tract neoplasia. Metastatic lesions are usually diffuse and distributed throughout all lung lobes, whereas primary respiratory neoplasia tends to present with a larger, solitary lesion.

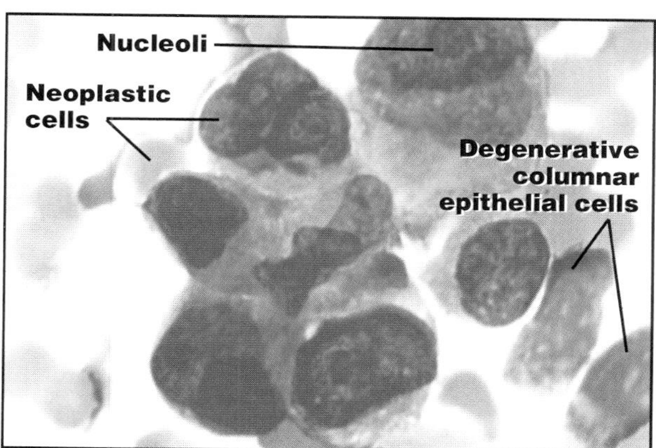

20.75 Metastatic pulmonary carcinoma in an unspayed 12-year-old bitch with a history of histologically confirmed mammary carcinoma. Note the presence of atypical features including anisokaryosis, nuclear moulding and large prominent nucleoli. (Wright's stain; original magnification X1000) (© Axiom Veterinary Laboratories.)

Carcinomas (both primary and secondary) are the most common form of neoplasia involving the respiratory tract. Squamous cell carcinoma of the lung may be difficult to distinguish from squamous metaplasia. The lung is also one of the primary sites of canine malignant histiocytosis.

Hyperplasia and dysplasia of respiratory epithelium may occur in response to chronic airway irritation and should not be mistaken for neoplasia.

References and further reading

Baker R and Lumsden JH (2000) *Color Atlas of Cytology of the Dog and Cat.* Mosby, St Louis

Bonfanti U, Bussadori C, Zatelli A, De Lorenzi D, Masserdotti C, Bertazzolo W, Faverzani S, Ghisleni G, Capobianco R and Caniatti M (2004). Percutaneous fine-needle biopsy of deep thoracic and abdominal masses in dogs and cats. *Journal of Small Animal Practice* **45**, 191–198

Chalita MC, Matera JM, Alves MT and Longatto Filho A (2001) Nonaspiration fine needle cytology and its histologic correlation in canine skin and soft tissue tumors. *Analytical and Quantitative Cytology and Histology* **23**, 395–399

Cowell RL, Tyler RD and Meinkoth JH (1999) *Diagnostic Cytology of the Dog and Cat, 2nd edition.* Mosby, St Louis

Dunn JK and Villiers EJ (1998) General principles of cytological interpretation. *In Practice* **20**, 429–437

Fournel-Fleury C, Magnol J and Guelfi J (1994) *Color Atlas of Cancer Cytology of the Dog and Cat.* Conférence Nationale des Véterinaires Specialisés en Petits Animaux, Paris

Fournel-Fleury C, Magnol JP, Bricaire P, Marchal T, Chabanne L, Delverdier A, Bryon PA and Felman P (1997) Cytohistological and immunological classification of canine malignant lymphomas: comparison with human non-Hodgkin's lymphomas. *Journal of Comparative Pathology* **117**, 35–59

Hawkins EC, Morrison WB, DeNicola DB and Blevins WE (1993) Cytological analysis of bronchoalveolar lavage fluid from 47 dogs with multicentric malignant lymphoma. *Journal of the American Veterinary Medical Association* **203**, 1418–1425

Kravis LD, Vail, DM, Kisseberth WC, Ogilvie GK and Volk LM (1996) Frequency of agyrophilic nucleolar organizer regions in fine needle aspirates and biopsy specimens from mast cell tumours in dogs. *Journal of the American Veterinary Medical Association* **209**, 1418–1420

Kristensen AT, Weiss DJ, Klausner JS and Hardy RM (1990) Liver cytology in canine and feline hepatic disease. *Compendium on Continuing Education for the Practicing Veterinarian* **12**, 797–808

Langenbach A, McManus PM, Hendrick MJ, Shofer FS and Sorenmo KU (2001) Sensitivity and specificity of methods of assessing the regional lymph nodes for evidence of metastasis in dogs and cats with solid tumours. *Journal of the American Veterinary Medical Association* **218**, 1424–1428

Obradovich J, Walshaw R and Goullaud E (1987) The influence of castration on the development of prostatic carcinoma in the dog: 43 cases (1978–1985). *Journal of Veterinary Internal Medicine* **1**, 183–187

Padrid PA, Feldman BF, Funk K, Samitz EM, Reil D and Cross CE (1991) Cytological, microbiological and biochemical analysis of bronchoalveolar lavage fluid obtained from 24 healthy cats. *American Journal of Veterinary Research* **52**, 1300–1307

Ponce F, Magnol JP, Ledieu D, Marchal T, Turinelli V, Chalvet Monfray K and Fournel-Fleury C (2004) Prognostic significance of morphological subtypes in canine malignant lymphoma during chemotherapy. *The Veterinary Journal* **167**, 158–166

Raskin RA (2001) Lymphoid system. In: Atlas of Canine and Feline Cytology, *ed. Raskin RA and Meyer DJ, pp.93–134.* WB Saunders, Philadelphia

Raskin RE and Meyer DJ (2001) *Atlas of Canine and Feline Cytology.* WB Saunders, Philadelphia

Roth L (2001) Comparison of liver cytology and biopsy diagnoses in dogs and cats: 56 cases. *Veterinary Clinical Pathology* **30**, 35–58

Teske E, Naan EC, van Dijk EM, Van Garderen E and Schalken JA (2002) Canine prostate carcinoma: epidemiological evidence of an increased risk in castrated dogs. *Molecular and Cellular Endocrinology* **197**, 251–255

Villiers EJ, Dunn JK, Jefferies AR and Nicholls PK (1995) A comparison of cytological and histopathological diagnosis of intrathoracic lesions. In: *BSAVA Congress Paper Synopses 1995*, ed. JV Davies, p.256

Villiers EJ and Dunn JK (1998) Collection and preparation of smears for cytological examination. *In Practice* **20**, 370–377

Wang KW, Panciera DL, Al-Rukibat RK and Radi ZA (2004) Accuracy of ultrasound-guided fine-needle aspiration of the liver and cytological findings in dogs and cats: 97 cases (1990–2000). *Journal of the American Veterinary Medical Association* **224**, 75–78

21

Body cavity effusions

Kostas Papasouliotis and Emma Dewhurst

Introduction

Body cavity effusions occur when there is abnormal accumulation of fluid in a body cavity. In dogs and cats, effusions occur commonly in the pleural, peritoneal or pericardial spaces. Clinical signs, such as dyspnoea, lethargy, exercise intolerance and abdominal distension, can be due to the presence of the effusion, the disease responsible for producing the effusion or both. Analysis of effusions is an important component of diagnosis: it can identify the pathological process responsible for the fluid accumulation and lead to a specific diagnosis; or it can indicate further investigative procedures which may be helpful.

Pathophysiology of effusion formation

In healthy animals, body cavities are lined by a single continuous layer of mesothelium that covers the inner body wall, the mediastinum and the viscera. Interstitial fluid (i.e. lymph) constantly permeates into the thoracic cavity through the pleural capillaries and into the abdominal cavity through the intestinal capillaries. This movement out of the capillary is favoured by the fact that the capillary hydrostatic pressure (dependent on the blood pressure) exceeds the oncotic pressure (dependent on the blood albumin concentration). However, most of the fluid is rapidly absorbed through the lymphatic capillaries, so that only a small amount remains in the cavities, where it acts to lubricate the abdominal and thoracic organs. The amount of fluid present in the cavity at any one time is determined by equilibration between the mechanisms governing the production (hydrostatic pressure, oncotic pressure) and resorption (lymphatic drainage) of the fluid.

In summary, effusions are formed due to one or more of the following primary pathophysiological mechanisms:

- Decreased plasma colloid oncotic pressure. Effusions occur because there is a loss of oncotic pull (hypoalbuminaemia), which is responsible for keeping fluid within the vasculature. As a result, fluid is lost from the capillaries at a rate that exceeds the absorption capacity of the lymphatics
- Increased hydrostatic pressure. Effusions occur because fluid is forced into the body cavity. Fluid production is increased, exceeding the transport capacity of the lymphatics
- Increased vascular permeability. Effusions occur because there is an excessive loss of fluid from abnormal vasculature into the body cavity
- Obstruction of lymphatic flow. Effusions occur because removal of fluid from the body cavity is impaired.

Collection of body cavity effusions

Equipment

Equipment for collection of body cavity effusions includes:

- Clippers
- Surgical scrub and alcohol spray
- Local anaesthetic (optional)
- Sterile needle, butterfly needle, or over-the-needle catheter (advantages and disadvantages are summarized in Figure 21.1)
- Sterile syringe
- Extension tube and three-way tap
- Scalpel blade and suture (for over-the-needle catheter only)
- Gloves
- Kidney dish (if collecting large volume of fluid for therapeutic reasons)
- Three sample tubes (EDTA, plain, plain sterile).

Drainage method	Suitable for	Advantages	Disadvantages
Simple needle	Abdominocentesis	Cheap and readily available	Needle may penetrate/damage adjacent organs (risk greater where fluid volume small or therapeutic drainage carried out) Very easily blocked by flocculent/fibrous material

21.1 Comparison of different methods of drainage available for effusions. (continues) ▶

Drainage method	Suitable for	Advantages	Disadvantages
Butterfly catheter (or assembled needle and extension tubing)	Thoracocentesis and pericardiocentesis in cats and very small dogs	Cheap Readily available Extension tubing allows for movement during drainage Good for harvesting diagnostic samples	Needle may penetrate lung/heart (risk greater where fluid volume small or therapeutic drainage carried out) Very easily blocked by flocculent/fibrous material
Over-the-needle intravenous catheter	Thoracocentesis, pericardiocentesis, abdominocentesis (suitable sizes available for all sizes of animals)	Cheap Readily available No sharp ends	Kinks easily (especially at hub) Easily blocked by flocculent/fibrous material Need to attach extension tube
Through-the-needle catheter (or passing a urinary catheter through an over-the-needle catheter)	Pericardiocentesis (see Figure 21.3)	Does not tend to kink at hub No sharp end exposed Blocks less readily than over-the-needle catheters	More costly Less readily available
Specialized fenestrated catheter	Thoracocentesis, pericardiocentesis, abdominocentesis (specialized catheters available for each site)	Effectively drains flocculant or fibrous effusions Blocks less easily No sharp ends	More costly Less readily available Need to attach extension tube (unless included)
Trocar chest drain	Thoracocentesis	Does not block easily Can be indwelling for therapeutic lavage	More costly General anaesthesia or sedation required for placement
Trocar peritoneal catheter	Abdominocentesis	Can be used for therapeutic drainage Can be used for diagnostic peritoneal lavage Tends not to block with omentum	More costly Less readily available

21.1 (continued) Comparison of different methods of drainage available for effusions.

Pleural effusion

Thoracocentesis is best performed with the patient standing or in sternal recumbency as this is safer than lateral recumbency, especially in severely dyspnoeic patients. The patient is restrained manually and the lateral thorax is clipped (either side) and surgically prepared from the fifth to the eleventh intercostal space. Drainage is generally carried out through the seventh or eighth intercostal space, just above the costochondral junction (Figure 21.2). If local anaesthetic is used, it should be injected in the appropriate rib space, infiltrating not only the subcutaneous tissue but also the pleura to avoid discomfort during thoracocentesis.

A needle, butterfly needle or over-the-needle catheter (18–20 gauge)(ideally fenestrated if available) is then advanced at an angle of 45 degrees next to the cranial aspect of the rib to avoid the intercostal vessels and nerve which are located parallel to the caudal aspect of the rib. If a catheter is used, a small stab incision through the skin can be made first using a scalpel blade. Drawing the skin forwards before penetrating the chest reduces the risk of pneumothorax, because after the needle is withdrawn the hole in the skin is not directly opposed to the hole into the pleural cavity. Once the pleural cavity is penetrated, an extension tube and three-way tap are placed between the needle (or catheter) and a 20–60 ml syringe. Pleural effusions are usually bilateral but occasionally can be unilateral and/or pocketed. In these situations, radiography or ultrasonography should be used to identify the site for thoracocentesis. If a large quantity of fluid is to be drained or the fluid is viscid, full of debris or fibrin clots then it may be necessary to place a chest drain (Figure 21.2).

Pericardial effusion

For pericardiocentesis, the patient is allowed to adopt a comfortable position, usually sternal recumbency. Manual restraint or light sedation may be required to minimize movement. A large area of the right or left hemithorax (sternum to mid thorax, third to eighth rib) is prepared surgically. Examination of thoracic radiographs may indicate where the heart is most closely associated with the body wall and thus determine the puncture site. The most common site is either the fourth or fifth intercostal space at the level of the costochondral junction (Figure 21.2).

The area is infiltrated with local anaesthetic in the same manner as for thoracocentesis. A skin incision is made with a scalpel blade and an over-the-needle catheter is passed into the chest. Medium- to large-size dogs may require a 14–16 gauge (7–15 cm long) catheter, while smaller dogs and cats usually require an 18–20 gauge (5–8 cm long) catheter. Alternatively, an over-the-needle catheter can be used and a suitably sized urinary catheter fed through the cannula after withdrawal of the stylet. This avoids kinking of the catheter, especially where large volumes are involved.

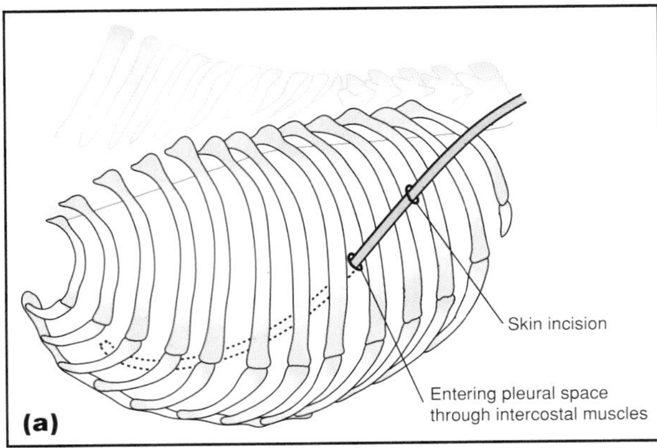

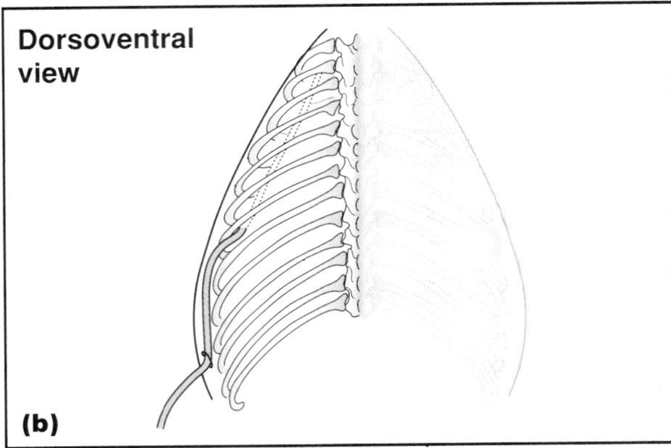

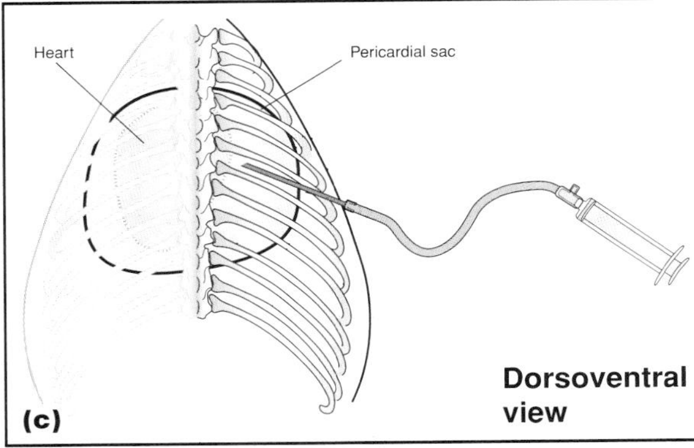

21.2 (a,b) Sites for thoracocentesis. A drain enters the pleural cavity through the eighth intercostal space, just above the costochondral junction. The drain is tunnelled subcutaneously (only required for indwelling drain). (c) Site for pericardiocentesis. Drainage is via the right sixth intercostal space.

The catheter is attached to extension tubing and a three-way tap, and a 20–60 ml syringe (Figure 21.3). Although dedicated pericardial catheters are available, the expense may be unjustifiable considering the low number of cases requiring pericardiocentesis in general practice.

The catheter is advanced into the chest towards the heart. As the needle contacts the pericardium a scratching sensation will be noticed, before the catheter penetrates the tense pericardial sac. Fluid can then be aspirated from the pericardium. Haemorrhagic pericardial effusion does not clot (except where haemorrhage has occurred acutely), while blood collected directly from the heart does.

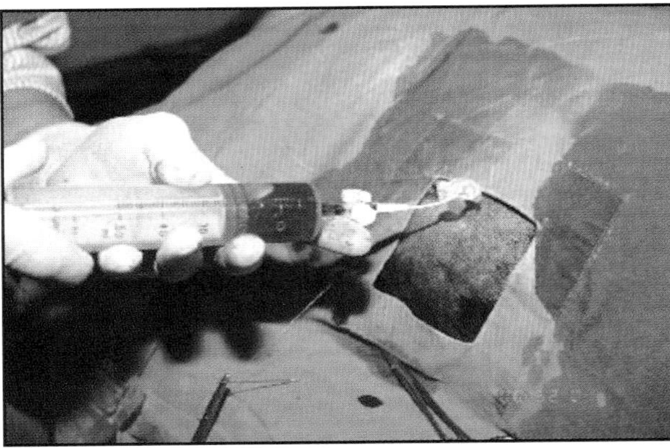

21.3 Pericardiocentesis being performed on an 11-year-old Labrador using a 16 gauge 'through-the-needle' catheter, three-way tap and syringe. The fluid being drawn is typical for a pericardial effusion being haemorrhagic in appearance. This animal was found to have a heart base mass on ultrasonography. (Courtesy of JK Dunn.)

Peritoneal effusions

Abdominocentesis can be performed with the patient standing or in lateral recumbency. If standing, an area of 5x5 cm at the point of maximal dependency (fluid accumulation) should be clipped and surgically prepared. If in lateral recumbency then an area between the bladder and umbilicus, just lateral to the midline should be clipped and surgically prepared. Emptying the bladder before attempting peritoneal drainage will reduce the risk of accidental cystocentesis. Some authors do not advocate performing abdominocentesis with the patient standing as this can increase the risk of omentum occluding the needle resulting in a dry tap. It has also been suggested that collection from the point of maximal dependency may increase the risk of seroma formation post drainage.

In most cases, sedation or local anaesthesia is not needed and the patient is restrained manually in order to minimize movement and avoid accidental bowel puncture. The usual site for abdominocentesis is on the ventral midline, 1–2 cm caudal to the umbilicus where an 18 or 20 gauge needle is inserted. Collection of fluid is more effective with the needle only, so a syringe usually is not attached. If a syringe is attached, only slight negative pressure (up to 3 ml) should be applied to minimize blockage of the needle by omentum. A fenestrated catheter can also be used for abdominocentesis. A 'dry' tap can occur when the effusion is localized or pocketed, and does not mean that there is no fluid present. In these situations, ultrasonography should be used to identify the site for abdominocentesis. Other approaches include performing abdominocentesis from each quadrant of the abdomen but this blind procedure is unlikely to harvest localized fluid.

Historically, diagnostic peritoneal lavage (DPL) was often recommended; it is very rarely indicated in small animals (the only indication being suspected diffuse peritonitis and a dry tap). DPL is absolutely contraindicated where neoplasia is suspected, and may result in extension of a localized peritonitis. It is generally carried out with the animal in lateral recumbency: the area around the umbilicus is clipped and aseptically prepared and a small 'nick' incision is made 1–2 cm caudal to the umbilicus. A large bore (10–14 gauge) over-the-needle catheter which has been fenestrated, or a trocar peritoneal catheter if available, is placed through the incision and into the peritoneal cavity in a caudal direction. The catheter is advanced and the trocar/stylet removed. The catheter is then sutured in place and 20 ml/kg of warm normal saline or Hartmann's solution instilled. The patient is rolled from side to side, and a few minutes later fluid is harvested (only a small proportion of the instilled fluid will be drained). Identification of fluid by ultrasonography often allows sampling without recourse to DPL.

Handling of samples

Fluid samples should be placed in EDTA, plain and sterile plain tubes. The EDTA tube is used for total nucleated cell count (TNCC) and cytology. EDTA anticoagulant is required to prevent the sample from clotting, which can lead to disruption of cell morphology and decreased TNCC (Conner *et al.*, 2003). The plain tube is used for measurement of total protein concentration (TP) and other biochemical tests, while the sterile plain tube is submitted for bacterial culture if necessary. Serological testing, including coronavirus antibody titres, can also be measured using plain samples, and effusions collected in plain tubes are also generally suitable for in-house biochemistry analysers.

Formalin is often added to samples that are submitted to diagnostic laboratories for cytology. Formalin is generally inappropriate for cytological samples as it interferes with the routine stains used for cytological preparations. However, some laboratories can perform specialized staining procedures which allow them to process some fluid samples with added formalin (e.g. CSF, in which EDTA does not provide adequate preservation of cells). It is therefore advisable to contact the laboratory and check if these procedures are available, before submitting samples with added formalin for cytological examination.

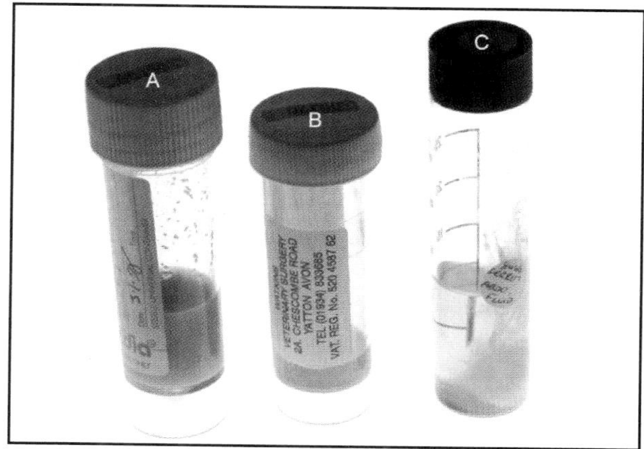

21.4 Gross appearance of effusions can vary markedly and may provide additional information. (A) This thoracic effusion is brown–green and opaque. This fluid was also foul smelling and therefore suggestive of a septic exudate (pyothorax). (B) This abdominal effusion was a pink–red colour suggestive of the presence of haemolysed red cells. This may have occurred at the time of sampling. If blood contamination occurs this may appear as a streak of red cells entering the sample, at which point sampling should be stopped. (C) This abdominal effusion is from a cat with histologically confirmed FIP. Note the proteinaceous (fibrin) material.

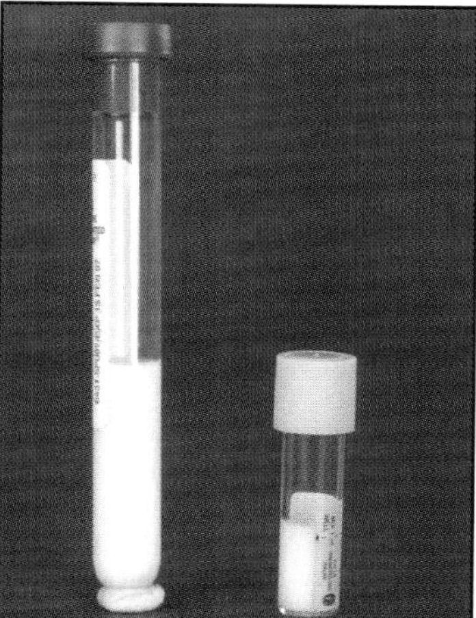

21.5 Chylous effusion. This effusion was collected from the thoracic cavity of a 13-year-old cat, which presented with tachypnoea and dyspnoea. This effusion is typical of a chylous effusion (milky-white colour and opaque). Chylous effusions may also appear more pink–red coloured, 'strawberry milkshake'.

Laboratory evaluation

Gross examination

Gross examination of an effusion is as important as any other examination procedure but is often overlooked. Colour, consistency and smell may all provide information on the possible pathological process. Septic effusions may have a green/brown opaque colour and be foul smelling, particularly if anaerobes are present (Figure 21.4A). Blood contamination at time of sampling may be evident by the presence of blood strands through the sample (Figure 21.4B), or there may be fibrin strands running through the sample. Flocculent material is suggestive of a high protein content (Figure 21.4C). A white milky fluid is pathognomonic for chylous effusion (Figure 21.5). The white milky appearance is due to the high concentration of triglycerides. In contrast, pseudochylous effusions contain high cholesterol levels which do not give a milky appearance, but appear opaque due to the presence of cell debris.

Total protein concentration

TP is used with TNCC to classify body cavity effusions as transudates, modified transudates or exudates (Figure 21.6). Very bloody or turbid fluids should be centrifuged (at 150–350 G for 5 minutes) and the supernatant used for TP measurement. Bloody fluids can be also centrifuged in a capillary tube using a microhaematocrit centrifuge (i.e. Hawksley microhaematocrit, StatSpin centrifuge). This will allow the determination of packed cell volume (PCV) while the supernatant fluid can be used for TP estimation by refractometry.

In the practice situation, TP can be measured by a refractometer, urine test strips (negative, 0.3–1, 1–3, 3–20, >20 g/l) or an in-house dry chemistry analyser (Braun *et al.*, 2001; George and O'Neill, 2001; Papasouliotis *et al.*, 2002). Peritoneal and pleural fluids from dogs and cats can be efficiently differentiated into transudates and modified transudates/exudates on the basis of TP less than or greater than 20 g/l, respectively.

Effusion	Appearance	TP	TNCC	Cytology	Other tests (see text for details)
Transudate	Clear, colourless or pale straw colour	<25 g/l (Often <15 g/l)	<1–1.5 x 10^9/l	Neutrophils and macrophages with some mesothelial cells	Serum albumin concentration
Modified transudate	Often yellow, blood-tinged, slighly turbid	Usually >25g/l (Variable reported values; 25–75 g/l)	<5–7 x 10^9/l	Macrophages and mesothelial cells, increasing numbers of neutrophils and small lymphocytes	Serum albumin concentration Liver enzymes Liver function tests Diagnostic imaging
Exudate	Typically turbid, various colours, may have clots	>25 g/l (Usually >30 g/l)	>7 x 10^9/l	Neutrophils and macrophages. (Degenerate neutrophils if septic exudate)	Culture and sensitivity. Glucose concentration in plasma and effusion

21.6 Criteria employed for the classification of effusions as transudates, modified transudates or exudates.

However, if the threshold of 25 g/l is applied to differentiate between transudates and modified transudates/exudates misclassifications can occur with the urine test strips (Braun *et al.*, 2001) and the refractometer (Papasouliotis *et al.*, 2002). In the authors' experience, dry chemistry analysers provide the most accurate in-house measurement of TP in body cavity effusions. In feline patients, in addition to TP measurement, albumin and globulin concentrations should always be determined because this can be helpful in diagnosing or ruling out certain diseases, especially feline infectious peritonitis (FIP) (see below and Chapter 26).

Total nucleated cell count

The combination of TP and TNCC is used to classify fluids as transudates, modified transudates or exudates. TNCC can be performed using a haematology cell counter or a haemocytometer. TNCC includes the mesothelial cells, macrophages, white blood cells and any other nucleated cells in the effusion.

Cytological examination

For rewarding cytological examination of effusion samples, good quality preparations are essential. Direct smears from the collected fluid should always be prepared as for peripheral blood smears. Fluid samples which do not appear turbid or purulent should be centrifuged (150–350 G for 5 minutes) and smears prepared from the resuspended pellet. Centrifugation of samples using microhaematocrit (PCV) or StatSpin centrifuges should be avoided because the generated speed is much higher than 350 G and causes cell damage. Approximate calculated G force for the StatSpin at the lower speed urinalysis setting (9,800 rpm) is 5,000 G, which is far greater than that recommended for cytological specimens. However, in an emergency situation it is often possible to gain diagnostically useful information (for example, to visualize debris from ingesta, degenerate neutrophils and intracellular bacteria in suspected peritonitis after intestinal surgery). Samples should always be submitted to the laboratory for confirmation.

Samples can also be processed using cytocentrifuges (e.g. Cytospin). These are cell preparation systems, distinct from a general purpose centrifuge, which use centrifugal force to deposit cells directly onto a microscope slide. These centrifuges offer programmable speed, centrifugation time and acceleration rate, thus maximizing cell concentration and preservation for microscopic examination. Although Cytospins are routinely employed by commercial diagnostic laboratories, the expense may be unjustifiable for general practice.

Cytological examination should always be performed irrespective of the TNCC. However, although a low TNCC does not exclude the possibility of the presence of diagnostically significant cells, such as neoplastic cells, cytological evaluation of samples with moderate to high TNCC is generally most rewarding.

Cells that are typically seen in the trace amount of fluid found in body cavities include a mixture of mature neutrophils, monocytes/macrophages in various stages of activation and mesothelial cells, with much lower numbers of small lymphocytes and very occasional eosinophils and mast cells.

The mesothelial cells line the pleural and peritoneal cavities and cover the visceral surfaces from where they are naturally exfoliated into the body cavity fluids. These cells are typically large (3–5 erythrocytes in diameter), mononuclear or binuclear, with uniformly sized round to oval nuclei and pale basophilic cytoplasm. Recently exfoliated mesothelial cells may have small cytoplasmic projections or a pink cytoplasmic brush border (glycocalyx halo) (Figure 21.7). Mesothelial cells can be problematic to evaluate due to their propensity to exhibit cytological criteria of malignancy in response to any inflammatory process.

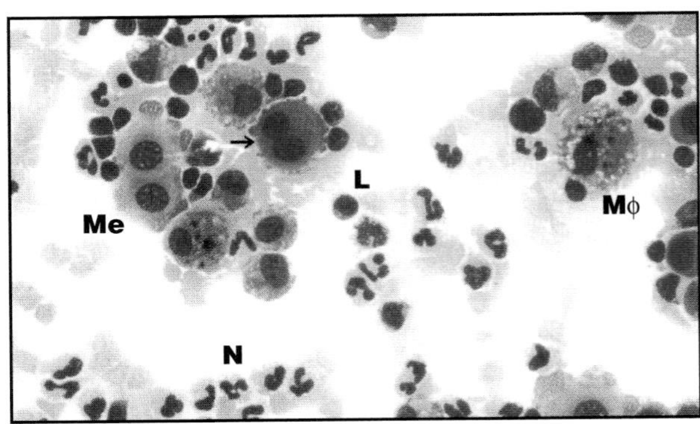

21.7 Reactive mesothelial cells: Cytospin preparation of pleural effusion from a dog. Moderate numbers of red cells present. The nucleated cells consist of neutrophils (N), small morphologically normal lymphocytes (L), occasional macrophages (Mϕ) and low numbers of reactive mesothelial cells. The reactive mesothelial cells have a basophilic cytoplasm, glycocalyx halo and may also be multinucleated (a binucleate form is seen here) (arrowed). (Romanowsky stain; original magnification X500.)

Classification of effusions

Classification of effusions is generally based on TP, TNCC and cytological findings. Classification aids in identifying the general pathological process responsible for the fluid accumulation. The most common general categories of effusions with their physical, biochemical and cytological characteristics are presented in Figure 21.6. However, there are some types of effusions that do not fall into any of these general categories and are presented in Figure 21.8. It is important to remember that different factors (e.g. sample ageing, chronicity of disease, repeated drainage of the effusion) can change these characteristics and that numerical TP and TNCC values reported for the different categories of effusions differ amongst different authors (Tyler and Cowell, 1989; Davies and Forrester, 1996; Dunn and Villiers, 1998; Canfield and Martin, 1998; Wright *et al.*, 1999). Therefore, these figures should be treated as general guidelines not as absolutes. Common underlying causes of canine and feline body cavity effusions are summarized in Figure 21.9.

Transudates

Transudates are usually the result of severe hypoalbuminaemia, which decreases the plasma colloid oncotic pressure, thus allowing fluid to accumulate in body cavities. The serum albumin concentration must fall at least below 15 g/l (in many cases <10 g/l) for spontaneous transudation to occur due to hypoalbuminaemia alone.

If hypertension is also present, then a transudate can develop with serum albumin concentrations >15 g/l: e.g. abdominal effusions in animals with hepatopathies resulting in reduced albumin production accompanied by portal hypertension. The most common causes of transudates due to hypoalbuminaemia are protein-losing nephropathy (e.g. glomerulonephropathy), hepatic failure and protein-losing enteropathy (e.g. primary intestinal lymphangiectesia). Severe malnutrition can also result in transudate effusion. Occasionally, transudates can occur in patients that are not hypoalbuminaemic. In these cases, venous and lymphatic drainage may be impaired due to a mechanical compression (e.g. diaphragmatic hernia) or, rarely, due to thromboembolism resulting in the formation of a transudate.

Grossly transudates are typically clear colourless fluids (Figure 21.10). Cytological findings are generally non-specific with low numbers (TNCC <1.5 x 10^9/l) of macrophages, mesothelial cells, neutrophils and occasional lymphocytes.

Effusion	Appearance	TP	TNCC	Cytology	Other tests (see text for details)
Chylous	Opaque, white to pink ('strawberry milk-shake')	Variable (reported values: 25–65 g/l)	Variable. Usually <10 x 10^9/l (reported values: 1–17 x 10^9/l)	Lymphocytes, neutrophils and variable numbers of macrophages	Triglycerides and cholesterol concentrations in serum and effusion
Haemorrhagic	Red	Variable (usually >30 g/l)	Variable. Usually 1.5–10 x 10^9/l	Erythrocytes, variable numbers of neutrophils and macrophages. Erythrophagocytosis and haemosiderophages if chronic	PCV/ haematocrit (HCT) of peripheral blood and effusion
Neoplastic	Variable	Variable (usually >25g/l)	Variable	Neoplastic cells, neutrophils, macrophages and reactive mesothelial cells	

21.8 Criteria employed for the classification of effusions as chylous, haemorrhagic or neoplastic.

Underlying cause	Dog		Cat	
	Pleural (n=168) (%)	*Peritoneal* (n=240) (%)	*Pleural* (n=216) (%)	*Peritoneal* (n=239) (%)
Neoplastic process	44	28	32	24
Cardiac disease	18	38	20	10
FIP	–	–	19	42
Bacterial infection	13	8	13	6
Haemorrhage	6	9	2	1
Hypoalbuminaemia	4	10	0	6
Tissue/organ inflammation	7	2	0.5	3

21.9 Common underlying causes of canine and feline body cavity effusions (Else and Simpson, 1988; Hirschberger and Koch, 1995; Davies and Forrester, 1996; Hirschberger and Koch, 1996, Hirschberger *et al.*, 1999; Wright *et al.*, 1999; Mellanby *et al.*, 2002). (Not all causes are given and therefore percentages do not total 100.)

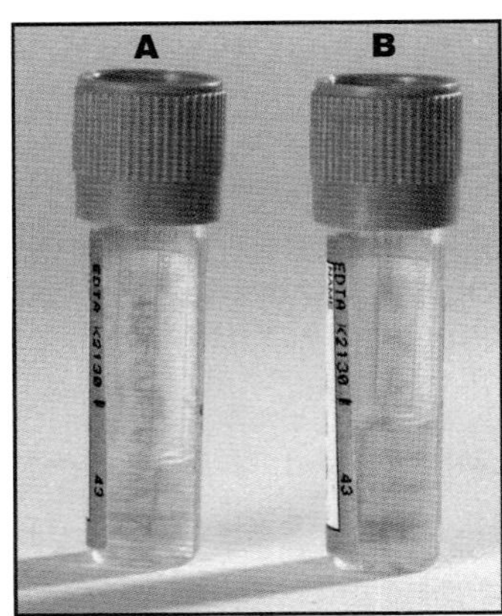

21.10 (A) Gross appearance of a transudate. Abdominal effusion collected from a dog with serum albumin concentration of 10 g/l. Note the clear, colourless appearance of the sample. (B) Gross appearance of a modified transudate.

Modified transudates

Modified transudates are usually the result of increased hydrostatic pressure within the blood and/or lymphatic circulation, or within the liver in abdominal effusions. Disorders that commonly result in modified transudates include neoplasia, lung lobe torsion, cardiovascular disease and hepatic insufficiency. Most neoplastic effusions are modified transudates. TP is the most important parameter in differentiating modified transudates from transudates, as TNCC is relatively low in both categories and counts may overlap: in transudates total protein is <25 g/l (often <15 g/l), while in modified transudates it is >25 g/l. It should be remembered that longstanding transudates may irritate the mesothelium, resulting in exfoliation of mesothelial cells and secondary inflammation, which will result in increased TP and TNCC. Therefore, transudates may become temporarily modified transudates as they progress to exudates.

Grossly, modified transudates are often yellow (see Figure 21.10). Cytological findings in modified transudates are generally non-specific unless overtly neoplastic cells are seen. Cell types identified can include macrophages, mesothelial cells, neutrophils, small morphologically normal lymphocytes and the occasional eosinophil (Figure 21.11).

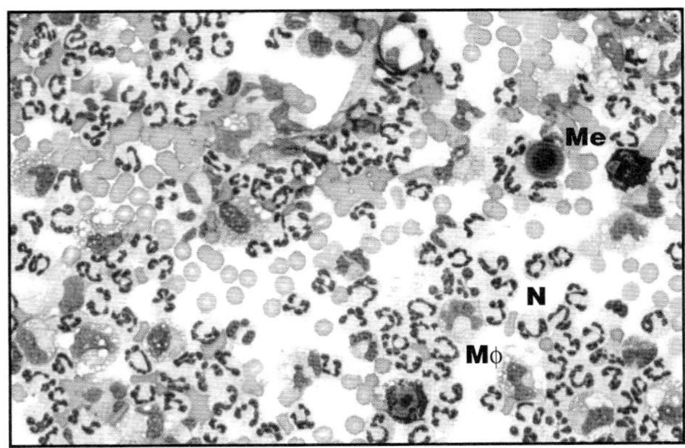

21.11 Modified transudate: Cytospin preparation of an abdominal effusion from a dog with hepatic dysfunction. A mixed population of cells including macrophages (Mϕ) and neutrophils (N) are commonly seen in a modified transudate. A mesothelial cell (Me) is also seen. (Romanowsky stain; original magnification X200.)

Exudates

Exudates are formed as a result of any infectious or non-infectious inflammatory process. During inflammation, there is release of chemotactants and vasoactive substances which attract inflammatory cells into the cavity and also cause increased vascular permeability. The result is the leakage of a high-protein fluid which can be rich in neutrophils and other phagocytic/inflammatory cells. TNCC is the most important parameter in differentiating modified transudates from exudates, as TP in both categories may overlap: in transudates and modified transudates TNCC is <7 x 10^9/l, while in exudates it is >7 x 10^9/l. Exudates can be classified as septic or non-septic. Septic exudates can be caused by aerobic or anaerobic bacteria, fungi or mycoplasmas.

Septic exudates

Septic exudates may arise from penetrating wounds, secondary to surgery, extension or rupture of an adjacent infected lesion and, uncommonly, from bacteraemia. They usually contain numerous degenerate neutrophils and intracellular and/or extracellular bacteria (Figure 21.12). Using haematological stains, bacteria can stain dark blue, red or pink depending on the stain and staining time. These stains cannot differentiate Gram-positive from Gram-negative bacteria but, in general, Gram-positive bacteria are larger than Gram-negative bacteria. Most cocci are Gram-positive bacteria, and staphylococci tend to form clusters while streptococci tend to form chains. Small rods are usually Gram-negative. However, cytology cannot reliably identify the bacterial species or indicate antibiotic sensitivities. Occasionally, effusions from body cavities infected by bacteria contain a high number of neutrophils, but no bacteria can be identified microscopically. This may be due to recent/ongoing antibiotic treatment, the presence of very low number of bacteria or bacteria that are not visible because they are too small (e.g. mycoplasmas) and/or poorly stained.

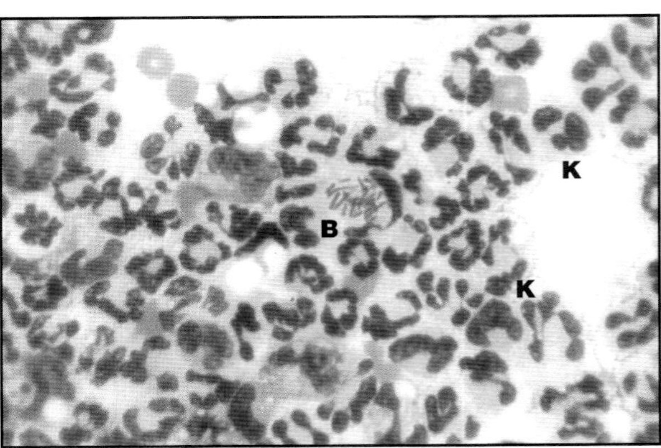

21.12 Septic exudate: Cytospin preparation of a thoracic effusion from a cat. Intracellular bacteria are identified here (B). Note that a number of the neutrophils appear karyolytic (K). Karyolysis is identified when the nucleus of the neutrophil swells and stains less intensely. It is believed to indicate rapid cell death due to the toxic environment. (Romanowsky stain; original magnification X1000.)

When bacteria are identified cytologically, or where there is suspicion of sepsis even in the absence of obvious bacteria, a fluid sample (avoid swabs) should be submitted for culture and antibiotic sensitivity testing (see Chapter 25). The most commonly isolated species of bacteria are anaerobes or facultative anaerobes (e.g. *Clostridium* spp., *Bacteroides* spp., *Fusobacterium* spp., *Pasteurella* spp., filamentous bacteria (*Nocardia* spp., *Actinomyces* spp.)). If only extracellular bacteria are seen and the neutrophils are low in number or appear non-degenerate, a possibility of *in vitro* contamination during collection of the sample or a peracute inflammatory process should be considered.

Apart from cytology and culture, it may be possible to identify septic exudates by simultaneous measurement of glucose concentration in plasma and fluid. A recent study in dogs concluded that a difference between blood and effusion glucose concentrations of >1 mmol/l was 100% sensitive and 100% specific for septic peritoneal effusion. This study also evaluated feline cases where it was reported that a difference between blood and effusion glucose concentrations of >1mmol/l was 86% sensitive and 100% specific for a diagnosis of septic peritonitis. All blood and effusion samples were collected into heparinized tubes and analysed for glucose within 15 minutes of collection using an in-house dry chemistry analyser (Bonczynski *et al.*, 2003).

Non-septic exudates

Apart from the progression of a modified transudate to exudate due to ongoing inflammation, non-septic exudates may develop from organ inflammation or neoplasia. Cytologically, non-septic exudates are characterized by a predominance of non-degenerate neutrophils and absence of bacteria, although the neutrophils may appear aged (i.e. hypersegmented, pyknotic) and the macrophages may exhibit neutrophilic phagocytosis (Figure 21.13).

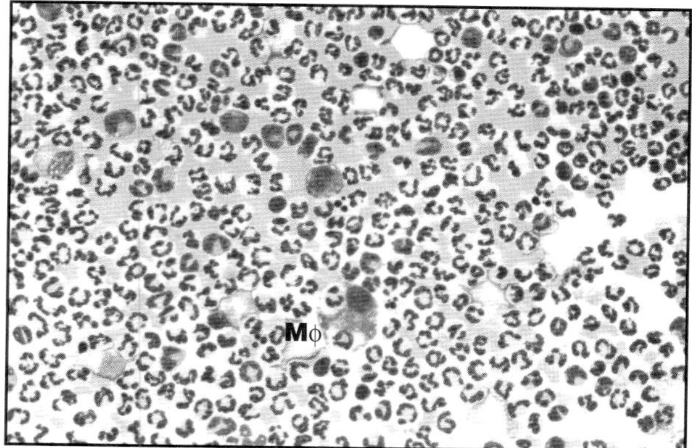

21.13 Non-septic exudate: Cytospin preparation of a thoracic effusion from a cat. There are markedly increased neutrophils (confirmed on an automated TNCC) consistent with an inflammatory process. There is no cytological evidence here for a septic process (presence of pathogenic microorganisms or changes in neutrophil morphology induced by sepsis) but many neutrophils appear hypersegmented. A macrophage which has phagocytosed neutrophils is seen (Mϕ). (Romanowsky stain; original magnification X200.)

Leakage of sterile irritants (urine, bile) can also cause non-septic exudates, which are diagnosed by biochemical tests. Uroperitoneum is easily diagnosed because it is characterized by higher concentrations of urea and creatinine in fluid than in blood. However, urea equilibrates rapidly (hours) between the effusion and blood and for this reason measurement of creatinine is a more reliable way to detect uroperitoneum as creatinine concentration remains elevated in the fluid for a longer period of time (days). These animals are commonly hyperkalaemic and may be hyponatraemic (see Chapter 8). Similarly, bile peritonitis can be diagnosed by demonstrating higher total bilirubin concentration in the effusion than in the serum (there is no diagnostic benefit in analysing conjugated and unconjugated fractions). Grossly, bile peritonitis is typically a green colour, but may equally be brown to deep yellow in colour. Microscopically it may be evident that there are macrophages present which contain blue–green to yellow coloured bile pigment.

Feline infectious peritonitis: Effusions due to FIP are the result of a non-septic inflammatory process which is characterized by deposition of immune complexes within vessels resulting in increased vascular permeability and chemotaxis of neutrophils. For this reason a FIP-associated effusion is a non-septic exudate which appears viscid, and straw to golden in colour with fibrin strands or flecks. TP is high (>35 g/l) and TNCC is typically <10 x 10^9/l, although counts >25 x 10^9/l have also been reported. Cytologically FIP effusions are characterized by a pink, protein-rich, granular background with non-degenerate neutrophils, lymphocytes, macrophages, mesothelial cells and, occasionally, plasma cells. Protein analysis of effusions has proven to be the most valuable of the laboratory tests for diagnosing FIP. Fluid electrophoresis results with γ-globulin concentration of >32% and an albumin:globulin ratio of <0.81 are highly suggestive of FIP (Shelly *et al.*, 1988). Duthie *et al.* (1997) reported effusion albumin:globulin ratios of <0.81 in 42 out of 43 FIP cases and in 19 of these cases the ratio was <0.4.

In addition, TP of >35 g/l with ≥50% globulins in feline effusions have been shown to have a sensitivity of 100% for FIP (Sparkes *et al.*, 1994). However, effusions due to lymphocytic–plasmacytic cholangiohepatitis may also have high globulins. It should be noted that estimation of globulin concentration (globulins = TP – albumin) by in-house dry chemistry analysers in feline effusions can be inaccurate as albumin concentration can be underestimated (Papasouliotis *et al.*, 2002).

The potential value of increased levels of α1-acid glycoprotein (AGP) in the diagnosis of FIP has also been studied. Although AGP concentrations can be increased in a variety of diseases, Duthie *et al.* (1997) have shown that effusion AGP concentrations >1.5 g/l (serum AGP reference interval: 0.1–0.48 g/l) can differentiate cats with FIP from cats with clinically similar conditions (sensitivity 85%, specificity 100%). Finally, coronavirus antibody titres can be measured by immunofluorescence or enzyme-linked immunosorbent assay (ELISA) and viral genome can be detected by polymerase chain reaction (PCR) in effusion samples from cats where FIP is suspected. Absolute confirmation of FIP requires histopathological examination.

Chylous effusions

Chylous effusions can result from any disorder that causes obstruction or destruction of lymphatics leading to leakage of chyle (lymph and lipids) into the body cavity. Because the major lipid in chyle is derived from triglyceride-rich chylomicrons, chylous effusions have a unique characteristic: the triglyceride concentration is higher and the cholesterol concentration lower than those of serum.

It has been suggested that most chylous effusions form a thick, white layer at the top of the tube on standing in the refrigerator, due to the presence of the triglyceride-rich chylomicrons. This has been disputed by a report which suggested that after a 16-hour stand in the fridge only 20% of samples which had chylomicrons detected by electrophoresis were positive (McNeely *et al.*, 1981). Another way to identify chyle is by centrifuging a microhaematocrit tube filled with the chylous fluid: the triglycerides create a white plug at the top of the fluid or a diffuse turbidity above the packed cells.

Chylous effusions occur most frequently in the thoracic cavity but occasionally can occur in the abdomen. Chylous effusions may be idiopathic or secondary to heart disease (believed most common cause in cats), neoplasia, thoracic trauma, thrombosis of the thoracic duct, diaphragmatic hernia, congenital defects in lymphatics and mediastinal fungal granulomas (Tyler and Cowell, 1989; Meadows and MacWilliams, 1994; Dunn and Villiers, 1998). Chylous abdominal effusions may be formed secondary to a number of processes, including cardiac and hepatic disease, neoplasia (e.g. lymphoma) and steatitis. Cytological examination typically reveals a predominance of morphologically normal small lymphocytes (Figure 21.14). However, lipid material can act as a significant irritant causing an increase of neutrophils and macrophages over time (days to weeks) such that neutrophils can eventually outnumber lymphocytes in the fluid. Macrophages, neutrophils and lymphocytes may also have small, clear cytoplasmic vacuoles which are most likely associated with lipid accumulation by the cells (Figure 21.15).

Pseudochylous effusions have a similar gross appearance to chylous fluid but are not related to lymph leakage and do not contain chylomicrons. They appear opaque due to the presence of large amounts of cell debris, which is high in cholesterol, and their lactescence frequently decreases with repeated drainage. Centrifugation of a microhaematocrit tube does not result in a white layer at the top of the tube and the supernatant is minimally turbid. Pseudochylous effusions are uncommon but can occur with inflammatory and neoplastic disorders of a chronic nature. Their cytological characteristics are variable depending on the underlying cause. It has been reported that in chylous effusion cases the cholesterol:triglyceride ratio (both in mg/dl) is <1 (Fossum *et al.*, 1986) and that all pleural effusions with triglyceride >2.6 mmol/l are chylous in origin (Waddle and Giger, 1990). However, the best way to differentiate chylous and pseudochylous effusions is to measure the

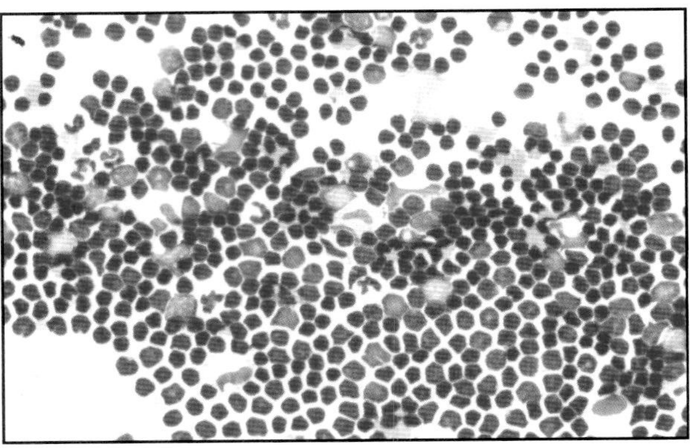

21.14 Chylous effusion: Cytospin preparation of a thoracic effusion from a cat. The nucleated cells are predominantly small, morphologically normal lymphocytes. This cat was found to have hypertrophic cardiomyopathy. (Romanowsky stain; original magnification X200.)

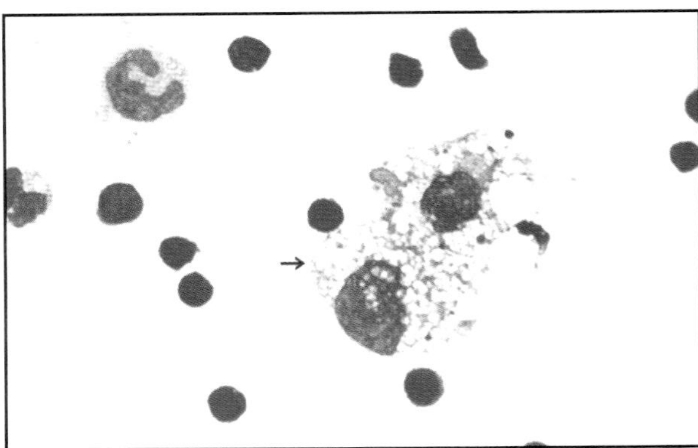

21.15 Lipid-filled macrophages: Cytospin preparation of a chylous thoracic effusion from a cat. Macrophages (arrowed) contain large numbers of small vacuoles consistent with phagocytosis of lipid. Lymphocytes are seen in the background. (Romanowsky stain; original magnification X400.)

triglyceride and cholesterol concentrations in the fluid and compare them to serum values. In chylous effusions the triglyceride concentration is higher and the cholesterol concentration lower than those of serum, while in pseudochylous effusions the triglyceride concentration is lower and the cholesterol concentration higher.

Haemorrhagic effusions

Haemorrhagic effusions occur with many disorders, including surgical and non-surgical trauma, haemostatic defects, neoplasia (especially haemangiosarcoma), vascular malformations and infections. Typically haemorrhagic effusions have a significant PCV (≥5%) while the TP is variable depending on the fluid dilution of the haemorrhage. In the majority of acute haemorrhagic effusions the PCV is comparable to that of peripheral blood, while PCV is often reduced by dilution in more chronic effusions.

Cytological examination can be useful in differentiating chronic from acute haemorrhage. Chronic haemorrhagic fluids typically reveal cytological evidence of erythrocyte and haemoglobin breakdown, such as erythrophagocytosis (Figure 21.16), presence of

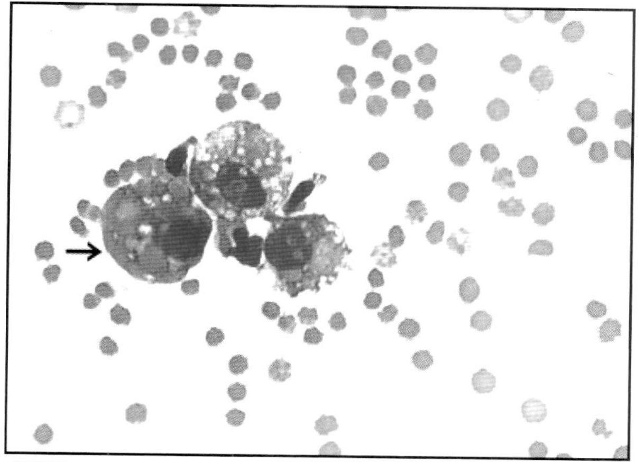

21.16 Erythrophagocytosis: Cytospin preparation of abdominal fluid from a dog. Red blood cells have been phagocytosed by macrophages (arrowed), suggesting that red cells are less likely to be due to blood contamination at time of sampling. (Romanowsky stain; original magnification X200.) (Courtesy of JK Dunn.)

haemosiderophages and haematoidin crystals. Haemosiderophages are macrophages which contain dark brown–black–green haemosiderin pigments (breakdown product of haemoglobin). Haematoidin crystals are rhomboid, yellow crystals which do not contain iron and represent anaerobic haemoglobin breakdown. In contrast, acute haemorrhagic fluids reveal no evidence of erythrocyte or haemoglobin breakdown.

In some cases, differentiation between true haemorrhage and iatrogenic blood contamination during sample collection may prove difficult. Probably the most important evidence that can help make this differentiation is to observe the appearance of the fluid during collection. In cases of peripheral blood contamination, blood appears as 'swirls' which are being added in a non-bloody fluid, while in true haemorrhage bloody fluid is seen continuously throughout the collection process. Once blood enters a body cavity, platelets aggregate, degranulate and disappear very quickly (<6 hours). Therefore the presence of clumped platelets will indicate intravascular sampling (or peracute haemorrhage) rather than true haemorrhage.

Neoplastic effusions

Neoplastic effusions are the most complicated of all categories of effusions. They occur due to any (or any combination) of the primary mechanisms of effusion formation and for this reason have variable appearance, TP and TNCC. Neoplastic effusions are typically modified transudates or exudates, although primary and metastatic neoplastic diseases of the kidney or liver can result in marked hypoalbuminaemia and formation of a transudate. Neoplasms affecting the intestines can cause septic exudates through leakage or rupture. Obstruction of lymphatic drainage due to a space-occupying neoplasm can result in a chylous effusion. In addition, invasion of neoplasms into vessels or tissues can cause a haemorrhagic effusion. Neoplastic cells are difficult to find in haemorrhagic fluids, especially those with a PCV of >20%. In these cases, cytological examination should be performed on a buffy coat smear following centrifugation of the fluid in a microhaematocrit tube (as for measurement of PCV in blood) (Canfield and Martin, 1998).

Cytology is essential for the detection of neoplastic cells but their presence or absence depends on the location and type of the neoplasm, and an apparent absence of neoplastic cells does not rule out neoplasia. However, cytological examination is a moderately sensitive tool in diagnosing malignant tumours in body cavity effusions. Hirschberger *et al.* (1999) reported 64% sensitivity in dogs and 61% in cats with malignant effusions. In general, lymphoma (Figure 21.17), carcinoma (Figure 21.18) and mesothelioma (Figure 21.19) are the most commonly identified neoplasms in body cavity fluids. Carcinomas and round cell tumours tend to exfoliate more readily than mesenchymal tumours. Most effusions associated with carcinomas are due to metastatic disease. It has been suggested that an underlying neoplastic process should be suspected in body cavity effusions where the eosinophils are ≥10% of the TNCC. It was found in a retrospective study of 14 cases of eosinophilic effusion in dogs and cats that over half of the cases had lymphoma or disseminated mast cell tumours (Fossum *et al.*, 1993). Eosinophilic effusions have also been associated with parasitic migration or disease, hypersensitivity and lymphomatoid granulomatosis.

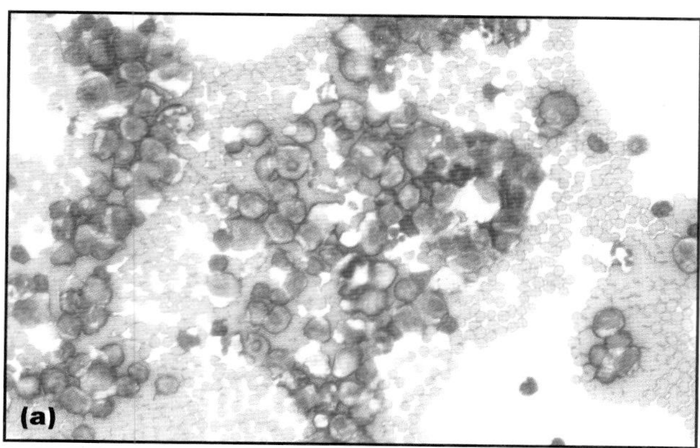

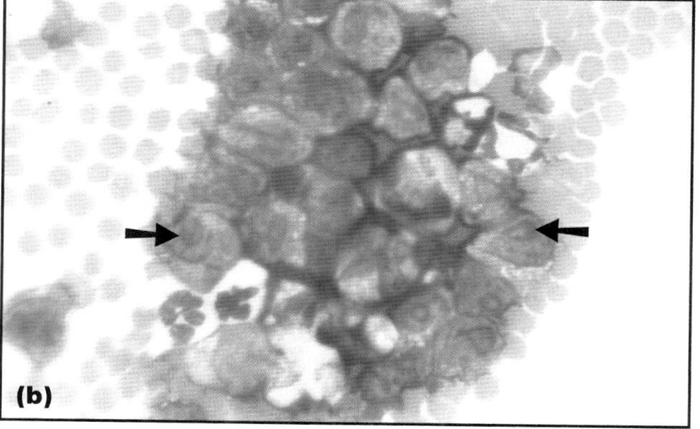

21.17 Neoplastic effusion, lymphoma: Cytospin preparation of a thoracic effusion from a cat. Moderate numbers of red blood cells are present. The nucleated cells consist of a population of large atypical lymphoid cells. These cells are approximately 4 to >6 red blood cells in diameter, with high nuclear:cytoplasmic ratio, fine chromatin and multiple, prominent, large, abnormally shaped nucleoli (arrowed). Note that some of the bizarre nuclear morphologies can be due to the cytospin preparation. (Romanowsky stain; original magnification (a) X200, (b) X400.)

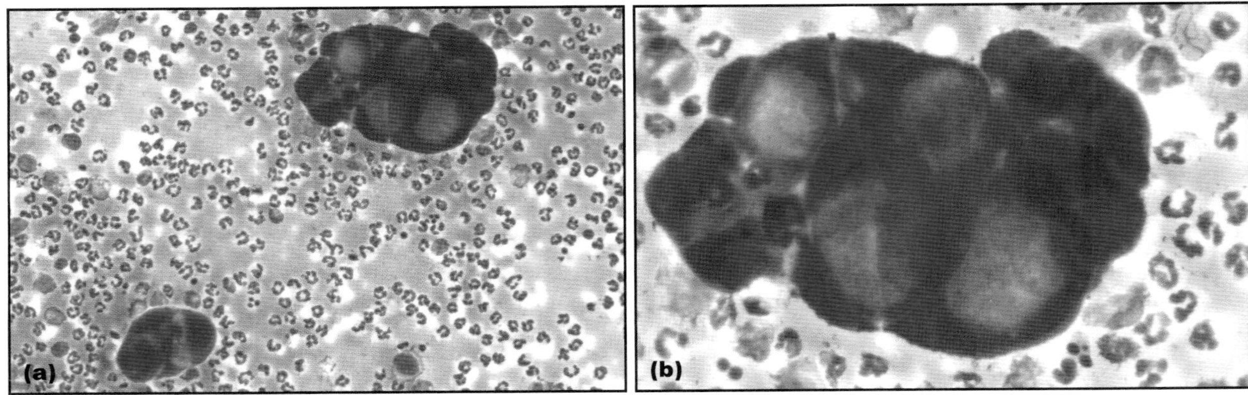

21.18 Neoplastic effusion, carcinoma: Cytospin preparation of a peritoneal effusion from a dog. Abundant red blood cells and neutrophils are present. There are cohesive clusters of very large mononuclear cells. These cells appear pleomorphic. Detailed examination is hampered by the extremely basophilic nature of these cells. Cytologically it is difficult to differentiate between reactive mesothelial cells and carcinoma. This animal was found to have a carcinoma on histology of lung tissue collected at thoracotomy. Atypical, large, round mononuclear cells present in a cohesive cluster which has an acinus-like formation; this is suggestive of carcinoma rather than mesothelioma. High nuclear:cytoplasmic ratio is also discernible at the higher magnification. (Romanowsky stain; original magnification (a) X200, (b) X400.)

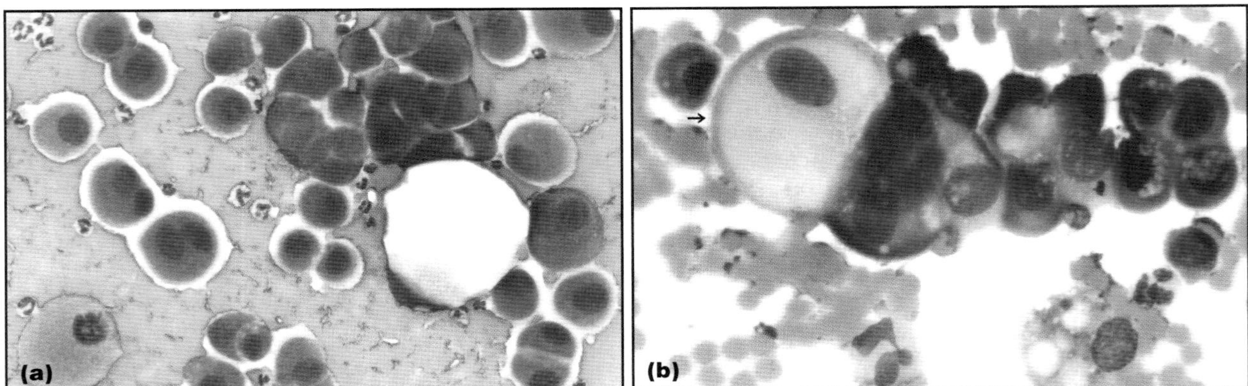

21.19 Neoplastic effusion, mesothelioma: Cytospin preparation of a thoracic effusion from a dog. Large numbers of red blood cells are present. Nucleated cells consist of a pleomorphic population of large, atypical mononuclear cells, which are mesothelial in origin. Anisokaryosis is also present. Prominent nucleoli are just visible. Note the bizarre signet ring form (arrowed) on the far left of the cohesive cluster of mononuclear cells. There is no cytological evidence of inflammation. (Romanowsky stain; original magnification (a) X200, (b) X400.)

Determining the origin of the neoplastic cells is not always straightforward because cells tend to appear round irrespective of their origin: epithelial and mesothelial cells appear round, though they are not of round cell origin. In addition, clumping of cells (a feature associated with epithelial tumours) tends to occur, not only with carcinoma and adenocarcinoma, but with mesothelioma as well. Another important problem in diagnosing neoplastic effusions occurs when there is significant inflammation present. The mesothelial surface of body cavities reacts by producing dysplastic/hyperplastic mesothelial cells which can exhibit cytological characteristics similar to those of malignant cells: increased cell numbers, anisocytosis, anisokaryosis, variation in nuclear:cytoplasmic ratio and presence of prominent multiple nucleoli (see Chapter 20). Despite these limitations, it has been shown that the specificity of cytology in diagnosing neoplastic effusions can be excellent (99% in dogs and 100% in cats) (Hirschberger *et al.*, 1999), although sensitivity is more limited. It is recommended that fluid cytology is carried out, or verified, by an experienced cytologist.

Pericardial effusions

Pericardial effusions are the most common type of pericardial abnormality in dogs but are uncommon in cats. They are typically haemorrhagic in appearance and classification, although, less frequently, they may be septic exudates or modified transudates.

In some haemorrhagic effusions the PCV of the pericardial fluid can exceed that of peripheral blood. Additional localized haemorrhage and increased pressure within the pericardial sac (development of tamponade) forcing fluid to egress at a more rapid rate than red blood cells may explain this.

Common diagnoses in cases of haemorrhagic pericardial effusions include neoplasia (mainly haemangiosarcoma, chemodectoma and mesothelioma), or benign idiopathic pericardial effusion. In one study 41% of canine pericardial effusions were neoplastic and 45% benign idiopathic (Kerstetter *et al.*, 1997). Other causes include infection (e.g. *Actinomyces* spp., *Mycobacterium* spp., *Bacteroides* spp.), trauma and haemostatic disorders. Hypoproteinaemia, congestive heart failure, uraemia and FIP can cause non-haemorrhagic pericardial effusions but are reported infrequently.

Haemorrhagic pericardial effusions

On cytology, erythrocytes predominate with variable numbers of neutrophils, macrophages exhibiting erythrophagocytosis, reactive mesothelial cells, lymphocytes and, rarely, neoplastic cells. Cytological evaluation may be an unreliable means of distinguishing between neoplastic and non-neoplastic pericardial effusions due to the difficulty in interpreting morphological changes associated with reactive mesothelial cells (Figure 21.20) (Sisson *et al.*, 1984). Therefore, the most important objective for cytological evaluation of pericardial fluid is to rule out infection or inflammation. The other causes should be investigated further using diagnostic modalities such as coagulation assessment (see Chapter 6), radiography, ultrasonography, pericardectomy and histopathology.

The pH of the pericardial effusion has been used to try to differentiate neoplastic from non-neoplastic effusions. One study reported that non-inflammatory (usually neoplastic) pericardial effusions typically had a pH >7.3 when measured using a calibrated pH meter and a pH >7.0 using a urine strip (Edwards, 1996). However, a recent study concluded that the discriminatory ability of pH to differentiate neoplastic from non-neoplastic pericardial effusions is not as great as previously perceived, and reported that 87% of effusions had overlapping pH values between the two groups (Fine *et al.*, 2003), so measurement of pH is not recommended as a screening technique.

Evaluating cardiac troponin I may also be useful for differentiating idiopathic pericardial effusions from those secondary to haemangiosarcoma (Shaw *et al.*, 2004). Cardiac troponin I was significantly greater in pericardial effusions where a diagnosis of haemangiosarcoma was made (2.77 ng/dl ; range: 0.09–47.18 ng/dl) than in idiopathic pericardial effusions (0.05 ng/dl; range: 0.03–0.09 ng/dL). Cardiac troponin I is expressed in cardiac myocytes and blood levels are found to increase in cases of cardiac ischaemia and necrosis (see Chapter 22).

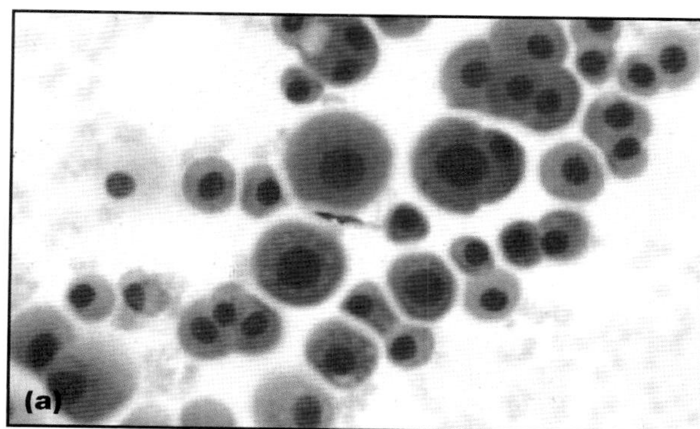

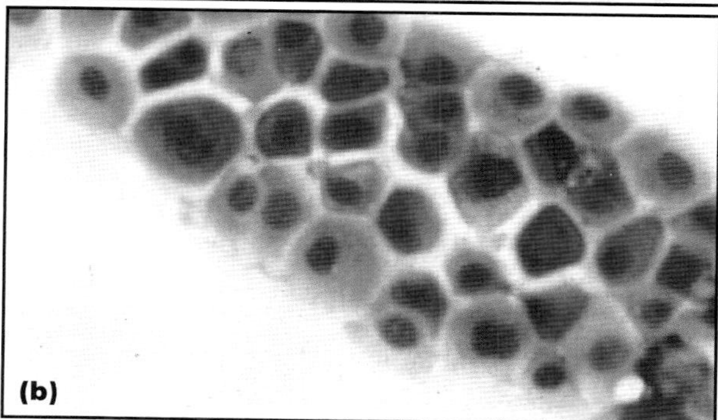

21.20 Pericardial effusion: Cytospin preparation of pericardial effusion from a dog. Abundant red blood cells are present. The mononuclear cells consist of a pleomorphic population of mesothelial cells. There is evidence of anisokaryosis here. This animal was believed to have an idiopathic pericardial effusion. Atypical mesothelial cells are shown at higher magnification. (Romanowsky stain; original magnification (a) X200, (b) X400.) (Courtesy of JK Dunn.)

In some cases, patient factors, such as time to recurrence of clinical signs and survival time, may help differentiate a non-neoplastic (idiopathic) from a neoplastic (mesothelioma) pericardial effusion (Stepien *et al.*, 2000).

Case examples

Case 1

Signalment

6-month-old male Siamese kitten.

History and clinical findings

History of ill thrift and intermittent diarrhoea. Not as well grown as sibling. Has been less active over last 48 hours, and the owner noted increased respiratory effort. On clinical examination, the cat was small and thin. There was obvious hyperpnoea. Thoracocentesis harvested fluid, shown in Figure 21.21.

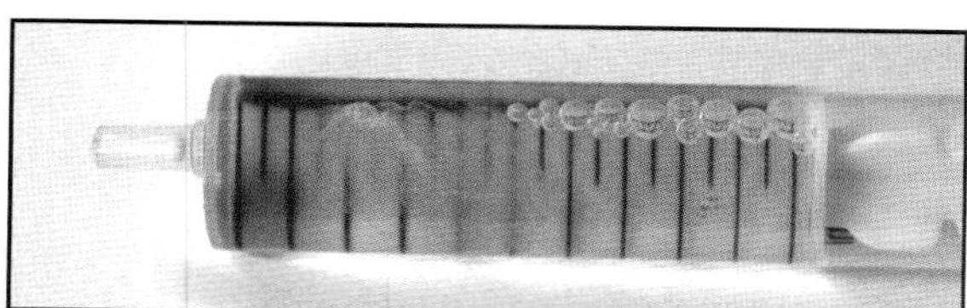

21.21 Fluid harvested by thoracocentesis.

Clinical pathology data

Fluid analysis	Result	Reference interval
RBC ($\times 10^{12}$/l)	0.005	
WBC ($\times 10^{9}$/l)	1.39	
Neutrophils ($\times 10^{9}$/l)	1.28	
Lymphocytes ($\times 10^{9}$/l)	0.11	
TP (g/l)	66	
Albumin (g/l)	17	
Globulin (g/l)	49	
A:G ratio	0.35	
FCoV antibodies	>1280	
Alpha-1 AGP (µg/ml)	1160	(100—480)

Case 1 continues ▶

Case 1 continued

Smear comment

Mild degenerative changes in neutrophils. No bacteria seen.

How would you describe and classify the effusion?

Grossly, this is a clear yellow fluid with clotted proteinaceous material within it (obscuring the syringe markings centrally). The cell count and protein levels would classify this as a modified transudate (see Figure 21.6).

How would you interpret the results and what are the likely differential diagnoses?

The gross appearance of the fluid is consistent with FIP, but the effusion could be due to lung lobe torsion, cardiovascular disease, neoplasia or hepatic disease. The high protein levels with the low A:G ratio are consistent with FIP, and ratios of <0.4 are considered suggestive of FIP, as is a TP of >35 g/l with >50% globulin. This is further supported by the very high anti-FCoV titre. Elevated AGP is also consistent with FIP, but may be elevated in many other conditions.

What further tests would you recommend?

- Haematology and biochemistry
- Anti-FCoV titre determination in sibling (to confirm exposure)
- Definitive diagnosis would require histopathological examination of affected tissue

(Case 1 courtesy of L Blackwood)

Case 2

Signalment

12-year-old, male entire Greyhound.

History and clinical findings

6-week history of weight loss and melaena. On clinical examination the dog was thin. Abdominal palpation revealed thickened intestines and moderate amount of free abdominal fluid.

Clinical pathology data

Abdominal effusion analysis	Result
TP (g/l)	38.4
RBC ($\times 10^{12}$/l)	0.05
Total nucleated cell count ($\times 10^{9}$/l)	9.2
Cytology	The majority of the nucleated cells were large cells as shown in Figure 21.22. In addition, small numbers of neutrophils and macrophages are seen

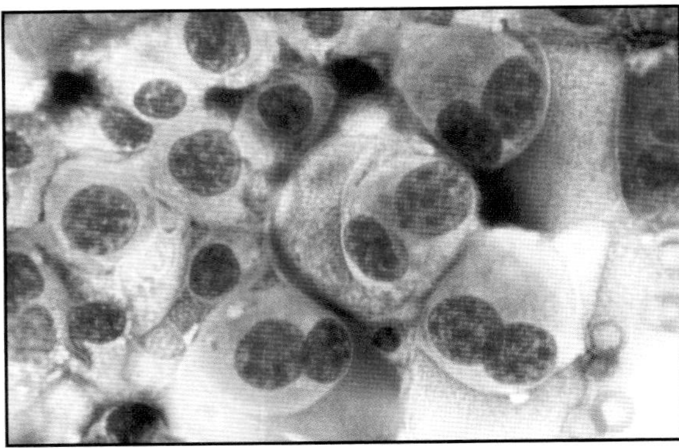

21.22 Cytology of abdominal effusion.

How would you classify the effusion?

The effusion has a high protein and moderately high cell count and so is classified as an exudate.

How would you describe the cells present and what are the likely differential diagnoses?

Clusters of large mononuclear and some binuclear cells are seen, showing criteria of malignancy: large variably sized nuclei; coarse chromatin; multiple nucleoli; binucleated cells; variable nuclear:cytoplasmic ratio. These cells are in clusters and may be epithelial or mesothelial in origin. The criteria of malignancy are marked; the effusion is very cellular and is dominated by these cells. Thus, the findings are consistent with a tumour effusion.

The two main differential diagnoses are carcinoma/adenocarcinoma and mesothelioma. The cell features are most consistent with carcinoma. In view of the melaena, the site of the primary tumour may be the GI tract. Carcinoma/adenocarcinoma cells can exfoliate from the affected organ(s) directly into the cavity, or more commonly from metastatic lesions affecting the surface of the body cavity. In these cases the prognosis is very poor.

What further tests would you recommend?

Thoracic radiography and abdominal ultrasonography could be carried out to identify the location of the primary neoplasm, and identify possible metastases. Abdominal ultrasonography is likely to be more useful than radiography due to the presence of the effusion. However, given the presence of the neoplastic effusion metastatic spread is likely, and the prognosis must be guarded.

Results of further tests

Chest radiographs revealed no abnormalities. Abdominal radiographs and ultrasonograms revealed intestinal thickening, abnormal splenic and hepatic architecture, and the presence of an intestinal mass.

Histopathological examination of Trucut biopsy specimens from the liver and intestinal mass confirmed extensive tissue infiltration by an adenocarcinoma.

Case 3

Signalment

4-year-old male Greyhound.

History

Initially presented with hindleg paresis and hypercalcaemia. Lymphoma (B cell phenotype) with CNS and bone marrow involvement was diagnosed. Responded well to initial chemotherapy, but at echocardiography prior to first dose of epirubicin (week 4 of treatment), a small volume of pleural fluid was detected and was harvested (Figures 21.23 and 21.24).

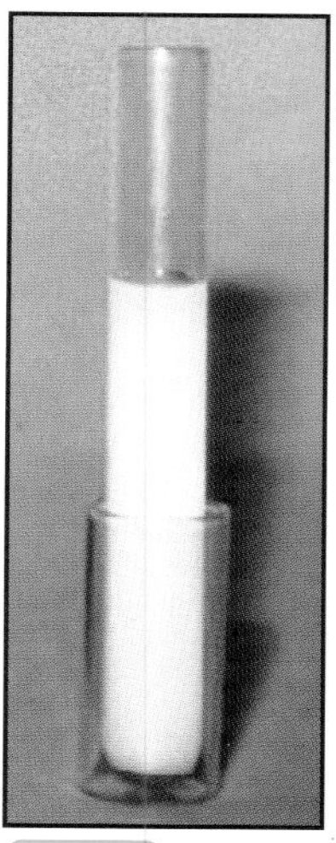

21.23 Harvested pleural fluid.

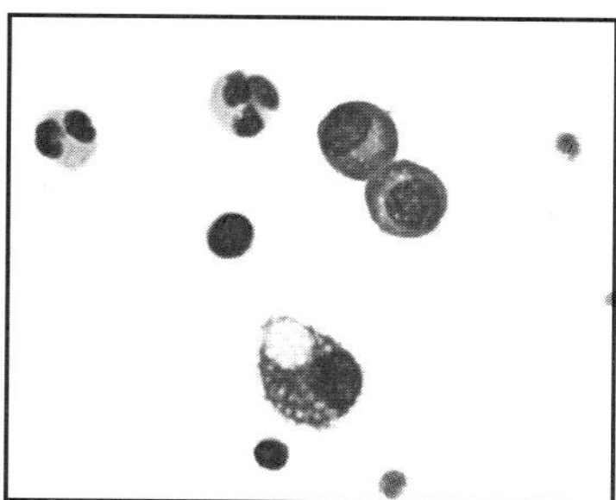

21.24 Sediment from pleural fluid. (Rapi-Diff II stain, original magnification X400.)

Clinical pathology data

Fluid analysis	Result
TP (g/l)	32
RBC ($x10^{12}$/l)	0.05
Total nucleated cell count ($x10^9$/l)	12.3
Cholesterol	3.2 mmol/l (123.52 mg/dl)
Triglycerides	24.4 mmol/l (2159.4 mg/dl)

Conversion factors:
cholesterol (mg/dl) = 38.61 x mmol/l
triglyceride (mg/dl) = 88.5 x mmol/l

Serum analysis	Result
Cholesterol (mmol/l)	3.5
Triglycerides (mmol/l)	1.77

How would you describe and classify the effusion?

Grossly, this is a white milky fluid with the appearance of chyle. The cell count and protein levels would classify this as an exudate (see Figure 21.6) but confirmation of the chylous nature is more important. The fluid triglyceride concentration is much greater than the serum triglyceride concentration, and this is the most reliable discriminatory test. Cholesterol concentration is also lower in the fluid than in the serum. The cholesterol:triglyceride ratio for both in mg/dl is far below 1 (actual value 0.06). These findings are also supportive of chyle.

How would you describe the cells present?

On cytological examination, there is a mixed population of cells including neutrophils, large round-to-oval cells, and lymphocytes. Neutrophils appear pyknotic and slightly degenerate. No bacteria are seen. There are moderate numbers of apparently normal small and medium lymphoid cells. The larger round-to-oval cells have round eccentric nuclei and some plasmacytoid features with open chromatin (nucleoli are not prominent). Cytoplasm is moderately abundant and basophilic and in some cells has a lacy or vacuolated appearance. (These are similar to the cells seen in the original bone marrow aspirate.)

How would you interpret these results and what are the likely differential diagnoses?

The fluid is chyle. Chylous effusions can result from any disorder that causes obstruction or destruction of lymphatics leading to leakage of chyle (lymph and lipids) into the body cavity. Neoplastic cells are also present within this effusion, and it is likely that the underlying lymphoid tumour is the cause of the chyle. The destruction of lymphoid vessels may have been a consequence of chemotherapy (and tumour being lysed) or residual disease causing obstruction or destruction of lymphatics.

What further tests would you recommend?

- Thoracic radiography and ultrasonography to identify residual disease and mass lesions (which can subsequently be monitored)
- Possibly repeat bone marrow aspiration, or further staging. As this was an incidental finding, and the presence of the effusion with neoplastic cells within shows that the dog is no longer in complete remission, a change in chemotherapeutic regime is warranted and bone marrow aspiration will not influence this decision.

(Case 3 courtesy of L Blackwood)

References and further reading

Baker R and Lumsden JH (2000) Pleural and peritoneal fluids. In: *Color atlas of cytology of the dog and cat*, ed. R Baker and JH Lumsden, pp. 159–176. Mosby, St. Louis

Braun JP, Guelfi JF and Pages JP (2001) Comparison of four methods for determination of total protein concentrations in pleural and peritoneal fluid from dogs. *American Journal of Veterinary Research* **62,** 294–296

Bonczynski JJ, Ludwig LL, Barton LJ, Loar A and Peterson ME (2003) Comparison of peritoneal fluid and peripheral blood pH, bicarbonate, glucose, and lactate concentration as a diagnostic tool for septic peritonitis in dogs and cats. *Veterinary Surgery* **32,** 161–166

Canfield P and Martin P (1998) Cytology and general fluid analysis of effusions in mesothelial-lined body cavities: peritoneal, pleural and pericardial cavities. In: *Veterinary Cytology. A bench manual for the feline and canine practitioner*, ed. P Canfield and P Martin, pp. 59–75. University of Sydney Publication, Sydney

Center SA (1999) Fluid accumulation disorders. In: *Small Animal Clinical Diagnosis by Laboratory Methods*, ed. M Willard *et al.*, pp. 208–228. WB Saunders, Philadelphia

Conner BD, Lee YCG, Branca P, Rogers JT, Rodriguez RM and Light RW (2003) Variations in pleural fluid WBC count and differential counts with different sample containers and different methods. *Chest* **123,** 1181–1187

Davies C and Forrester SD (1996) Pleural effusion in cats: 82 cases (1987–1995). *Journal of Small Animal Practice* 37, 217–224

Dunn J and Villiers E (1998) Cytological and biochemical assessment of pleural and peritoneal effusions. *In Practice* **20,** 501–505

Duthie S, Eckersall PD, Addie DD, Lawrence CE and Jarrett O (1997) Value of α1-acid glycoprotein in the diagnosis of feline infectious peritonitis. *Veterinary Record* **141,** 299–303

Edwards NJ (1996) The diagnostic value of pericardial fluid pH determination. *Journal of American Animal Hospital Association* **32,** 63–67

Else RW and Simpson JW (1988) Diagnostic value of exfoliative cytology of body fluids in dogs and cats. *The Veterinary Record* **123,** 70–76

Fine DM, Tobias AH and Jacob KA (2003) Use of pericardial fluid pH to distinguish between idiopathic and neoplastic effusions. *Journal of Veterinary Internal Medicine* **17,** 525–529

Fossum TW, Jacobs RM and Birchards SJ (1986) Evaluation of cholesterol and triglyceride concentrations in differentiating chylous and nonchylous pleural effusions in dogs and cats. *Journal of American Veterinary Medical Association* **188,** 49–51

Fossum TW, Wellman M, Relford RL and Slater MR (1993) Eosinophilic pleural or peritoneal effusions in dogs and cats: 14 cases (1986–1992). *Journal of American Veterinary Medical Association* **202,** 1873–1876

Fournel-Fleury C, Magnol J-P and Guelfi J-F (1994) Effusions in coelomic cavities. In: *Colr⁻ atlas of cancer cytology of the dog and cat*, ed. C Fournel-Fleury, J-P Magnol, J-F Guelfi, pp. 69–141. Conférence Nationale des Vétérinaires Spécialisés en Petits Animaux, Paris

George JW and O'Neill SL (2001) Comparison of refractometer and Biuret methods for total protein measurement in body cavity fluids. *Veterinary Clinical Pathology* **30,** 16–18

Hirschberger J, DeNicola DB, Hermanns W and Kraft W (1999) Sensitivity and specificity of cytological evaluation in the diagnosis of neoplasia in body fluids from cats and dogs. *Veterinary Clinical Pathology* **28,** 142–146

Hirschberger J and Koch S (1995) Validation of the determination of the activity of adenosine deaminase in the body effusions of cats. *Research in Veterinary Science* **59,** 226–229

Hirschberger J and Koch S (1996) Validation of an adenosine deaminase assay and its use in the evaluation of body fluid in dogs. *Veterinary Clinical Pathology* **25,** 100–104

Kerstetter KK, Krahwinkel DJ, Millis DL and Hahn K (1997) Pericardiectomy in dogs: 22 cases (1978–1994). *Journal of American Veterinary Medical Association* **211,** 736–740

Meadows RL and MacWilliams PS (1994) Chylous effusions revisited. *Veterinary Clinical Pathology* **23,** 54–62

Mellanby RJ, Villiers E and Herrtage ME (2002) Canine pleural and mediastinal effusions: a retrospective study of 81 cases. *Journal of Small Animal Practice* **43,** 446–451

McNeely S, Seatter K, Yuhaniak J and Kashyap ML (1981) The 16-hour standing test and lipoprotein electrophoresis compared for detection of chylomicrons in plasma. *Clinical Chemistry* **27,** 731–732

Papasouliotis K, Murphy K, Dodkin S and Torrance A (2002) Use of the Vettest 8008 and refractometry for determination of total protein, albumin, and globulin concentrations in feline effusions. *Veterinary Clinical Pathology* **4,** 162–166

Shaw SP, Rozanski EA and Rush JE (2004) Cardiac Troponins I and T in dogs with pericardial effusion. *Journal of Veterinary Internal Medicine* **18,** 322–324

Shelley SM, Scarlett-Kranz J and Blue JT (1988) Protein electrophoresis on effusions from cats as a diagnostic test for feline infectious peritonitis. *Journal of American Animal Hospital Association* **24,** 495–500

Shelley SM (2001) Body cavity fluids. In: *Atlas of canine and feline cytology*, ed. RE Raskin and DJ Meyer, pp. 187–205. WB Saunders, Philadelphia

Sisson D, Thomas WP, Ruehl WW and Zinkl JG (1984) Diagnostic value of pericardial fluid analysis in the dog. *Journal of American Veterinary Medical Association* **184,** 51–55

Sparkes AH, Gruffydd-Jones TJ and Harbour DA (1994) An appraisal of the value of laboratory tests in the diagnosis of feline infectious peritonitis. *Journal of the American Animal Hospital Association* **30,** 345–350

Stepien RL, Whitley NT and Dubielzig RR (2000) Idiopathic or mesothelioma-related pericardial effusion: clinical findings and survival in 17 dogs studied retrospectively. *Journal of Small Animal Practice* **41,** 342–347

Tyler RD and Cowell RL (1989) Evaluation of pleural and peritoneal effusions. *Veterinary Clinics of North America: Small Animal Practice* **19,** 743–768

Waddle JR and Giger U (1990) Lipoprotein electrophoresis differentiation of chylous and nonchylous pleural effusions in dogs and cats and its correlation with pleural effusion triglyceride concentration. *Veterinary Clinical Pathology* **19,** 80–85

Wright KN, Gompf RE and DeNovo RC (1999) Peritoneal effusion in cats: 65 cases (1981–1997). *Journal of American Veterinary Medical Association* **214,** 375–381

22a

Laboratory evaluation of joint disease

John F. Innes

Introduction

The evaluation of synovial fluid is an underused technique in animals with joint disease, and even when there are no overt clinical or radiological abnormalities within the joint, failure to examine joint fluid can result in important errors in case management. It is especially important when the cause of the joint disease is in doubt, but will often provide useful information in apparently straightforward cases. For example, some cases of cruciate ligament rupture are secondary to immune-mediated polyarthritis, which can only be detected by synovial fluid analysis. Similarly, patients with chronic osteoarthritis often present with an acute exacerbation of clinical signs, which might represent a 'flare' of osteoarthritis, but could be due to haematogenous infective arthritis or neoplasia.

The main types of arthritis are summarized in Figure 22.1. The most common form of arthritis in dogs and cats is osteoarthritis, which is often secondary to a primary initiating factor that can be identified clinically, radiograpically or by arthroscopy (Figure 22.2). However, in some cases, laboratory analysis of synovial fluid is required to differentiate non-inflammatory arthritis from inflammatory arthritis. Immune-mediated joint diseases are the commonest inflammatory arthropathies, followed by infective arthropathies, in which identification of infective organisms always relies on laboratory techniques. Articular neoplasia is uncommon, and usually requires biopsy for diagnosis, though non-specific changes in joint fluid are common.

Common causes of osteoarthritis in dogs
Hip dysplasia
Cranial cruciate ligament disease
Elbow dysplasia
Osteochondrosis (shoulder, elbow, stifle, tarsus)
Intra-articular fracture
Collateral ligament rupture
Causes of osteoarthritis in cats
Hip dysplasia
Cranial cruciate ligament rupture
Intra-articular fracture
Collateral ligament rupture

22.2 Common primary causes of secondary osteoarthritis in dogs and cats. Note: elbow osteoarthritis is a common finding in older cats but the cause of this disease is as yet unknown.

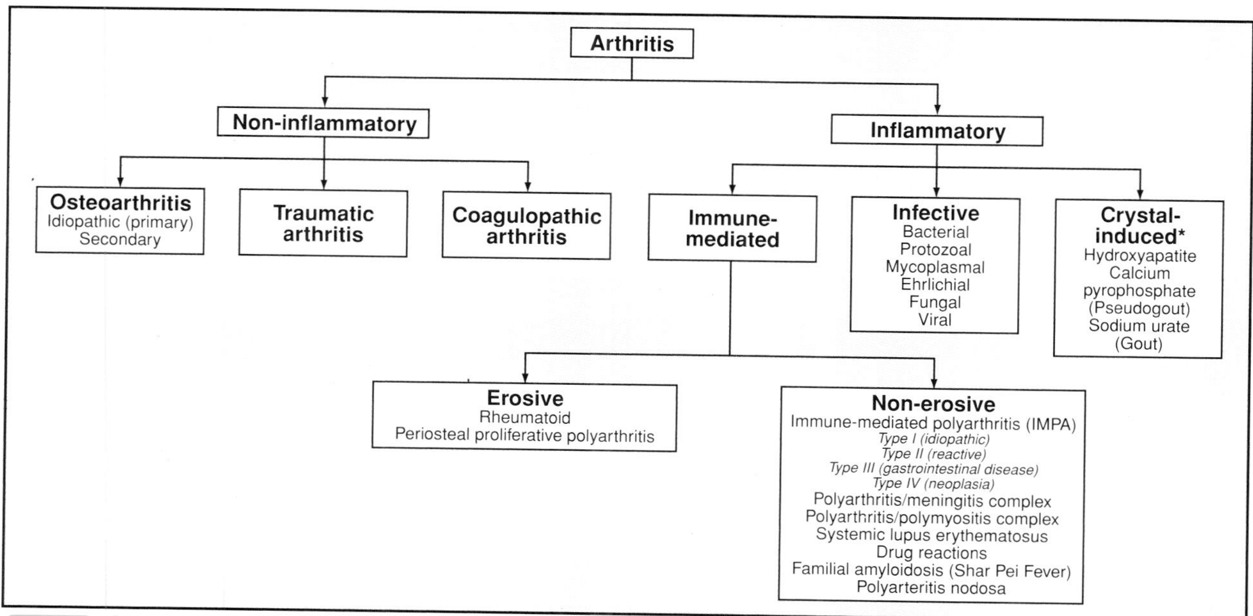

22.1 Classification of arthritis (adapted from Bennett, 1990). *Crystal-induced arthropathies are extremely rare in dogs and cats.

Indications for arthrocentesis

The main indications for arthrocentesis are:

- Joint disease of unknown aetiology
- Joint effusion
- Disease in multiple joints
- Suspected infective arthritis
- Pyrexia of unknown origin
- Monitoring response to therapy in infective arthritis and immune-mediated polyarthritis.

In cases of suspected polyarthritis, samples should be submitted from a minimum of three joints for cytology. Immune-mediated polyarthritis often affects the smaller joints (carpus and tarsus) and it can be difficult to obtain sufficient fluid from these: in this situation, other larger joints (shoulder, elbow, hip, stifle) should be sampled, as these will often also have inflammatory changes.

Technique for arthrocentesis

Arthrocentesis can be performed under general anaesthesia or heavy sedation. The sites for needle insertion are illustrated in Figure 22.3.

1. The hair over the site should be clipped and the site prepared aseptically. If the operator wishes to palpate the insertion site, sterile gloves are worn. If the operator is familiar with the landmarks, a 'no touch' technique can be used.
2. The needle should be of sufficient diameter to facilitate the flow of viscous synovial fluid (i.e. 0.6–0.9 mm (20–23 gauge)) and long enough to reach the joint cavity through the soft tissues. The length of the needle varies with the joint being sampled, with proximal joints requiring needles 25–63 mm (1–2½ inches) long and distal joints requiring 16–25 mm (5/8–1 inch) needles.
3. Typically, a 5 ml (or 2.5 ml in cats and small dogs) syringe is attached prior to insertion: gentle suction is applied to the syringe (normal joints have a pressure below that of the atmosphere, so joint fluid generally requires aspiration).
4. Once sufficient fluid has entered the syringe, suction is released to avoid inadvertent aspiration of blood, and the needle and syringe are withdrawn.
5. Fluid is then placed into appropriate containers, usually EDTA tubes and a blood culture bottle (Figure 22.4), and squash smears are made (see Chapter 20 for smearing techniques). Rapid air-drying reduces cell shrinkage artefact and can be achieved by directing a hair dryer on warm setting at the back of the slide held at a distance of about 15 cm. If the sample is to be mailed to a laboratory, smears are made immediately, at the time of sampling, and sent with the sample tube.

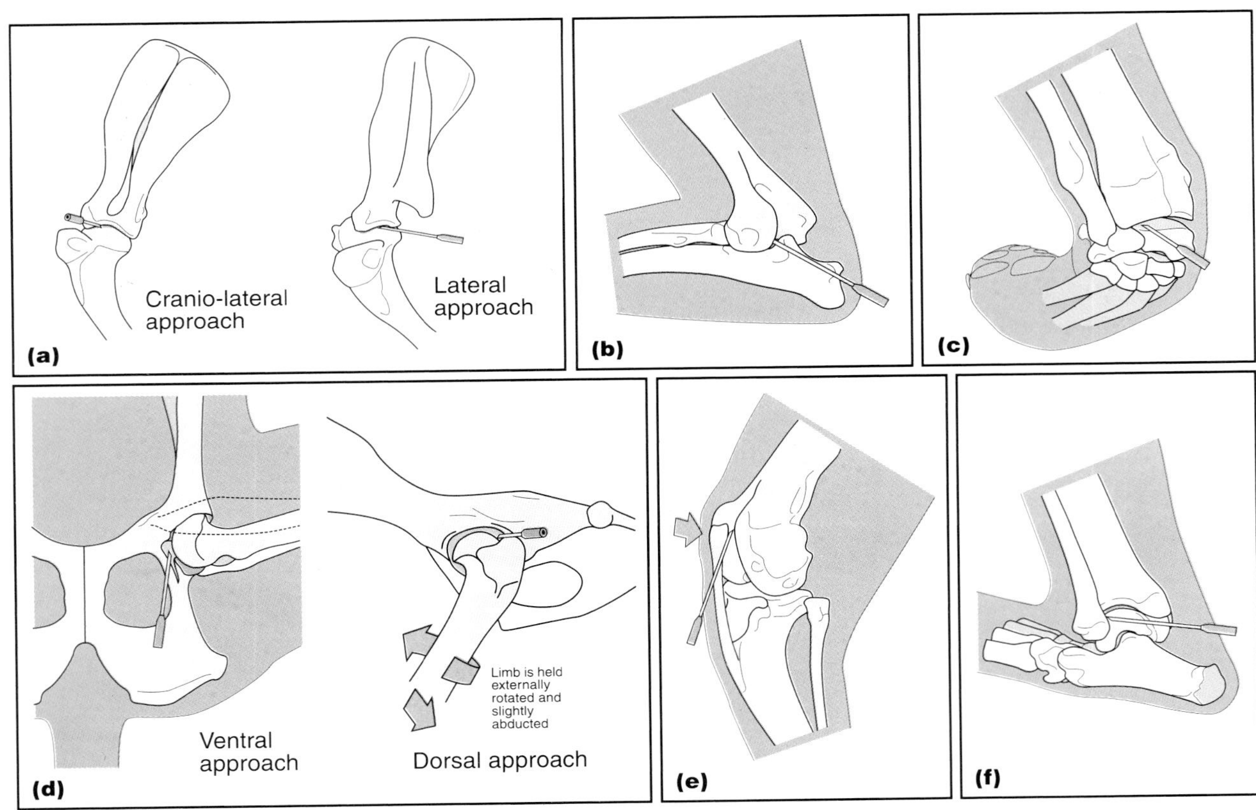

22.3 Sites for arthrocentesis. (a) Shoulder. (b) Elbow. (c) Carpus. (d) Hip. (e) Stifle. (f) Tarsus.

Test required	Preferred sample tube
Cytology	EDTA
Culture and sensitivity	Blood culture (or plain)
Biochemistry	Plain
Serology	Plain

22.4 Appropriate sample tubes for synovial fluid analyses.

Sample artefacts can develop rapidly as fluid samples age: for example, neutrophils may become lytic (mimicking degenerative change seen with infection) and synovial cells may become vacuolated (mimicking reactive change seen with osteoarthritis). If there is insufficient sample, then a direct smear should be made, although the examination of a smear alone is inferior without objective cell counts.

The volume of fluid aspirated is dependent on the size of the animal, the particular joint sampled, the health status of the joint and the technique of the operator. However, normal joints in the dog generally only have 0.1–1.0 ml of clear, viscous synovial fluid.

Evaluation of synovial fluid

Gross evaluation

Gross evaluation of synovial fluid can provide useful information, but further analyses are generally required.

Normal fluid

Synovial fluid is similar to eggwhite (*syn-ovia*). Normal synovial fluid can be clear or slightly yellow, with a high viscosity and a non-Newtonian (viscoelastic) behaviour. The viscosity is provided by the high content of the long chain polysaccharide hyaluronan.

Changes in gross appearance

Gross appearance of canine synovial fluid in different conditions is summarized in Figure 22.5.

Blood contamination during arthrocentesis is usually recognized as a streak of blood running through an otherwise clear fluid, whereas in true haemarthrosis the fluid is uniformly discoloured. An increase in the volume of synovial fluid indicates effusion. This is often accompanied by a reduction in the apparent viscosity of the fluid. However, this may be caused by a dilution of the hyaluronan by plasma dialysate. A true reduction in viscosity is caused by depolymerization of the hyaluronan and is usually associated with inflammatory changes within the joint. The mucin clot test can be used to differentiate effusion from a true decrease in viscosity, although this is rarely necessary for clinical decision-making.

Changes in colour can be associated with haemorrhage and inflammation. Recent haemorrhage within the joint (haemarthrosis) will produce a red colour (Figure 22.6a). Common causes of haemarthrosis are intra-articular injury (e.g. fracture or ligament rupture) and recent surgery or arthrocentesis. Haemarthrosis is also seen (less commonly) in haemostatic disorders (see Chapter 6). After an isolated intra-articular haemorrhage, the haemoglobin is gradually removed over 2–4 weeks and the colour of the joint fluid may become more orange or yellow because of residual haemosiderin.

Changes in the transparency of synovial fluid generally indicate inflammatory change, as high numbers of inflammatory cells will cause the fluid to become cloudy or turbid, and sometimes white–yellow or grey–red in colour (Figure 22.6b).

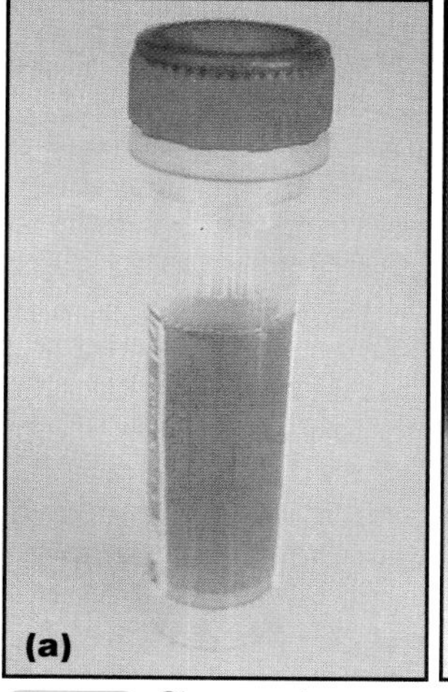

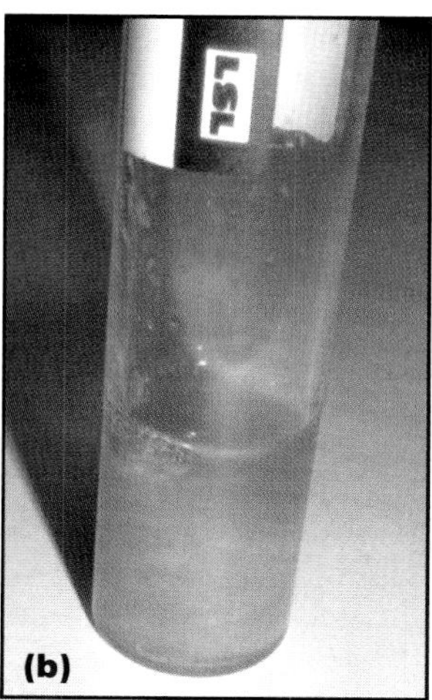

22.6 Changes in appearance of synovial fluid (a) Synovial fluid from a Labrador Retriever with recent cranial cruciate ligament rupture. Haemarthrosis and effusion indicate a recent haemorrhage within the joint. (b) Synovial fluid from a dog with bacterial infective arthritis. Note the turbidity and grey-red colour.

Classification of joint status	Gross appearance	Viscosity	Total cell count (x 10^9/l)	Neutrophils (%)
Normal	Clear	High	0.1–2.0	<3
Recent trauma	Red (haemarthrosis)	Low	2.0–15.0	2–15
Osteoarthritis	Clear/yellow	High	1.0–5.0	2–5
Infective arthritis (acute)	Turbid, yellow/grey/red	Low	>100	90–98
Infective arthritis (chronic)	Turbid, yellow/grey	Low	5–100	60–90
Immune-mediated arthritis	Clear–turbid, grey/yellow	Low	5–100	20–95

22.5 Typical features of canine synovial fluid. The clinician should interpret cytological results in the light of other clinical information. See text for additional information.

Mucin clot test

The mucin clot test is a crude test to evaluate the viscosity of synovial fluid. A small amount of fluid is dropped into a beaker of 5% acetic acid. Normal fluid should form a tight clot, but fluid with depolymerized hyaluronan will fail to do this. The test result is usually normal in osteoarthritis, but clot formation is sometimes poor. It is variable in inflammatory arthropathies, and fair to poor in acute haemarthroses. The variability of results limits the clinical usefulness of this test.

Cytology

Qualitative and quantitative cytological examination of synovial fluid is the most useful test to help classify the disease process within the joint. Examination of a smear is useful (Figure 22.7), but the sensitivity, specificity and reliability of qualitative assessment are poor (Gibson *et al.*, 1999). Whenever possible, a total and differential cell count should be performed. Some laboratories will not perform a total cell count because the viscosity of synovial fluid can make this technically demanding. However, appropriate dilution of the sample should facilitate this and the clinician should use a laboratory that is prepared to perform these analyses.

There is significant overlap in the cytological changes between different articular disease processes, and cytological results need to be interpreted in the light of patient history, clinical signs and results of other diagnostic modalities.

Guidelines for interpretation of synovial fluid analyses are summarized in Figure 22.5 and a flow chart of synovial fluid cytology interpretation is shown in Figure 22.8. It is generally possible to distinguish between 'inflammatory' and 'non-inflammatory' joint disease on the basis of total cell count and the percentage of neutrophils, but there is considerable overlap between the inflammatory conditions (infective arthritis and immune-mediated disease) and the results must be interpreted in the light of other clinical information. As a general principle, if multiple joints show evidence of inflammatory change in a symmetrical pattern with a predominance of neutrophils, the likely diagnosis is immune-mediated polyarthritis. Infective arthritis of multiple joints in dogs and cats is rare, particularly in adult animals, and is less likely to be symmetrical in distribution.

Normal joint fluid

Normal joint fluid has low cellularity ($<1.5 \times 10^9$/l). On a smear this equates to ≤2 nucleated cells per X40 field. Cells may be arranged in palisades or rows (windrowing), reflecting the viscous nature of the fluid. There is usually prominent background staining, consisting of pink granular material (not to be confused with bacteria) caused by the glycosaminoglycans (mostly hyaluronan) in the fluid (see Figure 22.7a). Red cells are absent unless blood contamination occurred at sampling. Nucleated cells are a mixture of large mononuclear cells (synovial lining cells and macrophages 60–90% of cells) and lymphocytes (3–30% of cells) with <3% neutrophils. Synovial lining cells are round cells with a single round nucleus and a moderate amount of basophilic cytoplasm. A small proportion of these may be activated with

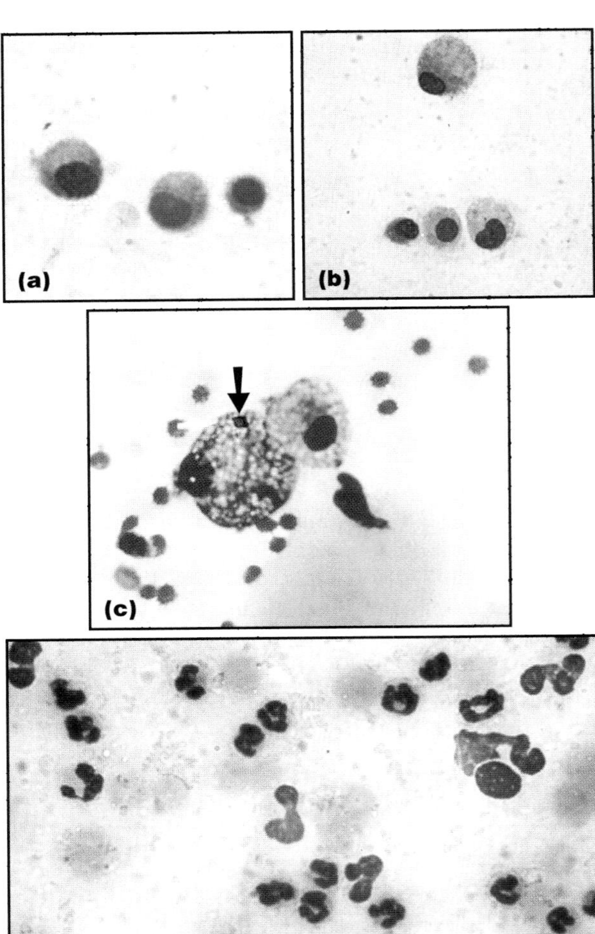

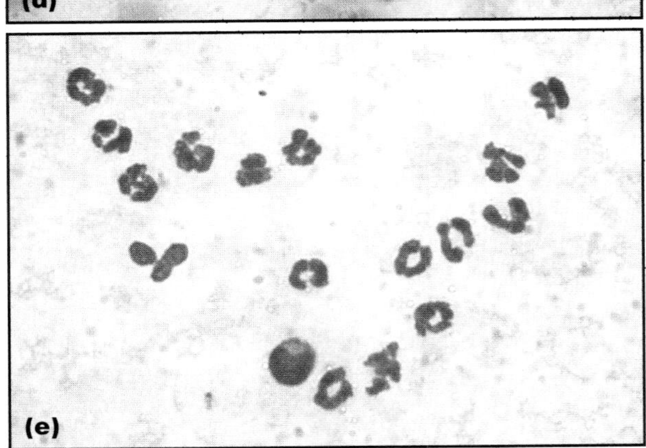

22.7 Synovial fluid cytology. (a) Normal canine synovial fluid showing a scant mononuclear population consisting of one lymphocyte and 2 larger mononuclear cells (synovial lining cells). (b) Synovial fluid from a stifle with osteoarthritis. Some of the mononuclear cells have abundant foamy cytoplasm. (c) Synovial fluid from an elbow joint with haemarthrosis. A haematoidin crystal (arrowed) is present within a macrophage, reflecting erythrophagocytosis. (d) Synovial fluid smear from a dog with infective arthritis. Numerous neutrophils are present, some showing degenerative change. Red cells are present in the background. (e) Synovial fluid smear from a dog with immune-mediated arthritis, consisting predominantly of neutrophils with a small proportion of mononuclear cells. (Giemsa stain, except (d) Wright's; original magnification X1000.)

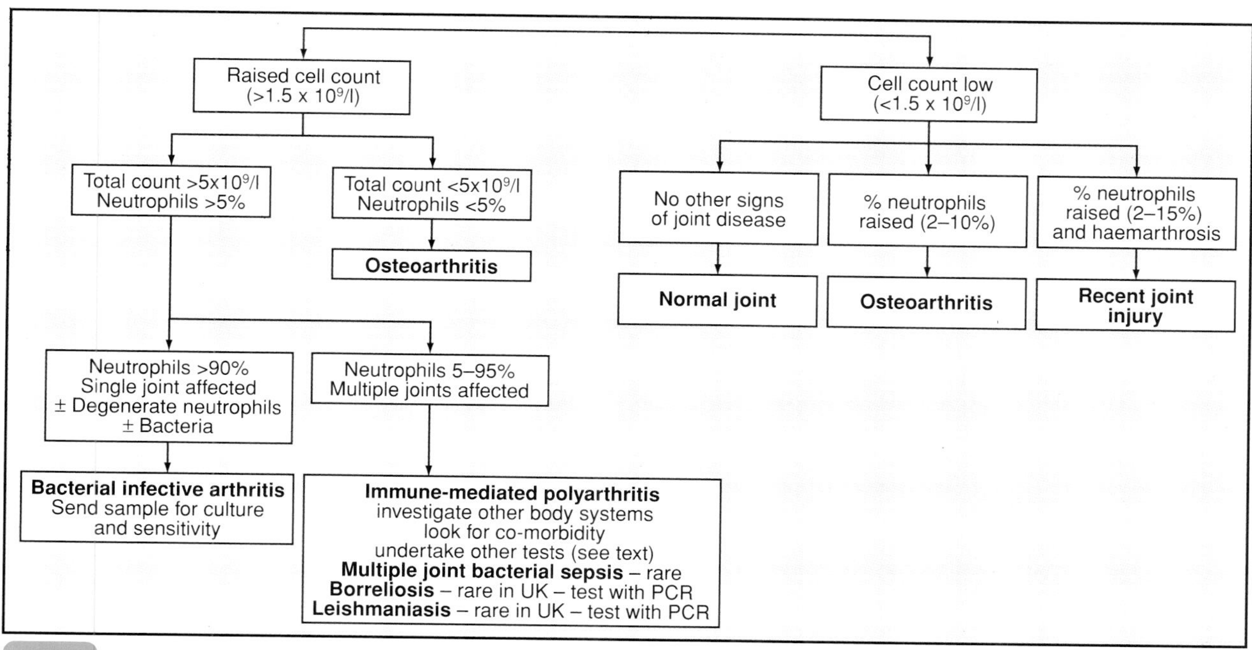

22.8 Flow chart to illustrate the interpretation of synovial fluid cytology.

increased amounts of vacuolated cytoplasm appearing very similar to macrophages. It is not clinically important to distinguish synovial cells and macrophages; they are classified together as large mononuclear cells, although the proportion of vacuolated (reactive) cells is important and in normal joints is <10%.

Non-inflammatory arthropathies

Osteoarthritis: Cytologically, there is significant overlap with normal joints, as cell numbers are usually normal or very slightly raised (up to 5 x 10^9/l) with <2–5% neutrophils. Thus the majority of cells observed on cytology are large mononuclear cells, with >10% of these having abundant foamy/vacuolated or phagocytic cytoplasm (see Figure 22.7b). Occasionally osteoarthritic joints have a moderately raised neutrophil count, accounting for up to 10% of cells. The reasons for this are often unclear but may involve recent joint trauma (sprain), crystal (hydroxyapatite) formation or an idiopathic inflammatory 'flare'. A repeat sample 2–3 weeks later should usually see a return to more typical cytological features.

Recent joint injury or haemorrhage: Joint injury or haemorrhage will cause a haemarthrosis, reflected as large numbers of red cells. In acute haemarthrosis the differential nucleated cell count may be similar to that of peripheral blood, and platelets may be present; with recent injury there is likely to be accompanying inflammation. With more long-standing haemorrhage there are increased numbers of neutrophils and macrophages but platelets are absent (these disintegrate rapidly within the fluid). Erythrophagocytosis and/or haemosiderin or haematoidin crystals in macrophages provide evidence of pre-existing haemorrhage into the joint (see Figure 22.7c); these features are not seen with iatrogenic blood contamination.

Inflammatory arthropathies

These can be divided into two main groups: infective and immune-mediated arthropathies. Both result in a moderate to marked increase in numbers of neutrophils with variable numbers of large mononuclear cells.

Arthritis associated with microorganisms: Bacterial infective arthritis in adult small animals is typically characterized by a severe suppurative inflammatory monoarthropathy and may occur following haematogenous spread, surgery or local penetration (e.g. cat bites). Multiple joint sepsis in adult small animals is rare, although it may result from seeding of infection from endocarditis (which can also trigger immune-mediated arthritis). In neonates, multiple joints may become infected following haematogenous spread from omphalophlebitis or pharyngeal infection with *Streptococcus canis*, or following mammary or uterine infections in the dam.

Bacterial infective arthritis generally causes a large increase in neutrophils in the synovial fluid. Red cell counts may also be raised with associated haemorrhage. In acute infection, neutrophils usually account for 90–98% of nucleated cells (see Figure 22.7d). With more chronic disease (weeks), neutrophil percentage may drop to the region of 60–90%. In bacterial infection, neutrophils may be degenerate with swollen 'ragged' pink-staining nuclei, and bacteria may be seen both extracellularly and within neutrophil cytoplasm. However, these classic cytological features of bacterial infection are often absent in septic synovial fluid. More typically the neutrophils are non-degenerate and no bacteria are identified; thus the cytological morphology is indistinguishable from immune-mediated arthritis and the cell counts, clinical history and presentation must be considered.

Borreliosis (Lyme disease) may cause infective polyarthritis, where a single joint or a small number of joints may be infected, or may trigger a more generalized immune-mediated polyarthritis (May and Bennett, 1994). In the former, synovial fluid cytology typically shows moderately high white cell counts with a high percentage of non-degenerate neutrophils. The organisms are not visible on smears. Serology (see Chapter 27) and polymerase chain reaction (PCR) tests (see below and Chapter 27) are helpful. The presence of antibody to *Borrelia burgdorferi* can support a diagnosis in the presence of other characteristic historical and clinical signs. However, since seroprevalance rates are often high in endemic areas (May *et al.*, 1991), the value of such a test is limited. PCR is to be preferred in such instances, in an attempt to demonstrate the presence of DNA from the relevant organism (see Chapter 27).

Leishmania donovani has been associated with an erosive arthritis in dogs, sometimes affecting multiple joints. Other clinical signs include pyrexia, malaise, weight loss, lymphadenopathy, dermatopathy and hepatosplenomegaly. Synovial fluid samples are generally normocellular to mildly hypercellular with a mixed population of neutrophils and large mononuclear cells and lymphocytes. The intracellular *Leishmania* organisms may be seen within macrophages, or within macrophages in lymph nodes or bone marrow. PCR (see below) and serology can be used for definitive diagnosis.

Ehrlichia spp. and *Anaplasma phagocytophilum* are tick-borne organisms associated with non-erosive polyarthritis, particularly in the acute forms of the diseases. Arthritis may be only one of a range of signs, including pyrexia, lymphadenopathy and thrombocytopenia. Synovial fluid samples are markedly hypercellular with >60% neutrophils. Morulae may be present in a small proportion of the neutrophils.

Other infections that may (rarely) cause infective arthritis include *Mycobacterium* spp., *Mycoplasma* spp., 'L forms' (cell wall-deficient bacteria), fungi (e.g. *Coccidioides immitis, Blastomyces dermatitidis, Histoplasma capsulatum, Cryptococcus neoformans*) and, in cats, calicivirus.

Immune-mediated polyarthritis: IMPA is characterized by inflammatory change, with a predominance of neutrophils, in multiple joints in a symmetrical pattern. IMPA may be non-erosive (most common) or erosive, and the latter occurs in rheumatoid arthritis. There are four subtypes of IMPA (May and Bennett, 1994):

- Type I idiopathic IMPA (Clements *et al.*, 2004), accounting for approximately 50% of all idiopathic IMPA
- Type II, associated with an identified infection elsewhere in the body (e.g. cystitis, pyometra, discospondylitis, osteomyelitis)
- Type III, associated with gastrointestinal disease
- Type IV, associated with neoplasia.

These IMPAs are defined by their associated comorbidity, which may produce a range of abnormalities on clinicopathological tests. Appropriate treatment of the underlying disease may resolve the IMPA. Polyarthritis may be one component of systemic lupus erythematosus (Figure 22.9) and may also occur in association with sterile suppurative corticosteroid-responsive meningitis (Webb *et al.*, 2002); analysis of cerebrospinal fluid is recommended (see Chapter 23) if spinal pain is a feature of a dog with suspect polyarthritis. Similarly, a polyarthritis/polymyositis complex is described, and appropriate investigation of muscle is indicated (see Chapter 22b). Rheumatoid arthritis is much less common than non-erosive polyarthritis; diagnostic criteria are summarized in Figure 22.10.

Evidence of immune-mediated disease of more than one body system
High titre of antinuclear antibody (ANA), e.g. >1:32
Clinical pathological or histological evidence of immunopathology, e.g. immune-mediated destruction of red cells, platelets or white cells; deposition of immune complexes in synovium, glomeruli, skin

22.9 Criteria for diagnosis of systemic lupus erythematosus in dogs.

Radiographic changes including bony destruction
Serological evidence of rheumatoid factor
Abnormal synovial fluids with high white cell counts
Inactivity stiffness (stiffness after rest)
Pain or tenderness on motion of at least one joint
Swelling of at least one joint
Swelling of at least one other joint within a 3-month period
Symmetrical joint swelling
Characteristic histological changes in the synovium

22.10 Criteria for the diagnosis of canine rheumatoid arthritis (adapted from May and Bennett, 1994). Seven criteria should be present to diagnose 'classical rheumatoid arthritis' and five for 'definite rheumatoid arthritis', but it is recommended that the criteria in bold are present.

The synovial fluid cytology for all types of IMPA varies between joints and between patients. Typically, the white cell count is 5–100 x 10^9/l with 20–95% neutrophils (non-degenerate) and varying proportions of lymphocytes and large mononuclear cells. The proteinaceous background material seen in normal synovial fluid is usually present, although it may be absent.

Confirmation of inflammatory polyarthritis is an indication for further diagnostic work to classify the polyarthritis (see above), and identify any underlying causes. Typically this would involve haematology, biochemistry, urinalysis, radiology of joints, thorax and abdomen, and echocardiography. The antinuclear antibody test is performed if systemic lupus is suspected, and the rheumatoid factor test if rheumatoid arthritis is suspected. These tests are not useful in the 'blanket' testing for autoimmune disease, as chronic inflammation of any sort can cause positive results, and the specificity of these tests is low.

Bacterial culture and sensitivity testing

Infective arthritis is usually caused by bacteria, but can also be associated with spirochaetes, protozoa, fungi, mycoplasmas and viruses (see above). In cases of suspect infective arthritis, synovial fluid should be submitted for bacterial culture and sensitivity. However, not all synovial fluids from such cases will yield a positive culture, and the initial handling of the sample may influence this. Placing the sample in a blood culture bottle, and initially incubating in this medium for 24 hours, can improve the sensitivity of synovial fluid culture (see Chapter 25). Alternatively, synovium obtained by needle biopsy, arthroscopy or arthrotomy may be cultured.

The common bacteria isolated from infected joints reflect the sources of infection. In dogs, the most common organisms are *Staphylococcus intermedius*, and β-haemolytic *Streptococcus*. Methicillin-resistant forms of *Staphylococcus aureus* (MRSA) have also been isolated, while coliform and anaerobic organisms are less commonly involved, as are *Pseudomonas aeruginosa*, *Nocardia asteroides* and *Bacillus* spp. In cats, *Pasteurella multocida*, *Bacteroides* spp. and *Escherichia coli* are more commonly isolated, as infection is a result of bites from other cats.

For further information on culture of bacteria, fungi, mycobacteria and mycoplasma see Chapter 25.

Polymerase chain reaction

Although a positive PCR result is strong evidence for the presence of a given organism within the sample, the relationship between the organism and the disease process may be complex. Recent investigations of synovial fluids of human patients with inflammatory polyarthritides have shown that PCR of synovial fluid can detect bacterial DNA or rRNA both from organisms associated with arthritis and from other skin and gut commensals (Pacheco-Tena *et al.*, 2001; Schnarr *et al.*, 2001). It is suggested that there may be trafficking of organisms not involved in initiating the disease process to inflamed joints. Thus a positive PCR needs to be interpreted with caution. Further discussion on PCR can be found in Chapter 27.

Biochemistry

Several simply measured biochemical parameters can be altered in synovial fluid during disease, e.g. glucose can be lowered and protein elevated in bacterial infective arthritis. However, the usefulness of these tests is very limited and the results do not alter clinical decision-making.

There is much ongoing research on the measurement of various macromolecules ('biomarkers') in joint disease. These biomarkers are released from joint tissues (cartilage, bone or synovium) and are measured in synovial fluid (or blood or urine). Typical markers are cartilage matrix molecules, or epitopes thereof, such as glycosaminoglycans (Innes *et al.*, 1998), chondroitin sulphate (Johnson *et al.*, 2001, 2002), keratan sulphate, and collagen (Chu *et al.*, 2002). These markers are not yet validated in the clinic.

Synovial fluid crystals

Crystal-induced arthropathies appear to be very rare in dogs and cats, although certain crystals have been reported in canine joint fluids. Crystals are identified in synovial fluid samples (in EDTA) using polarized light microscopy. Accurate identification requires skill and training and is based on morphology and birefringence characteristics. Staining with alizarin red can help detect calcium-containing crystals. Basic calcium phosphate crystals, such as hydroxyapatite crystals, are often seen in canine joint fluid, particularly with osteoarthritis. However, the significance of these crystals is unknown. Synovitis associated with calcium pyrophosphate ('pseudogout') has been reported in a few canine case reports. Although the Dalmatian might be expected to be at risk of urate crystal arthropathy (gout), high renal excretion of uric acid appears to prevent urate crystal precipitation. Intra-articular corticosteroid therapy may also result in crystal formation in synovial fluid (Singer and Gruber, 1983).

Serology

Rheumatoid factor

The detection of rheumatoid factor (RF) is one of the diagnostic criteria for canine rheumatoid arthritis (Bennett, 1987; Bennett and Kirkham, 1987; Bell *et al.*, 1993; May and Bennett, 1994). Typically an enzyme-linked immunosorbent assay (ELISA) is used. Rheumatoid factor (RF) is an IgM autoantibody with specificity for the Fc region of IgG (ie. an anti-IgG immunoglobulin). Because normal dogs and dogs with other arthritides will often have mildly positive results for RF, assays are usually interpreted in the light of results from confirmed cases of rheumatoid arthritis and dogs with other arthritides, and the laboratory performing the assay should advise what constitutes a positive result. A positive RF result does not constitute a diagnosis of rheumatoid arthritis; other diagnostic criteria must be satisfied (see Figure 22.10).

Antinuclear antibody

Antinuclear antibody (ANA) is anti-nuclear immunoglobulin and is associated with systemic lupus erythematosus (SLE). The test for ANA is an indirect immunofluorescence test (Bell *et al.*, 1997). ANA may be detected in normal individuals as well as those with chronic inflammatory disease and so a positive ANA test result is not diagnostic of SLE. Compared with humans, dogs and cats generally have low titres of ANA, and there is a high prevalence of low ANA titres in the normal population, especially in cats. For example, cats with feline leukaemia virus or feline immunodeficiency virus infections or feline infectious peritonitis can be positive for ANA. A positive ANA titre is only part of the diagnosis of SLE (May and Bennett, 1994) (Figure 22.9).

Case examples follow ▶

Case examples

Case 1

Signalment

2-year-old male Chow Chow.

History and clinical findings

Left cranial cruciate ligament rupture diagnosed 8 weeks ago. Treated with extracapsular suture of monofilament nylon. Lameness was improving but has now acutely deteriorated and the dog is 70% lame on the left hindlimb. Moderate effusion and pain on manipulation of the left stifle. Synovial fluid aspirated from both stifle joints.

Clinical pathology data

Synovial fluid cytology	Left stifle	Right stifle	Reference interval
RBC (x 10^{12}/l)	0.04	0.1	0
WBC (x 10^{9}/l)	80	3	0.1–2.0
Neutrophils (%)	95	3	<3
Large mononuclear cells (%)	5	97	60–90

Comment

- Left stifle: some neutrophils appear degenerate; no bacteria seen; some hydroxyapatite crystals seen
- Right stifle: normal cell morphology; no crystals seen

What abnormalities are present?

- Markedly raised total nucleated cell count in left stifle
- Marked increase in percentage of neutrophils in left stifle
- Degenerate neutrophils in left stifle
- Slight increase in total nucleated cell count in right stifle
- Hydroxyapatite crystals are relatively common in a cruciate-deficient stifle joint.

How would you interpret these results and what are the likely differential diagnoses?

This is most likely an infective arthritis associated with previous surgery. The nylon suture may have acted as a nidus for infection to spread to the joint or there may have been haematogenous spread of bacteria to an already hyperaemic post-surgical joint.

The near normal synovial fluid in the right stifle makes immune-mediated polyarthritis (IMPA) much less likely, as this tends to be symmetrical. In addition, the very high percentage of neutrophils in the left stifle is not typical of IMPA. However, the slight increase in total nucleated cell count in the right stifle may suggest early osteoarthritic changes consistent with cruciate disease in this joint also.

What further tests would you recommend?

- Culture and sensitivity of the synovial fluid from the left stifle (use blood culture bottle)
- Stability testing and radiography of the right stifle joint to check for early cruciate disease.

Case 2

Signalment

6-month-old male Bernese Mountain Dog.

History and clinical findings

Acute-onset reluctance to stand, of 24 hours' duration. There is pain on attempting to stand and also on manipulation of the hindlimbs and the cervical spine. Extension of both hips is very painful and extension of both elbows is also somewhat painful. No neurological deficits are present. The dog's temperature is 39.5°C.

Clinical pathology data

Synovial fluid cytology	Left hip	Right hip	Left elbow	Right elbow	Reference interval
RBC (x 10^{12}/l)	0.03	0.02	0.02	0.03	0
WBC (x 10^{9}/l)	20	16	26	18	0.1–2.0
Neutrophils (%)	60	35	57	36	<3
Macrophages (%)	40	65	43	64	60–90

Comment

No bacteria seen

What abnormalities are present?

Raised total cell counts in all joints sampled. The neutrophil count is moderately raised in all joints.

How would you interpret these results and what are the likely differential diagnoses?

Polyarthritis is present. The total cell counts and percentage of neutrophils is consistent with immune-mediated polyarthritis.

What further tests would you recommend?

- Haematology and blood biochemistry for evidence of co-morbidity or other immune-mediated disease.
- Urinanalysis for evidence of co-morbidity or other immune-mediated disease.
- Radiography of thorax and abdomen for evidence of co-morbidity.
- CSF analysis: in a young dog of this breed, meningitis–polyarthritis syndrome should be considered, as the cervical pain may relate to meningitis rather than vertebral column apophyseal joint inflammation.
- (Radiography of joints: unlikely to show changes at this early stage).
- (Serology for RF and ANA: may help classify the disease but unlikely to change clinical decision-making).

References and further reading

Bell SC, Carter SD, May C and Bennett D (1993) IgA and IgM rheumatoid factors in canine rheumatoid arthritis. *Journal of Small Animal Practice* **34,** 259–264

Bell SC, Hughes DE, Bennett D, Bari ASM, Kelly DF and Carter SD (1997) Analysis and significance of anti-nuclear antibodies in dogs. *Research in Veterinary Science* **62,** 83–84

Bennett D (1987) Immune-based erosive inflammatory joint disease of the dog – canine rheumatoid-arthritis .1. Clinical, radiological and laboratory investigations. *Journal of Small Animal Practice* **28,** 779–797

Bennett D and Kirkham D (1987) The laboratory identification of serum rheumatoid-factor in the dog. *Journal of Comparative Pathology* **97,** 541–550

Chu Q, Lopez M, Hayashi K, Ionescu M, Billinghurst RC, Johnson KA, Poole AR and Markel MD (2002) Elevation of a collagenase generated type II collagen neoepitope and proteoglycan epitopes in synovial fluid following induction of joint instability in the dog. *Osteoarthritis and Cartilage* **10,** 662–669

Clements DN, Gear RNA, Tattersall J, Carmichael S and Bennett D (2004) Type I immune-mediated polyarthritis in dogs: 39 cases (1997–2002). *Journal of the American Veterinary Medical Association* **224,** 1323–1327

Gibson NR, Carmichael S, Li A, Reid SWJ, Normand EH, Owen MR and Bennett D (1999) Value of direct smears of synovial fluid in the diagnosis of canine joint disease. *Veterinary Record* **144,** 463–465

Innes J, Sharif M and Barr A (1998) Relations between biochemical markers of osteoarthritis and other disease parameters in a population of dogs with naturally acquired osteoarthritis of the genual joint. *American Journal of Veterinary Research* **59,** 1530–1536

Johnson KA, Hart RC, Chu Q, Kochevar D and Hulse DA (2001) Concentrations of chondroitin sulfate epitopes 3B3 and 7D4 in synovial fluid after intra-articular and extracapsular reconstruction of the cranial cruciate ligament in dogs. *American Journal of Veterinary Research* **62,** 581–587

Johnson KA, Hay CW, Chu QL, Roe SC and Caterson B (2002) Cartilage-derived biomarkers of osteoarthritis in synovial fluid of dogs with naturally acquired rupture of the cranial cruciate ligament. *American Journal of Veterinary Research* **63,** 775–781

May C and Bennett D (1994) Immune mediated arthritides. In: *BSAVA Manual of Small Animal Arthrology,* ed. J Houlton and R Collinson, pp. 86–99. BSAVA Publications, Cheltenham

May C, Carter SD, Barnes A, Bell S and Bennett D (1991) Serodiagnosis of Lyme-Disease in UK Dogs. *Journal of Small Animal Practice* **32,** 170–174

Pacheco-Tena C, de la Barrera CA, Lopez-Vidal Y, Vazquez-Mellado J, Richaud-Patin Y, Amieva RI, Llorente L, Martinez A, Zuniga J, Cifuentes-Alvarado M and Burgos-Vargas R (2001) Bacterial DNA in synovial fluid cells of patients with juvenile onset spondyloarthropathies. Rheumatology **40,** 920–927

Schnarr S, Putschky N, Jendro MC, Zeidler H, Hammer M, Kuipers JG and Wollenhaupt J (2001) *Chlamydia* and *Borrelia* DNA in synovial fluid of patients with early undifferentiated oligoarthritis – Results of a prospective study. *Arthritis and Rheumatism* **44,** 2679–2685

Singer F and Gruber J (1983) Microscopic demonstration of crystal formations in synovial-fluid with a special regard to corticosteroid-crystals administered intra-articularly. *Aktuelle Rheumatologie* **8,** 105–111

Webb AA, Taylor SM and Muir GD (2002) Steroid-responsive meningitis-arteritis in dogs with noninfectious, nonerosive, idiopathic, immune-mediated polyarthritis. *Journal of Veterinary Internal Medicine* **16,** 269–273

22b

Laboratory evaluation of muscle disorders

Natasha Olby

Introduction

Muscle disease can affect skeletal (striated), cardiac and, more rarely, smooth muscle. It can be primary or secondary to other systemic disorders (Figure 22.11) but can be difficult to recognize clinically due to its non-specific signs. Even when suspected, the appropriate diagnostic work-up is often poorly understood and test results can be misinterpreted.

Systemic disorder	Myopathy
Hyperadrenocorticism	Profound muscle weakness and atrophy Myotonic type myopathy
Hypoadrenocorticism	Profound muscle weakness, megaoesophagus, muscle cramps
Hypothyroidism	Muscle weakness
Hyperthyroidism	Muscle weakness and elevated creatine kinase (CK)
Renal disease	Hypokalaemic myopathy
Sepsis, shock, DIC	Muscle weakness, elevated CK
Thromboembolic disease	Painful, oedematous extremity, markedly elevated CK

22.11 Systemic diseases that can cause muscle disease (DIC, disseminated intravascular coagulation).

Classic signs of muscle disease include: weakness, characterized by exercise intolerance and/or a stiff stilted gait; muscle atrophy or hypertrophy; muscle contractures (with associated skeletal deformities in growing animals); regurgitation and aspiration pneumonia (due to megaoesophagus), and myalgia (muscle pain). Dysphagia may be present if there is involvement of the pharyngeal muscles; and dysphonia can occur if laryngeal muscles are severely affected.

Weakness due to muscle disease can be profound and even cause recumbency, but can be differentiated from disease of the nervous system by the presence of intact myotactic reflexes (in the majority of cases) and intact conscious proprioception. However, in very weak animals, body weight must be supported carefully in order to evaluate conscious proprioception accurately. A distinction should be drawn between myotactic reflexes, such as the patellar reflex, and withdrawal (flexor) reflexes. To evaluate the flexor reflex, the leg is extended and the strength of the animal's ability to flex the leg is assessed in response to pinching its toes (see *BSAVA Manual of Canine and Feline Neurology*). Animals with myopathies severe enough to cause recumbency tend to have reduced withdrawal reflexes as this reflects muscle strength, but their myotactic reflexes are usually intact. Involvement of cardiac muscle may lead to heart failure or cardiac arrhythmias with resultant weakness.

Laboratory evaluation of muscle focuses on skeletal and cardiac muscle; although smooth muscle disorders exist they are poorly characterized at present. Routine markers of muscle disease are primarily limited to indicators of myocyte necrosis and measuring antibody titres specific to muscle and its receptors. Specific diagnosis of a primary myopathy usually requires histological evaluation of a muscle biopsy specimen and may then require additional specialized testing to characterize the disease more fully. However, myopathies can occur secondary to other systemic diseases, such as renal disease and hyperadrenocorticism, and so routine haematology and biochemistry and endocrine testing can play an important role. Cardiomyopathies can result from dietary deficiencies and the plasma concentrations of various substances should, therefore, be measured in cardiomyopathic animals (see below). Finally, genetic tests for primary muscle diseases are now emerging and will play an important role both in diagnosing inherited diseases and in identifying carriers of such diseases.

Skeletal (striated) muscle

Enzymes

Creatine kinase

Creatine kinase (CK) is made up of two subunits, denoted M (muscle) and B (brain). The various combinations of these subunits give rise to three different isoenzymes found in the nervous system (BB or CK_1), cardiac muscle (MB or CK_2) and skeletal muscle (MM or CK_3). CK activity is much lower elsewhere in the body, but can be detected in the kidney, intestinal tract, uterus, thyroid gland and urinary bladder. In practice, CK activity is much higher in skeletal muscle and it is a relatively specific marker of skeletal muscle injury. Although the isoenzymes can be separated by electrophoresis, specific isoenzyme measurements have not proven useful in veterinary medicine and are not routinely used.

CK is a cytosolic enzyme that is released into the interstitium when the sarcolemma (muscle cell membrane) becomes permeable. From there it passes via the lymphatic system to the venous system, causing an elevation in blood CK activity. The half-life of CK in blood is in the region of 2–4 hours. Plasma concentrations start to increase 4–6 hours after muscle injury, peak 12 hours after enzyme release into the circulation and decrease back to normal within 24–48 hours. An elevation in CK therefore reflects a recent process and persistent elevations imply that there is ongoing muscle damage occurring.

CK activity can be influenced by a variety of non-pathological circumstances (Figure 22.12). In addition, it is a very sensitive test and in general it is only taken as clinically significant if:

- There are more than 5–10-fold elevations in activity
- The elevation is persistent, even if it is lower
- There are accompanying, compatible clinical signs.

Diseases that cause an increase in CK activity are listed in Figure 22.13 and can be primary or secondary. Increased CK must be interpreted with the presenting clinical signs in mind. Only diseases that cause an increase in sarcolemmal permeability cause elevations in CK activity; normal CK values do not rule out muscle disease. In addition, CK activity may be reduced in end-stage disease associated with severe destruction of muscle, simply because there is little muscle mass left.

Haemolysis
Substances released from erythrocytes affect the assay
Age
CK activity is up to five times higher in day-old pups than adult dogs. It decreases to the adult level by 7 months of age. As dogs age, their CK activity gradually decreases, but not enough to change the reference range
Delayed assay
If the assay cannot be performed for 12 hours or more the sample should be stored at -20°C. CK is only stable for approximately 4 hours at room temperature and 8–12 hours at 4°C. This loss of activity can be reversed by using reducing agents in the assay
Recent surgery
Intramuscular injection
Exercise
Recumbency
Frequently cited as a cause of elevation in CK activity. While this is undoubtedly true in large animals, such as cows, it is unusual to see a significant or persistent elevation in CK in recumbent dogs and cats

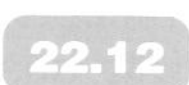
22.12 Non-pathological causes of creatine kinase elevation.

Aspartate aminotransferase

AST is found in the cytoplasm and mitochondria of many tissues and is therefore not a specific marker of disease. However, highest concentrations are present in liver and cardiac and skeletal muscle, and serum elevations usually reflect either a hepatic or a myopathic disease process in small animals. As AST has a much longer half-life than CK (approximately 12 hours) it will remain elevated for longer after an incident. Haemolysed samples are not useful because erythrocytes contain significant amounts of AST.

Alanine aminotransferase

ALT is present at high concentrations in hepatocyte cytoplasm in small animals and is generally considered to be a sensitive marker of hepatocellular damage. However, severe myonecrosis, such as that seen in X-linked muscular dystrophy, can cause an elevation in ALT in dogs concurrent with increases in CK and AST (Valentine *et al.*, 1990). The half-life is approximately 2.5 days, so concentrations remain elevated much longer than those of CK.

Others

Lactate dehydrogenase (LDH) and aldolase are rarely measured in small animals as they lack specificity and sensitivity, and LDH is artefactually elevated in even slight haemolysis.

Disease	Degree of CK elevation
Degenerative myopathy: X-linked muscular dystrophy Labrador Retriever myopathy	Marked elevation Mild to no elevation
Myositis – immune mediated or infectious	Value depends on extent of injury
Excessive muscular activity: exertional rhabdomyolysis; limber tail; seizures; tetanus; malignant hyperthermia; myokymia; myotonia	Value depends on extent of injury
Metabolic myopathies: hypokalaemic myopathy; mitochondrial myopathy; lipid storage myopathy	Value depends on the disease
Endocrine myopathies: hyper- and hypothyroidism; hyper- and hypoadrenocorticism	Value depends on the disease
Toxic and drug-induced myopathies, e.g. monensin (Wilson *et al.*, 1980)	Value depends on extent of injury
Trauma	Value depends on extent of injury
Vascular: hypotension; arterial thromboembolism	Marked elevation (thromboembolism)

22.13 Pathological causes of creatine kinase elevation.

Myoglobin

Myoglobin is a haem protein that transports and stores oxygen in muscle. Severe skeletal muscle necrosis, such as that seen after arterial thromboembolism and exertional rhabdomyolysis, results in release of myoglobin into the blood. This is a very specific indicator of severe muscle damage. At plasma concentrations >15–20 mg/dl (86–114 nmol/l), myoglobin is readily filtered at the glomerulus and is excreted in the urine. Myoglobinaemia can be differentiated from haemoglobinaemia by centrifuging plasma sample. As myoglobin is cleared rapidly, the plasma looks clear, in contrast to the pink appearance imparted by haemoglobin. Myoglobin produces a brown coloration of urine and is detected by standard urine dipsticks as occult blood. It can be differentiated from haemoglobin by the addition of ammonium sulphate to precipitate haemoglobin and leave myoglobin in solution. Unfortunately this is not a reliable test; more accurate detection of myoglobin can be accomplished by immunodiffusion. Myoglobinuria is always a serious finding because myoglobinaemia can cause acute renal failure.

Potassium concentration

Potassium ions play an important role in the maintenance of a polarized membrane in the nervous system and muscle, and are found at high concentrations intracellulary throughout the body. Muscle contains approximately 95% of total body potassium. If extensive muscle necrosis occurs, such as that seen after arterial thromboembolism in cats, a dangerous elevation in serum potassium concentration can occur (see Chapter 8). Conversely, hypokalaemia can cause a myopathy associated with generalized weakness and an increase in CK. This is a well established phenomenon in cats as a result of dietary insufficiency, renal loss, diuretics, hyperthyroidism and diabetic ketoacidosis, and occurs as an inherited disease in Burmese cats (Dow *et al.*, 1989). This syndrome is rare in dogs but has been reported in one dog treated with furosemide for congestive heart failure (Harrington *et al.*, 1996). Signs of weakness occur with potassium <4 mmol/l, although rhabdomyolysis usually occurs when concentrations are <3 mmol/l.

Antibody titres

Anti-type 2M antibodies

Masticatory myositis is an immune-mediated disease of the muscles of mastication in dogs (Shelton *et al.*, 1987). These muscles (temporal, masseter and digastricus) have a different embryonic origin to other skeletal muscles and have a unique isoform of myosin that can be detected in a subset of myofibres, termed type 2M fibres. Antibodies are produced specifically against these myofibres in masticatory myositis. Serum samples can be sent to the Comparative Neuromuscular Laboratory at the University of California, San Diego, for measurement of antibody titres to this myofibre type in dogs using an enzyme-linked immunosorbent assay (ELISA) test. This test is highly specific (100%) and sensitive (85–90%).

Infectious disease titres

Myositis can be caused by the protozoal organisms *Neospora caninum* (dogs), *Toxoplasma gondii* (dogs and cats), *Leishmania infantum* (dogs) and *Trypanosoma cruzi* (dogs). Less common causes of myositis include *Hepatozoon canis* and *H. americanum*, feline immunodeficiency virus (FIV), *Ehrlichia canis, Leptospira australis, L. icterohaemorrhagicae*, and clostridial infections. Many of these diseases are geographically specific, and rarely encountered. However, if a diagnosis of myositis is made on muscle biopsy, antibodies to protozoa should be measured (see Chapter 27).

Anti-acetylcholine receptor antibodies

There are acquired and congenital forms of myasthenia gravis (MG) but the acquired forms are prevalent. Acquired MG is caused by production of antibodies against the nicotinic acetylcholine receptor (ACHR). Clinical syndromes include generalized exercise intolerance, with or without regurgitation, or a more specific form involving just the oesophageal and pharyngeal muscle, causing regurgitation and aspiration. There is also a rare fulminant form that causes generalized lower motor neuron paralysis and is usually rapidly fatal. Antibody titres can be measured sensitively and specifically by immunoprecipitation radioimmunoassay. ACHR labelled with ^{125}I-α-bungarotoxin are used to quantitate circulating antibodies against these receptors from a serum sample (Comparative Neuromuscular Laboratory, University of California, San Diego; UK laboratories will forward samples). Antibody concentrations >0.6 nmol/l and >0.3 nmol/l are considered diagnostic of acquired MG in dogs and cats, respectively (Shelton, 2002). Approximately 2% of affected dogs are seronegative on this test. Possible explanations include a low circulating concentration of high affinity antibodies, antibodies directed against a different region of the endplate to the receptor, e.g. muscle-specific kinase (MuSK) (Evoli *et al.*, 2003), and damage to the test receptors used in the assay during their preparation. More recently, an ELISA assay has been developed based on a subunit of the canine acetylcholine receptor (Yoshioka *et al.*, 1999). However, the sensitivity and specificity of this test remain to be established.

Endocrine testing

Muscle disease can result from hypothyroidism, hyperthyroidism, hyperadrenocorticism and hypoadrenocorticism. Appropriate testing for these diseases is indicated if there are compatible clinical signs (see Chapters 17 and 18).

Metabolic testing

Inborn errors of metabolism are a rare but important cause of exercise intolerance, weakness and collapse. Such diseases cause progressive signs and can be fatal. If a metabolic myopathy is suspected, it is standard for a complete work-up to include an evaluation of plasma lactate concentrations. Further metabolic testing is undertaken based on the results of muscle biopsy (which may show characteristic changes in mitochondrial shape, size, distribution and numbers, see below) and measurement of lactate concentrations.

Lactate and pyruvate concentrations

Lactic acid is produced by anaerobic metabolism of pyruvate in a process dedicated to glucose metabolism, known as glycolysis. Lactic acidaemia can be a secondary consequence of extreme muscular activity (e.g. heavy anaerobic exercise, malignant hyperthermia, seizures) or the result of a primary enzyme defect (e.g. pyruvate dehydrogenase, pyruvate decarboxylase, enzymes of the respiratory chain or enzymes of the Krebs cycle). It can also result from generalized systemic disturbances, such as severe hypotension causing failure of perfusion and hence anaerobic metabolism. Measurement of serum lactate concentration is indicated in the evaluation of exercise intolerance in which an underlying metabolic myopathy is suspected. Resting samples may be useful, but frequently lactic acidaemia is only apparent when clinical signs are present. For optimal testing, the animal is exercised and blood samples are obtained both before and immediately after clinical signs appear. The blood sample must be collected in a tube containing a combined sodium fluoride/potassium oxalate anticoagulant, cooled and centrifuged within 15 minutes. Immediate analysis is preferable, but the plasma can be stored at –20°C for up to 30 days. Lactate concentration will increase in normal animals proportionate to the amount and type of exercise that they do: normal values of pre-and post-exercise lactate concentration have been reported for Labrador Retrievers (Figure 22.14) (Matwichuk *et al.*, 1999).

In order to determine the nature of lactic acidaemia, it is useful to measure pyruvate concentrations concurrently and compare the ratio of these two substances. Pyruvate is produced from glucose during aerobic glycolysis. Following entry into mitochondria, it is normally metabolized to acteyl-CoA (catalysed by pyruvate dehydrogenase), which then enters the Krebs cycle. In the absence of oxygen, pyruvate is reduced to lactate in a reversible reaction. Different enzyme defects produce characteristic changes in the ratio of lactate to pyruvate concentrations. For example, if both lactate and pyruvate concentrations are elevated while maintaining a normal ratio, there is a defect in pyruvate dehydrogenase. Conversely, pyruvate carboxylase deficiency is associated with lactic acidaemia and an increased lactate to pyruvate ratio; defects in the mitochondrial electron transport chain or other mitochondrial abnormalities can also produce this change. Pyruvate is difficult to measure because samples must be diluted with an equal volume of 10% perchloric acid prior to centrifugation. The plasma should be removed and frozen at –20°C until analysis although, as for lactate, prompt analysis is preferable. Normal pre- and post-exercise pyruvate concentrations have been reported for Labrador Retrievers (Figure 22.14) (Matwichuk *et al.*,1999).

Organic acid, amino acid and carnitine

Metabolic myopathies can result from a range of enzyme defects of oxidative phosphorylation, and β-oxidation. Dysfunction of an enzyme can result in accumulation of fatty acids and amino acids. These can be measured by specialist laboratories in urine and plasma using gas chromatography–mass spectrometry. Appropriate samples must be frozen immediately after they are obtained and shipped to the laboratory on dry ice. Many metabolic disorders are a result of carnitine deficiency. Total, free and esterified muscle, plasma and urine carnitine levels can be measured by some laboratories (hospital laboratories and Comparative Neuromuscular Laboratory, University of California, San Diego). Indications for such tests include unexplained exercise intolerance, lactic acidaemia and pathological changes consistent with a metabolic myopathy on biopsy examination.

Genetic tests

Tests that detect mutant alleles for a variety of diseases are emerging and are a sensitive and specific method of identifying carriers and affected animals; these are summarized in Figure 22.15.

Lactate concentrations (mmol/l)		Pyruvate concentrations (mmol/l)		Lactate: pyruvate ratio	
Pre-exercise	Post-exercise	Pre-exercise	Post-exercise	Pre-exercise	Post-exercise
1.31 (0.53–3.07)	3.57 (0.8–9.86)	0.082 (0.12–0.5)	0.192 (0.05–0.32)	17	20.5

22.14 Mean pre-and post-exercise plasma lactate and pyruvate concentrations in healthy working Labrador Retrievers (Matwichuk *et al.*, 1999). The dogs were exercised for 10 minutes doing retrieval work. The range is given in parentheses. The plasma lactate concentration returned to baseline in 60 minutes. The lactate to pyruvate ratio did not change significantly.

Disease	Breed	Clinical signs	Reference	Laboratory offering test
Myotonia congenita	Miniature Schnauzer	Stiff gait, muscle hypertrophy, dyspnoea, craniofacial and dental abnormalities (rare)	Bhalerao *et al.*, 2002	PennGenn Laboratories (ELISA)
Phosphofructokinase deficiency	Springer Spaniel	Haemolysis, exercise intolerance, muscle atrophy	Smith *et al.*, 1996	PennGenn Laboratories
Glycogenosis Type IV	Norwegian Forest Cat	Exercise intolerance, ataxia	Fyfe, 2002	PennGenn Laboratories

22.15 Genetic tests available for inherited muscle diseases in dogs and cats. See Resources section at end of the chapter for details of laboratories.

Muscle and nerve biopsy

Definitive diagnosis of primary myopathies and neuropathies usually requires evaluation of a biopsy specimen of the affected tissue. Muscle biopsy is a straightforward procedure that is minimally invasive. However, a specialist laboratory that can process frozen muscle is necessary to allow full interpretation of the sample. Nerve biopsy is technically more challenging and there is greater potential for causing permanent damage. It is also beneficial to have electrodiagnostic confirmation of nerve involvement prior to performing a biopsy, so this procedure is more appropriately performed by a specialist. As for muscle, it is preferable to use a laboratory experienced in the processing and interpretation of peripheral nerve biopsy specimens.

Muscle biopsy

Muscle biopsy is indicated in animals with unexplained muscle atrophy or hypertrophy, weakness or exercise intolerance, persistent or dramatic elevations in CK, or electromyographic evidence of myopathy. Although core biopsy can be performed under sedation and local anaesthesia, these are difficult to interpret and it is preferable to use an open dissection under general anaesthesia. In general it is prudent to harvest samples from more than one muscle. Sampling a muscle from both the thoracic and pelvic limbs and a proximal and distal site is desirable. The muscle to be sampled should not be end stage, as this will often only reveal fibrosis and the underlying disease may not be apparent. Appropriate muscles to sample include the biceps femoris, the quadriceps femoris, the cranial tibial and the gastrocnemius muscles in the pelvic limb, and the triceps brachii and extensor carpi radialis in the thoracic limb, although nearly any muscle can be sampled.

The technique is as follows:

1. Following surgical preparation, an incision approximately 2 cm long is made over the muscle.
2. The subcutaneous tissues are dissected to reveal the muscle to be sampled.
3. The direction of the myofibres is identified and the sample is taken parallel to them. The myotendinous junction should be avoided.
4. Parallel incisions about 1.5 cm long and 1 cm apart are made along the myofibres. These are joined at their proximal end by a transverse incision. The fibres are grasped with forceps just distal to this transverse incision and carefully dissected free from the muscle belly (Figure 22.16).
5. If possible, the sample is only handled at one end.
6. The incision is closed routinely.

Performing a muscle biopsy should not cause lameness: if this is occurring the sample is either too large or is being taken traumatically or from an inappropriate site. The sample can be frozen by immersion in precooled (using liquid nitrogen) isopentane but this is not available to the majority of practitioners. If precooled isopentane is not available, the sample can be placed in saline moistened gauze and shipped on ice immediately to arrive at an appropriate laboratory within 24–48 hours. Alternatively, if analysis of frozen muscle is not an option, the sample can be placed in 10% buffered formalin following fixation to a tongue depressor with needles.

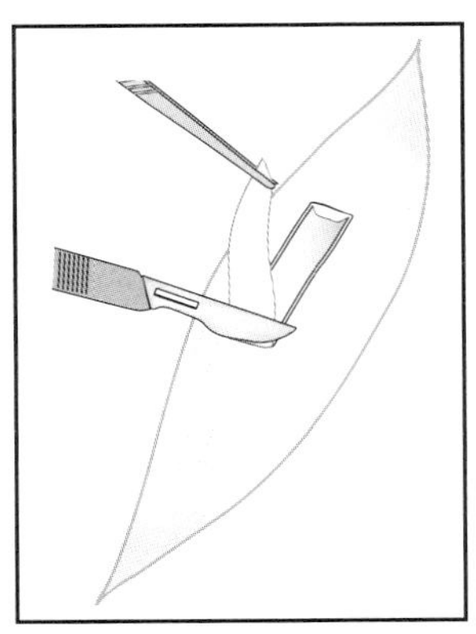

22.16 Muscle biopsy. The biopsy specimen is grasped at one end and carefully dissected away from the rest of the muscle without touching the body of the sample.

Muscle biopsy specimens are frozen and sections are cut with a cryostat. Processing includes (Figure 22.17):

- Haematoxylin and eosin staining to evaluate general histopathological features
- ATPases preincubated at acid and alkaline pHs (4.3, 4.6 and 9.8) to identify myofibre subtypes
- Periodic acid–Schiff (PAS) staining to identify glycogen
- Oil-Red-O staining to identify lipids
- NADH-reductase (NADH-TR) to identify oxidative activity
- Modified Gomori trichrome staining to identify general histopathological features and to highlight myelin and connective tissues.

Further histochemical and immunohistochemical stains can be performed depending on the initial findings. For example, if X-linked muscular dystrophy is suspected, immunostaining for the rod and c terminus of the dystrophin molecule can be undertaken.

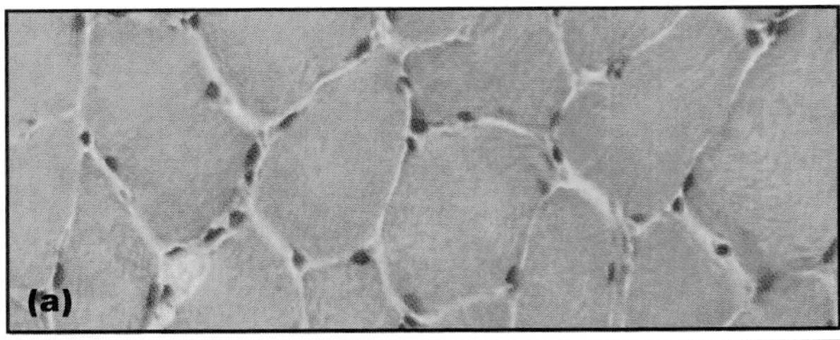

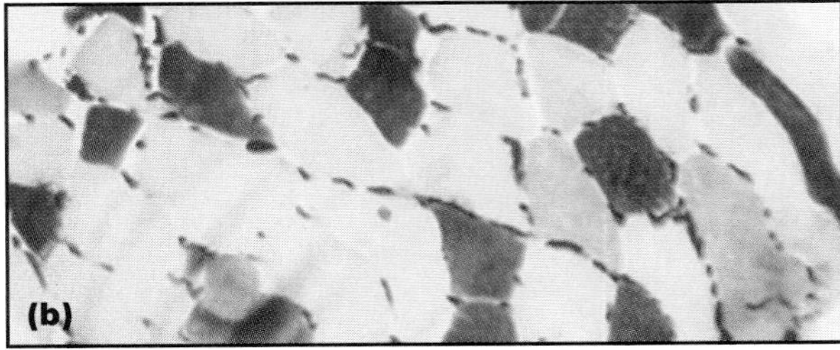

22.17 Histochemical staining of frozen muscle sections. (a) Hematoxylin and eosin: the muscle proteins are pink and the nuclei are purple. (Original magnification X180.) (b) ATPase, pH4.3. Three different staining intensities are present. Type 2A and B fibres are the palest, type 2 (dog) fibres are intermediate and type 1 fibres are the darkest. (Original magnification X150.) (continues) ▶

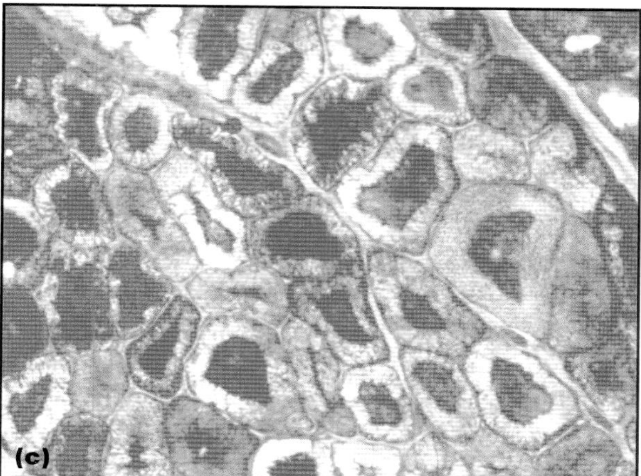

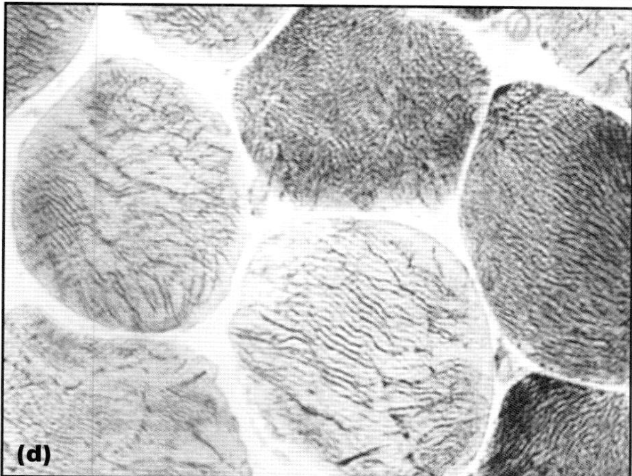

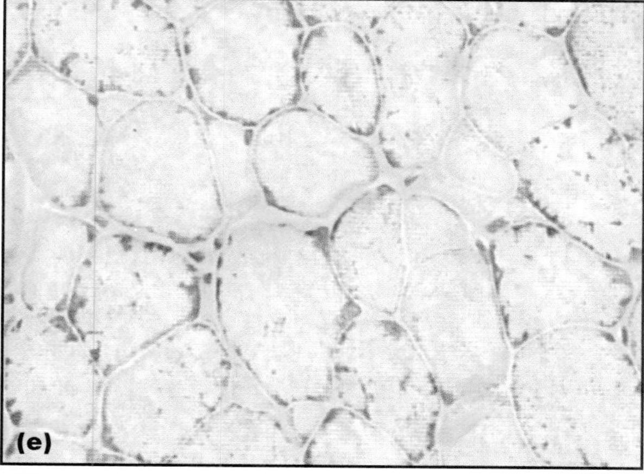

22.17 (continued) Histochemical staining of frozen muscle sections. (c) Periodic acid–Schiff (PAS). This muscle biopsy was taken from a young Great Dane with a central core-like myopathy. The central cores contain a lot of glycogen and therefore stain an intense pink colour with PAS. (Original magnification X150.) (d) NADH-TR. A section of normal muscle stained with NADH tetrazolium reductase (NADH-TR). This stain highlights oxidative activity in mitochondria and the endoplasmic reticulum. In normal muscle this produces a delicate pattern of staining of the intermyofibrillar network. (Original magnification X270.) (e) Modified Gomori trichrome. This section of muscle was taken from a young Jack Russell Terrier with a suspected mitochondrial cytopathy. The muscle proteins are stained green and the mitochondria stain red. The mitochondrial accumulations beneath the sarcolemma are clearly highlighted. (Original magnification X150.)

Cardiac muscle

Enzymes

CK, AST and ALT are all found in cardiac muscle and, indeed, severe, acute necrosis of cardiac muscle can be associated with elevation in CK-MB. However, levels of all of these enzymes are much lower in cardiac than in skeletal muscle and they are neither sensitive nor specific indicators of cardiac muscle disease. The cardiac isoform of CK (CK-MB or CK_2) can be measured individually but is not as sensitive or specific as measurement of troponin T and I concentrations.

Troponin

Troponin is a complex of three proteins, designated troponin C, I and T, that are found in cardiac and skeletal muscle. Troponin T (TnT) binds the complex to the myofibrillar protein tropomyosin; troponin C (TnC) binds calcium, producing a shape change. This shape change moves tropomyosin, revealing binding sites for myosin heads on actin filaments and producing contraction (Guyton and Hall, 2000). The third subunit, troponin I (TnI) is an inhibitory subunit. There are several isoforms of these proteins and the cardiac isoforms of TnT and TnI (cTnT and I) are specific to cardiac muscle, thus providing sensitive and specific markers of cardiac muscle damage. Cardiac TnI is more specific than CK-MB and more sensitive and specific than cTnT at detecting myocardial cell necrosis in humans. This high sensitivity and specificity, coupled with the advantage of rapid release into the bloodstream (increased concentrations are detected within 5–7 hours of injury) and persistence for up to 8 days after injury, have made this an invaluable marker of myocardial infarcts in humans.

The structure of these proteins is highly conserved across species and the human assays can be used to measure troponin concentration in companion animals. Normal concentrations of cTnT and I are extremely low in dogs and cats (Schober *et al.*, 1999; Sleeper *et al.*, 2001; DeFrancesco *et al.*, 2002). Concentrations of cTnT increase with doxorubicin cardiotoxicity and congestive heart failure (CHF) in dogs. However, two dogs with skeletal muscle trauma and no evidence of cardiac dysfunction also had elevations of cTnT (DeFrancesco *et al.*, 2002). A study on babesiosis in dogs showed an association between cTnI serum concentration and histological myocardial changes, clinical severity and survival, but no such association with cTnT serum concentrations (Lobetti *et al.*, 2002). CTnT was also shown to be less sensitive than cTnI in detecting myocardial damage following blunt trauma (Schober *et al.*, 1999). Conversely, a study on dogs with gastric dilatation–volvulus found that serum concentrations of both cTnT and I correlated with the presence of electrocardiogram (ECG) abnormalities and were significantly higher in dogs that died. Cats with hypertrophic cardiomyopathy have elevated cTnI serum concentrations (Connolly *et al.*, 2003), particularly in CHF (Herndon *et al.*, 2002). Both cTnT and I represent markers of myocardial necrosis superior to CK-MB (more specific) in dogs and cats. It is likely that cTnI is superior to cTnT, though this has not yet been fully evaluated.

Brain and atrial natriuretic peptides

The natriuretic peptides are endogenous hormones whose primary role, as their name suggests, is to promote natriuresis. Atrial natriuretic peptide (ANP) is produced in the atria of the heart and brain natriuretic peptide (BNP) is produced in both the ventricles and the atria. Synthesis of both hormones occurs in response to stretch of the walls of the heart and therefore can be expected to be increased in diseases that cause increased myocardial stretch.

In humans, both ANP and BNP are elevated in cardiac diseases, such as dilated cardiomyopathy, acute myocardial infarcts, regurgitant valvular disease and CHF. Both ANP and BNP concentrations have been shown to correlate well with pulmonary capillary wedge pressure (a measure of pressure within a pulmonary artery which reflects cardiac function: capillary wedge pressure increases as heart failure develops) although ANP has the closer correlation, particularly in CHF. Because of its ventricular origin, BNP is a better indicator of both diastolic and systolic ventricular dysfunction than ANP and has been shown to be predictive of premature death as a result of CHF.

Plasma levels of ANP and BNP have been measured in dogs with cardiac disease both with and without congestive heart failure (Takemura *et al.*, 1991; Vollmar *et al.*, 1991; Håggstrom *et al.*, 1994; Asano *et al.*, 1999; Boswood *et al.*, 2003; MacDonald *et al.*, 2003). Both peptides are elevated in response to cardiac disease and heart failure. ANP was found to correlate more closely than BNP with pulmonary capillary wedge pressure (and hence pulmonary oedema) (Asano *et al.*, 1999). The clinical utility of ANP as a diagnostic test for CHF and for cardiac disease has been limited by its short plasma half-life, its instability following collection due to proteolysis and the need for a radioimmunoassay (Boswood *et al.*, 2003). Boswood *et al.* (2003) evaluated the sensitivity and specificity of an ELISA test for the proANP 31–67 fragment at detecting heart failure. The sensitivity and specificity varied dependent on the cut-off value for proANP defined as diagnostic for heart failure, and were reported as 83.9% and 97.5%, respectively, when a cut-off value of 1750 fmol/l was used, and 93.5% and 72.5%, respectively, when the cut-off value was reduced to 1350 fmol/l.

Plasma levels of BNP can be measured using a commercially available radioimmunoassay kit (Canine BNP-32 radioimmunoassay, Peninsular Laboratories Inc). Using this kit, plasma levels of BNP have been measured in dogs with compensated and decompensated heart disease as a result of myxomatous mitral valve disease (MacDonald *et al.*, 2003). Plasma levels of BNP correlated to the severity of valvular disease and heart failure. Moreover, for every 10 pg/ml increase in BNP concentration, there was an increase in risk of mortality over the 4-month period after measurement of BNP concentrations of 44%. There is clear evidence that measurement of both ANP and BNP plasma concentrations has clinical utility, for example in distinguishing between primary lung disease and pulmonary oedema secondary to heart failure, and as a prognostic indicator in dogs with heart failure. Reliable, simple, safe and inexpensive tests are currently being developed.

Taurine

Taurine deficiency causes dilated cardiomyopathy (DCM) in cats (Pion *et al.*, 1987) and American Cocker Spaniels, and may play a role in the disease in a diverse group of dogs (Fascetti *et al.*, 2003). In cats, taurine deficiency results from feeding diets low in taurine. Because dogs, unlike cats, are able to synthesize taurine from cysteine and methionine, they were not believed to be at risk from dietary deficiency. However, recent studies have documented low plasma taurine in dogs with DCM fed lamb and rice diets. It is theorized that these diets have low bioavailable levels of the sulphur-containing amino acids that are precursors to taurine. When presented with a patient with DCM it is advisable to measure plasma taurine levels. Plasma levels <25 nmol/ml in cats and <40 nmol/ml in dogs are considered deficient.

Carnitine

Deficiency of L-carnitine can cause DCM in dogs. Unfortunately, the optimal method of detecting this deficiency is to measure levels in a myocardial biopsy specimen. Total, free and esterified plasma and urine carnitine levels can be measured but are a less sensitive means of detecting carnitine deficiency (Keene, 1990).

Case example

Signalment

6-month-old intact female Shar Pei.

History

Presented for tetraparesis. Previous history of being in a car in a road traffic accident. At the time the dog appeared to be unharmed, but she developed stiffness in one of her pelvic limbs 2 weeks later, and this was believed to be a result of the trauma. In spite of treatment with anti-inflammatory drugs, the dog's signs progressed to involve both pelvic limbs. Referral was precipitated by the sudden development of tetraparesis.

Physical examination

On admission the dog was febrile (40°C), tachypnoeic and tachycardic. The muscles of both pelvic limbs were severely atrophied and contractures had developed, restricting the range of motion of the tarsus and stifle bilaterally. On neurological examination the dog exhibited multifocal signs including central vestibular and cerebellar signs (vertical nystagmus, intention tremor and upper motor neuron paresis of the thoracic limbs) in addition to lower motor neuron signs of the pelvic limbs (muscle atrophy, loss of myotactic reflexes). An infectious process was suspected based on the age of the dog, the multifocal signs and the fever.

Clinical pathology data

Haematology	Result	Reference interval
RBC (x 10^{12}/l)	5.85	5–8
Hb (g/dl)	12.8	11.5–21
HCT (l/l)	0.36	0.33–0.56

▶

Case example continued

Haematology *(continued)*	Result	Reference interval
MCV (fl)	62.1	63–73
WBC (x 10^9/l)	24.4	5–18
Neutrophils (segmented) (x 10^9/l)	11.96	3–11.5
Neutrophils (band) (x 10^9/l)	0.24	0–0.3
Lymphocytes (x 10^9/l)	6.8	1–5
Monocytes (x 10^9/l)	0.98	0.15–1.35
Eosinophils (x 10^9/l)	4.36	0.1–0.75
Basophils (x 10^9/l)	0	0–0.1
Platelets (x 10^9/l)	279	200–450

Biochemistry	Result	Reference interval
Sodium (mmol/l)	147	141–155
Potassium (mmol/l)	4.3	4–5.6
Glucose mmol/l	4.1	3.4-6.4
Urea (mmol/l)	17	8–24
Creatinine (μmol/l)	53.4	20–160
Calcium (mmol/l)	2.45	2.15–2.85
Inorganic phosphate (mmol/l)	2.00	0.68–2.10
TP (g/l)	56	46–82
Albumin (g/l)	21	28–44
Globulin (g/l)	28	18–44
ALT (IU/l)	113	0–45
ALP (IU/l)	55	10–150
CK (IU/l)	4370	0–160

Urine analysis:
Specific gravity: 1.041; 3+ protein. No active sediment or bacteria.

What abnormalities are present?

- Eosinophilia
- Lymphocytosis
- Very mild neutrophilia
- Mild hypoalbuminaemia
- > 2-fold elevation in ALT
- Moderate elevation in CK (nearly 30-fold)
- Proteinuria.

How would you interpret these results and what are the likely differential diagnoses?

Very mild neutrophilia is non-specific and may be insignificant or caused by stress or inflammation. Eosinophilia could result from parasitic, protozoal or fungal infections or an allergic process. Lymphocytosis may reflect antigenic stimulation.

The hypoalbuminaemia is mild but could reflect urinary or GI loss or decreased production. When coupled with the proteinuria, it is possible that the dog has a protein-losing nephropathy.

The ALT elevation and CK elevation are significant.

The combination of above clinical pathological findings, coupled with the history, signalment, physical and neurological findings make a systemic infectious or inflammatory process the most likely differential. The involvement of muscle and peripheral and central nervous systems make protozoal disease the most likely differential diagnosis.

Results of further tests

CSF analysis

Cisternal CSF abnormalities included markedly elevated protein (0.327 g/l, reference range: <0.25 g/l) and mixed pleocytosis (108 white blood cells/μl, reference range <5/μl). Lumbar CSF had a protein concentration of 0.750 g/l (reference range <0.45 g/l) and 25 white blood cells/μl, again a mixed pleocytosis. Occasional eosinophils were seen in both CSF samples.

Electromyography and nerve conduction study

EMGs revealed marked spontaneous activity in the muscles of both pelvic limbs, but all other muscles were electrically silent. Nerve conduction studies in the thoracic limbs (ulnar nerve) were normal, but M waves could not be elicited on stimulation of the tibial nerves.

Muscle biopsy

A muscle biopsy was performed on the biceps femoris of the left pelvic limb. Pathological changes in the muscle included infiltration of plasma cells, neutrophils, eosinophils and monocytes, with marked variation of myofibre size and myofibre necrosis. Protozoal organisms (bradyzoites) could be identified (Figure 22.18). A diagnosis of a protozoal infection causing myositis, neuritis and meningoencephalomyelitis was made.

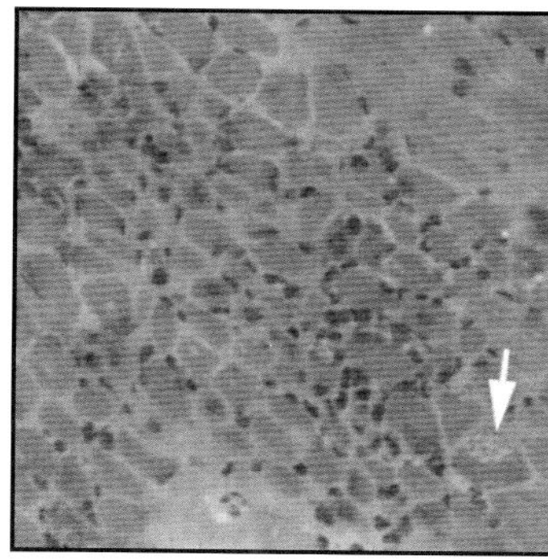

22.18 A section of the biceps femoris stained with haematoxylin and eosin. Note the presence of an inflammatory infiltrate and a bradyzoite cyst (arrowed). (Original magnification X40.)

Protozoal titres

Serum samples were submitted for measurement of anti-*Toxoplasma* and anti-*Neospora* titres. No anti-*Toxoplasma* antibodies were detected. Anti-*Neospora* titres were positive at 1:100.

Treatment and case outcome

Treatment with pyrimethamine and trimethoprim–sulphadiazine was instituted while serum antibody titres for *Toxoplasma* and *Neospora* were measured. Folic acid was administered daily to counteract the toxic effects of these two drugs. The dog's cerebellovestibular signs and thoracic limb strength improved for a month but her pelvic limb motor function made only minimal improvements. Her neurological signs then deteriorated acutely and her owners elected for euthanasia.

References and further reading

Asano K, Masuda K, Okumura M, Kadosawa T and Fujinaga T (1999) Plasma atrial and brain natriuretic peptide levels in dogs with congestive heart failure. *Journal of Veterinary Medical Science* **61,** 523–529

Bhalerao DP, Rajpurohit Y, Vite CH and Giger U (2002) Detection of a genetic mutation for myotonia congenita among Miniature Schnauzers and identification of a common carrier ancestor. *American Journal of Veterinary Research* **63,** 1443–1447

Boswood A, Attree S and Page K (2003) Clinical validation of a proANP 31-67 fragment ELISA in the diagnosis of heart failure in the dog. *Journal of Small Animal Practice* **44,** 104–108

Connolly DJ, Cannata J, Boswood A, Archer J, Groves EA and Neiger R (2003) Cardiac troponin I in cats with hypertrophic cardiomyopathy. *Journal of Feline Medicine and Surgery* **5,** 209–216

DeFrancesco TC, Atkins CE, Keene BW, Coats JR and Hauck ML (2002) Prospective clinical evaluation of serum cardiac troponin T in dogs admitted to a veterinary teaching hospital. *Journal of Veterinary Internal Medicine* **16,** 553–557

Dow SW, Fettman MJ, Curtis CR and LeCouteur RA (1989) Hypokalemia in cats: 186 cases (1984–1987) *Journal of the American Veterinary Medical Association* **194,** 1604–1608

Evoli A, Tonali PA, Padua L, Monaco ML, Scuderi F, Batocchi AP, Marino M and Bartoccioni E (2003) Clinical correlates with anti-MuSK antibodies in generalized seronegative myasthenia gravis. *Brain* **126,** 2304–2311

Fascetti AJ, Reed JR, Rogers QR and Backus RC (2003) Taurine deficiency in dogs with dilated cardiomyopathy: 12 cases (1997-2001). *Journal of the American Veterinary Medical Association* **223,** 1137–1141

Fyfe JC (2002) Molecular diagnosis of inherited neuromuscular disease. *Veterinary Clinics of North America, Small Animal Practice* **32,** 287–300

Guyton AC and Hall JE (2000) Contraction of skeletal muscle. In: *Textbook of Medical Physiology 10th edn,* pp. 67–72. WB Saunders, Philadelphia

Håggstrom J, Hansson K, Karlberg BE, Kvart C and Olsson K (1994) Plasma concentration of atrial natriuretic peptide in relation to severity of mitral regurgitation in Cavalier King Charles Spaniels. *American Journal of Veterinary Research* **55,** 698–703

Harrington ML, Bagley RS and Braund KG (1996) Suspect hypokalemic myopathy in a dog. *Progress in Veterinary Neurology* **7,** 130–132

Herndon WE, Kittleson MD, Sanderson K, Drobatz KJ, Clifford CA, Gelzer A, Summerfield NJ, Linde A and Sleeper MM (2002) Cardiac troponin I in feline hypertrophic cardiomyopathy. *Journal of Veterinary Internal Medicine* **16,** 558–564

Keene BW (1991) L-carnitine supplementation in the therapy of canine dilated cardiomyopathy. *Veterinary Clinics of North America: Small Animal Practice* **21,** 1005–1009

Keene BW, Kittleson ME, Atkins CE, Rush JE, Eicker SW, Pion P and Regitz V (1990) Modified transvenous endomyocardial biopsy technique in dogs. *American Journal of Veterinary Research* **51,** 1769–1772

Lobetti R, Dvir E and Pearson J (2002) Cardiac troponins in canine babesiosis. *Journal of Veterinary Internal Medicine* **16,** 63–68

MacDonald KA, Kittleson MD, Munro C and Kass P (2003) Brain natriuretic peptide concentration in dogs with heart disease and congestive heart failure. *Journal of Veterinary Internal Medicine* **17,** 172–177

Matwichuk CL, Taylor S, Shmon CL, Kass PH and Shelton GD (1999) Changes in rectal temperature and hematologic, biochemical, blood gas, and acid-base values in healthy Labrador Retrievers before and after strenuous exercise. *American Journal of Veterinary Research* **60,** 88–92

Pion PD, Kittleson MD, Rogers QR and Morris JG (1987) Myocardial failure in cats associated with low plasma taurine: a reversible cardiomyopathy. *Science* **237,** 764–768

Schober K, Kirbach B and Oechtering G (1999) Noninvasive assessment of myocardial cell injury in dogs with suspected cardiac contusion. *Journal of Veterinary Cardiology* **1,** 17–25

Schober KE, Cornand C, Kirbach B, Aupperle H and Oechtering G (2002) Serum cardiac troponin I and cardiac troponin T concentrations in dogs with gastric dilatation-volvulus. *Journal of the American Veterinary Medical Association* **221,** 381–388

Shelton GD, Cardinet GH III and Bandman E (1987) Canine masticatory muscle disorders: a study of 29 cases. *Muscle and Nerve* **10,** 753–766

Shelton GD (2002) Myasthenia gravis and disorders of neuromuscular transmission. *Veterinary Clinics of North America: Small Animal Practice* **32,** 189–206

Sleeper MM, Clifford CA and Laster LL (2001) Cardiac troponin I in the normal dog and cat. *Journal of Veterinary Internal Medicine* **15,** 501–503

Smith BF, Stedman H, Rajpurohit Y, Henthorn PS, Wolfe JH, Patterson DF and Giger U (1996) Molecular basis of canine muscle type phosphofructokinase deficiency. *Journal of Biological Chemistry* **271,** 20070–20074

Takemura N, Koyama H, Sako T, Ando K, Suzuki K, Motoyoshi S and Marumo F (1991) Atrial natriuretic peptide in the dog with mitral regurgitation. *Research in Veterinary Science* **50,** 86–88

Tiret L, Blot S, Kessler JL, Guillot H, Breen M and Panthier JJ (2003) The CNM locus, a canine homologue of human autosomal forms of centronuclear myopathy, maps to chromosome 2. *Human Genetics* **112,** 297–306

Valentine BA, Blue JT, Shelley SM and Cooper BJ (1990) Increased serum alanine aminotransferase activity associated with muscle necrosis in the dog. *Journal of Veterinary Internal Medicine* **4,** 140–143

Vollmar AM, Reusch C, Kraft W and Schulz R (1991) Atrial natriuretic peptide concentration in dogs with congestive heart failure, chronic renal failure, and hyperadrenocorticism. *American Journal of Veterinary Research* **52,** 1831–1834

Wilson JS (1980) Toxic myopathy in a dog associated with the presence of monensin in dry food. *Canadian Veterinary Journal* **21,** 30–31

Yoshioka T, Uzuka Y, Tanabe S *et al.* (1999) Molecular cloning of the canine nicotinic acetylcholine receptor alpha-subunit gene and development of the ELISA method to diagnose myasthenia gravis. *Veterinary Immunology and Immunopathology* **72,** 315–324

Resources

Laboratories relevant to muscle disease

Comparative Neuromuscular Laboratory
Basic Science Building, Room 2095
University of California, San Diego
La Jolla, CA 92093-0612
USA
Phone: 001-858-534-1537
Fax: 001-858-534-7319
http://medicine.ucsd.edu/vet_neuromuscular/geninfo.html

PennGenn Laboratories
3850 Spruce Street
Philadelphia, PA 19104-6010
USA
Phone: 001-215-898-3375
Fax:001-215-573-2162
e-mail: penngen@vet.upenn.edu
http:www.vet.upenn.edu/facultyanddepts/csphil/medicalgenetics/Services.cfm

23

Laboratory evaluation of cerebrospinal fluid

Kathleen Freeman

Introduction

Cerebrospinal fluid (CSF) collection and laboratory analysis are recommended as part of the investigation of central nervous system (CNS) disease of unknown cause. A definitive diagnosis on the basis of CSF laboratory evaluation alone is rare, but the laboratory evaluation of CSF may provide documentation of normal or abnormal findings and help make distinctions amongst various differential diagnoses.

CSF collection

Indications and contraindications

Collection and laboratory evaluation of CSF is indicated in the investigation of any CNS disease of unknown cause.

Anaesthesia is required for collection, so any condition that would contraindicate anaesthesia precludes collection of CSF. Other contraindications include causes of increased intracranial pressure (ICP), such as acute head trauma, active or decompensated hydrocephalus, or cerebral oedema. Expansile masses and unstable CNS or systemic conditions may cause increased ICP or decreases in the spinal compartment relative to the intracranial compartment. These conditions may result in herniation of the brainstem and severe compromise of brain function, coma and/or death. Physical and neurological examination, history, presentation and results of radiography or other imaging procedures may help determine whether the conditions that would contraindicate CSF collection are present. Anisocoria and papilloedema may be associated with increased ICP.

The risk of herniation may be reduced by administration of dexamethasone (0.25 mg/kg i.v.) prior to induction of anaesthesia, and by hyperventilation with oxygen during the procedure, as hypercarbia predisposes to herniation. However, unless herniation is considered likely, steroid administration should be avoided because of a potential alteration of CSF composition. Ketamine should not be used for anaesthesia for CSF collection in cats because it causes an increase in ICP and may induce seizures.

Requirements

Sterile preparation of the site of collection is required, with clipping of the hair, scrubbing and maintenance of a sterile field. Sterile gloves should be worn.

A sterile disposable or re-sterilizable spinal needle with a stylet is used. Usually a 20–22 gauge, 1.5-inch needle is recommended, although smaller needles may be needed in very small dogs and cats, and longer needles may be needed in large or giant breeds of dog. Several needles should be available, since replacement may be needed if there is contamination or if the needle is inserted off the midline and enters a venous sinus.

Several plain tubes should be reserved for collection of CSF. If bloody, collection into an EDTA tube may help prevent clotting of the specimen. A paediatric EDTA tube should be used, since the volume of CSF may be quite small and there may be significant dilution by EDTA if the volume does not fill the tube to the recommended level.

Sites

If the neurological examination localizes the CNS lesion to the head and/or neck, or the clinical signs involve seizures, generalized incoordination, head tilt or circling, collection from the cerebellomedullary cistern is recommended. Lumbar puncture may be preferred in cases with localized spinal disease because it may be more likely to confirm abnormality than a cerebellomedullary collection. However, lumbar cistern collections are more difficult than those from the cerebellomedullary cistern, may be of smaller volume, and are more likely to be contaminated with blood.

Volume and rate

- Approximately 1 ml of CSF per 5 kg of body weight can be collected safely.
- Collection of approximately 1 ml per 30 seconds is a safe rate of collection.
- Volume of CSF collected should not exceed 4–5 ml of CSF from a dog, 0.5–1.0 ml of CSF from an adult cat, or 10–20 drops from a kitten or puppy.

Techniques

Cerebellomedullary cistern

For collection from the cerebellomedullary cistern, the animal is placed in lateral recumbency, with the head and vertebral column positioned at a 90 degree angle. Excessive flexion of the neck may result in elevation of ICP and increased potential for brain herniation, or may result in occlusion of the endotracheal tube. The nose should be supported so that its long axis is parallel to the table (Figure 23.1).

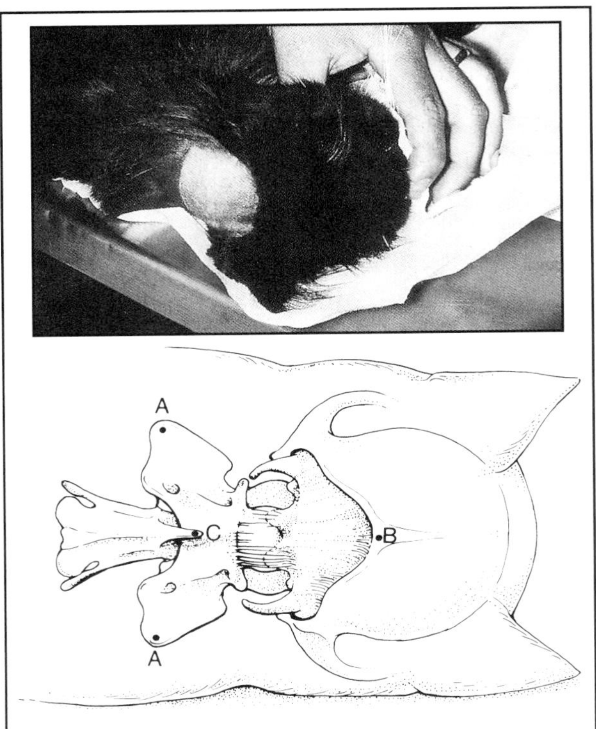

23.1 The correct site for collection of CSF from the cisterna magna is shown in the photograph. The drawing shows the important landmarks of the wings of the atlas vertebra (A), and the occipital protuberance (B) and the craniodorsal tip of the dorsal spine of the axis (C).

The needle should be inserted on the midline, approximately half way between the external occipital protuberance and the craniodorsal tip of the dorsal spine of the axis (C2) and just rostral to the anterior margins of the wings of the atlas vertebra (C1). An 18 gauge needle or scalpel blade can be used for initial puncture of the skin or the skin can be pinched and lifted so that the needle can be pushed through the skin with a twisting motion. The needle should be inserted with the bevel orientated cranially. It should be held perpendicular to the skin surface and gradually advanced, with the stylet in place. Periodically the needle can be stabilized and the stylet withdrawn to determine whether CSF is present.

A sudden loss of resistance may signal entry into the subarachnoid space, but may not be recognized in all cases. Passage of the needle through the spinal cord to underlying bone should be avoided, if possible, since it may cause damage to the spinal cord and/or blood contamination of the sample. If it is suspected that the needle may have been inserted too deeply, the stylet can be removed and the needle slowly withdrawn, a few millimetres at a time, watching for CSF to appear in the hub. If the needle hits bone during insertion, slight redirection cranially or caudally may be attempted.

CSF may be collected directly from the spinal needle hub by dripping into a test tube or by gentle aspiration of drops as they form at the hub, using a syringe held adjacent to the hub. Direct aspiration of CSF with an attached syringe is not recommended, since this may result in contamination with blood or may obstruct CSF flow by aspiration of meningeal trabeculae, although careful aspiration may be resorted to in some cases. The rate of flow of CSF may be increased by jugular compression.

Lumbar cistern

For collection of CSF from the lumbar cistern, the animal is placed in lateral recumbency, with the back flexed slightly to open the spaces between the dorsal laminae of the vertebrae. The L5–6 or L6–7 spaces are most commonly used in dogs because the subarachnoid space rarely extends to the lumbosacral junction. In cats, collection can be made from these sites or from the lumbosacral space.

To collect from the L5–6 space, the needle is inserted just off the midline at the caudal aspect of the L6 dorsal spinous process and advanced at an angle cranioventrally and slightly medially, to enter the spinal canal between the dorsal laminae of L5 and L6. Misdirection laterally into the paralumbar muscles or underestimation of the length of needle required may result in advancement of the needle to the hub without encountering bone. The needle may be passed into the dorsal subarachnoid space or advanced through the caudal nervous structures to the floor of the spinal canal for collection from the ventral subarachnoid space. The stylet is removed and the needle may be withdrawn carefully to encourage fluid flow. The rate of flow is usually slower than from the cerebellomedullary cistern, but may be increased by jugular compression.

Minimizing blood contamination

If the CSF appears to be bloody at the onset of collection, replacement of the stylet for 30–60 seconds may result in clearing of the CSF. If the first few drops are bloody, they can be collected separately from the following drops that are often clear. If the rate of flow of CSF is slow, slight rotation of the needle may be helpful. If abundant blood is present, venous sinus puncture should be suspected and a new approach with a fresh needle is recommended.

Handling CSF specimens

CSF is normally a low-protein fluid with rapid turnover. Cells lyse rapidly in CSF once it is removed, and unfixed fluid should be processed within 30–60 minutes of collection. Addition of an equal volume of 40–90% ethanol or 2 drops of 10% buffered formalin per ml of specimen may be used for fixation of fluids that cannot be delivered immediately to a laboratory or cannot be processed immediately. Some laboratories are prepared to use special techniques for cytological evaluation of fixed CSF. It is advisable to check with the laboratory regarding their requirements for CSF submissions. Cell counts may be affected by slight dilution when formalin fixation is used, but this is not usually clinically significant. Other techniques that may help retard cellular degeneration and/or increase cell stability include refrigeration, addition of fresh, frozen or thawed serum or plasma, or addition of 20% albumin.

Protein and enzyme concentrations in CSF are relatively stable and submission using routine methods is usually sufficient for accurate determinations.

Laboratory analysis of CSF

Usually 1–2 ml of CSF is available from dogs or cats. Routine analysis of CSF should include:

- Macroscopic evaluation (colour and transparency)
- Cell counts (red blood cells (RBC), nucleated cell count (NCC))
- Total protein (laboratory microprotein assay or commercial dipstick)
- Cytological evaluation.

General characteristics of normal and abnormal CSF are summarized in Figure 23.2.

Component of CSF evaluation	Normal	Abnormal
Colour	Colourless	Pink, red or xanthochromic, occasionally green to grey (slight, moderate or marked)
Transparency	Clear	Cloudy or turbid (slight, moderate or marked)
Erythrocyte count	Zero is considered to be normal but red cells are often present in small numbers (<250 per microlitre)	Variable
Nucleated cell count	Dogs: 0–6 cells per microlitre Cats: 0–8 cells per microlitre	Variable
Total protein	Microprotein (chemical determination): cerebellomedullary < 0.30 g/l; lumbar < 0.45 g/l	Microprotein (chemical determination): cerebellomedullary > 0.30 g/l; lumbar > 0.45 g/l

23.2 General characteristics of normal and abnormal CSF.

Macroscopic evaluation

Macroscopic evaluation should include evaluation of colour and transparency. Visible cloudiness or turbidity usually reflects a markedly elevated cell count, although moderate elevations in cellularity cannot be detected grossly. Yellow or orange discoloration is termed xanthochromia and indicates previous haemorrhage into the CSF, with resultant formation of haem pigments producing the colour change. Red discoloration indicates recent or current haemorrhage. Green to grey discoloration may result from various cellular and/or bacterial contents and is rarely observed. The macroscopic evaluation is aided by good, natural, non-fluorescent lighting and examining the tube containing the fluid against a piece of white paper.

Cell counts

Cell counts can be conducted using a standard haemocytometer (Figure 23.3). The haemocytometer should be clean and fully loaded on both sides, so that duplicate counts can be made. A clean coverslip should be used so that debris will not be confused with cells. The haemocytometer can be filled using well mixed CSF in a glass capillary tube. The cells should be allowed to settle for 5–10 minutes prior to counting. The cells in all nine large squares of the haemocytometer should be counted (Figure 23.3b). The condenser of the microscope should be lowered to provide contrast.

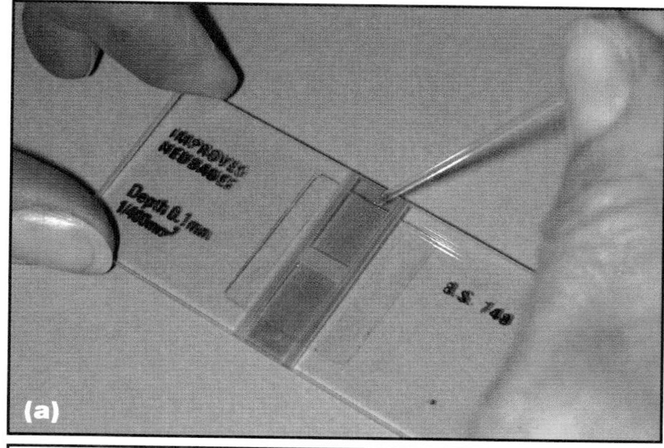

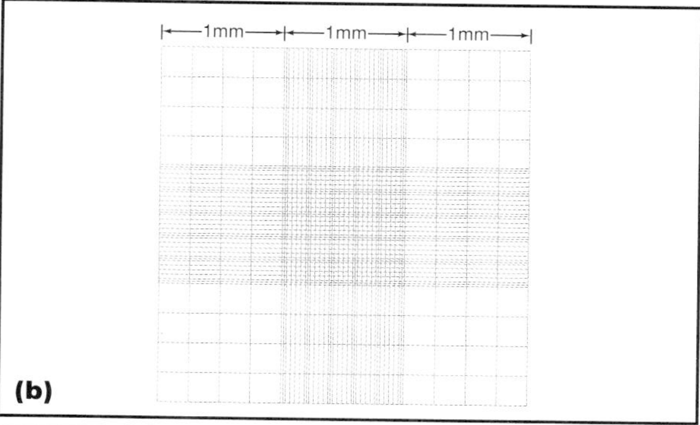

23.3 A haemocytometer is used for performing nucleated and red cell counts. (a) The haemocytometer is charged with undiluted fluid by gently touching the tip of a capillary tube containing CSF to the edge of the coverslip. (b) Diagrammatic representation of the grid lines seen microscopically in the haemocytometer. The cells in all nine large squares are counted. (Courtesy of E. Villiers)

Erythrocytes are recognized as small, clear, refractile disks without nuclei, while nucleated cells are larger, more refractile or appear granular and have recognizable nuclei. The total number of cells of each type (RBC and nucleated cells) should be divided by 9 (the number of squares counted) and multipled by 10 (depth of the haemocytometer) in order to obtain the cell count per microlitre. Cell counts obtained from each side of the haemocytometer should be within 10–20% of each other. If there is larger variation than this, a repeat count should be considered. Cell counts in normal CSF are <7 cells/μl in dogs and <9 cells/μl in cats. When the nucleated cell count is elevated, this is referred to as *pleocytosis*.

Various formulae have been applied to try to determine the possible contribution of blood contamination to CSF nucleated cell count. These formulae have been shown to be unreliable in 'correcting' for blood contamination and are not recommended. If the specimen contains a large amount of blood suspected to be due to contamination, repeat collection is recommended.

Total protein (microprotein assay)

Albumin makes up approximately 80–95% of the total protein in normal CSF. Reference intervals for total protein may vary slightly with laboratory and/or method used. Protein concentrations in cerebellomedullary CSF samples are usually <0.25–0.30 g/l and in lumbar cistern samples <0.45 g/l.

Reference laboratories use dye-binding spectrophotometric methods for quantitation of CSF protein levels (often referred to as microprotein assays). Refractometry is not suitable for evaluation of CSF protein and in-practice chemistry analysers are generally not suitable for evaluation of CSF microprotein levels.

In practice, the use of urine dipsticks for estimation of CSF protein provides a rapid assessment of protein levels. Ames Multistix urine dipsticks have been validated for this evaluation. Figure 23.4 summarizes the estimation of CSF protein using Ames Multistix urine dipsticks (N-Multistix SG, Bayer, Miles, Diagnostic Division, Elkhart, Indiana, USA). The dipsticks are most sensitive to albumin, and good correlation has been shown with standard dye-binding microprotein determinations.

Ames Multistix urine dipstick result	Estimated total protein	Interpretation
Trace	<3.0 g/l (< 30 mg/dl)	Within normal limits
1+	3.0 g/l (30 mg/dl)	Within normal limits
2+	10.0 g/l (100 mg/dl)	Abnormal
3+	30.0 g/l (300 mg/dl)	Abnormal
4+	200.0 g/l (>2000 mg/dl)	Abnormal

23.4 Estimation of CSF protein using Ames Multistix urine dipsticks.

Previously, Pandy's or Nonne–Apelt tests were used to determine whether globulins were present in CSF. These tests have fallen out of favour and are not now routinely used, because of difficulties in interpretation of the significance of globulins and the semiquantitative nature of the tests.

Sometimes there will be elevation in the total protein of CSF but no abnormalities are detected cytologically. This is referred to as 'albuminocytologic dissociation'. This is a relatively common finding and is non-specific, since it can occur with inflammatory, degenerative, compressive or neoplastic diseases. Elevated total protein may occur with increased permeability of the blood–brain barrier, necrosis, interruption of normal CSF flow or absorption and/or intrathecal globulin production.

Cytological preparations

Cytocentrifugation is commonly used for cytology preparations because CSF is of very low cellularity compared with other body fluids. Chamber sedimentation or membrane-filter techniques also may be used. Staining of air-dried preparations is usually by Romanowsky stains (Diff-Quik, Wright–Giemsa, May–Grünwald–Giemsa or others), while wet-fixed specimens may be stained using trichrome, Papanicolaou or haematoxylin and eosin (H&E).

Cytocentrifugation may be available at referral laboratories or specialized veterinary referral practices where extensive in-house laboratory facilities are justified by high case load. For in-practice use, a simple sedimentation chamber may be made using a 2.5 ml syringe with the barrel cut in half. The flanged end of the resulting cylinder can be attached to a microscope slide wrapped in filter paper with a hole cut in it (Figure 23.5). The barrel of the syringe is aligned over the hole and attached using a small amount of petroleum jelly around its edge. The filter paper and syringe are clipped to the slide using bulldog clips. An aliquot of well mixed CSF is placed in the cylinder and the cells allowed to settle on the slide for 30 minutes. The excess fluid is wicked away by the filter paper and the cells should settle on to the area of the glass slide defined by the hole in the filter paper. Following air-drying, the slide is stained by any of the Romanowsky stains used in practice.

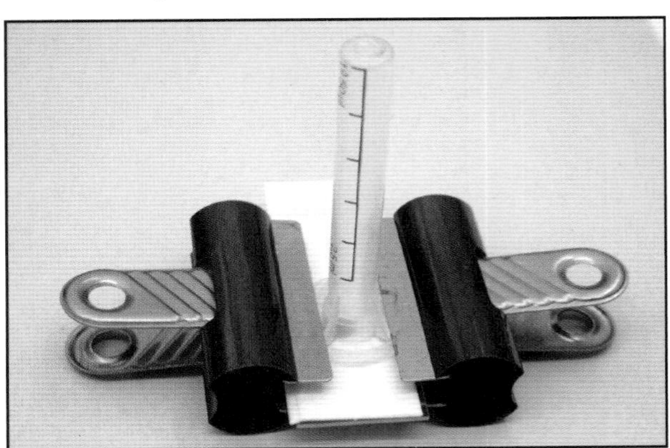

23.5 A sedimentation chamber constructed from a syringe barrel, filter paper, a slide and sticky tape. (Courtesy of R Powell)

Other assays

Creatine kinase (CK) assay has been recommended in the past, since damage to nervous tissue may result in elevation of the isoenzyme found in the CNS. However, there is difficulty in interpretation of elevated levels, particularly when blood contamination is present. CSF also may become contaminated with CK from skeletal muscle during collection. The difficulties in interpretation of the significance of elevated CK has resulted in discontinuance of its use in most laboratories.

Special stains or immunocytochemistry may be used to demonstrate bacteria, fungi, intracellular material or myelin. Specialized analyses, including electrophoresis, immunoelectrophoresis, antibody titres, fungal antigen tests, microbiological cultures or polymerase chain reaction amplification assays, may be used when particular conditions are suspected.

Normal and abnormal CSF

Cellular and non-cellular features of normal CSF

- **Small lymphocytes.** These are the predominant cell type in CSF from healthy dogs and cats. The appearance is similar to those of lymphocytes in peripheral blood: cells are usually 9–15 μm in diameter (canine and feline red blood cells have diameters of 7 μm and 5.5 μm, respectively), with a round to ovoid or slightly cleaved nucleus and a thin rim of palely basophilic cytoplasm.
- **Monocytoid cells.** These may be present in low numbers and are often slightly larger than small lymphocytes (12–15 μm diameter) with variable nuclear shape, open chromatin and moderate amounts of lightly basophilic cytoplasm that varies from homogenous to finely vacuolated.
- **Neutrophils and eosinophils.** A few neutrophils (up to 20% of the total nucleated cells when the nucleated cell count is within normal limits) may occasionally be seen in CSF from healthy animals and are similar to those seen in peripheral blood. Eosinophils are seen occasionally in very low numbers in CSF from healthy animals. In the absence of excessive blood contamination, neutrophil percentages >10–20% and eosinophils >1%, with or without elevations in total nucleated cell count, are considered abnormal and deserve further investigation.
- **Plasma cells.** These are not present in normal CSF, but may be seen with reactive or inflammatory processes with a response to antigenic stimulation.

Contaminants or unusual findings

Occasionally, ependymal or choroid plexus cells may be seen in CSF. These are round to cuboidal mononuclear cells, often occurring in cohesive groups. Subarachnoid (leptomeningeal) cells may be recognized as mononuclear cells with oval nuclei, delicate chromatin and elongated or indistinct cytoplasmic margins, and may be single or in small clusters. Haemopoietic precursor cells (immature cells of myeloid or erythroid origin; megakaryocytes) may be seen if bone marrow is accidentally punctured: they are most often seen in CSF from lumbar collections. Mitotic figures are occasionally seen in CSF from healthy animals, but their presence is more often associated with proliferative conditions, particularly neoplasia. Coiled 'ribbons' of basophilic non-cellular material have been reported in CSF obtained during post-mortem examination, and have been hypothesized to represent denatured myelin or myelin fragments.

Cellular findings in neurological disease

'Normal' CSF in the presence of disease

No abnormalities of CSF may be detected in many patients with neurological disease. The majority of cases of idiopathic epilepsy, congenital hydrocephalus, intoxication, metabolic or functional disorders, vertebral disease or myelomalacia do not have abnormalities detected. A significant proportion of cases with neurological disease due to feline infectious peritonitis (FIP), distemper encephalitis, neoplasia or granulomatous meningoencephalitis may also have CSF that is within normal limits.

Slight to moderate neutrophilic inflammation

Slight to moderate neutrophilic inflammation (25–50% neutrophils, with or without elevated microprotein, with or without pleocytosis) has been reported to occur with bacterial, fungal, protozoal, parasitic, rickettsial or viral infections, as well as with neoplasia or non-infectious conditions. Non-infectious conditions that may result in this appearance include traumatic, degenerative, immune-mediated, metabolic or ischaemic conditions.

Marked neutrophilic inflammation

Marked neutrophilic inflammation (>50% neutrophils, with pleocytosis, often with increased microprotein) has been reported to occur with bacterial meningitis and severe viral encephalitis, including FIP. It also may occur with steroid-responsive meningitis–arteritis, following myelography, with trauma, haemorrhage, acquired hydrocephalus or neoplasia.

Mixed cellular inflammation without a predominant type

Mixed cellular inflammation (mixed macrophages, lymphocytes and neutrophils, with or without plasma cells; with or without elevated microprotein; with or without pleocytosis) has been reported to occur with fungal, protozoal, parasitic or rickettsial infection. Some idiopathic inflammatory or degenerative diseases, and inadequately treated chronic bacterial infections also may result in this appearance. In addition, a mixed inflammatory response may be found in the early stages of therapy of bacterial meningitis.

Mononuclear inflammation

Mononuclear inflammation (predominantly monocytes, especially lymphocytes, usually with pleocytosis) has been reported to occur with necrotizing encephalitis of small-breed dogs, neoplasia, canine distemper virus infection and in a variety of non-infectious and degenerative conditions. Granulomatous meningoencephalitis should be considered.

Eosinophilic inflammation

Eosinophilic inflammation (predominantly eosinophils, usually with pleocytosis) has been reported to occur with parasitic, protozoal, bacterial, viral and rickettsial infections. It has also been reported with neoplasia, hypersensitivity reactions and as part of non-specific inflammatory reactions.

CSF findings in selected clinical conditions

Findings in CSF in selected clinical conditions are summarized in Figure 23.6.

Condition	CSF characteristics	Clinical features	Comments and differential diagnoses
Feline infectious peritonitis (FIP)	• Frequently see neutrophilic pleocytosis • TP usually > 2.0 g/l • NCC usually > 100 cells/μl • Neutrophils often > 50% • Mixed cell pleocytosis often present late in the course of disease	Often < 4 years of age. Multi-focal neurological signs referable to cerebellum and/or brainstem. Protracted course of illness	Need to rule out bacterial meningoencephalitis, non-FIP viral encephalomyelitis and other inflammatory conditions
Canine distemper	• Usually lymphocytic pleocytosis; may see mixed cell pleocytosis • NCC variable, but usually > 60% lymphocytes • TP usually increased	Usually young dog. History of absence of vaccination and/or exposure to other dogs with illness and/or death	Occasionally viral inclusions may be identified. Serum and CSF IgM antibodies to distemper virus in the absence of vaccination is supportive
Granulomatous meningoencephalitis (GME)	• Usually slight to moderate, lymphocytic or mixed cell pleocytosis; occasionally neutrophilic pleocytosis • NCC usually > 100 cells/μl; wide range reported, including 'within normal limits' • TP usually > 1.0 g/l (variable)	Usually young to middle-aged bitch. Toy and terrier breeds predisposed. Fever, ataxia, tetraparesis, seizures. May be localized as multifocal or focal (better prognosis)	Need to rule out necrotizing meningoencephalitis of small-breed dogs
Steroid-responsive suppurative meningitis–arteritis	• Neutrophilic pleocytosis • NCC often > 500 cells/μl • Usually > 75% non-degenerate neutrophils	Usually young to middle-aged dogs. Fever, cervical pain, hyperaesthesia, paresis	Improvement usually seen within 72 h of glucocorticoid. Need to rule out bacterial and ehrlichial meningoencephalitis
Steroid-responsive eosinophilic meningitis	• Eosinophilic pleocytosis with > 80% eosinophils • Slight to marked elevation in NCC	Reported in dogs and one cat. Golden retrievers predisposed. Usually respond to glucocorticoid therapy. Type I hypersensitivity reaction suspected	Need to rule out fungal, parasitic, protozoal and neoplastic conditions
Necrotizing encephalitis of small-breed dogs	• Lymphocytic pleocytosis; usually > 200 cells/μl; lymphocytes usually> 70% • TP often > 5.0 g/l	Pugs, Maltese and Yorkshire Terriers, usually < 4 years old. Seizures, depression, ataxia. Lack of response to steroids. Possibly immune-mediated	Multifocal to massive necrosis and non-suppurative inflammation. Fatal or leading to euthanasia. Need to rule out GME. Histology may be required to detect necrosis
Neoplasia	Variable NCC, TP and cytological findings	Lymphoma is the most common neoplasm found in CSF	Well differentiated or small-cell lymphoma may be difficult to differentiate from lymphocytic pleocytosis. Other tumour types, including primary brain tumours, rarely exfoliate into CSF; may require aspiration, crush preparations or imprint from biopsy sample for cytology

23.6 Characteristics of CSF in selected clinical conditions. NCC = nucleated cell count. TP = total protein.

Feline infectious peritonitis

FIP is a common cause of neutrophilic pleocytosis in the cat. Neutrophilic pleocytosis with a nucleated cell count >100 cells/μl and microprotein usually >2.0 g/l is often seen with FIP. A non-specific, mixed pleocytosis may occur later in disease. Cats with neurological disease due to FIP infection are usually <4 years old and have multifocal neurological signs referable to cerebellum and/or brainstem; they often have a history of a protracted course of illness. If the cat is >3 years of age and has <50 cells/μl and microprotein <1.0 g/l, FIP is unlikely, and other causes of viral meningoencephalitis should be considered. Common neurological signs associated with FIP include depression, head tilt, nystagmus, intentional tremor and tetraparesis (see also Chapter 26).

Canine distemper virus infection

Canine distemper virus often results in a lymphocytic pleocytosis. Cell counts may vary from within normal limits to >50 cells/μl. Lymphocytes usually account for >60% of the nucleated cells. Some cases have an increase in macrophages and increased microprotein. Intracellular viral inclusions are rarely seen. Positive CSF titres for canine distemper virus may be helpful in providing support for a diagnosis of distemper viral encephalomyelitis (see Chapter 26). Dogs with canine distemper virus are often young and are usually unvaccinated.

Granulomatous meningoencephalitis

Granulomatous meningoencephalitis (GME) is most often seen in young to middle-aged, small and medium-sized dogs, especially of toy or terrier breeds. Clinical signs include fever, ataxia, tetraparesis, cervical hypaesthesia and seizures. CSF may have slight to moderate lymphocytic inflammation, mixed cell pleocytosis (Figure 23.7), and/or occasionally neutrophilic pleocytosis. The majority of cases have nucleated cell counts >100 cells/μl. Microprotein levels are variable.

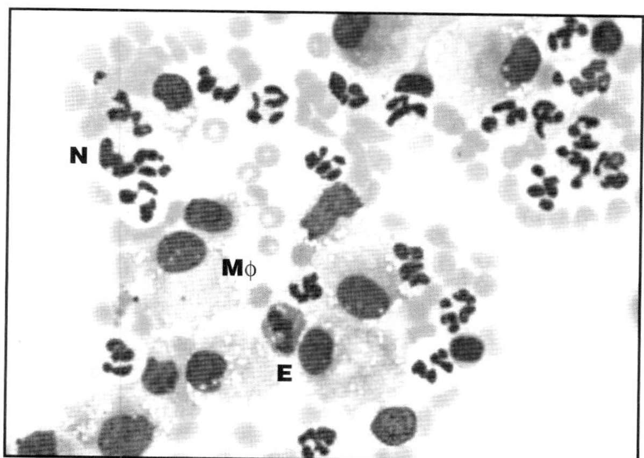

23.7 CSF from a dog with granulomatous meningoencephalitis. There is a mixed cell pleocytosis with moderate neutrophils (N) and macrophages (Mϕ). A single eosinophil (E) is seen. (Wright–Giemsa stain; original magnification X100)

Steroid-responsive suppurative meningitis–arteritis

Steroid-responsive, suppurative meningitis–arteritis is usually a condition of young to middle-aged, large-breed dogs, with fever, cervical pain, hyperaesthesia and paresis. CSF often contains >500 cells/μl, with >75% non-degenerate neutrophils (Figure 23.8). Bacteria are not present cytologically or on culture. A rapid response (improvement within 72 hours) is observed with glucocorticoid administration. *Anaplasma phagocytophilum* (*Ehrlichia phagocytophila*) infection can result in similar clinical signs and cytological findings (see Chapter 27).

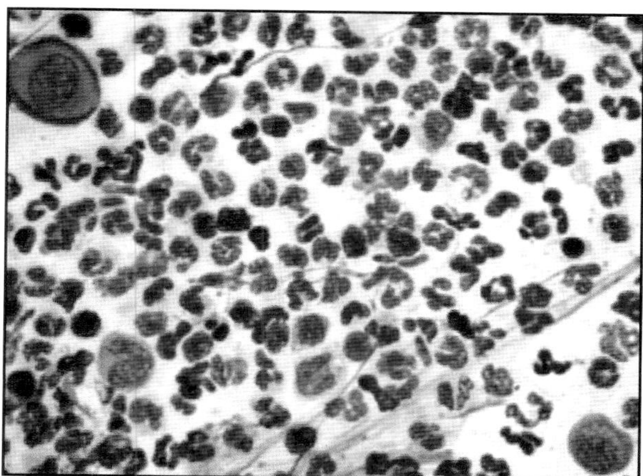

23.8 CSF from a dog with steroid-responsive meningitis-arteritis. There are numerous non-degenerate neutrophils as well as a few eosinophils and macrophages. Compare with Figure 23.9 showing degenerate and distorted neutrophils. (Wright's stain; orginal magnification X500.) (Courtesy of E Villiers)

Steroid-responsive eosinophilic meningitis

Steroid-responsive eosinophilic meningitis has been reported in dogs and cats. This has been hypothesized to be the result of an allergic (type I hypersensitivity) reaction. Slight to marked pleocytosis may be present, but usually >80% of the nucleated cells are eosinophils. Protozoal, parasitic or fungal infections need to be ruled out. Golden Retrievers may be predisposed to this condition. There is usually a good response to glucocorticoid treatment.

Necrotizing encephalitis in small-breed dogs

Necrotizing encephalitis in small-breed dogs has been primarily reported in young (<4 years old) Pugs and Maltese and Yorkshire Terriers. This condition has been hypothesized to be an immune-mediated disease with autoantibodies directed against astrocytes. Multifocal to massive necrosis and non-suppurative inflammation of the cerebrum and meninges occurs and may be fatal. Seizures, depression and ataxia are common presenting signs. The condition does not respond to glucocorticoid administration. Usually there is slight to moderate pleocytosis, often with >200 cells/μl, with lymphocytes predominating (usually >70%). Microprotein is often >5.0 g/l.

Bacterial meningoencephalomyelitis

This is also characterized by marked pleocytosis (usually >200 cells/μl) and is frequently accompanied by elevated microprotein. Neutrophils predominate (>70% of total nucleated cells). When intracellular bacteria are seen, this provides strong support for the presence of sepsis (Figure 23.9). Bacteria are not seen in all cases and correlation with the results of bacterial culture is important.

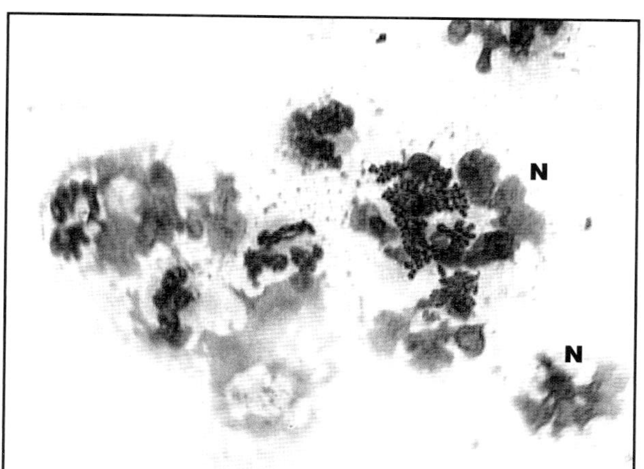

23.9 CSF from a dog with bacterial meningoencephalitis and sepsis. There are degenerate, smudged and distorted neutrophils (N) with blue-staining intracellullar bacterial cocci. Compare with Figure 23.8. (Wright–Giemsa stain; original magnification X1000)

Neoplasia

Primary or metastastic neoplasia may result in clinical neurological signs. These are often localized or focal signs, but may be more generalized. Findings on CSF evaluation are variable and neoplastic cells in CSF, although rarely present, may enable a positive diagnosis.

Lymphoma is the most commonly identified neoplasm in CSF (Figure 23.10). Well differentiated or small-cell lymphoma may be difficult to differentiate from lymphocytic pleocytosis. Encephalic plasma cell tumour has been reported. Other tumour types, including primary brain tumours, rarely exfoliate into CSF and may require aspiration, crush preparations or imprint from a biopsy specimen for cytological evaluation.

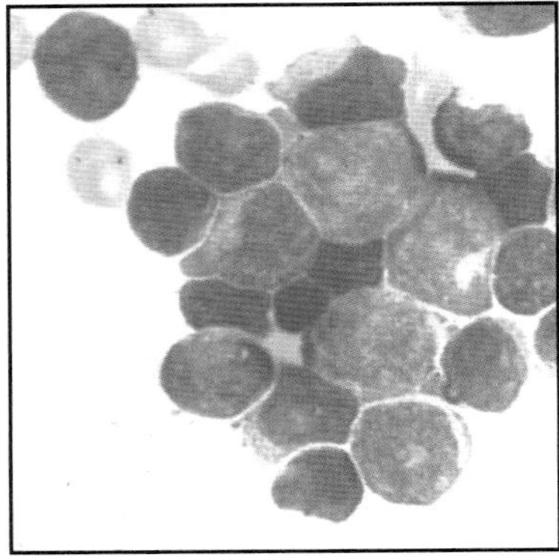

23.10 CSF from a dog with multicentric lymphoma and neurological signs. There are numerous large lymphoid cells and lymphoblasts with prominent nucleoli. (Wright–Giemsa stain; original magnification X1000)

References and further reading

Bailey CS and Higgins RJ (1986) Characteristics of cerebrospinal fluid associated with canine granulomatous meningoencephalomyelitis: a retrospective study. *Journal of the American Veterinary Medical Association* **188,** 418–421

Baroni M and Heinold Y (1995) A review of the clinical diagnosis of feline infectious peritonitis viral meningoencephalomyelitis. *Progress in Veterinary Neurology* **6,** 88–94

Chrisman CL (1992) Cerebrospinal fluid analysis. *Veterinary Clinics of North America: Small Animal Practice* **22,** 781–810

Cook, JR and Denicola, DB (1988), Cerebrospinal fluid. *Veterinary Clinics of North America: Small Animal Practice* **18,** 475–499

Freeman KP and Raskin RE (2001) Cytology of the central nervous system. In: *Atlas of Canine and Feline Cytology,* ed. RE Raskin and DJ Meyer, pp. 325–365. WB Saunders, London

Jamison EM and Lumsden JH (1988) Cerebrospinal fluid analysis in the dog: methodology and interpretation. *Seminars in Veterinary Medicine and Surgery (Small Animal)* **3,** 122–132

Meinkoth JH and Crystal MA (1999) Cerebrospinal fluid analysis. In: *Diagnostic Cytology and Hematology of the Dog and Cat,* ed. RL Cowell *et al.*, pp. 125–141. Mosby, St Louis

Parent JM and Rand JS (1994), Cerebrospinal fluid collection and analysis. In: *Consultations in Feline Internal Medicine 2,* ed. JR August, pp. 385–392. WB Saunders, Philadelphia

Tyler JW and Cullor JS (1989).Titers, tests and truisms: rational interpretation of diagnostic serologic testing. *Journal of the American Veterinary Medical Association* **194,** 1550–1558

Wamsley H and Alleman AR (2004) Clinical pathology. In: *BSAVA Manual of Canine and Feline Neurology, 3rd edition,* ed. S Platt and NJ Olby, pp. 35–53. BSAVA Publications, Gloucester

24

Laboratory evaluation of skin and ear disease

Tim Nuttall

Introduction

Very few skin disorders have an unequivocally pathognomic appearance and almost all require some form of laboratory investigation to confirm the diagnosis. Fortunately, the skin is readily accessible; most tests, furthermore, are straightforward and can be assessed in a practice laboratory. Any samples sent to external laboratories should be properly packaged with full clinical information. Any samples that are potentially zoonotic must be clearly labelled.

Equipment

A list of equipment required for skin evaluation is given in Figure 24.1.

- Good light
- Flea comb
- Hand lens
- Otoscope
- Wood's lamp
- Curved scissors and electric clippers
- Fine tipped forceps
- Liquid paraffin and potassium hydroxide
- No. 10 and no. 15 scalpel blades
- Cotton buds
- Bacteriology swabs
- Microscope slides
- Cover slips
- Rapid stain (e.g. Diff-Quik)
- Lactophenol cotton blue
- Light microscope
- Toothbrushes
- Dermatophyte test medium
- Biopsy punches (plus basic surgical kit and suture material)
- 10% neutral buffered formalin

24.1 A dermatologist's kitbag.

Good light is essential for proper examination of the skin, lesions and collected material. Good fluorescent room lighting is a minimal requirement and a high intensity spotlight is necessary for any serious examination. A hand lens is very useful for examining skin lesions and coat brushings for large parasites, such as fleas, lice, *Cheyletiella*, *Otodectes* and *Neotrombicula*. Large illuminated lenses (e.g. for map reading) are best.

Rapid stains

There are a number of rapid stains available (e.g. Diff-Quik). They are the most commonly used stains in practice by virtue of their ease of use and interpretation. There are three pots: fixer (pale blue to green), stain 1 (red) and stain 2 (purple). The procedure for staining is as follows:

1. Air-dried smears or tape-strips are dipped in each pot 5 to 10 times for a second each time. Staining time is longer for thicker or waxy preparations.
2. The slide is rinsed under a tap or with distilled water (directing the flow against the back of the slide stops the preparation being flushed down the sink).
3. The slide is gently blotted dry using textured paper towel without damaging the stained preparation.
4. Staining is checked under low power; if it is adequate a drop of oil and a coverslip are added; if not it is re-stained.

- Waxy or oily preparations are difficult to air dry and are soluble in the fixer. It is better to heat fix them and then use the red and purple stains only. Passing the slide through a Bunsen or spirit burner until it is hand hot suffices and avoids cooking the material.
- Staining efficiency declines over time and the pots will accumulate skin debris, *Malassezia* and bacteria that can contaminate slides. In a busy laboratory, they should be rinsed and replenished from the stock solutions at least every 2 weeks.
- To avoid evaporation (especially of fixer) lids should be replaced promptly.

Light microscope

No piece of equipment is so vital or subject to so much abuse as a microscope. Robust and inexpensive models with binocular lenses and integral light sources are easily mastered and give good results (Figure 24.2) (see also Chapter 2).

- The ideal microscope should have binocular eyepieces, an integral light source, a focusing condenser, a mechanical stage and four lenses: 4X, 10X, 40X and 100X oil immersion (eyepieces are usually 10X giving a final magnification of 40X–1000X)
- Adjust the eyepieces by focusing on a slide with one eye, then using the eyepiece to correct the focus for your other eye
- Close the light diaphragm and focus the condenser until there is a sharp image of the diaphragm. If there is no diaphragm, focus on a piece of card held against the light source
- Adjust the iris diaphragm to give the clearest image for each lens
- For parasites it is useful to close the iris diaphragm; the image is poorer but the increased contrast makes the parasites stand out better. For cytology open the diaphragm to reduce contrast and give a more detailed image
- Always use coverslips. They give a better image, a defined search area and protect the lenses
- Use the oil immersion lens last of all to avoid getting oil on the other lenses
- Clean the lenses and stage with lens cleaner and fine tissue or lens cloths immediately after use. Dried-on immersion oil and debris can be removed by carefully rubbing the lens on polystyrene soaked in lens cleaner

24.2 Use and abuse of the practice microscope.

Investigation of skin disease

Screening tests

Coat brushings

Surface debris can be collected with a flea comb or stiff brushes. The material can be brushed on to dark card or into a petri dish for examination with a hand lens. Alternatively, adhesive tape can be used to mount it on a microscope slide for examination under low power. Flea dirt, which is largely partly digested blood, leaves a reddish brown stain on moistened white paper or cotton wool.

Hair plucks and trichograms

Hairs are grasped with a pair of fine forceps (using rubber sleeves over the tips may reduce hair damage) and pulled in the direction of hair growth with a firm even pressure. The hairs are placed in some liquid paraffin on a microscope slide and a coverslip applied. Alternatively, hairs can be mounted on the slide with adhesive tape. Aligning the hairs makes interpretation easier. The slide is scanned under low power, and high power is then used to examine areas of interest in more detail (Figures 24.3–24.7).

Finding	Appearance	Significance
Anagen hairs (Figure 24.4)	Fat, active, moist bulbs	Growing phase
Telogen hairs (Figure 24.5)	Tapered, slightly frayed bulbs	Resting phase. Excess is suggestive of an endocrine or metabolic disorder. Most dogs and cats have predominantly telogen coats. Poodles and similar breeds have predominantly anagen coats
Shaft abnormalities	Twisted hairs, swellings, nodules, fractures, large melanin aggregates (macromelanosomes), etc.	Hereditary shaft abnormalities, deficiency diseases, trauma, colour dilution alopecia, follicular dysplasias
Tapered tips	Hair tips smoothly taper to a point	Normal hairs
Fractured tips	Blunt, frayed ends	Fractured hairs, self-trauma, dermatophytes
Follicular casts (Figure 24.6)	Collars of scale tightly adherent to the proximal hair shaft	Follicular hyperkeratosis, follicular dysplasias, sebaceous adenitis, keratinization disorders, demodicosis, dermatophytosis
Demodex	Adults, larvae, nymphs and eggs often associated with hair bulbs	Demodicosis; this is a particularly useful technique in pedal demodicosis especially if there is heavy scarring
Dermatophytes (Figure 24.7)	Disrupted and fractured hair shafts, small, bubble-like ectothrix spores surrounding affected hair shafts	Dermatophytosis; confirm with culture

24.3 Trichogram findings and their significance.

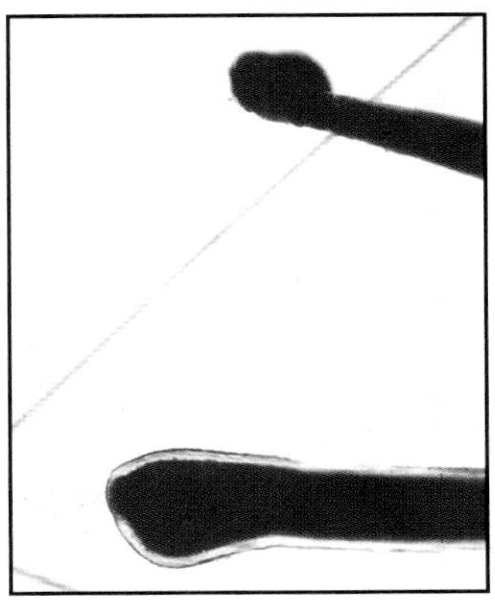

24.4 Anagen hairs from a German Shepherd Dog. (Original magnification X40.)

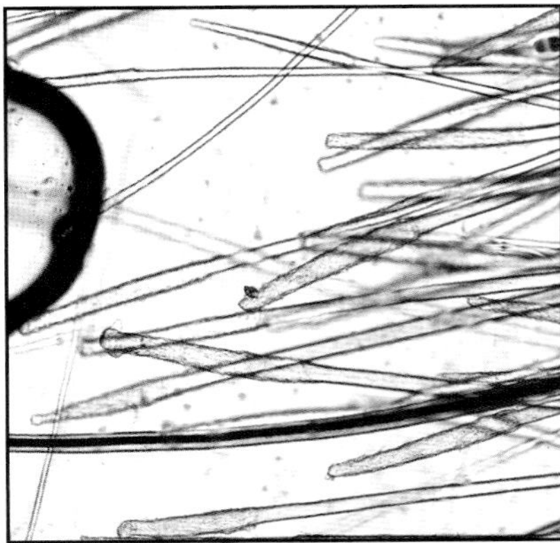

24.5 Telogen hairs from a crossbred dog with hyperadrenocorticism. (Original magnification X40.)

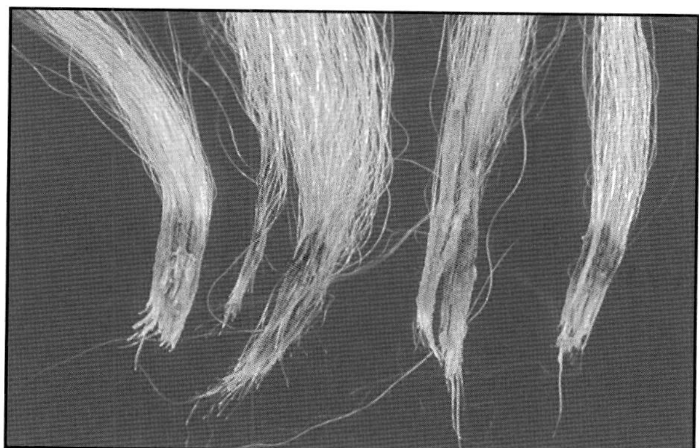

24.6 Follicular casts from a dog with sebaceous adenitis. (Courtesy of Dr B Kennis.)

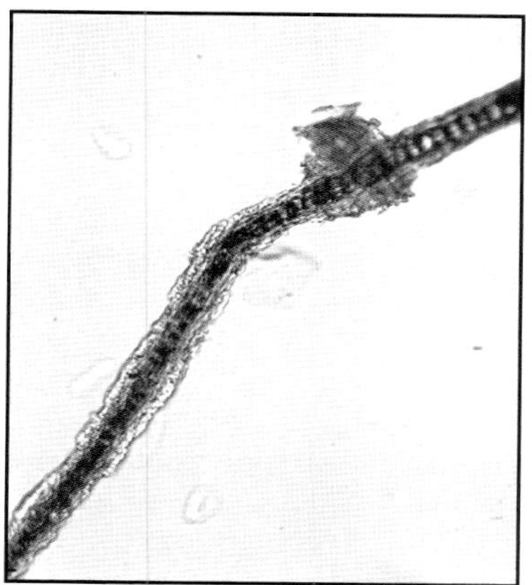

24.7 Ectothrix spores on a damaged hair from a cat with a *Microsporum canis* infection. The spores resemble tiny bubbles on the outside of the hair shaft. (Original magnification x100.)

Fungal examination

Wood's lamp

The Wood's lamp emits ultraviolet (UV) light of a wavelength that causes certain dermatophytes (including 50–70% of *Microsporum canis* strains) to fluoresce *in vivo*. It is more useful for cats, where 95% of infections are *M. canis*, than for dogs. Rare dermatophytes that may fluoresce include *M. equinum*, *M. audounii*, *M. distortum* and *Trichophyton schoenleinii*.

The best lamps have an integral magnifying glass. One should look for bright apple-green fluorescence of the hairs. Crusts and topical medications will glow a dull yellow green. Scale and fibres often shine blue-white. The lamp must warm up for 5–10 minutes and 5 minutes should be spent looking, as the fluorescence is sometimes delayed.

Hair plucks

Ectothrix spores (Figure 24.7) appear as tiny beads, particularly after clearing the hairs with potassium hydroxide (see Skin scrapes). Endothrix spores and hyphae may be visible inside cleared hairs.

Fungal cultures

Dermatophytes grow on two media:

- **Sabouraud's agar** is the best medium, but culture can take 3–4 weeks. Samples are usually sent away, although plates can be incubated at room temperature in practice laboratories
- **Dermatophyte test medium (DTM)** is a quick, easy in-practice alternative, but there are occasional false negatives. Dermatophytes utilize protein in the agar turning the indicator red as they grow (Figure 24.8). Saprophytes only use protein once the carbohydrate is exhausted and turn the agar red after profuse growth has already occurred. The medium is incubated in the dark at room temperature and checked daily to detect when the colour change occurs relative to fungal growth. Dermatophytes are usually evident by 5–7 days, but growth can take up to 14 days. They form fluffy whitish colonies but, unfortunately, DTM inhibits normal colony morphology, pigmentation and macroconidia production, which makes species identification difficult compared with using Sabouraud's agar. Results can be obtained more quickly by incubating above room temperature.

For examination, the colony is touched gently with adhesive tape, which is then attached to a microscope slide over a drop of lactophenol cotton blue. Identification is based on macroconidial morphology. *M. canis* forms rough, cigar-shaped macroconidia with more than six cells (Figure 24.9). N.B. Macroconidia are frequently found on skin scrapes and during cytology. These are saprophytes (usually environmental contaminants); dermatophytes only produce macroconidia in culture.

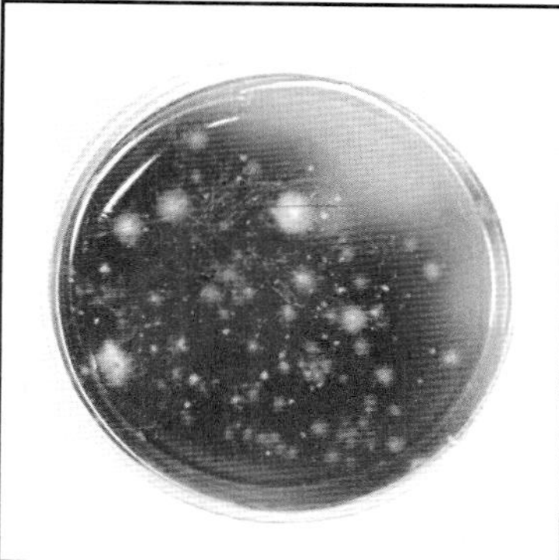

24.8 *Microsporum canis* on dermatophyte test medium. The red colour change coincides with early fungal growth.

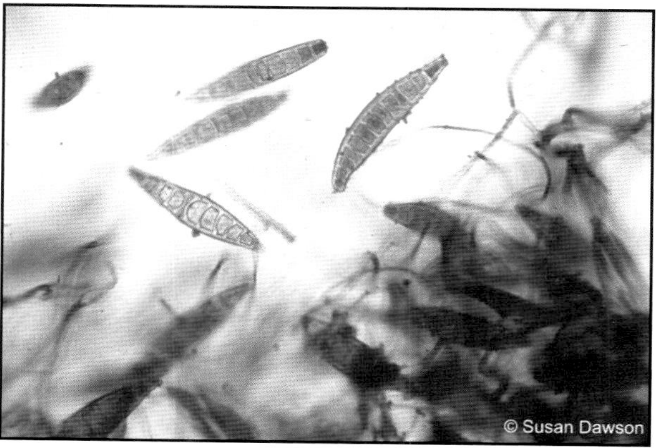

24.9 *Microsporum canis* macroconidia from *in vitro* culture; these are not produced *in vivo*. (New methylene blue stain; original magnification X400.) (© Susan Dawson.)

Sample collection for fungal culture is by:

- Hair plucks. Fluorescing hairs or hairs from the edge of lesions are picked
- Mackenzie brush technique. This allows sampling of many more hairs. The coat is combed vigorously with a toothbrush or plastic grooming brush, which is used directly to inoculate DTM or sent away.

Samples are submitted for culture in sealed but not airtight containers since bacteria will swamp fungi in moist anaerobic environments.

Deep fungal infections

Careful examination of cytology smears from sinus tracts and ulcerated lesions can reveal fungal elements but infection should be confirmed by fungal culture. This is best achieved by submitting a biopsy specimen (see below) of the affected tissues to a recognized mycology laboratory. Swabbing the skin with alcohol prior to performing the biopsy will reduce bacterial contamination.

Bacterial cultures

Bacterial culture and sensitivity is not necessary in every case. Staphylococci, which cause 95% of canine pyodermas, have predictable antibiotic sensitivity so an empirical choice of antibiotic can be made. Culture and sensitivity is advisable when:

- Cytology reveals rods or filamentous bacteria, as their antibiotic susceptibility is unpredictable and often limited
- Empirical antibiotic therapy does not resolve the infection as expected
- There have been multiple antibiotic courses
- There are nodules or draining sinuses
- Infection is severe and potentially life-threatening.

Samples should be taken from intact or freshly ruptured pustules, avoiding chronic and excoriated lesions. Pustules can be ruptured using a sterile needle and the pus absorbed on to a sterile swab. Material can also be expressed from furuncles and sinus tracts. Biopsies are more likely to recover representative organisms from deep pyodermas, especially heavily scarred lesions. The swab should be placed in transport medium and dispatched to a diagnostic laboratory. The laboratory should be warned if a Gram-negative or anaerobic species is suspected as these may require special handling.

Swabbing the skin with alcohol will reduce the risk of contamination from surface organisms. This can, however, result in false negative cultures from superficial lesions if the alcohol penetrates the pustule or contacts the swab. Sufficient time is needed for the alcohol to evaporate prior to sampling.

Another swab or impression smear should be taken for cytology. This will help to determine which is the most important if several species of bacteria are cultured. The smear should be examined carefully for intracellular bacteria. These may be scarce, especially in deep pyodermas.

Most canine and feline pyodermas are caused by *Staphylococcus intermedius* and *S. felis*, respectively; if the species cannot be identified, coagulase production is a good indicator of pathogenic potential. Antibacterial sensitivity will be reported either as Kirby–Bauer disc data (resistant, sensitive or intermediate) or the minimum inhibitory concentration (MIC); if available, the MIC is preferred (see Chapter 25). Ideally, antibiotics should attain 8–10 times the MIC at the target tissue. Some laboratories now provide MIC data. The product literature should state the peak plasma level and concentrations in various tissues as a percentage of the plasma level. This can be used to calculate the appropriate antibiotic dose. For example:

- MIC = 0.05 μg/ml
- Target tissue concentration (8–10 x MIC) = 0.4–0.5 μg/ml
- Peak plasma level at 10 mg/kg dose = 0.3 μg/ml
- Skin concentration as a percentage of plasma = 80% = 0.24 μg/ml
- Dose required = 20 mg/kg

Other bacteria

Biopsy specimens from granulomas, sinuses and non-healing wounds should be submitted for culture of filamentous bacteria and mycobacteria. Careful use of alcohol prior to performing the biopsy will reduce contamination from faster growing species. Lidocaine can inhibit bacterial growth, so ring or nerve blocks remote from the biopsy site or general anaesthesia are preferred. Mycobacteria are particularly difficult to grow and samples should be submitted to a mycobacterial reference laboratory. Polymerase chain reaction (PCR) detection of mycobacterial DNA may become the preferred method in the future.

Skin scrapes

Skin scrapes are usually performed to find ectoparasites (Figure 24.10). Primary lesions at the predilection sites should be sampled, avoiding excoriated skin. Different parasites live at different levels within the skin and it is important to collect material from each layer. The technique for skin scraping is as follows:

1. Any hair is clipped with scissors without disrupting the skin surface.
2. Liquid paraffin is applied to the skin.
3. Skin is scraped with a no. 10 blade (no. 15 blades are useful for difficult sites, such as the feet and ears).
4. Scraping is continued until capillary oozing appears but too much blood should not be collected; it obscures the view, making parasites very difficult to see.
5. Apply the material to a slide. (Too much hair and debris makes it difficult to find anything, so the collected material should be divided if necessary.)
6. The material is mixed evenly into more liquid paraffin on the slide and a coverslip is applied.
7. All ectoparasites are visible with the 4X lens, which makes for quick scanning. One should look for movement and check any suspicious objects with the 10X lens if unsure.

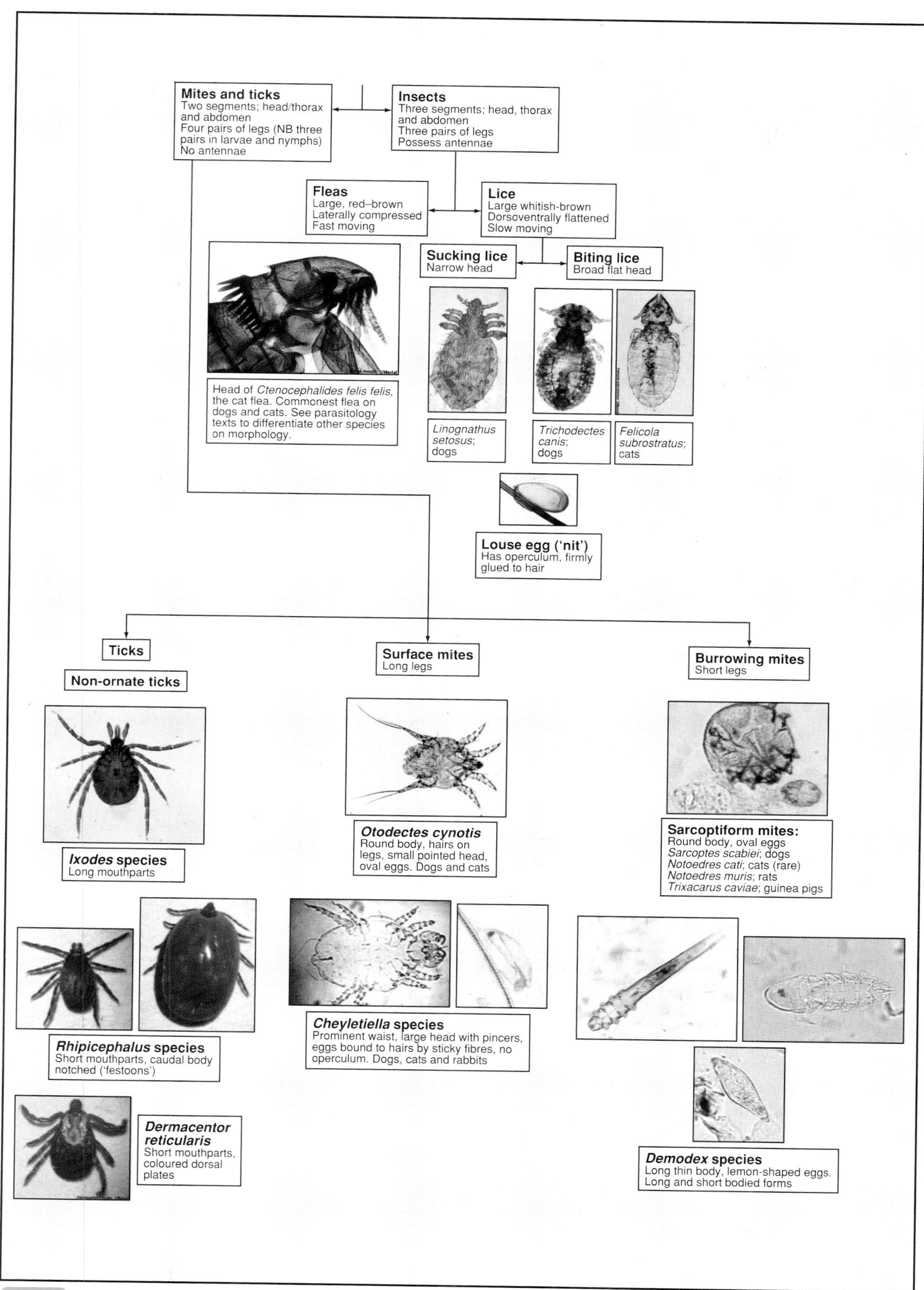

24.10 Ectoparasite identification key. This figure was produced with the assistance of Mérial Animal Health.

Potassium hydroxide* versus *liquid paraffin: Potassium hydroxide (KOH) is an alternative to liquid paraffin. It clears keratinaceous debris, making parasites easier to see, but it is caustic to the animal, humans and the microscope, and should be used with care. Nothing stronger than a 5% solution should be used on the skin but a drop of 10% or 20% KOH can be placed on the slide and gently warmed for 30–60 seconds to enhance clearing. This is lethal to mites, however, and the lack of movement can be a drawback. Mites will be alive and moving in a 5% solution but it takes up to 30 minutes to clear debris.

A 20% KOH solution can be mixed with material collected in liquid paraffin and left for 20–30 minutes to dissolve keratinaceous debris and the liquid paraffin. Using 20% KOH in 40% dimethyl sulphoxide, or after treatment with alcohol solvents, can aid removal of the oil. The solution is centrifuged, the supernatant is discarded and the pellet is transferred to a microscope slide. This method is time-consuming but has the advantage of concentrating material and avoids using KOH on the skin.

KOH should never be used near mucous membranes or delicate structures and the skin should be rinsed with water immediately after use.

Finding *Demodex*

Finding *Demodex* is usually straightforward provided that the scraping goes down to the dermis (i.e. capillary bleeding occurs). Squeezing the skin prior to scraping can force the mites out of the follicles on to the surface. Chronically inflamed, thickened skin can be difficult to scrape and hair plucks, material expressed from furuncles or even punch biopsies are more rewarding.

In clinical demodicosis there are usually large numbers of mites representing all stages of the life cycle. They are commensals, however, so one or two adults occasionally turn up as incidental findings. Clinical judgement is important; if necessary, the animal can be treated for demodicosis, the skin scrapes are repeated and any clinical improvement is carefully evaluated.

Repeated scrapes will help to assess the response to therapy. There should be an increasing ratio of dead and adult mites to live and immature mites. If not, the treatment regime should be re-evaluated and an underlying cause should be sought.

Finding *Sarcoptes*

Sarcoptes are not commensal, so any mites, eggs or faecal pellets are significant. Finding them can, however, be very difficult. Multiple scrapes should be taken from unexcoriated primary lesions (crusted papules) at the predilection sites (pinnal margins, elbows, hocks and ventral chest). Concentrating the collected material as above should be considered.

An enzyme-linked immunosorbent assay (ELISA) for specific anti-*Sarcoptes* IgG is a good alternative. The assay is very accurate, although false negatives (especially early on in the course of the disease) and false positives (particularly in atopic dogs sensitized to *Dermatophagoides* house dust mites) can occur. The pinnal scratch reflex (eliciting hind limb movements by rubbing the pinna against itself) has been shown to have good sensitivity and specificity. If all else fails, trial therapy with selamectin or amitraz should be tried.

Tape strips

Adhesive tape can be used to remove the outer layers of the stratum corneum and ectoparasites or microorganisms. Clear adhesive tape is applied repeatedly to the skin until skin debris is clearly stuck to it.

If one is looking for ectoparasites the tape is stuck to a microscope slide and examined with the 4X lens. Flea faeces (Figure 24.11), lice, *Cheyletiella*, *Otodectes* and their eggs are all easily seen. Short-tailed *Demodex*, which are more superficial, can also be found.

For cytology, the two ends of the tape are stuck to the slide to form a loop and then stained (Figure 24.12). Experimentation with locally available tape

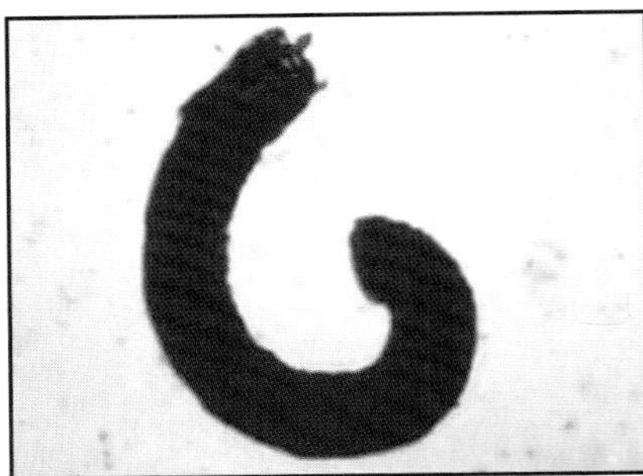

24.11 Flea faecal pellet. (Original magnification X100.) (© Peter J. Forsythe.)

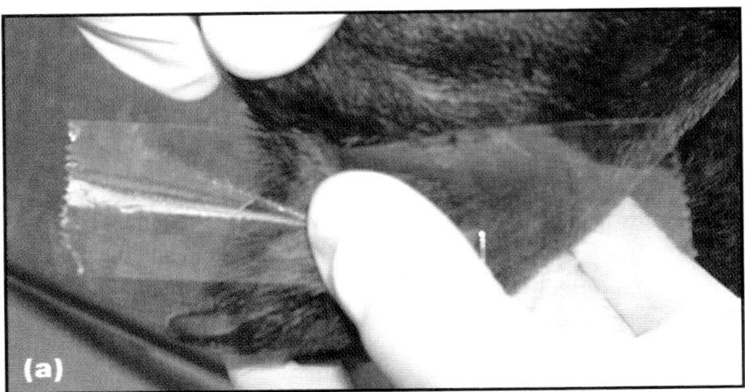

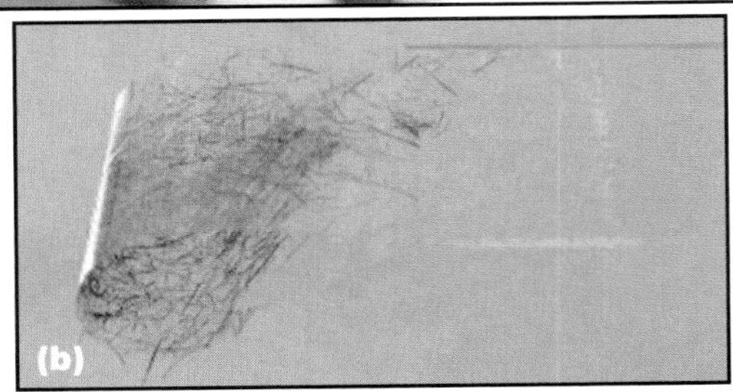

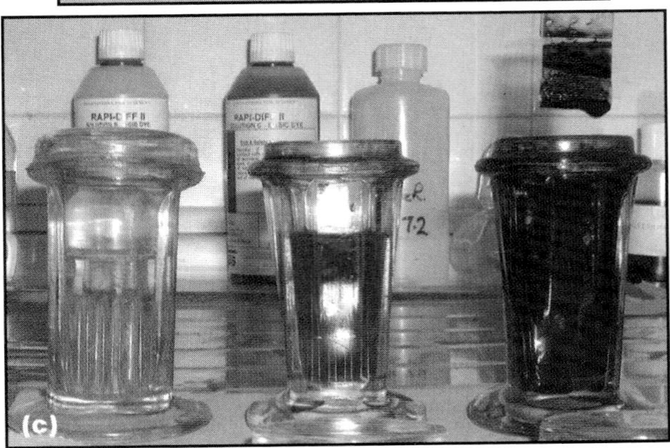

24.12 Tape strip cytology. (a) Tape-stripping from the skin. (b) Forming a loop on a microscope slide. (c) Staining with Diff-Quik.

and stains may be necessary, as not all are compatible. After rinsing, one end of the tape is detached and stuck down flat on to the slide. Any excess water is blotted. An alternative is to place a drop of the purple dye (Diff-Quik third pot) on a slide and stick the tape down over it. The slide is scanned with the 4X or 10X lens before examination of areas of interest with the 40X or 100X oil immersion lens. No cover slip is necessary. This is an excellent way to detect *Malassezia*, bacteria, inflammatory cells and exfoliated cells from eroded lesions, such as squamous cell carcinoma.

Cytology

Impression smears

Direct or indirect impression smears are especially useful for moist or seborrhoeic lesions that won't stick to adhesive tape. For direct smears a microscope slide is pressed firmly on to the lesions (ulcers, erosions, crusts, pustules, plaques, papules, nodules, sinus tracts). The surface is gently debrided to reveal representative cells first. Direct impression smears can also be made from the cut surfaces of excised lesions for quick identification of suspected tumours or inflammatory lesions (see Chapter 20).

Indirect smears are made using material collected by a swab or curette (Figure 24.13). The surface is debrided gently with the swab/curette and the harvested material transferred to a slide. A thin smear is made by rolling the swab on to the slide but great care must be taken to avoid rupturing the cells. Indirect smears are useful for more moist material and inaccessible areas of the skin (e.g. ears, feet).

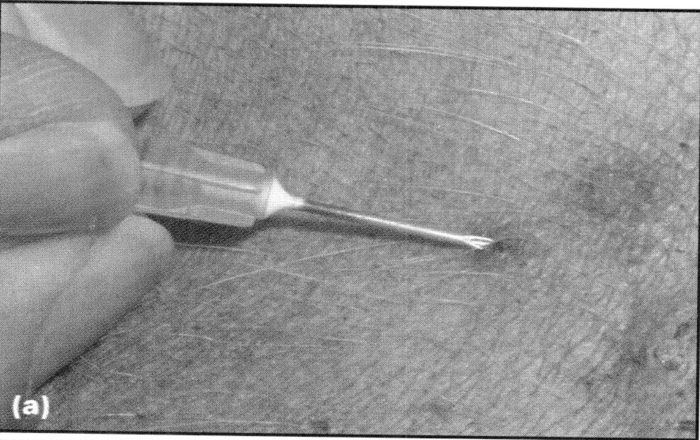

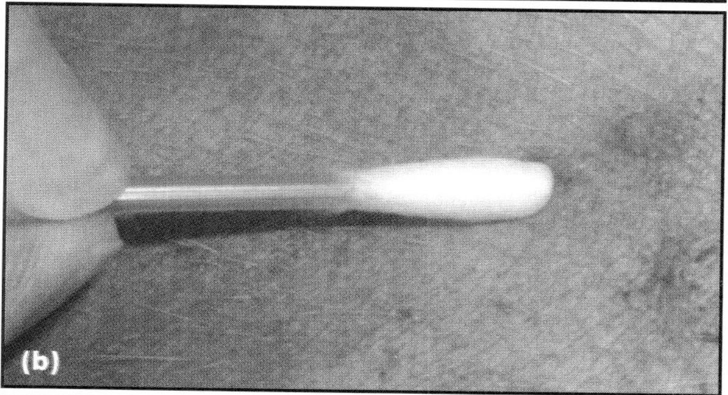

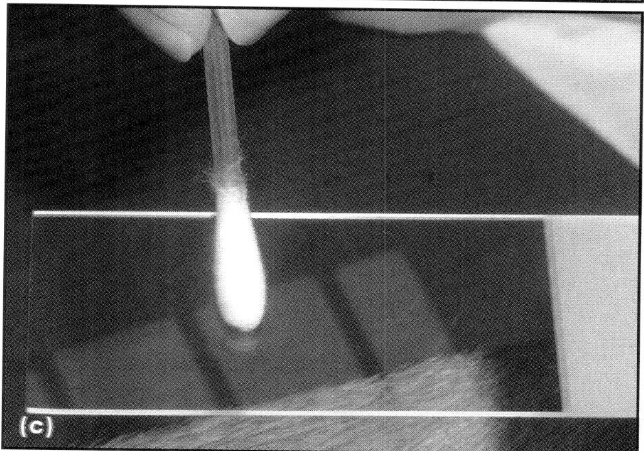

24.13 Impression smear from a pustule. (a) Rupture the pustule with a sterile needle. (b) Absorb the contents on to a swab. (c) Gently make a thin impression by rolling the swab on a microscope slide. Too much smearing will rupture the cells.

Fine needle aspirates

Fine needle aspirates (see Chapter 20) are a quick, cheap and minimally invasive way of investigating cutaneous masses and enlarged lymph nodes. They may only aspirate a few cells, however, which may not be representative and give no information about tissue architecture and invasiveness. Cytology is therefore a screening technique, not a replacement for biopsy and histopathology.

The technique for fine needle aspiration is as follows:

1. The hair over the site is clipped and the site is swabbed with alcohol.
2. The mass is fixed against the skin and a 21–23 gauge needle is inserted; larger needles recover more cells but cause more trauma and haemorrhage.
3. The needle is repositioned several times then withdrawn.
4. Firm lesions may need aspirating: a 2–10 ml syringe is attached to the needle, inserted into the lesion and the plunger pulled back. The needle is repositioned several times, the plunger is released and the needle is withdrawn. This harvests more cells but causes more trauma, damaged cells and haemorrhage.
5. A 2 ml syringe is filled with air, attached to the needle and the material in the needle hub is expressed on to a microscope slide. A second slide is used to make a smear (see Chapter 20). The aim is to make a cell monolayer without damaging the cells.
6. The slide is air-dried and fixed in methanol (or Diff-Quik fixative).
7. The slide can be sent to a cytologist or stained and interpreted in-house. Examining a duplicate slide and comparing one's findings to the cytologist's report is an excellent way to learn.

Interpretation of cytology preparations

An algorithm for interpreting cutaneous cytology is given in Figure 24.14 (see Chapter 20 for a more detailed discussion).

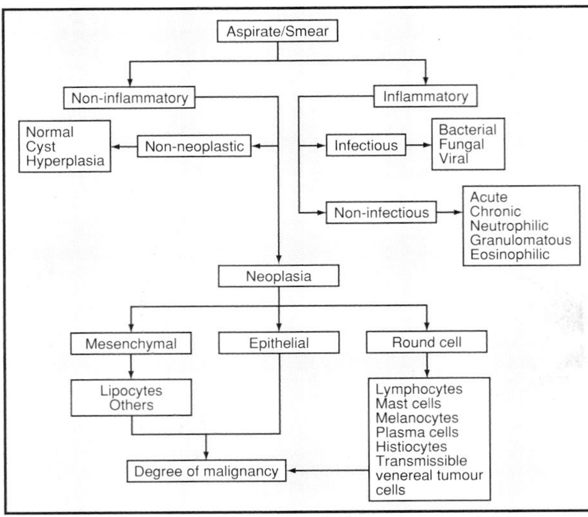

24.14 Algorithm for interpretation of cutaneous cytology.

Epithelial cell tumours: These have large, well defined cells with prominent cell adhesions (Figure 24.15). They aspirate well, forming sheets or gland-like arrangements. Glandular cells often have vacuolated cytoplasm.

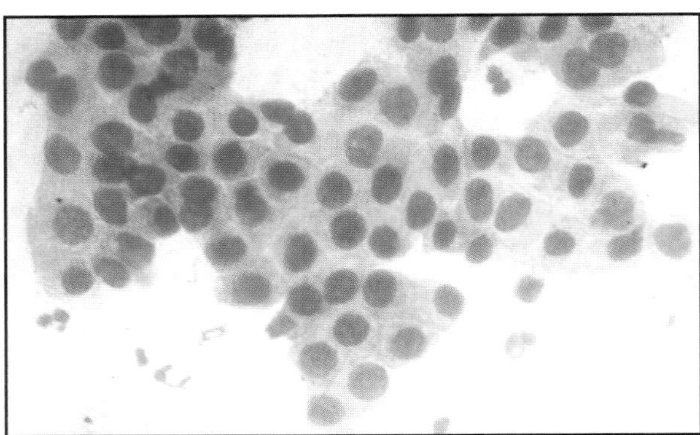

24.15 Epithelial cells from a feline ceruminous adenoma. (Diff-Quik stain; original magnification X400.)

Mesenchymal (spindle) cells: These are medium to large cells that aspirate poorly in unorganized clumps with no cell adhesions. They are spindle-shaped or irregular with poorly defined margins (Figure 24.16).

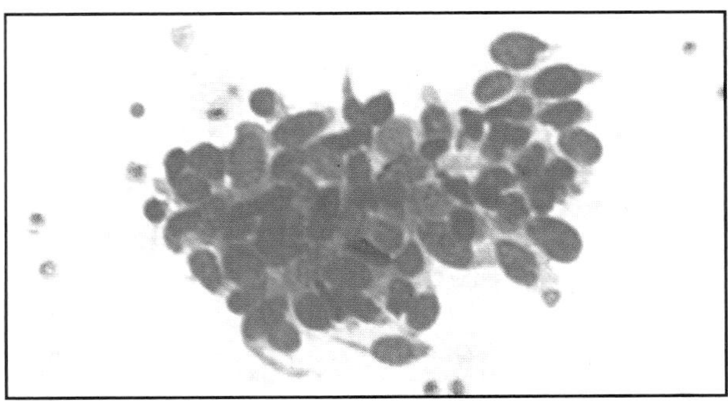

24.16 Spindle or mesenchymal cells from a rhabdomyosarcoma that metastasized to the skin. (Diff-Quik stain; original magnification X400.)

Round cell tumours: These exfoliate well as individual cells (Figure 24.17). They often have a distinct identity (e.g. lymphocytes, mast cells, plasma cells, monocytes, melanocytes).

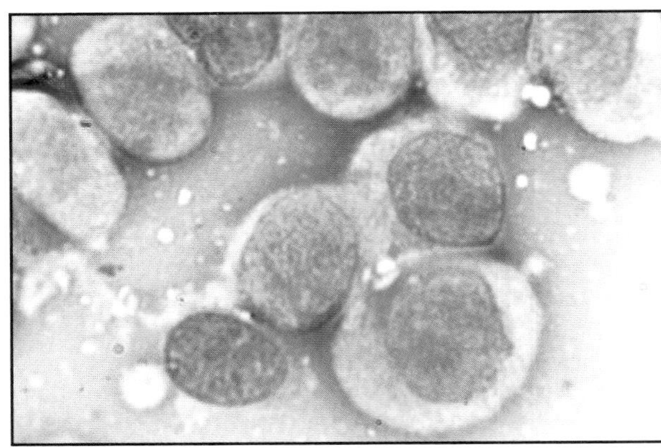

24.17 Round cells (histiocytes) from a histiocytoma in a young Boxer. (Rapi-Diff II stain; original magnification X1000.) (Courtesy of L Blackwood)

Lipomas: These are difficult to stain. The aspirate appears as oily drops on the slide that require heat fixing and thorough drying (Figure 24.18). Lipocytes form large, regular sheets of cells with prominent vacuoles and small, dark nuclei at the cell margin.

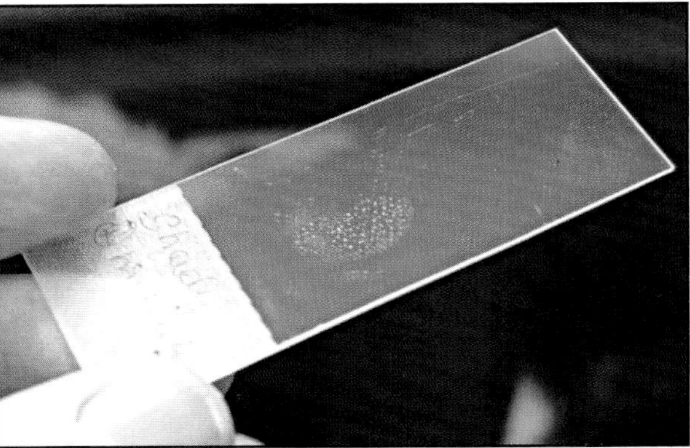

24.18 Fine needle aspirate from a lipoma, forming oily droplets on a microscope slide.

Malignancy: Malignancy should be considered as a sliding scale from highly aggressive, anaplastic tumours to benign, localized neoplasia. Features of malignancy are discussed in Chapter 20, and include:

- Increased nuclear to cytoplasmic ratio
- Variation in nuclear and cytoplasmic shape, size or staining
- Multiple or large nucleoli
- Multiple or abnormal mitotic figures
- Basophilic, granular cytoplasm
- Multinucleated and/or giant cells
- Anaplasia (i.e. lack of differentiation).

By convention, at least three features should be consistently present, but confirmation of malignancy is best carried out by an experienced cytologist.

Inflammatory lesions: See Figure 24.19. Characteristics of inflammatory lesions include:

- Mixed populations of neutrophils, eosinophils, lymphoid cells, monocytes/macrophages, epithelial cells and fibroblasts
- 70% or more granulocytes is suggestive of acute inflammation; 50% or more monocytes suggests chronic inflammation
- Reactive fibroblasts and epithelial cells may appear neoplastic; it is important to look at the whole picture
- Microorganisms. Free bacteria may be contaminants; ingested bacteria are more significant. Degenerate neutrophils (karyorrhexis; large, open, fragmenting nuclei) suggest infection whereas pyknotic (dark shrunken nuclei) non-degenerate neutrophils suggest sterile inflammation (Figure 24.20). All apparently non-infectious lesions should still be cultured
- Pyogranulomatous inflammation can be associated with less common bacterial and fungal infections: bluish staining hyphae suggest filamentous bacteria or a fungal mycetoma; thick-walled basophilic bodies suggest *Blastomyces* or *Cryptococcus* (with clear capsule); small, basophilic bodies with clear walls could be *Leishmania*, *Histoplasma* or *Sporothrix*. Mycobacteria rarely stain but can appear as clear, rod-shaped vacuoles in macrophages. This should be confirmed with a Ziehl–Neelsen stain
- Eosinophils suggest parasites, allergy, eosinophilic granuloma complex or foreign bodies (including free keratin and hair shafts in furunculosis) although a few can be found in almost any inflammatory dermatosis
- A few lymphocytes and plasma cells are often found in any inflammatory dermatosis but large numbers suggests neoplasia or lymphocytic–plasmacytic pododermatitis
- Acanthocytes are large, rounded and nucleated epidermal cells that are consistent with pemphigus foliaceus (Figure 24.21) although they can also occur in bacterial and fungal infections.

Skin biopsy

Skin biopsy is usually performed to obtain samples for histopathology or culture. Indications for biopsy include:

- Nodules and other possible neoplasia
- Ulcers
- Keratinization disorders
- Symmetrical alopecia with no obvious endocrine or metabolic cause
- Multifocal alopecia if skin scrapes and fungal culture prove negative
- Unexplained pigment changes
- Any suspected dermatosis that is most readily diagnosed by biopsy (e.g. sebaceous adenitis, follicular dysplasia or immune-mediated diseases)
- Unusual lesions or dermatoses
- Where a precise diagnosis is required for an accurate prognosis, suspect zoonosis or where treatment is expensive, long term or potentially hazardous.

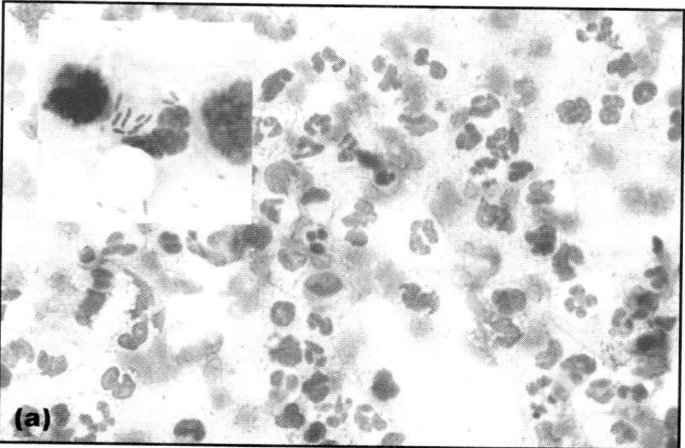

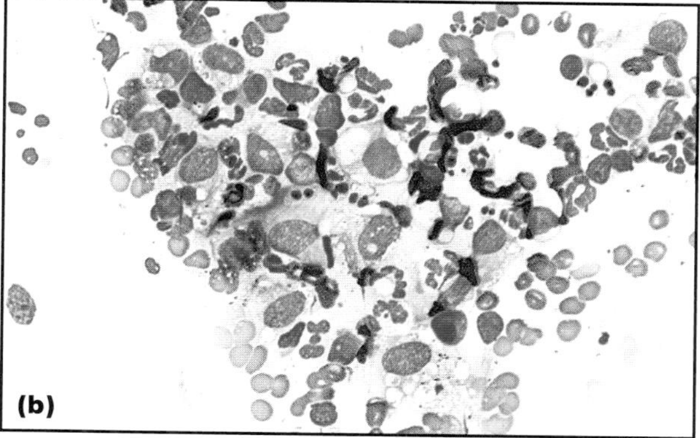

24.19 Inflammation. (a) Acute inflammation from a dog with otitis externa; note the preponderance of degenerate neutrophils. (b) Chronic inflammation in a dog with deep pyoderma; there is a mixture of neutrophils and macrophages. (Diff-Quik stain; (a) original magnification X400, inset X1000; (b) original magnification X400.)

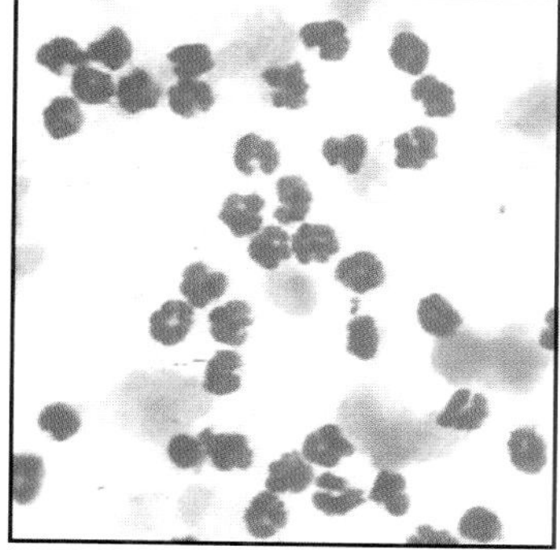

24.20 Non-degenerate neutrophils: note the shrunken, hypersegmented nuclei and cytoplasm. (Diff-Quik stain; original magnification X1000.) (Courtesy of E Villiers)

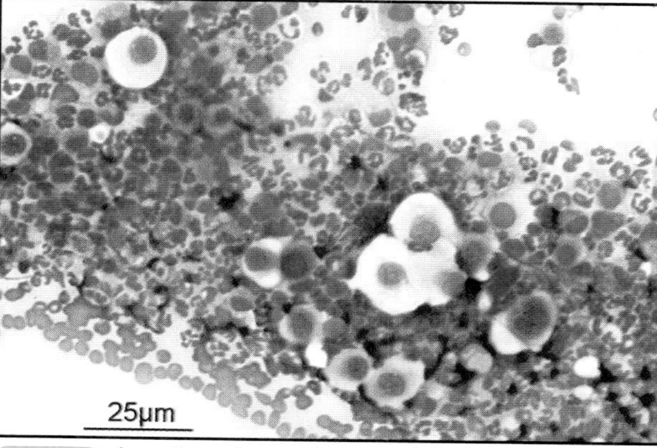

24.21 Acanthocytes and neutrophils in a smear from a pustule in a dog with pemphigus foliaceus. (Diff-Quik stain; original magnification X400.)

Glucocorticoid and other immunosuppressive therapy should be withdrawn and any secondary infection controlled prior to biopsy to avoid masking the pathological changes. In most dermatoses one should try to sample early lesions, such as pustules, vesicles and the leading edge of ulcers, avoiding chronic changes, infection, necrosis and excoriation. In contrast, endocrine or atrophic changes are most obvious in fully developed lesions. Selecting the right lesion takes some experience and if one is unsure a range of lesions should be sampled, including apparently healthy skin. There are a number of techniques that are used for different lesions and areas of the skin.

Punch biopsy

Punch biopsies are the quickest and easiest to perform. They are well suited to diffuse dermatoses but less so to ulcers and nodules as it is difficult to straddle the margin or encompass the lesion. Any lesions, such as pustules or papules, should be centred if possible, as, in processing, the biopsy specimen is sectioned through the centre. Punch biopsies only include the epidermis and dermis, not the subcutis.

Biopsy punches range from 4 to 8 mm diameter: 6 mm is most commonly used but 4 mm may be better in restricted sites, such as the face and feet; 4 mm punches only yield a small amount of skin and are more prone to shearing damage. Biopsies can be performed on most animals under light sedation and local anaesthesia. General anaesthesia is, however, preferred for sensitive sites where local anaesthesia is difficult.

Any hair is clipped with scissors without disturbing the skin surface. Some dermatologists advocate lightly swabbing the site with alcohol; others prefer not to disturb the skin at all, although an alcohol swab should be used before taking a biopsy sample for culture. A circle is drawn around the biopsy site in indelible pen and the subcutis is infiltrated with 1 ml of 2% lidocaine (without adrenaline to avoid inducing changes in the cutaneous blood flow). Inserting the needle outside the circle (Figure 24.22) will ensure that the biopsy specimen will not have a needle track through it. The biopsy punch is pressed firmly against the skin and rotated in one direction. Rotating the punch from side to side can cause separation of the epidermis and dermis. A cocktail stick, bent needle or fine forceps is used to lift the base clear and it is cut free. Grasping the biopsy itself will cause crush artefacts. If the biopsy specimen is firmly attached to the underlying tissues (e.g. on the ear pinna) one end should be grasped and it can be dissected free carefully.

Any blood is very gently blotted up and the biopsy specimen subcutis is placed down on a piece of card. A circle with an arrow through to indicate the direction of hair growth is drawn on the other end of the card. This helps the pathologist to section the sample along the length of the hair follicles. Alternatively a line can be drawn on the skin such that it is included in the biopsy specimen to indicate how the hairs lie. The completed biopsy specimen is placed in 10% formalin as quickly as possible and the skin is closed with tissue adhesive or a single suture. Where there is a risk of deforming the tissues (e.g. ear pinna) any haemorrhage should be controlled and the area is allowed to heal by secondary intention. Biopsy specimens for culture should be submitted fresh or with a single drop of saline to prevent drying in transit; the laboratory's preference should be checked. It is important to include full clinical details, the differential diagnosis and the biopsy sites on the submission form. Each biopsy specimen is submitted in a separate, clearly labelled pot to avoid any confusion. Most pathologists will read the biopsy specimen first, then the clinical history and re-evaluate their findings if the two are incompatible.

Complications are rare, although care should be exercised in animals with bleeding disorders, poor wound healing or immunosuppression. Lidocaine should be used with caution in very small or young animals and those with cardiac disease, seizures or receiving monoamine oxidase inhibitors (e.g. amitraz).

Wedge (incisional or excisional) biopsy

Scalpel blades can be used to take wedge-shaped biopsy specimens of varying size. If the whole lesion can be included then it is an excisional biopsy, if not it is incisional. In many situations, especially soft tissue sarcomas, attempting excisional biopsy can make future therapy more difficult, and have a detrimental effect on prognosis. With tumours, an excisional biopsy should not be regarded as the definitive surgery until the pathologist is satisfied the margins are adequate. If necessary the surgical site will have to be excised.

Wedge biopsies are useful for deeper lesions (e.g. subcutaneous fat, pads), where closure of a circular punch could deform tissues (e.g. nasal planum) and focal lesions, such as ulcers, where the active margin is of interest. The principles are otherwise similar to taking a punch biopsy except that it is often difficult to

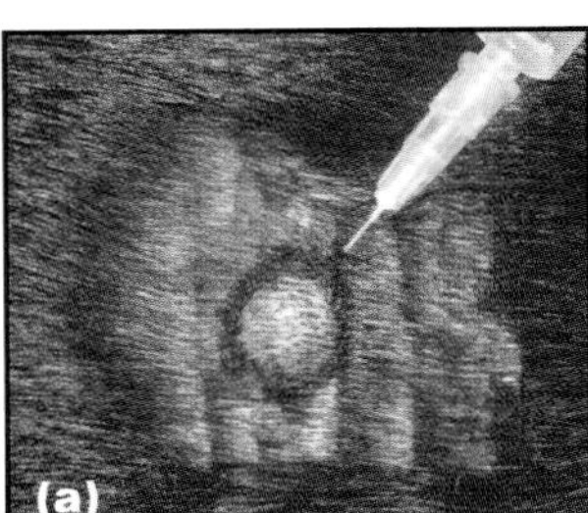

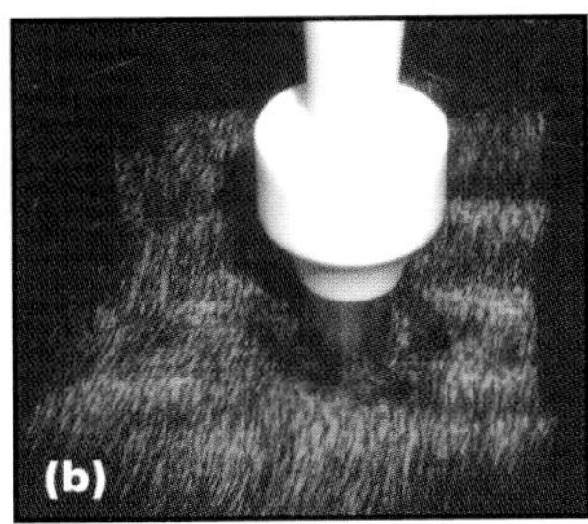

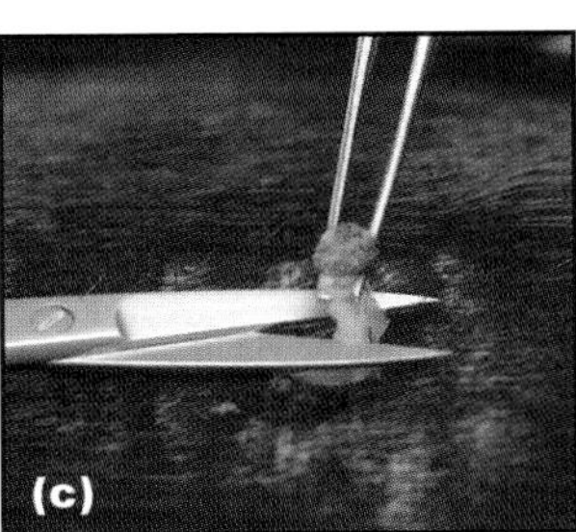

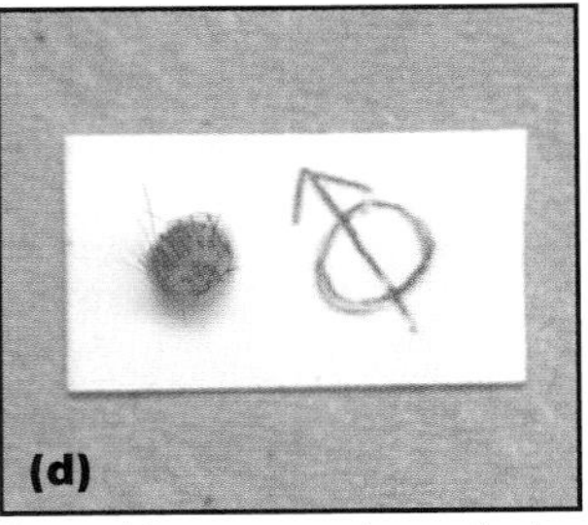

24.22 Performing a punch biopsy. (a) Infiltrate the skin with local anaesthetic. (b) Press a 6 mm biopsy punch against the skin and rotate in one direction. (c) Dissect free from the underlying tissues; note that the specimen is grasped below the skin itself. (d) Place on a piece of card, indicating the direction of hair growth, and fix in 10% neutral buffered formalin.

block these sites and local anaesthetic injected into subcutaneous tissues will distort them. A ring block, regional nerve block or general anaesthesia should be used instead.

Phalanx III (PIII) amputation

Most non-traumatic or infectious claw diseases are caused by lesions in the germinal tissues (nail bed) deep to the claw fold. It is impossible to perform a biopsy here by conventional means. PIII amputation is an invasive but effective technique that heals with minimal effect on function and appearance. It is a surgical procedure involving entry into a joint, however, and requires full asepsis. Dew claws (digit I) are preferred if present but, if not, digits II and V are the least weight bearing. A digit is chosen that is likely to give a diagnosis; affected claws without sloughing or secondary infection are best. An alternative technique that preserves PIII is described. A sharp 8 mm biopsy punch is used to strip off the lateral claw and underlying corium into the nail bed. This is difficult to master and, in the author's hands, often leads to fracture and tissue separation.

Allergy tests

Allergy tests should only be used to identify allergens for avoidance or specific immunotherapy in animals that have a clinical diagnosis of atopic dermatitis or rhinitis. They are not diagnostic for atopic disease, as positive tests can occur in healthy animals and clinically atopic animals can be persistently negative. Intradermal tests and serology both have a number of advantages and disadvantages. Most veterinary dermatologists prefer intradermal allergen tests (IDATs), which test the capacity of allergens to trigger a reaction in the skin. Serum IgE, in contrast, does not necessarily correlate with IgE levels in the skin. Intradermal tests, however, are time-consuming, require sedation and clipping, and cannot be performed on lichenified, hyperpigmented or inflamed skin. The allergens are expensive to maintain.

Intradermal allergen tests

Allergens should be selected for their local relevance by consulting botany texts, pollen charts, local dermatologists and allergists. They should be obtained from a reputable supplier that standardizes and validates the product. Allergens can be obtained in concentrated form, that requires regular dilution to testing strength, or ready diluted, although the latter have a short shelf-life. Experience with one source is important as there are differences between allergen extracts. Single allergens are preferred to mixes that may not contain the relevant allergens in sufficient concentration to elicit a reaction.

Sedation or anaesthesia will prevent struggling and reduce stress. Most dermatologists use xylazine, medetomidine or propofol in dogs, and ketamine or medetomidine/ketamine combinations in cats. The animal is placed in lateral recumbency. A patch on the chest is clipped gently but the skin is not prepared in any way; 0.05 ml of the positive control (0.01% histamine), negative control (buffered saline) and each allergen solution are injected into the dermis. Positive reactions, marked by erythema and swelling, are evident by 15–20 minutes (Figure 24.23). There are two ways to assess these:

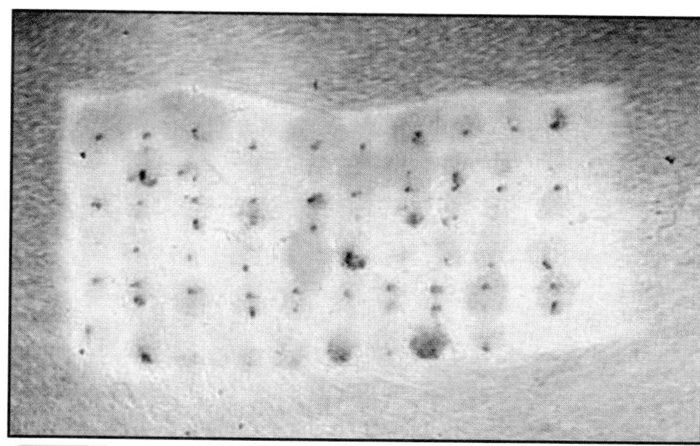

24.23 Multiple positive reactions to house dust mites and pollens in an atopic Shar Pei. Positive reactions are identified by erythema and swelling.

- Scores of 0 and 4 are assigned to the negative and positive control sites, respectively. The test sites are compared subjectively relative to these two; 2+ is considered positive
- The diameters of the negative and positive control sites are measured. A positive reaction is one with a diameter greater than the mean of these two values.

The clinical significance of late phase (6 hours) and delayed reactions (24 hours) is unclear. Pruritus at the test sites can be managed with topical emollients or glucocorticoids. Anaphylaxis is very rare.

False positive reactions can occur with irritant or contaminated allergen solutions, poor technique and trauma, dermatographism or urticaria. False negative reactions may result from out-of-date allergens, subcutaneous injections, stress and recent administration of anti-inflammatory drugs. Suggested withdrawal times prior to IDAT are:

- Antihistamines: 2 weeks
- Topical, oral or short-acting glucocorticoids: 3 weeks
- Depot glucocorticoids: 6–8 weeks
- Progestogens: 6–8 weeks.

Animals that have been on prolonged treatment may need considerably longer withdrawal times. Ciclosporin, essential fatty acids (EFAs) and high EFA diets do not appear to have a significant effect.

IDATs obviously require some experience in technique and interpretation. In particular, IDATs in cats are more difficult to perform than in dogs, as their skin is thinner and the reactions less obvious. Fluorescein (5 mg/kg i.v.) and UV light have been used to enhance recognition of positive reactions.

Serology

Serology is quicker and easier to perform than IDAT. It is also less vulnerable to prior anti-inflammatory therapy. There is, however, still some question over the specificity and sensitivity compared to IDATs. Polyclonal anti-IgE reagents can also detect IgG, leading to poor specificity. Monoclonal reagents are more specific but may be less sensitive. The most specific reagent is a recombinant high affinity IgE receptor molecule (FcεRIα; Allercept® detection system). The result of this test closely matches those of IDAT, although it may be slightly less sensitive for house dust mites and slightly more sensitive for pollens. As most cases of atopic dermatitis are sensitized to house dust mite allergens, IDATs are preferred but serology is useful in cases where an IDAT is not possible.

A screening test (E-Screen®) has recently been introduced. This is designed for rapid in-house detection of allergen specific IgE. Because it uses mixed allergens, however, it is useless for diagnosis or allergen selection. Its value is that its results closely match those from the full (and more expensive) Allercept® screen. Sera from animals with a positive test can be submitted for a full panel. Animals with a negative test should be referred for an IDAT, since approximately half of these will have a positive result.

Adverse food reactions

Serological tests for food allergens are also available. However, little information has been published about their usefulness and data comparing the results of commercially available tests to properly controlled food trials and provocation are lacking. A food trial with novel ingredients for at least 6 weeks, followed by provocative testing, remains the only reliable way to diagnose adverse food reactions.

Allergic contact dermatitis and patch tests

Allergic contact dermatitis (Figure 24.24) is uncommon and difficult to diagnose. Suspected cases can be hospitalized for 5–10 days on plain cotton or newspaper. The kennel should be thoroughly rinsed with water after cleaning, ceramic bowls should be used and the animal should be exercised on paved areas. If there is an improvement, patch testing can be used to identify the offending allergens.

The animal is sedated, the lateral chest is clipped and any suspected allergens are applied. These can be fixed in place using Opsite adhesive dressing or Finn chambers. Liquids can be absorbed on to gauze swabs or suspended in petroleum jelly. Blanks should be included as negative controls. The site should be covered for 48–72 hours. It is usually necessary to hospitalize the animal, bandage the feet and use an Elizabethan collar to prevent self-trauma. Positive reactions are marked by erythema and swelling. Patch testing kits for humans contain a wide variety of potential allergens but have not been validated in animals.

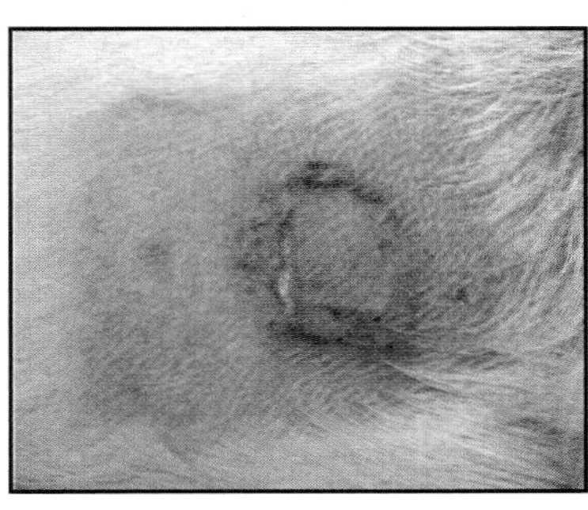

24.24 Contact reaction to an adhesive bandage in a dog.

Miscellaneous tests

Immune-mediated skin disease

Nearly 100% of systemic lupus erythematosus (SLE) cases have positive anti-nuclear antibody (ANA) titres. (The criteria for diagnosis of SLE are summarized in Chapter 22.) Positive titres, however, only support a clinical diagnosis of SLE as they are also seen in infectious diseases (especially *Leishmania* infection), neoplasia, other immune-mediated or inflammatory diseases and healthy animals. Other tests that may be used to demonstrate systemic involvement include the Coombs' test and anti-platelet antibody, rheumatoid factor and urinary protein assays. Cold agglutinin titres can be found in cases of cold agglutinin disease.

The pattern of antibody deposition and/or distribution of T-cell subsets can be used to support the diagnosis of immune-mediated diseases such as pemphigus, bullous pemphigoid, SLE, vasculitis, alopecia areata and others. Certain direct immunofluorescence studies can be performed on formalin-fixed sections, whilst others require Michel's medium or frozen tissues. If considering these tests the laboratory requirements should be checked first. Indirect immunofluorescence tests, using the patient's serum, are rarely performed in veterinary medicine except for research purposes, but they may become more widely available in the future.

Analysis of blood and urine

Routine haematology, biochemistry and urinalysis are not indicated in most dermatological conditions but may show:

- Abnormalities in certain endocrinopathies and metabolic conditions (see Chapters 16, 17 and 18)
- Neutrophilia in infection and inflammation
- Eosinophilia in hypersensitivity and parasitism.

Haematology and biochemistry may also be required for monitoring of animals that are undergoing immunosuppressive treatment. Other useful tests include:

- Feline immunodeficiency virus (FIV) and feline leukaemia virus (FeLV) testing in cats with recurrent pyoderma and other unusual dermatoses
- Serology to detect antibodies to *Sarcoptes*, *Leishmania*, *Cryptococcus* and *Aspergillus*.

Antibodies to infectious organisms do not necessarily indicate active infection unless rising titres are demonstrated. Polymerase chain reactions (PCRs) to amplify and detect microbial DNA are a specific and sensitive alternative for *Leishmania*, *Borrelia*, *Bartonella*, *Ehrlichia* and *Babesia* species (see Chapter 27). DNA can be detected in affected tissues, bone marrow aspirates and EDTA blood. Virus isolation is not commonly performed in dermatology but may be helpful if herpesvirus, calicivirus, poxviruses (cowpox or guinea pig orthopoxviruses) or papillomavirus are suspected. PCRs can also be used to identify the latter.

Sex hormone assays

Assays are available for a variety of sex hormones but the wide variation in normal ranges means that baseline levels are unhelpful in sex hormone dermatoses. Increased 17-hydroxyprogesterone post-ACTH administration can, however, be seen in cases of adrenal sex hormone imbalance.

Faecal examination

Faecal examination is not commonly performed in skin cases. It may, however, reveal fleas, lice and *Cheyletiella* in pruritic animals, hookworms in hookworm pododermatitis, or other endoparasites. Forage mites contaminating foodstuffs may also be ingested. Undigested food may be present in malabsorption syndromes associated with adverse food reactions and keratinization disorders. Identifying pollen grains in faeces may be useful in determining pollen exposure.

Diascopy

For differentiation of macular erythema from petechiae or ecchymoses a glass slide is pressed firmly against the skin. Erythema, caused by hyperaemia, will blanch, whilst haemorrhaged red blood cells will not.

Otoscopes and examination of the ears

Otoscopic examination is mandatory in any animal with otitis. The types of otoscope available are discussed in Figure 24.25. Gently pulling the pinna laterally and ventrally straightens the ear canals and allows access to the horizontal ear canal. One should not persist in fractious animals; struggling prevents a proper examination and can lead to injury. It is much better to sedate or anaesthetize these patients and flush out any obstructing debris if necessary. Careful examination will identify foreign bodies, *Otodectes*, inflammatory changes, ulceration, stenosis, condition of the tympanic membrane, amount and type of exudate, and chronic changes. Probing with a urinary catheter or feeding tube can assess the integrity of the tympanic membrane but it is important to be gentle! The tympanic membrane can heal, trapping infection in the middle ear. A taut, translucent grey–white appearance (Figure 24.26) is normal but myringotomy (the deliberate rupture of the tympanic membrane) should be considered if it appears opaque, discoloured or bulging. Under anaesthesia, the external ear canal is cleaned, then the otoscope cone is changed and the caudoventral portion of the membrane is pierced with a sterile spinal needle. ENT swabs (with small tips mounted on wire) are used to collect samples, the first for bacterial culture and sensitivity and the second for cytology. If the ear is kept free from infection the tympanic membrane should heal with 21–35 days.

Type	Features, advantages and disadvantages
Closed	Good view, limited access, can perform tympanometry
Open or operating	Slightly inferior view, excellent access, best choice if you are limited to one otoscope
Video otoscope	Excellent view and access, can record images
Rigid endoscope	Good view of deeper structures, reasonable access, prone to blockage by debris

24.25 Types of otoscope.

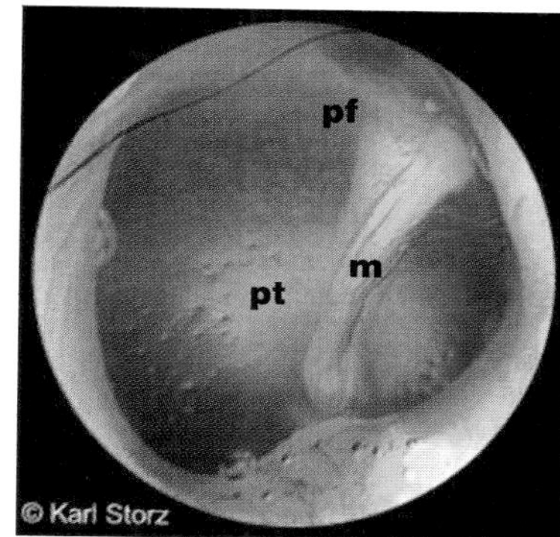

24.26 A normal tympanic membrane seen through a video otoscope. Note the taut and translucent pars tensa (pt), the dorsal, fleshy pars flaccida (pf) and the C-shaped manubrium (m) of the malleus. (© Karl Storz Endoscopy (UK) Ltd.)

Tympanometry

This is a technique using pressure to assess the integrity of the tympanic membrane and the contents of the middle ear. A closed head diagnostic or video otoscope is inserted into the ear to create a seal between the cone and ear canal. Air is introduced gently into the ear through the appropriate channel. A normal tympanic membrane should flex back and forth; abnormal rigidity, bulging or rupture indicates a diseased membrane and otitis media. Tympanometry is, however, a difficult technique to master and interpret.

Otic cytology

Samples are usually taken from ears to identify parasites or cells and microorganisms (Figures 24.27–24.29). They are collected after an initial otoscopic examination but before cleaning. A cotton bud is inserted down to the junction between the vertical and horizontal ear canals. The bud is rotated to collect debris then this is transferred to a slide with some liquid paraffin. A coverslip is applied and the slide is examined under low (4X objective) power. *Otodectes*, *Demodex*, their eggs and plant debris are easily visible. A second dry swab should be collected in the same way but the end is rolled gently on a microscope slide. The smear is air-dried or heat-fixed and stained in Diff-Quik. Otic cytology findings are discussed in Figures 24.27–24.29.

Finding	Appearance	Significance
Neutrophils (Figure 24.28)	Polymorphic nucleus and pale cytoplasm	Associated with infection, inflammation and ulceration (also see red blood cells)
	Large nucleus, open and disrupted chromatin pattern (karyorrhexis). Often see nuclear streaming	Degenerate (or toxic) neutrophils; a good indication of infection
	Dark, shrunken nucleus (pyknosis). Nuclear streaming uncommon	Non-degenerate neutrophils; an indication of sterile inflammation
	Intracytoplasmic bacteria	Definite indicator of infection rather than bacterial contamination
Bacteria (Figure 24.28)	Small cocci, often in groups. Blue to purple stain	Staphylococci; low numbers probably normal in most dogs, larger numbers suggest bacterial overgrowth and otitis. More serious infections associated with neutrophils
	Small, short rods; stain purple–red. Usually with degenerate neutrophils	Gram-negative rods, usually *Pseudomonas*
Red blood cells	Small, round anucleate cells	Haemorrhage, associated with trauma and ulceration
Keratinocytes (Figure 24.29)	Large flat and angular. Stain pale blue to pale purple. May have melanin or keratohyaline granules. Occasionally nucleated	Shed keratinocytes; normal
	Large trapezoid to cigar shapes. Stain deep purple–blue	Rolled keratinocytes; normal
	Large flat, angular to round, nucleated cells. Stain deep purple–blue	Acanthocytes; pemphigus foliaceus but also seen in severe bacterial infections
Malassezia (Figure 24.29)	Large ovoid to budding yeasts	Low numbers (<5 per high power field) probably normal in most dogs; larger numbers suggest *Malassezia* otitis

24.27 Otic cytology findings and their significance.

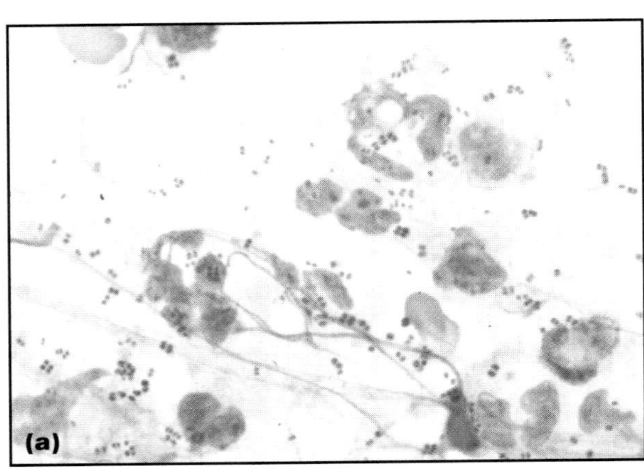

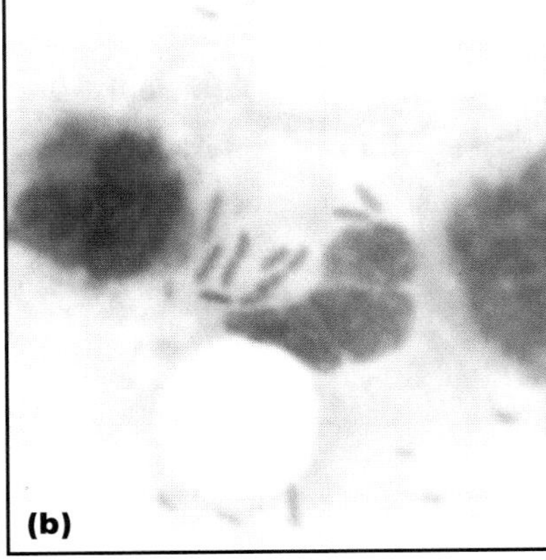

24.28 Numerous extra- and intracellular *Staphylococcus* (a), *Pseudomonas aeruginosa* (b) and degenerate neutrophils. Note the nuclear streaming from ruptured nuclei. (Diff-Quik stain; original magnification (a) X400, (b) X1000.)

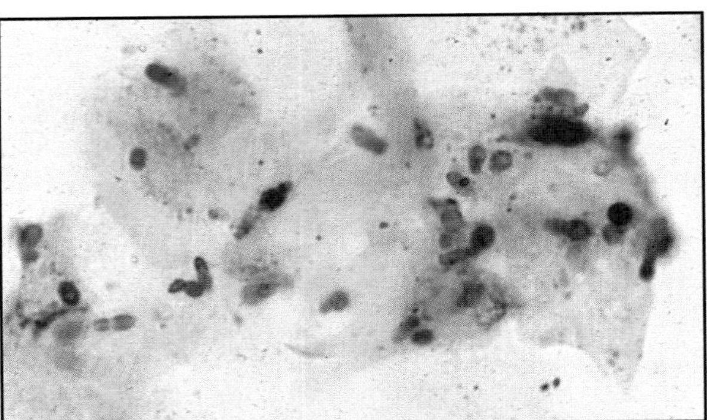

24.29 Oval and budding *Malassezia* yeasts overlying pale staining, angular keratinocytes. (Diff-Quik stain; original magnification X400.) Large numbers of *Malassezia* organisms, as seen here, suggest pathogenic significance (see Figure 24.27).

Further reading

Angus JC and Campbell KL (2001) Uses and indications for video-otoscopy in small animal practice. *Veterinary Clinics of North America: Small Animal Practice* **31,** 809–828

Barton CL (1987) Cytological diagnosis of cutaneous neoplasia – an algorithmic approach. *Compendium on Continuing Education for the Practicing Veterinarian* **9,** 20–33

Bowman DD, Eberhard ML and Lynn RC (2003) *Georgi's Parasitology for Veterinarians, 8th edn.* WB Saunders, Philadelphia

Curtis CF (2001) Evaluation of a commercially available enzyme-linked immunosorbant assay for the diagnosis of canine sarcoptic mange. *Veterinary Record* **148,** 238–239.

DeBoer DJ and Hillier A (2001a) The ACVD task force on canine atopic dermatitis (XV): fundamental concepts in clinical diagnosis. *Veterinary Immunology and Immunopathology* **81,** 271–276

DeBoer DJ and Hillier A (2001b) The ACVD task force on canine atopic dermatitis (XVI): laboratory evaluation of dogs with atopic dermatitis with serum-based 'allergy' tests. *Veterinary Immunology and Immunopathology* **81,** 277–287

Dunn J and Villiers E (1998) General principles of cytological interpretation. *In Practice* **20,** 429–437

Foster AP and Foil CS (2003) *BSAVA Manual of Small Animal Dermatology, 2nd edn.* BSAVA, Gloucester

Foster AP, Knowles TG, Moore AH, Cousins PDG, Day MJ and Hall EJ (2003) Serum IgE and IgG responses to food antigens in normal and atopic dogs, and dogs with gastrointestinal disease. *Veterinary Immunology and Immunopathology* **92,** 113–124

Foster AP, Littlewood JD, Webb P, Wood JLN, Rogers K and Shaw SE (2003) Comparison of intradermal and serum testing for allergen-specific IgE using a Fc epsilon RI alpha-based assay in atopic dogs in the UK. *Veterinary Immunology and Immunopathology* **93,** 51–60

Fraser MA, Caulton E and McNeil PE (2001) Examination of faecal samples as a method of identifying pollen exposure in dogs. *Veterinary Record* **149**, 424–426.

Hill PB (1999) Diagnosing cutaneous food allergies in dogs and cats - some practical considerations. *In Practice* **21,** 287–294

Hill PB (2002) *Small Animal Dermatology.* Butterworth Heinemann, Edinburgh.

Hillier A and DeBoer DJ (2001) The ACVD task force on canine atopic dermatitis (XVII): intradermal testing. *Veterinary Immunology and Immunopathology* **81,** 289–304

Ikonomopoulos J, Kokotas S, Gazouli M, Zavras A, Stoitsiou M and Gorgoulis VG (2003) Molecular diagnosis of leishmaniosis in dogs. Comparative application of traditional diagnostic methods and the proposed assay on clinical samples. *Veterinary Parasitology* **113,** 99–113

Kadoya-Minegishi M, Park SJ, Sekiguchi M, Nishifuji K, Momoi Y and Iwasaki T (2002) The use of fluorescein as a contrast medium to enhance intradermal skin tests in cats. *Australian Veterinary Journal* **80,** 702–703

Kipar A, Schiller I and Baumgartner W (2003) Immunopathological studies on feline cutaneous and (muco)cutaneous mycobacteriosis. *Veterinary Immunology and Immunopathology* **91,** 169–182

Malik R, Hunt GB, Goldsmid SE, Martin P, Wigney DI and Love DN (1994) Diagnosis and treatment of pyogranulmatous panniculitis due to *Mycobacterium smegmatis* in cats. *Journal of Small Animal Practice* **35,** 524–530

Morris DO (1999) *Malassezia* dermatitis and otitis. *Veterinary Clinics Of North America: Small Animal Practice* **29,** 1303–1310

Mueller RS (1999) Diagnosis and management of canine claw diseases. *Veterinary Clinics of North America: Small Animal Practice* **29,** 1357–1366

Mueller RS and Olivry T (1999) Onychobiopsy without onychectomy: description of a new biopsy technique for canine claws. *Veterinary Dermatology* **10,** 55–59

Nuttall TJ (2001) Current concepts in the diagnosis and management of canine atopic dermatitis. *In Practice* **23,** 442–452

Reedy LM, Miller WH and Willemse T (1997) *Allergic skin diseases of dogs and cats, 2nd edn.* W.B. Saunders, Philadelphia

Rosser EJ (1999) Advances in the diagnosis and treatment of atopy. *Veterinary Clinics Of North America: Small Animal Practice* **29,** 1437–1448

Scott DW, Miller WH and Griffin CE (2001) Diagnostic methods. In: *Muller and Kirk's Small Animal Dermatology, 6th edn,* pp. 71–206. WB Saunders, Philadelphia

Van Custem J and Rochette F (1991) *Mycoses in domestic animals.* Janssen Research Foundation, Beerse

Villiers E and Dunn J (1998) Collection and preparation of smears for cytological examination. *In Practice* **20,** 370–377

Wassom DL and Grieve RB (1998) *In vitro* measurement of canine and feline IgE: a review of Fc epsilon R1 alpha-based assays for detection of allergen-reactive IgE. *Veterinary Dermatology* **9,** 173–178

25

Diagnosis of bacterial, fungal and mycobacterial diseases

Tim Jagger

Introduction

Sampling for bacterial and, to a lesser extent, fungal and mycobacterial diseases, is common in veterinary practice. This chapter will review sampling procedures and the interpretation of results, including the significance of bacterial and mycotic isolates at different anatomical sites. For reasons of safety and expertise, most veterinary practices submit samples to veterinary laboratories. Laboratory methodology is included only where it promotes an understanding of the significance of the results obtained, for example in antibacterial susceptibility testing. Comments apply to both dogs and cats unless otherwise stated.

Direct microscopy

Direct microscopy of smears from pathological lesions and fluids is a useful but underutilized initial investigative tool. The goals of direct microscopy are:

- To detect bacteria and other microorganisms
- To determine bacterial morphology (and Gram staining characteristics)
- To identify any inflammatory response
- To predict the identification of the microorganisms detected
- To direct antimicrobial therapy pending the results of bacterial and other cultures.

Suitable samples include:

- Impression smears from cutaneous lesions or tissue biopsy specimens
- Smears from swabs of aural, vaginal or nasal discharges
- Direct smears from turbid peritoneal or pleural fluids and abscess material
- Concentrated sediment smears from urine, bronchoalveolar lavages, prostatic washes, and cellular cerebrospinal fluid (CSF) (see Chapters 10, 20, 21 and 23).

Staining techniques

The stains of choice for bacteria are Romanowsky stains (e.g. Leishman's and modified Wright–Giemsa) and the Gram stain. Pink-staining Gram-negative bacteria are often hard to visualize against background material (Figure 25.1). Bacteria are generally easier to visualize with Romanowsky stains as both Gram-negative and Gram-positive bacteria stain uniformly dark blue (Figures 25.2–25.5). Rapid Romanowsky stains, such as Diff-Quik, are not ideal as there is little contrast between the bacteria and background material. Stain precipitate, which is more common with this type of stain, can also easily be mistaken for bacteria.

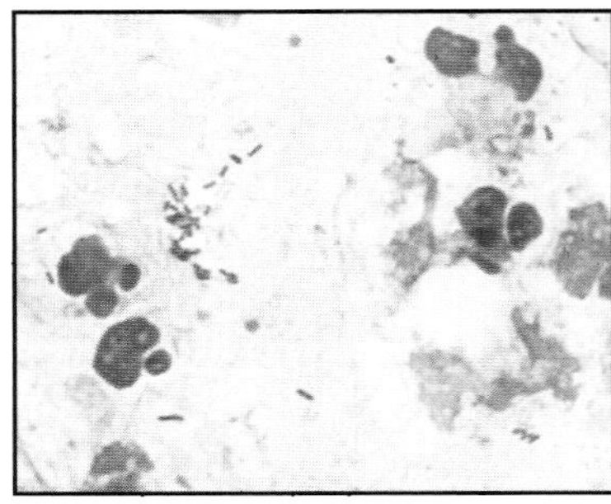

25.1 Nasal flush from a cat. *Pasteurella multocida*: Gram-negative bacilli stain pink against a pink background. (Gram stain; original magnification X1000.)

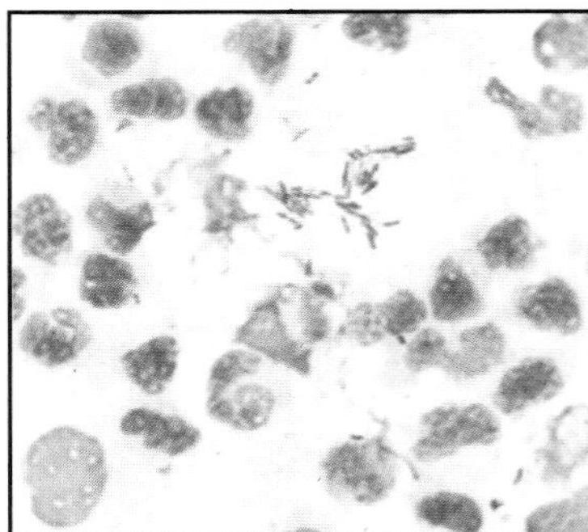

25.2 Nasal flush from a cat. *Pasteurella multocida*: bacterial bacilli stain dark blue with bipolar staining evident in some organisms. (Modified Wright–Giemsa stain; original magnification X1000.)

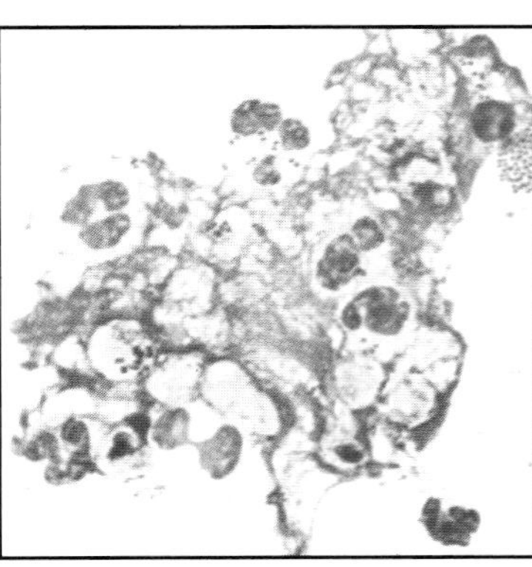

25.3 Nasal swab from a dog. *Staphylococcus aureus*: degenerate neutrophils with intracellular bacterial cocci in clusters ('bunches of grapes'), with background mucus. (Modified Wright–Giemsa stain; original magnification X1000.)

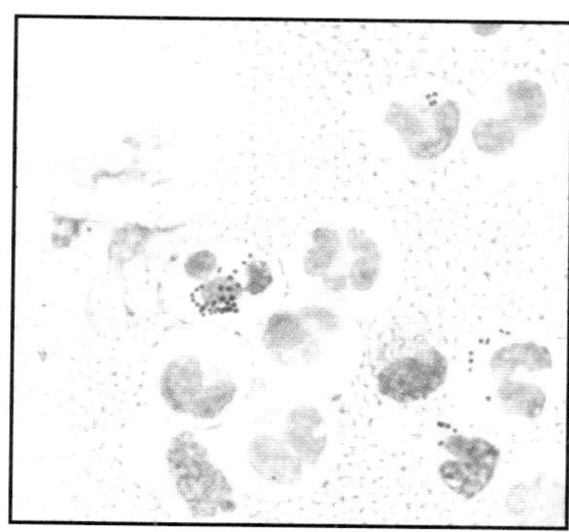

25.4 Material collected from a dog by a bronchoscope. β-haemolytic streptococci: bacterial cocci in pairs and short chains phagocytosed by neutrophils. (Modified Wright–Giemsa stain; original magnification X1000.)

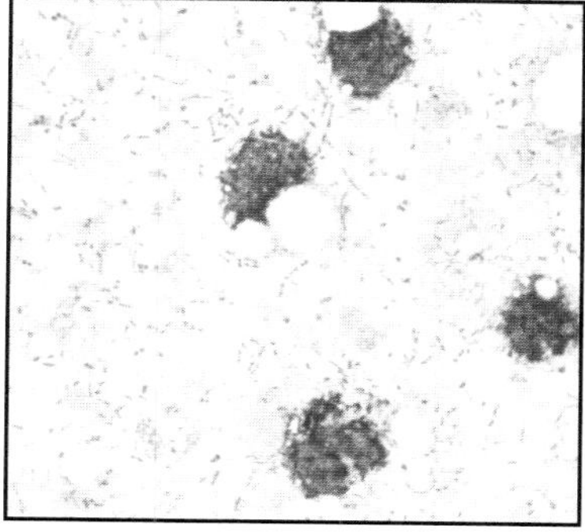

25.5 Aspirate from a subcutaneous abscess in a dog. *Bacteroides* sp. and *Escherichia coli*: pleomorphic mixed bacterial bacilli and degenerate neutrophils. (Modified Wright–Giemsa stain; original magnification X1000.)

Different protocols are available for Gram staining; the following protocol is in use in the author's laboratory (alternative materials in brackets):

1. The air-dried smear is passed through the top of a bunsen flame three times. **Do not overheat.**
2. The slide is allowed to cool and flooded with crystal violet (or *methyl violet* or *gentian violet*) for 1 minute.
3. The slide is washed **gently** with water.
4. The slide is flooded with Gram's iodine and left for 1 minute.
5. Iodine is washed from the slide with Gram's differentiator (*acetone*) until no more colour comes from the film: usually 2–5 seconds.
6. The slide is washed **gently** with water.
7. The slide is flooded with safranin (*dilute carbofuchsin, neutral red*) and left for 1 minute.
8. The slide is washed **gently** with water.
9. The slide is blotted with blotting paper.

Because of cell permeability the crystal violet–iodine complex will be washed from Gram-negative bacteria by the solvent but not from Gram-positive bacteria. Upon counter-staining with safranin, organisms that had been decolorized (Gram-negative) will stain pink. Gram-positive organisms that retain the crystal violet dye will appear blue–black/purple microscopically. Commercial kits are also available for Gram staining.

Further staining techniques are used to detect acid-fast organisms, such as *Mycobacterium* spp. (Ziehl–Neelsen stain) (Figure 25.6) or mycotic hyphae (periodic acid–Schiff, PAS).

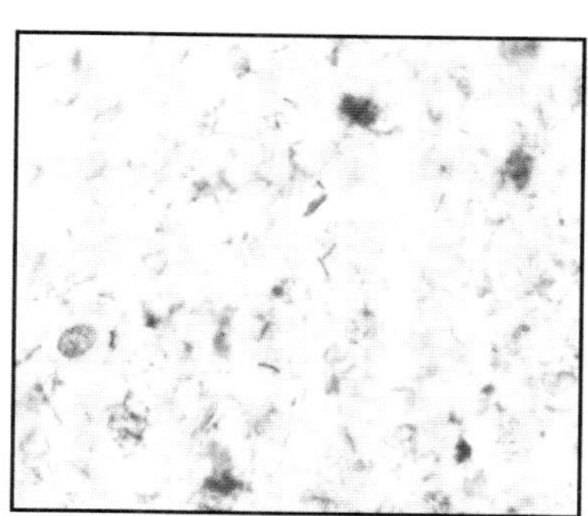

25.6 Abdominal abscess in a cat. *Mycobacterium tuberculosis* complex: acid-fast bacilli (red) and necrotic cellular material. (Ziehl–Neelsen stain; original magnification X1000.) (Courtesy of J Duncan.)

Sampling for bacterial cultures

Samples for bacterial cultures are ideally processed within 1–2 hours of collection, but this is rarely achieved in veterinary practice. Delays in processing, temperature changes and desiccation all combine to reduce bacterial survival, and rapidly growing contaminants readily overgrow more fastidious pathogenic species. Sampling techniques, sampling materials and sample storage methods must be selected carefully to optimize bacterial survival.

Sampling materials

A range of sampling materials is usually made available by veterinary laboratories.

- Anaerobic transport devices are commercially available but not commonly used by veterinary laboratories. They are designed to transport material containing obligate anaerobes but are also suitable for aerobes and facultative anaerobes.
- Blood culture medium is a nutrient type broth that commonly supports both aerobic and anaerobic bacterial growth. It can only be used for fluids aspirated from sterile body sites – usually blood, CSF or synovial fluid.
- Boric acid preservative is a crystalline material in a sterile universal tube. It is used only for urine; samples in boric acid preservative give culture results comparable to fresh urine when stored for up to 72 hours.
- All swabs are made of non-inhibitory material, such as viscose, and come with a sterile transport container. Swabs are usually immersed in a transport medium to prevent desiccation of the sample.
- Mini-tip swabs are suitable for sampling small sites, such as sinus tracts.
- Transport media are buffered, non-nutritive materials that limit the rate of replication of bacteria, preventing overgrowth by rapidly growing species. The most common example is Amies charcoal transport medium, usually supplied along with a sterile swab. Transport media are usually suitable for aerobic and anaerobic bacteria and for fungi. Some fastidious species will not survive in these nutritionally poor media.
- Sterile universal containers (20 ml volume) are suitable for a range of materials including fluids,

tissue, faeces and plain urine. These tubes should not contain preservatives or anticoagulants. Submission of samples in blood tubes, with or without anticoagulant, should be avoided where possible, as accurate information is not available for survival rates for bacteria in these tubes.

Principles of sampling

- Obtain samples from live animals before antibiotic treatment and as early in the disease process as possible.
- Take appropriate samples for the types of cultures required.
- Take all possible steps to minimize contamination.
- Do not use plain swabs. Inoculated swabs should be placed in bacterial transport medium to prevent desiccation and to maintain the viability of aerobic and anaerobic organisms.
- Pack samples for external laboratories safely and according to the carrier's regulations.
- Always include details of the anatomical site sampled, date of sampling, any antibiotic treatment and a clinical history with samples.

Specific sampling requirements depend upon the type of material and the likely pathogenic species at the anatomical site sampled.

Sample storage and processing

Even with the use of suitable transport media and sampling materials, bacterial cultures should be inoculated within 24 hours of collection where possible. Bacterial survival is optimized when samples are held at room temperature, making samples suitable for referral to external veterinary laboratories. Refrigeration is harmful to many species of bacteria.

Sampling for anaerobic cultures

Obligate anaerobic bacteria are unable to grow in the presence of oxygen. They form an important part of the normal flora of dogs and cats, e.g. at the gingival margin and in the intestines.

The most common clinical conditions involving anaerobic bacterial infections are:

- Abscesses
- Anal sacculitis
- Bacterial peritonitis
- Bacteraemia
- Enteritis/colitis
- Endometritis
- Fractures involving trauma to soft tissue
- Osteomyelitis
- Periodontal disease
- Postsurgical infection
- Pyothorax
- Skin granulomas
- Wounds

Anaerobic bacteria are most commonly isolated in mixed growths of two (or more) anaerobic species. Mixed infections with aerobes are also common (especially coagulase-negative and -positive staphylococci, β-haemolytic streptococci, *Escherichia coli, Pasteurella multocida, Enterococcus* spp. and *Arcanobacterium pyogenes*).

Common anaerobic bacterial pathogens (>10% of cases) include *Clostridium perfringens* and spp., and *Bacteroides melaninogenicus* and spp. Less common isolates (<10% of cases) include *Actinomyces* spp., *Eubacterium* spp., *Peptostreptococcus* spp., *Propionibacterium acnes, Bacteroides fragilis,* and *Fusobacterium necrophorum* and spp.

Obligate anaerobes do not survive for more than 20 minutes in air. Recovery is enhanced by avoiding all contact with atmospheric oxygen.

- Samples taken should be large enough to maintain anaerobic conditions (>2 ml of fluid or >2 cm^3 of tissue) or tissue should be immersed in a bacterial transport medium, such as Amies. Air should be excluded from liquid samples where possible. This can be achieved using an anaerobic transport device or by expelling air from the collection syringe and capping it. The use of swabs should be avoided where possible.
- Samples should be held in a cool place (about 15°C) but not refrigerated. Refrigeration (<4°C) kills anaerobes (oxygen absorption is greater at lower temperatures) whilst higher temperatures (25°C) favour overgrowth of aerobic bacteria.
- Tissue and fluid samples not protected by bacterial transport medium must be cultured within 24 hours.

Sampling for blood cultures

Blood cultures are indicated in any animal suspected of having a bacteraemia (e.g. endocarditis or pyrexia of unknown origin) and must be taken prior to treatment with antibiotics. Three samples are taken over a 24-hour period, except in acutely septic patients when three samples may be taken over a 30-minute period, prior to starting antimicrobial treatment.

- The skin is prepared as for surgery to avoid culture contamination.
- 10 ml of blood is collected using a sterile syringe and needle (or newly inserted jugular intravenous catheter).
- The culture medium bottle diaphragm is disinfected with 70% alcohol and allowed to dry.
- *Using a new sterile needle*, the blood is transferred to the blood culture medium bottle and mixed by inverting.
- The sample is incubated at approximately 37°C if possible and dispatched to the laboratory by next day delivery. Samples may be dispatched at room temperature; bacteria are unlikely to die once they are in the medium.

Significant isolates include all Enterobacteriaceae, *Bacteroides* spp., *Pseudomonas aeruginosa*, *Staphylococcus intermedius*, β-haemolytic streptococci and yeasts. Non-haemolytic streptococci and *Clostridium* spp. are significant in repeat cultures. Contaminants include *Corynebacterium* spp., *Bacillus* spp. and other skin commensals (see Figure 25.11).

Sampling for fluid cultures

Fluid samples are commonly collected for bacterial and fungal cultures in addition to cytological examination. These include:

- Tracheal, bronchial and prostatic washes – wash solution is collected for bacterial and mycotic cultures. Isotonic saline is most commonly used but better culture results will be obtained if a buffered solution, such as lactated Ringer's, is used. Anaerobic bacterial cultures are not indicated therefore the wash solution is collected into a sterile universal container
- Peritoneal and pleural fluid – fluid is collected aseptically from the unopened body cavity. Both aerobic and anaerobic cultures are indicated; therefore air should be excluded by expelling air from the syringe, being careful to remove the needle and to cap the end of the syringe. Fluid may be presented in a plain sterile tube if the tube is filled to exclude air. Alternatively, fluid may be transferred immediately to an anaerobic transport device
- Abscess material – again both aerobic and anaerobic cultures are indicated. Fluid is collected as for peritoneal and pleural fluid cultures
- CSF – bacterial infections are uncommon and usually involve one species. Sample contamination is usually not a problem. Fluid is collected into a sterile tube. Alternatively, CSF is inoculated into blood transport medium to maximize recovery of pathogenic species.

Significance of bacterial isolates

Bacteria that live in association with an animal but do not cause disease are called *commensals*, and most anatomical sites accessible for sampling have an established population of commensal species, referred to as *normal bacterial flora*. These include residents (which constantly inhabit an area and can re-establish themselves in that area) and transients (which originate from the environment or other anatomical sites and are carried passively).

Bacteria that cause disease are called *pathogens* and these may live in permanent association with animals or may be saprophytes (bacteria that normally inhabit the environment and obtain nutrients from non-living organic matter). *Opportunistic pathogens* are bacteria that are part of the normal bacterial flora but occasionally cause disease. *Opportunistic pathogens* may also be environmental bacteria that do not cause disease under normal circumstances.

Non-pathogenic bacteria isolated from clinical samples are occasionally described as *contaminants*. These may originate either from the environment or from the normal bacterial flora at that anatomical site. Voided or catheterized urine samples commonly contain bacterial contaminants.

The isolation of a bacterial species from diseased tissue is not proof of pathogenicity; the following factors must be considered when assessing the significance of a bacterial isolate:

- It is necessary to know which species are part of the normal bacterial flora and which species are pathogens at different anatomical sites
- Surveys of bacteria isolated in association with disease often do not establish the pathogenicity of the bacterial species isolated
- It can be difficult to distinguish between normal flora and opportunistic pathogens in clinical samples: either may multiply to occupy a new environmental niche created by disease or other factors
- The number of bacterial species isolated is important (multiple isolates suggest contamination or normal flora) as is the weight of bacterial growth (pure and profuse growth suggests a pathogenic bacterium).

In practice, samples from a limited number of clinical conditions give rise to the majority of submissions to veterinary laboratories for bacterial cultures; these conditions are considered below.

Otitis externa

Bacterial and fungal organisms are not considered to be primary causes of otitis externa, but secondary infections, often by more than one pathogen, are common (see also Chapter 24). Cats have similar normal bacterial flora and pathogenic bacteria to dogs.

Material is collected from the horizontal ear canal using a swab through an otoscope if possible, or from the vertical ear canal. Aerobic and yeast cultures should be requested. The significance of bacterial isolates is summarized in Figure 25.7.

Normal aerobic bacterial flora of the canine ear
Common (>10% of dogs sampled) *Staphylococcus* spp. (coagulase-positive); *Streptococcus* spp.
Others (<10% of dogs sampled) *Bacillus* spp.; Enterobacteriaceae; *Staphylococcus* spp. (coagulase-negative)
Aerobic bacteria associated with canine otitis externa
Common (>10% of affected dogs) *Escherichia coli*; *Proteus* spp.; *Pseudomonas aeruginosa*; *Staphylococcus intermedius*; *Streptococcus* spp. (β-haemolytic)
Others (<10% of affected dogs) *Bacillus* spp.; *Corynebacterium* spp.; *Enterobacter* spp.; *Enterococcus* spp.; *Klebsiella* spp.; *Pasteurella* spp.; *Staphylococcus aureus*; *Staphylococcus* spp. (coagulase-negative)

25.7 Canine otitis externa: significance of bacterial isolates.

Conjunctivitis

Conjunctivitis is the most common feline ophthalmic disorder and is often associated with non-bacterial infection (Feline herpesvirus-1, *Chlamydophila felis* and *Mycoplasma felis*). Bacteria isolated from cases of conjunctivitis are similar to the normal conjunctival bacterial flora.

A sample should be taken before instillation of local anaesthetic. The eyelid is reflected gently and a mini-tip swab is rolled across the conjunctiva. The swab is moistened as required with sterile saline (unnecessary in the presence of exudate) and then placed in bacterial transport medium. Aerobic bacterial cultures only are requested. The significance of bacterial isolates is summarized in Figure 25.8.

Normal aerobic bacterial flora of the conjunctiva
Dogs
Common (>10% of dogs sampled) *Bacillus* spp.; *Corynebacterium* spp.; *Neisseria* spp.; *Pseudomonas* spp.; *Staphylococcus* spp. (coagulase-positive and -negative); *Streptococcus* spp. (α- and non-haemolytic)
Others (<10% of dogs sampled) *Acinetobacter* spp.; *Alcaligenes* spp.; *Brahamella catarrhalis*; *Citrobacter spp.*; *Enterobacter* spp.; *Enterococcus* spp.; *Escherichia coli*; *Flavobacterium* spp.; *Haemophilus* spp.; *Klebsiella* spp.; *Micrococcus* spp.; *Moraxella* spp.; *Nocardia* spp.; *Pasteurella* spp.; *Proteus* spp.; *Streptococcus* spp. (β-haemolytic)
Cats
Common (>10% of cats sampled) *Staphylococcus* spp.
Others (<10% of cats sampled) *Bacillus* spp.; *Corynebacterium* spp.; *Streptococcus* spp. (α-haemolytic)
Aerobic bacteria associated with conjunctivitis
Dogs
Common (>10% of affected dogs) *Escherichia coli*; *Proteus mirabilis*; *Staphylococcus* spp. (coagulase-positive and -negative); *Streptococcus* spp. (α- and β-haemolytic)
Others (<10% of affected dogs) *Bacillus* spp.; *Corynebacterium* spp.; *Klebsiella* spp.; *Moraxella* spp.; *Neisseria* spp.; *Pasteurella* spp.; *Pseudomonas spp.*
Cats
Common (>10% of affected cats) *Staphylococcus* spp. (coagulase-negative); *Streptococcus* spp. (β- and non-haemolytic)

25.8 Conjunctivitis: significance of bacterial isolates.

Skin infections and wounds

Skin infections, particularly pyoderma, are very common in dogs but uncommon in cats, with the exception of subcutaneous bite wound abscesses. Underlying conditions, such as seborrhoeic skin disease, modify the microenvironment so that normal skin flora organisms multiply, increasing the supply of potentially pathogenic bacteria (see also Chapter 24).

Most cases of pyoderma are associated with coagulase-positive staphylococci, predominantly *Staphylococcus intermedius*, which is resident on the mucous membranes of dogs and forms part of the transient flora of the skin and hair coat. Opportunist Gram-negative pathogens tend to be isolated from chronic and deep pyodermas.

The coagulase test detects coagulase enzyme produced by pathogenic *Staphylococcus* species, such as *S. intermedius* or *S. aureus*. Coagulase-negative staphylococci tend to be non-pathogenic commensals. The rapid slide test used by many laboratories will not detect all pathogenic staphylococci; the tube test (Figure 25.9) is more sensitive.

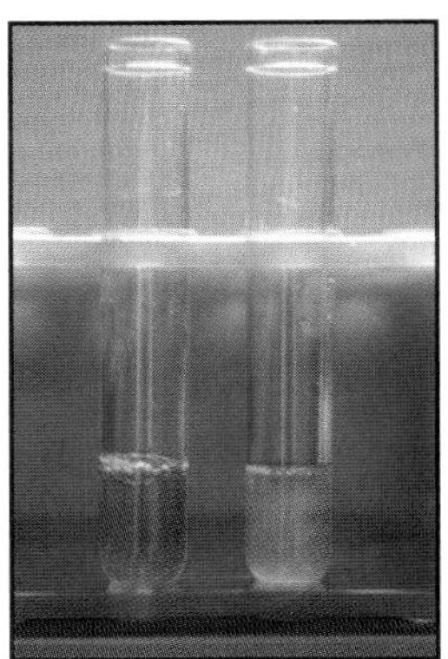

25.9 The tube coagulase test: rabbit plasma is incubated with a bacterial suspension. Fibrinogen is converted to fibrin by coagulase enzyme to give a weak clot in the right hand tube, which is coagulase-positive. The left hand tube shows a negative result.

The sampling technique depends upon the type of lesion (see Chapter 24). The type of culture requested also depends on the type of lesion:

- Intact pustules and superficial wounds – aerobic cultures only
- Surface pyoderma lesions – aerobic and yeast cultures
- Deep lesions or discharging sinus tracts (Figure 25.10) – aerobic culture of discharge; aerobic, anaerobic, fungal or mycobacterial culture of tissue (submit tissue collected by surgical biopsy in a plain sterile container or embedded in bacterial transport medium)
- Deep wounds – aerobic and anaerobic cultures.

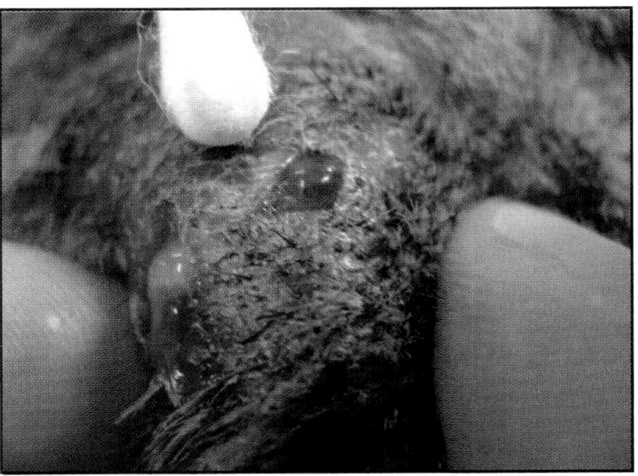

25.10 Pus expressed from a deep pyoderma lesion in a dog with concurrent demodicosis. (Courtesy of R Wilkinson.)

The significance of bacterial isolates from bacterial skin infections is summarized in Figure 25.11.

Normal aerobic bacterial flora of canine skin
Common (>10% of dogs sampled) *Acinetobacter* spp.; *Bacillus* spp.; *Corynebacterium* spp.; *Micrococcus* spp.; *Proteus* spp.; *Staphylococcus* spp. (coagulase-positive and negative); *Streptococcus* spp. (α-haemolytic)
Others (<10% of dogs sampled) *Enterococcus* spp.; *Escherichia coli*; *Nocardia* spp.; *Pseudomonas* spp.; *Streptococcus* spp. (β-haemolytic)
Bacterial pathogens associated with canine skin infections
Pathogens *Staphylococcus intermedius*; *Staphylococcus aureus*
Opportunist pathogens *Proteus* spp.; *Escherichia coli*; *Pasteurella multocida*; *Pseudomonas* spp.; *Streptococcus* spp. (α-, β- and non-haemolytic)
Granulomatous skin lesions *Actinomyces viscosus* (anaerobic); *Nocardia asteroides*

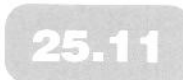
25.11 Canine skin infections: significance of bacterial isolates.

Bacterial enteritis

Faecal cultures largely reflect the bacterial flora of the caecum and colon. Anaerobes predominate but most laboratories do not routinely inoculate anaerobic cultures from faecal samples. The composition and distribution of the aerobic faecal flora are altered in enteric disease but faecal cultures are usually not quantitative and subtle changes in faecal flora may not be detected.

Normal aerobic faecal flora include *Escherichia coli*, other Enterobacteriaceae and *Enterococcus* spp. *Campylobacter* spp. have been isolated from 4–40% of asymptomatic dogs' faeces and from 4% of asymptomatic cats' faeces. *Salmonella* spp. have been isolated from 1–36% of healthy or hospitalized dogs' faeces and 1–18% of healthy or hospitalized cats' faeces.

Established enteric pathogens include *Escherichia coli*, *Campylobacter* spp., *Clostridium perfringens*, *Salmonella* spp., *Shigella* spp. (rare) and *Yersinia* spp. (rare). Pathogenic strains of *E. coli* are poorly characterized (see also Chapter 13); enteric infection is most common in neonates but haemorrhagic gastroenteritis has been reported in dogs over 3 months of age. Most *E.coli* isolated from faeces are likely to be normal faecal flora.

Fresh diarrhoeal faeces should be submitted in a sterile universal container. Rectal swabs should only be used in neonatal animals or animals acutely ill with diarrhoea. The swab is inserted beyond the anal sphincter and rotated. One should ensure that faeces is present before placing the swab in bacterial transport medium.

Urinary tract infection

Urinary tract infection (UTI) is defined as continuing bacterial multiplication within the urinary system detected by the presence of a bacteruria. UTIs are often asymptomatic.

There are four urine-sampling methods used in dogs and cats: midstream voided urine; assisted micturition; catheterization; and cystocentesis (see Chapter 10).

Urine in the bladder is considered sterile. Voided and catheterized urine samples are contaminated by resident bacterial flora from the mid-urethra to the external genitalia (vagina, vestibule and prepuce). In dogs, bacterial contamination occurs in up to 85% of voided midstream samples and up to 26% of catheterized samples. Contamination is greater in samples from bitches than from male dogs. Cystocentesis is the preferred collection method for urine culture. Contamination is uncommon but has been reported in up to 12% of cystocentesis samples, presumed to be from skin, transport or microbiological processing.

Fresh urine should be cultured within 2 hours or may be refrigerated for up to 6 hours. Urine samples in boric acid preservative for up to 72 hours give culture results comparable to fresh urine, whereas up to 65% of urine samples submitted to laboratories in plain tubes show a false positive bacteruria. The growth of more than three bacterial species is almost always attributable to contamination; most UTIs involve one bacterial species only.

Urine sediment microscopy

For details of this method see Chapter 10. Urine sediments should be prepared immediately after collection where possible. The number of white blood cells (WBCs) per X400 high power microscope field (per hpf) is a useful rule of thumb to help to diagnose UTI. The following guidelines relate to urine sediment prepared from 5 ml of urine (conical centrifuge tube, 1000–2000 rpm for 5 minutes, sediment resuspended in the fluid remaining after the supernatant is decanted). These guidelines do not apply when significantly smaller volumes of urine are sedimented, for example if a StatSpin centrifuge is used.

- Midstream voided: >8 WBCs per hpf associated with UTI
- Catheterized: >8 WBCs per hpf associated with UTI
- Cystocentesis: >3 WBCs per hpf associated with UTI.

The absence of WBCs does not rule out UTI; numbers may be suppressed due to glucocorticoid therapy, hyperadrenocorticism, immunosuppressive therapy or antibiotic treatment. WBCs may be increased in dogs with prostatitis or vaginitis.

The presence or absence of bacteria in the urine sediment gives a crude measure of the bacterial count. Bacilli are only visualized in urine sediment when there are at least 10^4/ml. Cocci are harder to see and are only visualized when there are at least 10^5/ml (see Figure 25.12 for the significance of these levels).

Looking at the number of WBCs *and* the presence of bacteria in urine sediment (Figure 25.13) increases the sensitivity for detection of UTI. Urine sediment examination may not, however, reveal any bacteria or WBCs in animals with significant UTIs, especially pyelonephritis. Negative results on sediment examination should not exclude urine culture.

Method of collection	Dog			Cat		
	UTI	*Equivocal*	*No UTI*	*UTI*	*Equivocal*	*No UTI*
Cystocentesis	$>10^3$		$<10^3$	$>10^3$		$<10^3$
Catheterized	$>10^5$	10^3–10^5	$<10^3$	$>10^3$	10^2–10^3	$<10^2$
Voided	$>10^6$	10^5–10^6	$<10^5$	$>10^5$	10^4–10^5	$<10^4$

25.12 Urine bacterial counts (per ml) associated with urinary tract infection.

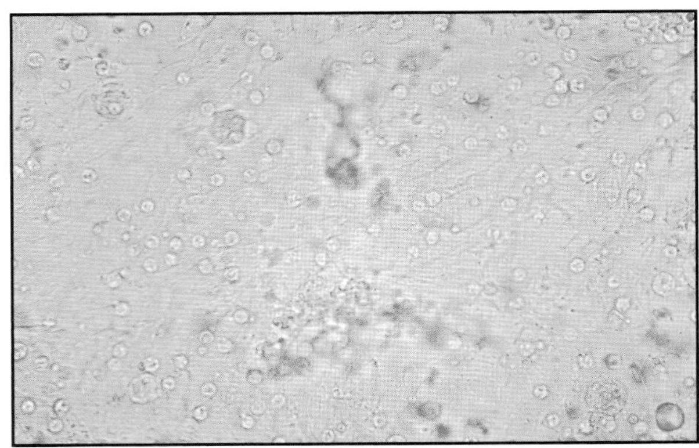

25.13 Urine sediment; numerous neutrophils with segmented nuclei and bacterial bacilli with occasional large uroepithelial cells. (Unstained; original magnification X400.)

Urine sample contaminants
Dogs
Male dog *Escherichia coli*; *Proteus mirabilis*; *Staphylococcus* spp. (coagulase-positive and -negative); *Streptococcus canis*
Bitch *Escherichia coli*; *Micrococcus* spp.; *Proteus* spp.; *Staphylococcus* spp. (coagulase-negative and -positive); *Streptococcus canis*
Cats
Corynebacterium spp.; *Escherichia coli*; *Flavobacterium* spp.; *Pasteurella* spp.; *Staphylococcus* spp.; *Streptococcus* spp.
Aerobic bacteria associated with urinary tract infection
Dogs
Common (>10% of affected dogs) *Escherichia coli* *; *Proteus* spp. *; *Staphylococcus* spp. (coagulase-positive) *; *Streptococcus* spp. (α- and β-haemolytic) *
Others (<10% of affected dogs) *Acinetobacter* spp.; *Bordetella bronchiseptica*; *Citrobacter* spp.; *Corynebacterium* spp.; *Enterobacter* spp. *; *Enterococcus* spp. *; *Klebsiella* spp. *; *Micrococcus* spp.; *Pasteurella* spp.; *Providencia* spp.; *Pseudomonas* spp. *; *Salmonella* spp.; *Staphylococcus* spp. (coagulase-negative)
Cats
Common (>10% of affected cats) *Escherichia coli* *; *Pasteurella* spp. *; *Proteus* spp. *; *Staphylococcus* spp. (coagulase-positive) *; *Streptococcus* spp. *
Others (<10% of affected cats) *Enterobacter* spp. *; *Enterococcus* spp. *; *Klebsiella* spp. *; *Pseudomonas* spp. *

25.14 Urinary tract infection: significance of bacterial isolates. Established urinary tract pathogens are asterisked.

Quantitative bacterial cultures

Bacteruria may be quantified and expressed as the number of colony forming units (CFUs) per ml of urine. Interpretation depends upon the collection method. Also the antibacterial properties of feline urine mean that a different level of significance should be taken compared with that for canine urine (see Figure 25.12). The significance of bacterial isolates is summarized in Figure 25.14.

Infective arthritis

Infective arthritis is usually caused by bacterial infection. Direct inoculation is the common route of infection (surgery or penetrating wound). Haematogenous spread is much less common but may be seen in neonates. Common bacterial isolates from infected joints in dogs include *Staphylococcus intermedius* and β-haemolytic streptococci. Less common isolates include Enterobacteriaceae, anaerobes, *Pasteurella multocida*, *Pseudomonas aeruginosa*, *Proteus* spp. and *Nocardia asteroides*. Joint infections in cats are uncommon and usually due to penetrating bite wounds, so oropharyngeal flora, including *Pasteurella multocida*, *Bacteroides* spp., *Streptococcus* spp. and spirochaetes, predominate.

Direct cultures of synovial fluid swabs only isolate bacteria from 50% of infected joints. The preferred technique is to use blood culture medium. Joint fluid is inoculated into blood culture medium that supports aerobic and anaerobic growth. The same technique as described for blood cultures is used. Approaches to arthrocentesis are illustrated in Chapter 22a. Figure 25.15 illustrates stifle arthrocentesis.

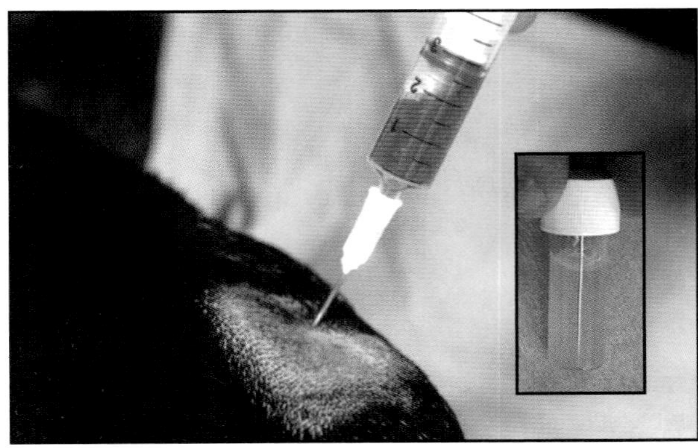

25.15 Stifle arthrocentesis. Bloody fluid consistent with joint trauma, inset shows turbid synovial fluid from a septic joint. (Courtesy of S Butterworth.)

Cytological examination of synovial fluid will usually identify an inflammatory arthritis but will not reliably distinguish between septic arthritis and immune-mediated arthritis (see Chapter 22a).

Vaginitis and infertility

Vaginal swabs are commonly submitted from bitches for the investigation of vaginitis and infertility, despite the fact that there are no known bacterial sexually transmitted diseases of dogs in the UK. The relationship between vaginitis and infertility is not a simple one (see Chapter 19) but vaginal bacteriological sampling of infertile bitches without clinical signs of genital infection is usually not indicated.

Concurrent urinary tract infection is seen in 20% of older bitches with vaginitis. Bacteria prevalent in vaginitis are also prevalent in the normal vaginal flora. Usually only one or two bacterial species will be isolated from cases of vaginitis but up to 18% of normal dogs also have only one bacterial species cultured from vaginal swabs.

Samples are taken from the anterior vagina where possible:

- The vulva is cleaned with surgical scrub, rinsed with 70% alcohol and allowed to dry
- A speculum (e.g. human nasal speculum) or guarded swab is introduced into the cranial vagina
- The dorsal and ventral vaginal walls are swabbed.

The significance of bacterial isolates from vaginal swabs is summarized in Figure 25.16.

Normal aerobic bacterial flora of the canine vagina
Common (>10% of dogs sampled) *Corynebacterium* spp.; *Escherichia coli*; *Moraxella* spp.; *Pasteurella multocida*; *Proteus* spp.; *Staphylococcus* spp. (coagulase-negative and -positive); *Streptococcus* spp. (α- and β-haemolytic)
Others (<10% of dogs sampled) *Acinetobacter* spp.; *Alcaligenes faecalis*; *Bacillus* spp.; *Citrobacter* spp.; *Enterobacter* spp.; *Enterococcus* spp.; *Flavobacterium* spp.; *Haemophilus* spp.; *Klebsiella* spp.; *Lactobacillus* spp.; *Micrococcus* spp.; *Neisseria* spp.; *Pseudomonas* spp.; *Streptococcus* spp. (non-haemolytic)
Aerobic bacteria associated with canine vaginitis
Bacillus spp.; *Citrobacter freundii*; *Corynebacterium* spp.; *Escherichia coli*; *Enterococcus* spp.; *Haemophilus* spp.; *Klebsiella* spp.; *Micrococcus* spp.; *Pasteurella multocida*; *Proteus mirabilis*; *Pseudomonas* spp.; *Staphylococcus aureus*; *Staphylococcus intermedius*; *Staphylococcus* spp. (coagulase-negative); *Streptococcus* spp. (β-haemolytic)

25.16 Canine vaginitis: significance of bacterial isolates.

Sampling for fungal cultures

Although there are some 250,000 species of fungi, fewer than 150 species are known to be pathogenic to animals and man. Many saprophytic fungi have been identified as normal flora, particularly of the hair and skin; most are contaminants from the air or soil.

Pathological fungal infections involve tissue invasion. Infections can be superficial, subcutaneous or systemic, but only superficial skin infections are common in the UK. These are divided into dermatophytoses, caused by dermatophytes (ringworm), and dermatomycoses, caused by commensals of the skin and mucous membranes, most commonly *Malassezia pachydermatis* and *Candida* spp. Nasal aspergillosis in dogs and *Cryptococcus neoformans* infections are encountered, but systemic mycoses (Figure 25.17) are rare.

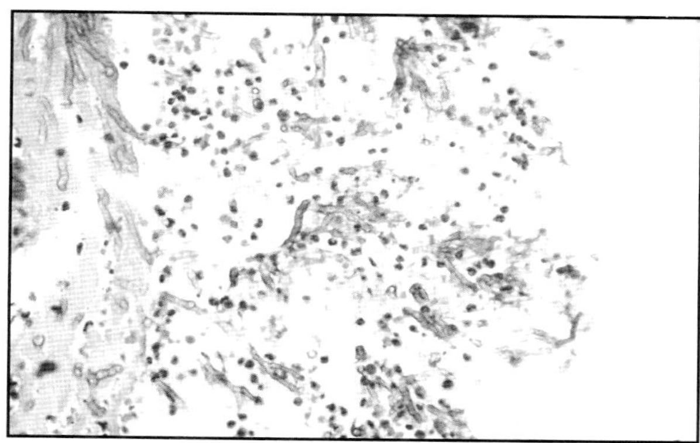

25.17 Fungal hyphae in a splenic capsule. Systemic mycosis in a 5-year-old Whippet secondary to azathioprine therapy. (H&E; original magnification X400.) (Courtesy of J Hargreaves.)

Dermatophytes

Dermatophytes are unique amongst fungi in that they can invade and maintain infection in keratinized tissues. The majority of infections are caused by *Microsporum canis*. *M. gypseum* and *Trichophyton mentagrophytes* are occasional pathogens in dogs and rare pathogens in cats. *T. erinacei* is an occasional pathogen in dogs. Other dermatophyte species are isolated only sporadically. Prevalence is low, with only 16% positive cultures from over 8000 samples from suspected dermatophyte infections in dogs and cats in one UK survey (Sparkes *et al.*, 1993).

M. canis infection is usually acquired from an infected cat and asymptomatic cats are an important reservoir. Carriage rates of 0–88% have been recorded in asymptomatic cats but one UK survey put the isolation rate at only 2.2% (Sparkes *et al.*, 1994). Asymptomatic culture-positive cats may be infected or may be transient carriers. In contrast to *M.canis*, *M. gypseum* is geophilic and infection is often acquired from digging.

Sampling procedures are described in Chapter 24.

Malassezia pachydermatis

M. pachydermatis is part of the normal bacterial skin flora and is commonly found in the ear canals, on the oral and anal mucosa, in the anal sacs and in the vagina. It is thought to have a symbiotic relationship with commensal staphylococci. It is also a common opportunist pathogen associated with otitis externa and skin disease in dogs. In contrast, in cats it is an uncommon cause of otitis externa and a rare cause of skin disease. Both culture and microscopy are utilized to identify infection:

- Culture: skin and external ear – swabs are submitted for yeast culture in bacterial transport medium
- Microscopy – impression smears are taken from affected skin, air dried and stained with a Romanowsky stain. More than one organism per X400 microscope field is significant. Smears may be prepared from swabs for ears and less accessible areas of skin. More than 10 organisms per X400 microscope field are considered significant in relation to otitis externa
- Do not send tape strippings to laboratories, as these are difficult to stain and examine.

Malassezia pachydermatis yeasts have a characteristic peanut shape and a broad-based apical bud (Figure 25.18).

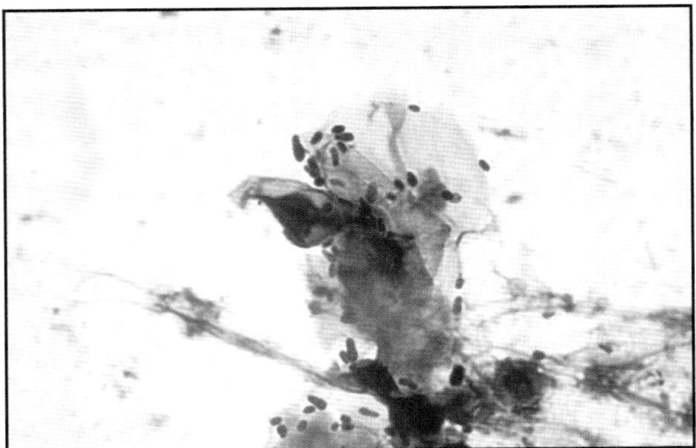

25.18 *Malassezia pachydermatis* yeasts, anucleate squamous epithelial cells and debris from a dog's ear. Several yeasts have broad-based apical buds. (Leishman's stain; original magnification X400.)

Candida species

Candida spp. yeasts are commensals of the ears, nose, oral cavity and anal mucosa. Prolonged antibiotic treatment, damage to mucosal surfaces, immunodeficiency and immunosuppression all predispose to infection. Infection is rare in both dogs and cats but may involve the ear, intertrigenous areas, nailbed and interdigital areas (dogs), paws and mucocutaneous junctions (cats), or the lower urinary tract (dogs and cats).

- Samples for culture and microscopy are taken as for *Malassezia pachydermatis*.
- Cytological preparations show narrow-based yeast cells with multilateral budding. Hyphae may be present.

Aspergillus species

Nasal aspergillosis in dogs is caused by *Aspergillus fumigatus*, and is much more common than infection with *Penicillium*, although clinically indistinguishable. Nasal infections with fungi are rare in the cat. Disseminated aspergillosis is rare.

- Cultures of nasal discharge are often negative for *Aspergillus* in cases of nasal aspergillosis and positive in randomly sampled normal dogs and dogs with nasal neoplasia.
- Microscopy: cytological examination of nasal discharges suffers the same inaccuracies as fungal culture.
- Serological examination: see later section on serological and other tests.
- Rhinoscopy may allow visualization of fungal plaques.
- Radiology typically demonstrates destruction of nasal turbinates with radiolucency.
- Histopathological examination is useful to confirm the significance of fungal isolates.

Cryptococcus neoformans

C. neoformans is a ubiquitous, saprophytic, yeast-like fungus. Infections are prevalent in areas of North America but infection is rarely diagnosed in the UK. Subacute or chronic infections of the CNS, respiratory system, skin and eye may be seen in cats. The organism is cultured from nasal discharges, CSF and biopsy specimens. Serology for circulating antigen is available (see later) and cytological examination of discharges and tissue aspirates may be diagnostic. Cryptococcosis is a serious potential zoonosis and suspected infected tissues should be handled in a microbiological safety cabinet.

Sampling for mycobacterial cultures

Mycobacterium spp. are uncommon pathogens in cats and sporadic pathogens in dogs. Classical tuberculosis (TB), feline leprosy and opportunist mycobacteriosis have all been reported in cats in the UK and produce primarily cutaneous lesions (Figure 25.19).

- *Mycobacterium tuberculosis* and *M. bovis* occasionally cause classical TB in dogs and cats.
- *M. lepraemurium* (feline leprosy) is contracted through rodent bites and does not grow on routine laboratory media. Infection can become generalized and is usually identified through histopathology. Recently, two different feline leprosy syndromes have been described with an unidentified *Mycobacterium* species responsible for infection in older cats (Malik *et al.*, 2002).
- Saprophytes, such as *M. chelonei*, *M. fortuitum*, *M. phlei*, *M. smegmatis*, *M. thermoresistable* and *M. xenopi*, cause infection through contamination of cutaneous wounds. These organisms are difficult to stain in histopathological sections but are relatively easy to culture.

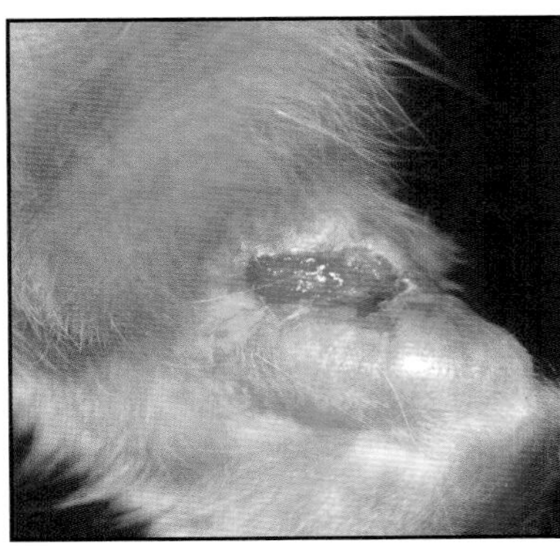

25.19 Cutaneous lesion in a cat due to a *Mycobacterium microti*-like organism. (Courtesy of D Gunn-Moore.)

Specialized culture techniques and containment facilities are essential to culture and identify the species involved. Details of mycobacterial reference laboratories are given in the Resources section at the end of this chapter; samples may also be submitted through any veterinary laboratory. The type of sample depends upon the site:

- Skin lesions – surgical biopsy is the sample of choice. Fresh tissue is submitted in a sterile universal tube
- Systemic disease – samples from surgical biopsies from intestinal tubercles, lymph nodes, pulmonary tubercles, bones and tonsils are submitted as appropriate. Again, fresh tissue is submitted in a sterile universal tube.

Samples should also be submitted for cytological and histopathological examination:

- Air-dried slides from fine needle aspirates and biopsy material in formal saline should be submitted
- Slides are stained with Ziehl–Neelsen stain to demonstrate characteristic acid-fast bacilli (see Figure 25.6)
- Biopsy samples may be divided at the time of sampling and one half frozen for possible culture pending the results of histopathological examination.

Sampling for mycoplasmal cultures

Mycoplasmas are the smallest free-living microorganisms. They include the genera *Mycoplasma*, *Ureaplasma* and *Acholeplasma*. These organisms form part of the normal flora on mucosal surfaces in the upper respiratory, genital and urinary tracts. They are occasionally associated with disease:

- Bite wound abscesses in cats
- Conjunctivitis in cats
- Genital tract infections in cats and dogs (possible association with infertility)
- Lower respiratory tract infection in cats and dogs (often in association with other pathogens)
- UTI in dogs.

Mycoplasmas may occasionally be isolated from bacterial swabs and fluids, and some veterinary laboratories will supply liquid-phase transport media. See Resources section at the end of this chapter.

Serological and other tests

Not all microorganisms are easily cultured; serological and other tests are also used to identify infection. Further advice regarding sample submission should be obtained from the veterinary laboratory.

- *Aspergillus fumigatus* – agar gel immunodiffusion is commonly used to detect antibodies to *Aspergillus* spp. in serum. A 6% false positive rate is reported, possibly due to frequent exposure to environmental aspergilli. Counterimmune electrophoresis (reported 0–15% false positives) and ELISA techniques may also be used.
- *Bartonella henselae* – a polymerase chain reaction (PCR) test is offered on EDTA blood by the Acarus Laboratory, University of Bristol.
- *Brucella canis* – slide agglutination, tube agglutination, agar-gel immunodiffusion, indirect fluorescent antibody and ELISA tests have all been used to detect antibodies in serum. All tests occasionally give false positive results, as antibodies to lipopolysaccharide antigens of several bacterial species cross react with *B. canis*. False negative reactions are less common.
- *Chlamydophila felis* – culture, antigen detection and serological tests have largely been superseded by the use of the PCR test. The conjunctiva (or other mucosal surface) is rubbed vigorously with a cotton swab to harvest epithelial cells containing the organism and the swab(s) is submitted *without transport medium* for PCR testing. N.B. The classification of Chlamydiaceae has recently changed. *Chlamydia psittaci* has been differentiated by 16S and 23S rRNA sequencing into a number of new species including *Chlamydophila psittaci*, *C. abortus*, *C. felis* and *C. caviae*. *C. felis* is an obligate intracellular parasite and is part of the normal flora of the feline conjunctiva and respiratory, gastrointestinal and urogenital systems. *C. felis* causes acute, chronic and recurrent conjunctivitis in cats. Nasal and lower respiratory tract infections are less common and the significance of genital infection is unclear. *Chlamydophila* infection in dogs is thought to be rare.
- *Clostridium perfringens* – tests for *C. perfringens* enterotoxin (reverse passive latex agglutination or ELISA) are not species-specific. Samples can therefore be tested by veterinary or medical laboratories; 1 g of faeces is required and may be refrigerated or frozen before analysis. False negative test results are seen with watery diarrhoea, interfering substances or sampling late in the course of the disease. Positive test results are obtained from affected animals and clinically healthy carrier animals and must therefore be correlated with clinical findings, endoscopy and histological examination of colonic biopsy samples.
- *Cryptococcus neoformans* – latex agglutination and ELISA tests are available for cryptococcal capsular antigen in serum, urine and CSF, where sensitivity is >90% and specificity >97% (cats and humans). Antigen may also be detected in pleural or bronchoalveolar lavage fluid.
- *Leptospira* spp. – the microscopic agglutination test (MAT), complement fixation and ELISA are all used to detect antibody to *Leptospira* spp. The MAT is most commonly used and is sensitive and serovar-specific. Titres may not rise significantly in acute infection; acute and convalescent sera may be required to identify active infection (4-fold increase in titre in 2–4 weeks). Titres in field infection are usually greater than vaccinal titres but may be reduced by early effective antibiotic treatment.

Antibacterial susceptibility

Testing techniques

In vitro susceptibility testing is indicated for any bacterial pathogen when the susceptibility cannot be reliably predicted and/or when the organism is capable of developing resistance to antimicrobial drugs. Until recently, only the agar gel disc diffusion technique was used in the UK. Now broth dilution minimum inhibitory concentration (MIC) testing is also used to generate information on *in vitro* susceptibility of bacterial pathogens. Whatever technique is used it is important to standardize the method and interpretation. The most commonly used standards are those approved by the National Committee for Clinical Laboratory Standards (NCCLS, 2001).

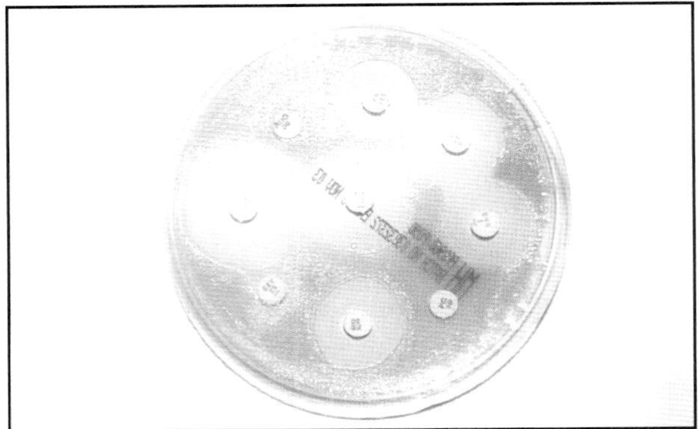

25.20 Agar gel disc diffusion; *Pseudomonas aeruginosa* showing *in vitro* resistance to fusidic acid (FC), trimethoprim/sulphonamide (SXT) and amoxicillin/clavulanate (AUG).

Agar gel disc diffusion

A uniform suspension of the bacterium is spread across an agar gel plate and paper discs impregnated with a known concentration of antibiotic are added. Typically six to eight discs are added to one plate. The plate is then incubated. If the bacterium is sensitive to an antibiotic, a zone of inhibition occurs around the disc. Zone diameters are compared to published figures to determine whether a bacterium is sensitive or resistant to an antibiotic (Figure 25.20). Results have been shown to be 95% reproducible between laboratories when standardized procedures are used.

Broth dilution MIC

The minimum inhibitory concentration (MIC) is the lowest concentration of an antibiotic that inhibits the growth of a given strain of bacterium. If the growth of a bacterial pathogen can be inhibited *in vivo* then a healthy immune system will complete the job of eliminating infection. MICs are determined by inoculating a bacterial isolate into a series of test wells, usually four to six, with doubling dilutions of the antibiotic to be tested against. After incubation the wells are examined for growth or inhibition of growth.

Interpretation of test results

Agar gel diffusion and broth dilution MIC results are compared in Figure 25.21. The list of antibiotics selected for testing is appropriate for the bacterial species and follows NCCLS recommendations. Both techniques classify the bacterial isolate as resistant (R), sensitive (S) or of intermediate resistance (I) *in vitro* to each antibiotic.

Agar gel disc diffusion		**Broth dilution MIC**					
Antibiotic	*Result*	*Antibiotic*	*Result*	*MIC*	*Antibiotic concentration range (µg/ml)*		
Penicillin	R	Penicillin	Resistant	>=16	0.03	sssrrrrrrR	16
Ampicillin	R	Ampicillin	Resistant	>=16	0.12	ssrrrrrR	16
Amoxicillin/clavulanate	S	Amoxicillin/clavulanate	SENSITIVE	<=2	2	Ssr	8
Cefalexin	S	Cefalexin	SENSITIVE	<=2	2	Sssir	32
Erythromycin	S	Erythromycin	SENSITIVE	<=0.5	0.5	Siiir	8
Clindamycin	S	Clindamycin	SENSITIVE	<=0.5	0.5	Siirr	8
Enrofloxacin	S	Enrofloxacin	SENSITIVE	<=0.25	0.25	Ssir	2
Marbofloxacin	S	Marbofloxacin	SENSITIVE	<=0.25	0.25	Ssir	2
Trimethoprim/ sulphonamide	S	Trimethoprim/ sulphonamide	SENSITIVE	<=10	10	Sssrrr	320
Tetracycline	S	Tetracycline	SENSITIVE	2	1	sSsrr	16
	S =Sensitive I = Intermediate R =Resistant					s =Sensitive i =Intermediate r =Resistant	

25.21 Agar gel disc diffusion and broth dilution MIC test results indicating *in vitro* susceptibility of an isolate of *Staphylococcus intermedius* to selected antibiotics. Agar gel disc diffusion classifies the bacterial isolate as simply resistant, sensitive or of intermediate resistance to each antibiotic. Broth dilution MIC also gives the lowest inhibitory concentration of antibiotic *in vitro* . For example, the MIC value for tetracycline = 2. If the bacterium is *sensitive* to the lowest antibiotic concentration tested, the MIC is reported as <= the lowest concentration (amoxicillin/clavulanate, cefalexin, erythromycin, clindamycin, enrofloxacin, marbofloxacin, trimethoprim/sulphonamide). If the bacterium is *resistant* to the highest concentration, the MIC is reported as >= the highest concentration of the antibiotic (penicillin, ampicillin). The range of antibiotic concentrations is given, and bacterial sensitivity at each concentration is reported as s (sensitive), r (resistant) or i (intermediate). The first concentration at which there is resistance, i.e. the first r on the scale, is the breakpoint. The point at which the MIC result falls on the s-i-r scale is given by the use of a capital letter, and corresponds to the the antibiotic concentration given in the MIC column (2 mg/ml in the case of tetracycline). See also Case 2.

Further interpretation of MIC test results follows a logical sequence:

- The MIC value in µg/ml is noted. If the bacterium is sensitive at the lowest antibiotic concentration tested, then the MIC will be given as <= the lowest concentration (amoxicillin/clavulanate, cefalexin, erythromycin, clindamycin, enrofloxacin, marbofloxacin and trimethoprim/sulphonamide in Figure 25.21). If the bacterium is resistant at the highest antibiotic concentration tested, then the MIC will be given as >= the highest concentration (penicillin and ampicillin).
- The range of antibiotic concentrations is given numerically as the lowest and highest concentration tested (0.03 and 16 µg/ml, respectively, in the case of penicillin). Each antibiotic concentration tested in this range is represented by a letter (s, i or r) on the scale reading from left (*highest concentration*) to right (*lowest concentration*). There are 10 concentrations or test wells for penicillin and 3 for potentiated amoxicillin.
- Each antibiotic concentration is classified as representing sensitivity (s), intermediate sensitivity (i) or resistance (r) based on *in vitro* studies. The 'breakpoint' is represented by the first letter r on the scale. The s-i-r scale is fixed for each combination of antibiotic and bacterial species.
- Finally, the point at which the MIC result falls on the s-i-r scale is given by the use of a capital letter, and corresponds to the antibiotic concentration given in the 'MIC' column (2 µg/ml in the case of tetracycline).

The interpretation of the results of MIC testing makes use of all these data:

- SENSITIVE (MIC <= any number) – The antibiotic is effective at the lowest concentration tested and should be effective in serum or urine
- SENSITIVE (MIC any number) – The antibiotic is effective, but not at the lowest concentration tested. Refer to the MIC range to determine where in the range it tested. The closer the MIC is to the breakpoint, the less likely it is that the bacterium will be susceptible *in vivo* to this antibiotic
- Intermediate (MIC any number) – The antibiotic may be effective in high dosages, or if it concentrates at the site
- Resistant (MIC any number) – The antibiotic will be unlikely to reach effective serum levels. Choose an antibiotic to which the organism is susceptible
- Resistant (MIC >= any number) – Choose an antibiotic to which the organism is susceptible.

The following points should also be considered when selecting an antibiotic:

- Safety, ease of use and cost
- Some antibiotics reach much higher tissue levels than the plasma levels on which the MIC dilutions are based
- If an organism shows resistance to all the antibiotics selected then this may be overcome by selecting one that reaches high tissue concentrations or by increasing the dose and/or frequency of administration
- Animals with compromised immune systems will require a higher drug concentration than the MIC number to achieve bactericidal concentrations of the antibiotic in tissues

Limitations to *in vitro* susceptibility testing

Only fast-growing aerobic bacteria, such as staphylococci and Enterobacteriaceae, are routinely tested. Susceptibility testing of slow-growing aerobic bacteria, obligate anaerobic bacteria, bacteria growing in a microaerophilic environment (e.g. *Campylobacter* spp.) and fungi is beyond the scope of most veterinary laboratories. Published guidelines for antibacterial susceptibility are considered more reliable for these organisms (Quinn *et al.*, 1994; Aucoin, 2002).

In vitro susceptibility tests assume an average serum concentration of the antimicrobial drug. Tissue levels may differ from these serum levels for a number of reasons:

- Use in species or ages of animals not covered by the data sheet applications
- Use of a different drug formulation to the class-representative example used in the tests
- Variable tissue penetration – usually low in CSF and high in urine
- Topical drug concentrations are usually much higher than serum concentrations. For this reason, some laboratories do not provide susceptibility testing for topical antibiotics.

Generally, *in vitro* antibacterial susceptibility testing is most successful at predicting failure of a drug to clear infection *in vivo*. The predictive value of *in vitro* testing for a good therapeutic response is moderate. A veterinary surgeon must always interpret susceptibility test results against a knowledge of which antibiotics are most effective at which anatomical sites.

Methicillin-resistant *Staphylococcus aureus*

The isolation of methicillin-resistant *Staphylococcus aureus* (MRSA) from companion animals has been reported recently in the press (Anon, 2003). MRSA is resistant to antibacterial agents available for the treatment of severe staphylococcal disease and is a continuing and increasing problem in many UK hospitals. Isolates from companion animals are typically from postoperative infections and open wounds. On the basis of the strain types involved it is thought that infection of companion animals with MRSA is likely to be the result of transmission from the human population (Rich *et al.*, 2004). Strict hygiene is important in reducing MRSA.

Case examples

Case 1

Signalment

5-year-old male neutered Springer Spaniel.

History

Dyspnoea.

Microscopy

Flocculent pus was collected from the pleural cavity. Gram-stained smears contained numerous neutrophils with pleomorphic Gram-positive bacilli (Figure 25.22) and Gram-positive cocci in short chains (Figure 25.23).

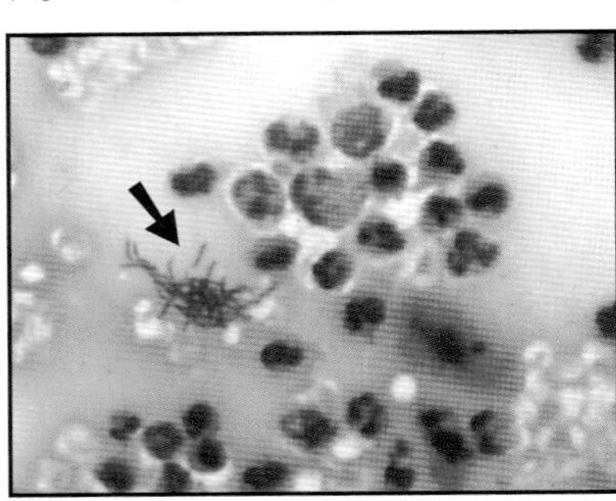

25.22 Canine pleural fluid, Gram-positive bacilli (arrowed) and neutrophils. (Gram stain; original magnification X1000.)

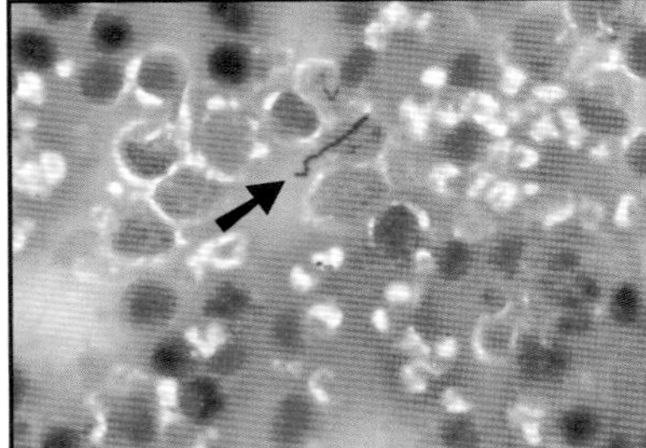

25.23 Canine pleural fluid, chain of Gram-positive cocci (arrowed) and neutrophils. (Gram stain; original magnification X1000.)

What are the likely bacterial species?

The most likely bacterial species, based on 47 published cases of pyothorax in dogs (Walker *et al.*, 2000) are:

Gram-positive cocci	*Peptostreptococcus* spp. (anaerobic, 27% of isolates) *Streptococcus canis* (aerobic, 11%) *Staphylococcus intermedius* (aerobic, 4%, not commonly in chains)
Gram-positive bacilli	*Actinomyces* spp. (aerobic, 19%) *Nocardia* spp. (aerobic, 4%) *Eubacterium* spp. (anaerobic, 3%) *Propionibacterium* spp. (anaerobic, 2%)

Should initial antibiotic therapy be directed against aerobic or anaerobic bacteria?

The balance of probabilities suggests a mixed anaerobic and aerobic infection, indicating that antibiotics should be selected with activity against both.

Bacterial cultures isolated *Bacteroides* and *Peptostreptococcus*. *Bacteroides* spp. are Gram-negative anaerobes that were not identified in the smears. No Gram-positive bacilli were isolated. This case illustrates some of the limitations and advantages of direct microscopy:

- Gram-negative bacilli can be difficult to visualize against background material on a Gram-stained smear (see Figure 25.1)
- Suboptimal sampling and storage conditions will affect the viability of fastidious bacteria, especially anaerobic bacterial species, but these bacteria may be recognized on microscopy
- A working knowledge of common bacterial isolates in different species at different anatomical sites is required to interpret the results of direct microscopy.

Case 2

Signalment

10-year-old female neutered West Highland White Terrier.

History

Polyuria/polydipsia.

Urine sediment examination and bacteriological cultures

- 20–30 WBCs per hpf
- 5–10 RBCs per hpf
- Bacterial cultures from the voided urine sample isolated >10^5 CFU/ml of *Enterococcus* spp.

MIC antibacterial susceptibility testing gave the following results:

Broth dilution MIC					
Antibiotic	**Result**	**MIC (µg/ml)**	**Reference range**		
Penicillin	SENSITIVE	4	0.03	sssssssSsr	16
Ampicillin	SENSITIVE	0.5	0.12	ssSssssr	16
Enrofloxacin	SENSITIVE	1	0.25	ssSr	2
Marbofloxacin	SENSITIVE	1	0.25	ssSr	2
Tetracycline	SENSITIVE	<=1	1	Sssir	16

Why are these results consistent with a urinary tract infection?

The significant numbers of WBCs present in the sediment, the significant bacterial count (see Figure 25.12), and the isolation and identification of a recognized urinary tract bacterial pathogen (see Figure 25.14) all point to a urinary tract infection.

How would you use the MIC data to help to select an appropriate antibiotic for use in this case?

The results indicate susceptibility of the isolate to all the antibiotics tested. However, only tetracycline is effective at the lowest dilution tested and it should therefore be effective in serum or urine. Tetracycline predicts the susceptibility of the isolate to related antimicrobials such as oxytetracycline and doxycycline. Oxytetracycline would be preferred on grounds of cost, is easily administered and is more likely than doxycycline to concentrate in the urine. Given the history of polyuria/polydipsia it would be important to rule out renal failure, as this would be a contraindication to the use of oxytetracycline.

The second choice antibiotic would be ampicillin, as the MIC falls furthest from the breakpoint on the s-i-r scale. Cost, ease of administration and safety are all satisfied by the use of this antibiotic. The decreased risk of adverse effects when compared with oxytetracycline may make this the preferred choice for some clinicians. Ampicillin predicts the *in vitro* susceptibility to amoxicillin, which may also therefore be used.

References and further reading

Addie D and Ramsay I (2001). The laboratory diagnosis of infectious diseases. In: *BSAVA Manual of Canine and Feline Infectious Diseases*, ed. I Ramsay and B Tennant, pp. 1–17. BSAVA Publications, Cheltenham

Anon (2003) Hospital superbug MRSA spreads to animals. *The Observer*, 14th December

Aucoin D (2002) *Target – The Antimicrobial Reference Guide to Effective Treatment, 2nd edn*. North American Compendiums Inc., Port Huron

Biberstein EL and Zee YC (1990) *Review of Veterinary Microbiology*. Blackwell Scientific, Boston

Dunning M and Stonehewer J (2002) Urinary tract infections in small animals: pathophysiology and diagnosis. *In Practice* **24,** 418–432

Duquette RA and Nuttall TJ (2004) Methicillin-resistant *Staphylococcus aureus* in dogs and cats: an emerging problem? *Journal of Small Animal Practice* **45,** 591–7

Greene CG (1998) *Infectious Diseases of the Dog and Cat, 2nd edn*. WB Saunders, Philadelphia

Gunn-Moore D and Shaw S (1997) Mycobacterial disease in the cat. *In Practice* **19,** 493–501

Houlton JEF (1994) Ancillary aids to the diagnosis of joint disease. In: *BSAVA Manual of Small Animal Arthrology*, ed. JEF Houlton and RW Collinson, pp. 22–38. BSAVA Publications, Cheltenham

Malik R, Hughes MS, James G, Martin P, Wigney DI, Canfield PJ, Chen SCA, Mitchell DH and Love DN (2002) Feline leprosy: two different clinical syndromes. *Journal of Feline Medicine and Surgery* **4,** 43–59

Miller JM (1996) *Specimen Management in Clinical Microbiology*. American Society for Microbiology, Washington DC

NCCLS (2001) *Performance Standards for Antimicrobial Disk and Dilution Susceptibility Tests for Bacteria Isolated from Animals, Approved Standard*. M31-A2. Wayne, PA

Quinn PJ, Carter ME, Markey B and Carter GR (1994) *Clinical Veterinary Microbiology*. Mosby, St Louis

Quinn PJ, Markey BK, Carter ME, Donnelly WJC, Leonard FC and Maguire D (2002) *Veterinary Microbiology and Microbial Disease*. Blackwell Science Ltd, Oxford

Rich M and Roberts L (2004). Methicillin-resistant *Staphylococcus aureus* isolated from companion animals. *Veterinary Record* **154,** 310

Sparkes AH, Gruffydd-Jones TJ, Shaw SE, Wright AI and Stokes CR (1993) Epidemiological and diagnostic features of canine and feline dermatophytosis in the United Kingdom from 1956 to 1991. *Veterinary Record* **133,** 57–61

Sparkes AH, Werrett G, Stokes CR and Gruffydd-Jones TJ (1994) *Microsporum canis*: inapparent carriage by cats and the viability of arthrospores. *Journal of Small Animal Practice* **35,** 397–401

Walker AL, Jang SS and Hirsh DC (2000) Bacteria associated with pyothorax of dogs and cats: 98 cases (1989–1998). *Journal of the American Veterinary Medical Association* **216,** 359–363

Resources

Mycobacterial reference laboratories

Health Protection Agency
Mycobacterium Reference Unit and Regional Centre for Mycobacteriology
Dulwich Hospital
East Dulwich Grove
London
SE22 8QF
Tel. 020 8693 2830

National Public Health Service of Wales
Regional Centre for Mycobacteriology
Llandough Hospital
Cardiff
CF64 2XX
Tel. 02920 716408

Scottish Mycobacteria Reference Laboratory
Edinburgh Royal Infirmary
51 Little France Crescent
Edinburgh
EH16 5SA
Tel. 0131 242 6022

Reference laboratories are also situated in Birmingham, Newcastle, the Royal Brompton Hospital, London, and the City Hospital, Belfast. These laboratories together form the UK Mycobacterial Network to monitor tuberculosis drug resistance in humans.

Mycoplasma

Specialist advice on *Mycoplasma* cultures can be obtained from:

Mycoplasma Experience
1 Norbury Road
Reigate
Surrey
RH2 9BY
Tel. 01737 226662
Fax. 01737 224751
E-mail. mexp@mycoplasma-exp.com

26

Diagnosis of viral infections

Alan Radford and Susan Dawson

Introduction

Viral infections of small animals are common and frequently represent an important cause of disease. Although precise diagnosis is not always necessary, it may be required to determine appropriate therapy and prognosis, and to give advice about the potential for disease in other susceptible animals sharing the same environment. In many cases, a presumptive diagnosis may be made without recourse to specific diagnostic tests, based on the signalment, history, clinical signs and more routine diagnostic assays, such as haematology and biochemistry. For example, lack of vaccination and panleucopenia suggest canine parvovirus; mouth ulcers and upper respiratory tract disease suggest feline calicivirus. However, a more definitive diagnosis may be facilitated by using one or more of a wide range of specific diagnostic tests.

This chapter will cover the theory of the most common diagnostic tests available for small animal viruses. In order to interpret any given result correctly, it is critical to understand both the biology of the virus in question and the principles of the test used. For a more detailed discussion of virus biology, readers are referred to other texts (e.g. Greene, 1998).

Viral diagnostic tests can be divided into two categories:

- Tests that detect parts of the virus, such as isolation, antigen detection, polymerase chain reaction (PCR) and both light and electron microscopy (EM)
- Tests that detect antibody produced by the immune response to the virus, following either infection or vaccination.

No single test is perfect: the advantages and disadvantages of various methodologies are discussed below. In addition, when interpreting test results it is important to consider the limitations of the test and the biological behaviour of specific viral infections.

Virus detection

These tests include historically well established tests, such as virus isolation (VI) and haemagglutination (HA), and much newer ones, such as those based on PCR. Some rely on the presence of the whole virus (e.g. isolation, electron microscopy) whereas others detect specific components or fractions of the virus (e.g. antigen detection). Currently, no one test consistently outperforms the others in all cases, and all methodologies are still used in routine diagnosis.

Virus isolation

Virus isolation relies on the ability of some viruses to replicate in cell cultures in the laboratory. Clinical samples are taken and placed into specialized virus transport medium (VTM), which restricts the growth of bacterial contaminants in the sample during transit to the laboratory. VI relies on having both functional virus particles and a cell line that supports the replication of the virus in the laboratory. It works best for viruses that are stable outside the host (e.g. canine parvovirus (CPV), feline calicivirus (FCV), cowpox virus), but works poorly for very fragile viruses that rapidly lose infectivity outside the host (e.g. feline coronavirus). The cell cultures used are generally semi-permanent cell lines grown as a monolayer on plastic. However, primary cell lines and organ explants may be used less commonly.

Virus replication is usually associated with cellular toxicity that is manifested as a cytopathic effect (cpe). In the cell culture common cpes include cell lysis, syncytium formation and inclusion body formation (Figure 26.1). Usually the combination of the cell type that supports virus growth and the nature or pattern of the cpe is sufficient to achieve a diagnosis. In some cases, the virus may be further characterized by fixing the cells and staining the viral antigens with virus-specific antisera.

The principal disadvantage of VI is the requirement for dedicated facilities to maintain the growth of cells in culture, limiting such tests to specialist laboratories. It is advisable to use the correct VTM supplied by the laboratory, as this medium will have been tested to ensure it is not harmful to the cell culture system being used. Despite the use of VTM, viruses can still be inactivated in transport or the VTM can become contaminated with bacteria from the sample, and this can render the sample unusable. Arguably, the major drawback of VI is the time taken to report samples as 'no virus isolated', which may be as long as 2–3 weeks, and may be too late to inform clinical decision making.

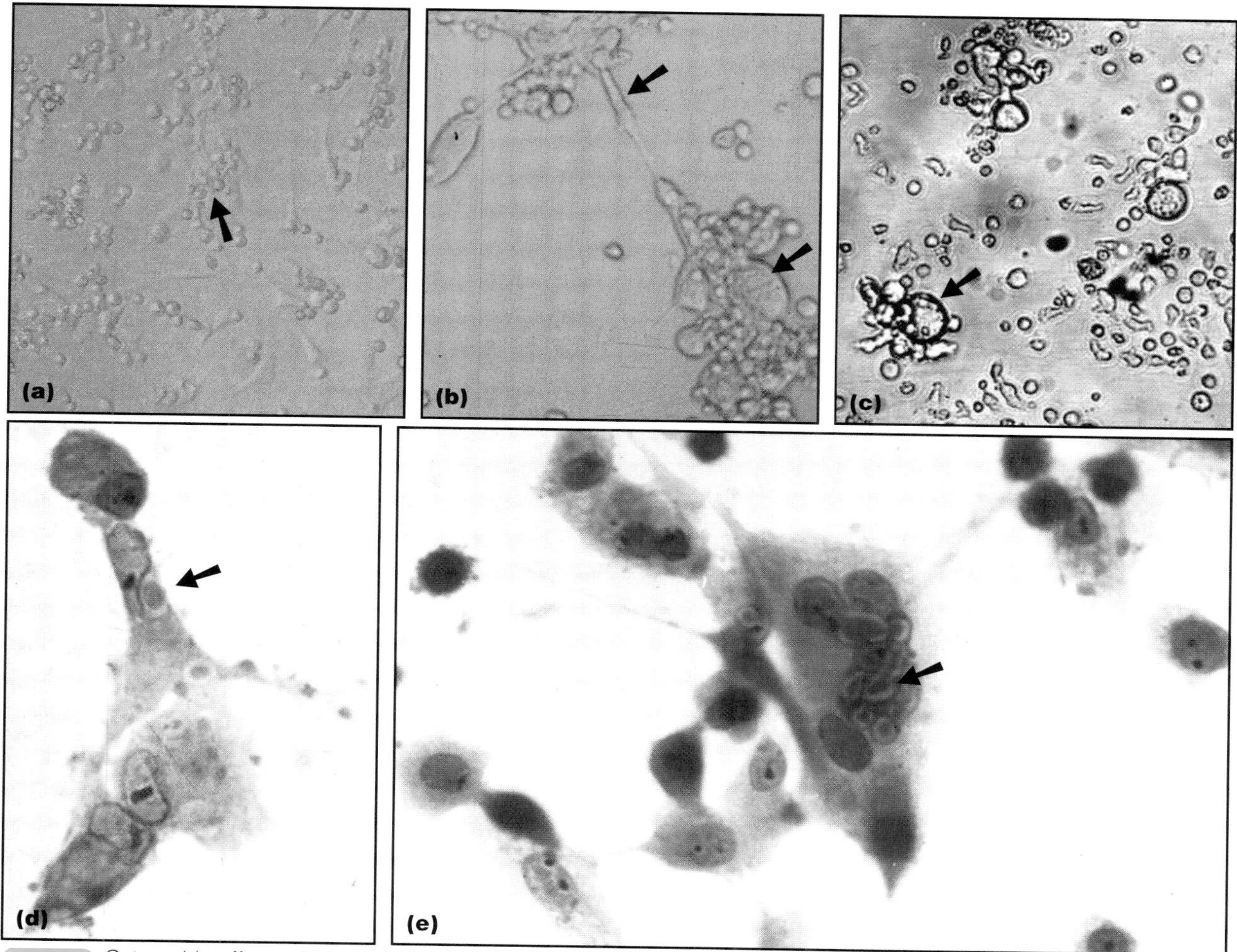

26.1 Cytopathic effects. (a) Feline calicivirus (FCV) cpe (in tissue culture) manifests as cell rounding and shrinkage (arrowed). (© Susan Dawson) (b) Feline herpesvirus (FHV) cpe (in tissue culture) manifests as ballooning of cells and long strands of cellular material (arrowed). (© Susan Dawson) (c) Feline immunodeficiency virus (FIV) cpe (in lymphocytes in liquid co-culture) manifests as ballooning of infected cells (arrowed). (Courtesy of O Jarrett) (d) Cowpox intracytoplasmic inclusion bodies (arrowed). (H&E stain) (Courtesy of M Bennett) (e) Feline herpesvirus syncytium and intranuclear inclusion bodies (arrow shows inclusion body within a syncytium). (H&E stain) (Courtesy of RM Gaskell)

Viral antigen detection in clinical specimens

Antigen detection relies on the ability of viral antigens present within clinical samples (e.g. blood and tissue sections) to react specifically with antibodies raised to that particular antigen. There are two common sources of these antigen-specific antibodies:

- Polyclonal antisera contain a range of antibodies to different epitopes from the virus and usually come from infected animals
- Monoclonal antibodies come from experimental mice; they are produced from a single clone of B-cells and therefore are specific for a single epitope.

In the first stage of the process, the antigen in question needs to be immobilized on a solid surface. In some clinical specimens, the viral antigen may already be immobilized on a glass slide within infected cells, such as in a tissue smear (feline leukaemia virus (FeLV), canine distemper virus) or tissue section (immunohistology) (Figure 26.2A,B). In other cases, where the antigen is free in a biological solution, such as in blood or serum, the antigen must first be captured. This can be achieved with a specific antibody which is bound to a solid surface (antigen capture or 'sandwich') (Figure 26.2C,D).

Once the antigen has been immobilized, it can be detected by incubation with a specific antibody. Sometimes this antibody has a coloured molecule directly attached to it, such as fluorescein or colloidal gold particles, to allow the direct visualization of bound antibody (immunofluorescence (Figure 26.3) and rapid immunomigration, RIM). Alternatively, the antibody may have an enzyme attached to it (commonly phosphatase or peroxidase; Figure 26.4) that catalyses the subsequent synthesis of a coloured product. However, more commonly, this antibody is unlabelled and its specific binding is detected with a second antibody that is labelled (Figure 26.2B,D). In such a two-antibody system the antibodies are referred to as the primary and secondary antibodies.

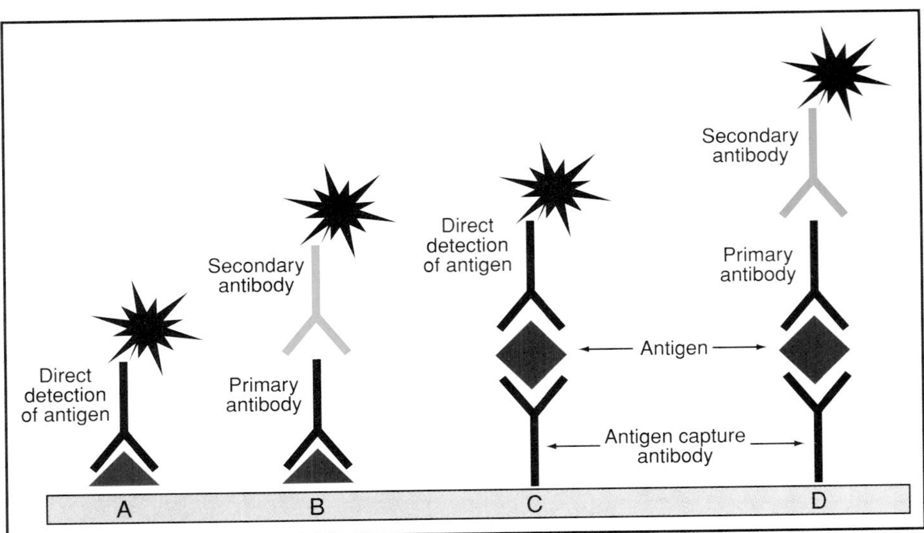

26.2 Viral antigen detection. Direct and indirect methods. The antigen to be detected is in red.

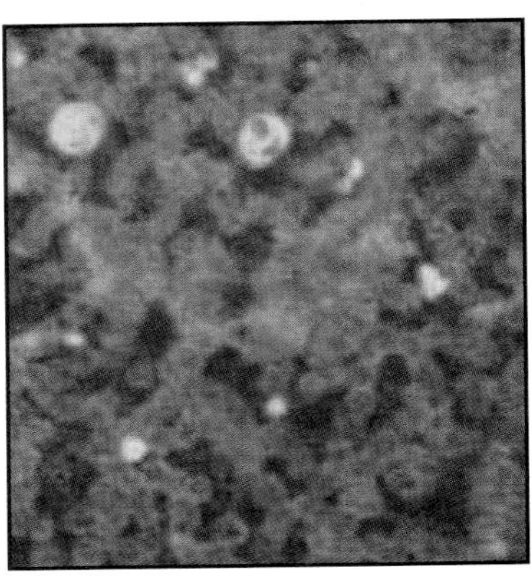

26.3 Immunofluorescence of FeLV antigens in a peripheral blood smear, showing green positive fluorescence in leucocytes and platelets. (Courtesy of O Jarrett)

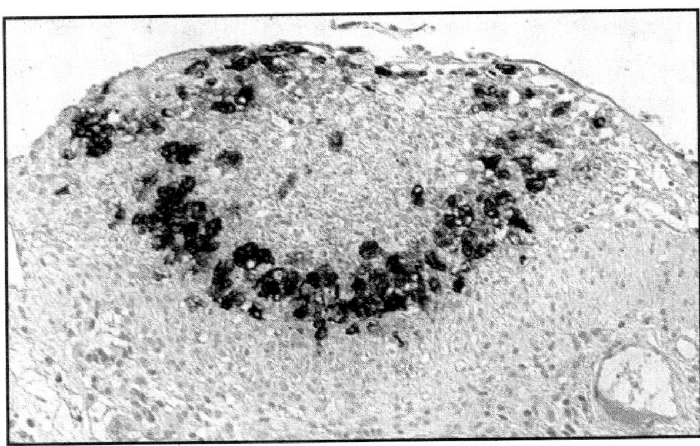

26.4 Immunoperoxidase method. Granulomatous inflammation of the intestinal serosa in a cat with feline infectious peritonitis (FIP), showing a central area of necrosis surrounded by macrophages expressing viral antigen (stained brown). (Courtesy of A. Kipar)

The best example of viral antigen detection from clinical specimens in small animals is probably FeLV, in which p27 is detected in the blood. This viral protein is produced in abundance in FeLV-infected animals within infected cells and spills out into the serum. The p27 protein may be detected directly on blood smears where antigen is present, particularly within white blood cells and platelets (immunofluorescence; Figure 26.3). Alternatively, it can be detected by antigen capture using either an enzyme-linked immunosorbent assay (ELISA) in the commercial laboratory, or the RIM kits most frequently used in general practice (Figure 26.5). The term ELISA refers to a wide range of tests that take place on a plastic surface and can be used either for the detection of antigen or antibody (see below).The principal advantage of direct viral antigen detection within infected cells is the ability to localize viral antigen expression to the appropriate cellular compartment, thereby reducing the number of false positives. This does not apply to RIM practice kits and may explain some of the false positives obtained with such tests.

Polymerase chain reaction

Unlike other methods for detecting virus, PCR is unique in detecting the viral genetic information rather than viral protein. PCR allows the specific multiplication (amplification) of small amounts of DNA to a level that can be readily detected. The amplification is specific, being limited to a particular region of DNA (target) by the use of short molecules of single-stranded DNA (primers) that are complementary to the DNA on either side of the target. Whilst the specifics of any given PCR may vary, the principles of each remain the same and consist of denaturation, annealing and extension phases, which are repeated multiple times in the same order.

- In the first stage of the PCR, the DNA double helix (template) is heated to around 94°C to separate (denature) the two strands of DNA (Figure 26.6a)
- In the second stage of the PCR, the DNA is cooled down to allow the single-stranded primers to bind (anneal) specifically to their target sequence in the single-stranded template. The annealing temperature is one of the most critical things in any PCR and depends on the sequence of the primer (Figure 26.6b; primers in red)
- In the third round of the PCR, the DNA is heated to approximately 72°C. At this temperature, the DNA polymerase extends the primers in the 5' to 3' direction (Figure 26.6c).

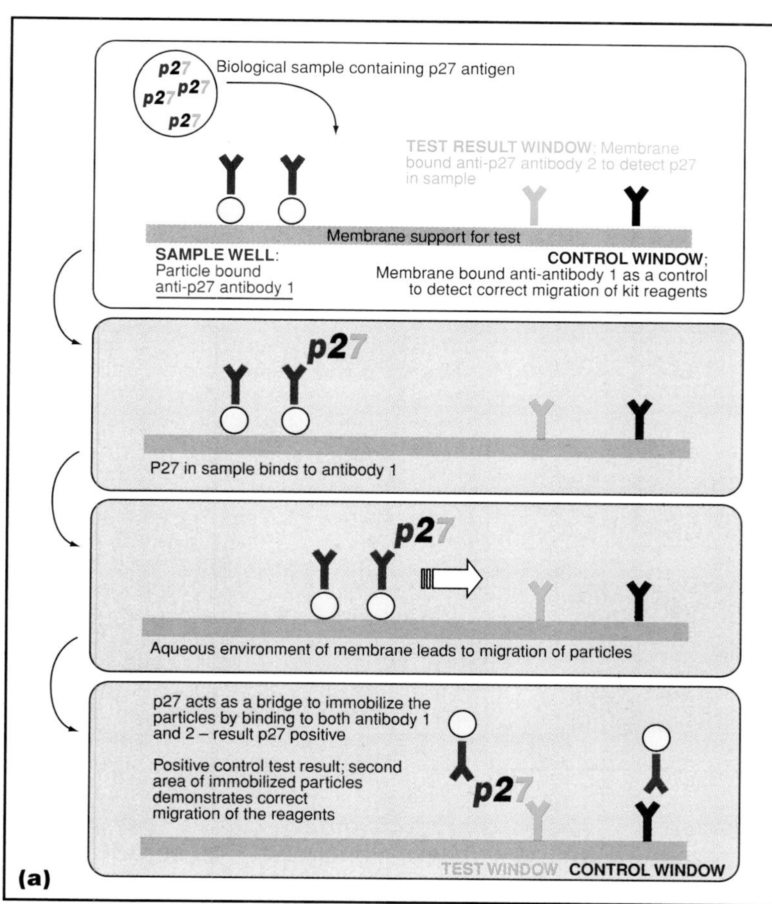

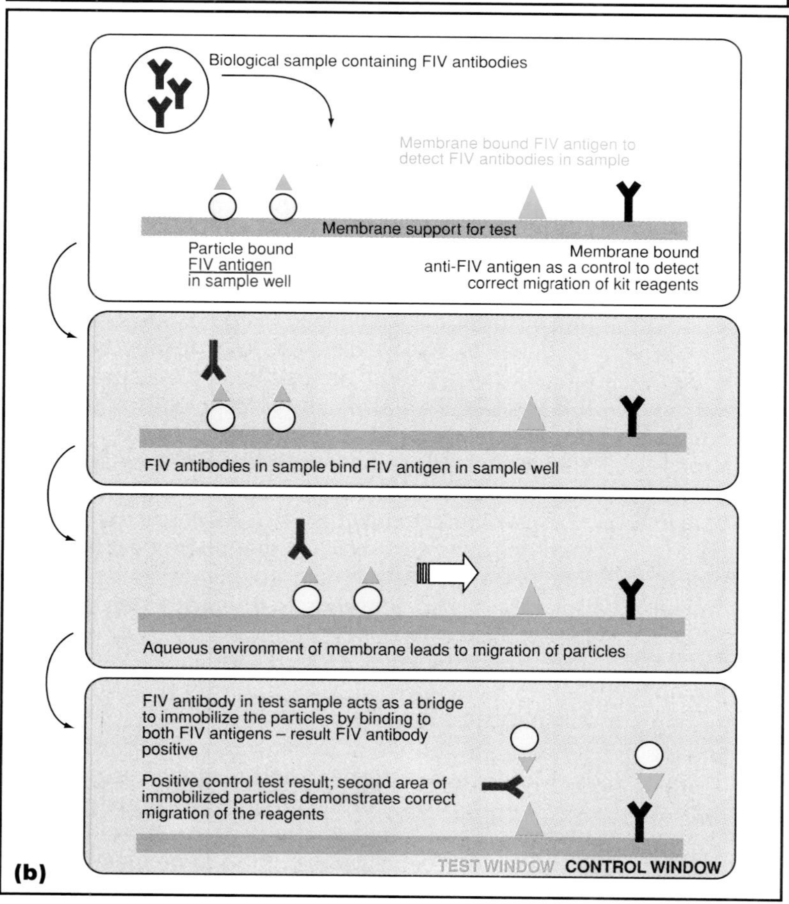

26.5 Examples of rapid immunomigration technology used for the detection of (a) FeLV p27 antigen and (b) FIV antibodies. (Based on pictures kindly supplied by Synbiotics Europe)

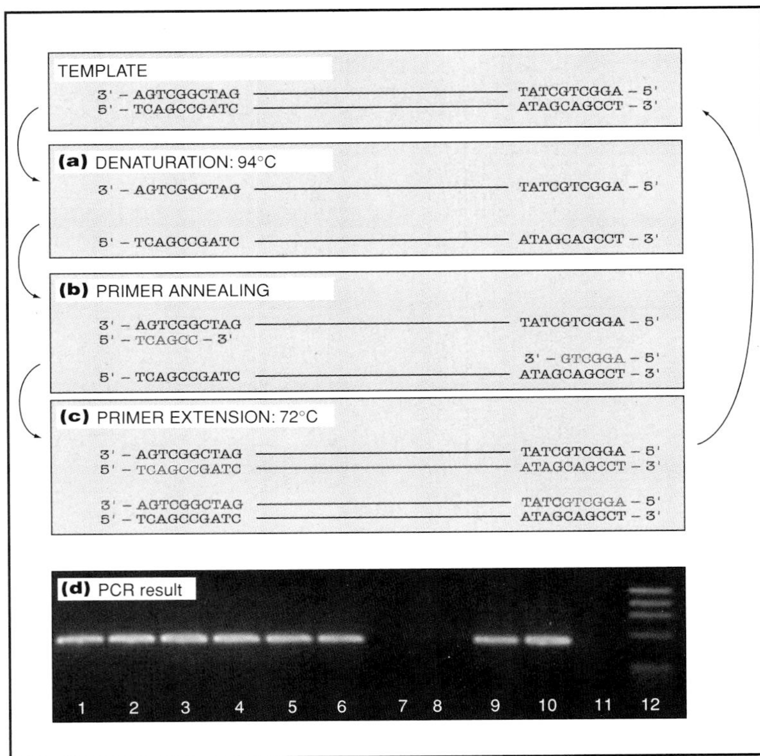

26.6 Polymerase chain reaction. Reactions occur in a solution containing the template DNA, the DNA polymerase enzyme and nucleotides. The template is double-stranded DNA, shown as two black lines with the nucleotides at each end specified. 3' and 5' refer to the different chemical ends of the DNA, and are shown because DNA polymerase extends the sequence only in the 5' to 3' direction. (a) Denaturation: the DNA template is heated, so the double strands separate, allowing access by the primers and enzyme. (b) Primer annealing: at a lower temperature, specially designed primers (short sequences of DNA shown in red) complementary to the DNA sequence flanking the area of interest bind (anneal) to their target sequence on the new single stranded template DNA. (c) Primer extension: DNA polymerase creates a complementary DNA strand (shown in blue) from the primer in a 5' to 3' direction. The result is double-stranded DNA that is a copy of the template DNA. These cycles are repeated, and DNA copies increase exponentially. (d) Results of typical PCR: lanes 1–6 are positive; lanes 7 and 8 are negative; lanes 9 and 10 are positive controls; lane 11 is the negative control; lane 12 is a molecular weight marker to identify the size of the amplified DNA product.

At the end of the extension phase, the DNA is again double-stranded and one cycle has been completed. An individual PCR will typically repeat this cycle 35–40 times, with the number of target molecules, in theory, doubling in each cycle. Amplified DNA molecules are detected by running them on an agarose gel, where an electric current separates them on the basis of their size (Figure 26.6d).

Since the DNA polymerases used in the reaction only replicate DNA and not RNA, the PCR reaction must be modified for RNA viruses. In this case, the viral RNA must first be converted to DNA by incubation with a reverse transcriptase enzyme; this DNA can then be amplified by PCR. The whole protocol is referred to as a reverse transcriptase PCR or RT-PCR.

The principal advantage of PCR is its speed (a result may be attainable in as little as 1 working day, whereas isolation may take up to 2–3 weeks). In addition, PCRs may be set up to detect more than one pathogen, saving on cost and time (e.g. feline herpesvirus and *Chlamydophila felis*) (Sykes *et al.*, 1999; Helps *et al.*, 2003). An exciting recent development in PCR technology is 'light-cycler' PCR. This system is even more rapid than conventional PCR and also allows the quantification of specific DNA in the original sample. In human medicine, this type of PCR is being used to quantify viral load in order to stage human immunodeficiency virus infection and monitor the response to antiviral therapy. Such quantification may become available in the future to allow the staging of feline immunodeficiency virus (FIV) infection.

As well as its speed, a well designed PCR is extremely sensitive, being capable of detecting very small quantities of DNA. In some cases, the sensitivity can be increased further by using a nested PCR, where the products of the PCR are re-amplified in a second reaction. With such high sensitivity, PCR may give a positive result when other tests, such as VI or EM, are negative (Mochizuki *et al.*, 1993; Schunck *et al.*, 1995).

Once viral DNA has been amplified, its nucleotide sequence can also be determined. This allows confirmation that the DNA amplified by the PCR is indeed the target DNA, and this is important for quality control. In addition, by sequencing a variable region of the virus genome, strains of virus can be compared and differentiated. This is particularly useful for typing studies, often allowing the source of infections to be identified. Whilst this is not always clinically necessary, it can prove useful in investigating the potential ability of live vaccines to cause disease (e.g. feline calicivirus) (Radford *et al.*, 2000). In the future, it may be possible to design PCRs that identify virulent forms of virus and distinguish them from less harmful types. In small animal virology such a test would be of great use in the diagnosis of feline infectious peritonitis (FIP).

The principal drawbacks of PCR are the requirement for specialist facilities (although most laboratories now have these available) and its sensitivity. Because it is so sensitive, PCR is extremely prone to false positives unless carried out in specially designed laboratories by highly trained staff.

Histopathology

Viruses are too small to allow direct visualization of individual virus particles by light microscopy. However, for some viruses, the pattern of the histopathological changes associated with the virus are so specific that it can allow a definitive diagnosis to be made (Figure 26.7). Another common diagnostic feature of some

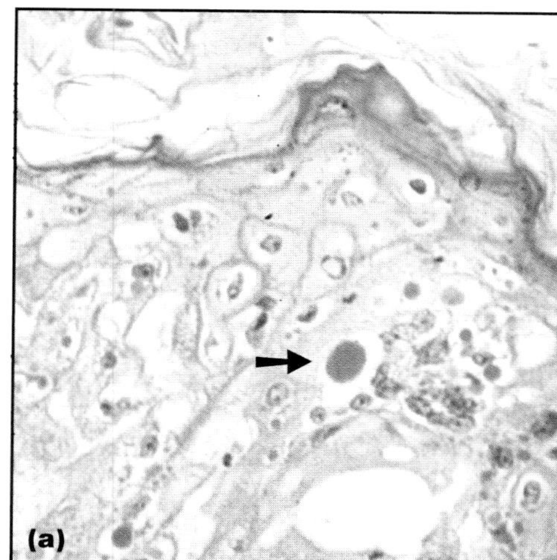

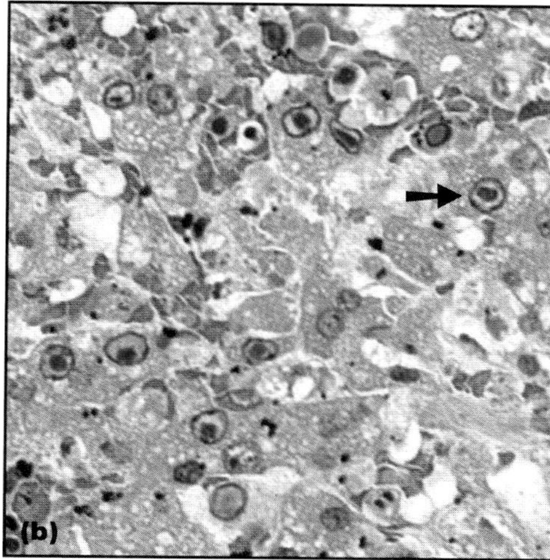

26.7 Histopathology. Lesions can sometimes be used to provide a diagnosis for viral infections. (a) Cowpox lesion in a cat. The arrow indicates an intracytoplasmic inclusion. (H&E stain; original magnification X400) (Courtesy of M Bennett.) (b) Infectious canine hepatitis, showing adenoviral inclusions (arrowed) in infected hepatocytes. (H&E stain; original magnification X1000) (Courtesy of A Kipar)

viruses are inclusion bodies, which represent aggregates of virus proteins within the cell. These may be intranuclear (herpesviruses, canine adenovirus) or intracytoplasmic (cowpox, rabies Negri bodies, canine distemper). In many cases, the presence of viral antigen within histological sections may be confirmed by immunohistology (see above). Such tests are fairly cumbersome and require specialist pathological interpretation. However, they still have their use in those cases where more definitive diagnosis cannot be achieved by other means (e.g. FIP).

Electron microscopy

Perhaps the purest example of virus antigen detection is direct visualization of the virus in clinical samples by electron microscopy (EM). However, virus particles are very small and can easily be missed, even with the electron microscope. EM is particularly suited to those cases where large amounts of virus are present within clinical samples. Visualization of virus particles can be enhanced by clumping them together with specific antisera (immune EM). Once seen, most viruses have a fairly distinctive appearance to the trained eye, and can be identified based on their morphological appearance and size (Figure 26.8). The use of EM is limited because of its expense, associated with the need for highly specialized equipment, and due to the availability of cheaper, more sensitive, assays for most viruses. It is still used for the demonstration of poxvirus particles in clinical specimens (cowpox), or for the demonstration of virus particles in faeces. It also remains a valuable tool in research for the investigation of outbreaks of disease caused by new viruses, where, by definition, specific tests will not be available.

Haemagglutination

For many years it has been recognized that some viruses have the seemingly peculiar ability to agglutinate (clump) red blood cells; this is termed haemagglutination (HA). Although the mechanism by which this occurs may not be known, HA can be used for diagnosis. The result can be confirmed by inhibiting the HA with specific antiserum raised against the virus: haemagglutination inhibition (HAI; Figure 26.9). The best examples of viruses in small animal virology that cause HA are the parvoviruses of cats and dogs.

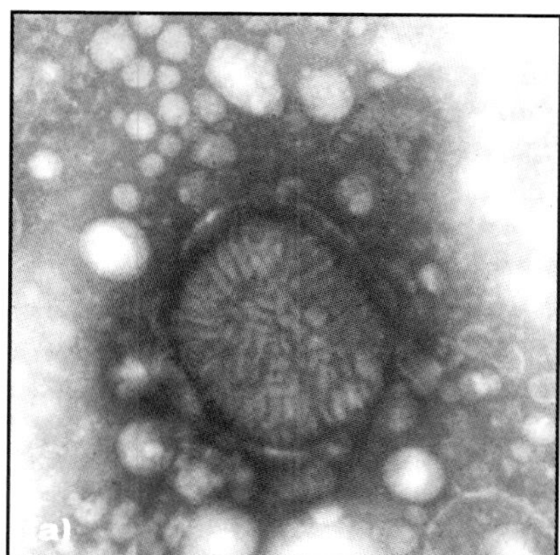

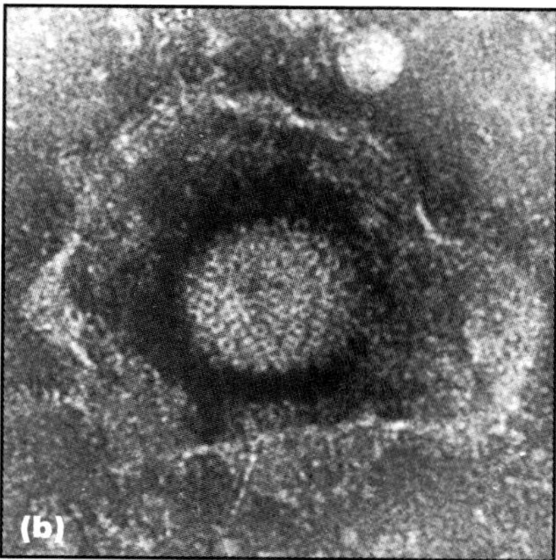

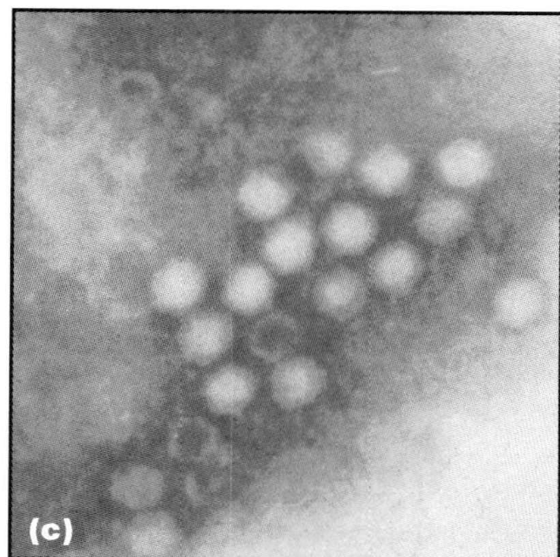

26.8 Electron microscopy. Although often difficult to find, most viruses have a very characteristic morphology which can allow a diagnosis to be made. (a) Cowpox virus with typical orthopoxvirus morphology. (Courtesy of M Bennett) (b) Feline herpesvirus particle with capsid morphology and envelope. (Courtesy of RM Gaskell) (c) Canine parvovirus particles in a faecal sample. (© Alan Radford)

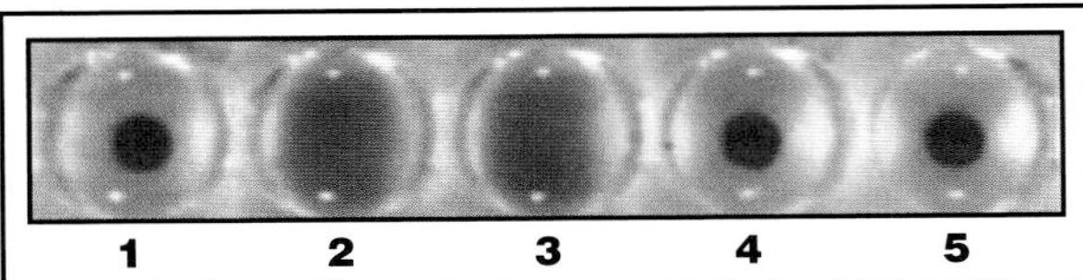

26.9 Haemagglutination inhibition. The presence of specific antibodies against virus is detected by inhibition of red cell agglutination. Where agglutination occurs, cells are clumped and remain in suspension; where agglutination is inhibited, cells settle to form a pellet. Wells 1, 4 and 5 are positive (agglutination is inhibited). Wells 2 and 3 are negative (no inhibition of agglutination). If this were a haemagglutination test, the opposite results would be reported. (Courtesy of DD Addie)

Antibody detection

In contrast to those tests that directly demonstrate part or whole of a specific virus to diagnose infection, antibody tests detect the host's immune response to viral antigens and use that to imply exposure to that particular virus. For all antibody tests there are some factors that must be considered.

- Antibodies may persist for a long time after acute viral infection and therefore detection of antibodies indicates previous as well as current infection. Where animals are able to mount an immune response but antibodies are unable to eliminate the virus, as with FIV infection, then the presence of antibodies can indicate current infection.
- As well as determining the simple presence or absence of a particular antibody, with many antibody tests (ELISA, immunofluorescence, virus neutralization, HAI), it is also possible to determine the amount (titre) of antibody against a particular virus. The test antiserum is serially diluted until it no longer produces a positive reaction in a given test. This point is called the end point and the antibody titre is usually given as the amount of times the test antiserum needs to be diluted to reach this end point. Thus, the higher the level of antibodies present in the test sample, the more the serum can be diluted before reaching the end point. Although not commonly used clinically, measuring antibody levels is required to indicate rising antibody titres suggestive of recent infection and is also used to demonstrate satisfactory response to vaccination (e.g. rabies).
- A rising antibody titre can be used to suggest recent infection. This usually means comparing the antibody titre in a sample during acute disease with that in a convalescent sample.
- If comparing antibody titres, it is important to use the same diagnostic method and laboratory for all titre comparisons. This is because there can be marked differences in titres between the same samples tested using different methodologies. Even with the same method in a single laboratory, differences in the titres may be observed for a given sample run on different days. Therefore, an allowance has to be made for experimental error. For many tests, up to 4-fold differences in titre are acceptable as experimental error, whereas differences of > 4-fold are taken as significant.
- Another method of differentiating acute and previous infection is to look for IgM class antibodies, which are only present early in infection. These IgM tests are not always available for individual viral infections. The majority of antibody tests used in small animal virology detect IgG class antibodies.
- Antibodies do not develop immediately after viral infection, so there is a lag phase where infection is present but antibodies cannot be detected. This may be the period of time when clinical signs are present and, therefore, diagnosis is required.
- Antibodies are also likely be present following vaccination and these can make the interpretation of test results difficult. For some viruses antibody titres would be expected to be higher after acute infection than following vaccination. However, in most cases it is not possible to differentiate between infection and vaccination based on antibody titres alone. Therefore, detection of antibody for diagnosing infection in animals that have been previously vaccinated is not appropriate. More recently, marker or DIVA (Differentiating Infected from Vaccinated Animals) vaccines have been produced, which allow the immune response in a vaccinated animal to be differentiated from that in an infected animal. Although no such vaccines are available currently for use in dogs and cats, these may become available in the future.
- The presence of maternally derived antibody (MDA) may interfere with antibody tests for diagnosis. The age of the animal may indicate whether the antibodies found are from the dam. However, some antibodies last longer than others, dependent on the levels acquired from the dam, and there are 'grey' areas where interpretation can be difficult. MDAs cause most problems when screening kittens for FIV infection. In this case, kittens can be tested at 12 weeks of age. However, there is some evidence that MDAs may last longer, for up to 6 months in occasional animals.

Broadly speaking, antibody tests can be divided into two groups:

- Detection using bound antigen (Figure 26.10); tests incorporating this methodology are antibody ELISA, IFT, Western blotting and rapid immunomigration
- Detection by inhibition of a detectable feature; such methods include virus neutralization tests and HAI.

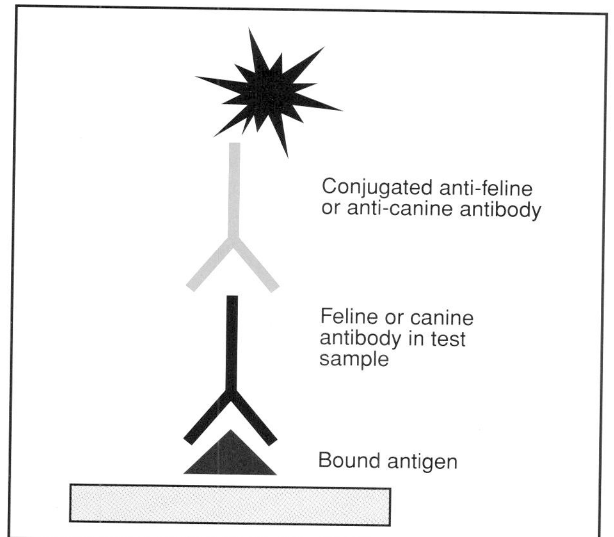

26.10 Detection of antibody using bound antigen. Antigen from the virus is immobilized on a solid surface to bind or capture any virus-specific antibodies present in the test sample. Unbound, non-specific antibodies are removed by washing. Subsequently, the presence of bound specific antibody is detected with a second species-specific antibody that reacts with any antibody from that species, i.e. anti-dog IgG or anti-cat IgG. This second antibody incorporates a marker system that allows its binding to be detected. This may be a directly visible product (e.g. fluorescein or colloidal gold particles) or, more commonly, an enzyme that catalyses a colour reaction with its substrate (e.g. peroxidase and alkaline phosphatase). The same format is essentially used for ELISA, immunofluorescence, Western blot and RIM tests.

Antibody ELISA

ELISA tests are most commonly carried out in plastic plates with small wells for each sample. Occasionally they can also be carried out on membranes. The most commonly used antibody ELISA test for small animal viruses is for anti-FIV antibodies. The ELISA format is particularly appropriate for processing large numbers of samples and also for measuring antibody titres.

Immunofluorescence

In immunofluorescence, the test serum (antiserum) is incubated on infected cell cultures. If specific antibody is present, it will bind to the specific viral antigens, and is then detected using a further species-specific antibody with a fluorescent molecule attached. The infected cells with the antibodies attached are then examined under a fluorescent microscope and apple-green fluorescence (more rarely orange) is seen where the antibody is present (Figure 26.11). The antibody only attaches to areas of the cell where virus is present; this localization within the cell helps to ensure the specificity of the test. The cell cultures should contain both infected and uninfected cells to improve the specificity of the test; in a true positive reaction only infected cells should fluoresce. The titre of antibodies can be determined by serially diluting the antiserum. Immunofluorescence is used commonly to determine anti-feline coronavirus antibody titres.

Western blotting

In Western blotting the virus against which antibodies are to be detected is first disrupted into its individual proteins (Figure 26.12). These proteins are then sepa-

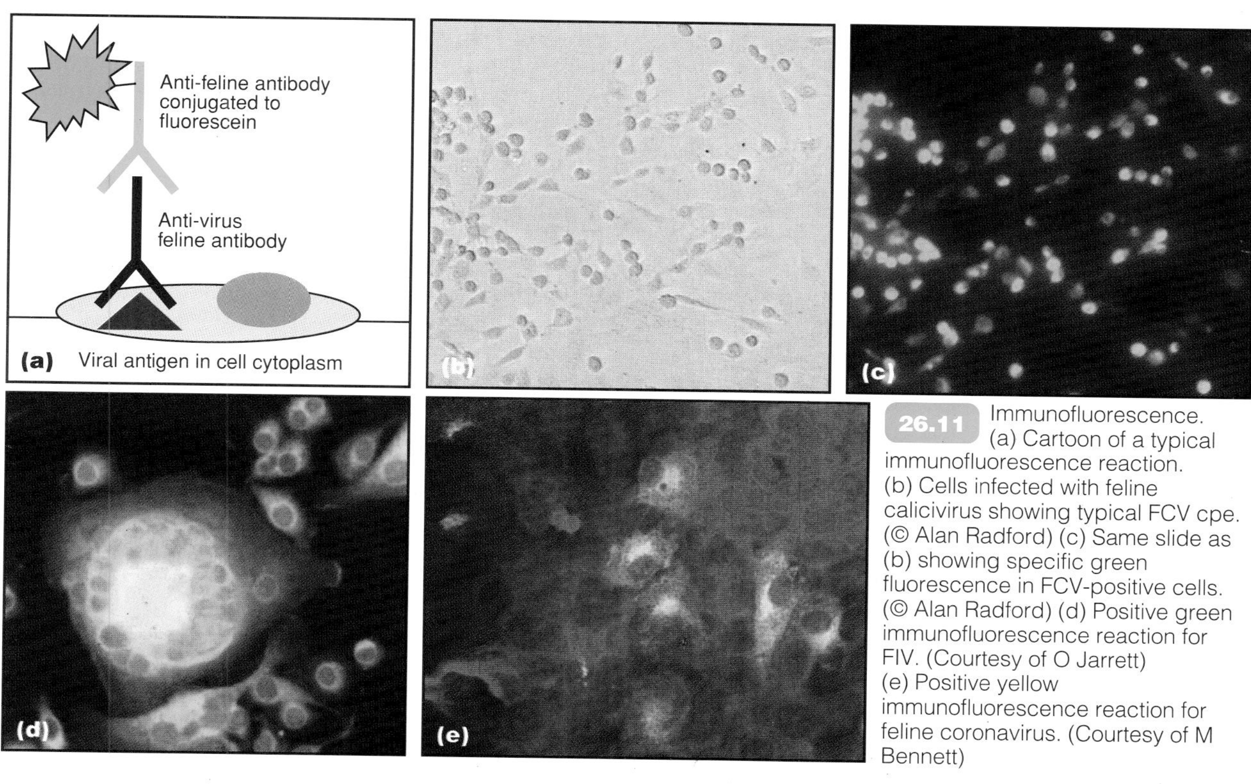

26.11 Immunofluorescence. (a) Cartoon of a typical immunofluorescence reaction. (b) Cells infected with feline calicivirus showing typical FCV cpe. (© Alan Radford) (c) Same slide as (b) showing specific green fluorescence in FCV-positive cells. (© Alan Radford) (d) Positive green immunofluorescence reaction for FIV. (Courtesy of O Jarrett) (e) Positive yellow immunofluorescence reaction for feline coronavirus. (Courtesy of M Bennett)

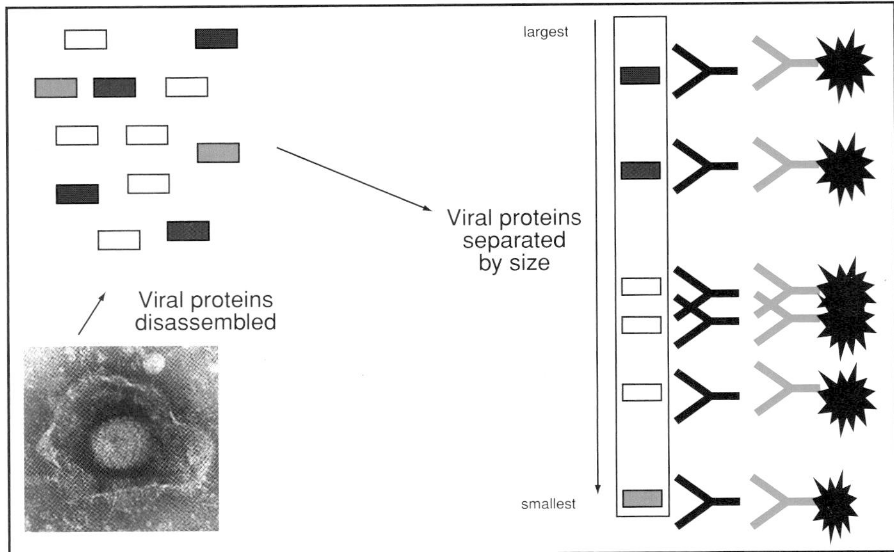

26.12 A typical Western blot reaction. The viral proteins are disassembled and separated on a gel according to their molecular weight. Specific antiviral antibodies from patient serum (black) are used as a target for subsequent antibody detection by the secondary antibody system (blue with black spiked star).

rated by size on a gel using an electric current, transferred (blotted) on to a membrane, and used to detect specific antibodies present in the test antiserum. If specific anti-virus antibodies are present they bind to the individual viral proteins on the membrane and are detected by a secondary antibody system. Positive results are seen as a series of bands on the membrane, corresponding to the individual viral proteins recognized by the immune response. This banding pattern is highly specific for each virus and makes the Western blot a highly specific test. Western blotting is used by some laboratories for the detection of anti-FIV antibodies. It is a fairly time-consuming and expensive test, so is not routinely used for the majority of viral diagnostics. It can be used to confirm positive FIV RIM tests. Because it detects antibodies to several viral proteins it may also be of use in 'end-stage' FIV infection where RIM tests may be falsely negative.

Rapid immunomigration

In this test the antigen–antibody complexes are captured on to colloidal gold particles and then diffuse along a membrane to be captured by the secondary antigen (see Figure 26.5b). Where they are captured, a colour change develops to indicate the test as positive. There is also a positive control band to confirm that the complexes have migrated sufficiently along the membrane. If this control reaction does not develop, the test should be repeated, otherwise a false negative result may occur.

The best examples of antibody RIM tests in small animal virology are for the detection of specific anti-FIV antibodies. These tests are commonly used within the practice situation and have the advantage of being easy to use and quick. They do, however, have limitations and in some cases positive results should be confirmed by other tests, particularly in low prevalence populations and where a positive result is unexpected (see below).

Virus neutralization

Specific antibody in the test sample is used to neutralize a set amount of a laboratory virus. Neutralization of the virus is detected by the lack of development of cytopathic effects in cell culture. Virus neutralization tests are relatively laborious and, for many viral infections, have been superceded by newer and quicker methods. A good example of their remaining use is the measurement of anti-rabies antibody titres following vaccination as part of the PETS travel scheme, where the antibody titre has to reach a certain level for the animal to be classified as responding to vaccination.

Haemagglutination inhibition

Where viruses are capable of HA, the presence of specific antibodies against these viruses can be detected by the inhibition of this agglutination (see Figure 26.9). Again, the test antiserum can be diluted until no further HAI occurs, giving a titre for the antibodies present. This methodology is relatively labour-intensive and is carried out only at specialist laboratories. HAI is only applicable for viruses that have HA activity (e.g. canine and feline parvoviruses).

Test accuracy

Sensitivity and specificity

No diagnostic test is perfect. In order to measure the accuracy of a test, the results of the test need to be compared to an accepted 'gold standard' or known true result. By comparing the result achieved with a given test to that achieved by the gold standard, it is possible to calculate two simple measures of the test's accuracy:

- The **sensitivity** of a test is the proportion of true positives detected by the test
- The **specificity** of a test is the proportion of true negatives detected by the test.

Example

A population of 1000 dogs is tested for virus X. According to the gold standard test, 100 dogs are positive for virus X and 900 are negative (equal to a prevalence of 10%).

A new test for virus X is applied to the same population. Of the 100 animals that really have the virus according to the gold standard test, 90 test positive (true positives) with the new test; the remainder test negative (false negatives). Of the 900 dogs that are actually negative for virus X by the gold standard test, 855 test negative (true negative) with the new test and 45 test positive (false positives).

These data can be tabulated in a grid (Figure 26.13a). Using this grid and calculating down the columns, it can be seen that this equates to a sensitivity of 90% and a specificity of 95% for the new test.

For most tests, sensitivity and specificity are inversely related: as sensitivity increases, the specificity decreases and *vice versa*. Therefore, it is very rare to get a test that has both 100% sensitivity and specificity.

		True status		
		Virus X positive	Virus X negative	
New test	Virus X positive	90	45	90 / 135 = 67% Positive predictive value
	Virus X positive	10	855	855 / 865 = 99% Negative predictive value
		90 / 100 = 90% sensitivity	855 / 900 = 95% specificity	

(a) Population size 1000; prevalence 10%

		True status		
		Virus X positive	Virus X negative	
New test	Virus X positive	9	49	9 / 58 = 16% Positive predictive value
	Virus X positive	1	941	941 / 942 = 99.9% Negative predictive value
		9 / 10 = 90% sensitivity	941 / 990 = 95% specificity	

(b) Population size 1000; prevalence 1%

26.13 Measurements of a test's accuracy.

Positive and negative predictive values

Using the same grid (Figure 26.13a), two further very useful measures of a test's accuracy can be calculated:

- The **positive predictive value (PPV)** is the likelihood of a positive test being genuine
- The **negative predictive value (NPV)** is the likelihood of a negative test being genuine.

These values can be calculated from Figure 26.13a by using the data in the rows. Of 135 positive results 90 are correct, giving a PPV of 67% (90/135 x 100). Of 865 negative results 855 are correct, giving a NPV of 99%. Thus, although this test appears to have relatively high values for both sensitivity and specificity, a positive test is only correct in two thirds of cases.

The critical feature of both the PPV and NPV is that, unlike the sensitivity and specificity which are inherent features of a given test, the PPV and NPV are affected by the prevalence of the condition in the population being tested.

Example

The same diagnostic test for virus X is applied to another population of 1000 dogs, in which the prevalence of the virus is only 1% (10 dogs positive and 990 dogs negative) (Figure 26.13b). The sensitivity and specificity remain the same (we have applied the same test). This time, of 942 negative results 941 are correct and only one is incorrect (false negative), giving a NPV of 99.9%. Critically, however, of 58 positive results only 9 are correct, with a massive 49 being incorrect (false positives), giving a PPV of only 16% (9/58 x 100). Put another way, this means that in this low-prevalence population, less than one of every five positive results is correct. In contrast, negative results are nearly always right.

Clinical significance

When trying to interpret the accuracy of a given test it is important to be aware of its sensitivity and specificity, and what gold standard was used to evaluate the test. Unfortunately, the answers to some, or even all, of these questions may be unknown!

In addition, when deciding how to interpret positive and negative results, it is important to consider the prevalence of infection and to be aware that this will vary depending on the population tested. For example, the prevalence of any virus is likely to be lower in a clinically normal population that is being screened for infection than it is in a population of sick animals being tested for disease. Therefore, the PPV is likely to be lower when screening for infection in healthy populations and higher when testing animals where there is a clinical index of suspicion for disease. This can be illustrated using FIV where, in clinically normal cats, the prevalence of infection is likely to be < 1% in the UK. In such cats, a test whose sensitivity and specificity are 95% would give a PPV of approximately 16%! These positive results must be treated with great caution and should be confirmed with a second independent test, especially as the consequences of a positive result may serious.

How does this compare to tests performed on clinically sick animals? It is certainly true that the prevalence of a given disease is likely to be higher in sick than in the healthy cats. However, this prevalence is often unknown, will by no means be 100% (otherwise we would not need to test), and it is likely to vary depending on the clinician (as will be seen if one considers the proportion of clinically sick cats one tests for FIV that actually test negative). Therefore, even in populations of sick animals, the PPV may still be low (and unacceptable) and test results may still need to be confirmed. For an interesting discussion of the sensitivity and specificity of the RIM tests for FeLV and FIV, see Hartmann *et al.*, 2001. (Sensitivity and specificity are also discussed in Chapter 2.)

False positives and false negatives

With most tests, false positives and false negatives will occur and represent failures of a given test. However, these may be compounded by placing the incorrect clinical interpretation upon what is actually a correct test result. Common causes of false positive and negative results are shown in Figure 26.14.

Test type	Causes of false positive results	Causes of false negative results
All tests		Poor sampling technique Sample deterioration in transit Operator error Incorrect reagent storage
Virus tests	Contamination (especially PCR)	Strain variation
Antibody tests	Cross reactive antibodies Anti-mouse antibodies: some cats have antibodies against mouse antibodies and these can cross-react with the mouse antibodies used in some diagnostic tests Anti-cell culture antibodies	Antigen excess: all antibody-bound and unavailable to be detected in the test

26.14 Causes of false positive and false negative test results.

Feline viruses

Diagnosis and interpretation of feline virus infections is often complicated. This reflects complex carrier states, and the frequent use of vaccines that often do not protect against infection.

Feline calicivirus

Feline calicivirus (FCV) is one of the viruses involved in upper respiratory tract disease. In addition, due to the large number of different strains of the virus, there can be variable clinical signs ranging from subclinical infection to a severe systemic disease with high mortality.

Diagnosis of FCV is usually made by VI from oropharyngeal swabs or other affected tissues (cpe shown in Figure 26.1a). A plain sterile cotton-tipped swab should be used to collect saliva from inside the cat's mouth and placed into a VTM. The VTM is best supplied by the laboratory that is carrying out the isolation. As FCV can be isolated from clinically normal carrier animals, care must be taken when interpreting positive virus isolations. Virus isolation does not necessarily equate to disease. In addition to VI, some laboratories have tried to develop RT-PCRs to detect the viral genome. These have the potential advantage of being quick. However, to the authors' knowledge, most PCRs suffer from the inability to detect some strains, which may lead to false negative results.

Tests based on detecting antibody titres (virus neutralization) are generally not used because of vaccination and the high prevalence of infection in the population. They have some use in determining whether a vaccine response is likely to neutralize a particular strain of virus.

Sequencing of portions of the FCV genome can be used as a method of molecular typing of FCV although this technique is only carried out in certain specialist laboratories and is expensive. For this test, the viral genome must first be amplified by RT-PCR, either from virus in a swab, or, more usually, from virus first grown in cell culture. This typing method has been used in the investigation of adverse vaccine reactions (Radford *et al.*, 2000).

Feline herpesvirus

Feline herpesvirus (FHV) is also associated with upper respiratory tract disease and, similarly to FCV, clinically recovered cats can become carriers. It is also frequently associated with ocular disease.

Diagnosis of FHV is most commonly made by VI from oropharyngeal swabs (cpe shown in Figure 26.1b). In addition, some specialist laboratories also offer PCR, which is quicker than VI, and may allow the detection of higher numbers of shedding cats. Some laboratories offer a combined PCR to detect FHV and another feline ocular/respiratory pathogen, *Chlamydophila felis* (so-called multiplex PCR). The DNA is usually amplified directly from oropharyngeal swab material. It is advisable to contact the laboratory prior to sample collection.

Once infected, it is likely that all cats become latently infected carriers. Shedding becomes intermittent and often follows a period of stress, so latently infected carriers may not be detected by single diagnostic tests.

As with FCV, tests based on detecting antibody titres (virus neutralization) are generally not used because of vaccination and the high prevalence of infection in the population.

Feline leukaemia virus

FeLV is associated with both malignant and non-malignant clinical conditions. The most common syndromes seen are lymphoma, leukaemia and anaemia. Not all cats infected with the virus go on to develop these clinical syndromes, and only persistently infected cats will succumb to most FeLV-related diseases; however, transient exposure increases the risk of later development of malignant disease.

Most cats clear viral infection and therefore any positive results should be followed up by re-testing in 12 weeks to determine whether persistent infection has been established. Initial screening tests available for FeLV rely on detection of free p27 antigen in heparinized blood by ELISA or RIM (see Figure 26.5a). FeLV antigen can also be detected in white blood cells by immunofluorescence, usually on smears of heparinized blood (see Figure 26.3). The sensitivity and specificity of these tests varies, and is likely to be reasonably high for the commercially available practice kits. However, because of the low prevalence of FeLV in some populations (approximately 1% of healthy cats), the PPV of in-house testing is low and more than half the positive results may be false positives. This is most important if a positive result is found in a healthy cat.

VI is also used to confirm positive results from p27 screening tests, and can be carried out using the same heparinized sample. VI is expected to be 100% specific but may give negative results if the cat is undergoing recent infection or recovery from infection. A very small number of cats may give discordant results, being p27 antigen-positive but VI-negative, due to localization of virus infection within a specific tissue, such as the mammary gland. The prognosis for these discordant cats is unclear. Depending on the test used, it may be more likely that the antigen result was a false positive.

Following on from initial infection some cats develop latent infection, with the virus present in bone marrow. In these cases VI from bone marrow may be positive. The role of latent infections in disease is uncertain, although most latently infected cats appear to have eliminated the virus within a few months. If one is considering sampling a cat to determine if it is latently infected with FeLV, it is advisable to first contact the laboratory to discuss the optimal sample collection procedure.

PCR can be used to detect FeLV viral genes, for example integrated retroviral elements in the DNA of some lymphoid tumours. The presence of these DNA fragments confirms that the animal has been exposed to FeLV but does not imply persistent infection. These are specialized techniques requiring cell or tissue samples.

Virus neutralizing (VN) antibodies can be detected in feline serum, and the presence of VN antibodies in the absence of viral antigen is an excellent indicator of a protected cat, which has previously been exposed to natural infection. Cats positive for VN antibodies do not require FeLV vaccination. Conversely, because the current vaccines may not induce VN antibodies the virus neutralization test does not give any indication of whether a cat has been previously vaccinated or whether vaccination has been protective. Finally, cats with persistent FeLV infection become immunotolerant to FeLV antigens and do not make antibodies.

Feline immunodeficiency virus

Infection with this retrovirus is characterized by a prolonged incubation period before the development of clinical signs. Once clinical signs develop they are associated with immunosuppression and accompanying secondary infections, so are very variable. Therefore, cats with a range of clinical signs may be tested for feline immunodeficiency virus (FIV) infection along with many healthy cats as part of routine testing.

Most diagnostic tests for FIV infection detect antibody. For FIV, the presence of antibody is indicative of persistent infection, as the immune response is not able to eliminate the virus. Most samples are tested with in-house RIM kits (see Figure 26.5b), but antibodies can also be detected in laboratories with immunofluorescence (Figure 26.11a), ELISA tests or Western blotting (see Figure 26.12).

Where diagnosis relies on detection of antibody it is important to be aware that:

- Maternally derived antibody may last up to 6 months in some individuals
- The time to seroconversion means that infected animals will be antibody-negative early in disease. Seroconversion typically takes around 8 weeks but may be longer (up to 6 months) in some cats
- Loss of antibody may occur in terminal disease due to a combination of immunosuppression and antigen excess. If there is a high clinical suspicion that a cat has terminal FIV-related disease and it is antibody-negative by RIM, it should be retested using a different method, such as Western blotting, VI or PCR
- An FIV vaccine has been marketed in the USA. Vaccinated cats will test positive for antibody.

Because of these limitations with antibody tests, it may be appropriate to try VI (cpe is shown in Figure 26.1c) or PCR in certain circumstances. However, these test are not as widely available.

Feline coronavirus

Feline coronavirus (FCoV) infection is common in cats, especially where grouped together. Infection is most commonly subclinical or associated with mild diarrhoea. However, in occasional cats infection leads to feline infectious peritonitis, a usually fatal disease. It is not completely understood why some cats develop FIP, although the immune status and genetics of the cat, the strain of the coronavirus and mutation of the virus within the cat are all thought to play a role.

It is not possible categorically to diagnose FIP clinically, and definitive diagnosis is based on histopathology of affected tissues (see Figure 26.4). There are no definitive diagnostic tests available for FIP and diagnosis is often based on a combination of laboratory tests and clinical examinations.

Diagnosis of FCoV infection may be easier, although the results still have to be interpreted with care. Antibody titres can be measured by immunofluorescence (Figure 26.11e) or ELISA, and viral genome can be detected by PCR. If antibody or viral antigen is present in blood samples this may indicate infection with FCoV but does not diagnose FIP. There is still no way to distinguish those feline coronaviruses that cause FIP from those that do not. Examination of effusions (e.g. abdominal fluid) by PCR or immunofluorescent staining of cells is a more useful test for diagnosing FIP, although still is not completely specific. Cats should not be euthanased on the grounds of a positive FCoV test result alone. Although not routinely performed, PCR has also been used to monitor FCoV shedding patterns (Addie and Jarrett, 2001).

Other tests helpful as an aid to diagnosis of FIP include:

- Routine haematology – lymphopenia, neutrophilic leucocytosis, non-regenerative anaemia
- Routine biochemistry – hyperproteinaemia (hypergammaglobulinaemia), low albumin:globulin ratio

- Acute-phase proteins – elevated α_1-acid glycoprotein (AGP) and haptoglobin
- Examination of effusions – high protein content (>35 g/l or as evaluated by Rivalta's test (Hartmann *et al.*, 2003)), low albumin:globulin ratio, low total cell count.

Cowpox virus

Cowpox virus circulates in wild rodents and can occasionally infect cats causing skin lesions. It is a zoonotic infection and more severe disease is seen in both human and feline immunocompromised patients. Therefore, care should be taken when handling infected cats and samples.

The virus survives for long periods in the environment and samples of scab material can be transported to the laboratory without specialist transport media. VI (see Figure 26.1d) or electron microscopy (see Figure 26.8a) can identify the virus. If tissue samples have been fixed, eosinophilic intracytoplasmic inclusion bodies can be seen histopathologically (Figure 26.7a).

Feline panleucopenia virus

Feline panleucopenia virus (FPV; also called feline parvovirus) multiplies in rapidly dividing cells and the clinical signs reflect this propensity. The clinical signs range in severity from subclinical to sudden death, with enteritis, panleucopenia and cerebellar hypoplasia.

Where cerebellar hypoplasia is present in kittens, diagnosis may be based on clinical signs. However, diagnostic tests are required where enteritis or sudden death are the main clinical signs. Virus isolation or detection (HA or ELISA/RIM tests) from faecal samples is often unsuccessful, as many animals will have ceased to shed detectable viral antigen by the time overt clinical disease develops. PCR may be a more sensitive method of viral detection in faecal and tissue samples.

Antibody titres can be measured, although many cats will have antibodies present due to vaccination or previous infection. Rising antibody titres may be difficult to demonstrate over the course of infection.

As the name of the virus suggests, affected cats are usually severely panleucopenic and this can help diagnosis.

Canine viruses

Diagnosis of disease associated with viral infections is generally more straightforward in the dog than in the cat because, in general, canine viruses do not have complex carrier states, and canine vaccines appear to be much more efficient in blocking infection and disease. As such, vaccination history is an important part of the diagnostic work-up for canine viral infections.

Canine distemper virus

The clinical signs of acute distemper are varied and depend on the epithelial surface most infected. Possible clinical signs include nasal discharge, conjunctivitis, coughing, dyspnoea, vomiting, diarrhoea and hyperkeratosis. Some dogs go on to develop acute and/or chronic neurological signs.

Ante-mortem diagnosis of canine distemper virus (CDV)-associated disease is not always straightforward. VI can be difficult but may be possible, and is most likely to succeed from the buffy coat. Some laboratories may use immunofluorescence to demonstrate viral antigen directly in acetone-fixed cytological smears. Suitable samples include conjunctiva, tonsil, buffy coat, respiratory epithelium, cerebrospinal fluid (CSF), bone marrow or urine sediment. As these tests are not routinely performed, it is recommended to contact the diagnostic laboratory to discuss the most suitable samples for collection.

Paired virus neutralization tests (carried out using serum samples) may demonstrate rising antibody titres, but often antibody levels have already peaked by the time clinical samples are first taken. Antibody levels may also be measured in the CSF and this may be more specific in cases of neurological disease. Anti-CDV antibodies are produced locally in the central nervous system (CNS) in animals with neurological disease and are not usually present in vaccinated dogs or dogs with distemper but without CNS signs. In order to rule out iatrogenic contamination of CSF with blood-derived antibodies, a serum:CSF antibody ratio can be performed and compared to another infectious agent.

Characteristic histopathological changes found on post-mortem examination include eosinophilic intracytoplasmic inclusion bodies and detection of viral antigen in infected cells by immunohistology.

Virus neutralization tests to measure serum antibody can be used to characterize the immune response to vaccination and inform the decision on the requirement for booster vaccinations. RT-PCRs have been developed to detect viral genome but are not readily available.

Canine parvovirus

Canine parvovirus-1 (CPV-1) (also called minute virus) has been suggested to be a rare cause of diarrhoea. The clinical signs associated with CPV-2 are variable and range from inapparent to severe gastrointestinal disease with vomiting and diarrhoea; severely affected puppies may die within 72 hours of the onset of clinical signs.

CPV-2 can be detected in the faeces of clinically affected animals by isolation, EM (see Figure 26.8c), HA, antigen capture assays and PCR. The latter is likely to be most sensitive, but, in all cases, the amount of virus shed in faeces has often severely declined by the time clinical signs develop and so false negatives are a possibility. Animals that have recently received a live CPV-2 vaccine may also test false positive on some faecal virus tests.

Antibody levels can be measured against CPV-2 but may be difficult to interpret in some cases. High antibody titres in animals that have been sick for 3 or more days are highly suggestive of CPV infection. Since antibody levels are often high by the time clinical signs develop, it is often not possible to demonstrate rising antibody titres. The measurement of IgM levels may be offered by some laboratories and is likely to be more useful in cases of acute disease.

HAI (see Figure 26.9) to measure serum antibody can be used to characterize the immune response to vaccination and inform the decision on the requirement for booster vaccinations. PCR has been shown experimentally to be more sensitive than other methods for detecting CPV-2 in faeces, but is not readily available.

Canine coronavirus

Canine coronavirus infection is generally associated with only mild diarrhoea. Virus can be isolated from fresh faecal samples providing they arrive at the laboratory quickly.

Canine herpesvirus

The clinical signs associated with canine herpesvirus are varied and depend on the age of infection, ranging from abortion and stillbirths, to fading puppy syndrome and mild respiratory disease in puppies; more rarely, canine herpesvirus causes vesicular genital lesions in adults.

Virus can be isolated from many tissues in cases of fading puppy syndrome including kidneys and adrenal glands, lungs, spleen, liver and lymph nodes. In adult dogs, the virus can normally only be isolated from the oral mucosa and the respiratory and genital tracts. On post-mortem examination intranuclear inclusion bodies are evident.

Canine adenovirus

The clinical signs associated with canine adenovirus (CAV) type 1 infection are variable and range from mild pyrexia to acute abdominal catastrophe and death. CAV-2 is one of the pathogens associated with the 'kennel cough' complex.

In the more severe cases of CAV-1-associated disease, biochemical changes associated with hepatic necrosis and disseminated intravascular coagulopathy are suggestive of infection.

Virus isolation from throat swabs in laboratory VTM can be used to demonstrate infection, the virus growing readily in several cell types from different species. On post-mortem examination, liver changes are often quite specific for CAV-1 infection and include intranuclear inclusion bodies (see Figure 26.7). Similar inclusion bodies are evident in the respiratory epithelium of dogs with CAV-2-associated kennel cough. Immunohistology may also be available at some laboratories, and may be performed on acetone-fixed impressions for rapid diagnosis.

Virus neutralization tests are available to measure anti-CAV-1 serum antibody and can be used to characterize the immune response to vaccination.

Canine parainfluenza virus

Like CAV-2, canine parainfluenza virus is one of the pathogens associated with the 'kennel cough' complex. Diagnosis is by virus isolation of virus from a throat swab in VTM.

Rabies virus

Rabies virus is a neurotropic virus capable of infecting many animal species worldwide, including humans. Although clinical signs can be variable, a progression is often described through prodromal (behavioural changes), excitative (nervousness, aggression, tremors, spasms, vocalization) and paralytic (incoordination, convulsions, paralysis, coma) phases. Infection is usually fatal in the absence of specific postexposure immune therapy. Rabies is a notifiable disease.

Veterinary surgeons suspecting a case of rabies based on history and clinical signs should detain the animal and notify the local veterinary officer. Specific diagnosis is coordinated by government agencies (DEFRA in the UK), and carried out by a specialist laboratory. Possible tests used to detect virus include VI (initially in mice but mostly now replaced by cell culture) or PCR. Histopathological examination shows characteristic Negri inclusion bodies in the brain. Immunological techniques can be used to confirm the specificity of antigen in cell cultures or fixed tissues.

Whilst it is hoped that veterinary surgeons in the UK are unlikely to be involved in diagnosing rabies infection, it is now common for owners to request vaccination under the UK PETS Travel Scheme. In order to be certified, animals must show an adequate response to vaccination. Serum samples for this purpose must be sent to an approved laboratory where a fluorescent antibody virus neutralization test is usually carried out.

References and further reading

Addie DD and Jarrett O (2001) Use of a reverse-transcriptase polymerase chain reaction for monitoring the shedding of feline coronavirus by healthy cats. *Veterinary Record* **148,** 649–653

Greene CE (1998) *Infectious Diseases of the Dog and Cat, 2nd edn.* WB Saunders, Philadelphia

Hartmann K, Werner RM, Egberink H and Jarrett O (2001) Comparison of six in-house diagnostic tests for the rapid diagnosis of feline immunodeficiency virus and feline leukaemia virus infections. *Veterinary Record* **149,** 317–320

Hartmann K, Binder C, Hirschberger J, Cole D, Reinacher M, Schroo S, Frost J, Egbenik H, Lutz H and Hermanns W (2003) Comparison of different tests to diagnose feline infectious peritonitis. *Journal of Veterinary Internal Medicine* **17,** 781–790

Helps C, Reeves N, Egan K, Howard P and Harbour D (2003) Detection of *Chlamydophila felis* and feline herpesvirus by multiplex real-time PCR analysis. *Journal of Clinical Microbiology* **41,** 2734–2736

Mochizuki M, San Gabriel MC, Nakatani H, Yoshida M and Harasawa R (1993) Comparison of polymerase chain reaction with virus isolation and haemagglutination assays for the detection of canine parvoviruses in faecal specimens. *Research in Veterinary Science* **55,** 60–63

Radford AD, Dawson S, Wharmby C, Ryvar R and Gaskell RM (2000) Comparison of serological and sequence-based methods for typing feline calicivirus isolates from vaccine failures. *Veterinary Record* **146,** 117–123

Schunck B, Kraft W and Truyen U (1995) A simple touch-down polymerase chain reaction for the detection of canine parvovirus and feline panleukopenia virus in feces. *Journal of Virology Methods* **55,** 427–433

Sykes JE, Anderson GA, Studdert VP and Browning GF (1999) Prevalence of feline *Chlamydia psittaci* and feline herpesvirus 1 in cats with upper respiratory tract disease. *Journal of Veterinary Internal Medicine* **13,** 153–162

27

Diagnosis of protozoal and arthropod-borne disease

Kate Murphy and Kostas Papasouliotis

Introduction

Since the introduction of the Pet Travel Scheme (PETS) an increasing number of animals are travelling abroad. Despite the requirements of the scheme for vaccination, worming and acaricidal therapy, these animals can return to the UK with clinically important exotic diseases and more virulent types of already endemic arthropod-borne diseases. The arthropod-borne bacterial and protozoal infections that are currently endemic in the UK are *Anaplasma phagocytophilum*, *Bartonella*, *Borrelia*, *Haemoplasma*, *Neospora* and *Toxoplasma* (see also *BSAVA Manual of Canine and Feline Infectious Diseases*).

Laboratory diagnosis

There are a number of different laboratory tests available for the diagnosis of arthropod-borne bacterial and protozoal diseases. Diagnosis is based on a combination of compatible clinical signs and clinicopathological abnormalities, and more specific diagnostic tests. Some of these tests detect the organism itself (direct identification, culture, polymerase chain reaction (PCR)) while other tests detect the host's immune response to the organism (serology).

Detection of the organism or components

Microscopic examination

Haemoparasites can be identified using routine haematological and cytological stains on blood smears and fine needle aspirates from appropriate tissue. In some cases definitive diagnosis can be reached, based on the morphology of the organism, cellular tropism and staining characteristics. Organisms that can be observed during routine examination of a blood smear include *Mycoplasma haemofelis*, '*Candidatus* Mycoplasma haemominutum' (both previously classified as *Haemobartonella felis*), *Mycoplasma haemocanis* (previously *Haemobartonella canis*), *Babesia* spp., *Leishmania* spp. and *Ehrlichia/Anaplasma* spp. There is increased sensitivity for the detection of some organisms using peripheral (capillary) blood smears, e.g. ear tip samples for identification of *Babesia gibsoni*. Standard differential stains (Giemsa) are used for microscopic identification of the majority of these organisms (e.g. *Ehrlichia*, *Leishmania*, *Babesia* and *Anaplasma*), but for organisms such as *Bartonella,* more advanced staining methods are required, e.g. Warthin–Starry silver stain in biopsy material. *Borrelia* spp. are motile bacteria, which can be seen in fresh body fluid specimens, such as blood and urine, using dark field microscopy.

Some organisms may be evident on histological or cytological examination of specimens such as in bronchoalveolar lavage fluid (*Toxoplasma gondii*), faeces (*T. gondii*) or tissue from biopsy (*T. gondii* and *Neospora caninum*). The use of direct immunohistochemical or immunocytochemical methods may increase the sensitivity of direct identification, but this is not commercially available in the UK. (This is similar to the detection of viral antigen described in Chapter 26.)

Culture

The majority of these organisms have very exacting culture requirements and are generally very difficult to grow *in vitro*. In cases where growth is possible, it is usually very slow and therefore impractical in clinical cases where rapid diagnosis is necessary. *Borrelia burgdorferi* and *Bartonella henselae* can be grown in culture, but it takes approximately 1 month between inoculation and identification.

Polymerase chain reaction

PCR is an enzymatic technique that allows amplification of specific nucleic acid sequences (see Chapter 26). As well as detecting organisms, PCR can allow accurate diagnosis by amplifying species- or strain-specific DNA. Conventional PCR provides information regarding the presence or absence of DNA, but no quantitative analysis. For this reason, in some diseases where the presence of an organism in low numbers may not be clinically significant, over-diagnosis of disease can occur.

PCR can be used in a quantitative assay. Real-time PCR has fluorescent dyes incorporated into the reaction mixture. The fluorescence increases proportionally to the amount of the DNA product, providing quantitative results that reflect the number of organisms present in the sample; this can be used to assess the pathogen load and response to treatment. The reaction and quantitation all occurs within the PCR tube, which minimizes the risk of cross-contamination. In addition, newer real-time PCR machines can monitor fluorescence at different wavelengths simultaneously, enabling the concurrent measurement of DNA from a number of different organisms. The ACARUS laboratory (University of Bristol) is currently the only UK laboratory to offer PCR-based diagnostics for some of the infections discussed in this chapter (*Ehrlichia*, *Leishmania*, *Babesia*, *Borrelia*, *Bartonella* and *Anaplasma*). PCR-based diagnosis of *Mycoplasma haemofelis* and '*Candidatus* Mycoplasma haemominutum' is also available through the Langford Veterinary Diagnostic laboratories at the University of Bristol.

The main advantages of PCR are its rapidity and its sensitivity to small amounts of target DNA. Conversely, the major limitation of PCR is also due to its high sensitivity: it is prone to false-positive results if sample contamination occurs; specialized laboratory facilities and staff are also required. Reputable diagnostic laboratories include steps to minimize the risk of contamination by running appropriate controls to ensure that any contamination is detected. However, it is possible that contamination can occur in the veterinary practice during sample collection.

It should be remembered that a positive PCR does not necessarily indicate clinical disease, since PCR will amplify DNA from both live and dead organisms.

Detection of the host immune response

There are five laboratory techniques that are commonly used for the detection of antibodies (described in more detail in Chapter 26):

- Enzyme-linked immunosorbent assay (ELISA)
- Immunofluorescent assay (IFA)
- Agglutination/haemagglutination
- Rapid immunomigration (RIM)
- Immuno-blotting (Western blotting).

These techniques are mainly employed in commercial/specialist diagnostic laboratories, although ELISA and RIM have been adapted for in-practice use.

Serology

The measurement of serum antibody titres is commonly available for many diseases. To interpret serology, it is important to understand that the antibody response changes during infection. In the early stages the response is dominated by immunoglobulin M (IgM) but, within days to weeks, a switch to the production of IgG occurs. Second and subsequent exposure to the organism can result in a more rapid increase in IgG. Typically, the IgM response is evident within 1 week following exposure and does not usually persist after elimination of infection. The IgG response usually peaks at about 14 days but persists for a long period post infection.

In clinical practice, there are two main approaches in the use of serology for the diagnosis of infection:

- Single measurement of IgM or IgG titres
- Measurement of IgM or IgG titres in paired blood samples.

Single measurement of IgM or IgG titres: High titres of antigen-specific IgM are believed to indicate active or recent infection. IgM is of particular value in the diagnosis of endemic diseases when a high proportion of the animal population may have been exposed to the organism and therefore may have antigen-specific IgG detectable. Certain arthropod-borne pathogens, such as *Leishmania* and *Ehrlichia canis*, cause dysregulation of the immune response and induce non-specific IgG, which can interfere with diagnostic serology. Others, such as *Anaplasma phagocytophilum*, cause immunosuppression, leading to the generation of a weak antibody response. Other limitations of single measurement of antibodies include:

- The prevalence of seroconversion exceeds the presence of clinical disease
- Detection of IgG antibodies can reflect exposure to the organism and not necessarily active infection
- Cross-reaction of antibodies against closely related species of organisms can lead to false positives, due to antibodies reacting non-specifically with antigens other than those against which the immune response was generated e.g. *Ehrlichia canis* and *Anaplasma phagocytophilum*
- Antibody responses require time to develop and therefore serology has limited value in the diagnosis of acute infections
- Vaccination induces antibodies and these may be detected by certain assays, so that vaccinated animals may be falsely identified as diseased, e.g. *Borrelia burgdorferi* where one must ensure that the assay does not detect vaccinal antibodies to *Borrelia* or other spirochaetes (including *Leptospira* and non-pathogenic related spirochaetes).

Measurement of IgM or IgG titres in paired blood samples: The presence of relevant clinical signs and a 4-fold or greater increase in antibody titre in two samples collected over a 2-week period has been suggested to indicate active infection. The limitations of a rising antibody titre as a diagnostic criterion include:

- Maximum antibody levels may have been reached by the time clinical signs develop, which limits the utility of serology in samples for the demonstration of rising antibody titres
- Antibody titres may not increase in immunocompromised animals
- Laboratory variation in titres: titres from different laboratories may vary, and should not be directly compared. In addition, there may be variations in titre between assays carried out on different days; ideally paired samples should be assayed together (i.e. repeat assay on the first samples). A 4-fold or greater increase is unlikely to be due to laboratory variability.

Diagnostic tests for specific diseases

Babesiosis

Babesia is an intraerythrocytic protozoan parasite, transmitted by the ticks *Dermacentor reticulatus* and *Rhipicephalus sanguineus*. Although these vectors are not endemic in the UK, they have been identified on dogs and cats entering UK quarantine kennels and in their transport containers. There are different species and strains of *Babesia* and therefore its pathogenicity can vary.

Large *Babesia*

Babesia canis is the large *Babesia* in dogs and has variable pathogenicity.

- *B. canis* var. *canis* – moderate pathogenicity, endemic in central and southern Europe
- *B. canis* var. *vogeli* – causes only mild disease, worldwide distribution
- *B. canis* var. *rossi* – highly pathogenic, found in South Africa and has a different vector, *Haemaphysalis leachi*.

Small *Babesia*

Babesia gibsoni and the new 'small *Babesia*' have high pathogenicity. *B. gibsoni* is found widely throughout Asia and focally in Europe, North America and Australia. The other small *Babesia* are found in North America and Europe but the distribution is uncertain.

Babesiosis has been reported in domestic cats but less is known about the infection in this species: *B. felis* has been identified in southern Africa; a new subspecies of *B. canis* has been identified in cats in Israel; and one case of *Babesia* was identified on morphological grounds in India and called *B. cati*. All species identified so far are pathogenic but the vectors are unknown.

Babesiosis in Europe typically causes haemolytic anaemia, anorexia, fever, lethargy, hepatosplenomegaly, haemoglobinuria, icterus and sometimes hypotensive shock. This can be seen with both *B. canis* and *B. gibsoni* infection. Details of clinicopathological abnormalities and diagnostic tests for *Babesia* are given in Figure 27.1. *Babesia* can be observed on blood smears (Figure 27.2).

Clinicopathological abnormalities
Haematology
Regenerative anaemia, thrombocytopenia, leucocytosis, positive Coombs' test, autoagglutination
Biochemistry
Hyperglobulinaemia, electrolyte abnormalities (rare), azotaemia, hyperbilirubinaemia and increased liver enzymes
Urinalysis
Bilirubinuria, haemoglobinuria, proteinuria, granular casts
Specific diagnostic tests
Microscopic examination (fresh peripheral blood smear, e.g. ear tip sample)
Blood smear evaluation can reveal intraerythrocytic parasites *B. canis* (large and in pairs) and *B. gibsoni* (small and single)
PCR (whole blood in EDTA)
PCR on blood samples has good sensitivity using the 18s rRNA PCR target. Specific primers are available to detect different *Babesia* species and strains; however, DNA sequencing is currently the preferred method for speciation
Serology (separated serum)
A variety of serological tests have been developed: currently in the UK, *B. canis* IFA is available. Seropositive animals have antibody titres >1:80 False negatives have been reported in peracute or acute cases Can be used to identify subclinically or chronically affected animals. The commonly used tests cannot distinguish between *B. canis* and *B. gibsoni* due to antigenic cross reactivity and antibody to *B. gibsoni* may cross react with *Toxoplasma gondii* and *Neospora caninum*
Common co-infections
Ehrlichia, Leishmania, Anaplasma phagocytophilum
Zoonotic potential
Large *Babesia*: none Small *Babesia*: undetermined

27.1 Diagnosis of *Babesia* infection.

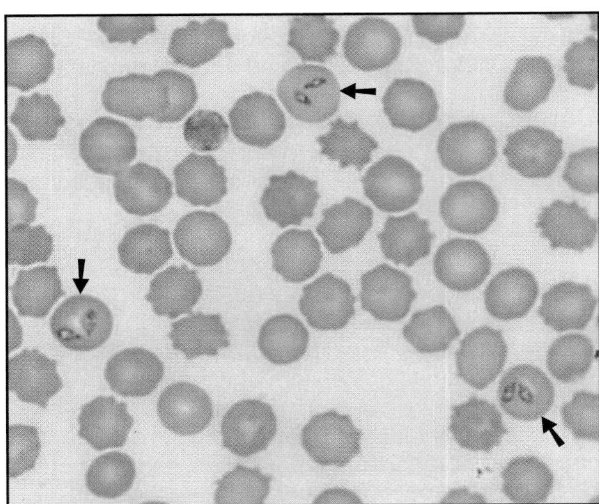

27.2 Blood smear from a dog showing *Babesia canis* in three erythrocytes (arrowed). (Giemsa; original magnification X400.) (Courtesy of Drs Caldin and Furlanello, Veterinary Clinic San Marco, Padua, Italy.)

Bartonellosis

Bartonella spp. are fastidious Gram-negative intraerythrocytic bacteria with worldwide distribution. *Bartonella henselae* has worldwide distribution in cats; the geographical distribution of *B. vinsonii* var. *berkhoffii* requires further work. *Bartonella* is found in cats and sometimes in dogs and is of zoonotic importance as the causative agent of cat scratch disease in humans. Cats are reservoirs for *Bartonella*, and arthropod vectors are involved in transmission. Asymptomatic infection is common in cats; a recent UK survey reported 41% seropositivity. If symptomatic infection develops, the clinical signs may include fever, anorexia, stomatitis, lymphadenopathy, lethargy, transient anaemia and neuromuscular or urogenital disease. Uveitis has also been associated with *Bartonella* infection. Bartonellosis in dogs has been associated with vasculoproliferative disorders, such as peliosis hepatis, granulomatous lymphadenitis, dermatitis, endocarditis and myocarditis. Diagnosis of *Bartonella* infection is described in Figure 27.3.

Clinicopathological abnormalities
Haematology and biochemistry
Non-specific
Specific diagnostic tests
Culture (blood: contact laboratory for sample handling requirements)
B. henselae can be grown after prolonged culture on specialized media. Colonies may be seen within 7–21 days, but can take up to 56 days to develop. Low level bacteraemia can result in false-negative cultures. *B. vinsonii* is very difficult to culture
PCR (whole blood in EDTA, fresh/frozen tissue from lesion)
PCR can be performed on blood or tissue samples. It is particularly indicated in cases where pyogranulomatous inflammation or peliosis hepatis is diagnosed. The PCR target used is a fragment of the citrate synthase gene (gltA)
Serology (separated serum)
ELISA is available in the UK and results are reported on a 1–9 matrix scale (9 = strongly positive, 1 = negative). A matrix reading >5.5 is considered a significant increase. It is valuable as a screening test, since negative serology would be unexpected in an infected animal. Up to 40% of normal UK cats are seropositive. Seropositivity is likely to be more clinically significant in dogs
Common co-infections
Ehrlichia, Babesia canis, Borrelia, Anaplasma phagocytophilum
Zoonotic potential
Agent of cat scratch disease in humans

27.3 Diagnosis of *Bartonella* infection.

Borreliosis

Borreliosis or Lyme disease is caused by the tick-borne extracellular spirochaete *Borrelia burgdorferi sensu lato* (Figure 27.4). It is transmitted by ticks of the genus *Ixodes*. *B. burgdorferi* is reported from Europe and America. Both the vector and organism are endemic in the UK. There are geographical variations in the severity of disease but serious morbidity is considered rare in dogs in the UK. Borreliosis causes recurrent fever, lethargy or weakness, inappetence, lymphadenopathy and inflammatory polyarthritis. It has also been associated with myocarditis and arrhythmias, neurological disease, glomerulonephritis and uveitis. Skin lesions, which are seen in humans, have not been definitively identified in dogs. More virulent disease exists in Europe. Diagnosis of borreliosis is described in Figure 27.5.

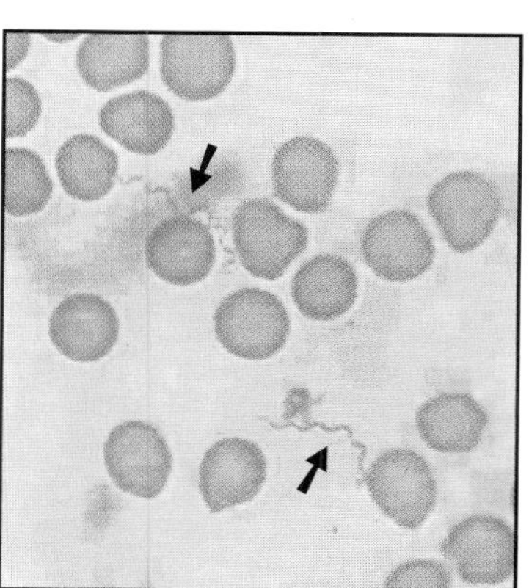

27.4 Blood smear from a dog showing *Borrelia* spp. (arrowed) seen on direct microscopy. These organisms are rarely visualized in this way; dark field microscopy is usually utilized. (Giemsa; original magnification X1000.) (Courtesy of G. Baneth, Hebrew University of Israel, Jerusalem.)

Clinicopathological abnormalities
Non-specific haematological and biochemical changes Increased volume of synovial fluid. Synovial fluid analysis shows neutrophilic inflammation
Specific diagnostic tests
Microscopic examination or culture (fluid and fresh tissues)
B. burgdorferi can be identified by dark field microscopy in blood, urine, synovial fluid, CSF or tissues. It can also be cultured from fluid specimens and from tissue, e.g. skin, but this is very difficult
PCR (EDTA whole blood, fluid and fresh tissue)
PCR can identify the organism even when it is present in low numbers using the PCR target outer surface protein A (OspA)
Serology (separated serum)
In the UK an ELISA is available which detects IgG antibodies. Results are expressed on a 1–9 matrix (9 = positive, 1 = negative). A test result >4.5 is considered positive. Antibody titres increase within 4–6 weeks post-exposure to infected ticks. The IgG response peaks after 90–120 days and can remain elevated for over 1 year. A high antibody titre does not necessarily indicate active infection. There may be cross reactivity with non-pathogenic *Borrelia* spp. A negative antibody titre is unlikely in animals with clinical signs unless they are in the acute phase of disease There is an in-house combination ELISA test for *E. canis* and *B. burgdorferi* antibody and heartworm antigen. This test is able to distinguish between natural exposure and vaccinal antibody to *Borrelia*
Common co-infections
Anaplasma phagocytophilum
Zoonotic potential
Potential zoonotic agent, though the mode of transmission is unclear

27.5 Diagnosis of *Borrelia* infection.

Ehrlichiosis

Ehrlichia organisms are Gram-negative, intracellular bacteria (Figure 27.6, 27.7, 27.8), which have recently been reclassified based on molecular studies. *E. platys* has been reclassified as *Anaplasma platys* and *E. phagocytophila* as *A. phagocytophilum*. *Ehrlichia* organisms have tropism for different cells (Figure 27.9). *E. canis* has worldwide distribution except Australia

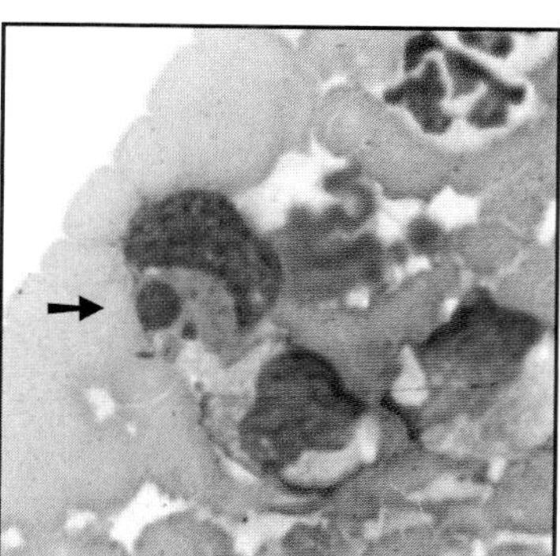

27.6 Blood smear from a dog showing *Ehrlichia canis* morula in a monocyte (arrowed). (Giemsa; original magnification X1000.) (Courtesy of G. Baneth, Hebrew University of Israel, Jerusalem.)

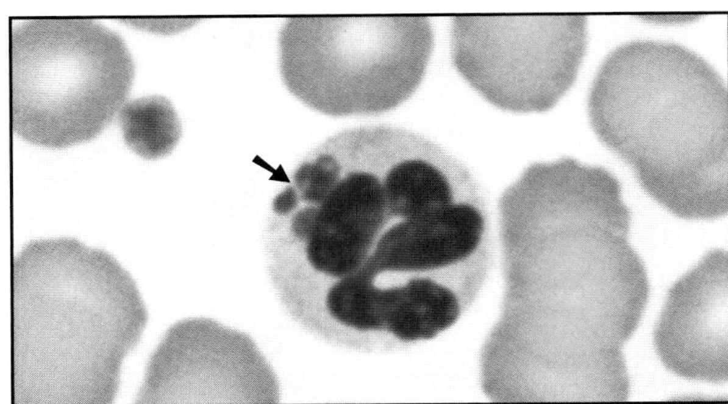

27.7 Blood smear from a dog showing *Anaplasma phagocytophilum* in a neutrophil (arrowed). (Giemsa; original magnification X1000.) (Courtesy of Drs Caldin and Furlanello, Veterinary Clinic San Marco, Padua, Italy.)

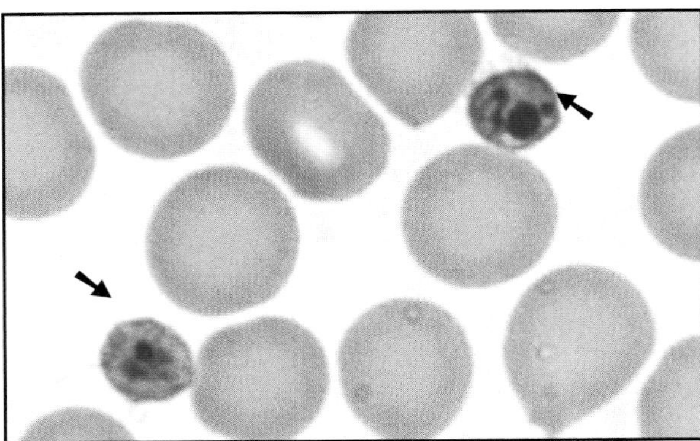

27.8 Blood smear from a dog showing *Anaplasma platys* in the platelets (arrowed). (Giemsa; original magnification X1000.) (Courtesy of Drs Caldin and Furlanello, Veterinary Clinic San Marco, Padua, Italy.)

Ehrlichia organism	Cell tropism	Tick vector	Pathogenicity
E. canis (exotic)	Monocytes	*Rhipicephalus sanguineus*	Moderate to severe
A. platys (exotic)	Platelets	Unknown, likely to be *Rhipicephalus sanguineus*	Mild unless co-infection with *E. canis* or *Babesia canis*
A. phagocytophilum (endemic)	Granulocytes	*Ixodes* species	Variable

27.9 Tropism, vectors and pathogenicity of *Ehrlichia*. (Exotic and endemic refer to the UK)

and New Zealand, *A. phagocytophilum* is reported in North America and Europe (including the UK) and *A. platys* has been reported in the USA, Japan, Venezuela, Thailand, Europe, Taiwan, Israel and Australia.

E. canis infection has acute, subclinical and chronic phases. The acute phase is characterized by fever, anorexia, lymphadenopathy, oculonasal discharge, uveitis, central nervous system signs, vasculitis, petechiae/ecchymoses and bleeding (epistaxis). The chronic phase is typically associated with vague signs of illness and weight loss. Diagnosis of *E. canis* infection is described in Figure 27.10.

Clinicopathological abnormalities

Haematology

Acute: thrombocytopenia, leucopenia, variable anaemia
Chronic: pancytopenia, lymphocytosis

Biochemistry

Hyperglobulinaemia, which may be polyclonal or monoclonal/oligoclonal, and hypoalbuminaemia
Increased liver enzymes, azotaemia

Urinalysis

Proteinuria, low specific gravity, bacteriuria

Coagulation

Abnormalities (e.g. platelet dysfunction)

CSF analysis

Increased proteins and pleocytosis

Bone marrow examination

Hyper- or hypocellular, often with increased numbers of plasma cells due to antigenic stimulation

Synovial fluid analysis

Increased numbers of non-degenerate neutrophils

Specific diagnostic tests

Microscopic examination (fluids or tissues)

Ehrlichia morulae may be seen in blood, bone marrow, synovial fluid and CSF or in tissue aspirates (e.g. spleen, lung, lymph nodes) in the acute phase

PCR (EDTA whole blood, fluid and splenic aspirate)

The PCR target is 16s rRNA. PCR may be positive within 4–10 days post infection. It is the preferred method for speciation, using species-specific primers. EDTA blood, synovial fluid, aqueous humour, CSF and tissue can be used. PCR can be positive before antibody levels are detected, is useful for the diagnosis of acute or peracute disease, and also for monitoring response to treatment:

- If PCR is positive 2 weeks after cessation of treatment, then treatment for a further 4 weeks and retesting is recommended. If the PCR remains positive, the use of alternative therapy should be considered
- If PCR is negative 2 weeks after cessation of therapy retesting after 8 weeks is advised: if then negative, it can be assumed that the infection has been cleared

Serology (separated serum)

IFA is available commercially in the UK. IgG antibodies, detected by the IFA, increase within 7 days post infection, peak at 2–5 months, and are persistent. Positive results will be found in asymptomatic animals from endemic areas. There is cross reaction between *E. canis* and *Neorickettsia helminthoeca* and *E. ruminantum*. IFA for *E. canis* does not detect *A. platys*, *A. phagocytophilum* or *N. risticci*.
Interpretation of IFA titres:

- Antibody titre ≥1:40 indicates exposure
- A 4-fold increase in titre, on samples taken 1–2 weeks apart, indicates active infection. IgG is usually detectable by 20 days post infection; some dogs show clinical signs within 7 days, but at this time they will be seronegative
- Some dogs remain seropositive after therapy and this may represent a persistent carrier state
- Cross-reactions with *A. phagocytophilum* may occur

An in-house ELISA is available and there is a combination test for *E. canis*, and *B. burgdorferi* antibody and heartworm antigen. There is good correlation between the in-house ELISA and the IFA when IFA titres are >1:320

Common co-infections

Babesia spp., *Leishmania infantum*

Zoonotic potential

None currently known. A closely related organism named *E. chaffeensis* is zoonotic, causing human monocytic ehrlichiosis

27.10 Diagnosis of *Ehrlichia canis* infection.

Clinicopathological abnormalities
Haematology
Thrombocytopenia, mild leucopenia followed by a transient leucocytosis
Biochemistry
Mild increases in liver enzymes
Specific diagnostic tests
Microscopic examination (fresh blood smear)
Inclusions may seen in neutrophils, but there is variation in the number of neutrophils affected
PCR (EDTA whole blood)
Species-specific primers are available
Serology (separated serum)
Serological tests are not readily available for *A. phagocytophilum*. Serology using *A. equi* (previously *Ehrlichia equi*) antigen is used but only shows evidence of exposure
Common co-infections
Borrelia, also *Ehrlichia, Bartonella, Rickettsia, Babesia*
Zoonotic potential
Yes, causative agent of human granulocytic ehrlichiosis

27.11 Diagnosis of *Anaplasma phagocytophilum* infection.

Clinicopathological abnormalities
Haematology
Thrombocytopenia with macrothrombocytes, anaemia and monocytosis
Biochemistry
Hypoalbuminaemia
Specific diagnostic tests
Microscopic examination (fresh blood smear)
Basophilic inclusions inside the platelets can be seen on Giemsa-stained blood smears. The bacteraemia is cyclic so negative microscopy does not exclude the diagnosis
PCR (EDTA blood)
A generic ehrlichial PCR will identify *A. platys*. There are species-specific primers available for the diagnosis of *A. platys*
Serology (separated serum)
IFA has been developed but is not commercially available. A positive titre is >1:40. There is no cross reactivity between *A. platys* and *E. canis*
Common co-infections
Babesia, Ehrlichia
Zoonotic potential
None known

27.12 Diagnosis of *Anaplasma platys* infection.

Infection with *A. phagocytophilum* has been associated with fever, weakness, lymphadenopathy, muscle stiffness and pain, polyarthritis, thrombocytopenia and meningitis. Diagnosis of *A. phagocytophilum* is described in Figure 27.11.

A. platys is an organism of generally low pathogenicity causing mild to moderate cyclical thrombocytopenia, which is often asymptomatic. Infection can become symptomatic if the dog has surgery or is co-infected with *Babesia* or other *Ehrlichia* species. A more pathogenic strain is reported from Greece and the Middle East. Diagnosis of *A. platys* is described in Figure 27.12.

Haemoplasmosis

Feline infectious anaemia (FIA) is caused by *Haemobartonella felis*, which has recently been reclassified as a *Mycoplasma*. There are two species, which can be identified by PCR, *Mycoplasma haemofelis* (large form) and '*Candidatus* Mycoplasma haemominutum' (small form) (Figure 27.13). *M. haemofelis* appears to be more pathogenic than '*Candidatus* Mycoplasma haemominutum'. The mode of transmission is unknown but is believed to be associated with blood-sucking arthropods. FIA is associated with depression, weakness, anorexia, weight loss, pallor, splenomegaly and pyrexia. Diagnosis of infection with *Mycoplasma haemofelis or* '*Candidatus* Mycoplasma haemominutum' is described in Figure 27.14.

Haemobartonella canis infects dogs but is rarely associated with disease. It has been reclassified as *Mycoplasma haemocanis*. It can be detected using the *Mycoplasma haemofelis* PCR.

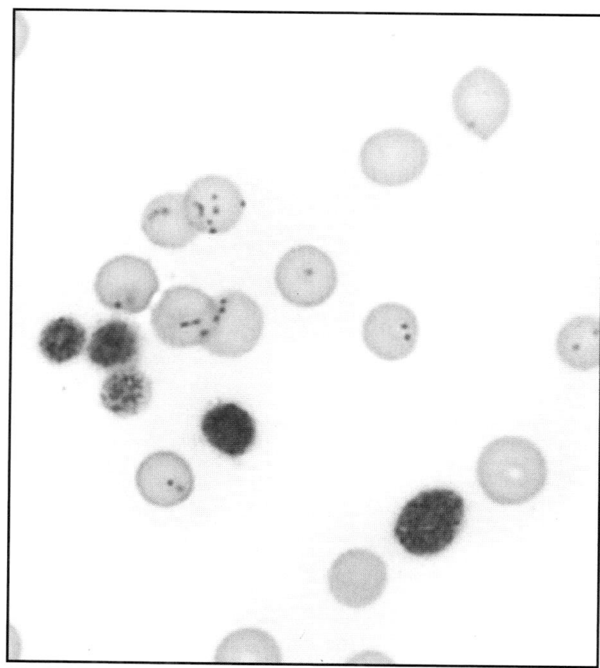

27.13 Blood smear from a cat showing haemoplasmas on the erythrocytes. Large and small haemoplasmas cannot be differentiated reliably based on size/appearance, unless both forms are present concurrently. (Giemsa; original magnification X1000.) (Courtesy of Drs Caldin and Furlanello, Veterinary Clinic San Marco, Padua, Italy.)

Clinicopathological abnormalities
Haematology
Regenerative anaemia, positive Coombs' test (some cases), neutrophilia and monocytosis
Specific diagnostic tests
Microscopic examination (fresh blood smear)
Giemsa-stained blood smear: the organisms are seen as small, blue-staining cocci, rings or rods attached to the surface of the erythrocytes. False-positive diagnosis is common because Howell-Jolly bodies or stain precipitate can be misidentified as epi-erythrocytic parasites. The parasite may detach from the erythrocyte during storage and therefore it is recommended to prepare the blood smears as soon as possible after collection of the blood sample. The absence of organisms on blood smear evaluation does not exclude the diagnosis. Acridine orange stains are used in some commercial laboratories.
PCR (EDTA whole blood)
Performed on blood samples. Enables identification of the two species. PCR positivity does not equate with clinical disease and therefore the PCR result should be interpreted in conjunction with the clinical findings and the species identified Real-time quantitative PCR is now available and allows quantification of the bacterial load and monitoring of the response to treatment
Common co-infections
None known
Zoonotic potential
None known

27.14 Diagnosis of *Mycoplasma haemofelis* or '*Candidatus* Mycoplasma haemominutum' infection.

Leishmaniasis

Leishmania is a protozoan parasite transmitted by sandflies (*Phlebotomus* and *Lutzomyia*). In Europe, leishmaniasis is caused by *Leishmania infantum* and the sandfly vector is *Phlebotomus. L. infantum* has an almost worldwide distribution (not Australia, New Zealand or Asia) and is an important disease in dogs in the Mediterranean areas of Europe, the Middle East, and South and Central America. Leishmaniasis is a disease of public health importance. The parasite infects macrophages and other cells in many tissues but particularly in lymphoid tissue, skin and viscera (Figure 27.15). It causes chronic infection with an incubation time varying from 1 month to several years. Clinical signs commonly reported include pyrexia, weight loss, lymphadenopathy, pallor, shifting lameness, panophthalmitis, exfoliative dermatitis, periocular alopecia and overgrowth of claws. Diagnosis of leishmaniasis is described in Figure 27.16.

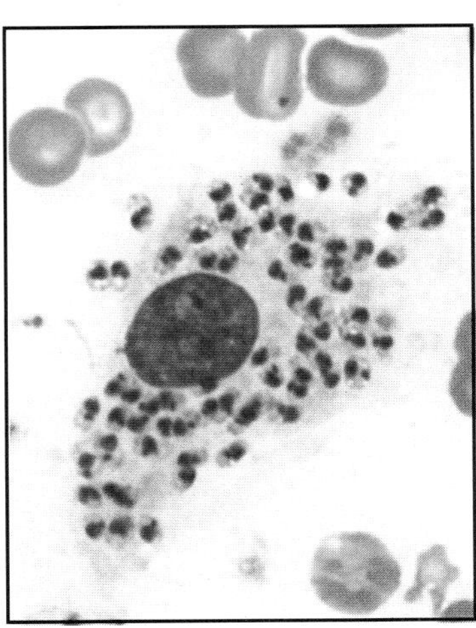

27.15 Blood smear from a dog showing *Leishmania* amastigotes associated with a macrophage. (Giemsa; original magnification X1000.) (Courtesy of Drs Caldin and Furlanello, Veterinary Clinic San Marco, Padua, Italy.)

Clinicopathological abnormalities
Haematology
Anaemia, thrombocytopenia, leucopenia, lymphocytosis or lymphopenia. Coombs' test positive (some cases).
Coagulation
Prolonged clotting times
Biochemistry
Hyperglobulinaemia (polyclonal or monoclonal/oligoclonal gammopathy), hypoalbuminaemia, increased liver enzymes, azotaemia
Urinalysis
Proteinuria
Specific diagnostic tests
Microscopic examination (blood, bone marrow, lymph nodes or skin biopsies)
The amastigotes (round to oval, with a basophilic round nucleus and a small rod-like kinetoplast) can be seen in blood smears and aspirates of lymph nodes and bone marrow or in Giemsa-stained biopsy specimens of cutaneous lesions. The amastigotes are seen within macrophages or free in cytological preparations from ruptured cells. Immunohistochemistry can be used to increase the sensitivity of parasite detection but it is not available in the UK
PCR (EDTA blood, bone marrow, lymph nodes or skin biopsies)
Highly sensitive and specific test using the kinetoplast PCR target. Can be performed on blood, bone marrow, skin biopsy specimens or lymph node aspirates. It is helpful in asymptomatic cases or those with an IFA <1:80
Serology (separated serum)
Antinuclear antibody-positive (some cases). IFA is the preferred method and is available in the UK. Due to the long incubation period, the majority of infected animals with clinical signs are seropositive. However there are also seropositive asymptomatic carriers. IgG develops within 2–3 weeks after infection and decreases within 45–80 days after treatment, although in many cases it remains high. If negative titres are obtained, repeat 1 month later to avoid false negatives. An IFA >1:80 is usually considered positive, but, as there are many serological tests available (including an in-house ELISA), the reader is advised to refer to the titres recommended for the test being used
Common co-infections
Ehrlichia, Babesia, Dirofilaria immitis
Zoonotic potential
Low zoonotic potential, but must be considered. Particular concern with immunosuppressed humans

27.16 Diagnosis of *Leishmania* infection.

Neosporosis

Neospora caninum is a protozoan parasite with a structure similar to that of *Toxoplasma gondii*. It is associated with clinically significant disease in dogs. Puppies with neosporosis develop ascending paralysis, resulting in faecal and urinary incontinence. In older dogs a variety of clinical signs have been reported including polymyositis (hindlimb extensor rigidity, muscle atrophy and hyporeflexia), pneumonia, myocarditis, hepatitis, pancreatitis, dermatitis, chorioretinitis and extraocular myositis. To date there are no documented feline cases. Diagnosis of *Neospora caninum* infection is described in Figure 27.17.

Clinicopathological abnormalities
Haematology
Eosinophilia (occasionally)
Biochemistry
Increased creatine kinase, aspartate aminotransferase, alanine aminotransferase and bile acids
CSF analysis
Increased white blood cells (often neutrophils or eosinophils). Increased total protein concentration
Specific diagnostic tests
Microscopic examination (CSF, lavages, tissues)
Tachyzoites can be seen in CSF, tracheal wash or bronchoalveolar lavage fluid, lung aspirate, tissue biopsy specimen or skin impression smears. Immunohistochemistry is required to differentiate *Neospora* from *Toxoplasma* but this is not commercially available in the UK
PCR
Potentially useful diagnostic tool but currently its availability is limited
Serology (separated serum)
IFA is available and titres of >1:800 are considered clinically significant. Titres of <1:50 have been reported in some dogs with histologically confirmed neosporosis. Titres can remain persistently increased despite successful therapy
Common co-infections
Leishmania
Zoonotic potential
None known

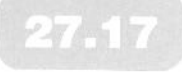
27.17 Diagnosis of *Neospora caninum* infection.

Toxoplasmosis

Toxoplasma gondii is a protozoan parasite with an intestinal sexual stage in cats and an extraintestinal asexual tissue stage in mammals and birds. Clinical disease is related to the extraintestinal stage. Figure 27.18 shows *Toxoplasma* in a blood smear. Tissue cysts survive for the life of the organism and clinical disease occurs if the cysts are reactivated. Infection occurs after ingestion of infected tissues, contaminated water or food or via infective faeces. Clinical signs include pyrexia, anorexia, uveitis, chorioretinitis, optic neuritis, pneumonia, hepatitis, polymyositis, hyperaesthesia (cat), pancreatitis, myocarditis and a variety of neurological signs. Diagnosis of *Toxoplasma gondii* is described in Figure 27.19.

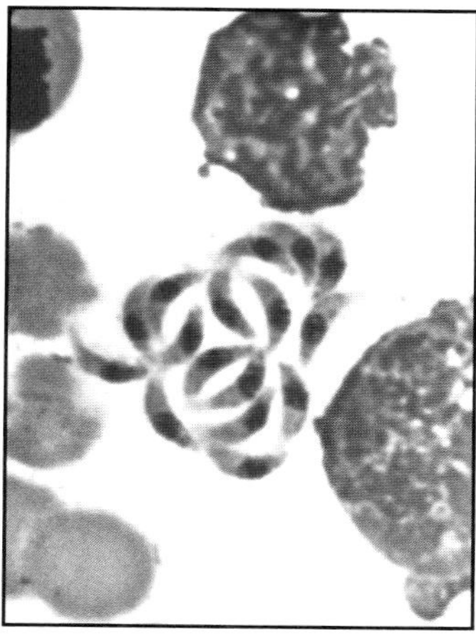
27.18 Blood smear showing *Toxoplasma* tachyzoites. (Giemsa; original magnification X1000.) (Courtesy of Drs Caldin and Furlanello, Veterinary Clinic San Marco, Padua, Italy.)

Clinicopathological abnormalities
Haematology
Non-specific
Biochemistry
Increased liver enzymes, bilirubin and bile acids, creatine kinase, hypoalbuminaemia and hyperglobulinaemia
CSF analysis
Mixed pleocytosis and increased total protein concentration
Specific diagnostic tests
Microscopic examination (samples required below)
Demonstration of tachyzoites in tissue aspirates or biopsy specimen, CSF, bronchoalveolar lavage fluid, aqueous humour and blood. In the cat faecal examination may be positive for oocysts
PCR (tissue, CSF, aqueous humour)
PCR can be performed on tissue, CSF or aqueous humour samples. It has been suggested that high IgM titres and positive PCR in CSF or aqueous humour are good indicators of clinical disease. Many clinically healthy animals are blood PCR positive
Serology (separated serum, CSF, aqueous humour)
IgG and IgM assays are available for blood, CSF and aqueous humour. The modified agglutination test is reported to be superior to other methodologies. IgG titres can be low or negative in acute toxoplasmosis. High IgG titres can persist for months to years post infection. IgG titre <1:50 is not consistent with a diagnosis of *Toxoplasma* infection. IgG >1:50 confirms exposure to *Toxoplasma*. IgG titres >1:400 are more consistent with but do not prove active infection. A 4-fold increase in an IgG titre on two samples collected 2–4 weeks apart is indicative of recent or active infection, but not all animals show such an increase. If IgG is >1:800 it can cause a false-positive IgM titre. A high IgM titre is the best indicator of clinical disease. IgM titres develop within 2–3 weeks post infection and generally become negative within 16 weeks. IgM titre >1:64 is suggestive of recent or active infection. IgM titres not supported by IgG titres should be interpreted with caution and re-testing 2 weeks later to assess for development of an IgG titre is recommended. CSF or aqueous humour antibody titres, higher than those in blood, indicate local production and active infection. It has been suggested that high IgM titres and positive PCR in CSF or aqueous humour are good indicators of clinical disease. High IgG or IgA titres in CSF or aqueous humour do not correlate with clinical disease and are found in many clinically healthy animals

27.19 Diagnosis of *Toxoplasma gondii* infection. (continues) ▶

Common co-infections
Possibly *Dirofilaria immitis*
Zoonotic potential
High in humans. Congenital infection can cause blindness and mental retardation and so pregnant women should exercise care in handling cats that might be excreting oocysts. Main sources of infection for humans are soil, contaminated litter trays and undercooked meat. Immunocompromised adults are at risk

27.19 (continued) Diagnosis of *Toxoplasma gondii* infection.

References and further reading

Barber JS and Trees AJ (1996) Clinical aspects of 27 cases of neosporosis in dogs. *Veterinary Record* **139,** 439–443

Barnes A, Bell SC, Isherwood DR, Bennett M and Carter SD (2000) Evidence of *Bartonella henselae* infection in cats and dogs in the United Kingdom. *Veterinary Record* **147,** 673–677

Birtles RJ, Laycock G, Kenny MJ, Shaw SE and Day MJ (2002) Prevalence of *Bartonella* species causing bacteraemia in domesticated and companion animals in the United Kingdom. *Veterinary Record* **151,** 225–229

Burney DP, Chavkin MJ, Dow SW, Potter TA and Lappin MR (1998) Polymerase chain reaction for the detection of *Toxoplasma gondii* within aqueous humour of experimentally-inoculated cats. *Veterinary Parasitology* **79,** 181–186.

Ciaramella P and Corona M (2003) Canine leishmaniasis: clinical and diagnostic aspects. *Compendium on Continuing Education for the Practicing Veterinarian* **25,** 358–375

Egenvall AE, Hedhammar AA and Bjoersdorff AI (1997) Clinical features and serology of 14 dogs affected by granulocytic ehrlichiosis in Sweden. *Veterinary Record* **140,** 222–226

Ferrer L, Aisa MJ, Roura X and Portus M (1995) Serological diagnosis and treatment of canine leishmaniasis. *Veterinary Record* **136,** 514–516

Greene CE (1998) *Infectious Diseases of the Dog and Cat, 2nd edn,* WB Saunders, Philadelphia.

Harrus S, Waner T, Strauss-Ayali D, Bark H, Jongejan F, Hecht G and Baneth G (2001) Dynamics of IgG1 and IgG2 subclass response in dogs naturally and experimentally infected with *Ehrlichia canis. Veterinary Parasitology* **99,** 63–71

Harrus S, Aroch I, Lavy E and Bark H (1997) Clinical manifestations of infectious canine cyclic thrombocytopenia. *Veterinary Record* **141,** 247–250

Kraje AC (2001) Canine haemobartonellosis and babesiosis. *Compendium on Continuing Education for the Practicing Veterinarian* **23,** 310–318

Lappin MR (1996) Feline toxoplasmosis: interpretation of diagnostic test results. *Seminars in Veterinary Medicine and Surgery* **11,** 154–160

Lutz H, Leutenegger C and Hofmann-Lehmann R (1999) The role of polymerase chain reaction and its newer developments in feline medicine. *Journal of Feline Medicine and Surgery* **1,** 89–100

Macintire DK and Breitschwerdt EB (2003) Emerging and re-emerging infectious diseases. *Veterinary Clinics of North America: Small Animal Practice* **33**

Morgan RV, Bright RS and Swartoot MS (2003) *Handbook of Small Animal Practice, 4th edn,* pp. 1121–1144. WB Saunders, Philadelphia

Nelson RW and Couto CG (2003) *Small Animal Internal Medicine, 3rd edn,* pp. 1265–1305. Mosby, St Louis

Preziosi DE and Cohn LA (2002) The increasingly complicated story of *Ehrlichia. Compendium on Continuing Education for the Practicing Veterinarian* **24,** 277–287

Ramsey IK and Tennant BJ (2001) *Manual of Canine and Feline Infectious Diseases.* BSAVA, Cheltenham

Roura X, Sanchez A and Ferrer L (1999) Diagnosis of canine leishmaniasis by a polymerase chain reaction technique. *Veterinary Record* **144,** 262–264

Shaw SE, Day MJ, Birtles RJ and Breitschwerdt E (2001) Tick transmitted infectious diseases of dogs. *Trends in Parasitology* **17,** 74–80

Tasker S, Helps CR, Day MJ, Gruffydd-Jones TJ and Harbour DA (2003) Use of real-time PCR to detect and quantify *Mycoplasma haemofelis* and '*Candidatus* Mycoplasma haemominutum' DNA. *Journal of Clinical Microbiology* **41,** 439–441

Tasker S and Lappin MR (2002) *Haemobartonella felis*: recent developments in diagnosis and treatment. *Journal of Feline Medicine and Surgery* **4,** 3–11

Trees A and Shaw SE (1999) Imported diseases in small animals. *In Practice* **10,** 482–491

Appendix 1

Common laboratory abnormalities and differential diagnoses

These tables indicate the major differential diagnoses for abnormalities of parameters discussed throughout the Manual. Square brackets denote rare causes.

Haematology

Abnormality	Differential diagnoses
Anaemia (regenerative)	Immune-mediated haemolytic anaemia (especially in dogs) Haemotrophic *Mycoplasma* infection Babesiosis Onion toxicity Zinc toxicity Acute or chronic haemorrhage Microangiopathic haemolytic anaemia associated with e.g. neoplasia, disseminated intravascular coagulation
Anaemia (non-regenerative)	Anaemia of chronic/inflammatory disease Anaemia of renal failure Iron deficiency Aplastic anaemia (aplastic pancytopenia) Pure red cell aplasia Myelofibrosis Myelopthisis Myelo/lymphoproliferative disease Myelodysplasia FeLV-related Ehrlichiosis Severe malnutrition
Erythrocytosis	Dehydration Primary erythrocytosis (polycythaemia rubra vera) Secondary to renal neoplasia, extra-renal neoplasia, other renal diseases Secondary to hypoxia
Neutrophilia	Physiological response Stress/corticosteroid-induced Acute inflammatory response: • Bacterial infection (localized or general) • Immune-mediated disease; polyarthritis • Neoplasia, especially tumour necrosis [Neutrophil dysfunction:] • [Acquired (diabetes, occasionally neoplasia)] • [Congenital] [Chronic granulocytic leukaemia] [Paraneoplastic syndromes]
Neutropenia	Overwhelming demand (e.g. sepsis) Reduced granulopoiesis: • Myeloproliferative and lymphoproliferative disease • Myelophthisis • Cytotoxic drug-related myelosuppression • Idiosyncratic drug reactions • Endogenous or exogenous oestrogens (N.B. neutrophilia early) • Some infections (e.g. canine parvovirus) Ineffective granulopoiesis: • Myeloproliferative and myelodysplastic diseases • [Cyclic haemopoiesis] [Immune-mediated neutropenia]

Abnormality	Differential diagnoses
Monocytosis	Acute, in trauma Stress Chronic inflammation: • Infection • Malignancy • Internal haemorrhage • Pyogranulomatous inflammation • Necrosis Immune-mediated disease Compensatory, secondary to neutropenia Haemolysis [Monocytic or myelomonocytic leukaemia]
Lymphocytosis	Physiological: stress (especially cats) Reactive: • Chronic infection • Transient post-vaccination Lymphoproliferative disease
Lymphopenia	Corticosteroids: • Endogenous (hyperadrenocorticism) • Exogenous Loss: • Chylothorax • Lymphangiectasia Decreased production: • Immunosuppressive drug therapy • [Myelophthisis] [Obstruction of lymph flow: inflammation/neoplasia]
Eosinophilia	Parasitic infection Inflammatory/hypersensitivity: • Allergic skin disease • Eosinophilic enteritis or myositis • Eosinophilic bronchopneumopathy (pulmonary infiltrate with eosinophils, PIE) • Panosteitis • Allergic respiratory disease Mast cell tumours [Inconsistently in hypoadrenocorticism]
Eosinopenia	Corticosteroids: • Endogenous (hyperadrenocorticism) • Exogenous Acute infection
Thrombocytopenia	Immune-mediated thrombocytopenia (primary and secondary) Aplastic anaemia (aplastic pancytopenia) Ehrlichiosis/*Anaplasma phagocytophilum* Babesiosis Splenomegaly Disseminated intravascular coagulation

continues ▶

Haematology *continued*

Abnormality	Differential diagnoses
Thrombocytopenia *continued*	Acute blood loss Myelopthisis Myelo/lymphoproliferative disease Vasculitis Breed-related: Cavalier King Charles Spaniel
Thrombocytosis	Rebound following acute haemorrhage Chronic gastrointestinal bleeding/iron deficiency Secondary to inflammation (e.g. infection, immune-mediated) Secondary to neoplasia Following vincristine Primary (essential) thrombocythaemia Acute megakaryoblastic leukaemia

Features of stress/steroid-induced haemogram

Feature	Dogs	Cats
Neutrophilia	Yes	Slight
Monocytosis	Yes	No
Lymphopenia	Yes	Yes
Eosinopenia	Yes	Yes

Biochemistry

Electrolytes

Analyte	Increased	Decreased
Bicarbonate	**ALKALOSIS** Metabolic alkalosis due to 'gastric' vomiting Compensatory response to respiratory acidosis	**ACIDOSIS** Metabolic acidosis: • Loss of bicarbonate in diarrhoea, renal tubular acidosis • Accumulation of unmeasured anions (e.g. lactate (shock), phosphate, sulphate, citrate (renal failure), ketone bodies (ketoacidosis) • Toxins (e.g. ethylene glycol) • Decreased renal excretion of H^+ in renal failure, hypoadrenocorticism, uroabdomen Compensatory response to respiratory alkalosis Spurious: delay in analysis
Calcium	**HYPERCALCAEMIA** Growing animals Malignancy-associated (e.g. lymphoma, anal sac adenocarcinoma, multiple myeloma) Hyperparathyroidism Hypoadrenocorticism Chronic renal failure Acute renal failure – diuretic phase Osteolytic bone lesions Vitamin D intoxification Granulomatous disease Excessive calcium supplementation [Chronic dietary phosphate restriction]	**HYPOCALCAEMIA** Low albumin (hypocalcaemia not clinically significant) Eclampsia (lactation tetany) Acute pancreatitis Hypoparathyroidism following thyroidectomy (common) or lymphocytic parathyroiditis (rare) Chronic renal failure Malabsorption, especially lymphangiectasia Ethylene glycol toxicity Post-transfusion (excess anticoagulant) Spurious: EDTA contamination
Chloride	**HYPERCHLORAEMIA** In parallel with hypernatraemia (e.g. due to dehydration, diabetes insipidus) Hyperchloraemic metabolic acidosis (e.g. due to alimentary loss of bicarbonate) Spurious: bromide therapy (interferes with assay)	**HYPOCHLORAEMIA** In association with hyponatraemia (see sodium) Hypoadrenocorticism Metabolic alkalosis due to loss of HCl in gastric vomiting High anion gap metabolic acidosis (e.g. ketoacidosis) Lactic acidosis associated with hypovolaemia
Magnesium	**HYPERMAGNESAEMIA** Renal failure (pre-renal, renal or post-renal azotaemia) Intravascular haemolysis	**HYPOMAGNESAEMIA** Hypoproteinaemia Acute or chronic diarrhoea Diabetes mellitus, especially with ketoacidosis
Phosphate	**HYPERPHOSPHATAEMIA** Young animals Reduced glomerular filtration rate (due to pre-renal, renal or post-renal causes) Ruptured urinary bladder Vitamin D toxicity Diabetic ketoacidosis Tumour lysis syndrome Acute severe myopathy Osteolytic bone lesions Hyperthyroidism (cats)	**HYPOPHOSPHATAEMIA** Hyperparathyroidism Malignancy-associated hypercalcaemia with release of PTH-rP Hypovitaminosis D (e.g. intestinal malabsorption, dietary deficiency) Following insulin therapy Re-feeding syndrome (cats) Prolonged anorexia Fanconi syndrome

Analyte	Increased	Decreased
Potassium	**HYPERKALAEMIA** Acute oliguric or anuric renal failure Urinary tract obstruction or rupture Hypoadrenocorticism Metabolic acidosis Tumour lysis syndrome Rhabdomyolysis or tissue necrosis Drug therapy: Spironolactone, ACE-inhibitors Heparin Mitotane Transfusions Spurious: marked thrombocytosis or leucocytosis; haemolysis (Japanese Akitas); EDTA contamination of sample	**HYPOKALAEMIA** Anorexia Fluid therapy using potassium-free fluids Vomiting and/or diarrhoea Chronic renal failure Diabetic ketoacidosis Initial insulin therapy of diabetes mellitus (especially ketoacidotic) Hyperaldosteronism (Conn's syndrome) Acute hyperventilation (respiratory alkalosis) Following insulin therapy Hypokalaemic myopathy of Burmese cats
Sodium	**HYPERNATRAEMIA** Gastrointestinal disease: vomiting and diarrhoea Diabetes mellitus Diuretic therapy Central diabetes insipidus Nephrogenic diabetes insipidus Primary adipsia Heatstroke Burns or extensive degloving injury Water deprivation Hypertonic intravenous fluid therapy Hyperaldosteronism Hyperadrenocorticism Sodium bicarbonate therapy	**HYPONATRAEMIA** Hypoadrenocorticism Third-space loss of fluid: pleural effusion or peritoneal effusion Volume overload associated with congestive heart failure, liver disease, end-stage renal failure, nephrotic syndrome, hypotonic fluid administration Diuretics (e.g. thiazide) Diabetes mellitus Mannitol infusion [GI losses] [Syndrome of inappropriate antidiuretic hormone secretion (SIADH) (v. rare)] Spurious: lipaemia

Enzymes

Enzyme	Increased in:
Alanine aminotransferase (ALT)	Hepatocyte damage in primary liver disease: • Inflammatory hepatic disease (e.g. chronic active hepatitis, cholangiohepatitis, feline infectious peritonitis, infectious canine hepatitis) • Drug-related, due to phenobarbital, carprofen, glucocorticoids • Trauma • Toxic damage • Hepatic neoplasia Hepatocyte damage secondary to extra-hepatic disease: • Pancreatitis • Gastrointestinal disease • Endocrine disease (e.g. diabetes mellitus, hyperadrenocorticism, hyperthyroidism) • Hypoxia due to anaemia or reduced blood flow (e.g. in thromboembolism) • Congestive heart failure
Alkaline phosphatase (ALP)	Cholestasis: • Intrahepatic (e.g. cholangiohepatitis, hepatic lipidosis, neoplasia) • Post-hepatic (e.g. pancreatitis, cholangitis, cholelithiasis) Steroid induction – *dogs only:* • Hyperadrenocorticism • Steroid therapy Drug induction: • Phenobarbital • Primidone Bone remodelling: • Young animal • Fracture • Neoplasia • Osteomyelitis • Hyperthyroidism Secondary to extra-hepatic disease: • Gastrointestinal disease • Endocrine disease (e.g. diabetes mellitus, hyperadrenocorticism, hyperthyroidism)

Enzyme	Increased in:
Amylase	Pancreatitis Pancreatic neoplasia Azotaemia (2–3 x upper reference limit) Intestinal disease
Aspartate aminotransferase (AST)	Hepatocyte damage: *see* ALT Muscle damage Haemolysis
Creatine kinase (CK)	Myopathies Myositis Muscle ischaemia Trauma
Gamma glutamyl transferase (GGT)	Cholestasis: • Intrahepatic (e.g cholangiohepatitis, hepatic lipidosis, neoplasia) • Post-hepatic (e.g. pancreatitis, cholangitis, cholelithiasis) Drug-induced: • Corticosteroids • Phenobarbital • Primidone
Lipase	Pancreatitis Pancreatic neoplasia Azotaemia Glucocorticoids Hepatic disease (especially neoplasia) Enteritis (?)

Other

Analyte	Increased	Decreased
Bile acids	Biliary obstruction/cholestasis Reduced hepatic function (e.g. chronic active hepatitis, cirrhosis) Portosystemic shunt	
Bilirubin	**HYPERBILIRUBINAEMIA** Pre-hepatic: haemolysis (e.g. immune-mediated haemolytic anaemia, oxidant toxicity, haemotrophic mycoplasmosis, babesiosis) Intra-hepatic (e.g. cirrhosis, hepatic lipidosis, cholangiohepatitis, neoplasia) Post-hepatic (e.g. pancreatitis, cholangitis, cholelithiasis, biliary neoplasia)	
Cholesterol	**HYPERCHOLESTEROLAEMIA** Post-prandial Diabetes mellitus Hyperadrenocorticism Hypothyroidism Pancreatitis Cholestasis (many liver diseases) Protein-losing nephropathy with nephrotic syndrome Primary hyperlipidaemia	**HYPOCHOLESTEROLAEMIA** Severe liver disease Portosystemic shunts Protein-losing enteropathy (especially lymphangiectasia)
Creatinine	Reduced glomerular filtration rate due to renal, pre-renal and post-renal causes	Decreased muscle mass
Glucose	**HYPERGLYCAEMIA** Stress (especially cats) Diabetes mellitus Hyperadrenocorticism Growth hormone excess Pancreatitis Drugs: intravenous glucose; alpha-2 agonists (e.g. medetomidine); progestogens Post-prandial (mild) Spurious: lipaemia	**HYPOGLYCAEMIA** Toy breeds Neonates Starvation Bacteraemia/septicaemia Parvovirus and other severe GI infections Hypoadrenocorticism Insulinoma Hepatic tumours GI smooth muscle tumours Renal failure Liver failure (severe) Cachexia (cardiac or neoplastic) Drugs: ethanol, salicylates, propanolol Artefact: delay in processing
Protein (A = albumin; G = globulin)	**HYPERPROTEINAEMIA** Dehydration (A and G) Inflammation, particularly of liver (G) Neoplasia (G) Plasma cell myeloma (monoclonal G) Spurious: lipaemia (A and G)	**HYPOPROTEINAEMIA** Haemorrhage (A and G) Protein-losing nephropathy (A) Protein-losing enteropathy (A and G) Third-space loss of fluid (A>G) Severe liver disease (A and G) Young animals Starvation Diuresis Acute phase response (A>G, mild)
Urea	High-protein diet GI bleeding Renal failure (acute or chronic) Pre-renal azotaemia Urinary obstruction Rupture of ureter, bladder or urethra	Severe starvation Diuresis Portosystemic shunts Hepatic disease/insufficiency Diabetes insipidus

Urine analysis

Specific gravity

Increased (>1.030 in dog, >1.035 in cat)
Hypovolaemia
Marked increase in glucose or protein content

Decreased (1.015–1.030 in dog, 1.105–1.035 in cat)
Early renal failure
Diabetes mellitus
Hyperadrenocorticism
May be normal (dog)

Isosthenuria (1.007–1.015) or
Hyposthenuria (< 1.007)
Renal failure (I, H)
Hyperadrenocorticism (I, H)
Steroid therapy (I, H)
Hypercalcaemia (I, H)
Pyometra (I, H)
Pyelonephritis (I, H)
Renal medullary washout (e.g. post-obstruction) (I, H)
Hyperthyroidism (I, rarely H)
Psychogenic polydipsia (I, H)
Fluid therapy (I, H)
Liver disease (I, H)
Partial central diabetes insipidus (I, H)
Central or nephrogenic diabetes insipidus (usually H)

pH (Normal 6.0–7.5)

Increased: ALKALURIA
Urease-containing bacteria
Aged sample
Transient (post-prandial)
Renal tubular acidosis
Metabolic alkalosis
Diet rich in vegetable protein

Decreased: ACIDURIA
Acidifying diet
Metabolic acidosis
Hypochloraemic metabolic alkalosis (gastric vomiting)
Hypokalaemia

Sediment

White blood cell count
Increased: LEUCOCYTOSIS
Urinary tract inflammation
Urinary tract infection
N.B. Absence of WBCs does not rule out urinary tract infection

Dipstick

Glucose
Positive: GLUCOSURIA
Diabetes mellitus
Stress hyperglycaemia (cats)
Renal tubular disease: idiopathic
Fanconi syndrome
Primary renal glucosuria
[Aminoglycosides]
[Hyperadrenocorticism]

Ketones
Positive: KETONURIA
Diabetes mellitus
Very young animals
[Starvation]

Protein
Increased (>trace): PROTEINURIA
Pyuria
Protein-losing nephropathy (glomerulonephritis, amyloidosis)
Haemorrhage
[Genital tract secretions if voided]

Bilirubin
Increased (>trace in cats, >2+ in dogs): BILIRUBINURIA
Haemolytic anaemia
Hepatobiliary disease (especially cats)
[Very concentrated urine can give false increase]

Blood
Positive: HAEMATURIA
Urolithiasis
Inflammation (any cause including urinary tract infection, neoplasia)
Iatrogenic

Haemoglobin
Positive: HAEMOGLOBINURIA
Immune-mediated haemolytic anaemia
In vitro lysis of red blood cells from haematuria

Myoglobin:
Positive: MYOGLOBINURIA
Muscle damage

Urobilinogen
(Normal trace to 1+)
Increased: Hyperbilirubinaemia
Negative: Complete biliary obstruction

Appendix 2

Test sample requirements

Haematology

Test	Sample requirements
Complete blood count	EDTA–blood Air-dried blood smears
Erythropoietin	Serum
Blood typing	EDTA–blood

Haemostasis

Platelet count	EDTA–blood
von Willebrand factor antigen	Sodium citrate– (or EDTA–)plasma (fill tube exactly to line; mix gently but thoroughly)
Prothrombin time Activated partial thromboplastin time Fibrin(ogen) degradation products	Sodium citrate–plasma (fill tube exactly to line; mix gently but thoroughly)
D-dimer	EDTA– or sodium citrate–plasma (fill tube exactly to line; mix gently but thoroughly)

Bone marrow

Test	Sample requirements
Bone marrow cytology/histology	Air-dried bone marrow smears EDTA–blood Air-dried blood smears ± Core biopsy in formalin
Flow cytometry (for immunophenotyping leukaemia)	EDTA–blood ± ACD-anticoagulated bone marrow

Immunology (general)

Test	Sample requirements
Coombs' test	EDTA–blood
Anti-platelet antibody	EDTA–blood
Antinuclear antibody	Serum
Rheumatoid factor	Serum

Biochemistry and endocrinology

Test	Sample requirements
Routine analytes (enzymes, proteins, electrolytes)	Serum (preferably) or heparinized plasma
Glucose	Separated fluoride oxalate plasma
Fructosamine	Serum
Iron	Serum
Bile acids	Serum
Drug levels (phenobarbital, digoxin, potassium bromide)	Serum (gel tubes interfere with analysis of many drug levels)
Adrenocorticotropic hormone (ACTH)	Sample into cooled plastic EDTA tube and separate plasma immediately. Transfer plasma into cooled plastic plain tube on ice. Freeze and send in freezer transport pack
Aldosterone	Heparinized or EDTA–plasma or serum
Cortisol	Heparinized plasma or serum
17-Hydroxy-progesterone	Heparinized plasma or serum
Insulin	Serum
Insulin antibodies	Serum
Parathyroid hormone (PTH) PTH-related protein	Sample into cooled plastic EDTA tube and separate plasma immediately. Transfer plasma into cooled plastic plain tube on ice. Freeze and send in freezer transport pack
Thyroxine	Heparinized plasma or serum
TSH	Heparinized plasma or serum
Free T4 by equilibrium dialysis	Serum
Thyroglobulin autoantibody	Serum
Reproductive hormones	Most either heparin plasma or serum
Canine relaxin	Heparinized plasma or serum

Miscellaneous tests

Test	Sample requirements
Genetic testing (DNA)	EDTA–blood or mucosal swab
Blood gas analysis	Fresh or heparinized blood that has not been in contact with air
Cerebrospinal fluid (CSF):	
Cell counts, culture, serology	Plain CSF
Cytology	Plain CSF plus one drop of formalin (contact laboratory)
Effusions:	
Cell counts, cytology, PCR	EDTA–effusion
Biochemistry	Plain effusion
Culture	Plain sterile effusion
FIP profiles	Heparin–effusion

Tests for gastrointestinal disease

Test	Sample requirements
Trypsin-like immunoreactivity (cTLI, fTLI)	Serum
Folate	Serum
Cobalamin (Vitamin B12)	Serum
Canine pancreatic-lipase immunoreactivity	Serum
Faecal α_1-proteinase inhibitor	Three fresh faecal samples, pooled and shipped on ice

Tests for infectious diseases

Test or method	Infectious agent	Sample requirements
α_1-Acid glycoprotein	Feline coronavirus	Heparinized plasma
Electron microscopy	Cowpox virus	Scab or skin biopsy material
ELISA	FeLV (p27 antigen)	Heparinized blood
	Feline coronavirus (antibody)	Heparinized blood or effusion
	FIV (antibody)	Heparinized blood or serum
	Feline parvovirus (antigen)	Faeces or gut contents
Haemagglutination	Feline parvovirus (antigen)	Faeces or gut contents
Immunofluorescence	Feline coronavirus	Heparinized blood or effusion
	FeLV	Smear of whole blood
Polymerase chain reaction (PCR)	Feline herpesvirus	Oropharyngeal swab into VTM
	Canine parvovirus, feline parvovirus	Faeces or gut contents
	Anaplasma phagocytophilum, Babesia canis, Ehrlichia spp., *Mycoplasma haemofelis*/ '*Candidatus* Mycoplasma haemominutum'	EDTA–blood
	Bartonella spp.	EDTA–blood; lesional tissue (fresh/frozen)
	Borrelia spp.	EDTA–whole blood; fluid and fresh tissue
	Leishmania spp.	EDTA–blood, fresh bone marrow, lymph node or skin biopsy tissue
	Toxoplasma gondii	Fresh tissue; CSF; aqueous humour
Reverse transcriptase PCR (RT-PCR)	Feline calicivirus	Oropharyngeal swab into VTM
	Feline coronavirus	Heparinized blood or effusion
Rapid immunomigration (RIM)	FeLV (p27 antigen)	Heparinized blood
	FIV (antibody)	Heparinized blood or serum
	Feline parvovirus (antigen)	Faeces or gut contents
Serology	Canine adenovirus	Heparinized blood or serum
	Canine distemper virus	Heparinized plasma or serum or CSF
	Canine parainfluenza virus	Serum
	Canine parvovirus	Heparinized plasma or serum
	Feline parvovirus	Heparinized or EDTA–plasma/serum

Test or method	Infectious agent	Sample requirements
Serology *continued*	*Anaplasma phagocytophilum*, *Babesia canis*, *Bartonella* spp., *Borrelia* spp., *Ehrlichia* spp., *Leishmania* spp., *Leptospira*, *Neospora caninum*, *Toxoplasma gondii*	Serum
Virus isolation	Canine adenovirus, canine parainfluenza virus	Throat swab in VTM
	Cowpox virus	Scab material
	Feline calicivirus, feline herpesvirus	Oropharyngeal swab into VTM
	FeLV	Heparinized blood or bone marrow
	Feline parvovirus	Faeces or gut contents
Western blot	Anti-FIV antibody	Heparinized blood or serum

Urine analysis

Test	Sample requirements
Urine culture	Boric acid/borate–urine (plain if fresh)
Dipstick analysis and sediment examination	Plain urine

Abbreviations: ACD = acid citrate dextrose; ELISA = enzyme-linked immunosorbent assay; FeLV = feline leukaemia virus; FIP = feline infectious peritonitis; FIV = feline immunodeficiency virus; VTM = virus transport medium

Appendix 3

Conversion tables

Biochemistry

	SI unit	Conversion	Non-SI unit
Adrenocorticotropic hormone (ACTH)	pmol / l	x 4.54	pg / ml
Alanine aminotransferase	IU / l	x 1	IU / l
Albumin	g / l	x 0.1	g / dl
Alkaline phosphatase	IU / l	x 1	IU / l
Ammonia	µmol / l	X 1.703	µg / dl
Aspartate aminotransferase	IU / l	x 1	IU / l
Bicarbonate	mmol / l	x .0005	mEq / l
Bile acids	mmol / l	x 0.393	mg / ml
Bilirubin	µmol / l	x 0.0584	mg / dl
Calcium	mmol / l	x 4	mg / dl
Carbon dioxide (total)	mmol / l	x 1	mEq / l
Chloride	mmol / l	x 1	mEq / l
Cholesterol	mmol / l	x 38.61	mg / dl
Cortisol	nmol / l	x 0.362	ng / ml
Creatine kinase	IU / l	x 1	IU / l
Creatinine	µmol / l	x 0.0113	mg / dl
Fibrinogen	g / l	x 100	mg / dl
Folate	nmol / l	x 0.44	µg / l
Globulin	g / l	x 0.1	g / dl
Glucose	mmol / l	x 18.02	mg / dl
Insulin	pmol / l	x 0.1394	µIU / ml
Iron	µmol / l	x 5.587	µg / dl
Lactate	mmol / l	x 9	mg / dl
Magnesium	mmol / l	x 2	mEq / l
Inorganic phosphate	mmol / l	x 3.1	mg / dl
Potassium	mmol / l	x 1	mEq / l
Sodium	mmol / l	x 1	mEq / l
Total protein	g / l	x 0.1	g / dl
Thyroxine (T4) (free)	pmol / l	x 0.0775	ng / dl
Thyroxine (T4) (total)	nmol / l	x 0.0775	µg / dl
Tri-iodothyronine (T3)	nmol / l	x 65.1	ng / dl
Triglyceride	mmol / l	x 88.5	mg / dl
Urea nitrogen	mmol / l	x 2.80	mg / dl
Urea	mmol / l	x 6	mg/dl

Haematology

	SI unit	Conversion	Non-SI unit
Red blood cell count	10^{12} / l	x 1	10^{6} / µl
Haemoglobin	g / l	x 0.1	g / dl
Haematocrit	l / l	x 1	l / l
MCH	pg / cell	x 1	pg / cell
MCHC	g / l	x 0.1	g / dl
MCV	fl	x 1	µm^{3}
Platelet count	10^{9} / l	x 1000	/ µl
White blood cell count	10^{9} / l	x 1000	/ µl

Temperature

SI unit	Conversion	Non-SI unit
°C	(x 9/5) + 32	°F

Pressure

SI unit	Conversion	Non-SI unit
kPa	x 7.5	mmHg

Hypodermic needles

	Metric	Non-metric
Needle gauge	0.8 mm	21 G
	0.6 mm	23 G
	0.5 mm	25 G
	0.4 mm	27 G
Needle length	12 mm	½ inch
	16 mm	5/8 inch
	25 mm	1 inch
	30 mm	1.25 inch
	40 mm	1.5 inch

Index

Page numbers in italic type refer to illustrations

Index

Index

Index

Index